Joints and Vertebral Connections

Clinical Radiology

Wolfgang Dihlmann

Translated by Dr. Gottfried Stiasny

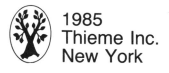

1985
Thieme Inc.
New York

Georg Thieme Verlag
Stuttgart • New York

Thieme Inc.
381 Park Avenue South
New York, New York 10016

Library of Congress Cataloging in Publication Data

Dihlmann, Wolfgang.
  Joints and vertebral connections.

  Translation of: Gelenke—Wirbelverbindungen.
  Bibliography: p. 523
  Includes index.
  1. Joints—Diseases. 2. Joints—Radiography.
3. Spine—Diseases. 4. Spine—Radiography. I. Title.
RC932.D5413   1985   616.7′2   84-16327
ISBN 0-86577-161-8

Cover design by Patrice Giusto

Printed in the United States of America

JOINTS AND VERTEBRAL CONNECTIONS
Wolfgang Dihlmann

TI ISBN 0-86577-161-8
GTV ISBN 3-13-660401-6

5 4 3 2 1

Contents

Preface

Roentgen diagnosis should be exercised only by those physicians who possess sufficient specialized knowledge (insight and experience) or who are striving to acquire it. The second prerequisite for efficient roentgen diagnosis is the ability and possibility of applying the modern methods and techniques of radiologic examination. This second prerequisite has been the subject of much debate—it suffices to consider the advances made in angiography. I have gladly accepted the invitation by the late Mr. Rolf Glauner, the former editor of Thieme's textbooks on radiology, to write a contribution to roentgen diagnosis which should primarily convey to the reader practical knowledge and not the results of sophisticated applied technology. The roentgen diagnosis of the diseases of the joints has been chosen to this end not by chance but by taking into consideration the fact that an abundant literature on other fields is available, whereas up to now no comprehensive description of the radiographic diagnosis of the gliding tissues has been published. Personal experience, extensive study of the literature, and fruitful discussions with colleagues who are particularly familiar with certain branches of the radiology of the joints have enabled the composition of the present work, which is intended to interest a large readership: the students who in their various clinical studies see patients with diseases of the joints and the accompanying radiologic pictures, as well as the referring physicians who also will find in these pages the indications for examining the joints radiologically. With the aid of this book they will learn how to interpret the roentgen findings they encounter in their practice. The specialized radiologic examiner, whether he or she be a general surgeon, an orthopedic surgeon, an internist, a rheumatologist, a pediatrician, a dermatologist, a neurologist, or—last but not least—a radiologist can consult this book to find detailed information about the general and special problems of radiologic arthrology from a practical point of view. Deduction as well as induction are the didactic principles that govern the text, which is accompanied by personally drawn sketches. Radiologic sketches offer advantages as well as disadvantages. One of their advantages is that they promote abstraction (the formation of concepts). Radiologic sketches show no disturbing shadows. To the contrary, particular emphasis can be placed on important diagnostic details—black on white, white on black, or whatever. The eye for essential features thus becomes sharpened and engrams are created. It is a disadvantage or—rather a matter of course—that a roentgenologic textbook that presents sketches cannot and should not replace a textbook or an atlas dealing with the roentgenologic diagnosis of the gliding tissue and containing reproductions of roentgenograms. On the other hand, the textbook character promises detailed information, a handy size, and a convenient price. In any event, critical readers are invited to form their own opinions about these matters. In addition, it should be emphasized that the book interprets facts—diseases of the connections between bones—from the viewpoint of the radiologist. It could be that these interpretations will not always be satisfactory to the representatives of other medical specialties. Suggestions from readers will be gladly accepted.

WOLFGANG DIHLMANN
Hamburg, Spring 1985

General Radiographic Diagnosis of the Gliding Tissues

Natural differences of the gliding and supporting tissues in attenuating radiographs allow one to make a radiographic diagnosis in studying the diarthroses, synchondroses, and syndesmoses.

The *effective ordinal numeral* is one of the variables on which the attenuation of the radiographs depends. Mainly because of its calcium content, bone has a higher effective ordinal numeral than the synovial membrane, the synovia, the fibrous joint capsule, the articular cartilage, and the ligaments (Table 1). Moreover, the attenuation of the radiographs depends on the *thickness* and *density* of the radiographed substance as well as on the selected *wave length* of the rays. Therefore, periarticular fatty bodies—for example, the infrapatellar fat pad—can sometimes be differentiated from the water-equivalent components of the joint, owing to its lesser density and its lower effective ordinal numeral (Table 1). The diminished attenuation of the roentgen beam by the infrapatellar fat pad manifests itself as increased blackening of the film (Fig. 1). *Artificial* differences in attenuation may provide information about the inner structures of the joint. To this end, air may be insufflated into a joint cavity or an iodinated water-soluble contrast medium may be injected (Table 1). "Artificial" contrast may also be produced by the double-contrast technique (insufflation of air or an elemental gas, combined with a small quantity of an iodinated water-soluble contrast medium). Roentgenograms convey a two-dimensional impression of a spatial structure. The absent third dimension, extension in depth, may be assessed in different ways:

1. Roentgenograms are routinely taken in two planes, one perpendicular to the other. Exceptions must be made in the following situations: (a) if taking a roentgenogram in a second plane *perpendicular* to the first one is impracticable (for example, the sacroiliac joint), (b) if the planes of the two roentgenograms must form an acute angle to provide additional information (for example, the hand). (c) Furthermore, experience shows that the technique of projection for the second roentgenogram sometimes depends on the clinical problem (for example, the hip joint). The so-called axial view of this joint or the head and neck of the femur is the preferred view when a fracture of the femoral neck is suspected or when the position of such a fracture must be checked. The Lauenstein projection (frog position, Fig. 343) is preferred when a slipped fem-

Table 1   Parameters of the attenuation of x-rays

	Effective ordinal numeral	Density (g/cm³)
Water	7.4[b]	1.0[b] [b]
Soft tissues (including gliding tissues)	7.42[a]; 7.5[b]	0.92–1.06[a]; 1.0[b]
Fat	6.0[b]	0.92[b]
Bone	8.7–11.6[a]; 15.0[b]	1.13–1.19[a]; 1.9[b]
Air	7.64[a]; 7.7[b]	0.0013[a]
Iodine	53[a]	4.94[a]

[a] = after Schinz et al. (1965); [b] = after Grashey and Birkner (1964)

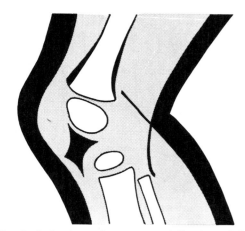

Fig. 1   Lateral roentgenogram of the knee joint (small child). Hoffa's infrapatellar fat pad, the anterior and posterior fat pad of the distal metaphysis of the femur, and the subcutaneous adipose tissue do not stand out against the water-equivalent soft tissues (hyaline cartilage, joint capsule, menisci, musculature etc.), which cannot be differentiated from one another.

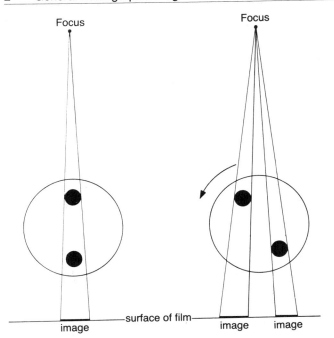

Fig. 2 Principle of parallactic motion and its application to radiographic diagnosis. A shadow-forming region *close to the film*—e.g., a foreign body—is depicted with but little magnification. When the portion of the body being filmed is rotated counterclockwise, it moves to the right. An area of increased density *remote from the film* appears in higher magnification, and when the part of the body is rotated in a counterclockwise direction, it moves to the left.

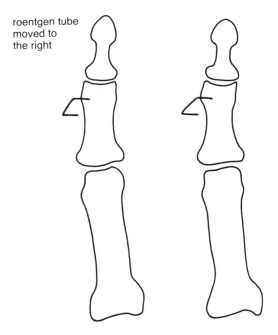

Fig. 3 Drawing after two stereoscopic roentgenograms of the right index finger. With some practice one can see the subjective (three-dimensional) spatial impression by examining the drawings with the eyes convergent (strabismus), even without the aid of a stereoscope. A third drawing then appears between the other two and gives a sharp, plastic impression. On *convergent* spatial inspection, the two roentgenograms must be hung laterally inverted; i.e., the roentgenogram taken after displacing lhe tube to the right is hung on the left side and the other one correspondingly on the right side. Focusing technique: see text.

Question: Does the part of the metal staple directed toward the fingertips lie anterior (dorsal) or posterior (volar) to the middle phalanx? (Answer on p. 395).

oral epiphysis or early Legg-Calvé-Perthes disease is suspected (Fig. 340 B). The various types of congenital dislocation of the hip require a "false profile" view. (d) Polyhedral objects or objects with approximately symmetrical rotation (i.e., most of the joints) should be radiographed at more than two sites to exploit the full possibilities of roentgenologic study. This is especially necessary when giving expert opinion and when forensic problems are involved. (e) Finally, the following *technical* prerequisites are indispensable for the optimal radiographic diagnosis of affections of the joints and the vertebral column:

· Reducing geometrical haziness by selecting a fine focus with adequate film-focus distance.
· Using *finely recording* amplification foils—so-called running foils.
· Providing object-correct exposure of the roentgen film and selecting a gradation that reproduces all the important details of the object in the range of blackening that can be visually analyzed.
· Although the foil-less film has been called a matter of history (Rausch and Frik, 1970), its great capacity to reveal the smallest details makes its use mandatory for early diagnosis of inflammatory and certain endocrine (hyperparathyroid) affections of bones and joints and in searching for discrete injuries of bone, at least in the hands and feet.

2.   The position of a contour near to or remote from the film, a structural change, or a foreign body can also be ascertained with use of the *parallactic motion* (Fig. 2).

3.   *Tomographs,* including computed tomographs (of the sacroiliac or the hip joint) can provide information about the depth and extension in depth of a pathologic finding.

4.   The spatial impression of *stereoscopic roentgenograms,* for instance, facilitates the accurate localization of a loose body ("joint mouse") or a foreign body that may be visible in the roentgenogram.

Focusing technique: The so-called central beam is directed toward the usual centering point of the joint. Subsequently, the roentgen tube is displaced 3.5 cm to the right, parallel to the surface of the film, and the first roentgenogram is then taken. A second film is exposed 7.0 cm to the left of the first. The two roentgenograms (half pictures) are hung side by side for inspection (Fig. 3).

Rules for the Radiographic Study of the Gliding Tissues

Paired joints must, as a matter of principle, be radiographed in paired fashion under identical conditions (positioning, focusing technique, exposure time, etc.).

Advantages: the decrease in calcium content of the bones surrounding a diseased joint can be recognized sooner and more easily by comparison with the sound side. Such abnormalities as persistent ossification centers, disturbed (delayed or accelerated) development of bone, detached apophyses, avulsions, supernumerary ossicles, and slight malpositions of joints can be identified more confidently by comparison with the unaffected contralateral joint and its surroundings. When a roentgenogram is taken with the joint held in a certain position (see below), the roentgenogram of the sound joint held in the same position may indicate the normal range of passive motion.

The (assumed to be) diseased portion of the joint should be positioned as close as possible to the film because the shorter the distance from film to object, the sharper are the contours, according to the laws of central projection; the magnification decreases and the number of identifiable details increases.

Example: When a fracture of the patella is suspected, a posteroanterior roentgenogram of the knee joint with the patella close to the film is preferable to the conventional anteroposterior roentgenogram.

When there is clinical reason to suspect a polyarticular affection—e.g., rheumatoid arthritis—the radiologist should not be influenced by the site of greatest pain. Instead, the views chosen should depict the greatest number of painful affected joints with the least possible exposure to radiation; hence, films should be taken of the hands and the feet. Moreover, pain is not always experienced at the site of its origin. Diseases of the sacroiliac joint, for instance, sometimes give rise to pain in the inguinal region, near the hip joint. Diseases of the hip joint often produce pain referred to the knee. If, in such cases, only the painful regions were radiographed, erroneous diagnoses would likely result. Conversely, when the activity of an already diagnosed polyarticular affection has to be judged, one will film the joints that give the greatest discomfort.

Roentgenograms taken in the lying position depict the *morphology* (the shape, the contours, and the structures) of the gliding and supporting tissues.

Roentgenograms taken with the patient standing provide *additional* information about the *static situation* of a joint. Particularly in the *spine*, they are preferable to roentgenograms in the lying position. They can, however, also be of advantage in the *lower extremities*. For example, the extent of destruction of the articular cartilage can be estimated by the narrowing of the roentgenographic joint space, and the condition of the capsuloligamentous apparatus can be judged by the comparative position of the articulating bones. This can be recognized more accurately in roentgenograms of the knee joint with the patient standing (Ahlbäck, 1968) than in roentgenograms with the patient lying down. For comparison of the right and left side, both knee joints should be exposed *concomitantly* in an anteroposterior roentgenogram. Conversely, the thickness of the articular cartilage and the condition of the capsuloligamentous apparatus can be still better estimated when the roentgenogram is taken with the patient standing on one leg so that the load of the entire body rests on the joint to be tested. Similar considerations are applicable to the talocrural joint and the plantar arch. The radiographic technique should therefore be flexible and adapted to the individual case.

Roentgenograms with the limb held in a certain position are indicated when abnormal mobility—mostly instability following a ligament injury—is suspected in the joint of an extremity and shall be evidenced in the position of the greatest possible displacement. Similarly, roentgenograms made when weight is borne in the standing position give information about the stability of the capsule and ligaments in the acromioclavicular joints, the symphysis pubis, and the sacroiliac joints. To test the acromioclavicular joints, both sides are weighted with from 3 to 4 kg each. In addition, radiologic examination of the acromioclavicular joint in the overload posture can illustrate instability of this joint (Usadel, 1940). To this end, the patient is asked to assume the following position: standing on both legs, he extends the cervical spine and *lowers* his shoulders forward as far as possible, with both upper arms rotated inward. In this posture, the clavicles are pulled maximally upward by the tensing of their elevating muscles while the shoulder blades are pulled downward, principally by the action of the pectoralis and serratus anterior muscles. Rupture of the acromioclavicular joint causes the clavicle to be displaced cranially. For testing the stability of the pelvic joints see Figure 737.

The chief function of the joints is motion. In the peripheral joints this can best be tested clinically as active and passive mobility. In the axial skeleton, however, *functional roentgenograms* compete successfully with the clinical study of mobility. On making functional roentgenograms in the end position of motion (e.g., in maximal anteflexion and retroflexion), less attention is paid to the *global* mobility of the spinal segment tested than to the mobility and stability of the *individual* moving segments. Functional roentgenograms are definitely indicated in the following situations:

1. *Functional roentgenograms of the cervical spine in maximal anteflexion* should be made in whiplash injuries to avoid overlooking a fresh injury of the in-

tervertebral disk and/or a capsular tear of the intervertebral joints.[1] (Fig. 4). When mobility is greatly impaired by pain, an assistant may support the part examined.

2. *Functional roentgenograms in maximal ante-flexion and retroflexion* provide information about the stability of the atlantoodontoid joint, the atlantoaxial intervertebral joints, and the transverse ligament of the atlas when patients with *juvenile* or *adult rheumatoid arthritis* complain of discomfort in the upper spinal segment or when they present neurologic def-

icits referable to the upper spine. Widening of the atlantoodontoid cleft to more than 3 mm in adults and to more than 4 mm in children and adolescents is evidence of *ventral dislocation of the atlas* (Fig. 5), involving the danger of compression myelopathy. The critical atlas-dens interval exceeds 10 mm. In addition to this, any major ventral slipping of the atlas causes the tip of the dens to rise above the level of the foramen magnum, with serious threat to the medulla. Finally, ventral dislocation of the atlas can intermittently block circulation in the vertebral arteries. Additional causes of ventral dislocation of the atlas are psoriatic arthritis, Reiter's syndrome, ankylosing spondylitis, chronic arthritis in disseminated lupus erythematosus, gout, lipoid dermoarthritis, articular chondrocalcinosis, tuberculosis ("malum suboccipitale"), nonspecific bacterial infections, and certain types of osteochondrodysplasia; e.g., chondrodysplasia punctata. Additional possibilities are mucopolysaccharidosis I (Hurler) and IV (Morquio), Win-

---

[1] Hypermobility of the second cervical vertebra (less frequently also the third) has been observed as a variant of normal in children, e.g., in 19 percent of those between the ages of 1 and 7 (Cattell and Flitzer, 1965). It is manifested on functional roentgenograms taken in ante- and retroflexion by ventral, sometimes also dorsal, displacement of C2 upon C3 or C3 upon C4. This possibility should be considered when the *radiologist* has to form an opinion about a possible traumatic or inflammatory loosening of the cervical structure in children.

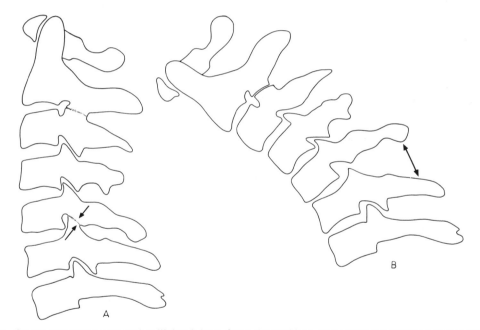

Fig. 4 **Status following rear-end collision injury.** Since the accident, patient has experienced nuchal discomfort, especially on bending forward.

A = Lateral roentgenogram of the cervical spine in normal posture. The interosseous space of the paired intervertebral joints C5/C6 is not shown in the illustration *(arrows)*. In lateral roentgenograms of the cervical spine, usually only the interosseous spaces C2/C3 are *not* freely projected because the two joint planes in this segment converge slightly forward, whereas in the other segments the joint planes either lie in the frontal plane or converge slightly backward. *The following rule is therefore applicable:* If in the normal posture any cleft of the paired intervertebral joints C3/C4 to C6/C7 is not freely projected on the lateral roentgenogram, or if—conversely—the interosseous space of the intervertebral joint C2/C3 is projected as a free cleft, a malposition of the joint or a malformation of the articular processes should be suspected (take an anteroposterior film of the cervical spine or a roentgenogram in anteflexion—see Fig. 617—or possibly a lateral tomograph).

B = The functional roentgenogram in anteflexion shows structural loosening of C5/C6, which manifests itself by an unphysiologic mutual mobility and increased distance of the articular processes, by ventral displacement of the vertebral body C5, and by conspicuous "gaping" of the spinous processes C5 and C6 *(arrow).*

Roentgenographic diagnosis: Capsular tear of the intervertebral joints, rupture of the interspinous ligament, and trauma to the disk C5/C6 (whiplash injury).

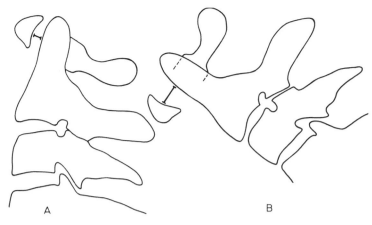

A   B

Fig. 5 A = **Lateral roentgeno-gram of the cervical spine with the patient standing** (Normal posture, detail).

Atlas-dens interval *possibly* increased; therefore roentgeno-gram B.

B = **Functional roentgeno-gram in anteflexion.** Atlas-dens interval considerably increased, hence unequivocal *ventral dislo-cation of the atlas;* in addition, el-evation of the tip of the dens (see text).

chester's syndrome, and Down's syndrome (trisomy 21, mongolism). Traumas with rupture of joint cap-sule and ligaments, may also be a cause, as may de-velopmental anomalies of neck and occiput. These may include hypoplasia of the dens, aplasia of the dens (Freiberger et al., 1965) or the os odontoideum, or a supernumerary skeletal element interposed be-tween the dens and the anterior arch of the atlas (Kammerer and Traupe, 1978), or aplasia of the an-terior arch of the atlas).

Grisel's syndrome, also called infectious torti-collis or nasopharyngeal torticollis (Fig. 6), consti-tutes, in principle, the combination of a transverse[2] (Figs. 7 and 8) and a ventral dislocation of the atlas (Wackenheim, 1974). The nature of the faulty posi-tion of the atlas depends on the site of the inflamma-tion (atlantoodontoid joint, transverse ligament of the atlas, *and* unilateral *or* bilateral involvement of the lateral atlantoaxial joints) as well as on the extent of damage to the articular and ligamental structures (possibly also on the involvement of the interverte-bral joints C2/C3). This painful torticollis occurs par-ticularly in nasopharyngeal infections in childhood and adolescence, and following a tonsillectomy. Apart from this, infectious ventral dislocation of the atlas has also been observed in hematogeneous nonspecific bacterial affections of the upper cervical spine; e.g., in *Salmonella* infections (Pilger et al., 1977).

3.   For the *cervical motion diagram* and *functional roentgenograms* to test the *lateral inclination* and the *rotation* of the entire cervical spine see Figures 651 to 653.

4.   *Cervical* and *lumbar functional roentgenograms in maximal anteflexion and retroflexion* may indicate whether an injury to the spine has healed with good stability or whether there is a residual instability. Such

functional roentgenograms are indispensable in forming an expert opinion.

5.   In *functional roentgenograms of the lumbar spine* it is possible to discern whether an anterior or poste-rior spondylolisthesis is mobile or fixed (Figs. 632 A and B). *Mobile* ventral displacements of vertebrae are usually prone to further slippage. In addition, even with normal activities, the gliding back and forth of the displaced vertebra can give rise to discomfort.

6.   *Functional roentgenograms of the lumbar spine in maximal* anteflexion,[3] retroflexion,[4] and lateral in-clination to the left and right[5] reveal pain-induced *segmental* reflex locking of movements that cannot

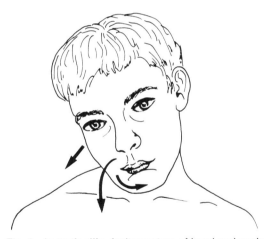

Fig. 6   In **torticollis,** faulty posture of head and neck (lateral inclination, rotation toward the opposite side, slight anterior flexion) is frequently observed.

---

[2] A "genuine" transverse dislocation of the atlas (without a rotary component) occurs, for example, in rheumatoid arthritis (Fig. 8).

[3] Arched back without flexion at the hip and knee joints, hands at the level of the knee joints.

[4] Hollow back without flexion at the knee joints.

[5] Both feet together on the floor, knee joints fully extended. On the flexor side, fingertips on the outer aspect of the knee joints.

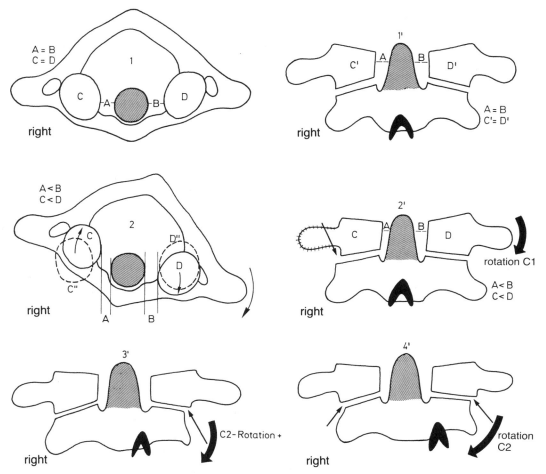

Fig. 7 For anatomic reasons, **any rotation of the atlas**—whether physiologic or pathologic—shows in the roentgenogram a concomitant "transverse dislocation" of the atlas with respect to the odontoid process of the axis.

1 = Top view of atlas. For better understanding, however, the *inferior* articular surfaces (C and D) have also been sketched in. Atlas-dens interval equal on both sides (A = B). Odontoid process *shaded*.

1' = C' and D' = Massive lateral parts of atlas. Spinous process black.

2, 2' = Atlas rotated to the right. C" and D" = Inferior articular surfaces in their normal position (not rotated) sketched for comparison.

Right transverse process of atlas projected hazily in tomographic plane of section. The *long arrow* points to a step, as the lateral mass that moves dorsally is projected with a shortened transverse diameter. A *pathologic* rotation of the atlas with respect to the axis must be presumed when both vestibules of the inner ear appear in the same section in the anteroposterior tomographic picture of the occipitocervical junction or when the axis is projected symmetrically (hence the patient has been positioned correctly [Wackenheim, 1974]) and, despite this, the roentgen findings sketched under 2' have been obtained.

Note: The *nonrotated vertebra* (atlas or axis) "surmounts" the rotated vertebra laterally *(long* arrow in 2' and 3'). With *marked* rotation of the axis, *both* lateral masses *(long arrows* in 4') surmount *both* articular surfaces of the axis. The direction of rotation of the axis is also indicated by the spinous process moving laterally.

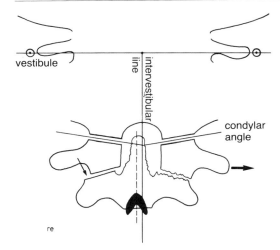

Fig. 8 Transverse dislocation of the atlas is most frequently observed in inflammatory rheumatic affections (Dirheimer, 1977). Furthermore, the sketch shows erosion of the odontoid process and erosions of the left atlantoaxial joint in rheumatoid arthritis.
Roentgenologic criteria in the tomograph:
1. The intervestibular line (Wackenheim, 1974) is displaced to the side of the transverse dislocation of the atlas, more or less parallel to the longitudinal axis of the odontoid process of the axis *(dashed line).*
2. The tip of condylar angle (angle of the articular axis) lies on the intervestibular line.
3. Step formation between the articular surfaces of atlas and axis *(arrow,* step also on the opposite side).
4. Both transverse processes of the atlas are represented with sharp contours in the tomograph.
5. Lateral atlas-dens intervals different on the two sides.

Note: Ventral and transverse dislocations of the atlas are the most frequent faulty positions in the occipitocervical junction. Additional malpositions include dorsal dislocation of the atlas in lesions of the odontoid process or the anterior arch of the atlas. Furthermore, transverse, ventral, or dorsal dislocations may occur at the atlantooccipital joints, with and without a rotary component. Combinations of all these malpositions, which are hard to differentiate, also occur.

be so confidently identified on roentgenograms taken in the normal posture. With the aid of a potent x-ray generator (film-to-focus distance 150 cm) and a Potter-Bucky device attached to the wall, it is possible—even without myelography—to identify a root compression responsible for the locking (commonly dorsal herniation of an intervertebral disk) and to determine the side and the segmental level of the lesion. When the findings on physical examination *and* the result of functional radiography of the lumbar spine suggest a dorsal dislocation of the disk, the surgeon

called into consultation must decide whether a preoperative myelogram is necessary. Such will usually be the case (compare p. 426).

The interpretation of functional roentgenograms of the *lumbar spine* is based on the following *rules:*

• With ante- and retroflexion, the excursion is greatest in the segment L4/L5; with lateral flexion it is smallest in L5/S1.
• With lateral flexion to the opposite side, a posterolateral prolapse of the intervertebral disk permits a harmonious movement. In the involved segment, however, it blocks the normal flexion toward the side of the prolapse (Fig. 9) or may even cause the vertebral interspace on the side of the prolapse to gape. This finding is particularly conspicuous in and above the segment L4/L5.
• When, in a single segment, lateral flexion to *both sides* is restricted or lost, this finding indicates a completely disintegrated functionless intervertebral disk, a postdiscectomy condition, or a posteromedial prolapse of the disk. An intraspinal tumor, also, should be considered in the differential diagnosis.
• The following finding (Fig. 10) also raises a well-founded suspicion of posterolateral prolapse of the disk, especially in the segment L5/S1: a *left-sided* posterolateral prolapse in the segment L5/S1, for instance, sometimes impedes lateral flexion *to the right* in the next segment superiorly (L4/L5) and, as expected, restricts lateral flexion *to the left* in the segment of the prolapse (L5/S1). In the next segment superiorly (L4/L5), however, flexion to the left (the side of the prolapse) proceeds normally. With lateral flexion to the side opposite the prolapse, the fourth (or fifth) lumbar vertebra rotates slightly around its longitudinal axis so that its spinous process moves to the side of the prolapse—in the case mentioned thus, to the left.
• With anteflexion and retroflexion, the intervertebral disk space becomes deformed. As this takes place, the tangents of the opposite endplates converge in the direction of flexion. If, in the end position of anteflexion, the tangents fail to converge ventrally in a particular segment, this suggests a reflex locking of movement, usually in consequence of a dorsal prolapse of a disk (Fig. 11). If there is no narrowing of the intervertebral space, locking of movement with maximal anteflexion *and* retroflexion is also a sign of dorsal prolapse of a disk (Fig. 12) or an intraspinal tumor, which may be of the hour-glass type.

Radiocinematography of the joints is reserved for scientific research. For practical purposes it is too complicated. Also complicated are *roentgenograms of the entire spine.* One of the prerequisites for taking usable roentgenograms of the entire spine *with the patient standing* is a potent x-ray generator that permits making roentgenograms with a focal distance of up to 3 m. In this way the spine, together with parts of the pelvic girdle and the shoulder girdle, can be reproduced on a film of 20 × 96 cm or 30 × 90 cm. The variable attenuation of the x-rays by the different segments of the spine requires, as a rule, compensation for thickness. To this end, one can make use of a unit that has been developed by Edinger and associates (1956). This unit, together with a special support, is supplied by Siemens Corporation (Erlangen) and has been termed "collimator with light beam and rotating compensatory mask." With use of the *oscil-*

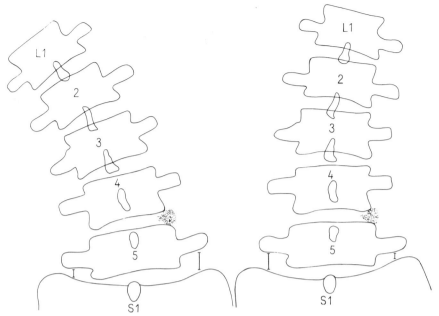

Fig. 9 **Left-sided posterolateral prolapse of the disk between L4 and L5.** Unimpeded lateral flexion toward the side opposite to the prolapse (right side). In the involved segment, flexion toward the side of the prolapse is obstructed. Since the disk space between L5 and S1 cannot usually be confidently estimated in the anteroposterior roentgenogram, one must concentrate on the distance between the inferior transverse process of L5 and the superior border of the sacrum *(marked)*.

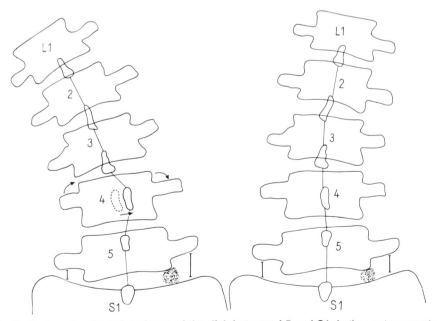

Fig. 10 **Left-sided posterolateral prolapse of the disk between L5 and S1.** In the next segment superiorly (L4/L5), lateral flexion to the right (to the side opposite to the prolapse) is impeded. Additional slight rotation of L4 so that its spinous process moves to the side of the prolapse (to the left) *(schematically)*. Lateral flexion to the side of the prolapse (left side) blocked in the 5th lumbar segment, normal in the 4th segment.

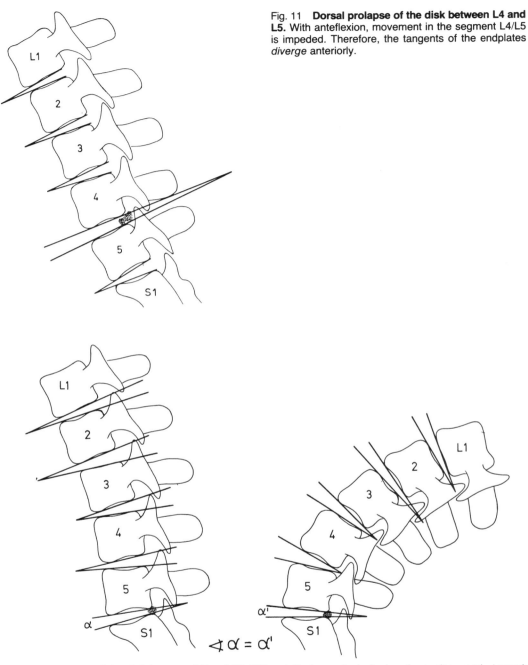

Fig. 11 **Dorsal prolapse of the disk between L4 and L5.** With anteflexion, movement in the segment L4/L5 is impeded. Therefore, the tangents of the endplates *diverge* anteriorly.

Fig. 12 **Prolapse of the disk between L5 and S1.** With anteflexion and retroflexion, the angles α and α' remain unchanged (movement of L5/S1 blocked).

lating diaphragm designed by Raspe in 1956 (F. Hofmann, Ltd., Erlangen), the roentgenogram of the total spine consists of three single exposures in sections. Overlaps are blotted out by the oscillating movements of the diaphragm. For this radiographic technique one can employ automatic exposure.

Arthritis

Arthritis occurs as the consequence of damage to the joint to which the synovial membrane reacts with hyperemia, exudation (effusion into the joint, capsular and periarticular edema), and proliferation (hypertrophy of the synovial membrane, thickening of the fibrous capsule).

The histologic processes of arthritis are reflected *by the roentgenogram* as follows: the **soft-tissue signs of arthritis** appear, at the earliest, a number of *days or weeks* after the onset of the disease. The **(inflammatory) collateral phenomena of arthritis** become manifest roentgenologically a number of *weeks or months* after onset.

The **direct signs of arthritis,** depending on the activity of the inflammation, usually become visible in the roentgenogram only a number of *months or years* after the onset of arthritis.

It is true, however, that each of these roentgen signs can be imitated by other diseases. *On the one hand,* the roentgen signs of arthritis are part of a mosaic into which the history, the physical findings, and the results of serologic, hematologic, and biochemical studies must fit. *On the other hand,* any *combination* of the roentgen signs listed below is sufficient to make a presumptive diagnosis or even to settle the diagnosis:

* Soft-tissue signs *plus* collateral phenomena *plus* direct signs
 = arthritis + +
* Soft-tissue signs *plus* collateral phenomena
 = arthritis (+) or +
* Soft-tissue signs *plus* direct signs
 = arthritis(+) or +
* Collateral phenomena *plus* direct signs
 = arthritis +
* Soft-tissue signs
 = arthritis − or (+)
* Collateral phenomena
 = arthritis − or (+)
* *One* direct sign only
 = arthritis − or (+)
* Several direct signs (see Fig. 20)
 = arthritis (+), +, or + +

The *soft-tissue signs of arthritis* appear in connection with an increase in volume of the synovia and edema of the synovial membrane, the fibrous joint capsule, and the periarticular tissue. They may, however, be attributable to an increase in volume of the synovial membrane (cellular infiltration and proliferation).

The *collateral phenomena of arthritis* make their appearance in the subchondral bone. They are consequent upon a local impairment of circulation produced at this site by the arthritis (Rutishausel and Jacqueline 1959; Aufdermaur 1974). This local disturbance leads to roentgenologically demonstrable processes of remodeling in the cancellous trabeculae and the compacta;[6] i.e., demineralization. In addition to this, disuse or immobilization of the inflamed joint contributes to the demineralization that accompanies the arthritis (Burkhart and Jowsey, 1967).

The *direct signs of arthritis,* finally, reveal the destructive action of the effusion into the joint and the inflammatory proliferation of the synovial membrane on the articular supporting and gliding tissue, including the articular cartilage. However, it is also true of the direct signs of arthritis that processes that are not directly connected with the arthritic reaction can influence the appearance, the extent, and the radiographic morphology of the direct signs. One of these factors, particularly in chronic arthritis, is the often inevitable, though only reduced, restriction of motion. *Examples:*

An arthritis accompanied by a *serous* effusion into the joint may manifest itself by the soft-tissue signs and the collateral phenomena. The nutrition of the articular cartilage is disturbed concomitantly by the serous effusion. The articular cartilage, which is damaged in this way, may no longer be capable of withstanding the normal stress of motion and load. With time, a *paraarthritic* or *postarthritic osteoarthrosis* then develops, the signs of which dominate the radiographic diagnosis.

Also, in a *slowly progressive chronic arthritis* (e.g., a coxarthritis developing during the course of an ankylosing spondylitis), the paraarthritic osteoarthrosis can completely overshadow the radiologic signs of inflammation. This osteoarthrosis likewise develops as a result of the traumatic influence of motion on the articular cartilage, which has been previously damaged by the inflammation. The articulating bones of an inflamed joint assume by reflex that position in which the joint capsule is "relaxed" to the maximum. The slightly flexed metacarpophalangeal and/or interphalangeal joints then mimic a narrowing of the interosseous space in the roentgenogram, thus giving a direct sign of arthritis (Fig. 39). In addition, inactivity from immobilization causes the articular cartilage to suffer a (reversible) loss of fluid, which also manifests itself in the roentgenogram as a (reversible) narrowing of the interosseous space. In polyarthritis, inflammatory involvement of one or the other small joint, especially of the hands and feet, can thus be mimicked.

Soft-Tissue Signs of Arthritis and Their Differential Diagnosis

The soft-tissue signs of arthritis indicate, *quite generally,* an increase in volume of the joint cavity and/or the synovial membrane, and the fibrous joint capsule and/or the immediate vicinity of the joint. The in-

---

[6] *Note:* In the Anglo-American literature, the term "cortex" is used synonymously with "compacta." In German, cortex denotes only the narrow layer of bone that covers the meshes of cancellous bone.

flammatory origin of such an increase in volume can therefore, as a rule, be recognized roentgenologically only in connection with collateral phenomena and/or direct signs of arthritis. Similarly, consideration of the anamnesis, the physical findings, and the result of laboratory examinations aid in differentiating, for example, between an inflammatory, a traumatic, or a neoplastic effusion, or between an inflammatory and a neoplastic proliferation of the synovium. The roentgenologic morphology of the (arthritic) soft-tissue signs depends on the *local* anatomic conditions. There are joints in which no (arthritic) soft-tissue signs whatsoever are observed.

Examples are the acromioclavicular, the sternoclavicular, and the sacroiliac joints. Other joints show *certain* soft-tissue signs of arthritis only in a definite period of life; namely, in early childhood. *Examples* are the shoulder and the hip joint. Finally, certain joints are known in which an intraarticular increase in volume of a few millimeters becomes visible in the roentgenogram. *Examples* are the elbow, the knee, and the talocrural joint. In addition, an articular and periarticular increase in volume manifests itself at a particularly early date in joints whose soft-tissue con-

tours stand out normally in the roentgenogram. (*Example:* the phalangeal joints.)

The soft-tissue signs of arthritis manifest themselves in the following joints: Distal and proximal interphalangeal joints of the hands and feet (Figs. 92 and 491); metacarpophalangeal and metatarsophalangeal joints (Figs. 92, 97, and 491); carpal joints and carporadial joint (Fig. 124); distal radioulnar joint (under certain morphologic conditions; see Fig. 98); elbow joint (Fig. 189), shoulder joint (Fig. 235); hip joint (Figs. 291 and 292); knee joint (Figs. 399, 400, and 402); talocrural joint; and possibly also subtalar joint (Fig. 490).

Collateral Phenomena of Arthritis and Their Differential Diagnosis

In the bones surrounding an inflamed joint, increased radiolucency usually appears as early as within a few weeks or months of onset. This increased radiolucency can show a sharp or a hazy structure. It may

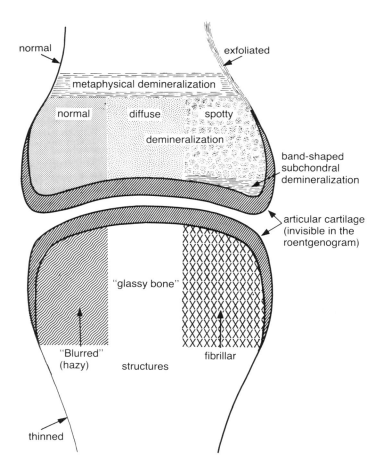

Fig. 13 **Diagram of the collateral phenomena of arthritis (see text) in the juxtaarticular bone.** The symbol "normal" signifies regular structure of the cancellous bone and regular thickness and structure of the cortical bone (see Fig. 14). "Demineralization" means increased translucence of bone. "Glassy bone" denotes such a high degree of decalcification that differences in roentgen beam attenuation between the bone and the surrounding soft tissues are hardly demonstrable. Band-shaped demineralization of the metaphysis is observed only after closure of the epiphysis in the region of the former epiphyseal plate. A special feature of demineralization developing in the growth period—of either inflammatory or noninflammatory origin (due, for example to immobilization; see text)—is its *fibrillar* character. This fibrillar structure of the juxtaarticular cancellous bone (so-called hypertrophic atrophy of bone) persists after cure of the arthritis or after remobilization, in contrast to the other collateral phenomena of arthritis or the sequelae of immobilization. It is thus irreversible (Dihlmann, 1976).

be spotty or—in the immediate sucbchondral area and the metaphysis—band-shaped. At times it is fibrillar or else homogeneous. In the literature, this manifestation has been termed *juxtaarticular osteoporosis, inflammatory atrophy of bone,* or *inflammatory demineralization.* This decalcification, associated with the soft-tissue signs of arthritis, is often one of the first pathologic roentgen signs, particularly if it develops in an arthritis of acute or subacute onset, or in fresh episodes of chronic (poly-)arthritis. Accurate analysis of the radiographic picture of juxtaarticular decalcification is helpful in the specification and differentiation of this roentgen finding, which is composed of different roentgen signs (Figs. 13 and 14). The totality of these roentgen signs has been termed *(inflammatory) collateral phenomena of arthritis.* As already noted, these signs develop (1) as the result of a local circulatory disturbance in the juxtaarticular bone marrow, which is triggered by the arthritis. This disorder, together with (2) the immobilization of the diseased joint induced by the pain and/or the therapeutic measures compromises the physiologic remodeling of bone. In some arthropathies—e.g., rheumatoid arthritis and tuberculosis of joints—it is a matter of debate whether or not (3) the function of the osteoblasts, in addition, becomes directly damaged by the basic disorder. These three factors, depending on the degree of their involvement, influence the bone structure in the vicinity of inflamed joints (Figs. 13 and 14).

Demineralization of disuse (Jones, 1969) follows prolonged immobilization of a skeletal part; for example, after an injury or an operation. This disorder cannot be differentiated radiologically from the collateral phenomena of arthritis (Figs. 13 and 14), especially since it is part of these phenomena, as mentioned above. Demineralization of disuse, however, is *not accompanied by pain!* This circumstance facilitates its *clinical* differentiation from arthritis as well as from the reflex dystrophies (Sudeck's syndrome, etc.; *vide infra*). Another posttraumatic phenomenon may be mentioned here, namely **posttraumatic pagetoid remodeling of bone** (Fig. 15). This disorder is probably to be regarded as a special form of Sudeck's reflex dystrophy (Rohner 1957; Aufdermaur 1977). The *roentgen findings* obtained in the decalcification and the structural changes of cancellous and cortical bone described above as collateral phenomena of arthritis are not fundamentally different from those in **Sudeck's syndrome** and in causalgia. The swelling of soft tissues in Sudeck's syndrome, however, is more evenly developed and not, like an arthritic soft-tissue swelling, limited to the joints and their surroundings. The latter disorder is also visible in the roentgenogram. On the other hand in Sudeck's syndrome one also sees juxtaarticular

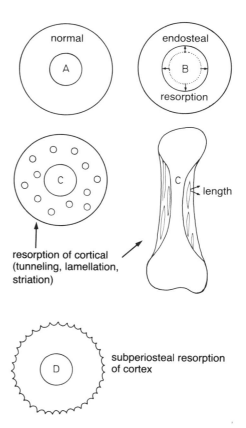

Fig. 14 *Schematic display of resorptive cortical reactions.* B and C = Diseases of bone with increased remodeling (accelerated turnover), namely hyperparathyroidism, hyperthyroidism, acromegaly. B alone, however, suggests decelerated remodeling of bone; e.g., in involutional osteoporosis (Meema et al., 1978).

C = Collateral striation (small tubular bone) in arthritis, but also in reflex dystrophies and hyperparathyroidism.

D = Hyperparathyroidism (here, C often precedes D).

Note: In the adult, striation (intracortical resorption) is always pathologic if at least half of the surveyable cortical bone (of the 2nd metacarpal) shows such widening of the haversian canals (Meema, 1977). B and D can be recognized early if mammography films (fine-grained films for material testing with a high silver content) are used and studied with a loupe at 6× to 8× magnification ("microradioscopy" after Meema, 1977). This radiographic technique makes use of low tube voltage and a high mAs value for exposure. Sites of predilection for B and C are the metacarpals, for D and C the middle phalanges of the fingers.

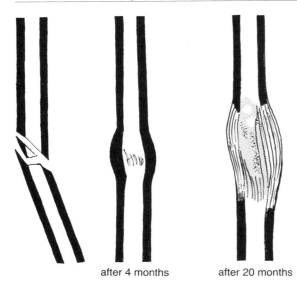

after 4 months   after 20 months

Fig. 15 **Development of posttraumatic pagetoid remodeling of bone** (see text).

Radiographic diagnosis: Bone structure normal at the moment of fracture. The fracture heals uneventfully. The pagetoid remodeling of bone manifests itself after months or years by pain and dysfunction in the region of the former fracture.

periosteal reactions, striation of the cortical bone (Fig. 14), delicate erosions, partial wasting of the marginal subchondral lamella, and decreased thickness of the articular cartilage. Anomalous flexion of the finger joints, similar to that observed in the different types of arthritis (p. 11), can mimic narrowing of the radiographic joint space. Some of these roentgen signs suggest that reflex dystrophies lead not only to osteopathy but also to arthropathy. This supposition has been corroborated by histologic studies by Genant et al. (1975). These workers described proliferation of epithelial cells, increase of collagenous fibrils, proliferation of vessels, hyperemia, edema, and inflammatory cellular infiltration in the synovial membrane in reflex dystrophies.

The diagnosis of Sudeck's syndrome is therefore based on the skeletal findings *and* on the well-known manifestations in the soft tissues ("atypical of arthritis"): edematous swelling that extends distally, cyanosis, muscle wasting, contractures or at least impaired mobility of joints that are not affected by the precipitating cause, hyperhidrosis, trophic lesions of skin and nails, and pain. By careful clinical study (note, for example, the absence of systemic humoral signs of inflammation) and detailed notation of the history the physician will succeed in making the correct diagnosis, even in cases where Sudeck's syndrome did not occur as an aftermath of a mechanical injury but followed, for example, an infection of the soft tissues, a frostbite, a burn, or an electric injury. Diagnosis will also be successful when the syndrome accompanies a disease of the central nervous system, the thoracic organs (pleuropulmonary and cardioaortal disorders), or the peripheral vessels, or when it follows the use of certain drugs (Lequesne 1967, 1968 a,b; Kaiser 1976; Bensasson et al., 1977).

Causalgia, similarly to the syndrome named after Paul Sudeck, belongs among the reflex dystrophies.

It occurs after partial nerve injuries and concerns principally the tibial, median, and ulnar nerves. Its leading clinical symptom is the "burning pain" that is triggered by acoustic or visual stimuli, by imagination, and also by emotion.

The shoulder-hand syndrome—clinically an association of periarthritis of the shoulder and Sudeck's syndrome of the hand—is also a reflex dystrophy, hence a neurovascular disorder with vasomotor dysregulation and dystrophic sequelae. This syndrome of multifactorial etiology makes its appearance a few weeks or months after the precipitating event, which may be a myocardial infarction, a massive cerebral hemorrhage, a trauma, or a pleuropulmonary disease. At times, the anamnesis is unproductive (idiopathic shoulder-hand syndrome). The roentgenogram *may,* as in the other reflex dystrophies, reveal spotty or diffuse demineralization in the regions of the shoulder and the hand.

A *variant of Sudeck's syndrome* is a disorder known variously as **transient osteoporosis** (of the hip), transient painful osteoporosis (of the lower extremities), idiopathic algodystrophy (of the hip), and migratory transient osteoporosis (Duncan et al. 1967; Lequesne 1968b; Swezey 1970; Schilling 1973; Langloh et al. 1973; Hasche and Meyer 1974; and other writers).

Clinical Features of Transient Osteoporosis

It is a painful monoarticular movement disorder (principally on weightbearing), which sometimes is accompanied by a roentgenologically demonstrable effusion into the joint. It develops spontaneously or following an inadequate trauma and, occasionally, even in connection with pregnancy (Cayla et al., 1978). Most frequently affected are the joints of the foot and the knee joint; the hip joints and the joints of the upper extremities are less often involved. The disorder clears spontaneously if the diseased joint does not bear weight for several months. A characteristic, though not essential, feature of the disorder is its tendency to *successive* involvement of other joints of the ipsilateral or contralateral side; hence the term "migratory" transient osteoporosis. The erythrocyte sedimentation rate is usually normal; sometimes it is slightly increased. The soft-tissue findings listed in discussing Sudeck's syndrome are absent or inconspicuous. This is why the diagnosis sometimes offers difficulties (the most frequent erroneous diagnosis: arthritis) and why this reflex dystrophy has become known much later than the classic Sudeck's syndrome.

Roentgen Findings in Transient Osteoporosis (Figs. 16, 17 and 18)

Between a few weeks and 1 month—at most 2 months—after the onset of pain, demineralization is demonstrable in the subchondral layer of the involved joint. The radiographic joint space does *not* appear to be narrowed, whereas the marginal subchondral lamella *may* become decalcified and thereby invisible. *Sometimes* demineralization begins in a rather circumscribed area of the subchondral bone; e.g., in a femoral condyle, in the patella, in one digit of the foot or the hand, or in a tarsal or carpal bone. The latter is called the zonal type of transient osteoporosis (Lequesne et al., 1977; Figs. 16, 17, and 18). After a few weeks or up to several months, the totality of the osseous subchondral layer (the entire skeleton of the hand or the foot) becomes decalcified. Remineralization takes place between about 6 and 12 months after the onset of pain.

Differential Diagnosis of Transient Osteoporosis

A "rheumatic" or bacterial monoarthritis must be ruled out by clinical and roentgenologic study (sedimentation rate in transient osteoporosis normal or slightly increased; absence of direct signs of arthritis, except for possible decalcification of the marginal lamella; and an equally possible minor periosteal reaction). The zonal type of transient osteoporosis must also be differentiated from a *metastatic malignancy*, a fibrosarcoma, reticulum cell sarcoma and lymphosarcoma of bone, and from an aseptic necrosis of bone.

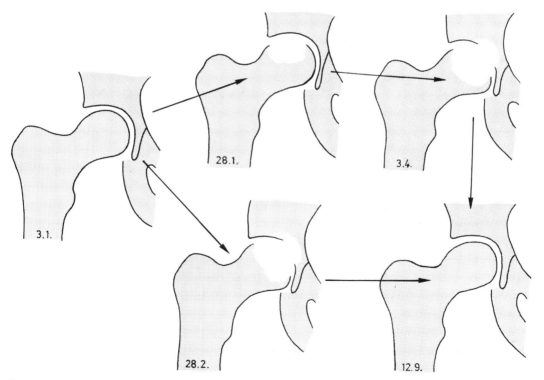

Fig. 16   **Follow-up studies in transient osteoporosis of the hip joint.** Onset of pain (initial radiologic examination) on January 3. "Upper pathway" = zonal type of transient osteoporosis. "Lower pathway" = classic type of transient osteoporosis (with reversible wasting of the marginal subchondral lamella). September 12 = remineralization (disease episode finished). This circumstance, however, does not rule out the possibility of another ipsilateral or contralateral joint being affected before long (see text). *(Decalcification = "white")*.

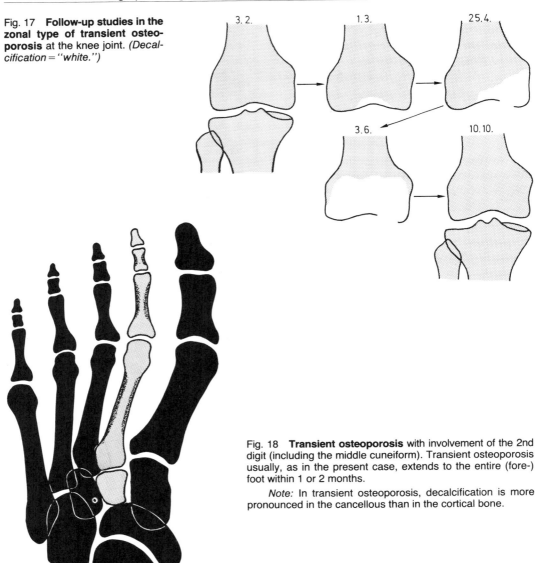

Fig. 17 **Follow-up studies in the zonal type of transient osteoporosis** at the knee joint. *(Decalcification = "white.")*

Fig. 18 **Transient osteoporosis** with involvement of the 2nd digit (including the middle cuneiform). Transient osteoporosis usually, as in the present case, extends to the entire (fore-) foot within 1 or 2 months.

Note: In transient osteoporosis, decalcification is more pronounced in the cancellous than in the cortical bone.

Fig. 19 **Diagram of the histologic findings in the inflamed joint,** as far as they can be reflected in the roentgenogram.

Obliquely dashed: Articular cartilage.

Dotted: Effusion into the joint or inflammatory edema of the capsule and its surroundings.

Arrows: Pannus (highly cellular, fibrovascular resorption tissue) originating in the recesses of the joint where the synovial membrane inserts into the cartilage-bone interface. The pannus spreads inside the joint cavity; it coats the articular cartilage, penetrates it, and thus extends to the subchondral bone. The pannus, however, also may—from the recesses—invade the bone directly, sometimes by way of so-called "naked" areas (Martel et al., 1965); i.e., free surfaces of bone between the insertion of the capsule and the border of the articular cartilage. The most important example of pannus formation in an inflamed joint is rheumatoid arthritis.

Black bulges, bilaterally vertical to the joint space: Proliferated synovial membrane.

Crossed dashes or stripes sketched in the junction between metaphysis and diaphysis: Periosteal reactions.

Spotty decalcifications of bone have also been observed in lymph stasis following radical resection of a mammary cancer and after a thrombosis. They must therefore be differentiated from the collateral phenomena of arthritis. Generalized disorders of the metabolism of bone similarly involve the juxta-articular segments and modify radiotranslucence there: e.g., osteoporosis,[7] rickets, osteomalacia, and hyperparathyroidism. Genuine articular disturbances occurring with these diseases will be discussed and illustrated under the heading of "Topographic radiologic diagnosis of the gliding tissue."

***

[7] In about 50 percent of osteoporosis patients treated with sodium fluoride joint pains occur occasionally, accompanied by periarticular edematous swelling (Kruse et al., 1978).

Direct Signs of Arthritis and Their Differential Diagnosis

The direct signs of arthritis can be traced to the histologic processes in the inflamed joint (Fig. 19). In this figure, the inflammatory exudation is indicated by dots. It forms an effusion and impregnates the synovia, the fibrous joint capsule, and possibly also the periarticular soft tissues. The effusion gives rise to circumscribed chondroosteolytic processes that—by enzymic destruction?—produce rounded (spherical) translucences in the subchondral spongiosa. These translucences are termed arthritic *signal cysts (signal geodes)* and *attendant cysts (attendant geodes)* (Fig. 20A, page 19 ff). Such cystic subchondral osteo-

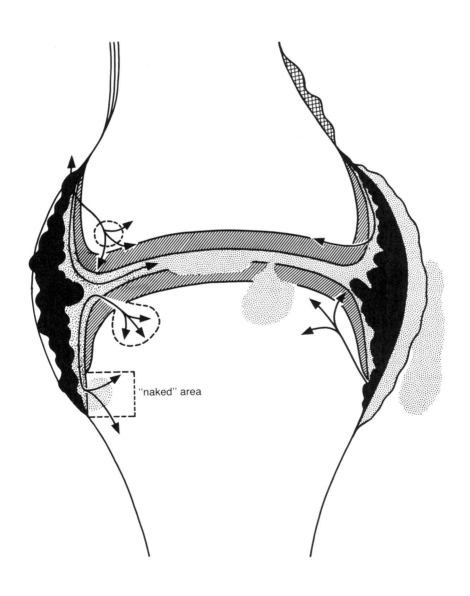

"naked" area

lyses, however, are also produced by a highly cellular, fibrovascular resorption tissue, the so-called *pannus*. The pannus develops in the recesses of the joint. From there it invades the surroundings, accompanied by destruction of cartilage, bone, and soft tissues (*arrows* in Fig. 19). In rheumatoid arthritis two additional histologic processes occur: rheumatoid nodules and focal rheumatoid necrosis of bone. These lead to subchondral spherical osteolyses (cysts, geodes).

Rheumatoid Nodules

The subcutaneous rheumatoid nodule has been known as the prototype of the rheumatoid granuloma. It presents a characteristic zonal structure comprising central necrosis, a perinecrotic radial palisade of connective tissue cells, and a highly cellular and fibrotic marginal area. Subcutaneous rheumatic nodules develop preferentially at sites exposed to mechanical stress; e.g., over the olecranon. Moreover, rheumatoid granulomas manifesting themselves in the roentgenogram as cystic structures have also been observed in vertebral bodies, in the proximal end of the femur, in the ulna, and in the metatarsals (Magyar et al., 1974; Aufdermaur 1974). Intravertebral rheumatoid granulomas of sufficient size can lead to collapse of the vertebra (Baggenstoss et al., 1952).

Focal Rheumatoid Necrosis of Bone (Uehlinger, 1971)

This necrosis of bone sometimes develops during the evolution of rheumatoid arthritis. It consists of necrotic bone and bone marrow as well as of deposits of fibrin which are enclosed by a hyaline membrane and collagenous fibrils. Their histologic structure thus distinguishes them unequivocally from the rheumatoid granuloma (Mather, 1954). The spherical osteolysis produced by focal rheumatoid necrosis of bone can generally be distinguished from its surroundings by a delicate seam of increased density visible in the roentgenogram. Focal rheumatoid necroses of bone are also seen in the subchondral layer of joints that present no other direct signs of arthritis. In such cases, however, contiguous joints in which no subchondral focal necroses may yet have developed do present definite arthritic destruction.

Pannus and purulent effusion into the joint and collateral arthritic processes in the subchondral bone marrow (see p. 13)—can, through decalcification or resorption, lead to *disappearance of the marginal subchondral lamella*. This is demonstrable in the roentgenogram primarily by the convexity of the articular contours (Fig. 20A).

In addition, pannus and purulent effusion into the joint lead to destruction of the articulating bones, which is designated as *erosion, destruction, mutilation,* and *dissection*. Apart from this, erosions sometimes are the local result of inflammatory hyperemia which shifts the balance between osteoblasts and osteoclastic cells against the former. Finally, mechanical forces—particularly muscular contraction and gravitation—participate in the destruction of a joint affected by arthritis. With a faulty position of the joint, for instance, parts of the articulating bones which otherwise have no contact are sometimes pressed against each other during motion. When the cartilage cover in these places is already lacking and the subchondral layer has become largely demineralized, either the marginal lamella and the subjacent spongiosa break down or the persistent pressure leads to resorption of bone. The roentenogram then shows erosion or destruction.

Smoothed erosion (Fig. 20 B) is the term applied to defects of bone with smooth contours and often even a cortex-like marginal zone. Smoothed erosions are suggestive evidence of a local stationary or a healed arthritic process.

Erosion and *destruction* are not synonyms but indicate quantitative differences of destruction in a joint-bearing bone. Erosion is a small loss in continuity which often is marginal, hence at the cartilage/bone interface. Destruction, by contrast, affects larger parts of the articulating bones (Fig. 20 A).

Mutilation (Figs. 20 A and 38) is an arthritic destruction of the articular gliding and supporting tissues that extends to parts of bone remote from the joint. Similarly to ankylosis, mutilation is encountered in the final stage of arthritis. The term "mutilating arthritis" was introduced decades ago (Stursberg, 1935) to characterize an "extreme degree of arthritis involving numerous joints, accompanied by abundant resorption of calcium from bone." The process in question, however, is *not* a specific clinical picture but only an advanced stage of *any* (poly-) arthritis. The activity of a (poly-)arthritis, the duration of the disease, and of course the therapy govern the progression of the disease and the extent of joint destruction. These factors therefore determine whether or not the stage of mutilation is reached. In rheumatoid arthritis, for instance, mutilations occur only after a few decades, whereas in psoriatic arthritis and in lipoid dermatoarthritis (see p. 131) it often occurs much earlier. True, the extent of mutilation is limited by the range of capillaries budding in the inflammatory granulation tissue and the possibility of capillaries being transformed into arterioles or even still larger vessels (Dihlmann et al., 1961). This is why arthritic mutilation is encountered preferentially in the small joints (hands, feet, acromioclavicular and temporomandibular joint) as well as in flat (thin) bones (distal ulna, region of the elbow).

In chronic rheumatoid polyarthritis of many years' standing one sometimes sees *extraarticular mutilations;* for example, in the spinous processes of the vertebrae, the bone ends in the phalanges, or the ribs (Elke 1963; Peter et al., 1964; Dihlmann 1977).

The term *"arthritic dissection"* denotes the disconnection of a necrotic portion of the joint-forming bone. The type of cartilage resorption characteristic of arthritis—whether of humoral nature or triggered by tissue proliferation and/or lack of oxygen[8]—leads to *concentric (even) narrowing of the radiologic joint*

---

[8] The *inflamed* synovial membrane "steals" oxygen from the upper layer of the articular cartilage (Tillmann and Binzus, 1969).

Fig. 20 A **The direct roentgen signs of arthritis.**

Explanation of terms: erosion = small (often marginal) defect of contour. Destruction = extensive breakdown. Mutilation = extreme degree of deformation of the articulating bones. Mutilation and ankylosis form the final stage of arthritis. Signal cyst = spherical osteolysis as the first direct sign of arthritis. Attendant cyst = spherical osteolysis occurring in conjunction with other direct signs of arthritis.

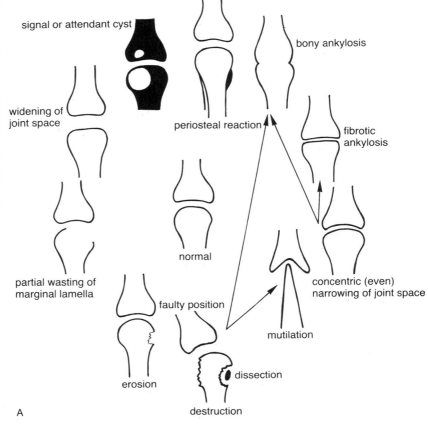

Fig. 20 B **Basic roentgenographic aspect of the florid arthritic erosion** *(arrow).* **This lesion, following local healing of the arthritis, is remodeled into a smoothed erosion** *(tailed arrow i.e., covered by a cortex like marginal seam).*
(t = time = follow-up study.)

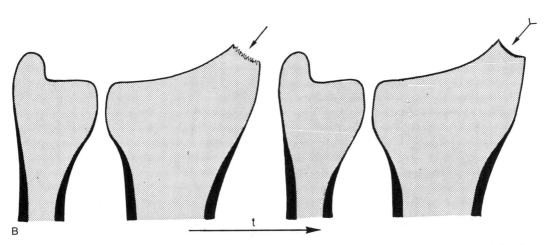

space. The inevitable movements of the diseased joints also have an injurious effect on the articular cartilage, which can no longer cope with the physiologic strain and wears away.

Fibrotic and *bony ankylosis* (Fig. 20 A) are final stages of arthritis. The articular cartilage has been resorbed, and fibrotic cicatricious connective tissue forms between the articulating bones, or osseous trabeculae grow across the obliterated joint and stiffen the articulating bones irreversibly. The result is a more or less pronounced malposition of the joint.

Malpositions of the joint—deviation, subluxation, dislocation (Fig. 20 A)—are sequelae of arthritic loosening of destruction of the capsuloligamentous apparatus and eccentric capsular shrinking. Their direction is influenced by the static load on the joint and the pull of tendons and muscles. Malpositions may, at times, also develop as the result of a reflex position of comfort.

Juxtaarticular, lamellar, or irregularly structured *periosteal new bone formations* (Fig. 20) probably occur in connection with periosteal edema. Marked arthritic periosteal reactions are observed particularly in childhood. In addition, they are apt, at any age, to accompany psoriatic arthritis, Reiter's syndrome, peripheral arthritis in ankylosing spondylitis, and Crohn's disease.

At times an effusion into a nonweightbearing joint can lead to spacing of the articular surfaces, hence to *widening of the radiologic joint space* (Fig. 20 A). This, however, presupposes additional relaxation of the collateral ligaments.

A *spontaneous* accumulation of gas in joints ("pneumarthrosis," see Fig. 307) that exceeds the so-called vacuum phenomenon suggests an anaerobic infection, an *E. coli* infection, or diabetes mellitus with enzymic glucose dissimilation in infected tissues (Meredith and Rittenberg, 1978).

The phenomenon "arthritis" produces the roentgen findings sketched in Figure 20. Their association strongly suggests or even settles the diagnosis. As single findings, the direct signs are not convincing enough to dispense with the following differential diagnostic considerations:

Cystic[9] defects of bone in the immediate vicinity of a joint occur in numerous pathologic conditions. Among all bodies with the same volume, the sphere has the smallest surface, and among all surfaces with the same area that of the sphere encloses the largest volume. A spherical osteolysis can therefore be regarded as the "biological compromise" between the local defense reaction and the osteolytic agent.

In joints exposed to static load, *osteoarthrotic cysts* develop prevalently in the pressure-absorbing zone. Depending on their content, one speaks of hemorrhagic, debris, or detritus cysts; depending on their mode of development, a distinction is made between compression and insufficiency cysts. The osteoarthrotic cysts thus are indicators of diminished or absent elasticity of the articular cartilage. They result in focal necroses of the cancellous bone, which are removed. Experience shows that a "quantitative" balance exists between the other roentgen signs of osteoarthrosis and the osteoarthrotic cysts. This balance becomes disturbed when, for example, a *minor* narrowing of the radiologic joint space, a *minor* sclerosis of the subchondral cancellous bone, and only *delicate* arthrotic osteophytes are demonstrable next to *very large* subchondral cysts or when the cysts appear without any other signs of osteoarthrosis and/or they have not developed in the pressure-absorbing area. In this instance, the following causes of *subchondral* cystic structures should also be taken into consideration:

1. **Intraosseous ganglion** (Fig. 21 A and B). This has the following distinctive features: young or middle-aged individuals, local pain. The ganglion is located in the epiphysis or metaphysis. It is well demarcated, round or oval, and sometimes trabeculated. In about 50 percent of cases, it presents a narrow, sclerotic marginal seam. The lesion is more frequently solitary than multiple. Its diameter varies from a few millimeters to a number of centimeters. The seat of the lesion is often eccentric; its topographic relationships to the pressure-absorbing area of the joint are not definite but are at most incidental. Tomography does not, as a rule, reveal a connection with the joint space. No calcium shadows are demonstrable in the osteolytic area, and there is no lamellar reaction on the part of the periosteum. Extremely rare findings are expansion of bone, breaks, and increased density of soft tissues outside the bone (to be differentiated from ganglion in the soft tissues with pressure erosion of bone). The preferential seat is in the tubular bones, whereas the carpal and tarsal bones are seldom affected. Sites of predilection are: the bones surrounding the talocrural joint (particularly the medial malleolus), the knee, the hip, and the shoulder joint. Contents of the ganglion are: a yellowish, mucoid, or gelatinous fluid enclosed by a fibrous wall with partly loosened structures (note the histologic similarity of this finding to cysts in arthrosis [Salzer and Salzer-Kuntschik, 1968]).

2. **Benign chondroblastoma** (Fig. 22 A and B): The majority of patients between the ages of 10 and 25, have painful lesion. Pain referred to the contiguous joint (pain on motion; effusion into the joint may occur). Lesion almost consistently located in the epiphyses of the long tubular bones (particularly the proximal humerus, femur, and tibia), possible spread to the metaphysis. In the latter case, the typical roentgenogram that is observed exclusively in chon-

---

[9] The term "cyst" (synonyms: pseudocyst, geode) is applied *here* universally to any defect of bone that produces a rounded projection, without considering its "content," its lining, or its origin. However, cyst-shaped translucences in juxtaarticular regions of bone can, particularly in small bones, also be mimicked by (arthritic) erosions that are projected marginally. This underlines our postulate (p. 1) that all roentgenograms of joints be taken in at least two planes.

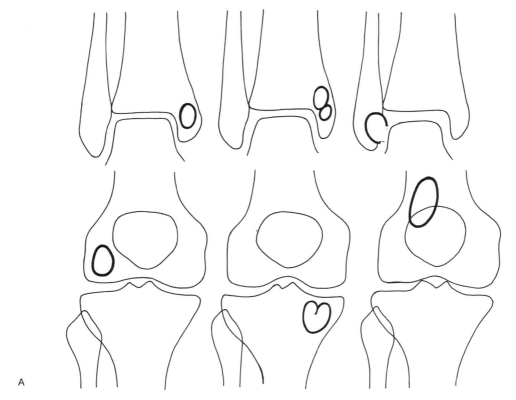

Fig. 21 A   **Radiographic morphology of an intraosseous ganglion** (see text).

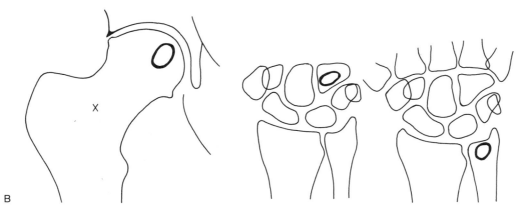

Fig. 21 B   **Intraosseous ganglion** (continued). x = the differential diagnosis between osteoarthrosis of the hip and a (somewhat atypically located) detritus cyst and the *incidental* combination of intraosseous ganglion and osteoarthrosis of the hip cannot be determined radiologically.

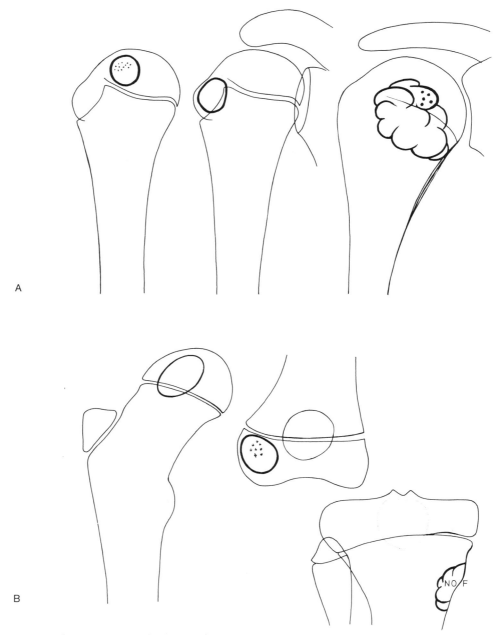

Fig. 22 A and B **Benign chondroblastroma.** NOF = incidental association of a chondroblastoma with a non-ossifying fibroma of bone.

Note: Benign chondroblastoma is a tumor that (though infrequently) not only spreads to the surrounding soft tissues but also develops successively in multiple centers of the neighboring bones (Hull et al., 1976). "Aggressive" variants of *benign* chondroblastoma are even liable to metastasize although histologically they present "benign" features (Riddell et al., 1973; Green and Whittaker, 1975).

droblastoma and in cystic tuberculosis of bone (Nelson, 1966) is seen: the rounded or oval osteolysis (Fig. 22) extends on both sides of the epiphyseal plate, which has not yet closed (Fig. 22 A and B). Sometimes septate osteolysis, frequently a sclerotic marginal seam, and equally often focal calcium deposits occur inside the osteolytic area. Discrete lamellar reaction on the part of the periosteum, particularly when the tumor is located in the epiphysis and the epiphyseal plate is already closed (Braunstein et al., 1979) or when the tumor also spreads to the metaphysis or (infrequently) has its origin in the metaphysis. Expansion of the cortex ("ballooning") and spread to the soft tissues may occur. Differential diagnosis by radiography *after closure* of the epiphysis: osteoclastoma, chondromyxoid fibroma, "brown tumor" in hyperparathyroidism.

3. **Osteoclastoma** (Fig. 23 A and B): Approximately 90 per cent of osteoclastomas develop after the age of 20. Prior to puberty this tumor is a rarity.

Sites of predilection are the epiphyses of the tubular bones on both sides of the knee joint, the proximal end of the femur, and the distal end of ulna and radius. When this tumor develops in a tubular bone, it is usually located eccentrically in the epiphyses, although it may spread to the metaphyseal region. With time, the growing tumor leads to thinning of the cortex and expansion ("ballooning") of the end of the bone. Lamellar and spicular reactions on the part of the periosteum are lacking. The so-called "soap bubble picture" is rather exceptional.

Inflammatory spherical osteolyses (cysts, pseudocysts, geodes) in the subchondral layer of joints, have already been described as *arthritic* signal or attendant cysts (p. 17). Occasionally they are even in the forefront of arthritic destruction, attracting attention either by their great number or by their size ("macrogeodes," Cabanel et al., 1973; "giant cysts," Magyar et al., 1974) (Fig. 24). There is apparently a

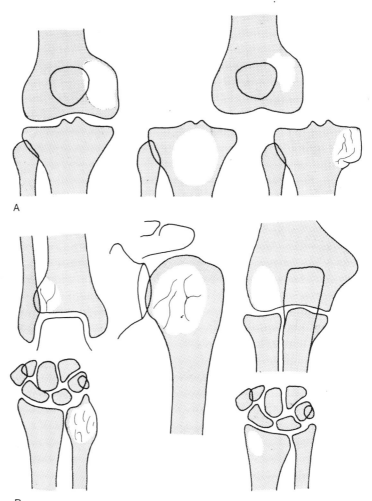

A

B

Fig. 23 A and B   **Projections in osteoclastoma.**

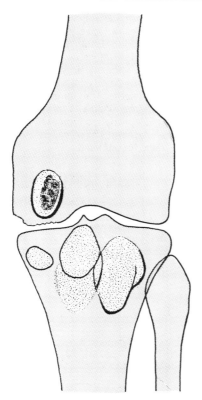

Fig. 24   Rheumatoid arthritis that has existed for 6 years. Roentgenologically demonstrable involvement of both hands, the right hip joint, and both knees. The latter (only *left* joint sketched) reveal strikingly large cysts *(macrogeodes)* in the head of the tibia and the medial condyle of the femur. In addition, narrowing of the radiologic joint space and delicate erosions in the medial condyle of the femur. Such macrogeodes sometimes contain calcified detritus that is visible in the roentgenogram as opacity of the cyst contents (Jayson et al., 1972). Note the macrogeode in the medial femoral condyle.

connection between the level of the intraarticular pressure on the one hand and the size and number of the arthritic cysts on the other. Castillo et al., (1965) therefore hold the extent of "physical activity" (of hands affected by rheumatoid arthritis) responsible for the number and size of arthritic cysts. Their argument is convincing because the (inflammatory) effusion, on the one hand, increases the intraarticular pressure and on the other, being a liquid, it is not compressible. A spherical osteolysis that develops in the subchondral layer and communicates with the joint cavity (Jayson et al., 1972) therefore acts as a decompression valve, for its volume rises to the third power of its radius. Incidentally, such a decompressing valve action has also been ascribed to the synovial cysts (Resnick et al., 1977).

When juxta-articular cystic osteolyses (1) are accompanied by discomfort in the joint, (2) appear in

larger numbers, and (3) do not exceed a diameter of 5 mm in *small* bones (phalanges, metacarpals, metatarsals, carpal and tarsal bones), the serum level of uric acid should always be determined! This is a rule in the radiographic diagnosis of gout; its principal exception is rheumatoid arthritis (Fig. 25 A).

Affections of the subchondral layer without a primary relationship to the contiguous joints may also give rise to cystic osteolyses.

Jüngling's ostitis multiplex cystoides (Figs. 117 to 120) is a skeletal manifestation of sarcoidosis. Its cystic osteolyses sometimes extend to (small) joints which are destroyed: mutilating type of Jüngling's disease.

Bacterial infections of the epiphyses and metaphyses of long tubular bones, short bones and, above all, flat bones can present cystic features in the roentgenogram. Among them are "cystic" tuberculosis of bone (Edeiken et al., 1963; Fig. 127) and leprosy. The changing clinical picture of pyogenic osteomyelitis in the era of antibiotics has also led to modifications of its radiographic morphology. With a Brodie abscess and in plasma cell osteomyelitis (albuminous osteomyelitis), a rounded or oval zone of osteolysis is at present more frequently encountered than a delicate zone of reactive sclerosis (Fig. 26). The periosteal reaction is also generally lacking, leading to difficulty in differentiating these conditions from benign and malignant tumors of the epiphysis or metaphysis, which expand with destruction of bone!

Parasitic colonization in the bones, for example by cystic echinococcus and fungal infections (coccidiodomycosis, blastomycosis, cryptococcosis [torulosis]) present conspicuous cystic osteolyses. The fungal diseases listed lead to development of inflammatory granulomas which are generally known to form spherical osteolyses.

Among the *disorders of metabolism* which are accompanied by (subchondral) cystic osteolyses belongs also ("brown tumor"; Fig. 150).

Intraosseous hemorrages in *hemophilia* can lead to necrosis of bone. When such a necrosis is resorbed, a cystic osteolysis develops. The same applies to necroses of bone of different etiology. *Epiphyseal aseptic osteonecroses* that do not extend to the surface of the bone involved are, in fact, either resorbed *or* revascularized and thereby reossified, *or* they calcify. Mixed pictures of these histologic processes are also observed.

In small bones, the carpals, for instance, cystic translucences are occasionally the result of *herniation of the synovium.* Sometimes they are also *vascular channels radiographed in orthograde alignment* (Ravelli, 1955a), or they develop as a consequence of *local disorders of circulation* (Rutishauser and Bugnion, 1951). Such carpal cysts increase in frequency with advancing age (Bugnion, 1951).

Posttraumatic cysts can, in principle, occur in any bone. Multiple "cystic" translucences in the epiphyses of tubular bones reflect *disorders of ossi-*

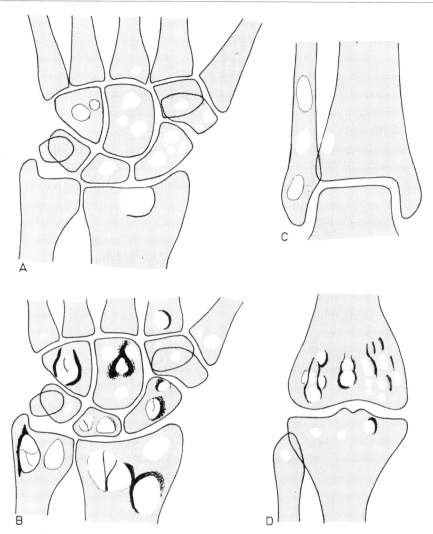

Fig 25   A = **Arthritic signal cysts.** 46-year-old gardener (manual worker). For about 6 months pain (in the night, but also during the day) and morning stiffness of the joints in both hands, lasting about half an hour.

Roentgen finding: In the region of both wrists (only *left* wrist sketched) numerous *cystic osteolyses,* mostly without sclerotic marginal seam. The majority of the cysts exceed 5 mm in diameter. Bilaterally symmetrical swelling of the proximal interphalangeal joints, which is also visible in the roentenogram *(not* sketched).

Radiologic differential diagnosis: Rheumatoid arthritis ("signal cysts"; see under this heading) more probable than gout and sarcoidosis. Adjunctive simple diagnostic procedures that most probably will settle the diagnosis: rheumatoid factors, serum concentration of uric acid, sedimentation rate, radiologic study of thorax.

B, C, D = **Diffuse skeletal angiomatosis** (this patient had no discomfort referable to the skeleton).

Roentgen finding: Numerous sharply defined rounded or oval cystic osteolyses in the epiphyses with a tendency to spread to the diaphyses. The size of the osteolyses varies from a few millimeters to a number of centimeters. Sometimes the cysts have a sclerotic marginal seam. The short bones (the carpals, for instance) and the flat bones (the pelvis and the skull, for instance) also become affected. The compact bone substance is but rarely involved. No periosteal reaction. Follow-up studies may show an increase in size of the cysts or even the development of new osteolyses.

Differential diagnosis: Hyperparathyroidism, fibrous dysplasia, histiocytosis X, bone metastases, plasmacytoma of the so-called peripheral type (Mieheke and Brandt 1979), non-Hodgkin's lymphomas.

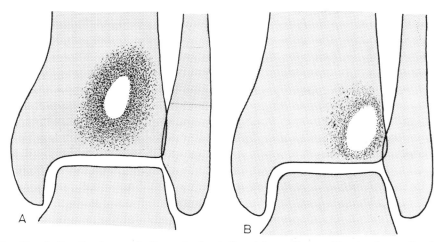

Fig. 26   A = **Classic Brodie abscess in the metaphysis** (breakdown of bone with extensive perifocal sclerosis).
   B = Brodie abscess without massive perifocal sclerosis of the cancellous bone (hypovirulent bacteria? see text).

fication (Fig. 334), e.g., in mucopolysaccharidoses. They have also been observed in *tuberous sclerosis* (Kämmerer et al., 1971).

Enchondromas in small tubular bones likewise produce cystic defects that often expand the bone. The subchondral region, however, is generally not involved (Fig. 27 A).

Electrical accidents (Kolár and Vrabec, 1976) and *frostbite* (Šváb, 1976) of the phalanges manifest themselves among other signs by small, rounded juxtaarticular translucences.

Basal cell nevus syndrome (Gorlin-Goltz syndrome) is a hereditary disease that is characterized by multiple basal cell carcinomas, mandibular cysts, anomalies of ribs and spine,

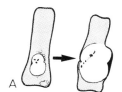

Fig. 27   A = **Enchondroma of the phalanx** (follow-up over 4 years).
   Note: In the small bones, the enchondroma generally spares the immediate subchondral region and gradually expands the portion of bone involved.
   B = Flame-shaped or oval translucences in the structure of the phalanges in the **basal cell nevus syndrome** (see text).

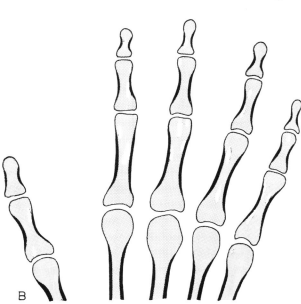

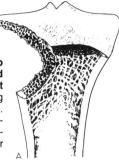
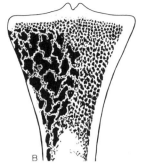
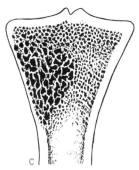

Fig. 28 **Relationship between size and growth of malignant bone tumors** according to *Lodwick* (see text). *From left to right:* Geographic osteolysis, moth-eaten appearance, tumor penetration.

a short metacarpal (of the 4th digit), dural calcifications and diverse neurologic and ophthalmologic anomalies. In 46 percent of cases (Dunnick et al., 1978), peculiar flame-shaped obliterations of the skeletal structure are found in the phalanges and occasionally in the distal radius and the metatarsals (Fig. 27 B).

Kaposi's sarcoma presents, in the hands and feet, the following constellation of roentgen findings: marked increase in soft-tissue density immediately next to erosions or extensive osteolyses in the small tubular bones; the spongiosa and compacta of these bones also presents cystic translucences. Metastases of malignant tumors can also affect the subchondral layer and are recognized there as (rounded) osteolyses. Regarding the identification and prognosis of **solid skeletal metastases,** attention is called to the following established facts:

1. **Relationship between shape and growth of malignant tumors of bone** (Lodwick, 1966; Figs. 28 and 29). This relationship has been described for primary tumors of bone but it is almost equally applicable to metastases. There are three basic radiographic patterns of malignancy-induced osteolysis; these patterns indicate a different growth rate of the tumor cells. *Geographic osteolysis* occurs with a *slow* rate of tumor growth. It forms a continuous bone defect that stands out sharply against its bony surroundings. The *"moth-eaten appearance"* created by numerous partly confluent "holes" of greatly variable size. The marginal contour is uneven, sometimes also hazy. This radiographic picture suggests an *acceler-* *ated* growth rate of the tumor. *Permeation* of the tumor cells is manifested by innumerable small osteolyses. The number and size of these decrease centrifugally. The marginal zone has dull borders. The tumor penetration resembles the normal structure of the spongiosa but the meshes are somewhat larger. In addition to this, the meshes are rounded or at least oval, whereas in the normal spongiosa their diameter is in alignment with the longitudinal axis of the bone. Tumor penetration occurs with *very rapidly growing* types of tumor. The different *periosteal reactions* indicate the growth rate of the tumor. As a rule, Codman's triangle accompanies permeation of the tumor cells and thus points to its aggressive, very rapid growth. Periosteal lamellae ("onion skins") probably reflect the alternation of exacerbation and remission (phasic tumor growth?—e.g., in Ewing's sarcoma). The periosteal spicules present three different formations (Fig. 29), *first* the radial sunray type; *second* the parallel brush type; and *third* the velvet type. The brush type and the sunray type frequently accompany tumor permeation. Since the velvet type can, with moderate probability, be correlated with chondrosarcoma of the tubular bones (Lodwick, 1966), its presence suggests that the rate of tumor growth is relatively slow.

2. **Isotopic isomorphism of malignant bone tumors** (Holtz and Gerstenberg, 1975). Certain observations suggest that, in primary sarcoma of bone and with skeletal metastases, the reaction of the bony elements may be radiologically identical. Therefore, not

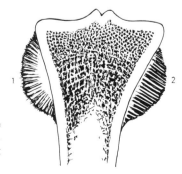
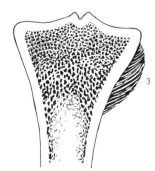

Fig. 29 **The three different types of projection of periosteal spicules:** Sunray type (1), brush type (2), and velvet type (3). See Text.

only the analysis of the roentgenogram but also the tumor history of the patient, his or her age, and the location of the finding are considered in making the differential diagnosis. The typical age peak of osteosarcoma, for instance, is in the second decade. In contrast, skeletal metastases occur prevalently beyond the fourth decade. The predominant localization of osteosarcomas is in the bones of the extremities. Bone metastases are encountered mostly in skeletal segments that contain a great deal of blood-forming (red) bone marrow, probably because of the better perfusion of the red bone marrow. This is why bone metastases are encountered principally in the vertebrae, the ribs, the sternum, the pelvis, in the proximal humerus, and in the ends of the femur. Bone metastases develop, for hemodynamic reasons, prevalently in the bone marrow. Hemodynamic reasons (small luminal size of the arteries) probably are also responsible for the infrequent occurrence of periosteal metastases. When, however, a periosteal (subperiosteal) metastasis of an extraosseous malignancy develops, it leads to the formation of spicules, periosteal lamellae or Codman's triangle, depending on the growth rate such as in osteosarcomas.

3. **For differential location of primary tumors in the tubular bones,** see Figure 30 (in the German literature: Poppe 1965, Adler and Klümper 1977).

The following paragraphs present a list of rare diseases that include *cystic osteolyses* among their typical radiographic features:

• (Probably) **hereditary polycystic osteodysplasia with progressive dementia** (Laasonen, 1975).

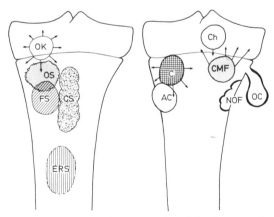

Fig. 30 Differential topography of benign, semimalignant, and malignant bone tumors as well as tumorlike affections. AC = Aneurysmatic bone cyst. C = Solitary juvenile bone cyst. CH = Benign chondroblastoma. CMF = Chondromyxoid fibroma. CS = Chondrosarcoma. ERS = Ewing's sarcoma, reticulum cell sarcoma. FS = Fibrosarcoma. NOF = Nonossifying fibroma of bone. OC = Osteochondroma (cartilaginous exostosis). OK = Osteoclastoma. OS = Osteosarcoma with osteolytic or osteoblastic growth.

• **Congenital (generalized) lipodystrophy (lipatrophic diabetes)** (Güell-González et al., 1971) with epiphyseal cystic lesions.
• **Focal medullary dystrophy** (Masshoff and Träger, 1975) shows cyst-like osteolyses that are indefinite in outline, or (marginal) erosions in small bones (hand, forefoot). In large bones this finding can, *roentgenologically,* be misdiagnosed as metastases of a malignant tumor or as foci of a plasmacytoma.
• **Diffuse skeletal angiomatosis** (Graham et al., 1978; Fig. 25 B to D) is frequently associated with visceral angiomas. Clinically and roentgenologically it is impossible to say whether a hemangiomatosis or a lymphangiomatosis is present; hence the neutral term "angiomatosis." The disease sometimes manifests itself by a pathologic fracture, occasionally also by low back pain (vertebral involvement). In principle, any part of the skeleton can be affected. The following combinations of bones occur most frequently: femur and humerus; humerus and ribs; femur, humerus, and ribs; femur, humerus, ribs, and pelvic bones; femur, humerus, ribs, pelvic bones, and skull.

After the various causes of more or less *circular* pathologic translucences in the subchondral bone have been listed, it should be pointed out that in certain—often juxtaarticular—parts of the supporting tissue one can, even *normally,* observe rounded translucent areas that have nothing to do with cysts in the sense used here. Ignorance of these roentgen findings leads to misinterpretations (Fig. 31). Such translucences usually originate with variations of skeletal thickness or structure. Thus, the insertion of the rectus femoris tendon in the tuberosity of the tibia often presents "hills and valleys." The "valleys" may appear in the anteroposterior roentgenogram (of the knee joint) as circumscribed translucences. Translucences of similar origin in the tendinous insertions on the ischiuum can be mistaken for osteolytic metastases. Finally, one should mention a *normal roentgen finding,* which especially in tomographs, is plainly visible; namely, orthograde projections of vascular channels above the intercondylar fossa (Fig. 39). Likewise, orthograde projections of drilled canals following traction therapy of fractures—e.g., in the posterior segment of the calcaneus—can persist as rounded translucences.

The *marginal subchondral lamella* is composed of a strip of calcified cartilage and the supporting cortex (Fig. 33). The calcified cartilage corresponds to the borderline of calcification and thus to the boundary of growth of the originally cartilaginous part of the skeleton. When the marginal lamella is no longer visible in the roentgenogram, one may conclude that it has either been decalcified or resorbed. Since the original thickness of the marginal lamella in the different joints is variable, a pathologic narrowing or dissolution of this structure should be diagnosed only after comparison with the (sound) contralateral joint! In generalized disorders of calcium metabolism (hyperparathyroidism, osteomalacia, rickets) and in lo-

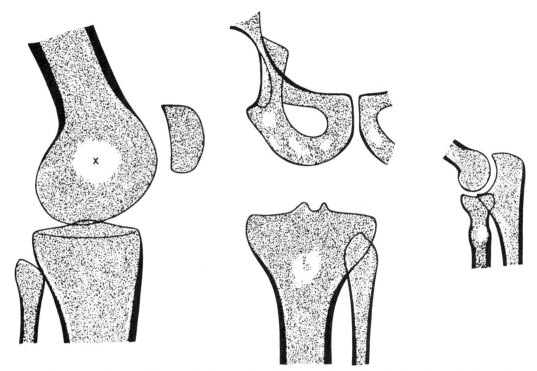

Fig. 31 **Instances of normal juxtaarticular translucent zones in bone** (see text). Their anatomic substrates occur in varying degree and may give rise to misinterpretations. x = Ludloff spot.

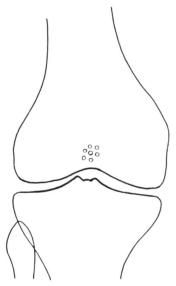

Fig. 32 **Orthograde projection of normal vascular channels above the intercondylar fossa,** particularly clearly visible in tomographs.

calized noninflammatory conditions such as aseptic necrosis of the femoral head, the marginal subchondral lamella may also be wasting or absent.

Defects in the contours of the articulating surfaces, hence *erosions* and *destructions,* point to resorption of bone which, however, need not be of inflammatory origin. Flat-arched, juxtaarticular *pressure erosions* may be produced by subcutaneous rheumatoid nodules in rheumatoid arthritis, by gouty tophi in the soft tissues, by hypercholesterolemic xanthomas, or by juxaarticular nodules in reticulohistiocytosis (lipoid dermatoarthritis). Occasionally, pressure erosions are also the result of lipomas developing between tightly connected bones (the metacarpals, for instance), of multiple hemangiomas[10] and the Klippel-Trenaunay syndrome, Kaposi's sarcoma, neuro-

---

[10] Suspicion of a skeletal lesion (pressure erosion in the outer contour) from angimatous malformations, including the Klippel-Trenaunay syndrome, is particularly justified when concomitant widening of the nutrient canal is present. Such *dilatations of the nutrient canal* are seen in the short tubular bones but they also occur in leprosy (Fig. 55), in hemoglobinopathies with sickle cell formation, in arteriovenous fistulas, and in the Camurati-Engelmann disease (hereditary [diaphyseal] hyperostosis without pachyderma).

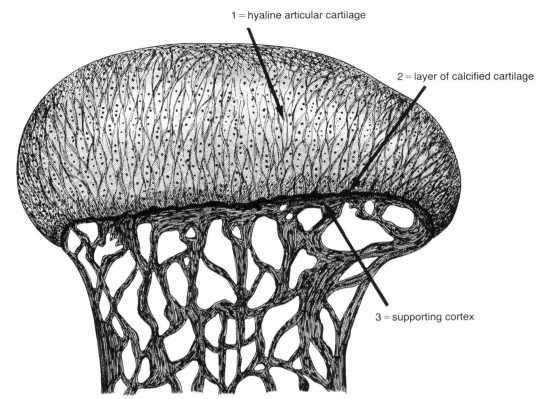

1 = hyaline articular cartilage

2 = layer of calcified cartilage

3 = supporting cortex

Fig. 33   The marginal subchondral lamella is made up of the delicate layer of calcified cartilage (2) and the supporting cortex (3).

fibromas in von Recklinghausen's neurofibromatosis, fibromas in tuberous sclerosis, and pigmented villon-odular synovitis involving the tendon sheaths and the bursae. Pigmented villonodular synovitis and early stages of malignant synovialoma developing close to a joint sometimes cause erosions in the immediate vicinity of the capsular insertion, particularly in larger joints. Finally, contour defects from *subchondral* and subperiosteal resorption of bone occur in hyperparathyroidism, whereas those due to *subchondral* resorption of bone are observed in storage diseases (Ansell and Bywaters, 1957), in the early stage of neurogenic osteoarthropathies, in hemophilia, following frostbite, in late irradiation damage to the joint, and as a result of trauma.

The so-called *condylar grooves of the femur* (Fig. 34) are variants of the normal condylar shape (Harrison et al., 1976). They are identified in lateral roentgenograms of the knee joint and in axial views of the patella as contour defects or flat depressions. They must be differentiated initially from the bed of a loose body in osteochondrosis dissecans, the lesions of spontaneous osteonecrosis in the distal femur (Fig. 429), and from depressed fracture.

In the vicinity of the knee joint, particularly the

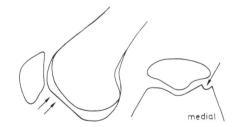

medial

Fig. 34   **The *arrows* point to the so-called condylar grooves of the femur.** These grooves can be seen on lateral roentgenograms, both in the medial *(illustrated)* and the lateral condyle. They are variants of normal.

distal femur, certain osteolytic *(erosive)* lesions are observed in children and young adults, which offer a favorable prognosis and mostly are incidental findings; namely, the fibrous cortical defect, the nonossifying fibroma of bone, and the periosteal or cortical desmoid.

The fibrous cortical defect (Fig. 35 A) is detected in childhood, mostly between the ages of 2 and 14 (Edeiken and Hodes, 1973). It lies eccentrically in the metaphysis, most often posteromedially and

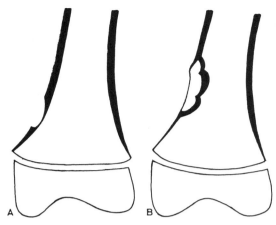

Fig. 35   A = **Fibrous cortical defect** (see text).
B = **Nonossifying fibroma of bone** (see text).

Note: The fibrous cortical defect is located in the cortical bone only. The nonossifying fibroma of bone also penetrates the marrow cavity. Chief localizations of both lesions are, in decreasing frequency, the distal metaphysis of the femur, the proximal metaphysis of the tibia, and the distal metaphyses of the tibia and the fibula. The nonossifying fibroma of bone is a roentgen finding in adolescents and young adults.

much less frequently posterolaterally, particularly in the distal femur. Histologic studies have shown that the defect is probably produced by periosteal fibrous tissue that grows into the subjacent cortical bone. The lesion is evidently due to a local disturbance of the formation and modeling of the metaphyseal shaft.

Nonossifying fibroma of bone (Figs. 22 B, 30, and 35 B) is caused by a fibroblastic lesion that penetrates the marrow cavity from the cortical bone and can bulge the overlying cortex. In the roentgenogram this new growth appears as an osteolysis that lies eccentrically with respect to the longitudinal axis of the tubular bone; it is often lobulated and is demarcated from the marrow cavity by a sclerotic border. Some writers consider the fibrous cortical defect and

the nonossifying fibroma of bone to be identical. Others, such as the Dutch Committee for Bone Tumors (1973), presume that the nonossifying fibroma of bone develops as a nonmalignant tumor from the fibrous cortical defect.

The periosteal or **cortical desmoid** (Kimmelstiel and Rapp 1951, Fig. 36) also shows histologically a fibrous tissue that often encloses small islets of bone. The tumor is located in the metaphysis *on the dorsal aspect of the medial femoral condyle,* above the insertion of the capsule of the knee joint. The roentgenogram reveals at that site a flat, sometimes uneven defect which often shows a surrounding sclerosis and, less frequently, a periosteal reaction. Small bone shadows are sometimes visible in the soft tissues that form the immediate neighborhood of the lesion (Bufkin, 1971). If the examiner is ignorant of the typical location, the equivocal roentgenogram can raise suspicion of an early malignant bone tumor or an inflammatory bacterial process in the bone! It is very likely that sometimes a bilateral cortical desmoid is produced by microtraumas to the insertion of the adductor magnus muscle on the medial labrum of the linea aspera; such microtraumas are apt to be followed by local proliferation of vessels and connective tissue, which leads to resorption of bone. Some writers use the terms cortical desmoid, fibrous cortical defect, and nonossifying fibroma of bone synonymously.

For the **distal anterior defect of the femoral metaphysis** (Keats, 1974), see Figure 454.

Form variants or ligament insertion furrows on the convexity of the scaphoid, the capitate, the trapezium, the triquetrum, and the articulating surface of the 5th metacarpal are sometimes mistaken for arthritic erosions (Fig. 37). Particularly on inspection with a magnifying loupe, these notches show a delicate cortical seam. Only when this seam disappears and when these notches deepen and present delicate irregularities of contour, have pathologic (e.g., inflammatory) lesions been superimposed on the normal findings.

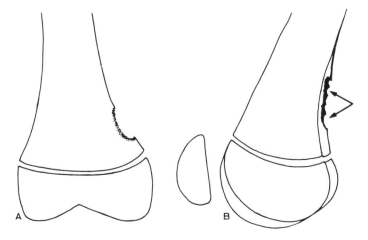

Fig. 36   **Cortical desmoid** (see text) on the posteromedial metaphysis of the distal femur. The finding in A (anteroposterior view) is not always as distinctly identifiable as in the present sketch.

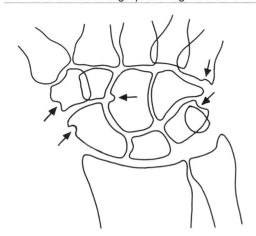

Fig. 37 **Normal (Variable) notches or hollows in the carpal region.**

Arthritic *mutilation* must be differentiated from the so-called osteolysis syndrome, which has a varied etiology (p. 49 ff), and from advanced tumorous destruction. To differentiate arthritic mutilation from neurogenic or other osteolyses (the osteolysis syndrome), the established rule is to search in the neighboring joints for additional direct signs of arthritis, particularly bony ankylosis (Fig. 38). It is true that neurogenic osteolyses may be accompanied by indolent ulcers in the soft tissues. Such ulcers are apt to develop in tabes dorsalis as pressure sores or without a recognizable etiology, or in syringomyelia as the result of local heat-induced damage. Such ulcers fre-

quently lead to infection of the neighboring bones and joints. In these cases, therefore, bony ankyloses and other direct signs of arthritis can also be seen in neurogenic osteolyses. *In addition,* ossifying periostitis and osteitis may be present. These processes, however, do *not* belong to the stage of arthritic mutilation. Finally, it should be mentioned that the well-known increased fragility of bone in the neurogenic osteoarthropathies (see under this heading) is at times the cause of exuberant reparative reactions on the part of the periosteum, particularly in tubular bones, even without an infection of bone. This should be considered in undertaking the differential diagnosis by radiography.

The differential diagnosis of *arthritic dissections* includes juxtaarticular osteomyelitic sequestra, osteochondrosis dissecans, calcified capsular chondromas, and capsular osteomas, as well as persistent apophyseal centers of ossification, so-called supernumerary ossicles, and (old) traumatic avulsions and breaks.

Narrowing of the radiographic joint space should prompt the following differential considerations: in arthritis, the entire joint space is mostly involved in the *concentric* narrowing from the outset (but see also Fig. 298). In osteoarthrosis, the narrowing of the joint space—in joints exposed to uneven strain—is usually limited to the pressure-absorbing area (*eccentric narrowing of the joint space,* Fig. 310). Concentric narrowing may also occur with prolonged immobilization, flaccid paralysis (Pool, Jr., 1974), or following amputation of a skeletal part. In this instance, the bone *and* the articular cartilage present an atrophy of disuse. Finally, atrophy of the articular cartilage has been observed in reflex dystrophies and in trophic

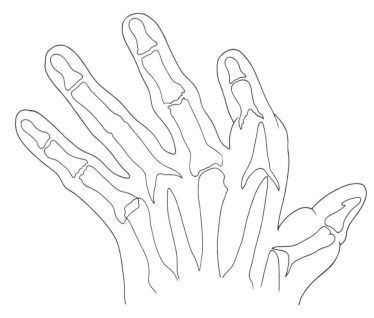

Fig. 38 **Stage of mutilation** in rheumatoid arthritis of many years' standing. The distal joint-forming bone is typically "cupped," and the proximal is "sucked on" (see 1st, 2nd, and 4th metacarpophalangeal joint and 2nd proximal interphalangeal joint). The soft tissues of the thumb and the index finger are telescoped. Arthritic erosions in the 3rd metacarpophalangeal joint and in the 3rd and 5th proximal interphalangeal joint. Arthritic *bony ankylosis* (see text) of the 4th proximal interphalangeal joint. Ulnar deviation of the metacarpophalangeal joints II–V.

disorders. For *chondrolysis,* which also is accompanied by concentric narrowing of the joint space, see page 250 ff.

Postarthritic bony ankylosis has to be differentiated from congenital synostosis (articular aplasia) and from arthrodesis. Also in pachydermoperiostosis (for *forme fruste* cases and synonyms see p. 133 ff, Uehlinger 1942; Schilling et al. 1961; Vogl and Goldfischer, 1962; Shawarby and Ibrahim, 1962) extensive synostoses sometimes develop in the hands, the connections of the pelvic bones, the costovertebral joints, etc.

Arthrogryposis multiplex (congenital tight joints) presents the leading clinical signs of "absence of motion" and "muscle wasting." This fibrotic tightness of joints (Ruiz-Torres et al., 1976) manifests itself in the upper and the lower extremities. *Carpal synostoses* are seldom observed (Jacobs, 1975). Similarly, the involvement of a single joint is infrequent. Usually, two and more (even all) joints of the extremities are affected. Radiographic examination is sometimes ordered because of the cylindrical or fusiform deformation of the (involved) elbow and/or knee joints. In other patients, the stiffening of the joints themselves and/or the possible attendant manifestations of arthrogryposis (unilateral or bilateral dislocation of the hip, hypoplasia or aplasia of the patella, clubfoot) prompt a radiologic examination or differentiation; for example, from dystrophic dwarfism or the various mucopoly-saccharidoses.

Rosenbloom and Frias (1974) have described the syndrome of "chiroarthropathy in *juvenile* [type I] diabetics" (Heim et al., 1976). This syndrome, in which *stiffening of joints,* particularly the interphalangeal joints of hands and feet but also the other joints of the extremities and even the spine have been observed, develops a number of years after onset of the diabetes. The joints with disturbed motion and their immediate periarticular surroundings present *normal* roentgen findings.

In the setting of *alcoholic embryopathy* (Leiber, 1978), a certain complex of dysplasia and dysmorphism develops. It is the result of alcohol abuse by the mother during (early) pregnancy. In alcholic embryopathy, anomalies of the joints, the hands, and the feet occur, among them *impaired motion* of the elbow joint (absent extensibility), limited pronation and supination of the hand, and limited flexibility of the metacarpophalangeal joints. In the newborn period, malposition of the fingers is often conspicuous: when a fist is made, the index finger overlaps the middle finger.

Faulty positions of joints also occur in degenerative and neurogenic arthropathies, after an injury, and in congenital as well as acquired affections of the tendons, tendon sheaths, muscles, skin, and subcutaneous tissues. They also can be the attendant or cardinal signs of certain hereditary diseases; e.g., Ehlers-Danlos syndrome (see legend accompanying Fig. 111). Finally, Figure 39 demonstrates that an arthritis-dependent reflex malposition of a joint can mimic a narrowing of the radiologic joint space, hence destruction of the articular cartilage.

In small tubular bones, *new formations of periosteal bone* triggered by an arthritis often extend to the diaphysis. This can be observed particularly in children. In (small) children, arthritic narrowing of the joint space is a relatively late manifestation. Therefore, when the presence of periosteal bone reactions raises the suspicion of arthritis at this age, it

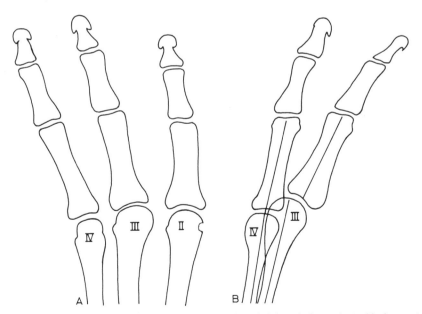

Fig. 39 A = **Detail from the dorsovolar roentgenogram of the left hand** of a patient with rheumatoid arthritis. *Pathologic roentgen findings:* Erosion in the head of the 2nd metacarpal, ulnar deviation of the metacarpophalangeal joints. *Narrowing of the roentgenologic joint space of the 3rd metacarpophalangeal joint.*

B = **Detail from the oblique roentgenogram in the so-called zither player's position.** The joint space of the 3rd metacarpophalangeal joint is of normal width. The *volar subluxation at this joint in the dorsovolar view hence only mimics a narrowing of the joint space!*

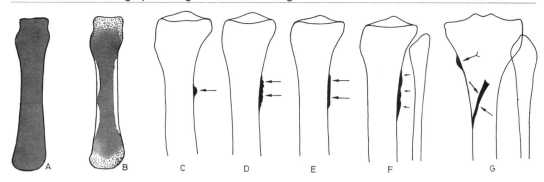

Fig. 40   A = **Normal metatarsus.**
   B = **Pseudoperiostitis** (Forrester and Kirkpatrick, 1976) due to rapid band-shaped subperiosteal resorption of the diaphysis (in reflex dystrophies, immobilization, arthritis). C–G = **Pseudoperiostitis** (soleus line = bulging of the contour of variable shape at the insertion of the soleus muscle in the proximal shaft of the tibia, *arrows*). *Tailed arrow* in G = tuberosity of the tibia (Ravelli, 1955). The concept "pseudoperiostitis" in C–G is used in the sense of Grashey-Birkner (1964), Köhler-Zimmer (1967), and Levine et al. (1976).

is necessary to include bacterial osteomyelitis (also of tuberculous origin or due to congenital syphilis), primary bacterial periostitis, and osteitis, as well as infantile cortical hyperostosis (Caffey's syndrome) in the diagnostic considerations. One should also think of periosteal reactions to malignant tumors (including nonsecretory plasmacytoma), benign tumors, and to vitamin deficiency diseases (rickets, scurvy). Periosteal reactions have also been observed in overdosage of vitamin A or D, in sickle cell anemia (following infarction of the diaphysis), in Gaucher's disease, in Crohn's disease (Streuli and Puliadis, 1978) and in acute leukemia. Periosteal lesions may also follow an electrical accident. Furthermore, the following conditions have to be differentiated from arthritis-induced new bone formation, particularly in adults: the periosteal consequences of venous stasis (varicosis) and disorders of arterial circulation,[11] (pulmonary) hypertrophic osteoarthropathy, hyperparathyroidism, fluorosis, tuberous sclerosis, Gardner's syndrome, progressive scleroderma, osteopoikilosis[12] with hyperostosis, melorheostosis, idiopathic pachydermoperiostosis, thyroid acropachy, and the even less frequent periosteal hyperostosis with dysproteinemia (Goldbloom et al., 1966). The periosteum thus reveals itself as an extremely reactive part of bone!

The form in which the periosteal reactions are projected, e.g., lamellae, "onion skins," radiate spikes (spicules), irregular (e.g., clustered or undulating) appositions of bone, offer no certain clues about the underlying disorder. Of greater importance to the no-

sological classification is to determine whether (1) the roentgen finding is localized or extensive, perhaps bilaterally symmetric in the extremities, *or* (2) signs of destruction or new bone formation are present in the subperiosteal bone, *or* (3) the neighboring joint presents pathologic lesions in the roentgenogram.

As a postscript, one should mention the term "**pseudoperiostitis**": *on the one hand,* this concept denotes a rapid subperiosteal resorption of bone in reflex dystrophies, immobilization for fracture, and in the vicinity of an acute arthritis (Forrester and Kirkpatrick, 1976). One then sees a delicate, *band-shaped* translucent line running parallel to the (total) surface of the diaphysis (Fig. 40 B). On superficial inspection, this line can mimic a lamellar periosteal reaction. *On the other hand,* some writers (Grashey-Birkner 1964; Köhler-Zimmer 1967) speak of periostitis when variously shaped physiologic irregularities are encountered in specific parts of the skeleton; e.g., the deltoid tuberosity, the neck of the scapula, the surgical neck of the humerus, the distal metaphysis of the humerus, the linea aspera of the femur, the linea terminalis at the level of the acetabulum, the tibial tubercle (Ravelli, 1955), the tibial insertion of the soleus muscle (Levine et al., 1976), the proximal metaphysis of the fibula or the distal metaphysis of the tibia (Fig. 40 C to G).

In concluding the general discussion of arthritis, it should be pointed out that not only the soft-tissue signs of arthritis at any age and the collateral phenomena of arthritis in adulthood (see the legend accompanying Fig. 13) but also most of the direct signs of arthritis are, in principle, reversible roentgen findings (Dihlmann, 1969a). Figure 41, for instance, shows a follow-up study of a case of rheumatoid arthritis. In this figure, destructive lesions have been "repaired." In addition to this, it is known that a narrowing of the roentgenologic space can return (largely) to normal. In chronic rheumatoid arthritis, this process takes place, as a rule, through *fibrocar-*

---

[11] A circumscribed painful periosteal new bone formation has also been described as the consequence of periosteal arteritis in polyarteritis (nodosa) and in disseminated lupus erythematosus (Ball and Grayzel, 1964).
[12] It should be mentioned here that in osteopoikilosis pain and even articular swelling are observed (Jonasch, 1955).

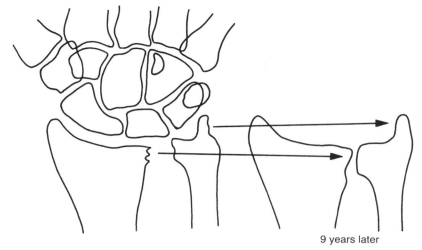

9 years later

Fig. 41   **Roentgenologic follow-up study in rheumatoid arthritis**
During the period of observation the styloid processes of the ulna and the distal radioulnar joint have been *reconstructed*. (Hence, not only resorption of the effusion into this joint but also regression of erosions has taken place.)

tilaginous metaplasia of the pannus. The effectiveness of therapeutic procedures in arthritis has so far been estimated by the improvement in function and the diminution of the serologic signs of inflammation. The search for roetgenologic signs of repair and reconstruction and their description therefore gives additional information about the influence of therapy and the healing quality in a case of arthritis.

Osteoarthrosis

In old age, the efficiency of the gliding tissues diminishes because its reactive power and its ability to function are reduced, as are muscular strength and the incentive to move. The aging joint is basically an atrophic joint. Osteoarthrosis, on the other hand, is a *disease process* caused by wear and tear. It develops, together with its characteristic roentgenologic manifestations, only when there is a disproportion between load and load capacity of the articular cartilage. Such a disproportion can result from a congenital, developmental, or acquired incongruity of the articulating surfaces in faulty positions, ligament instability, and malalignment **(preosteoarthrotic deformity)** (Hackenbroch 1943, see p. 226).

Chondrotropic disorders of metabolism, hormonal dysregulations, inflammatory arthropathies, and inherited functional inferiority of the articular cartilage are likewise known to be causes of osteoarthrosis. Repeated direct injuries of the articular cartilage can also reduce its resistance to such a degree that it can no longer withstand the normal strain. Finally, investigations have shown that peak demands or excessive persistent strains on the gliding tissues (e.g., in competitive athletes) can also, under certain circumstances, lead to signs of attrition in the articular cartilage (Schneider and Lichte, 1970). When the pressure between the two layers of the articular cartilage exceeds a critical value, the synovial fluid (the physiologic lubricant) is forced from the joint space into the recess of the capsule. The joint is then no longer lubricated, the friction between the layers of the articular cartilage increases precipitously, and the result is mechanical abrasion of the cartilage (hence wear and tear) with *degeneration of the cartilage.*

The histologic findings in osteoarthrosis must be classified, from the anatomic point of view, as pathologic. Initially, the roentgen signs of osteoarthrosis signify only a *potential disease* **(latent osteoarthrosis)** which is not experienced subjectively by the patient until pains and dysfunction of the involved joint supervene. This stage has been described as **activated osteoarthrosis** (Otte, 1971). The symptoms in activated osteoarthrosis are principally the result of a reactive synovitis that is occasioned and maintained by the abraded and exfoliated detritus of the articular cartilage. The increasing abrasion of the cartilage ultimately also involves the marginal subchondral lamella, and the marrow cavity is opened (Fig. 42). This gives rise to "wounds of the marrow cavity" (Otte, 1976). Through these wounds (gaps in the bone), fibrous bone marrow invades the joint cavity and tends to coat the exposed trabeculae in the form of a grass-like cover. The fate of these medullary proliferations—which of course are invisible in the roentgenogram—is of particular importance to the further evolution of the osteoarthritis. The vascular connective tissue in the pressure-absorbing area is largely crushed by the motion of the joint. This leads to release of enzymes and molecules of another kind in the joint cavity. These elements are derived from the pulverized connective tissue components, the blood, and its cells. Not only do they further damage the hyaline cartilage, but they exacerbate the reactive synovitis and thus intensify the patient's discomfort. However, the medullary proliferations also may have "positive" consequences. For example, the hanging hip operation first described by Voss lowers the intraarticular pressure and thereby often slows down

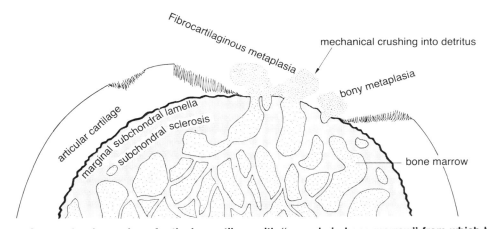

Fig. 42 Osteoarthrotic erosion of articular cartilage with "wounds in bone marrow" from which bone marrow tissue invades the joint cavity (see text). Outcome of these connective tissue proliferations:
(1)   Motion of the joint crushes them for the most part into detritus which maintains the reactive synovitis.
(2)   They can ossify and thus contribute to the osteoarthrotic remodeling of bone.
(3)   Fibrocartilaginous metaplasia (following, for instance, operative reduction of the intraarticular pressure) may give rise to the development of a "new" articular cartilage.

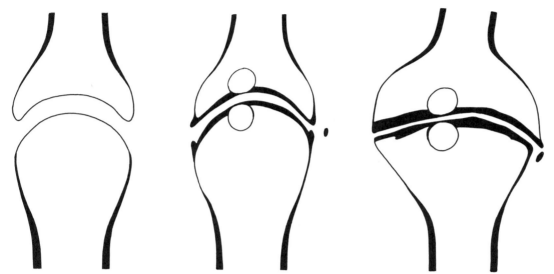

Fig. 43   *Left:* **Normal projection** of an *evenly loaded* joint. *Center:* **Solitary signs of osteoarthrosis** (see text). *Right:* **Osteoarthrotic remodeling completed.**

the crushing of the medullar proliferations. These can thus expand across the denuded, previously subchondral, bone and—through fibrocartilaginous metaplasia—are capable of forming a "new" articular cartilage. The latter, however, will be of inferior quality as compared with hyaline cartilage. The roentgenogram then shows increasing widening of the joint space, and the function of motion will improve!

The *roentgen signs of osteoarthrosis* indicate the damage to the articular cartilage and the corresponding lesions in the subchondral bone as well as processes that govern the deforming character of the osteoarthrosis (Figs. 43 and 44).

In osteoarthrosis, the *narrowing of the radiologic joint space* (which, in unevenly stressed joints, very often is initially demonstrable in the pressure-absorbing area) reveals the loss of substance of the articular cartilage, the osseous metaplasia of the medullary tissue (see Fig. 42), and the reversible dehydration of the articular cartilage as a consequence of impaired joint motion (Otte, 1968). *Increased density of the subchondral spongiosa* indicates loss

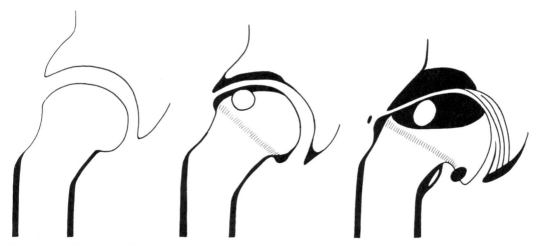

Fig. 44   *Left:* **Normal projection** of an *unevenly* loaded joint. *Center:* **Solitary signs of osteoarthrosis.** In the pressure-absorbing zone one recognizes narrowing of the joint space, increased density of the cancellous bone, and detritus cysts. Osteophytes form in the *nonweight-bearing areas.*

Right: **Osteoarthrotic remodeling completed.** Among other manifestations, duplication of the acetabular floor which renders the faulty position irreversible (Fig. 312).

of elasticity of the articular cartilage. The subchondral cancellous trabeculae thicken in response to increased compression stress.

The osteoarthrotic *debris cyst* is the sign of functional collapse of the cancellous trabeculae due to excessive strain (generally demonstrable in the pressure-absorbing area of the joint) and thereby the sign of focal devitalization of bone. Such osteoarthrotic cysts (synonyms: debris cysts, hemorrhagic cysts, detritus cysts, pressure cysts, insufficiency cysts) develop after the removal of dead bone. They sometimes are located symmetrically on both sides of the joint space and commonly have a bony cover (marginal sclerosis).

Marginal osteophytes (hypertrophic lipping) in the area of pressure relief of an osteoarthrotic joint frequently are early roentgen manifestations. The epithet "marginal" emphasizes that they prevalently arise at the cartilage/bone interface. Mechanical forces, particularly joint motion, contribute to the morphology of the osteoarthrotic osteophytes.

Abrasions of bone are observed when corresponding areas of two articulating bones have been completely denuded of their cartilage cover so that the bones, which have undergone reactive sclerosis (eburnation), are abraded by motion (Fig. 45). Sesamoid bones and osteoarthrotic lippings can also present such abrasions.

The roentgenogram of *advanced osteoarthrosis* initially shows processes of remodeling in the articulating bones (Figs. 43, 44, and 45). The articulating bones lose their roundness and become straightened, coarsened, and enlarged. The initial morphology and

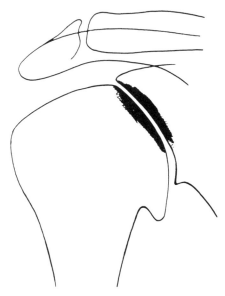

Fig. 45 **Abrasions of bone** in the humeral head and the glenoid of the scapula in advanced osteoarthrosis of the right shoulder joint.

the (still preserved) function of motion influence the degree of this deformation.

The reactive synovitis in (activated) osteoarthrosis gradually gives rise to cicatricious fibrosis and irregular shrinking of the capsule. This can lead to faulty positioning and additional limitation of motion. These processes can be intensified by reflex increases in muscle tone, or they develop in combination with extraarticular sequelae to osteoarthrosis; e.g., muscular atrophies.

In the morphologically altered joint capsule there sometimes develop circumscribed cartilaginous or osseous metaplasias that are termed *capsular chondromas* and *capsular osteomas* (Fig. 72).

Any of the bone connections with a cartilage cover may develop osteoarthrosis, as may the epiphyses and the large joints of the spine. The latter are formed by the intervertebral disk, the adjacent endplates, and the contiguous vertebral bodies. Certain terms referring to the *qualitative* and *quantitative* assessment of disk degeneration serve to characterize the roentgenologically recognizable sequelae to the degenerative lesions in these vertebral connections: spondylosis deformans, spondylosis uncovertebralis, chondrosis, intervertebral osteochondrosis, and so on.

Crain, in 1961, described the clinical picture of polyosteoarthrosis of the finger joints characterized by unusually violent inflammatory episodes that even lead to bony ankylosis of one or the other finger joint. In Crain's cases, the reactive synovitis—i.e., the activation of this osteoarthrosis *(vide supra)*—reached proportions that had theretofore been unknown. This observation and its confirmation by other workers eventually led to the concept of **erosive osteoarthrosis** (Peter, 1966; Peter et al., 1966; Kidd and Peter, 1966; McEwen, 1968; Radi, 1970; Smukler et al., 1971; Munoz Gomez et al., 1972; Schacherl and Schilling, 1973, Dihlmann, 1977; and other writers) (Fig. 46). Between 4 and 5 percent of patients (males being more often affected than females) with polyosteoarthrosis of the fingers develop not only the typical signs of osteoarthrosis *(vide supra)* but also destructive phenomena, particularly in the distal and proximal interphalangeal joint and infrequently also in the first carpometacarpal joint.

Among "erosive" roentgen signs one encounters *large* subchondral cystic osteolyses (often as an initial finding), erosions of the articulating bones (sometimes with consecutive malpositions) and, in the final stage, even bony ankyloses. Juxtaarticular demineralization, however, does not develop. This is an important roentgenologic criterion in distinguishing this condition from arthritis.

The pathogenesis of erosive osteoarthrosis is still a matter of dispute: Excessive (and therefore destructive) reactive synovitis? Abnormally aggressive synovium? Subchondral disorder of circulation? In some cases the destruction was preceded by intraarticular injections of corticosteroids (Alarcón-Segovia and Ward, 1966); hence, crystal-induced erosive synovitis (see under this heading)? Aseptic necrosis of bone?

Erosive polyosteoarthrosis is a diagnosis of exclusion! Prior to diagnosing this disorder, the following diseases must be ruled out clinically and roentgenologically:

• Rheumatoid arthritis, especially so-called **superimposed arthritis** (Wagenhäuser, 1967). This term is intended to emphasize that in patients with known polyosteoarthrosis of the fingers, rheumatoid arthritis

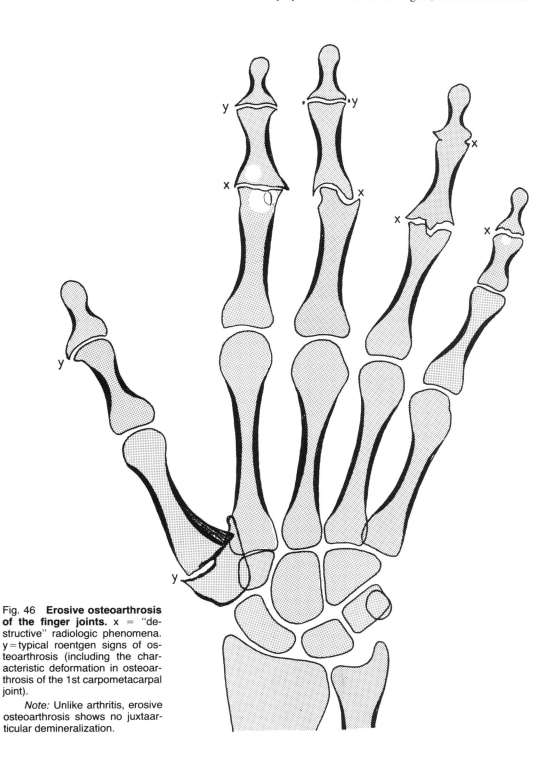

Fig. 46 Erosive osteoarthrosis of the finger joints. x = "destructive" radiologic phenomena. y = typical roentgen signs of osteoarthrosis (including the characteristic deformation in osteoarthrosis of the 1st carpometacarpal joint).

Note: Unlike arthritis, erosive osteoarthrosis shows no juxtaarticular demineralization.

has supervened incidentally as a secondary disease. In such cases it also attacks finger joints that already have been affected then by osteoarthrosis (Ehrlich, 1972a,b, 1975).
· Gout, similarly to erosive polyosteoarthrosis, can present subchondral cystic osteolyses with a diameter of 5 mm or more.
· Psoriatic arthritis, especially so-called *psoriatic arthritis without psoriasis* (see under this heading).

By analogy with the concept of erosive osteoarthrosis of the fingers the term **erosive osteoarthrosis** **of the hip** has been coined (Lequesne et al., 1970; Puls, 1974; Abelanet et al., 1974; and other writers). In this particular evolution of osteoarthrosis of the hip, painful chondroosteolytic destruction of the femoral head (in the majority of cases) takes place in less than a year's time. Therefore, the condition has also been termed ''rapid erosive osteoarthrosis of the hip.'' In these cases, also, the pathogenesis of the short-term chondroosteolysis has not been established. Neurogenic arthropathy and (idiopathic) avascular necrosis of the femoral head, especially, will come up for diagnostic differentiation.

Arthropathies and Osteoarthropathies

Arthropathy is defined here as a joint disease with more or less pronounced involvement of the juxtaarticular bones (hence the term osteoarthropathy) in which the clinical manifestations and roentgen signs depart from the *typical* pattern of arthritis and osteoarthrosis. Frequently, however, this definition does not include all the joints but refers only to specific joints that are known to become affected frequently and early in the disease (the so-called *test joints*). Certain arthropathies can also be defined as affections which in one patient follows the course of a pure arthritis and in another that of a pure osteoarthrosis; they are thus ambivalent in character. This ambivalence reveals itself occasionally in the same patient when one joint, for instance, is affected by arthritis whereas in another joint the same arthropathy is present as osteoarthrosis.

The best known arthropathy is the involvement of joints in gout: **gouty osteoarthropathy.** Under the heading of gout are grouped disorders of purine metabolism concerning prevalently males, which manifest themselves by hyperuricemia *and* deposition of urates in the tissues, *principally* the joints and their bony surroundings, the tendon sheaths, the bursae, and the kidneys. Gout is thus the clinical manifestation of chronic hyperuricemia. Beyond this, it is a genetically *and* environmentally conditioned disease. The genetic determination shows itself in about 20 percent of the patients by the familial incidence of the disorder. (Schilling, 1967). The most important environmental—hence extrinsic—factor that governs the manifestation of the disease is probably overnutrition. This is true of *primary* gout.

Secondary gout, or *secondary* hyperuricemia, also develops, however, through increased formation of uric acid and/or diminished renal excretion of uric acid in the presence of a *known* underlying disease; e.g., one of the hemoblastoses or myeloproliferative diseases associated with the breakdown of cells, and in the hemolytic anemias. It is known, however, that secondary gout with involvement of joints can be present for years before the diagnosis of polycythemia vera is established (Calabro, 1969).

Psoriasis, and therefore also psoriatic arthritis, is sometimes accompanied by hyperuricemia, and very infrequently even by typical gout (Watt and Middlemiss, 1975). The significance of these observations, however, has been questioned (Lambert and Wright, 1977). Secondary gout is rarely encountered in chronic renal diseases. Hyperuricemia likewise does not occur very frequently in chronic renal insufficiency. Finally, it should be borne in mind that not only does (secondary) gout occur as a complication of chronic renal disease, but (primary) gout can lead to gouty nephropathy and thereby to renal insuffi-

ciency. There exist both *renal gout* and *gouty nephropathy!* Renal as well as extrarenal factors (enzyme deficiency) cause hyperuricemia in certain types of glycogen storage disease (Mertz, 1973). It should also be mentioned that "iatrogenic" hyperuricemia and gout have been observed as a complication of treatment with thiazide duiretics in hypertension (Mertz, 1959, and other writers).

Formally, gouty osteoarthropathy develops as a consequence of limited solubility of uric acid and its salts in the blood. The pH of blood (plasma) and the normal body temperature admit a solubility of uric acid in the form of monosodium urate up to a concentration of 6.4 mg/dL. The risk of falling ill with manifest gout therefore parallels the serum concentration of uric acid. When, for instance, the level of serum uric acid exceeds 8 mg/dL, manifest gout develops in 36 percent of cases. With a uric acid level above 9 mg/dL, manifest gout becomes "almost certain" (Mertz, 1973). Apart from this, the sex, age, and body constitution of the patient also play a part in the "conversion" of asymptomatic hyperuricemia into the clinical picture of gout; the prevalent incidence of gout in males has already been mentioned; the older a patient is, the lower is the threshold between hyperuricemia and gout; more than two thirds of gouty patients have a pyknic constitution (Mertz, 1972, 1973, and other writers).

The precipitation of crystalline monosodium urate in the tissues acts as a foreign substance and triggers a number of local reactions in the gliding tissue, the clinical *and* roentgenologic picture of which depends on the **quantity-time ratio of urate precipitation** (Fig. 47; Dihlmann and Fernholz, 1969).

A high quantity-time quotient (i.e., *massive* precipitation of urates in a *short time*) leads to hyperacute gouty arthritis; for example, inflammation of the metatarsophalangeal joint of the great toe with swelling and erythema of the surrounding tissues ("podagra"), or to the development of gouty polyarthritis with, generally, asymmetrical involvement of joints (Hadler et al., 1974). The *metatarsophalangeal joint of the great toe* is affected in about 75 percent of gouty patients (Schilling, 1967). It is therefore the *test joint* for gouty arthropathy. In the first attacks of podagra, the roentgenogram reveals at most a nondescript edema of the periarticular soft tissues, which often extends beyond the immediate vicinity of the joint (see Fig. 530 A). In the long run, however, gouty arthritis produces roentgenologically demonstrable lesions of the gliding tissue because the inflamed synovium does not come to rest but reacts with chronic irritation on which intermittent phases of acute inflammation are superimposed. At this stage it is possible to demonstrate disappearance of the

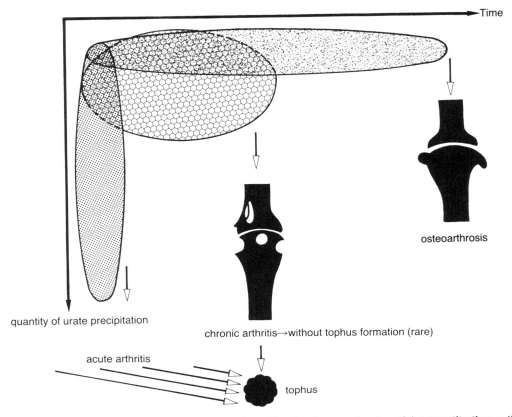

Fig. 47 **The roentgen findings in gouty osteoarthropathy** develop as a function of the **quantity-time ratio of urate precipitation in the gliding tissue** (see text).

marginal subchondral lamella, narrowing of the interosseous space, erosions, and other anomalies in the roentgenogram. On the other hand, apart from the roentgen signs of chronic joint inflammation, recurrent gouty (poly-)arthritis presents an additional peculiarity: at the sites where deposits of monosodium urate monohydrate (the tophi) that can no longer be absorbed extend into the subchondral bone, the bone substance is resorbed. This resorption brings about the development of slowly growing, sharply demarcated, rounded osteolyses which are capable of destroying the joint as well as the metaphyseal and diaphyseal segment of the bone. These osteolyses are termed "punched-out defects." But this designation characterizes the typical radiographic features of the urate tophus rather superficially, for such sharply demarcated, rounded osteolyses are encountered in rheumatoid arthritis with much greater frequency than in gout. A more dependable rule for differentiating these lesions in the roentgenogram says: The more irregularly rounded a juxtaarticular osteolysis is *and* the farther it extends beyond the epiphysis of a small tubular bone to the diaphysis, the greater is the probability that a gouty tophus is present (Fig. 48).

Tophaceous urate deposits—the signs of chronic gout—form *in the joint* and *in the subchondral layer* even when the precipitation of monosodium urate monohydrate is *protracted* but still takes place in *higher concentration*. The quantity-time quotient is then smaller than in the first-named instance, and therefore the onset of this type of gouty arthropathy is not so dramatic and hyperacute. Rather, from the beginning it runs a chronic insidious course. It is not the exudative reaction of the synovium but the proliferative phase of arthritis that is in the forefront of the clinical picture.

With *protracted* sedimentation of urate *in low concentration,* the quantity-time quotient is still smaller than in the first and even in the second instance. The threshold for an inflammatory reaction of the synovium is no longer reached, but the articular cartilage becomes damaged. With time, osteoarthrosis develops in the involved joint.

Additional peculiarities of the roentgenologic morphology of gout to be mentioned are the *spicular tophus* (Figs. 135, 138, 139, 531, and 532; Dihlmann and Fernholz 1969, 1974), the *overhanging bone edge* (Figs. 136, 138, 139, and 531; Martel, 1968), and osteoplastic deformations of small tubular bones *(bulbous enlargement of a phalanx)* (Fig. 138) and

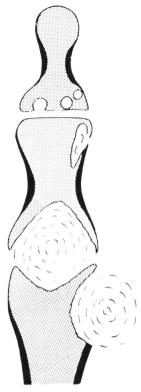

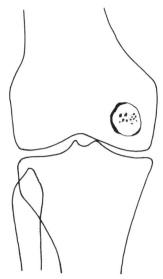

Fig. 49 **Infrequent intraosseous gouty tophus,** (in this case) with calcifications **in the vicinity of a roentgenologically normal joint**—here the knee joint. *Radiologic differential diagnosis:* Benign chondroblastoma, enchondroma, bone infarct. In the case illustrated, the calcifications permit the lesion to be differentiated from an intraosseous ganglion (see Fig. 21 A and B), which does not calcify. Monostotic fibrous dysplasia, however, must enter into the roentgenologic differential diagnosis because, on the one hand, it also occurs in the epiphysis and, on the other, calcifications may appear in the "osteolytic area."

Fig. 48 **Projection of a tophus in the roentgenogram.** The tophaceous "cupping" (mutilation) is a characteristic finding in long-standing gout of small joints. Marginal tophi appear as semicircular erosions. *(Dashed:* The concentrically grown, roentgenologically *invisible* gouty tophus). Elongated, oval subchondral osteolyses extending as far as the diaphysis are much more suggestive of tophi than (rounded) punched-out defects in the immediate subchondral layer! Despite this, a safe rule to follow in practice is to consider gout in the differentiation of any rounded osteolysis in *small bones* that exceeds a diameter of 5 mm *and* is associated with discomfort referable to a joint.

mushroomed shape of the first metatarsal head (Fig. 533; Dihlmann and Fernholz, 1974).

The possible arthritic and osteoarthrotic reactions described and the consequences of the deposition of tophaceous urate in the joint and the subchondral bone marrow govern the multifaceted radiographic picture of gouty arthritis which therefore has to be classified as gouty osteoarthropathy.

Extraarticular depositions of urate can occur in the bone, mostly close to a joint, but do not necessarily present pathologic roentgen findings in the joint *(intraosseous gouty tophus)* (Fig. 49). The extremely infrequent solitary intraosseous gouty tophus has been termed by Bauer (1968a) *uric osteomyelitis.* This lesion may, particularly in small bones, occur as the primary manifestation of gout and may mimic the picture of a circumscribed osteomyelitis (Brodie abscess; see Fig. 26). In small bones, intraosseous gouty tophi have even been observed to produce total osteolysis (e.g., of a phalanx): *gouty pseudotumor* (Murray, 1977). The development of certain cases of (idiopathic) necrosis of the femoral head (see p. 254) has also been ascribed to gout. Finally, mention should be made of pressure erosions in the olecranon due to *gouty olecranon bursitis* and pressure erosions in the calcaneus (Gerster et al., 1975) due to *gouty Achilles bursitis* (Fig. 563).

When hyperuricemia or gout is diagnosed in boys after unremarkable development in early childhood but prior to puberty, the (sex-linked) *Lesch-Nyhan syndrome* must be taken into consideration. This syndrome originates with a hereditary enzyme deficiency that (largely) impedes the metabolic recycling of purine bases, leading to an excessive increase in purine neosynthesis. In addition to gout, the Lesch-Nyhan syndrome includes central nervous disorders (spastic cerebral paresis, choreoathetosis), impaired intelligence and, in the majority of sufferers, a psychopathic (compulsory, autoaggressive) behavior with proneness to self-mutilation of fingers and lips.

Ochronosis (alcaptonuria) is the consequence of an inborn enzyme defect that leads to a disorder of tyrosine and phenylalanine metabolism. Homogentisic acid oxidase is absent in affected persons so that an increased amount of homogentisic acid is excreted in their urine. A brown-black polymerized oxidation product is deposited in mesenchymal tissues, among them the articular cartilage and the intervertebral disks. This foreign substance interferes with the cartilage metabolism by inhibiting the energy turnover (Dihlmann et al., 1970); it renders the cartilage brittle and vulnerable to shearing forces and ultimately leads to osteoarthrosis. It may be mentioned here that ochronotic deposits in the cardiovascular system and the kidneys can produce death (Pageaut et al., 1971).

The roentgenogram of **ochronotic osteoarthropathy** in the peripheral joints—the knee joint seems to be particularly prone to ochronosis—is identical to that of osteoarthrosis. The osteoarthrotic joint lesions in ochronosis frequently occur at an age when manifestations of joint attrition are, as a rule, not yet to be expected and often are more rapidly progressive than in nonochronotic osteoarthrosis. Ossification of tendon insertions occurs in ochronosis patients; these roentgen findings do not differ from the usual degenerative spurs (fibroosteoses) at the insertions. At most, they appear to be thicker and occur more frequently than in patients not suffering from ochronosis (see Fig. 357). The "test joints" of ochronotic arthropathy are the thoracic, and particularly the lumbar, intervertebral disks (Fig. 50). The ochronotic disks collapse and with time become calcified. *Small* bony intervertebral hooks are formed. Lateral roentgenograms often reveal increased thickness underneath the disks and hazy translucences near the endplates of the vertebral bodies. These translucences (Bauer-Kienböck foci, 1929) are also demonstrable in the nearer and more remote subchondral layer of larger joints; e.g., in the ischium, of ochronosis patients. In lateral lumbar roentgenograms of the intervertebral disks, the so-called vacuum phenomenon can very often be demonstrated. This phenomenon is seldom observed in roentgeologically normal joints of adults; it is seen with somewhat greater frequency in osteoarthrotic joints and synarthroses (e.g., the symphysis pubis) but never with such frequency and to such an extent as in ochronotic discopathy.

Advanced *ochronotic spondylopathy* is a characteristic roentgen finding (see Fig. 50 C, C'). However, a similar roentgen picture, which therefore must be differentiated, has been described and illustrated by Ballou et al. (1976) in *primary amyloidosis* with massive deposition of amyloid and secondary calcification in intervertebral disks. In addition to this, calcifications of disks such as those sketched in Figures 50 B and B' are also known to occur in (hereditary, sporadic, and symptomatic) chondrocalcinosis (see under this heading).

Congenital *coagulopathies* can lead to osteoarthropathy **(coagulopathic osteoarthropathy)** which has clinical and radiodiagnostic significance. Among them are hemophilia A (diminished activity of antihemophilic factor VIII), hemophilia B (diminished activity of antihemophilic factor IX, the so-called Christmas factor), and hemophilia C (factor XI deficiency). *Congenital* deficiency of factor VII (hypoproconvertinemia; Vignon et al., 1979), but also *acquired* deficiency of factor VII; for example in anticoagulant therapy with discoumarol, in damage to the parenchymal cells of the liver, or in thrombopathies, have been described as causes of hemorrhage into the joints and bones.

Ordinarily, the genetically determined decrease of activity or the percentile residual activity of the coagulation factors governs the severity of the coagulopathy, the age of manifestation, and the extent of the osteoarthropathy. For example, in hemophilia with a residual activity of the coagulation factors varying between 0 and 5 percent, hemorrhages into joints form a regular part of the clinical picture. With residual activities between 5 and 15 percent, hemorrhages into joints are also to be expected.

Involvement of the skeleton in hemophilia has been the most thoroughly studied; the terms *hemophilic osteoarthropathy* and *hemophilic joint* are therefore in common use.

The pathogenesis of the hemophilic joint may be described as follows: The blood in the joint cavity has as its initial origin an intrasynovial hemorrhage that penetrates the joint. Blood in the joint is "hostile to the cartilage." Particularly, recurrent hemorrhages into the joint lead to degenerative lesions of the cartilage, increasing to necrosis. In addition blood, being a fluid, is not compressible and therefore intensifies the intraarticular pressure. With time, this increase in pressure has an adverse effect on those articular surfaces that are not covered with cartilage; e.g., the olecranon fossa in the elbow and the intercondylar fossa in the knee. At these sites, but also at the insertion of the joint capsule, the increase in intraarticular pressure leads to resorption of bone; i.e., pressure erosions and/or localized disorders of growth (Fig. 51).

In addition, repeated accumulations of blood in the joint cavity, the synovial membrane, the fibrous joint capsule, and the immediate pericapsular soft tissues give rise to a reaction on the part of the vascular and connective tissue; hence, chronic arthritis. The histologic picture of this *inflammatory* synovial reaction shows proliferation of synovial cells, cellular infiltration, increase of connective tissue, macrophages storing hemosiderin, and conglutination of villi. Thickening of the capsule with proneness to later shrinking supervenes. Ultimately, granulation tissue grows from the articular recesses. This granulation tissue, similarly to the pannus (the fibrovascular resorption tissue in any kind of chronic arthritis), expands with destruction of cartilage and bone. In time, the gliding tissue becomes increasingly damaged by the described association of degeneration and inflammation, with the recurrent hemorrhages igniting the morbid processes again and again.

Finally, the joint can—at worst—undergo fibrous or bony ankylosis, mostly in a faulty position. Prior to this, however, the mobility of the chronic

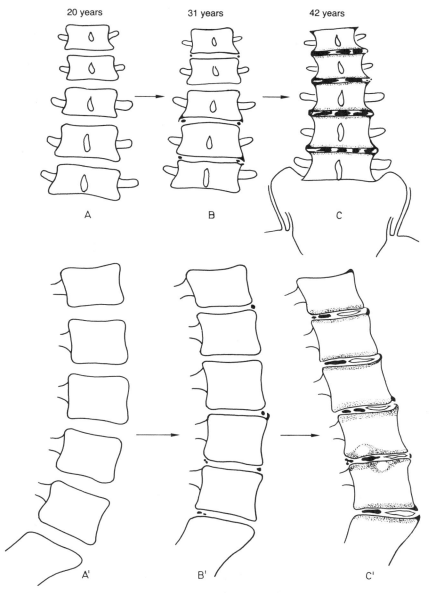

20 years   31 years   42 years

Fig. 50 **The lumbar intervertebral disks are the "test joints" of ochronotic (alcaptonuric) arthropathy.**

A, A' = 20-year-old male, no lumbar complaints. Normal roentgenogram of the lumbar spine (taken on the occasion of an accident).

B, B' = 11 years later (at age 31), considerable "low back pain" for several years. Roentgen findings in lumbar spine pathologic: *conspicuous decrease in height ("narrowing") of all intervertebral disk spaces with slight or absent reactive formation of osteophytes on the vertebral bodies!* Delicate calcifications in the annulus fibrosus of some of the intervertebral disks. Retrograde spondylolisthesis of L3 (see Figs. 632 A and B).

C, C' = The patient is now 42 years old. The lumbar roentgenograms in two planes show the characteristic appearance of *advanced ochronotic discopathy;* namely, an appearance resembling a gnarled stick, due to the collapse and calcification of the intervertebral disks. In addition, there are numerous vacuum phenomena *(marked with a light edge)* and calcifications of disks *(sketched dark).* In the surroundings of the caudal endplate L4 and the cranial endplate L5 one sees an irregularly rounded translucence in the vertebral body with delicate marginal sclerosis (so-called Bauer-Kienböck focus). Sacroiliac joints normal.

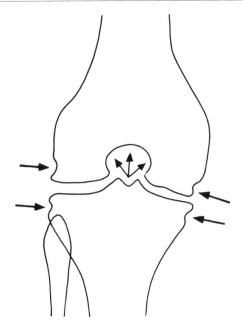

Fig. 51 Hemophilic joint (knee, *schematically*). The *arrows* point to those places on the joint-forming bones in which the recurrent hemorrhages into the joint first lead to an increase in the intraarticular pressure and thereby precipitates resorption of bone and growth disorders.

hemorrhage into the joint and as a result of immobilization of the hemophilic joint.

Fractures in hemophiliacs, especially intraarticular fractures and those in the vicinity of the joint, have a poor healing quality. Either the callus formation is impaired (hazard of pseudoarthrosis) or the progression of the previously existing destruction of joint and bones is stimulated. Another, infrequent, consequence of trauma is the *hemophilic pseudotumor*. It develops following recurrent subperiosteal and intraosseous hemorrhages within months or years and has been observed predominantly in the small bones of the hand (Figs. 52 and 140) and the foot, and in the mandible, the pelvis and the large tubular bones. Its cystic-trabecular radiologic appearance and the often grotesque expansion of the bone or part of it are the

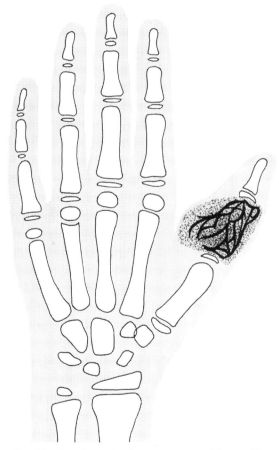

hemophilic joint becomes impaired by shrinking of the thickened fibrous joint capsule and the sequelae of recurrent bleeding into the muscles. Extraarticular hemorrhages into the soft tissues, among them recurrent muscle hematomas, give rise not only to contractures but sometimes also to heterotopic formation of new bone (Hutcheson, 1973; Fig. 360). Massive hemorrhages into the joint can increase the intracavitary pressure to such a degree that the blood supply to the intracapsular epiphyses (e.g., the head of the femur) is no longer ensured. The consequence is avascular necrosis of bone. In addition to this, the repeated hemorrhages into the joint interfere with the growth of the epiphyses and apophyses. Epiphyseal and apophyseal growth then follow a disharmonious course with acceleration or retardation, or epiphyseal closure occurs prematurely.

Among the best known skeletal deformations are widening of the intercondylar fossa (Fig. 51), rectangular shape of the patella (Fig. 437) and humerus varus (Fig. 260). These deformations, however, are not specific roentgen signs of hemophilia. Widening of the intercondylar fossa, for instance, has also been described in tuberculosis and in juvenile rheumatoid arthritis (Bohrer, 1969). Particularly in younger patients, the cancellous bone in the vicinity of affected joints is frequently remodeled to fibrillar (hypertrophic) atrophy. The latter develops both in connection with episodes of arthritic resorption following a

Fig. 52 Roentgenologic appearance of the cystic-trabecular hemophilic pseudotumor in the proximal phalanx of the thumb of an 8-year-old boy with hemophilia A. The cystic-trabecular appearance is the result of alternating resorption of bone and formation of new bone. Note also the increased density of soft tissues produced by a hematoma which is enclosed by a fibrous capsule. The hydraulic pressure exerted by the hematoma contributes to the resorption of bone.

results of hematoma-induced remodeling. The pseudotumor can give rise to a pathologic fracture. The hemophilic pseudotumor[13] is consistently associated with a periosteal reaction, pressure necrosis of the bone, and a soft-tissue mass with or without calcium deposits (hematoma with a thick fibrous capsule).

Experience has shown that in hemophiliacs only a small proportion of subperiosteal and intraosseous hematomas are transformed into pseudotumors. It is much more common for these hematomas, the presence of which may be suggested by bone-forming elevations of the periosteum with or without calcifications, to be reabsorbed during their further evolution. Intraosseous hematomas (hemorrhages into the bone marrow) sometimes manifest themselves by rounded translucences of the skeletal structure in the close or remote subchondral layer of a joint (to be differentiated from an osteoarthrotic debris cyst, an osteitis, or a tumor, see Fig. 260).

The description of the pathogenesis and the pathologic features of a hemophilic joint allows conclusions to be drawn about its *radiographic morphology:*

1. In larger joints with a thin cover of soft tissues, the synovial membrane is particularly prone to being traumatized. The knee, the talocrural, and the elbow joints are therefore the test joints of coagulopathic (hemophilic) osteoarthropathy.
2. The articular hematoma is reflected in the roentgenogram by the soft-tissue signs (p. 11); the resorptive processes in the synovium manifest themselves by the collateral phenomena (Dihlmann, 1974) and the consequences of immobilization (Fig. 13), that are known to occur in arthritis; the reactive proliferation of the synovium (pannus) leads to the direct signs of arthritis that have already been described (see Fig. 20) and which may be accompanied by signs of secondary osteoarthrosis (Figs. 43 and 44).
3. The disturbed growth and development of the joint-bearing bones contribute to the pathologic roentgenogram, depending on the patient's age.

The following conditions must enter into the *clinicoradiologic* differential diagnosis of hemarthrosis: congenital and acquired coagulopathies (including acute hemorrhage into the joint produced by long-term oral anticoagulant therapy [McLaughlin et al., 1966]); trauma; synovial tumors, including hemangiomas (calcified thrombi!); pigmented villonodular synovitis; infection, neurogenic osteoarthropathies; sickle cell anemia; myeloproliferative diseases (Harris and Ross, 1974); and chondrocalcinosis (pseudogout).

The roentgenologic *differential diagnosis* of the coagulopathic (hemophilic) pseudotumor in the *pelvic bones* must consider: osteoclastoma, aneurysmatic bone cysts, malignant tumors, massive osteo-

lysis (Gorham and Stout, 1955), and posttraumatic osteolysis due to an intraosseous hematoma or a large (posttraumatic) aneurysm of the pelvic arteries.

The roentgenologic characteristic of the **neurogenic (neuropathic) osteoarthropathies** is the *anarchic transformation and disintegration* of the joint involved, which in the articular soft tissues, the articular cartilage, and the joint-bearing bones by far exceeds the extent known in arthritis and osteoarthrosis. This applies to the resorption and apposition of bone, to the calcification and ossification of the articular and periarticular soft tissues, and to the degree of malposition in statically loaded joints.

Fried (1970) distinguishes three stages in the evolution of the neurogenic osteoarthropathies:

1. In the *first stage of the disease (chondro-osteonecrosis),* the roentenogram shows destruction of cartilage and bone, which *initially* may only manifest itself by a more or less distinct narrowing of the joint space and/or by erosions; hence, roentgen signs of "arthritis." The features atypical of arthritis, however, make their appearance before long: the joint-bearing bone breaks off at the border of the joint; it is detached, "*crumbles,*" or becomes abraded by motion. Small bones (the carpals, for instance) become necrotic and reveal an increase in density. Other bones (e.g., the tarsals) are "crushed" or "mashed." The developing bone debris disperses in the joint cavity, or, in the case of the shoulder joint, accumulates in the subdeltoid bursa. The flaked-off bone fragments either are dissolved or form centers from which the articular or periarticular formation of new bone starts. Finally, fatigue fracture (of the metatarsals or the femoral neck, for instance) also form part of the first stage of neurogenic osteoarthropathy. *Clinically,* neurogenic arthropathy may begin insidiously with a *painless* effusion into the joint, edematous impregnation of the articular soft tissues, instability of the joint, and malposition of the articulating bones. Conversely, the onset may be *painful* or even may *mimic cellulitis* (Fried, 1970) with increased heat and erythema of the joint involved, extensive periarticular edema, serologic signs of inflammation, and an elevation in temperature. It is rare for neurogenic osteopathy to be the *first* manifestation of the underlying nervous disease noticed by the patient. This explains why extremities affected by a neurogenic osteoarthropathy with predominant osteolysis have— incomprehensibly—been amputated following the erroneous diagnosis of osteolytic osteosarcoma.
2. *In the second, reactive, stage* of neurogenic osteoarthropathy, precipitous and disharmonious formation of new bone in the articular soft tissues and their surroundings takes place concurrently with osteolytic processes; i.e., crumbly disintegration of bone (in the presence of intraarticular fractures) and/or nonreactive dissolution of bone. In the small tubular bones—of the hands and feet, for instance—resorption of bone prevails so that they appear to be "sucked on" (Figs. 53 and 543). In the knee joint, formation

---

[13] Eichler (1966) has reported a coagulopathic pseudotumor in afibrinogenemia.

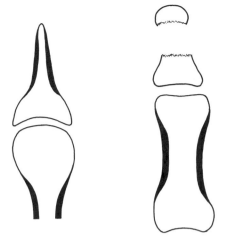

Fig. 53 *Left:* **Typical roentgenogram of nonreactive (acral) osteolysis** in a small tubular bone. The bone appears to be "sucked off." *Right:* **Picture of band-shaped (transverse) osteolysis** between the terminal tuft and the shaft of the phalanx; e.g., in vinyl chloride disease (here potentially reversible), in the Hajdu-Cheney syndrome, and in osteomalacia (reversible).

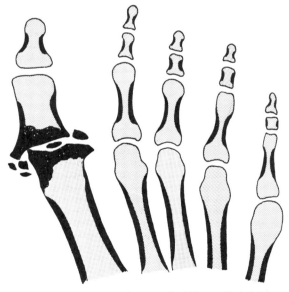

Fig. 54   **Example of a so-called Charcot's joint** (see text), sketched here in the metatarsophalangeal joint! *Major roentgen findings:* Fragmentation of bone, osteolysis; dense, irregularly shaped cancellous sclerosis, malposition of joint.

Note: In rare cases, typical Charcot's joints—of whatever location—appear without any recognizable neurologic findings. These cases are termed "idiopathic Charcot's joints" (Blanford et al., 1978).

of new bone is usually in the forefront, whereas in the shoulder and the hip joint osteolysis predominates.

3. The *third stage* of neurogenic osteoarthropathy has been designated by Fried as the *stabilization phase:* The skeletal findings hardly change for years; they have stabilized. At most, improved harmoniousness—e.g., rounding of contours in the bones involved—is demonstrable. Infrequently one even notes (partial) reconstruction. Such stabilization with more or less complete reconstruction is, of course, the objective of therapy in neurogenic osteoarthropathies.

Fried's division of the neurogenic osteoarthropathies into three stages describes the dynamics of these diseases. In practice, however, the *static* approach has proved its value because these disorders show two "faces" that the physician engaged in roentgen diagnosis must commit to memory. The first face is *nonreactive osteolysis* ("partly sucked candy bar") prevalent in small tubular bones. The second face is *Charcot's joint*—a term used for reasons of medical history—with osteolysis; dense, irregularly shaped, subchondral sclerosis of cancellous bone; pathologic proneness to fragmentation of the joint-bearing bones (the bone crumbles away) juxtaarticular focal calcifications; and formation of new bone and roentgen signs of capsuloligamentous instability (in weight-bearing joints). Lesions corresponding to Charcot's joint develop primarily in the epiphyses of the long tubular bones, and furthermore in the tarsal and carpal joints as well as in the spine (for exceptions to this rule see Fig. 54).

A concomitant finding of diagnostic significance in some neurogenic osteopathies is the *perforating ulcer*, which is encountered most often in the feet and less frequently in the hands. The term suggests the poor healing quality of these lesions, which generally are painless. On the one hand, detached parts of bone can be extruded through these ulcers and, on the other, the ulcers favor the development of secondary infections which are demonstrable in the roentgenogram as periostitis and osteomyelitis. These infections, likewise, can give rise to the extrusion of sequestra through the perforating ulcer (compare p. 49).

It is obvious that different pathogenetic factors must take effect for the picture of neurogenic osteopathy to develop:

The initial intraarticular fracture that is sometimes demonstrable (see Fig. 540), e.g., fracture of the femoral neck in neurogenic osteoarthropathy of the hip, suggests anomalous (trophic?) fragility of the joint-forming bones. (Trophic disturbance could be compared with what Fried and Kalna [1980] define as "regressive changes in a biologically abnormal soil.") The decreased sensibility to pain associated with the underlying disease and the muscular hypotonicity favor overloading of the articular gliding and supporting tissues and inconsiderate use of the joint. Vasomotor disorders and organic vascular lesions are also subjects of debate. Finally, there exist diseases and syndromes without any known relationship to the nervous system, which nevertheless present "neuropathic" roentgen findings, especially *nonreactive osteolyses* and *acral osteolysis* (see Fig. 53). Therefore, the term **osteolysis syndrome**[14] has been proposed by Sommer and Reinhardt (1959). Under this heuristic term, therefore, are grouped all those disorders that present "neuropathic characteristics" in the roentgenogram *(vide supra),* regardless of whether these diseases are connected with disorders of the central or peripheral, or the autonomous nervous system.

The osteolysis syndrome is characteristic of the following disorders.

Classic Neurogenic Osteoarthropathies

Tabes Dorsalis

Tabetic osteoarthropathy sometimes antedates the neurologic symptoms by years or may even remain the only clinical manifestation of this late syphilitic affection. The joints of the lower extremities are more frequently involved than those of the arms. Clinical peculiarities: tabetic flatfoot, tabetic spondylopathy (primarily) involving the lumbar spine, tabetic fractures (posttraumatic or spontaneous, often followed by excessive or retarded callus formation and sometimes by resorptive processes in the fractured bones).

Syringomelia

This dysraphia, which develops in early embryonic life, is most frequently located in the cervical or the upper thoracic cord. Therefore, the corresponding osteoarthropathy occurs predominantly in the upper extremities and the cervical spine. The pathologic substrate of the dysraphia is a cystic gliomatosis of the gray matter, which generally manifests itself between the ages of 20 and 40; it is slowly progressive. Syringomyelia patients present with variable frequency the following signs of dysraphia: macrosomatia, (thoracic) kyphoscoliosis, funnel chest, spina bifida occulta, arachnodactyly.

Generally, patients with dysraphia in the caudal end of the cord, its meninges, and the spine seem prone to suffer osteoarthropathies of the lower extremities: *trophopathia pedis*

---

[14] This concept, however, does not refer to the stage of articular and extraarticular mutilation in rheumatoid arthritis (see Figs. 38 and 710). This disease also presents osteolyses of the type illustrated in Fig. 53, but these are unequivocally associated with direct roentgen signs of arthritis (see under this heading). In addition, the clinical history in these cases reveals the presence of a (painful) arthritis that has been treated for years or decades. This diagnostic clue aids in avoiding confusion with the neurogenic osteoarthropathies or the osteolysis syndrome. Nor does the osteolysis syndrome include the total osteolysis of small bones (e.g., the carpals, tarsals, and phalanges) due to malignant tumors, metastases, or gouty tophi, and as an accompaniment of juvenile rheumatoid arthritis.

myelodysplastica (Kienböck, 1930) or *myelodysplasia* (Fuchs, 1909). The writers describing dysraphia-dependent neurogenic osteoarthropathies point to the occurrence in these patients of spina bifida occulta, anomalous hair growth, and lipomas, myomas, angiomas, and meningoceles in the sacrolumbar region, as well as pes cavus and talipes (Crasselet 1960, 1961, and other workers).

In syringomyelic osteoarthropathy, especially of the shoulder joint, one generally observes a preponderance of osteolytic processes, associated with crumbling of bone, calcifications, and local formations of new bone in the articular soft tissues and in the periarticular surroundings.

Hereditary Neuropathic Osteoarthropathies

Individuals with *congenital analgesia* lack sensibility to pain and the subjective experience of pain from the time of birth. In these patients, osteoarthropathies occur in the upper and lower extremities and in the spine. Francillon (1970) saw an interarticular neurogenic spondylolysis with spondylolisthesis in congenital analgesia. Fractures and traumatic epiphysiolyses as well as neglected infections of bones and joints contribute to the development of skeletal deformations. For the rest, epiphysiolyses and fractures of the metaphysis and diaphysis of long tubular bones are consistent roentgen findings in the neurogenic osteoarthropathies of *childhood* (Schneider et al., 1978).

Heredofamilial osteolysis (acroosteolysis) is a concept that has been dealt with and studied from many different perspectives. It is therefore not surprising that Partsch alone (1970) has encountered 16 synonyms in the literature for familial osteolysis (acroosteolysis) inherited in a dominant mode. Apart from this, there are recessively inherited, sporadic, and abortive cases with identical or at least very similar basic signs; namely, the association of skin lesions, neurogenic osteoarthropathy, and neurologic deficits in the lower (and infrequently also in the upper) extremities.

• **Skin lesions:** Trophic calluses, edematous and verrucous thickening of skin and subcutaneous tissues progressing to elephantiasis-like swelling of the foot, painless ulcers (perforating ulcers of the foot), and disturbed growth of nails.
• **Neurogenic osteoarthropathy:** Osteolyses involving principally the forefoot and metatarsus— "sucked-on bones"—especially in the proximal phalanges and metatarsals; malposition of toes. Together with the skin lesions described, osteoarthropathy leads to serious deformation, coarsening, and mutilation of the feet. The neurogenic lesions in the skin, the joints, and the bones are overshadowed by the clinical and roentgenologic findings of secondary infection, swelling of the inguinal lymph nodes, fever, paronychia, ossifying periostitis, osteomyelitis, and sequestra which may be extruded through the perforating ulcers. It should be borne in mind that the

formation of bone debris—''sequestra''—and of new bone is associated with the neurogenic disease picture itself, even in the absence of infection.

· **Neurologic deficits of the sensory (peripheral) type:** The sensory disturbance in the feet sometimes spreads to the lower leg in the form of a ''stocking paresthesia.'' By analogy, one speaks of ''glove paresthesia'' in the hands and forearms. Sensation of pain and temperature is more significantly impaired than sensibility to touch and vibration. Motor deficits are manifested by disturbances of the reflexes. The Achilles tendon reflex, for instance, is destroyed or can hardly be elicited. In advanced cases, muscular atrophies are conspicuous. The involvement of autonomous nerves is evidenced by hyperhidrosis of the feet.

Since the neurogenic affections are not only heritable but also can occur sporadically (as mentioned above), the following classification has been suggested, principally by French workers:

· **Familial ulceromutilating acropathy** *(Thévenard's syndrome)*. No sex preponderance, onset in early youth, involvement of the lower (infrequently also the upper) extremities
· **Nonfamilial ulceromutilating acropaty (Bureau-Barrière syndrome).** Males are almost exclusively affected; onset in middle age; lower extremities involved. The patients are mostly chronic alcoholics. A local noxious agent is generally demonstrable (e.g., humidity, slight frostbite). It should be mentioned here that Scott et al. (1973) have observed Charcot's joints (talocrural and knee joint) developing in Waldenström's macroglobulinemia with amyloidosis. The amyloidosis evidently gave rise to a peripheral neuropathy, which in turn led to a neurogenic osteoarthropathy. Similar though less pronounced destructions of the forefoot and hindfoot have been described by Lithner (1976) in familial amyloidosis with polyneuropathy. Fried and Kalná (1980) observed neurogenic osteoarthropathies of large joints as an aftermath of *infectious* polyneuritis plus myelitis.

Diabetic Osteoarthropathy

Generalized osteoporosis is a frequent complication of long-term diabetes mellitus (occurring in about one third of patients, according to Ringe et al., 1976). Calcification of the arterial walls, likewise, is a familiar finding in diabetics. Diabetic osteoarthropathy, in contrast, is an infrequent event (0.2 to 0.5 percent of diabetics, Forgács 1977; 2.4 percent, Fochem, 1971; 7.5 percent, Klümper et al., 1968b). Experience has shown diabetics with compromised metabolism related to *long-term disease* and those with neurologic disturbances (diminished sensibility, motor deficits such as reflex anomalies) are prone to developing osteoarthropathies. Diabetic osteoarthropathy is observed most commonly in the region of the

(fore-)foot and infrequently involves the talocrural joint. Occurrence in the remaining parts of the skeleton (e.g., in the proximal interphalangeal joints, the carpus, the elbows, the shoulder and the (lumbar) spine is exceptional (Feldman et al., 1960, Feldman et al., 1974, Campbell and Feldman, 1975).

Diabetic osteoarthropathy manifests itself in the forefoot principally as a nonreactive osteolysis. In the hindfoot, the roentgenogram is governed by the tarsometatarsal and intertarsal instability (that depends on the soft tissues) and increased susceptibility to fragmentation of the small bones. These processes lead to anomalous shearing and grinding movements which at once favor the dislocation of the small bones of the foot and abet their being crushed and crumbled. The description of diabetic osteoarthropathy shows that this disorder of joints and bones presents the above-mentioned two ''faces'' of a neurogenic osteoarthropathy.

The *clinical differentiation of diabetic osteoarthropathy*, therefore, must in the first place take into consideration tabes dorsalis syringomyelia, the hereditary neurogenic osteoarthropathies, leprous osteoarthropathy, and the sequelae of traumatic injuries to the nerves of the leg. Similarly *diabetic spondylopathy* must be differentiated clinically from spondylopathy in tabes dorsalis, in syringomyelia, and in congenital analgesia. Important manifestations of the spondylopathies mentioned are the increased thickness of the vertebral cancellous bone which can progress to eburnation, the crumbling and abrasion of the vertebrae, and an instability of the soft tissues that allows the vertebrae to be displaced in all directions. Vertebral osteophytes of bizarre shape complete the picture of anarchic remodeling *(vide supra)* of the spinal part involved (Fig. 638).

Neurogenic Osteoarthropathies Following Injury to the Peripheral Nerves

Such articular lesions have been described principally as an aftermath of injuries to the sciatic nerve or one of its main branches. However, an injury to the femoral nerve (severance) also can give rise to a neurogenic osteoarthropathy (Fried, 1969). Nonreactive osteolyses in the forefoot region then govern the roentgenologic picture. Clinically, trophic skin lesions in the feet (hyperkeratosis, perforating ulcers) may be conspicuous. Such ulcers sometimes pave the way for infection of the bone *(vide supra)* and pyogenic arthritis of the tarsal joints, which can terminate in bony ankylosis (Fried, 1969).

In individual patients with extensive poliomyelitic pareses, nonreactive osteolyses and trophic ulcers in the (fore-)foot region have been observed (Ott, 1957). Secondary infections of bone by way of perforating ulcers occur, and these manifest themselves roentgenologically by ossifying periostitis and chronic osteomyelitis (compare above).

Leprous osteoarthropathy

The mycobacterial disease leprosy is, as a rule, characterized by a very prolonged incubation period (extending over years and decades). Therefore, the patient often has forgotten about his stay in endemic areas (tropics, Far East). Moreover, physicians in the industrially advanced countries of the temperate zone have little practical experience in diagnosing this disease. There are two types of leprosy: the *Lepromatous (granulomatous, nodular)* and the *neural (anesthetic) type*. In addition, there are so-called *mixed types* (transitions between the two categories).

The lepromatous type attacks the skin and the mucous membranes of the respiratory tract. However, the specific granulation tissue can, in principle, appear anywhere in the body; for example, in the testes, the anterior segment of the eye, the visceral organs, the bone marrow, and the synovial membrane. In the latter instance, the (infrequent) leprous arthritis[15] develops, accompanied by a painful, often profuse effusion into the joint.

The skeletal lesions that may, but by no means always do, occur in leprosy, develop either directly by way of the bloodstream or indirectly by spread of the infection from the diseased skin and mucosa. Therefore, the phalanges and the bones of the skull are the most frequent sites of skeletal manifestations of lepromatous leprosy. Various types of periostitis and osteomyelitis develop (Fig. 55); contribute substantially to their extension, activity, and radiographic morphology.

Neural leprosy reflects the involvement of peripheral nerves. The specific granulation tissue develops in and around the nerve cords. The clinical consequences are sensory disturbances ("anesthesia"), muscular atrophies, and neurogenic (neuropathic, neurotrophic) skeletal lesions. These findings are particularly striking in the hands and the forefeet. Nonreactive osteolyses—"sucked-on bones"—dominate the roentgenogram. These neurogenic lesions are overshadowed by the consequences of secondary infections of bone that develop by way of the ulcers in the skin. The radiologic picture of Charcot's joint (see p. 48) is seen infrequently in neural leprosy but occurs occasionally in larger joints (Fig. 56) and in the tarsal region, which is exposed to heavy static load. The latter localization underlines once more the significance of repetitive everyday traumas to the development of neurogenic osteoarthropathy in denervated tissues. Finally, Edeiken and Hodes (1973) present illustrations of roentgenologically identifiable nerve calcifications in the vicinity of neurogenic leprous osteoarthropathies.

Chronic fungal infections of the skeleton (see p. 108) usually show the radiologic picture of chronic osteomyelitis;

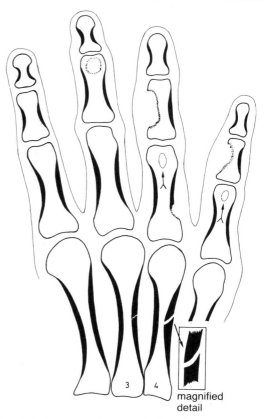

magnified detail

Fig. 55   Leprous osteomyelitis (lepromatous granulomatous leprosy) from bloodstream dissemination of the mycobacteria. The specific granulation tissue has led to cystlike skeletal defects (middle phalanx of 3rd finger) and to excentric osteolyses (middle phalanx of 4th and 5th finger) as to widening of the nutrient foramina in the proximal phalanges IV and V *(tailed arrows)* (Hirschberg and Biehler, 1909; Patersen and Job, 1964; Enna et al., 1971). The osteoporosis of the cancellous and cortical bone which, during the acute phase of inflammation, is often pronounced in the short tubular bones, the carpals, and the tarsals, has not been illustrated. The leprous periostitis has also not been reproduced.

The 3rd metacarpal shows a *normal* nutrient canal, whereas the 4th metacarpal shows a *widened* nutrient canal such as occurs in various diseases (see footnote on p. 29). The *arrow* points to a magnified detail that shows the slightly *arched* course of the *widened* nutrient canal (Beyer and Stecken, 1962).

i.e., inflammatory remodeling of bone (resorption, formation of new bone) with sequestrations. Clinically conspicuous features are swelling of soft tissues and (sometimes) fistulas in the skin (which often are conducive to pyogenic superinfection). Granulomatous fungal infections of the skeleton—e.g., in mycetoma (maduromycosis, Madura foot; Cockshott and Braband 1966)—are occasionally accompanied by extensive osteolyses that *radiologically* are reminiscent of neurogenic osteoarthropathy.

---

[15] Leprous arthritis develops hematogenously or by spread from infectious foci in the bone marrow and in the periarticular soft tissues.

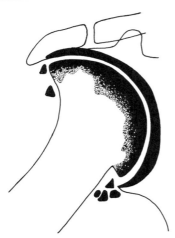

Fig. 56   Humeroscapular Charcot's joint in neural leprosy. Roentgenologic differentiation from other neurogenic osteoarthropathies (see Fig. 263) and from far advanced osteoarthrosis with abraded surfaces. A plain osteoarthrosis, however, shows *no* tendency to fragmentation but may present capsular osteomas and calcified capsular chondromas (Fig. 249). In addition, sclerosis of the cancellous bone in osteoarthrosis tends to *band-shaped* development in the subchondral area, whereas in neurogenic osteoarthropathy (such as sketched here in the head of the humerus) it need not be limited to the immediate subchondral cancellous bone.

event, sometimes with the classic local signs of inflammation and a rise in temperature (Rossak, 1961). They appear, however, only in sites where nerve deficits exist!

Neurogenic paraosteoarthropathies occur most often in the regions of the hip and shoulder. They occur less frequently in the knee and the vicinity of the elbow and are hardly ever observed in small joints; e.g., the metacarpophalangeal joints.

Neurogenic paraosteoarthropathies as well as the lesions and diseases of the central nervous system mentioned above can also be followed by bony ankyloses; for example, in the sacroiliac joints. Prior to the development of ankylosis, erosive changes in the contour of the joint are apt to occur (Dihlmann, 1978). Besides these pathologic lesions, such patients are prone to heterotopic formation of new bone in the paralumbar area. Erosive changes of contour are also observed outside the joints; e.g. (as an accompaniment to paraplegia), in the trochanters, the tuberosities of the ischium, and the sacrum. Only rarely do these contour defects develop into osteolyses involving more or less large portions of the bony pelvis, possibly even including the hip joints (Abel and Smith, 1974; Fig. 57). The joint lesions described, as well as extraarticular defects of bone, have been related by some writers to secondary infections originating in decubital ulcers or the urogenital tract. This hypothesis, however, is not universally tenable (Catterall et al., 1967; Rosin, 1975; Dihlmann, 1978).

Neurogenic Paraosteoarthropathies

The term *neurogenic paraosteoarthropathies* indicates that trauma and disease incurred by the central nervous system can give rise to certain pathologic changes in the *immediate* neighborhood of a joint (*para* = beside). These changes concern more or less extensive *calcifications* and *ossifications* of soft tissues adjacent to the joint and the (lumbar) spine (joint capsules, ligaments, fasciae, tendons, muscles). On the one hand, these lesions lead to complete immobilization of the joint when large "hooks," "cases," or "shells" are formed. On the other hand, *reversible subperiosteal* calcifications and new bone formations have also been observed (Rosin, 1975). The following disorders underlying the development of neurogenic paraosteoarthropathies in the upper and lower extremities and in the neighborhood of the spine have been reported: tetra-, para-, and hemiplegia; severe traumatic brain damage including the apallic syndrome; (suicidal) thallium intoxication; an overdose of insulin (Balzereit and Tänzer, 1968); tetanus infection; epidemic encephalitis; general paralysis (Heuck and Enchenhofer, 1974); brain tumor; multiple sclerosis, and lesion of the cauda equina from a prolapsed disk (Rosin, 1975). The calcifications and ossifications develop weeks or months after the causal

Idiopathic Osteolyses (Acroosteolyses)

The attribute "neurogenic" ("neuropathic") is meant to emphasize that these skeletal lesions in the neurogenic (neuropathic) osteoarthropathies and paraosteoarthropathies develop in connection with diseases and lesions of the central and/or peripheral, and/or autonomic nervous system. Moreover, there are many diseases and syndromes where nonreactive osteolyses are demonstrable in the roentgenogram although a causal connection with neurologic disorders of whatever kind has at most been suspected but never demonstrated. These are the idiopathic osteolyses and the idiopathic acroosteolyses. They will be listed summarily, without any claim to completeness:

• Various idiopathic osteolyses lead preferentially to resorption of the carpal and tarsal bones *("carpal or tarsal osteolyses")* and may, in addition, involve the contiguous parts of the metacarpals and metatarsals, which become "sharpened," slimmed, and "deflected" (Figs. 58 and 102). Apart from this, additional osteolyses occasionally develop in the neighborhood of the elbow, in the proximal humerus, and in the terminal tufts of the toes. These osteolyses are known to occur sporadically or as a hereditary disorder, with or without chronic glomerulonephritis.

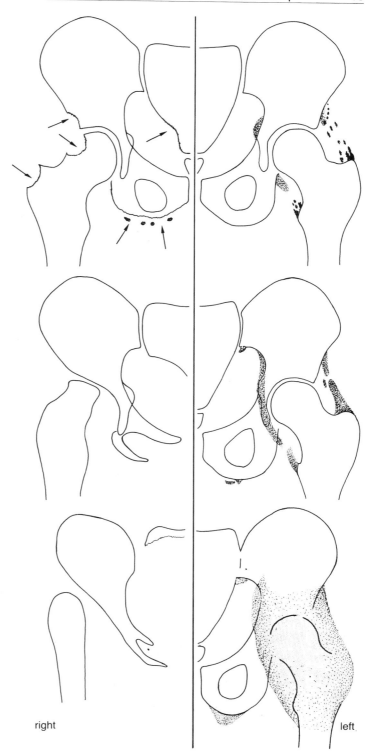

Fig. 57 **Sequelae of paraplegia. Excessive findings.** *Right half of pelvis:* Follow-up study of a neurogenic pelvic osteolysis over 10 years. *Arrows* point to the early stages of erosive lesions in the contours (about 3 years after the occurrence of traumatic paraplegia). Actually, both halves of the pelvis and the proximal ends of the femurs were involved.

Left half of pelvis: Bony encasement of the hip joint by paraplegic neurogenic paraosteoarthropathy developing in the course of 6 years. The cavities of the hip and sacroilicac joint undergo obliteration. In this case, also, ossification of soft tissues occurred bilaterally.

right

left

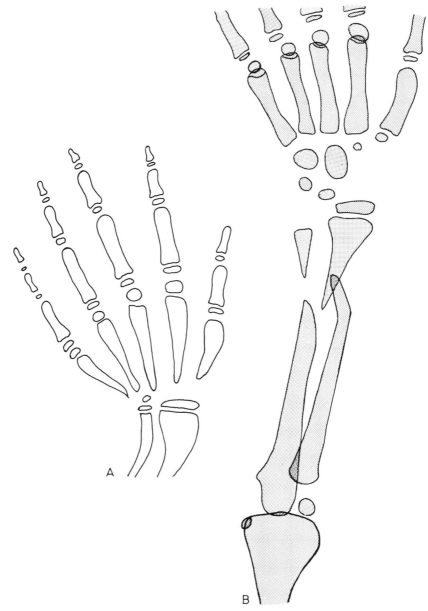

Fig. 58 **Principal radiographic aspect of a carpal (tarsal) osteolysis** (A). Clinical and roentgenologic *differential diagnosis* from B **(congenital pseudoarthrosis)** of both bones of the forearm—for example, in von Recklinghausen's neurofibromatosis, in fibrous dysplasia, or without any associated disease—and from juvenile rheumatoid arthritis (Fig. 102).

Note: Congenital pseudoarthrosis occurs principally in the tibia and fibula, less frequently in one bone of the forearm and—still less frequently—in both (Richin et al., 1976). About 50 percent of patients with congenital pseudoarthrosis present signs of von Recklinghausen's neurofibromatosis (Cleveland et al., 1978); for example, at least six café-au-lait spots with a diameter of at least 15 mm. In the region of the pseudoarthrosis, however, neurofibromatous tissue is absent (Brown et al., 1977).

They are sometimes associated with pain and edema[16] (Torg and Steel, 1968; Kohler et al., 1973; Tyler and Rosenbaum, 1976). During adolescence the condition is more or less arrested, but in adulthood, the residues become apparent by deformation and physical disability.

• *Progressive carpotarsal osteolysis (François syndrome)* is accompanied by corneal opacities and dermal xanthomas.

• *Idiopathic multicentric osteolysis with craniodysplasia and oligophrenia* (Mathias and Ludwig, 1977). Resorption of the carpal, tarsal, metacarpal, and metatarsal bones.

• *Winchester syndrome* (Winchester et al., 1969; Hollister et al., 1974) begins in childhood. Here, the polytopic osteolyses also affect the carpal and tarsal bones (Fig. 58). The resorbed bone and cartilage are replaced by fibrous connective tissue. The disorder is characterized by joint discomfort; erosions in the interphalangeal, metacarpal, and metatarsal joints; and sometimes also ankyloses of these joints. Progressive flexion contractures, dwarfism, and generalized osteoporosis may require roentgenologic differentiation from juvenile rheumatoid arthritis.

• The *Hadju-Cheney syndrome (hereditary arthrodento-osteodysplasia)* manifests itself by band-shaped resorption of acral bones (see Fig. 53, *right*), with osteolyses in the carpal bones, the distal end of the ulna, the head of the radius, the trochlea humeri, and the distal femur. Hypermobility of the interphalangeal joints, dental anomalies (dental aplasia, aplasia of the alveolar processes in the upper and lower jaw, partial resorption of teeth, hypoplasia of dental roots, premature loss of teeth), cranial malformations (aplasia of the frontal sinus, broad sutures, wormian bones, and bathmocephaly) also are associated with this syndrome.

• *Nonfamilial acro-osteolysis with cortical defects* (Gilula et al., 1976) leads to (band-shaped) acro-osteolyses of the phalanges, osteolysis of the ramus of the mandible, and flat, concave defects in the contours of the short and long tubular bones, the clavicle, and the scapula (see Fig. 264).

• Osteolyses of the terminal tufts of the fingers also occur in *Sézary's syndrome* (McCormick, 1977). This extremely rare disease is regarded as a malignant erythrodermal reticulosis with reticulocytemia.

• In *Osteopetrosis (Albers-Schönberg disease, marble bone disease)*, the terminal phalanges of the fingers and toes sometimes show deformations (Palmer and Thomas, 1958; Moss and Mainzer, 1970). The proximal parts of the distal phalanges assume the shape of triangular stumps. Distally to them, small bone shadows may be visible in the soft tissues. In pyknodysostosis, hypoplasia of (individual) distal phalanges has been described. Both hereditary diseases

present increased density of bone as a characteristic feature. In pyknodysostosis, the density is diffuse, whereas in osteopetrosis the degree and extent of increased density may be variable. The "bone in bone" picture is sometimes demonstrable in the hand (Fig. 59).

• A certain type of *familial acro-osteolysis* described by Lamy and Maroteaux (1961) is inherited in an autosomal dominant mode. It affects the phalanges, the metacarpals, and the metatarsals.

• *Progeria (Hutchinson-Gilford syndrome)* manifests itself by high-grade premature senility of the entire body *in childhood* (senile atrophic skin, loss of hair, arteriosclerosis, etc.). Acro-osteolyses in the terminal tufts of the fingers and in the clavicle have been observed (Ozonoff and Clemett, 1967).

• In *Rothmund's syndrome* (Maurer and Langford, 1967), acro-osteolyses in the hands and feet as well as soft-tissue calcifications are known to occur. Bilateral infantile cataract, atrophy, hyperpigmentation and depigmentation of the hair, premature graying of the hair, early baldness, and genital infantilism form part of the polymorphic syndrome, which becomes apparent in early childhood.

• In the *van Bogaert-Hozay syndrome,* a complex hereditary mesodermal and ectodermal dysplasia, acral disorders of circulation with absence of peripheral pulses and acrocyanosis are known to occur, as well as acro-osteolyses. Additional differential characteristics are anomalous shape of the face and intellectual impairment.

• *Apert's syndrome* belongs to the acrocephalosyndactylies (see Fig. 146). It shows not only progressive fusion of the phalangeal, metacarpal, carpal, metatarsal, and tarsal joints but also to "pointing" of the distal phalanges. In other cases, synostoses or pseudoarthroses of the *contiguous* distal phalanges are apt to develop.

• The *pincer-nail syndrome* is a painful dystrophy of the nails of the hands and feet (Cornelius III and Shelley, 1968) in which acro-osteolysis of the terminal tufts may occur.

Dactylolysis spontanea (Ainhum) is a tropical disease that affects the dark-skinned races. In the majority of patients, the noninflammatory disease picture (Cole, 1965) is accompanied by pain, which can be intensified by local infection and pathologic fracture. A deep, circular constriction at the base of the fifth toe (sometimes also another toe) gradually leads to spontaneous amputation (Fig. 60).

Nonreactive acro-osteolyses are also apt to occur during the course of Pick-Herzheime's *acrodermatitis chronica atrophicans* (Raschke, 1958).

Epidermolysis bullosa (Brinn and Khilnani, 1967), leads to distal osteolyses in the fingers, flexion contractures of the finger joints (claw hand), atrophy of soft tissues, and acquired webbing of the fingers. Calcinoses are observed in the fingertips.

In *pachydermoperiostosis* (see Fig. 159), resorption of the distal phalanges has been observed in

---

[16] The possible painful "arthritic" episodes at the onset and during the course of certain carpal (tarsal) osteolyses should not be confused with juvenile rheumatoid arthritis in which dissolution of carpal (tarsal) bones can also occur (see Fig. 102).

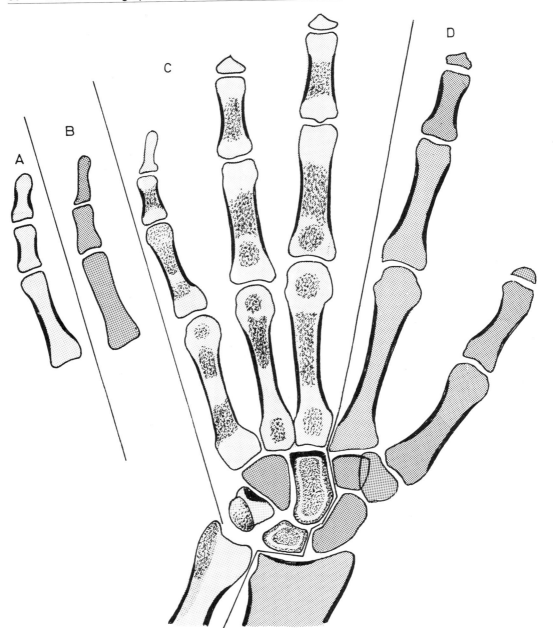

Fig. 59 **Roentgen findings in the hand in osteopetrosis (Albers-Schönberg disease, marble bone disease)** (B, C) and in **pyknodysostosis** (D).

A = Normal finger (the *shading* depicts the normal density of bone). B = Osteopetrosis tarda ("adult type," "late manifestation type") with *uniform* density of phalanges (marrow cavities are obliterated). C = Osteopetrosis tarda with *variable* bone density, "bone in bone" characteristic (note especially the capitate and the lunate). The distal phalanges III and IV in this case impress one as "triangular stumps." D = pyknodysostosis with increased density and stumpy terminal phalanges (no "bone in bone" appearance).

Note: The "bone in bone" appearance occurs in osteopetrosis, cleidocranial dysplasia, Gaucher's disease, chronic osteomyelitis, and hemoglobinopathies with sickle cell formation.

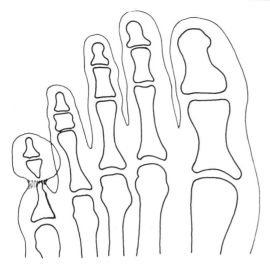

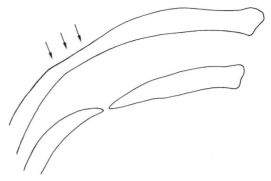

Fig. 61 **Lesions in the upper border of the rib in progressive scleroderma** *(arrows)*. Advanced involvement of ribs in progressive scleroderma (below). For the differential diagnosis see Figure 247.

Fig. 60 **Radiographic appearance of the Ainhum syndrome in the fifth toe** (see text).

association with multiple other roentgen findings (Krosch, 1955; Guyer et al., 1978).

Vinyl chloride disease (Wilson, et al., 1967; Dodson et al., 1971, Stein et al., 1973; and other writers) is an occupational acro-osteolysis. It occurs in workers charged with the cleaning of autoclaves for the polymerization of polyvinyl chloride. Clinically, the disorder manifests itself by Raynaud-like complaints in the fingers, less frequently in the toes. The fingers appear shortened and present a bulbous enlargement. The roentgenogram shows a more or less broad, band-shaped osteolysis between the terminal tuft and the diaphysis of the distal phalanx (Fig. 53, *right*). Less frequently, the terminal tuft is completely resorbed. After the worker has changed his job, the osteolyses of the phalanx are capable of partial or complete regression, sometimes with deformation (shortening) of the phalanx. A number of observations suggest that vinyl chloride intoxication leads to a systemic affection of the skeleton which—similarly to systemic endocrine and medullary osteopathies (Dihlmann, 1978)—manifests itself particularly at sites exposed to increased physiologic compressive and tensile stress. In this way it would also be possible to explain the defects in tendinous insertions and the so-called pseudodilatation of the sacroiliac joints observed in vinyl chloride disease.

Nonreactive (acro-) osteolyses occur in the late stage of *congenital porphyria,* a progressive photodermatosis, in Raynaud's syndrome, in *obliterating vascular diseases,* and in *progressive scleroderma.* In the latter disease, these lesions are encountered primarily in the phalanges, the distal end of radius and ulna (see Fig. 113), the ribs (Figs. 61 and 247), the acromion (Fig. 248) and, very infrequently, also in the cervical spine (concentric slimming of the vertebral arches, narrowing of the intervertebral disk

space, vertebral subluxation, calcification of soft tissues; Haverbusch et al., 1974).

Idiopathic as well as secondary *hyperparathyroidism* and *osteomalacia* (due to dietary or other vitamin D deficiency; for example, in renal osteopathy) can produce therapeutically reversible osteolyses of the terminal tufts of the fingers, band-shaped (transverse) osteolyses of the distal phalanges (in osteomalacia), resorption of bone in the upper border of the ribs (in hyperparathyroidism and in renal osteopathy), and osteolyses in the region of the acromioclavicular joints. Greenfield (1969) interprets the band-shaped osteolyses of the distal phalanges in osteomalacia or renal osteopathy as Looser's zones. In primary as well as secondary hyperparathyroidism, in which the roentgenogram shows pronounced resorptive processes in the terminal tufts of the fingers, subperiosteal resorption of bone (at least) on the radial aspects of the middle phalanges is, as a rule, also demonstrable (Johnson et al., 1967). This facilitates the differential classification.

Finally, mention will be made of *(acro-) osteolyses* following *frostbite* and *heat-induced damage, electrical accidents,* and *chronic occupational damage from ionizing rays.* Heat-induced damage can, infrequently, manifest itself by by nonreactive osteolyses of the phalanges without a heat injury to the bone (necrotic demarcation or local inflammatory bone lesions) being demonstrable in the roentgenogram (Rabinov 1961, Šváb 1976). However, it is more usual for nonreactive osteolysis following an electrical injury to be manifested by resorption of previously demarcated necrotic parts of bone. Major parts of devitalized bone are sometimes sequestrated through open soft-tissue necroses, or small limbs may even be cast off spontaneously. It is a remarkable fact that electrical injuries are seldom followed by infection of bone. This kind of trauma apparently provides no favorable medium for bacteria (Kolář and Vrabec, 1976).

Radiogenic acro-osteolyses can, as a rule, be distinguished roentgenographically from bone destructions due to a spreading infection and from radiation-induced malignancies. Radiogenic acro-osteolyses present the typical picture of nonreactive "sharpening" of the distal phalanx. A bacterial infection, which extends from a chronic radiation dermatitis to the bone, not only produces destruction but it also gives rise to reactive changes; for example, sequestrations. Radiogenic malignancies can originate in the bone, or they can arise in a chronic radiation dermatitis as a squamous cell carcinoma, invading the bone extensively, and destroying it erratically without producing a reaction.

Posttraumatic osteolysis occurs primarily in the acromial end of the clavicle, the distal radius, the distal end of the ulna (the styloid process), and the proximal humerus. However, a distinction should be made, also radiographically, between nonreactive posttraumatic osteolyses and the sequelae of traumatic disorders of circulation; for example in the hip, shoulder, and knee joints. **Ischemia of part of a bone,** gives rise, in principle, to three reactions : (1) fracture, (2) resorption (osteolysis), and (3) insidious

reossification (increased density) of the necrotic area. The coexistence and succession as well as the prevalence of one or the other of these biologic processes can lead to roentgen findings such as are reproduced in Figure 62.

The differential diagnosis of a posttraumatic osteolysis in the acromial end of the clavicle—e.g., one following a major injury or chronic occupational microtraumas (air drill damage; Ehricht, 1959)—must first consider a metastatic malignancy and a primary malignant bone tumor (particularly Ewing's sarcoma), as well as primary and secondary hyperparathyroidism. Especially with these diseases, osteolysis in the clavicle may be the first morbid manifestation noticed by the patient.

In athletes (handball players; Seymour, 1977), an osteolysis in the acromial end of the clavicle infrequently develops, probably as the result of excessive strain and repetitive microtraumas. Such an osteolysis usually becomes reconstructed over months or years. The case of acro-osteolysis in the finger of a

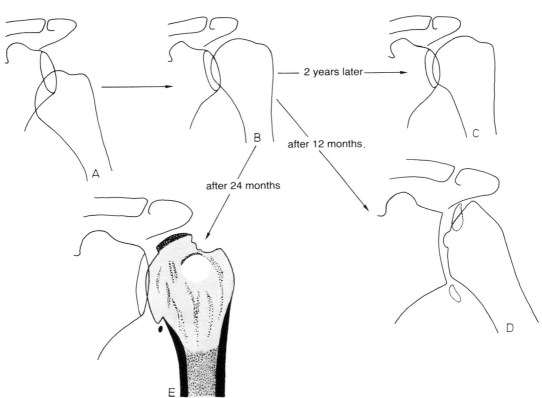

Fig. 62 **Follow-up study in traumatic anterior dislocation of the shoulder joint** (A = roentgenogram taken immediately after the accident and B = after resetting).
C = No posttraumatic sequelae demonstrable
D = *Advanced posttraumatic osteolysis of the proximal end of the humerus* has developed within a year (Neurologic diseases have been ruled out clinically; the patient does not have diabetes mellitus).
E = *Posttraumatic necrosis of the head and humerus* with resorption, fragmentation, insidious reossification and fibrillar osteoporosis (of disuse). The findings sketched in E (posttraumatic necrosis of the humeral head) also occur after subcapital fractures of the humerus and fractures of the humeral head. (The complaints usually start 1 or 2 years after the trauma; Fourrier and Martini, 1977).

Fig. 63 **Massive osteolysis (Gorham and Stout, 1955)** radiographic diagnosis begins in flat bones with *nondescript* "holes" (= numerous translucent intramedullary foci without marginal reaction) before it manifests its later tendency to massive osteolysis. In the present case the tendency to osteolysis first becomes apparent by thinning of the supra-acetabular portion of the ilium and the ischium *(arrows).*

Note: In addition, the wasting of cortical bone in the osteolytic area *(arrows; the normal cortex has been set off for didactic reasons).*

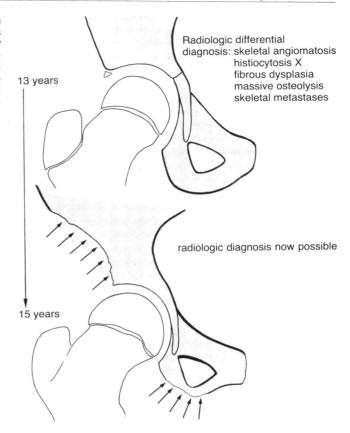

13 years

Radiologic differential diagnosis: skeletal angiomatosis
histiocytosis X
fibrous dysplasia
massive osteolysis
skeletal metastases

radiologic diagnosis now possible

15 years

violinist reported by Stecken (1954) can probably also be traced to excessive occupational strain.

The following conditions enter into the differential diagnosis of *posttraumatic* osteolysis in the pelvis (which commonly is precipitated by the pressure of a large subperiosteal and intraosseous hematoma): hemophilic pseudotumor, osteolysis from a large (posttraumatic) aneurysm of the pelvic arteries (Marx et al., 1962), massive osteolysis (Gorham and Stout, 1955), and malignant tumor.

In the majority of cases, **massive osteolysis (Gorham and Stout, 1955)** affects children and young adults. By skipping joints, intervertebral disks, and soft tissues it can attack several bones. The osteolytic process often sets in insidiously and causes little pain, unless it is complicated by pathologic fractures. Early roentgen findings in this disease have therefore seldom been reported (Torg and Steel, 1969; Heyden et al., 1977; Fig. 63). Massive osteolysis usually is spontaneously arrested; it "burns out." Complications, however, can lead to death, particularly when involvement of the ribs or vertebrae is followed by thoracic empyema or paraplegia. A characteristic roentgen finding in massive osteolysis is "pointing" of the small and *large* tubular bones involved, and of flat bones (Fig. 265). Histologic study reveals hemangiomatosis (less frequently lymphangiomatosis) and fibrosis instead of bone tissue. It is quite con-

ceivable, however, that vascular proliferation and fibrosis are not the primary cause of the disease but constitute an attempt on the part of the body to repair the morbid condition (Edeiken and Hodes, 1973). This supposition is justified because skeletal hemangiomas and diffuse skeletal hemangiomatosis (see Fig. 25 B, C, and D) produce a circumscribed destruction of the involved bone but do not dissolve it completely.

Pseudo-Charcot's Joint (Corticosteroid Arthropathy)

Adverse skeletal side effects of corticosteroid therapy depend on the duration of treatment, the dosage, and the mode of administration. Such undesirable sequelae of corticosteroid therapy include partial or total avascular necrosis of joint-bearing bones. Although such necroses do occur, even without this medication, in association with various diseases that at present are treated with steroids, the corticosteroid etiology of such osteonecroses cannot be doubted when they develop in patients whose diseases are not usually accompanied by necrosis of bones; e.g., bronchial asthma (Bouillet and Vermeulen, 1963), pemphigus and other skin diseases (Bloch-Michel et al., 1959; Heimann and Freiberger, 1960; Jansen, 1967; Canigiani and Pusch, 1969) and blood diseases (Uehlinger, 1964; Klümper, et al. 1967). Avascular osteonecroses following kidney transplantation (Aichroth et al., 1971; Murray 1976) should also be mentioned in this connection.

In some cases, however, the pathologic findings in bones and joints encountered during and following corticosteroid therapy, go beyond the usual picture of avascular epiphyseal osteonecrosis. The entire joint then displays disintegration involving the bones, the articular cartilage, and the soft tissues: a so-called *pseudo-Charcot's joint* develops (Chandler et al., 1959; Murray, 1961, 1976). On the one hand, this term designates disintegration of the joint; on the other, it emphasizes that in the light of present knowledge it is not the nervous system but the steroid administered that plays a causative role. The current ideas about the pathogenesis of the pseudo-Charcot's joint are as follows:

Corticosteroids are employed for their anti-inflammatory effect in the treatment of inflammatory rheumatic arthropathies and activated osteoarthrosis, particularly of larger joints. When the treatment is effective, the local complaints subside. In spite of this, the morbid process remains in a smoldering stage or may even become aggravated by the catabolic effect of the steroids; for example, in osteoarthrosis.

As pain is reduced or eliminated and function of the involved joint improves, increased use, in conjunction with the above-mentioned favoring of avascular epiphyseal osteonecrosis, can lead to overloading of the gliding tissue. In individual cases, especially in joints exposed to static load, overloading is followed by extensive disintegration (Fig. 64).

Amyloid osteoarthropathy develops as the result of the deposition of amyloid in the gliding tissue and the joint-bearing supporting tissue. Amyloid is a pathologic, fibril-forming protein produced by mesenchymal cells. Its deposition takes place at the site of origin in an intercellular pattern, either generalized—perireticular and pericollagenous—or localized (Missmahl, 1967). Amyloidosis may be *primary* (without preceding or attendant disease) or *secondary,* as accompaniment of chronic diseases; e.g., inflammations and tumors. Other forms of the disorder include *tumorous* amyloidosis—solitary or multiple massive deposits of amyloid, commonly in a single organ; *amyloidosis accompanying the paraproteinemias* (multiple myeloma, Waldenstöm's macroglobulinemia); *senile amyloidosis* occuring as the result of aging processes, and *hereditary amyloidosis* (Koletsky and Stecher, 1939; Goldberg et al., 1969; Hannon et al., 1975). Amyloid osteoarthropathy oc-

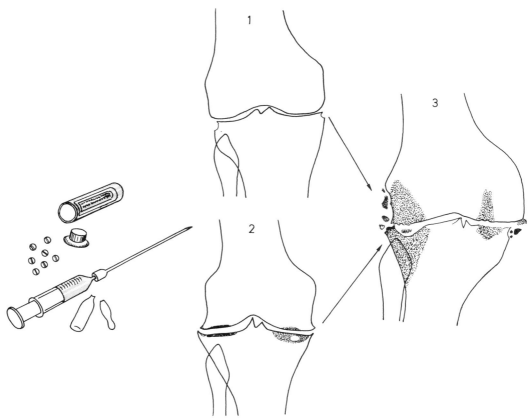

Fig. 64 **Corticosteroid therapy** of chronic rheumatoid arthritis (1) or activated osteoarthrosis (2) (compare Fig. 418) may lead to the development of **pseudo-Charcot's joint** (3); (see text) 3 to 18 months after 1 or 2.

curs in primary amyloidosis and in paraproteinemic amyloidosis (Wiernik, 1972).

Clinically, deposition of amyloid in the synovial membrane, the fibrous joint capsule, the joint cavity, and the periarticular soft tissues manifests itself by a mostly bilateral painful or painless swelling, a sensation of stiffness, and limitation of motion in small and large joints. The condition, therefore, must be differentiated from rheumatoid arthritis, particularly since subcutaneous amyloid deposits can be misdiagnosed as rheumatoid nodules, and amyloid deposits also may give rise to the carpal tunnel syndrome.

Deposition of amyloid in the subchondral marrow cavity causes cystic osteolyses and sometimes even pathologic fractures; e.g., of the femoral neck (Koletsky and Stecher, 1939; Kavanaugh, 1978) or the odontoid process of the axis (Hannon et al., 1975).

The following roentgen findings should arouse the suspicion of amyloid osteoarthropathy: Cystic osteolyses in the subchondral layer with or without marginal sclerosis (sites of predilection: head of the humerus, head and neck of the femur); erosions in the region of the capsular insertion; absent narrowing of the radiographic joint space; swelling and increased density of the surrounding soft tissues (Fig. 65).

Hemochromatosis is defined as deposition of excess iron in body tissues associated with identifiable damage to organs. *Hemosiderosis* likewise is a deposition of excess iron, but not associated with damage to organs. Idiopathic (primary) hemochromatosis is an innate (genetically determined) disorder of metabolism. Depositions of iron occur primarily in the liver, the pancreas, the myocardium and the glands of internal secretion. The resulting clinical picture includes: Grayish-brown skin pigmentation, hepatic fibrosis, hepatic cirrhosis, diabetes mellitus

("bronze diabetes"), hypogonadism (sterility, sexual impotence), and heart failure. Secondary (acquired) hemochromatosis can develop as a result of excessive iron intake (iron medication prolonged for years, numerous blood transfusions) and during the course of hepatic cirrhosis and porphyria cutanea tarda.

Kashin-Beck disease (see p. 114) is *probably* the consequence of iron overload from drinking water (Twersky, 1975); it occurs endemically in Eastern Siberia, Northern China, and North Korea. About 50 percent of patients with (idiopathic) hemochromatosis complain of joint discomfort (Dymock et al., 1970; de Sèze et al., 1972). The joint complaints *either* follow the clinical findings of hemochromatosis, *or* they occur concomitantly, *or* they even antedate the clinical findings listed above.

The spectrum of hematochromatosis-dependent osteoarthropathy ranges from polyarticular pain to positive roentgen findings. The latter are, in principle, an association of osteoarthrosis and chondrocalcinosis (p. 62 ff). The osteoarthrosis here has a predilection for the hand (Fig. 91). The second and third metacarpophalangeal joints are affected most frequently and most early by hematochromatosis-dependent osteoarthropathy though, of course, any other joint may be involved (Dymock et al., 1970; de Sèze et al., 1972; Sella et al., 1973; Twersky, 1975; Hirsch et al., 1976). Surgical exploration of metacarpophalangeal joints has confirmed the degenerative lesions of the articular cartilage identified by radiography in hemochromatosis-dependent osteoarthropathy (Laborde et al., 1977). Early radiographic studies in hemochromatosis-dependent osteoarthropathies show that initially cysts measuring between 1 and 6 mm in diameter are apt to occur in the subchondral layer of the (small) joints involved, as well as marginal erosions as the result of infractions of the delicate cyst

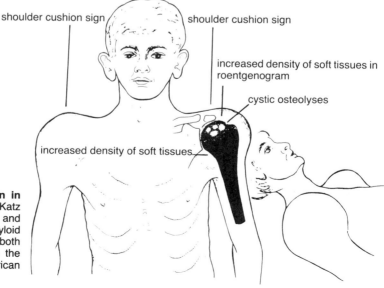

shoulder cushion sign   shoulder cushion sign

increased density of soft tissues in roentgenogram

cystic osteolyses

increased density of soft tissues

Fig. 65 Shoulder pad sign in amyloid osteoarthropathy (Katz et al., 1973). The articular and periarticular deposition of amyloid leads to massive bulging of both shoulder regions (similar to the shoulder pads used by American football players).

wall. In addition, the marginal subchondral lamella is resorbed and the subchondral spongiosa then is "opened" and appears to be "nibbled" (Dymock et al., 1970; Figs. 148 and 268). These findings reveal that the radiographic aspect of *early* hemochromatosis-dependent osteoarthropathy differs but little from that of ordinary osteoarthrosis. During the further evolution, however, the osteoarthrotic character dominates the radiographic picture, also.

Chondrocalcinosis manifests itself in the menisci, the articular disks, and the hyaline articular cartilage. Therefore, the finding of a strikingly pronounced osteoarthritis of the second and third metacarpophalangeal joints—test joints!—*and* the concomitant evidence of chondrocalcinosis in the distal articular disk and/or in the metacarpophalangeal articular cartilage should always raise the suspicion of hemochromatosis—whether or not this underlying disease has already been diagnosed. Finally, a generalized skeletal osteoporosis without predilection for the juxtaarticular parts of bone occurs in hemochromatosis.

Hereditary *hepatolenticular degeneration (Wilson's disease)* is also accompanied by osteoarthropathy. Wilson's disease is the result of chronic copper intoxication of the organism, which is caused by an enzyme deficiency. This deficiency leads to considerable accumulation of copper which produces serious damage to the internal organs, in the first place the liver, the brain, the kidneys and—to a lesser extent—the myocardium. Of diagnostic importance is the golden-brown or green-brown Kayser-Fleischer ring at the periphery of the cornea. In **osteoarthropathy related to Wilson's disease,** the following roentgen findings are to be expected:

1. Clues to damage of the articular cartilage as early as the third or fourth decade—hence premature osteoarthrosis.
2. Subchondral fragmentation of bone, similar to osteochondrosis dissecans, or osseous metaplasia of articular soft tissues.
3. Chondrocalcinosis.
4. Generalized skeletal osteoporosis. The characteristic roentgen signs of rickets or osteomalacia are often present. They can be interpreted as consequences of toxic damage to the renal tubules, which is liable to develop in Wilson's disease (see footnote on p. 25).

Articular and Periarticular Calcifications and Ossifications of Soft Tissues

Radiographically visible calcium shadows in the soft tissues and in the surroundings of a joint give grounds for the following considerations and questions:

1. Is one dealing with an osseous body or a calcium deposit? Calcium shadows have no regular structures, whereas ossifications present delicate trabecular markings and a thin cortex. This possibility of differentiation, however, depends upon the size of the calcification or ossification. The smaller such a radiographic shadow is, the more difficult it will be to discriminate between the two alternatives.
2. Is it an intraarticular or an extraarticular calcification or ossification? Which parts of the gliding tissue are calcified or ossified? The answer to these questions depends on accurate anatomic information, on roentgenograms taken in two or more planes, on tomographs and, if necessary, fluoroscopic spot films.
3. Is a juxtaarticular bone shadow in fact a pathologic formation or does it reflect physiologic structures or variants; for example, a sesamoid bone or a so-called supernumerary ossicle?

Calcifications of the Hyaline Articular Cartilage and the Fibrocartilaginous Menisci and Disks

In calcified menisci, calcium pyrophosphate dihydrate, dicalcium phosphate dihydrate, and hydroxyl apatite have been demonstrated (McCarty Jr. et al., 1966). Of nosological importance is the deposition of calcium pyrophosphate, which indicates a metabolic disorder that, according to its localization, has been termed **articular chondrocalcinosis** (Žitňan and Sitaj, 1963) often also pyrophosphate arthropathy and, after its clinical picture, **pseudogout** (McCarty Jr. et al., 1962). The calcium deposits are encountered not only in fibrocartilage (menisci, articular disks, annulus fibrosus of the intervertebral disks, the acetabular and glenoidal lip) but also in the hyaline articular cartilage and, less frequently, in the synovial membrane, the fibrous joint capsule, and the ligaments and tendons. The test joint for chondrocalcinosis is the knee joint (Fig. 66) because it is there that the deposition of calcium pyrophosphate most frequently takes place in the menisci, the hyaline articular cartilage and the periarticular soft tissues. In principle, however, the deposits of calcium prophosphate can be encountered in any joint (often in bilateral symmetrical fashion), among them the symphysis pubis; the distal radioulnar disk; the hyaline cartilage of the shoulder, hip, elbow and talocrural joint; and the carpal and the metacarpophalangeal joints. The deposition of calcium pyrophosphate is, in general, irreversible. In individual cases, however, partial or complete regression of meniscus calcifications has been observed (Luska et al., 1974). The calcium pyrophosphate is located in the intermediate layers of the articular cartilage and therefore contrasts with the marginal subchondral lamella. In the roentgenogram it appears as a delicate linear or dotted shadow (Fig. 66) running parallel to the sur-

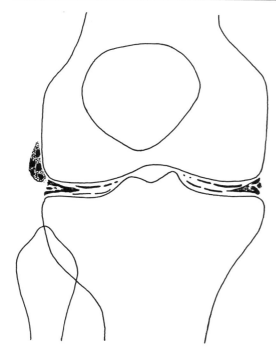

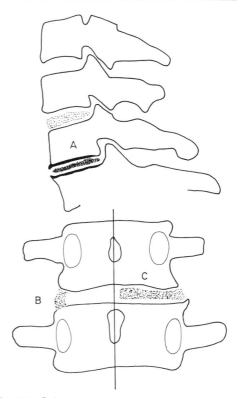

Fig. 66 **Principal radiographic appearance of articular chondrocalcinosis** (in the knee joint) with calcium pyrophosphate impregnation of the menisci, the hyaline cartilage, and (less frequently) the periarticular soft tissues. The knee is the test joint of chondrocalcinosis (see p. 41).

Note: There are two formal pathophysiologic prerequisites for the development of chondrocalcinosis: (1) the extra-cellular appearance of pyrophosphate, and (2) its crystalline deposition as a calcium salt (Mohr et al., 1981).

Fig. 67 **Spinal chondrocalcinosis** (compare Fig. 677).

A = Incipient and advanced calcification in two cervical disks. In the lower segment with heavier disk calcification there are roentgen signs of disk degeneration (osteochondrosis).

B = Early roentgen signs of lumbar chondrocalcinosis in the annulus fibrosus.

C = Advanced chondrocalcinosis of disks.

face of the bone. In fibrocartilaginous structures, the deposits of pyrophosphate produce a striated granular and/or coarse lumpy pattern (Figs. 66 and 67).

Chondrocalcinosis occurs as a *heredofamilial, sporadic,* or *symptomatic (secondary, associated)* disorder. Hereditary chondrocalcinosis mostly becomes manifest as early as the third or fourth decade of life. The course of secondary chondrocalcinosis is more frequently asymptomatic than the hereditary type *(vide infra)* and often manifests itself as late as the sixth or seventh decade. Symptomatic chondrocalcinosis has been described as an associated finding in various, mostly endocrine or metabolic, diseases, such as hyperparathyroidism—sometimes aggravation or initial occurrence following parathyroidectomy (Bilezikian et al., 1973; Glass and Grahame, 1976), hemochromatosis, (renal) hypomagnesemia, Wilson's disease, hypophosphatasia, hypothyroidism, diabetes mellitus or glucose intolerance, acromegaly, ochronosis (deposition of calcium pyrophosphate in the periarticular soft tissues and menisci but absent calcification of the articular cartilage in the roentgen-

ogram, Reginato et al., 1973), gout or hyperuricemia, Paget's disease of bone, vitamin D intoxication, and as an aftermath of infantile osteomyelitis. *Coincidental* association with chondrocalcinosis cannot be ruled out in all the above disorders collected from the literature. Still it is an established fact that (symptomatic) chondrocalcinosis can occur during the course of manifold endocrine and metabolic disorders and can even be an indirect sign of their presence. Therefore when chondrocalcinosis is demonstrated in the roentgenogram, some writers have recommended with good reason that serum levels of calcium and alkaline phosphatase, as well as blood levels of glucose, uric acid, iron, and copper, be determined and that renal and thyroid functions be studied.

Chondrocalcinosis presents different *clinical* pictures: it may be asymptomatic (clinically latent) or it may manifest itself by *joint pains* (without effusion and without clinical signs of inflammation). In other cases an acute *attack of arthritis*—pseudo-

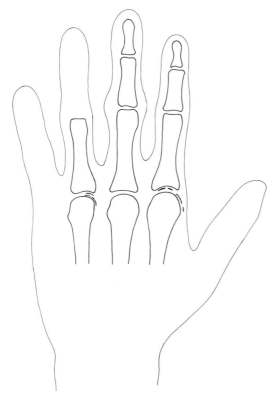

Fig. 68 So-called distant type of chondrocalcinosis. The patient is taken ill with an acute arthritis of the proximal interphalangeal joint III (painful fusiform expansion, erythema). The roentgenogram shows *asymptomatic* chondrocalcinosis of the metacarpophalangeal joints III and IV, raising suspicion of crystal-induced pyrophosphate synovitis (chondrocalcinosis, pseudogout) of the interphalangeal joint (see text). The suspicion was corroborated by study of the joint aspirate under a polarizing miscroscope (see text).

Note: Concentrations of pyrophosphate crystals that are not yet demonstrable in the roentgenogram may trigger an inflammatory synovial reaction!

neighboring joints (the metacarpophalangeal joints, for instance) show typical radiographic signs of chondrocalcinosis (Fig. 68). Such a suspicion is corroborated by the microscopic demonstration of pyrophosphate in the aspirated effusion.

Phagocytized calcium pyrophosphate crystals do not project from the leukocytes. There are triclinic (slab-shaped) crystals and monoclinic (needle- and rod-shaped) dimorphic forms. Under polarized light they are weakly positively birefringent. In contrast, the urate crystals of gout project from the phagocytizing leukocytes. These monoclinic crystals are strongly negatively birefringent. They appear *yellow* when the long axis of the crystal *parallels* the compensator axis, and they appear *blue* when they are directed *vertically* to the compensator axis of the polarizing microscope (Phelps et al., 1968; Schilling, 1971). With calcium pyrophosphate crystals it is exactly the opposite so far as colors are concerned.

On the one hand, chondrocalcinosis leads gradually to osteoarthrosis. *On the other hand*, one occasionally sees that chondrocalcinosis supervenes during the course of osteoarthrosis. For example, meniscus calcifications sometimes develop in osteoarthrosis of the knee. These meniscus calcifications probably signal a *local* (attritional) damage. In contrast, chondrocalcinosis as a systemic disease manifests itself at least by calcifications of the fibrocartilage *and* the hyaline articular cartilage.

The peculiar features of chondrocalcinosis in the hand (Bensasson et al., 1975) can be described as follows:

About half the chondrocalcinosis patients present calcification of the distal radioulnar disk. Calcifications of the cartilage in the triquetroulnar joint are somewhat less frequent, and about one fifth of the patients show calcifications in the metacarpophalangeal joints. The frequency of isolated osteoarthrosis of the scaphoidotrapezium joint (hence without involvement of the carpometacarpal joint of the thumb) is higher in patients with chondrocalcinosis than among the "normal population." Unless a calcified distal radioulnar disk already indicates the presence of chondrocalcinosis, isolated osteoarthrosis of the scaphoidotrapezium joint should therefore prompt a search for this disorder (radiologic study of the knee joints and the pelvis) and its clinical implications!

It is rare for chondrocalcinosis to produce a *destructive osteoarthropathy* in the involved joints; this is reminiscent of a neurogenic arthropathy (Charcot's joint). Evidently in these cases an osteonecrotic process is added to the attrition of the articular cartilage and its sequelae in the juxtaarticular bone, particularly in the knee, the shoulder, and the hip (Menkes et al., 1973; Villiaumey, et al., 1974; Richards and Hamilton, 1974; and other writers). Disintegration of the joint or the spinal segment then develops (with fragmentation, resorption, and malposition; see Fig. 69), without the presence of neurologic deficits in these patients. It should be mentioned, however, that chondrocalcinosis has been seen in tabetic osteoarthropathies—hence "genuine" neurogenic arthropathies with neurologic deficits (Jacobelli et al., 1973). This observation underscores that a great variety of

gout!—heralds the chondrocalcinosis.[17] Such an acute arthritis can regress completely and recur after an asymptomatic interval. On the other hand, a new attack can occur before the complaints have completely subsided. Apart from these manifestations, chondrocalcinosis sometimes presents the picture of a *chronic arthropathy* (pain, swelling, chronic effusion, hemarthrosis). Its chronic course may be interrupted by acute episodes, or it may continue smoldering without any exacerbations. Finally, there are acute or subacute types of arthritis—e.g., in an interphalangeal joint—that *roentgenologically* present no pathologic calcifications whatsoever. Despite this, such cases arouse the suspicion of pseudogout when

---

[17] An attack of pseudogout in the symphysis pubis may be the initial clinical manifestation of chondrocalcinosis (Djian et al., 1978).

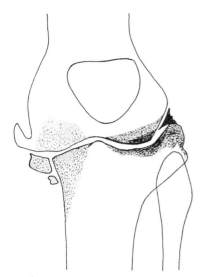

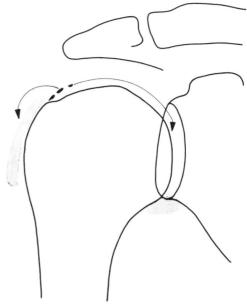

Fig. 69 **Destructive osteoarthropathy** of the left knee **similar to Charcot's joint** in *chondrocalcinosis* (see text) with anarchic remodeling of the joint (compare Fig. 54). In contrast to "genuine" Charcot's joint (see under this heading), the patient has *no neurologic deficits* and complains of *considerable pain.* Other joints present typical calcifications of the hyaline articular cartilage. There are calcifications in the menisci and the disks. In the left knee joint illustrated, the only indication of chondrocalcinosis is the calcification of the partially disinserted lateral meniscus.

Note: The further advanced the osteoarthrosis or the destructive osteoarthropathy in a joint affected by chondrocalcinosis, the less typical is the roentgeno-graphic aspect of chondrocalcinosis (as the result of extensive destruction of the fibrocartilaginous internal structures).

Fig. 70 **Perforation and evacuation of a calcium deposit of the rotator cuff into the subdeltoid bursa and into the cavity of the shoulder joint.** Only rem-nants of calcium are visible in the tendinous covering. The liquefied calcium, much like a contrast medium, has formed a cast of the bursa so that it has become demonstrable. The calcium mass invading the shoul-der joint has accumulated in the axillar recess. Clini-cally, a hyperacute, extremely painful inflammatory re-action of the synovial membrane has developed in both structures *(crystal-induced synovitis).*

Note: The subdeltoid bursa is sometimes also the "waste trap" in neurogenic osteoarthropathies of the shoulder joint (see Fig. 262).

factors is capable of interfering with the metabolism of the hyaline and fibrocartilage and thus can give rise to the development of chondrocalcinosis.

The observations in gout and pseudogout have led to a pathogenetic concept that has become known as *crystal-induced synovitis (crystal synovitis):* the presence of crystals in a cavity lined by a synovial membrane (hence in a joint, a bursa, or a tendon sheath) triggers an acute synovitis; for example, an attack of gout or pseudogout. The cause of such an acute, extremely painful arthritis may be iatrogenic, for instance the result of *intraarticular* injection of a crystalline corticosteroid (not to be misdiagnosed as inoculation of a pyogenic infection of the joint!). So-called periarthritis of the shoulder, also, *may* be the manifestation of an acute crystal-induced synovitis. This will be the case when the pasty calcium deposits leave the rotator cuff and perforate the immediately contiguous subdeltoid bursa (Fig. 70), giving rise to an acute, extremely painful bursitis (bursal synovi-

tis). On the other hand, the calcium deposits (hy-droxyl apatite, Swannell et al., 1970) may be dis-charged into the cavity of the shoulder joint and may precipitate an acute arthritis. In addition to urate- and pyrophosphate-induced arthritis, Dieppe et al. (1977) and Schumacher et al. (1977) have described hy-droxyl-apatite-induced arthritis as another pathophy-siologic type of crystal-induced synovitis. These writers encountered hydroxyl apatite crystals in the joint capsules of patients with acute arthritis of un-determined origin and during acute episodes of estab-lished osteoarthrosis (gout and pseudogout being ruled out). They also produced acute arthritis in an animal experiment by intraarticular injection of this crystal-line calcium phosphate compound. Finally, Štěpán and his colleagues (1976) observed crystal-induced synovitis in cystinosis, and Hug and Mihatsch (1975) described cases of aseptic arthritis in familial oxal-osis.

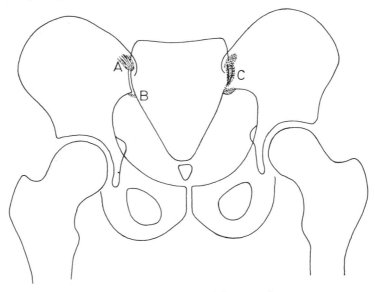

Fig. 71 Reparative ossification of the anterior sacroiliac joint capsule.
A = The site of predilection is the upper reflection of the joint capsule from its anterior to its posterior aspect. Why "site of predilection"? Because the axis for the slight physiologic tilting of the sacroiliac joint passes between 5 and 10 cm below the promontory of the sacrum. The greatest excursions are therefore to be expected in the upper region of the sacroiliac joint, and the joint capsule with its reinforcing ligaments there is exposed to the greatest strain. These strains lead, particularly in this location, to tears and avulsions which subsequently undergo reparative ossification.
   B = Reparative ossification of the capsule, projected into the soft tissues in the form of a hook.
   C = (Reparative) ossification of the *entire* sacroiliac joint capsule, which may reach a thickness of 1 cm, sometimes leads to partial or complete "obliteration" of the radiographic joint space. In the tomograph, however, a joint space is demonstrable behind the ossified joint capsule. Marked capsular ossifications also occur in diffuse idiopathic skeletal hyperstosis (see p. 458 ff).

Calcifications and Ossifications of the Synovial Membrane and the Fibrous Joint Capsule

In osteoarthrosis, the joint capsule can, starting from its insertion, become ossified in continuous or discontinuous fashion. In the plain roentgenogram, such bone plates can be identified primarily in lateral views. Capsular ossifications in osteoarthrosis occur preferentially in the hip joint and in the apophyseal joints of the spine. The sacroiliac joints, also, are a frequent site of capsular ossifications which develop during the course of repair processes after abnormal strain upon the capsuloligamentous apparatus and following injuries (Fig. 71). In addition, capsular ossifications are encountered with particular frequency in patients suffering from diffuse idiopathic skeletal hyperstosis; for example of the hip joint. This disorder is the expression of an *osteoplastic diathesis* of the body (Dihlmann, 1967) that manifests itself by ossifying processes in tight fibrous structures (ligaments, tendons, aponeuroses, joint capsules, etc.) and their insertions. *Circumscribed* cartilaginous meta-plasias are apt to develop in the synovial membrane of an (osteoarthrotic) joint, in (communicating) bursae, and in tendon sheaths. They become visible in the roentgenogram as soon as these metaplasias calcify and ossify. Such (calcified) capsular chondromas or osteomas (Fig. 72) gain clinical importance particularly when they are detached from the synovial membrane and become *loose bodies*. Loose bodies are formed during the course of various pathologic processes:

1.   The osteocartilaginous metaplasias in the synovial membrane of osteoarthrotic joints mentioned above and the damage produced by compressed air work—*metaplastic synovial chondromas and osteomas*—are among the causes of loose bodies.
2.   So-called *neoplastic synovial chondromas* develop in neoplastic synovial chondromatosis. It almost always affects one or two joints only. Less frequent are synovial chondromatoses of bursae and tendon sheaths (Fig. 73; Sim et al., 1977). They initially affect the knee, elbow, and hip joints. Chondromatous proliferation of the synovial membrane occurs polytopically in joints, giving rise to a great number of smaller and larger chondromas that fill the joint cavity and may conglomerate into a clustered

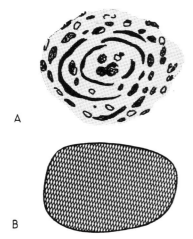

A

B

Fig. 72 Capsular chondroma and capsular osteoma.

A = Type of articulating cartilage with stippled and concentrically stratified *calcification;* e.g., fixed or mobile capsular chondroma.

B = Type of articulating bone; e.g., capsular osteoma, with regular cancellous structure and thin cortex.

mass. The impressive radiographic picture of neoplastic synovial chondromatosis is the result of calcification and ossification of the chondromas (see Fig. 197). Chondromatosis of joints leads to the following articular disorders: Individual chondromas may become detached, i.e., become loose bodies, and may cause symptoms of locking. Articular chondromatosis is a space-occupying process that impairs the function of the joint and, through pressure, leads to erosions of cartilage and bone and ultimately to osteoarthrosis. Diagnostic difficulties arise in synovial chondromatosis when the chondromas *do not calcify;* i.e., remain invisible in the roentgenogram, and

manifest themselves only by pain, swelling, and impairment of motion. The roentgenogram may then reveal only a decalcification of disuse in the immediate vicinity of the joint. In joints with a thin cover of soft tissues and in bursae or tendon sheaths, the synovial chondromas become a palpable mass. This mass must be differentiated from the rice bodies (melon-seed bodies) formed by precipitated fibrin, which also are radiotranslucent and appear in great numbers. In joints with a thin or thick soft-tissue cover, possible pressure erosions (for their radiographic appearance see Fig. 73) can provide guiding roentgenologic information. Articular chondromas degenerate into chondrosarcomas only very rarely.

3. Fragments of cartilage can become detached from a cartilage erosion; e.g. in chondromalacia of the patella; they are resorbed in the joint cavity or are nourished by the synovia. These loose bodies then increase in size, calcify, and ossify. When such cartilage particles unite with the synovium, they increase in size and sometimes also undergo calcification and ossification. Ultimately they again lose contact with the synovium.

4. Osteoarthrotic lippings occasionally break off and thus become loose bodies.

5. In avascular epiphyseal osteonecroses, the tendency to fragmentation of the necrotic subchondral bone leads to formation of loose bodies. The same is true of the tendency to fragmentation of bones with "trophic" disorders in neurogenic osteoarthropathies and the heterotopic bone formations in the periarticular soft tissues observed in this group of diseases.

6. Meniscus fragments—whether calcified or uncalcified—occur as loose bodies in the knee joint. They must be distinguished radiographically from circumscribed calcifications and ossifications in the cruciate ligaments which, because of their extrasynovial location, cannot become loose bodies!

7. Osteochondral fractures or isolated cartilage

Fig. 73 Extra-articular synovial chondromatosis in a tendon sheath.

A = *Equivocal* increased density of soft tissues with pressure erosion in the tibia. Biopsy necessary.

B = Increased density of soft tissues with numerous calcaneous foci and pressure erosion. *Radiologic differential diagnosis:* Synovial chondromatosis, malignant synovialoma (see Fig. 162 C), soft-tissue chondroma (see Fig. 164, no. 5), peripheral chondrosarcoma (see Fig. 164, no. 8).

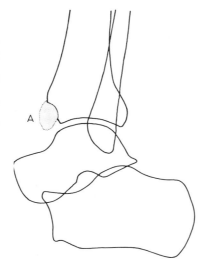

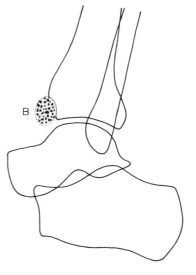

fractures also may give rise to the formation of a loose body ("joint mouse"). Osteochondrosis dissecans—the detachment of a subchondral part of bone from the convex articular surface—is currently classified by many writers from the pathogenetic point of view among the fatigue fractures (stress fractures) (Milgram, 1978). Only loose bodies with an adherent part of bone are recognizable in the plain roentgenogram. When the cartilage cap of the detached loose body is nourished by the synovia, it may increase in size and presents, particularly in the latter instance, stippled and stratified calcification. The loose body and its bed, therefore, will not always fit snugly. In joints with untreated, displaced osteochondrosis dissecans, osteoarthrosis develops in time.

8.   Damage to the elbow joint from compressed air work presents three characteristics. The *first* characteristic is the typical deformation of the joint whose concave surfaces become deepened and whose convex surfaces are flattened. In the *second* characteristic, a great number of loose bodies make their appearance. Their development is due to the processes described under items 1, 3, 4, and 7. A *third* characteristic consists in ossifications of the capsular insertions (Fig. 199).

The monotopic, monoarticular *osteomas of joints* are benign neoplasms that occur preferentially in the knee joint and can occasionally reach a considerable size. In the knee joint, they mostly develop close below the patella (see Fig. 453). In this location they must be differentiated from posttraumatic ossifications (calcifications) of the infrapatellar fat pad.

Periarticular (Paraarticular) Calcifications and Ossifications

The following considerations will be helpful in the *nosological classification* of periarticular (paraarticular) calcifications and ossifications.

Eliciting the patients's *history* sometimes facilitates the correct interpretation of juxtaarticular calcifications and ossifications. Thus, it may be possible to identify pleomorphic calcium deposits or structured new bone in a hematoma (due, for example, to hemophilia); those following tears of the capsule, the ligaments or the tendons; and those occurring in scars, in tumors of the skin (Parkash and Kumar, 1972), or following thermal injuries. Further to be mentioned are calcium deposits and formation of new bone in inspissated pus from (mostly tuberculous) bacterial arthritis and osteitis, and periarticular ossification of soft tissues in diseases and injuries of the central nervous system and the peripheral nerves. This statement is also applicable to **localized traumatic** (or **atraumatic,** Schulze et al., 1978) **myositis ossificans** and to **posttraumatic intraarticular calcifications** and ossifications of internal ligaments of joints, of fat pads, etc. In thallium poisoning, findings have

been observed that sometimes resemble the picture of myositis ossificans and sometimes that of the neurogenic paraosteoarthropathies (Klages, 1941).

Traumatic and atraumatic localized myositis ossificans, in which ossification of connective tissue usually prevails, presents at the outset delicate, cloudy, ill-defined calcium shadows. In this stage it may be extremely difficult to differentiate traumatic (or atraumatic) myositis ossificans in the roentgenogram from a hematoma just undergoing calcification and a cartilage- or bone-forming sarcoma of the soft tissues. Juxtacortical (parosteal) chondroma and juxtacortical (parosteal) osteosarcoma also enter into the differential diagnosis. The following clue may serve to distinguish between traumatic myositis ossificans and juxtacortical osteosarcoma, even in cases in which (atypically) the posttraumatic soft-tissue ossification rests directly on the periosteum and in which additionally a calcified or ossified hematoma or only an elevated periosteal lamella is demonstrable in the rentgenogram. Localized traumatic or atraumatic myositis ossificans presents the most intense shadow in its periphery, whereas the radiodensity of (metaphyseal) juxtacortical osteosarcoma is greatest in its center (Fig. 74). The differential diagnosis between the prevalently juxtaepiphyseal localized traumatic or atraumatic myositis ossificans and the juxtacortical sarcoma must also take into consideration the rare disease picture of **nodular (parosteal) fasciitis.** This palpable swelling of soft tissues, which is either painful or painless, can increase in size within a few weeks. It is a nodular, nonmalignant lesion that originates in superficial or deep fasciae. Cartilage, osteoid, and bone are apt to develop in fasciitis (Hutter et al., 1962). Therefore, the disorder must be differentiated roentgenologically from localized myositis ossificans and from juxtacortical osteosarcoma. On the other hand, nodular fasciitis frequently develops in the vicinity of the diaphysis of tubular bones; it sometimes erodes the bone from outside and produces a periosteal reaction. It then has to be differentiated radiographically from Ewing's sarcoma.

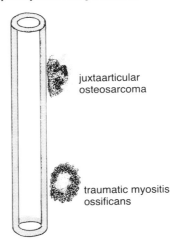

juxtaarticular
osteosarcoma

traumatic myositis
ossificans

Fig. 74   Radiologic differential diagnosis between so-called traumatic (atraumatic) myositis ossificans and juxtaarticular (parosteal) osteosarcoma. In traumatic (atraumatic) myositis ossificans, the most radiopaque shadow lies in the periphery, whereas in juxtaarticular osteosarcoma it is encountered at the base near the bone (the metaphysis). Lamellar periosteal reactions also occur occasionally in myositis ossificans!

The results of *physical examination* or *laboratory data* also can contribute to the correct assessment of *symptomatic* periarticular (paraarticular) calcifications. This is in the first place true of disorders of calcium and phosphate metabolism in hyperparathyroidism and renal osteopathia, of the milk-alkali syndrome (Burnett's syndrome) following long-term intake of easily absorbable alkaline earths in anti-ulcer regimens, also of overdoses of vitamin D, hypoparathyroidism, pseudohypoparathyroidism, Cushing's disease, sarcoidosis, idiopathic infantile hypercalcemia with osteosclerosis, and hypercalcemia in skeletal carcinoma or multiple myeloma. In infants, thickened *subcutaneous* calcareous lumps, which sometimes are fluctuating, and calcified veins have been observed in temporal connection with *intravenous* injections of calcium gluconate. (Ramamurthy et al., 1978).

The calcifications designated here as symptomatic have also been classified as **dystrophic** and **metastatic soft-tissue calcifications.** Dystrophic calcifications develop in necrobiotic and necrotic parts of tissue. Metastatic calcifications of soft structures occur in primarily (?) normal tissues as the result of disordered calcium and phosphate metabolism. Finally, there exists an additional kind of pathologic soft-tissue calcifications in the skin, the hypoderm, and the deeper connective tissue structures, the **calcinoses.** In these soft-tissue calcifications, calcium metabolism is generally normal. The following varieties are distinguished:

1. *Localized interstitial calcinosis (calcinosis circumscripta); so-called calcium gout.*
2. *Universal interstitial calcinosis (calcinosis universalis)*
3. *Lipocalcinogranulomatosis* (Teutschländer). Synonym: pseudotumorous calcinosis.

The initially clear separation and rigorous discrimination of these three types of calcinosis as an expression of different systemic mesenchymal diseases of unknown etiology have been largely abandoned because shadings between the different types are demonstrable. The concept of calcinosis, therefore, is at present used only as a *descriptive* term (for characterization and gross classification). This is true in the first place of calcinoses developing as an aftermath of progressive scleroderma (Thibierge-Weisrisenbach syndrome), dermatomyositis, and polyarteritis nodosa; of Raynaud's syndrome; and, occasionally, also (as a reversible disorder) of disseminated lupus erythematosus (Weinberger et al., 1979) and the consequence of injury to major arteries and nerves (Krasemann, 1965; Kohlmann, 1955). Further to be mentioned in this connection are advanced (juvenile and adult) rheumatoid arthritis and acrodermatitis chronica atrophicans (Pick-Herzheimer). Apart from these disorders, there occur cases with all three calcinoses which are unrelated to the listed or other diseases. The crumbly and spotty, reticular, striated or band-shaped, cloudy or homogeneus, lumpy calcium

deposits then are, in the current stage of our knowledge, the only demonstrable morbid substrate.

The morphology of the calcified tissue can influence the form in which the calcium shadows are projected. Striated or flat calcifications usually are located in the muscular interstices, the fasciae, and the tendons. Subcutaneous calcifications mostly form stippled, reticular, sometimes also striated or band-shaped structures that run in a direction different from that of the neighboring muscles.

In pseudotumorous calcinosis, the cystic calcium deposits contain an abundance of lipoids. They are located in the *juxtaarticular* bursae which become matted with their surroundings, but also in the muscles, tendons, tendon sheaths, and even the periosteum—hence not interstitially in the narrow sense of the term. However, pseudotumorous calcinosis develops not only in the surroundings of a joint (particularly the hip, elbow, shoulder, and acromioclavicular joints) but also in areas exposed to increased mechanical load (pressure areas) such as the vicinity of the scapulae, the ischial tuberosities, the gluteal region, and the lateral aspect of the foot. The disorder often begins in childhood, adolescence, or early adulthood. Pseudotumorous calcinosis is sometimes observed in uremic patients on long-term hemodialysis; it sometimes occurs in individuals with an elevated blood phosphate level without signs of renal insufficiency (Slavin et al., 1973). In the majority of cases, as mentioned above, no clinical, biochemical, or other anomalies are found which could be the cause of pseudotumorous calcinosis. The mostly painless calcifications seldom give rise to inflammation associated with pain, reddening of the skin, and swelling; still more infrequently do they damage the contiguous (small) joint or rupture to the surface through fistulas. Within the radiopaque oval or rounded, sometimes lobulated, shadows one sometimes discerns fluid levels which, with the patient erect (Fig. 75), indicate sedimentation of the liquefied pasty contents.

Periarticular (paraarticular) calcifications occur besides in gouty tophi, in ochronosis, in the Ehlers-Danlos syndrome (subcutaneous, resembling phleboliths, in superficial scars), in hereditary Werner's syndrome (progeria adultorum), in the similar Rothmund's syndrome, in (pseudo-) pseudohypoparathyroidism, in malignant synovialoma and other malignant and benign soft-tissue tumors. They also are observed following traumatic fat necrosis. Calcified animal parasites (nematodes or tapeworms in their larval stage), which by chance are located near a joint, also are visible in roentgenograms of the joint. The same is true of phleboliths calcified in layers inside a juxtaarticular (cavernous, arteriovenous) hemangioma. In chronic venous insufficieny—for example, accompanying or following thrombophlebitis, in extensive varicose veins, in arteriovenous fistulas, and congenital vascular anomalies—a number of sequelae occur, including edema; discoloration and ulcerations of the skin; calcifications of the vein wall, the

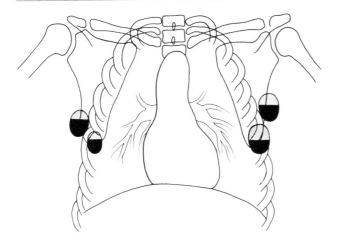

Fig. 75 **Pseudotumorous calcinosis.** Roentgenogram of the thorax with the patient standing. Near the inferior parts of the scapula one recognizes "cystic" structures with radiopaque contents, which present "fluid levels" (stratification phenomenon).

perivenous connective, and adipose tissues; and *subcutaneous* stasis calcifications in the upper and lower leg. These stasis calcifications form extensive cufflike reticular structures (Frössler and Osmers, 1976).

Progressive myositis ossificans (synonym: progressive ossifying fibrodysplasia) is a hereditary connective tissue disease characterized by congenital skeletal deformities *and* progressive ossification of soft-tissue structures. Among the frequent skeletal deformities are absence of fingers; single phalanx or microdactyly of the thumb and the great toe (Fig. 76); hallux valgus; clinodactyly of the little finger;

microdactyly of other fingers, toes and metatarsals; and cartilaginous exostoses. Ectopic ossification generally starts in the first years of life and very infrequently beyond the age of 20. The classical evolution of the disease begins with fever and a painful swelling and induration of the soft tissues at the nape of the neck ("torticollis") and in the surroundings of the scapulae. The acute complaints subside after a number of weeks, when the first ectopic ossifications of soft tissues make their appearance in the paravertebral region of the neck (Fig. 77), in the shoulder girdle, and in the soft tissue of the proximal arm.

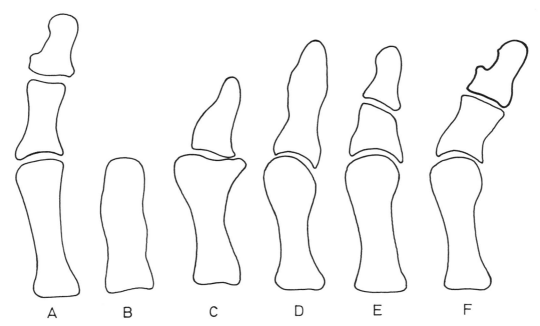

Fig. 76 **Skeletal anomalies in progressive myositis ossificans.**
A = Normal projection of the first digit of the foot.
B to F = Deformities and faulty position (hallux valgus) of the first digit. (D = interphalangeal synostosis; Kübler, 1954).

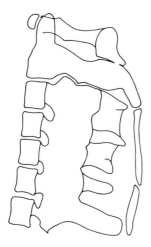

Fig. 77 **Progressive myositis ossificans** of 20 years' evolution (classic onset in 2nd year of life; see text). Extensive ossification of the ligamenta flava, the capsules of the apophyseal joints of the spine, partly also the interspinous ligaments and the ligamentum nuchae. The hypoplasia of the disks and the developmental anomalies of the vertebral bodies and the vertebral arches of C1 and C2 point to the onset of the disease in the (early) growth period. Compare this radiographic appearance with the Klippel-Feil syndrome and cervical spine of an adult individual who experienced juvenile rheumatoid arthritis in childhood or who is still suffering from this disease (see Figs. 662, 664, and 715).

During the subsequent craniocaudal course, the back, the pelvic girdle, and other structures become involved. The process extends in an episodic manner over years until, in the majority of cases, it ceases entirely with the completion of growth.

Disorders of the Fibroosseous Junction (Fig. 78)

The clinical terms epicondylitis (tennis elbow), styloiditis, and coracoiditis denote painful processes in the region of juxtaarticular epiphyseal or apophyseal insertions of tendons or ligaments. In accordance with the supposed histologic substrate one also speaks of tendinoperiosteitis or tendinoperiostosis. Lately, histologic studies of normal and diseased insertions of tendons and ligaments have improved our knowledge of these disorders (Schneider 1959; Niepel et al., 1966; Dihlmann, 1974):

In the region of the tubercles, surfaces and grooves where the insertion takes place, there is *no periosteum!* However, a zone of fibrocartilage—hence collagen fibers and chondrocytes—is interposed. It is less frequent for the fibers to pass directly into the bone. Since *absent* periosteum cannot react pathologically, terms such as tendinoperiosteitis and tendinoperiostosis are incorrect in this connection.

The interposition of cartilage tissue between the tendon or ligament and the bone reduces the mechanical strain on the zone of insertion because, for example, the fibrous strands are prevented from kinking by being embedded in cartilage. Moreover, the morphologic structure of the zone of insertion explains the way in which the insertions of the tendons and ligaments react biologically.

Phenomena of attrition and excessive strain on the insertions and their surroundings manifest themselves by the deposition of lipids, and calcium salts, by hyalinization, as necroses, etc. Hence, degenerative lesions also occur in the interposed cartilage zone. However, cartilage degeneration in the joint, in synchondroses, and also in the insertions of tendons and ligaments gives rise to a reaction that starts from the subchondral bone marrow: blood vessels invade the cartilage. Multipotential connective tissue cells degrade the degenerated portions of tissue and form scar tissue. In addition, they are transformed into osteoblastic cells. These processes lead to the development of osteoarthrotic osteophytes in the articular cartilage and to the formation of osseous spurs in the insertions

of tendons and ligaments. The latter have been termed **fibroostosis** (Dihlmann, 1974). In the roentgenogram, fibroostosis presents the appearance of a *pin* or a *spur,* a *knob* or a *bulge.* It has *smooth contours* and the regular structure of *cancellous bone* (Fig. 79). On the one hand, therefore, fibroostosis constitutes the degenerative spur in the zone of insertion. On the other hand, a particularly great number of large spurs in the zones of insertion are formed in diseases that reflect a constitutional peculiarity; namely, the tendency to excessive pathologic ossification of tight fibrous connective tissue; i.e., an *osteoblastic diathesis.* Among these diseases are diffuse idiopathic skeletal hyperstosis and pachydermoperiostosis (Uehlinger, 1942). Chronic endemic and industrial fluorine poisoning—fluorosis—also gives rise to the development of fibroostoses and even partial or complete ligamentous ossifications (Singh et al., 1962; Kumar and Kemp Harper, 1963; Lányi and Geryk, 1970; Dominok, 1975).

An important radiographic criterion in the diagnosis of fluorosis is the ossification of the insertion of the interosseous membrane of the lower arm (radius) (Fig. 218). Endocrine disorders such as acromegaly, (idiopathic) hypoparathyroidism (Jimenea et al., 1971; Patton, 1976; Adam and Davies, 1977), hyperphosphatasia (McNulty and Pim, 1972), familial tubular hyperphosphaturia (so-called vitamin D-resistant rickets or osteomalacia; Steinbach et al. 1959) and ochronosis also are among the diseases that induce large fibroostoses and/or extensive ligamentous ossifications. *Partial* ligamentous ossifications often have the appearance of stalactites. *Total* ligamentous ossifications also develop as a posttraumatic event and as the consequence of permanent overloading. In just as many cases, however, the cause of ossification of a solitary ligament—for example, in the pelvic region—can not be identified.

From the *clinical* point of view, fibroostoses can remain silent. Sometimes, however, the patients

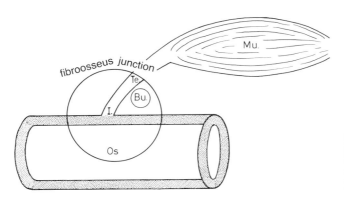

Fig. 78 **Definition of the fibroosseous junction.** The *circle* surrounds the structures of the fibroosseous junction (I = tendinous insertion, Te = tendon, Bu = bursa). Os = bone, Mu = muscle.

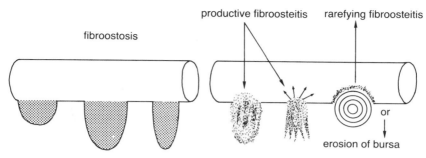

productive fibroosteitis   rarefying fibroosteitis

fibroostosis

or

erosion of bursa

Fig. 79 **Fibroostosis—fibroosteitis.** Lateral roentgenogram of *fibroostosis* (knob-shaped, bulb-shaped, or pin-shaped, smooth contours, regular structure of cancellous bone). *Productive fibroosteitis* (irregular shape, often "frayed" contours, irregular density. More pronounced [small arrows] or less pronounced increase in density of the cancellous bone near the spur). *Rarefying fibroosteitis* (hazy contours, defect in tendinous insertion mostly presenting slight increase in marginal density). Radiographic findings in bursitis identical.

Note: Fibroostosis = degenerative or otherwise noninflammatory bone spur (see text). *Fibroosteitis* = primarly inflammatory bone spur or insertion defect of inflammatory rheumatic or infectious origin (see text).

complain of discomfort produced by the regressive changes described and the mechanical impairment (pressure effect), which lead to reactive inflammation of the neighboring soft tissues and the contiguous bursae.

In spastic paralyses of the growth period (e.g., spastic infantile displegia, or Little's disease), the tubercles of tendinous insertions may become deformed (elongated). These are growth disturbances produced by permanently increased muscle pull—a *general* pathogenetic principle—and not fibroostoses.

Apart from the fibroostoses, there occur bony spurs in the fibroosseous junction which present a quite different radiographic picture. Their shape is *irregular,* often *vesicular;* sometimes they appear to be *frayed*. At times their contours are *ill-defined*. The cancellous bone and its surroundings mostly shows *increased density*. In addition, the spur is occasionally conspicuous by its *irregular thickness*. The formation of the spur may be preceded or paralleled by a "destructive phase." When *resorption* of bone prevails, the lateral roentgenogram shows *excavated* defects of the insertions, which present hazy contours and mostly a moderate marginal density increase. The top view reveals *translucences* with a *sclerotic marginal seam*. These roentgen findings are the result of primary inflammatory reactions at the sites of insertion (Hsien-Chi Fang, 1948; Guest and Jacobson, 1951; Niepel et al., 1966) which either give rise to a "precipitate" and therefore irregular formation of new bone or to resorption of bone. This disease picture, therefore, has been termed **productive or rarefying fibroosteitis** (Fig. 79; Dihlmann 1974). Fibroostitic lesions of ligament and tendon insertions have great importance in differential diagnosis. Particularly when they occur bilaterally in paired insertions, they are quite frequently an *extraarticular accompaniment* or, less often, even the *initial roentgenographic sign* of inflammatory rheumatic arthropathies. In this case,

the finding of fibroosteitis should prompt a clinical- and roentgenologic "chain reaction," i.e., the search for psoriatic arthritis, Reiter's syndrome, ankylosing spondylitis, rheumatoid arthritis, or Jaccoud's arthritis (see under this heading), listed in the order of incidence. With *unilateral* fibroosteitis, bacterial or other local infections also should enter into the differential diagnosis. Regarding the morphologic differential diagnosis of rarefying fibroosteitis by radiography it should be pointed out that ligaments and joint capsules are apt to insert in sharply contoured bony sulci and grooves. Well-known examples of variable grooves for the insertion of capsules and ligaments are the paraglenoidal (juxtaarticular) sulcus at the sacroiliac joint and the groove for the costoclavicular ligament on the inferior border of the clavicle (Fig. 80).

In psoriatic arthritis there exists—besides the typical fibroosteitis—a particular type of ossification of the tendinous insertions which, beyond the site of insertion, can involve the entire tendon and project into the musculature (Jansen, 1967; Wright, 1967). These spurs extend via cartilage islets that develop in the tendon tissue without inflammatory processes (Jansen, 1963).

The pathologic lesions of the fibroosseous junction also include *calcium deposits* which develop in tendons and ligaments at a distance varying between a few millimeters and about 1 cm from the sites of insertion. The nomenclature of these lesions (**calcareous tendinosis, calcareous tendinitis, calcareous peritendinitis, calcareous bursitis, periarthritis, periarthrosis, periarthropathy**) indicates that these calcium deposits occur not only in tendons and ligaments but also in tendon sheaths, bursae (Fig. 81), and in the fibrous joint capsule. Most familiar are circumscribed calcium deposits in the rotator cuff, the shoulder joint, and the immediate vicinity of the greater trochanter. These circumscribed calcifications are sometimes completely *asymptomatic* or cause the patient but *little pain*. In other cases they are ac-

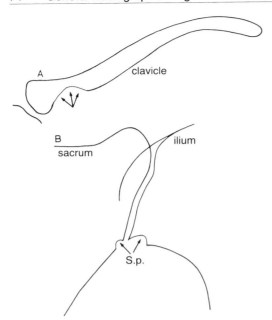

Fig. 80 **Roentgenologic differentiation of rarefying fibroosteitis** from grooves for the insertion of ligaments and the fibrous joint capsule.
  A = Variable groove for the insertion of the costoclavicular ligament *(arrows)*.
  B = The paraglenoidal (juxta-auricular) sulcus (S.p.) in the ilium and/or the sacrum is the variable groove for the insertion of the sacroiliac joint capsule.

erythema are apt to appear. Even fever and an elevated sedimentation rate have been observed. Moreover, cases have been described in which a painful calcareous (peri-) tendinitis successively involved various fibrous structures in the body. These patients, hence, were afflicted with a migratory type of calcareous (peri-) tendinitis (McCarty Jr. and Gatter, 1966). Besides this, *synchronous polytopic* tendon calcifications and periarticular calcium deposits have been reported (Bléry and Barré, 1978). Calcareous tendinitis of the longus colli muscle (Fig. 82) manifests itself by swelling of the prevertebral soft tissues of the *upper* cervical spine and amorphous calcium shadows below the anterior arch of the atlas (Newmark III et al., 1978). It is one of the causes of acute pain and limitation of motion in the (upper) cervical spine. Sometimes it is also responsible for dysphagia.

   The *etiology* of these depositions of calcium is so far not understood. The diverse generalizing theories and hypotheses have not been accepted, as they do not stand up to unbiased criticism (Reischauer, 1958). There probably exist different causes for these depositions of calcium. For example, they have been observed with greater frequency in patients with diabetes mellitus than in the "normal population" (Campbell and Feldman, 1975). Hereditary occurrence has also been described (Bahous and Müller, 1979).

   The *pathogenesis* of the acute inflammatory reactions is more likely to be explained by the fact that the calcium is deposited in crystalline form (generally as hydroxyl apatite, Swannell et al., 1970). These crystals, being foreign bodies, are capable of causing an inflammation (hydroxyl apatite-induced rheumatism). Sometimes, when such calcium deposits are completely asymptomatic or give rise to slight discomfort (generally on motion), one also speaks of *calcareous tendinosis* or (humeroscaplar, coxal, etc.)

companied by *acute discomfort.* The motion of the neighboring joint then is limited by pain. The calcium deposit in these patients triggers an inflammatory reaction which often spreads farther afield. Particularly in the region of the hand, swelling and

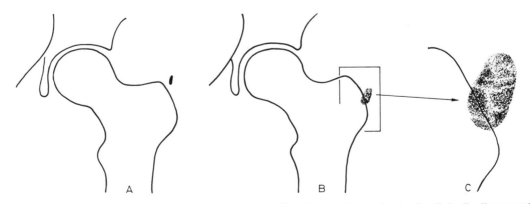

Fig. 81 **Roentgen findings in the soft tissues surrounding the greater trochanter in clinically diagnosed periarthritis coxae.**
A = Calcified tendon (pin-shaped homogeneous calcium shadow).
B = Calcified bursa (area of possible bursal calcification marked).
C = Magnified detail from B to demonstrate the lobulated lumpy appearance of the bursal calcification.

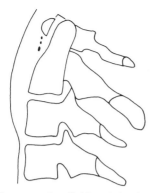

Fig. 82   Calcareous tendinitis of the longus colli muscle.

Roentgen finding: The prevertebral soft-tissue shadow in front of C2/C3, which normally has a thickness of 3 to 4 mm, is enlarged. In addition, amorphous calcium shadows are present below the anterior arch of the atlas.

Roentgenologic differential diagnosis: Fragment of fracture. Ossicle as the result of a developmental anomaly of the upper cervical region.

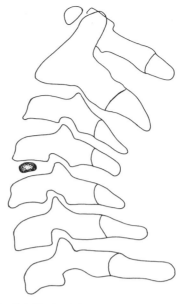

Fig. 83   Calcified nucleus pulposus C4/C5 —spinal analogue of calcareous tendinitis (?), then: *"calcareous discitis"* in a 5-year-old boy. Clinically: pain and limitation of motion. The calcification was resorbed within 3 months. The regression of the calcification was probably encouraged by the physiologic vascularization of the disk in childhood.

periarthrosis. Following therapeutic measures (e.g., antiinflammatory roentgen irradiation) but even without any treatment, the calcium deposits are resorbed within a short time and the discomfort subsides. This observation argues against the supposition that one always has to do with dystrophic calcifications occurring in degenerated or necrotic parts of tissue. Their *complete* cellular resorption would either take much more time or probably would not be possible at all.

In *children,* reversible calcifications of disks occur (Melnick and Silverman, 1963; Leichner-Weil, 1966; Klaus and Nekula, 1975; and other writers) which are considered to be spinal analogues of calcareous tendinitis (**"calcareous discitis"**). In one nucleus pulposus or in several of them one sees rounded, oval, flat, or fragmented calcium shadows (Fig. 83). The cervical and the thoracic spine are more frequently affected than the lumbar spine. Calcification of the sacral and coccygeal disks is a rarity. The calcifications of the nucleus pulposus either remain asymptomatic or they give rise to pain and limitation of motion, for example torticollis. Fever and leukocytosis are occasionally added to the complaints. The calcified nucleus pulposus can even prolapse anteriorly or posteriorly (Coventry 1970, Mainzer 1973). Growth disturbances (platyspondylia) have been observed as the result of disk calcifications (Klaus and Nekula, 1975). The cause of reversible infantile disk calcifications is not known. The reversibility of infantile and juvenile disk calcifications argues against a causal dystrophic process such as underlies, for example, the monotopic or oligotopic calcification of the nucleus pulposus in adulthood (see also the legend accompanying Fig. 83).

Topographic Radiologic Diagnosis of the Gliding Tissues

Imitate it
but imitate it exactly.

CH. F. SAMUEL HAHNEMANN   (1755–1843)

Arthritis, osteoarthrosis, and other kinds of arthropathies can occur in any joint. Although the histologic processes in the different joints follow the same basic principle, the shape, structure, and function of the joint involved influence the pathologic morphology and thus its reproduction in the roentgenogram. The topographic radiologic diagnosis described on the following pages takes into consideration these possible articular reactions, which depend on their location.

Joints of the Hand

Embryologic Errors

In the adult individual, the diagnosis of hereditary *aplasias* and *hypoplasias* can be readily established. The natural creasing over the aplastic joint is absent. In phalangeal synostosis, the roentgenogram (Fig. 84) shows a regular continuous structure of the trabeculae with slight or absent fusiform bulging. The involved finger is usually extended or slightly flexed; hyperextension is an infrequent finding. Developmental anomalies of the finger joints are more often encountered in the ulnar digits than on the radial side. These anomalies frequently occur symmetrically in both sides of the body, in association with other skeletal developmental disorders of the hand. This fact especially facilitates the diagnosis of hypoplasia of the interphalangeal joints with preservation of the contours of the contiguous phalanges.

In the *growing* skeleton, the clinical and roentgenologic findings in aplasia of the finger joints are less clear-cut because the ''synchondrosis'' that initially connects the fingers still permits a slight resilience and cannot be differentiated roentgenologically from a normal joint space. Figure 85 shows the roentgenogram of interphalangeal aplasia in the growth period.

Aplasias of joints in the region of the carpal bones

are observed primarily between the lunate and the triquetrum (Fig. 86). Fusion of the capitate with the trapezoid (Fig. 86) or between the capitate and the hamate is a rather frequent (incidental) finding. In general, synostoses are more frequently encountered in the transverse axis of the carpus than in its longitudinal axis. More than two carpal bones may be synostotic, and the synostosis may involve the radius and the metacarpals.

Differentiation between *congenital* and *acquired* fusions of carpal bones may be difficult if the roentgenogram is the only factor in the diagnosis (Schacherl and Schilling, 1965). In congenital synostoses, the basic shape of the involved bones is usually preserved, and the cancellous trabeculae present a normal pattern. Congenital synostoses frequently occur in bilateral symmetric fashion and sometimes are associated with embryonal defects of contiguous small tubular bones. Congenital synostoses of carpal and tarsal bones sometimes occur concomitantly in the same individual. Occasionally one also encounters regular cancellous structures and symmetrical occurrence in arthritic synostoses of the intercarpal, carpometacarpal, and carporadial regions acquired during the growth period. In addition to this, it is well known that, *in childhood*, rheumatoid arthritis does not produce pain in every joint involved. Moreover, a bacterial arthritis—for example, one following a trivial injury to the hand—can run a very mild course and therefore may have been forgotten by the patient. A distinction between congenital and ac-

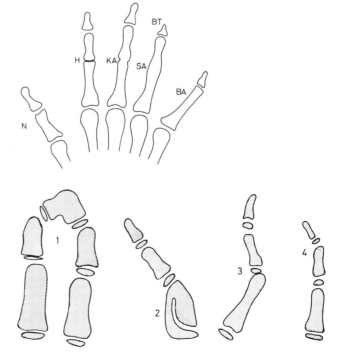

Fig. 84 Malformations of the finger joints. *Upper row:* **Aplasias and hypoplasias of the finger joints in the adult** (Sketched in the proximal interphalangeal joints). N = Normal picture. H = Hypoplasia. Marginal contours of the phalanges just visible; joints however are ankylosed. KA = Aplasia with delicate indentation of the marginal zone. SA = Aplasia with slight fusiform bulging of the marginal zone. BT = Incidental finding: brachytelephalangia (to be differentiated from acroosteolysis!). BA = Aplasia with brachymesophalangia associated with cylindrical coarsening of the synostotic proximal and middle phalanges.

Lower row: **Congenital malpositions of the fingers in the child.**

1 = Osseous distal syndactyly.

2 = Deltoid phalanx (Wood and Reading, 1977).

3 = Camptodactyly (flexion contracture at the 5th proximal interphalangeal joint, mostly bilateral, more frequently congenital than acquired).

4 = Klinodactyly (4th and 5th fingers).

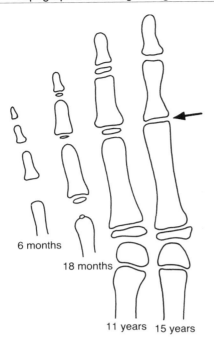

6 months

18 months

11 years   15 years

Fig. 85 **Aplasia of the proximal interphalangeal joint in the growing skeleton.** In the instances referring to the ages of 6 months, 18 months, and 11 years, the diagnosis can be based only on the clinical finding. In the instance referring to the age of 15, the transformation of the "synchondrosis" into a "synostosis" has taken place. This process may occur at an even earlier age. The open epiphysis of the middle phalanx *(arrow)* may mimic an "interosseous space." In the distal phalanx, the epiphysis has closed according to age. The cleft between the distal and the middle phalanx, therefore, corresponds here to the articular cartilage of the normally constituted distal interphalangeal joint.

quired synostoses of the carpus based exclusively on the patient's history is therefore not absolutely dependable.

In the adult, arthritic bony ankyloses are the result of complete destruction of the articular cartilage. In children, in small joints capable of limited motion, arthritic damage to the zone of endochondral ossification alone sometimes produces growth disturbance, that later can give the impression of synostoses.

Congenital total synostosis of the carpal bones, so-called *congenital os carpale,* occurs only in association with other embryonal malformations in bones and joints. *(Acquired) arthritic os carpale* occurs as the result of arthritic destruction of the carpal articular cartilage and is, for example, a frequent finding in advanced rheumatoid arthritis.

Unilateral or bilateral *aplasia of the carpal scaphoid* (Srivastava and Kochhar, 1972) is some-

times encountered in association with a developmental anomaly of the styloid process of the radius and/or the first metacarpal. Instead of the scaphoid, a small radiopaque shadow (rudimental scaphoid) is visible in Figure 86.

Recurrent subluxation at the carpometacarpal joint of the thumb is generally the result of an abnormal shape of the trapezium and flattening of the wrist. The radial aspect of the trapezium is mostly beveled (Fig. 87). The transverse curvature of the hand normally causes the trapezium to project farthest into the hollow of the hand. As a consequence, the first digit can be better opposed at the carpometacarpal saddle joint. When the curvature of the hand flattens (so-called *flat hand),* the first digit comes to lie in the same plane as the other digits. Opposition of the thumb, which is necessary for prehensile movements, thereby becomes impaired, and with time the base of the first metacarpal partially slips out from the atypically shaped distal articular surface of the trapezium (Hopf, 1959). This subluxation becomes habitual and ultimately leads to osteoarthrosis of the first metacarpophalangeal joint with the characteristic discomfort on prehension. The subluxation is particularly well demonstrable in a semi-oblique dorsovolar roentgenogram of the hand (zither player's position).

Madelung's deformity, which often occurs bilaterally, develops with growth disturbance of the distal epiphysis of the radius. The latter may be familial or may be the consequence of a system disorder of endochondral ossification, or (if unilateral) may be the

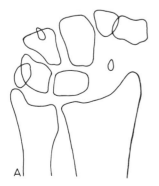
A

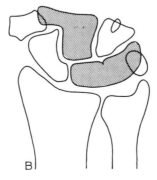
B

Fig. 86 A = (Unilateral) **aplasia of the carpal scaphoid.** The small radiopaque shadow in place of the scaphoid is probably a rudimentary scaphoid (hence, strictly speaking, hypoplasia of the scaphoid is present).

B = **Congenital synostosis** between the lunate and the triquetrum and between the capitate and the trapezoid *(hatched).*

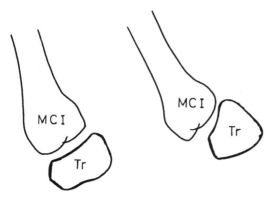

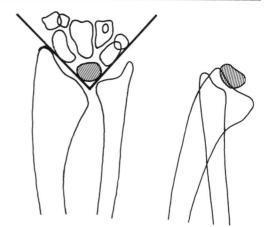

Fig. 87 *Left:* **Typical pentagonal projected shape of the trapezium** in a dorsovolar roentgenogram. *Right:* **Radial flattening of the trapezium** which, together with the flattened curvature of the hand, favors the development of habitual subluxation at the carpometacarpal joint.

Fig. 88 **Madelung's deformity,** dorsovolar and lateral view *(lunate hatched)*. Typical angulation of the proximal row of carpal bones (positive carpal sign; see text).

result of trauma (''pseudo-Madelung''). The disorder commonly becomes manifest in prepuberty. The hand presents a volar bayonet bend in the region of the carpus and the forearm. Sometimes there is also a radial or ulnar angulation, and the head of the ulna is subluxated dorsally at the distal radioulnar joint. This deformity causes the styloid process of the ulna to project dorsally. On lateral inspection, the dorsum of the hand and the flexor surface of the forearm lie approximately in the same plane. In the dorsovolar view, the distal articular surfaces of radius and ulna lie face to face; the distal surface of the radius slopes more strongly in the direction of the ulna than the distal surface of the ulna slopes in the direction of the radius. In addition, the articular surface of the radius is inclined volarward; the shaft of the radius presents a slight medial (radial) convexity. The position of the proximal row of carpal bones adapts itself to the deformed distal ends of radius and ulna. The roentgenogram (Fig. 88) evidences the unfavorable influence exerted by Madelung's deformity on the function of

the joints in the junction between carpus and forearm. When tangents are drawn from the radial and the ulnar side to the *proximal* contours of the scaphoid, lunate and triquetrum, they form a distally open angle. When this angle is less than 117°, one speaks of a positive *carpal sign* (Kosowicz 1962; Fig. 88). The carpal sign is encountered as an associated finding in various clinical types of gonadal dysgenesis and other developmental anomalies.

The *metacarpal sign* (compare Willich and Englert 1973; Fig. 89) is a clue to a metacarpal growth disturbance. This sign is negative (i.e., a normal finding) when the tangent to the *distal* metacarpal contours IV and V moves along distally to the contour of the metacarpal III or at most meets it (the later instance being a borderline finding between normal and pathologic). A positive metacarpal sign is present in all those cases where the tangent to the metacarpals IV and V intersects the distal end of the metacarpal III and hence becomes a secant. A positive metacarpal sign is encountered in endocrine anoma-

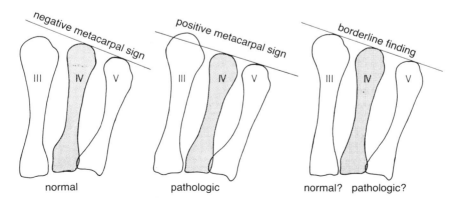

Fig. 89 The **positive metacarpal sign** indicates a growth disturbance of the 4th metacarpal (see text).

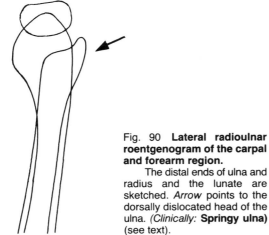

Fig. 90 Lateral radioulnar roentgenogram of the carpal and forearm region.
The distal ends of ulna and radius and the lunate are sketched. *Arrow* points to the dorsally dislocated head of the ulna. *(Clinically:* **Springy ulna)** (see text).

lies; for example, in pituitary dwarfism, giantism, gonadal dysgenesis, delayed sexual maturation, pseudohypoparathyroidism and pseudopseudohypoparathyroidism. Apart from these disorders, *familial* occurrence of a positive metacarpal sign has been observed in individuals who have no endocrine disorder. In addition, it has been reported in cases of achondroplasia, arthrogryposis multiplex, enchondromas, and juvenile chronic arthritis. When, besides the fourth metacarpal, the neighboring metacarpals also are shortened, the metacarpal sign cannot, of course, be tested (see Fig. 168).

Springy ulna is a subluxation at the distal radioulnar joint which is favored by a constitutional weakness of the capsule and the ligaments. This disorder can be the cause of discomfort. In lateral roentgenograms of the carpus one often recognizes an increased *dorsal* projection of the head of the ulna (see also the Caput ulnae syndrome, p. 83, Fig. 90). On physical examination, the ulna can be pressed volarward but, when released, it instantly springs back to the position of subluxation.

Arthritis

Dorsovolar roentgenograms of the hand give a view of more than twenty joints whose articular cartilages are only between 1 and 2 mm thick. An inflammatory or degenerative narrowing (decrease in substance) of the cartilage cover, therefore, can be detected early. For this reason, roentgenograms of the hand are of great diagnostic importance in systemic disease of the synovial tissue—*polyarthritis*—and the articular cartilage—*polyosteoarthrosis*. The classic polyarthritis of the (peripheral) joints is **rheumatoid arthritis.** (The most widely employed synonyms are chronic

rheumatic[1] polyarthritis, primary chronic polyarthritis, idiopathic arthritis, and progressive chronic polyarthritis.) Classic polyarthritis is regarded as a systemic disease of the connective tissue with a predilection for the synovial membrane in the joints, the tendon sheaths, and the bursae. It is classified as the most common of the inflammatory rheumatic diseases. Its incidence shows geographic differences; in Central Europe it varies between 0.5 and 2.0 percent. Females are affected from two to three times more frequently than males. In about two thirds of the patients the *onset of the disease is typical* (Wagenhäuser, 1968):

1. Following an indistinct prodromal stage, the joints are involved *insidiously. Possible prodromal symptoms* of rheumatoid arthritis, which can set in prior to any clinically or roentgenologically demonstrable involvement of joints, are as follows: general malaise, easy fatigability, weakness, lack of appetite, weight loss, transient subfebrile temperature, perspiration of hands and feet, vasomotor disturbances (acrocyanosis, cutis marmorata, pain on immersion of the hands in cold water, blanching of individual fingers, paresthesias [particularly nocturnal burning and tingling in hands and feet.]), nonobjectifiable joint symptoms (morning stiffness lasting longer than 30 minutes, pains in joints and muscles), mental disturbances (irritability, "nervousness," depressive mood).
2. The disease follows a *polyarticular* course from the beginning.
3. The disease affects *small* joints while the large joints are only involved during the course of the characteristic centripetal progression.
4. The joints (of the extremities) are affected in *bilateral symmetrical* fashion.

In about one third of the patients, however, the *onset of the disease is atypical*. Rheumatoid arthritis then sets in *acutely,* or the initial involvement of joints is *asymmetrical-polyarticular, monoarticular, or oligoarticular,* or *large* joints are affected first. Incidentally, prior to making the diagnosis of "rheumatoid arthritis with an atypical onset," one should—in a younger male—always consider the peripheral manifestation of a so far undiagnosed ankylosing spondylitis (hence, take an roentgenogram of the sacroiliac joints) or—in an elderly individual—the possibility of a paraneoplastic arthritis.

---

[1] The comprehensive concept of "rheumatic diseases" is at present exclusively used in a symptomatologic sense, without considering the etiology, the pathogenesis and the histologic findings, etc. A disease is called "rheumatic" when it is accompanied by migratory pains which often are precipitated by movement or by cold and humidity, and whose most conspicuous feature is the impairment of motion. However, the conventional term "rheumatoid arthritis," which is also employed in this book, owes its origin to illogical thinking. The suffix "-oid" actually classifies the **principal** rheumatic disease as **resembling rheumatism**. Illogical thinking, however, is not solely a privilege of the medical profession!

Fig. 91 **Pattern of manual involvement in poly-articular diseases.** The pattern of manual involvement in a polyarticular disease is spoken of when this disease *manifests itself in its early stage* (1) *with great regularity* (2) in *certain sites* (3) *in the hand.*

Red = Pattern of involvement in *adult* rheumatoid arthritis.

Blue = Pattern of involvement in psoriatic arthritis. Transverse and axial type.

Green = Heberden's polyosteoarthrosis, often associated with osteoarthrosis of the carpometacarpal joint of the thumb. Additional involvements (osteoarthrosis of trapezium and scaphoid) are possible.

Yellow = Polyosteoarthrosis of the proximal interphalangeal joints (so-called Bouchard's type of polyosteoarthrosis).

Black squares = Polyosteoarthrosis of the metacarpophalangeal joints. Combination of "green," "yellow," and "black" is possible. Marked metacarpophalangeal osteoarthrosis ("black"), however, occurs more frequently in an isolated form than in combination with the other types of osteoarthrosis.

Black rings = Pattern of involvement in osteoarthropathy related to hemochromatosis (see under this heading).

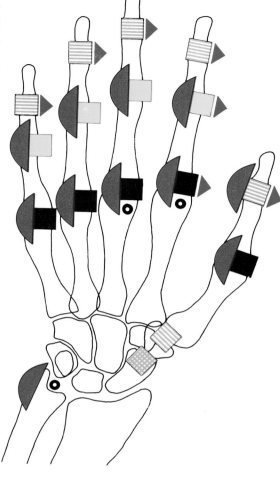

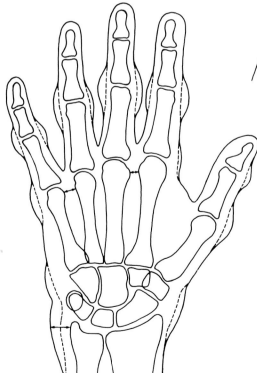

Fig. 92 **Pattern of manual involvement in adult rheumatoid arthritis, illustrated by the soft-tissue signs of arthritis.** In addition, the sequelae of a pericarpal inflammatory edema and the inflammatory proliferations of the synovial membrane in tendon sheaths and joints are illustrated; namely, the increased distance between the surface of the skin and the medial and lateral borders of the carpus and the border of the corresponding carpal bones, which is directed toward the skin. The edema additionally homogenizes the carpal soft-tissue shadow, which normally is structured as the result of delicate layers of adipose tissue between the muscles, tendons, and tendon sheaths (see under the heading of scaphoid fat stripes).

↔ = Increased distance between the metacarpal heads IV and V due to effusion into the 5th metacarpophalangeal joint and/or synovial proliferation (see text).

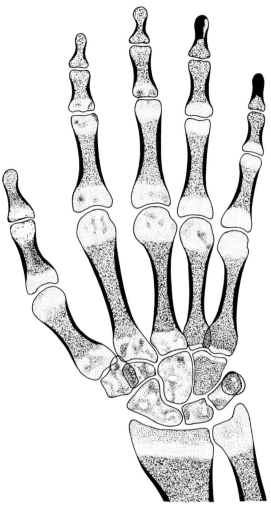

Fig. 93   **Pattern of manual involvement in adult rheumatoid arthritis, demonstrated by the collateral phenomena of arthritis.**

Note the juxtaarticular *spotty* demineralization (speckled, marbled appearance) and the *even* subchondral demineralization. An additional type of collateral arthritic phenomena with hazy, blurred juxtaarticular structures of cancellous bone cannot be reproduced as a radiographic sketch. The shafts of the small tubular bones involved show, as the result of juxtaarticular decalcification, an apparent sclerosis (increased density) of the diaphysis. The distal radius presents a transverse band-shaped zone of demineralization which appears in the region of the former epiphysis. In addition, a narrow band-shaped zone of subchondral decalcification has been illustrated in the bases of the 4th and 5th metacarpals and in the hamate.

Secondary finding: Distal phalanges IV and V reveal so-called *acroosteosclerosis* (Deák, 1958). It has no relation to rheumatoid arthritis but is encountered in women who historically and clinically raise the suspicion of hormonal dysfunction (estrogens?). Compare also the legend to Figure 120.

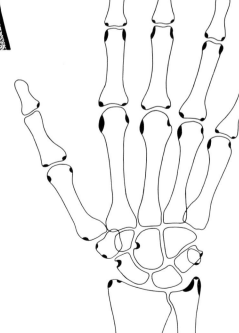

Fig. 94   **Favorite sites for erosions of adult rheumatoid arthritis in the hand.** Erosions in the carpal bones occur also in places where, even normally, (variable) indentations are demonstrable (Fig. 37); for example, in the groove for the insertion of the radial collateral ligament of the carpus (Fig. 169) on the convex side of the scaphoid. Normal indentations have smooth contours and a delicate cortex, whereas erosive indentations have irregular, ill-defined contours and a discontinuous cortex (study under a loupe!). Erosions in the distal interphalangeal joints II to V are not part of the typical pattern of involvement in rheumatoid arthritis. Generally, if these joints are attacked at all, it is only in advanced stages of the disease.

Experience has shown that in most patients with *adult* rheumatoid arthritis the proximal interphalangeal and the metocarpophalangeal joints are the first to be affected and that, together with the carpal joints, they retain their "leading position" during the further evolution of the disease. However, the radiologist should not direct attention exclusively to these joints in diagnosing rheumatoid arthritis but should also consider the styloid process of the ulna and its surrounding soft tissues. These three locations form the so-called *pattern of manual involvement in rheumatoid arthritis* (Fig. 91). This pattern is applicable to the *soft-tissue signs of arthritis* (Fig. 92), to the *collateral phenomena of arthritis* (Fig. 93), and to the *direct signs of arthritis* (Fig. 94). In rheumatoid arthritis, the carpal joints ("the joints of the hand") are also attacked quite early on. In the differential diagnosis of rheumatoid arthritis, however, this matter of experience is *only* important in connection with the radiographic findings in the proximal interphalangeal joints, the metacarpophalangeal joints, and the styloid process of the ulna. The carpal joints are also quite frequently affected in the early stages of different inflammatory rheumatic types of arthritis; they likewise are often the seat of hematogenous bacterial infections. On the one hand, therefore, involvement of the carpal joints does *not* belong to the pattern of manual involvement in rheumatoid arthritis. On the other, however, it is well known (Larsen, 1976) that the degree of the destruction in the carpal joints and in the *metatarsal* joints II to V provides comparatively the most precise reflection of the activity and progressiveness of rheumatoid arthritis.

Radiographic soft-tissue findings of the pattern of manual involvement in rheumatoid arthritis are:

1. Fusiform soft-tissue swelling around the interphalangeal joints due to the joint effusion (widening of the capsule); to thickening of the synovial membrane by hyperemia, edema and proliferation; and to inflammatory edema of the fibrous joint capsule and the periarticular tissues.
2. In the metacarpophalangeal joints, the soft-tissue lesions listed under item 1 are more difficult to identify. Soft-tissue swelling is demonstrable on the radial side of the first and second metacarpophalangeal joint and on the ulnar side of the fifth metacarpophalangeal joint. The articular and periarticular inflammatory increase in volume of the remaining metacarpophalangeal joints is mostly demonstrable by the increased distance between the individual heads of the metacarpals. It should be remembered that *normally* this distance is 2/3>4/5≥3/4 (compare Fig. 93). *In addition,* the effusion and/or the proliferation of the synovium in the metacarpophalangeal joints may manifest itself by increased density and bulging of the periarticular soft tissues (see Fig. 97).
3. The tendon and the tendon sheath of the extensor carpi ulnaris muscle become apposed to the convex side and the posterolateral surface of the styloid process of the ulna. The mostly painless tenosynovitis

of the extensor carpi ulnaris muscle is one of the early manifestations of rheumatoid arthritis of the hand (Dihlmann, 1968a).[2] In normally exposed roentgenograms, this tenosynovitis is recognizable by a radiopaque swelling of the soft tissues immediately apposed to the styloid process of the ulna. During the further course of the disease, the tenosynovitis produces modifications in the contour of the styloid process (Fig. 95). In addition, a small capsular recess on the ulnar side of the radiocarpal joint has intimate relations with the styloid process of the ulna (Kessler and Silverman 1961, Haage 1966). Inflammatory lesions in this joint, therefore, are also capable of eroding the styloid process of the ulna, particularly the region of its tip (Fig. 95).

In advanced rheumatoid arthritis, tenosynovitis of the extensor carpi ulnaris muscle and arthritic destruction of the distal radioulnar joint produce the *Caput ulnae syndrome.* Palmar dislocation of the carpal bones and dorsal projection of the head of the ulna are the principal manifestations of this syndrome in lateral roentgenograms of the carpus. The *collateral phenomena of arthritis* (Fig. 93, p. 12), hence demineralization, are initially limited to the juxtaarticular segments of the tubular bones. Since, early in the disease, the shafts of the small tubular bones do not reveal radiographic signs of decalcification, one often has the impression of an (apparent) *diaphyseal sclerosis.*

Depending on the activity of rheumatoid arthritis and its amenability to treatment, radiographically identifiable defects in the contours of the articulating bones occur only after months, sometimes even after a year or even longer. The same is true of the *concentric (even) narrowing of the radiographic joint space,* which indicates homogeneous resorption of the articular cartilage or—to be mentioned once again—only a (reversible) loss of fluid from the articular cartilage, due to pain-induced inactivity of the joint. Finally, a minor malposition of the joint (flexion of fingers) can mimic a narrowing of the joint space in the roentgenogram (see Fig. 39).

---

[2] Other tendon sheaths of the hand also are liable to be affected by rheumatoid arthritis. Tendovaginitis of the abductor pollicis longus and the extensor pollicis brevis, for instance, produces swelling of the soft tissues posteromedially to the styloid process of the radius. Independently from rheumatoid arthritis, a stenosing fibrous tendovaginitis of the above tendons, affecting principally females is known as *de Quervain's disease.* It, too, leads to roentgenologically demonstrable swelling of the soft tissues near the radial styloid process. The disorder is evidently the result of excessive strain. Finally, a hematogenous bacterial (e.g., tuberculous) tenosynovitis manifests itself by roentgenologically identifiable swelling of soft tissues. It may even occur in association with a hematogenous arthritis of the carpal bones. (It can be differentiated from rheumatoid arthritis by attention to the pattern of manual involvement. See Fig. 91). The association of bacterial arthritis of the carpal bones with bacterial tenosynovitis of the extensor carpi ulnaris muscle is probably the result of a physiologically variable communication between the two synovial cavities (Palmer, 1969). This communication might also be the cause of the early manifestation of rheumatoid arthritis in the tendon sheath of the extensor carpi ulnaris muscle.

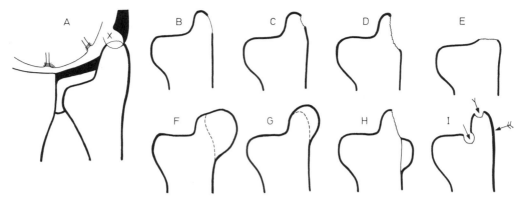

Fig. 95 **Contour changes in the styloid process of the ulna** in rheumatoid arthritis, possibly also in other types of rheumatic arthritis.

A = Anatomy of the distal radioulnar and the radiocarpal joint. Note particularly the course of the articular disk and the small prestyloid capsular recess of the radiocarpal joint (x), which is topographically related to the tip of the ulnar styloid process. B to E = Thinned cortex. Erosion in the convex side of the styloid process prior to its "amputation" (E). F, G = "Ballooning" of the styloid process following erosions (F) and without erosions (G). H = Periosteal new bone formation ("tubercle") proximal to the eroded styloid process. I = Erosion in arthritis of the distal radioulnar joint *(arrow);* erosion of the tip in radiocarpal arthritis *(tailed arrow). Double-tailed arrow* points to the convexity of the styloid process, where tenosynovitis of the extensor carpi ulnaris manifests itself by erosive (B–E) and osteoproliferative processes (F–H).

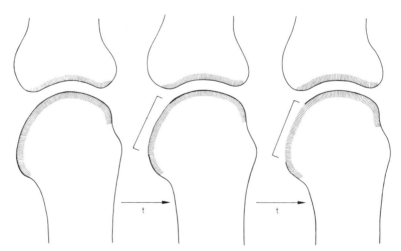

Fig. 96 **Partial wasting of the marginal subchondral lamella** illustrated by a follow-up study (t) of the right hand.

Notes: 1.   As a general rule, the marginal subchondral lamella can be better assessed in convex than in concave joint contours.

2.   In the region of the hand, changes of the marginal subchondral lamella are most readily demonstrable in roentgenograms of the radial side of the metacarpal heads II to V.

3.   The normal thickness of the marginal lamella is individually variable. Its bilaterally symmetrical thinning or wasting—for example, in the metacarpal head of the same digit of the left *and* right hand—is therefore less convincing than a difference (asymmetry) between left and right. (t = time [follow-up study]).

In the heads of the metacarpals, the same as is generally the case in convex articular surfaces, *thinning and wasting of the* marginal subchondral lamella (Dihlmann, 1968b) is recognizable early (Fig. 96), particularly when the roentgenogram is compared with that of the contralateral metacarpals.

A delicate *periosteal lamellar reaction* in rheumatoid arthritis in adult individuals is encountered— if at all—in the distal shaft of the metacarpal bones (Fig. 97 B).

Erosions are, as a rule, first demonstrable on the radial side of the metacarpal heads where they become manifest as small defects in the contours near the capsular insertion, hence *marginally* or, less frequently, more toward the *center* of the joint; or they appear in the lateral view, as cystlike or crescent-shaped translucences (Fig. 97). Figure 94 shows the sites of predilection for erosions in the joints of the hand produced by rheumatoid arthritis.

The joints of the hand are assessed in the dorsovolar roentgenogram. When a second roentgenogram in a different plane is required in arthropathies,

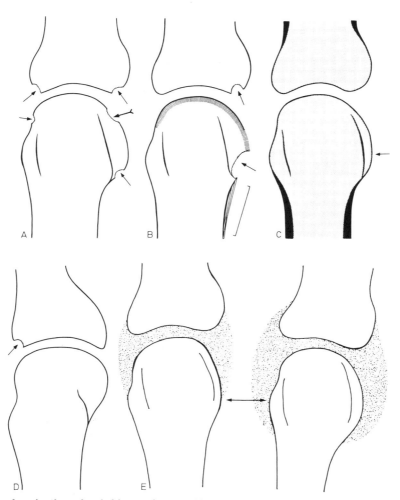

Fig. 97   **Type of projection of arthritic erosions and increased density of soft tissues in the metacarpophalangeal joints of the left hand.** A to C, E = Dorsovolar projection.

D = Roentgenogram in volodorsal, semisupinated (45°) position of hand with fingers spread apart. A = *Arrows* point to delicate marginal erosions; *tailed arrow* points to a so-called central erosion. B = Erosion of somewhat increased size. Distally to the erosion, the metacarpal head also shows wasting of the marginal subchondral lamella (loupe!). In addition, a delicate periosteal lamellar new bone formation is visible in the typical site of the distal metacarpal shaft *(marked)*. C = *Arrow* points to a crescent-shaped erosion which, in the dorsovolar view, appears nonmarginal. D = Typical Nørgaard's erosion *(arrow)* on the dorsoradial side of the proximal phalanx (see text). E = The arthritic involvement of the metacarpophalangeal joints is manifested not only by the increased distance between the metacarpal heads *(marked)* but also by the increased density and the bulging of the soft tissues. *(left* = normal finding; *right* = arthritis or other increase of volume in the joint cavity).

it should be taken in the volodorsal view with the hand in semisupination (45°) and the fingers *maximally spread apart*.

Advantages:
1. The joint between the pisiform and the triquetrum can be additionally assessed (see Fig. 131).
2. The so-called Nørgaard's erosions (Fig. 97D) sometimes appear early in rheumatoid arthritis on the dorsoradial side of the proximal phalanges II to V. Their diagnostic value, however, is considerably modified by the observation that such small contour defects in the place named above sometimes also occur in other diseases or as a variant of normal (Dihlmann 1970a).

With further progression of rheumatoid arthritis the partly discrete roentgen findings in the joints of the hand pass into lesions indicating complete destruction of the joints involved. Figure 98 depicts such an advanced finding in which the typical pattern of manual involvement can no longer be identified because in the meantime most of the distal interphalangeal joints have additionally been affected.

The best known malpositions of diseased metacarpophalangeal joints are *volar subluxation* and *ulnar deviation*. They give the hand of the rheumatoid arthritis patient its characteristic appearance which also is conspicuous in the roentgenogram.

Buttonhole deformity and *swan-neck deformity* denote malpositions at the proximal and distal interphalangeal joints, which primarily are of clinical interest (Fig. 99); the same applies to the so-called 90/90 deformity of the thumb. These deformations, together with the *subcutaneous rheumatoid nodules* (for example, over the extensor surfaces of the finger joints), impair the functional capacity of the hand. Displacement of the carpal bones, including perilunar dislocation and dislocation at the distal radioulnar

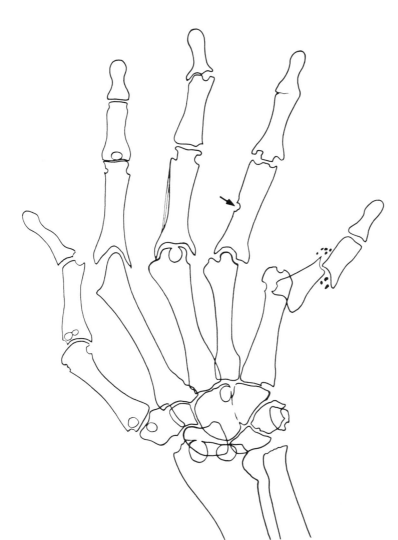

Fig. 98 **Advanced inflammatory destruction in the region of the hand** in rheumatoid arthritis of 15 years' duration (see also Fig. 38). *Identifiable lesions:* Erosions; destructions; mutilations; narrowing of joint spaces but also gaping of the joint space (distal radioulnar joint, see text); bony ankyloses; attendant cysts; periosteal reactions (infrequent; see proximal phalanx III); malposition of joints (note particularly the ulnar deviation of the metacarpophalangeal joints II to V, the volar malposition at the carporadial joint, the subluxation at the metacarpophalangeal joint of the thumb, and the hyperextension at the interphalangeal joint of the thumb). The marked narrowing of the joint space in the carpal region heralds the forthcoming development of a so-called arthritic os carpale. *Arrow* points to an erosion that very likely has been caused by inflammatory granulation tissue that, originating in the corresponding fibrous tendon sheath of the fingers (pars anularis), initiates the resorption of bone. In advanced rheumatoid arthritis one also encounters, very infrequently, spotty periarticular calcifications (localized interstitial calcinosis). See proximal interphalangeal joint V.

joint, occur following destruction of the capsule and the ligaments (Figs. 98 and 100). Their initial manifestation is "widening" of the radiographic joint space (Collins et al., 1972).

Decalcification of the hand skeleton and *malpositions* characterize the picture of the hand in Parkinson's syndrome (*"Parkinson hand"*). Changes in the contours of the articulating bones, however, do not accompany the disorder (Karagevrekis et al., 1972).

Additional Comments on Rheumatoid Arthritis

1. The pattern of manual involvement and the radiographic morphology of adult rheumatoid arthritis are also encountered in the following diseases:

Sjögren's syndrome is considered to be an autoimmune disorder. It preferentially affects menopausal women and, systemically it involves the exocrine glands. In about 50 percent of patients the syndrome is accompanied by a seropositive[3] polyarthritis and occasionally also by one of the classic collagen diseases (see p. 99 ff). With respect to the most frequent and most conspicuous findings one speaks of a Sjögren triad: *xerophthalmia* (keratoconjunctivitis sicca as the result of decreased lacrimal secretion), *xerostomia* from decreased salivary secretion),

---

[3] Rheumatoid arthritis is called seropositive when the so-called *rheumatoid factors* are present in the patient's serum. The rheumatoid factors belong among the immunoglobulins. They are antigammaglobulins, hence autoantibodies directed against other immunoglobulins. Depending on the tests employed, these immunoglobulins are encountered in up to 90 percent of patients with rheumatoid arthritis during the course of the disease. In addition, rheumatoid factors can be demonstrated with varying frequency in certain patients with a classic collagen disease, and in various internal disorders (e.g., chronic aggressive hepatitis, cirrhosis of the liver, sarcoidosis, syphilis, tuberculosis, leprosy). Finally, positive tests for the rheumatoid factors are obtained in from 2 to 4 percent of clinically healthy individuals of young and middle age. In clinically healthy persons beyond the age of 60 these figures are even higher. In patients with rheumatoid arthritis, the demonstration of the rheumatoid factors is of importance not only to the diagnosis but also to the prognosis. The latter is said to be more favorable in seronegative than in seropositive cases (Müller, 1976).

and *polyarthritis*. The combination of xerophthalmia, xerostomia and possibly insufficiency of other exocrine glands, but *without* chronic polyarthritis, has been termed *sicca's syndrome*. Patients with Sjögren's syndrome (sicca's syndrome) are said to become victims of neoplasms of the lymphatic tissue and Waldenström's macroglobulinemia with above average frequency (Talal et al., 1967).

In **Felty's syndrome,** a commonly seropositive polyarthritis is associated with pronounced activation of the lymphoreticular system, so that the disorder may be considered a reactive variant of rheumatoid arthritis. On physical examination, splenomegaly and enlarged lymph nodes are encountered; the hemato-

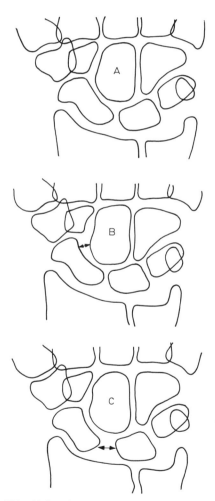

Fig. 100 **Malposition of individual carpal bones** during the course of rheumatoid arthritis.
A = Normal position of carpal bones. B = *Widening* of the radiographic joint space between the scaphoid and the capitate *(marked)* indicates subluxation of these carpal bones. C = Subluxation of scaphoid and lunate with *widening* of the corresponding joint space in the dorsovolar roentgenogram.

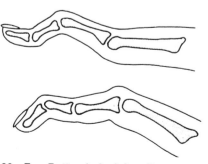

Fig. 99 *Top:* **Button-hole deformity.**
Bottom: **Swan-neck deformity** (see text).

logic picture shows leukopenia (granulocytopenia) and sometimes even pancytopenia.

Seronegative chronic polyarthritis in the antibody deficiency syndrome (agammaglobulinemia, hypogammaglobulinemia) also yields roentgen findings similar to rheumatoid arthritis. However, it often occurs in an oligoarthritic, asymmetric form and preferentially attacks large joints, particularly the knee joint. The condition then must be differentiated from oligotopic joint *infections,* since the immunologic deficiency paves the way for the colonization of pathogens.

Caplan's syndrome is the term applied to a combination of a pneumoconiosis presenting rounded foci with a seropositive chronic polyarthritis. Commonly, pneumoconiosis develops simultaneously or after the polyarthritis. Less commonly, the pulmonary affection manifests itself prior to the arthritis. This particular type of pneumoconiosis as well as the affection of the synovium obviously reflects a "rheumatic responsiveness" of the connective tissue (Fritze et al., 1962). Caplan's syndrome must be differentiated from the following *pleuropulmonary manifestations of rheumatoid arthritis* (Dihlmann, 1967):

- interstitial pneumonitis, pulmonary fibrosis, to acquired honeycomb lung
- Pulmonary rheumatoid nodules
- Pleurisy and its residues (adhesions)

Hashimoto's autoimmune thyroiditis may be accompanied by chronic polyarthritis, Sjögren's syndrome, acquired hemolytic anemia, disseminated lupus erythematosus, or chronic hepatitis. These associations can be regarded as signs of a systemic disturbance of the immunologic homeostasis (Hennemann, 1969).

2. In adult rheumatoid arthritis (see also p. 89) one encounters *asymptomatic joints* (Berens et al., 1967) which present roentgen signs of arthritis although they cause no discomfort to the patient. This is especially true of the metacarpophalangeal joints (metacarpal heads) and the metatarsophalangeal joints (metatarsal heads); among extraarticular structures, this observation is also applicable to the styloid process of the ulna and, occasionally, to the calcaneus. When the diagnosis is not clear in monarticular arthritis of a larger joint, additional roentgenograms of the hands *and* feet can at times facilitate the nosological classification and thus clarify the diagnosis.

3. In paralyzed extremities—for example, in hemiplegia or following poliomyelitis—the lesions of rheumatoid arthritis either fail to develop at all or are very poorly pronounced (Thompson and Bywaters, 1962; Glick, 1967; Bland and Eddy, 1968). This protective effect of paralysis of the limbs is also noticeable in polyosteoarthrosis.

4. *Attendant cysts* in the immediate juxtaarticular cancellous bone originate the more frequently the more the hand of the diseased person is moved (e.g., on occupational grounds). Attendant arthritic cysts, therefore, give information on the motor activity of the diseased hand (Castillo et al., 1965; see pages 23 and 24).

5. Joints afflicted by rheumatoid arthritis show diminished resistance to bacterial infections. This is true whether or not the patients have been treated with corticosteroids. An undiagnosed pyogenic arthritis involves the danger of a (fatal) generalized infection. The suspicion of a secondary bacterial arthritis, which mostly follows an insidious course, is raised by the following roentgen findings: striking progressive destruction of a joint while, in other diseased joints, therapy is subjectively effective, or rapid deterioration of the local condition and *continuously increasing* discomfort following the intraarticular administrations of a steroid.

6. The joint cavities of the distal radioulnar joint, the radiocarpal joint, the intercarpal joints including the joint between the triquetrum and the pisiforme, the mediocarpal joint, and the carpometacarpal joints II to V frequently communicate with each other (Fick, 1904). An arthritis of these joints has therefore to be classified *clinically* as a monarthritis. These cases then require the same differential diagnostic considerations as a monarthritis—bacterial arthritis? (see Fig. 123)—and not the general supposition that one is dealing with the initial manifestation of a beginning polyarticular arthritis.

7. Detached fragments ("seque") also occur in rheumatoid arthritis. The arthritic pannus is capable of detaching small fragments of bone from their connections, or such fragments are the result of pathologic fractures in the inflamed joint. Finally, the dissection may be the consequence of secondary bacterial infection of a joint affected by rheumatoid arthritis. Detached fragments either remain in the destroyed gliding tissue as dead (radiopaque) parts of bone or they are resorbed. They are infrequently discharged to the outside through fistulas ("fistulating rheumatism," Bywater, 1953; Resnick and Gmelich, 1975; Shapiro et al., 1975).

Juvenile Rheumatoid Arthritis—Juvenile Chronic Arthritis

The classic chronic rheumatic disease of children and adolescents differs from adult rheumatoid arthritis regarding the clinical manifestations, the roentgen findings, and the laboratory data. The following considerations should therefore be made and the following diagnostic insights and differential criteria are required:

1. The disease begins prior to the completion of the 16th year of life *and* the joint complaints have continued for at least 3 months after their onset.

2. The disease *begins* as a systemic disorder *or* as a chronic polyarthritis *or* as a polyarthritis *or* as an oligoarthritis (involving between two and four

joints), *or* as a monarthritis. Kölle therefore has proposed the following classification (1971, 1975, 1976):

The systemic type of evolution is termed *"complete Still's syndrome."* Remittent fever, hepatomegaly, splenomegaly, enlarged lymph nodes, xanthemas, myocarditis and pericarditis, hypochromic anemia, and leukocytosis are the prominent systemic manifestations and visceral findings. In principle, any joint may be affected by arthritis. Certain joints, however—the hand, the knee, and the talocrural joints—are preferentially attacked. In about two thirds of patients, the spine is concomitantly involved. In more than 50 percent of cases the disease begins prior to the age of 4. Among all the various types of evolution in juvenile rheumatoid arthritis, the fatality rate is highest in complete Still's syndrome.

In *juvenile rheumatoid arthritis (in the narrow sense of the term),* just as in adult rheumatoid arthritis, involvement of joints far exceeds visceral involvement. The joints of the hands, the knees, and the talocrural joints are prevalently affected. The spine is involved in about one third of the patients. Iridocyclitis occurs less frequently in the complete Still's syndrome than in the other types of juvenile rheumatoid arthritis. In the complete Still's syndrome, the joint manifestations usually are polyarticular from the outset. In contrast, juvenile rheumatoid arthritis in the narrow sense of the term starts in about one third of patients as a monoarticular disorder and remains as such for at least 3 months; in about 10 percent its onset is oligoarticular. Monoarticular onset of the disease carries a less favorable prognosis than oligoarticular onset of the disease: more than three quarters of the patients with initial monarthritis eventually develop a polyarthritis (involving more than four joints). Kölle speaks of an *incomplete Still's syndrome* when a mixed symptomatology develops in juvenile rheumatoid arthritis; for example, monarthritic onset with fever, lymph node enlargement, and hepatomegaly.

Subsepsis allergica (Wissler, 1944, 1965), as an additional type of evolution in juvenile rheumatoid arthritis, is still under debate. It is probably an inflammatory-hyperergic extreme variant of this disorder (Hornstein, 1967) which manifests itself clinically by a nonbacterial septic disease picture with remittent fever, polymorphous xanthemas, arthralgia and even arthritis, and elevated leukocytosis. The joint symptomatology is fleeting and, as a rule is not followed by permanent joint damage. It is very uncommon for this disorder to develop into a destructive polyarthritis.

In differentiating roentgenologically between monarthritis, oligoarthritis (two to four joints involved), and polyarthritis (more than four joints involved), it should be borne in mind that about every fourth patient with juvenile rheumatoid arthritis has individual *asymptomatic joints* (Grokoest et al., 1957). These joints are not painful but, clinically as well as roentgenologically, are affected by arthritis. This is an additional reason why every patient suspected of suffering from juvenile rheumatoid arthritis and juvenile chronic arthritis respectively (see p. 90) should

be subjected to a *minimal program of radiographic diagnosis* (Fig. 101).

3. The diagnosis "juvenile chronic arthritis" is, for the following reasons, initially only a diagnosis of differentiation:

The rheumatoid factors in this disease are much less frequently demonstrable than in adult rheumatoid arthritis (in only 20 to 30 percent of cases). Approximately 20 to 25 percent of the patients present involvement of the sacroiliac joints (Grokoest et al., 1957; Carter, 1962). According to Carter (1962), patients with juvenile chronic arthritis particularly prone to involvement of the sacroiliac joints are those in whom the rheumatoid factors are demonstrable, whose hip joints are diseased, and who are confined to bed because of polyarthritis. The majority of these patients develop a sacroiliitis of the "variegated picture" (see p. 490 ff) type such as is known to occur in ankylosing spondylitis and certain other inflammatory rheumatic diseases, *excepting adult rheumatoid arthritis.* Ankylosing spondylitis starting before the age of 16 is termed *juvenile ankylosing spondylitis.* In this disorder, complaints and clinical findings in the joints of the extremities are very often in the forefront (Schilling, 1968). In more than 90 percent of Caucasoid and patients with ankylosing spondylitis, the histocompatibility antigen $HLA-B_{27}$ (see p. 347 ff) is demonstrable on the surfaces of nucleated cells and thrombocytes. Therefore, the search for this antigen and the rheumatoid factors forms part of the clinicodiagnostic program in juvenile chronic arthritis. The following differential diagnostic constellations then result (Veys et al., 1976). *The case in question may be:*

a. Juvenile rheumatoid arthritis with a positive test for rheumatoid factors (= seropositive); $HLA-B_{27}$ is not demonstrable. Further evolution with or without sacroiliitis.
b. Juvenile rheumatoid arthritis *or* juvenile ankylosing spondylitis, seronegative, $HLA-B_{27}$ negative. Further evolution with or without sacroiliitis.
c. Juvenile ankylosing spondylitis, seronegative, $HLA-B_{27}$ positive, evolution with sacroiliitis *and* clinically (as well as roentgenologically) recognizable by stiffening of the spine.
d. Juvenile chronic arthritis, seronegative, $HLA-B_{27}$ positive, evolution with sacroiliitis. These patients are at high risk of developing definite ankylosing spondylitis during the further course of the disease. In these cases it would be incorrect to speak of a juvenile rheumatoid arthritis that develops, or is apt to develop, into ankylosing spondylitis.

The constellations listed under (b) are equivocal and therefore of questionable diagnostic value because about 5 percent of the cases with ankylosing spondylitis are $HLA-B_{27}$ negative and precisely in juveniles—approximately between the ages of 14 and 18—the sometimes irregular ossification of the lateral apophysis of the sacrum makes it difficult for the radiologist to assess the sacroiliac joints. Therefore

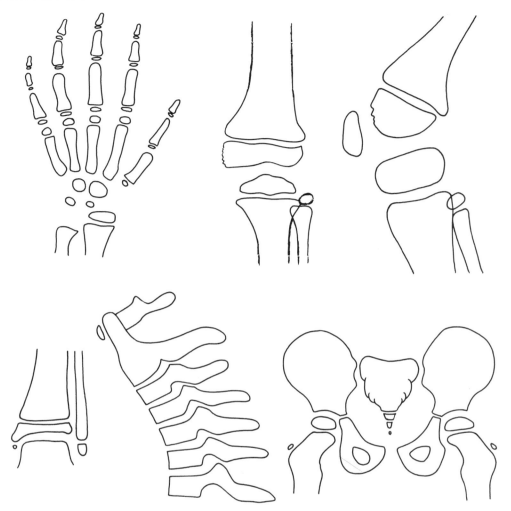

Fig. 101 **Minimal program of radiographic diagnosis in juvenile chronic arthritis:** Dorsovolar roentgeno-gram of both hands, roentgenogram of both knee joints in two planes, anteroposterior roentgenograms of both talocrural joints, lateral roentgenogram of the *anteflexed* cervical spine, survey film of pelvis.

Ansell (1978) has suggested that the designations "Still's syndrome" (a historical eponym) or "juve-nile rheumatoid arthritis" be abandoned and that the terms *"chronic juvenile"* or *"juvenile chronic ar-thritis"* be used. These designations leave temporar-ily unanswered the question of whether a chronic rheumatic arthropathy in childhood and adolescence is a rheumatoid arthritis, an ankylosing spondylitis, a secondary arthritis in ulcerative colitis or Crohn's disease, Reiter's syndrome, a psoriatic arthritis, or an arthritis accompanying one of the classic collagen diseases. These terms, therefore, do not anticipate the definitive diagnosis, which may result only from the further evolution (over years).

Figures 102 and 103 illustrate the possible radi-ographic findings in the hand that accompany and

follow juvenile chronic arthritis. To be mentioned in this connection are, *first,* the proneness of the juve-nile organism to develop periosteal reactions, and *second,* the simultaneous occurrence of arthritis *and* growth processes. Such simultaneous occurrence of a pathologic and a physiologic process precipitates, *irrespective of the etiology of the arthritis,* distur-bances of growth and development as well as defor-mations of the articulating bones. These pathologic manifestations will be the more pronounced the younger the patient is. The concept **"arthritis of the growth period"** therefore refers to the following radiologic findings:

• Delayed or premature appearance of the ossifica-tion centers, accelerated maturation of the ossifica-

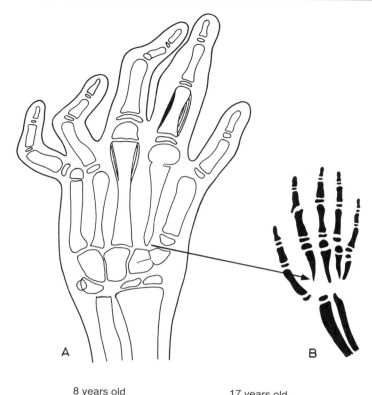

8 years old   17 years old

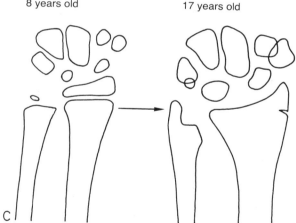

Fig. 102 **Possible roentgen findings in the hand in juvenile chronic arthritis** (A).

B shows by way of comparison a case of hereditary or sporadic carpal osteolysis (see also Fig. 58 and under osteolysis syndrome). C illustrates the growth disturbances following cured juvenile rheumatoid arthritis in the region of the left carpus and forearm. Carpal arthritis at the age of 8; Roentgen finding: Moderate swelling of soft tissues, no direct signs of arthritis, minor demineralization *(not set off in the figure)*. At age 17, malformation and malposition of the distal radius and ulna.

Note regarding analysis of roentgenogram A: Malpositions are frequently recognizable in joints without presenting erosions in the contours of the joint. The younger the patient, the more pronounced is the swelling of the soft tissues. Lamellar periosteal reactions in the diaphysis and metaphysis (see radial side of the 2nd proximal phalanx and the 3rd metacarpal) are more frequent and more pronounced in preschool age than later on. The periosteal new bone formation may lead to uniform thickening of the shaft (see ulnar side of the 2nd proximal phalanx). Endosteal resorptive processes produce a column-shaped deformation of the diaphysis of small tubular bones (see 1st metacarpal). Ossification centers of the carpal bones may be dissolved ("absence" of the lunate); the destroyed ends of the tubular bones have a "sucked-off" or "frayed" appearance (arthritic mutilation; see the base of the 2nd metacarpal and the distal end of the ulna). The condition then must be *differentiated* from the painless François syndrome (B) (see also p. 55) in which, in addition to the carpofugal osteolysis, xanthomatous dermal nodules and opacity of the cornea are apt to occur, or from idiopathic carpal and tarsal osteolyses (see p. 55) which sometimes are painful. Erosions and narrowing of joint spaces are late radiographic manifestations of juvenile rheumatoid arthritis, which occur more of frequently in adolescents than in children. Ankyloses are to be expected primarily in the carpal region. The transverse curvature of the hand flattens. The bones present marked demineralization.

Local disturbances of growth and maturation: Shortening and slimming of the 4th metacarpal, brachydactyly *(not illustrated)*. Excessive longitudinal growth of the metaphysis (see 3rd metacarpal). Premature epiphyseal closure with oversize of the epiphysis (see 2nd metacarpal). Deformation of the epiphyses ("compression"; see proximal phalanges II and III). Separation of ossification centers (see radius).

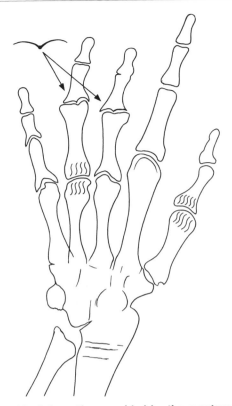

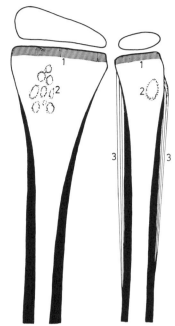

Fig. 103 **Information provided by the roentgeno-gram of an adult hand** (without knowledge of the an-amnesis and the clinical findings).

1. Chronic polyarthritis with the pattern of in-volvement characteristic of rheumatoid arthritis.

2. Growth disorders (in the digits III to V and the distal ulna) evidence the onset of the disease in the growth period (so-called arthritis of the growth period).

3. The disease either has been of many years' duration or has pursued a particularly active (progres-sive) course. (Ankylosis of the carpal joints, the radi-ocarpal joint, and the carpometacarpal joints II to V).

4. The "wing shape" of the eroded bases of the middle phalanges III and IV *(arrows)* indicates the preservation of mobility in these joints; it allows the in-ference that the arthritic process there has largely sub-sided (become inactive). The "wing shape" is a *gen-eral* radiographic sign of preserved mobility in an interphalangeal joint affected by arthritis or osteoarthri-tis but which is hardly any longer painful!

5. The duplicated marginal lamella in the 2nd metacarpal head corresponds to the so-called growth lines in the metaphysis of the distal radius and points to a period of disordered growth.

6. So-called hypertrophic atrophy of bone with *fi-brillar* subchondral structures of cancellous bone (see the legend to Fig. 13), sketched only in the metacar-pophalangeal joints I and IV.

Clinical finding: (Juvenile) chronic arthritis starting at age 5, which now, in adulthood, has become inac-tive.

Fig. 104 **Roentgenographic findings in childhood leukemia** which may be associated with joint discom-fort.

1 = *Metaphyseal* (but also subapophyseal and subdiscal) *band-shaped translucences.* These are not only the consequence of leukemia cell infiltration in the amply vascularized metaphysis but, in *small children,* they also occur in wasting diseases, among them ju-venile rheumatoid arthritis.

2 = *Osteolyses of cancellous bone,* often bilat-erally symmetrical extending from coarsened cancel-lous meshes through the "moth-eaten" appearance to circumscribed major osteolyses. To be differentiated from metastatic neuroblastoma! *Findings 1 and 2 = * Justified suspicion of leukemia (hemologic data necessary!). *3 = * one or more layers of *lamellar bony periosteal reaction* in tubular bones.

Additional roentgen findings in childhood leuke-mia: Evidence of effusion into joints in which this is an-atomically possible, generalized osteoporosis, osteo-scleroses, roentgen manifestations of bone infarction (Ansele, 1977), so-called growth arrest lines.

Note: Roentgen signs of leukemia occur most fre-quently in sites where longitudinal growth proceeds most rapidly (vicinity of the knee joint). In addition, the skel-eton of the hand and the foot, the elbow joint, and the talocrural joint are sites of predilection for the manifes-tation of leukemia.

tion centers, disturbed modeling of these centers and of the articulating epiphyses.

• Resorption of smaller bones (and their ossification centers).

• Shortening of the tubular bones through premature closure of the epiphyses.

• Enhancement of longitudinal growth.

The disturbances of growth, development, and modeling of bones are, in addition, intensified by prolonged inactivity or therapeutic immobilization of the diseased joint. Experience has shown that this is true not only of juvenile arthritis but equally of hemophilic joints. It is even true of intrinsically healthy joints whose mobility has been impaired by disordered muscle function and by calcification of soft tissues developing during the course of infantile dermatomyositis whose victims have survived (Canigiani and Zweymüller, 1972) (see Fig. 242 B). These disturbances are also encountered in paretic and paralytic joints (immobilized joints, Figs. 290, 398) whose motor muscles have been paralyzed in childhood.

Arthritis of the growth period in small children sometimes is followed by such severe disturbances of skeletal growth, modeling, and maturation that later on, when the condition may have been cured, *and when there is no awareness of polyarthritis in the history* a constitutional skeletal disease enters into the *differential diagnosis.* Among such diseases are, for instance, the osteochondrodysplasias *(systemic* disorders of osteochondral development) and the dysostoses (malformations of *individual* parts of the skeleton). Long-term corticosteroid therapy sometimes has an additional adverse effect on the localized arthritic disorders of development in juvenile rheumatoid arthritis. These include deceleration of longitudinal growth and demineralization that extends beyond the region of the joint and which, in the spine, becomes generalized; especially in the thoracic spine it involves the danger of compressed fractures. Furthermore, it gives rise to avascular necroses of bone which, particularly in weight-bearing epiphyses, are liable to produce extremely severe mutilations. On the other hand, the findings mentioned have been observed *prior to* the corticosteroid era. In those days they were interpreted as direct manifestations of the disease. Since the introduction of long-term steroid therapy, however, they have increased in frequency (Kölle, 1975).

In cases of juvenile chronic arthritis in which the roentgenogram is equivocal, the differential diagnostic considerations should—with full appreciation of the significance of the radiographic findings—be based on clinical findings.

Examples: Among the morbid manifestations of *disseminated lipogranulomatosis (Farber's disease)* are periarticular (nodular) swelling of soft tissues, impaired joint mobility, and juxtaarticular (juxtaepiphyseal) necroses of bone (Dihlmann, 1972). Without taking into consideration the clinical symptoms of this disease, which usually terminates fatally before the end of early childhood, the radiologic findings could be misinterpreted as manifestations of juvenile rheumatoid arthritis. Rheumatoid arthritis, however, is exceedingly rare in the first months of life, whereas Farber's disease occurs in the immediate postnatal period or at least in the first weeks or months of life. For the differential diagnosis between Farber's disease and congenital syphilis, see Fig. 405.

Childhood leukemias frequently give rise to monoarticular, oligoarticular, or polyarticular joint manifestations. The erroneous diagnosis of juvenile chronic arthritis suggests itself particularly in acute leukemias because the joint manifestations are usually among the first clinical signs and symptoms of this group of diseases (Spilberg and Meyer, 1972). The pathogenesis of the findings in the joints (pain, effusion, increased heat of the skin over the joint), in acute as well as in chronic leukemia, is referable to leukemic infiltrations in the synovial membrane, to hemorrhages into the joint capsule, and to subperiosteal infiltrates in the metaphysis. Figure 104 shows the *essential* roentgen findings in childhood leukemias inasmuch as they can give rise to joint complaints.

Patients with *psoriasis* are more frequently afflicted with chronic polyarthritis than the average population, the incidence of arthritis increasing with the duration of the disease. Such polyarthritis can clinically, serologically, and roentgenologically present the aspect of rheumatoid arthritis. Apart from this, psoriasis is associated with a specific reaction of the supporting and gliding tissues that has been termed **psoriatic arthritis.** This type differs clinically and roentgenologically from rheumatoid arthritis.

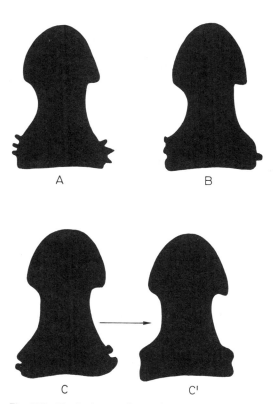

Fig. 105   Typical capsular and extracapsular "protuberances" in psoriatic arthritis (sketched in the base of the distal phalanx, A to C). C′ = Occasionally, protuberances are capable of regression or remodeling of the articulating parts of bone (in the case illustrated: base of the distal phalanx). Such remodeling is reminiscent of the deformations in osteoarthrosis.

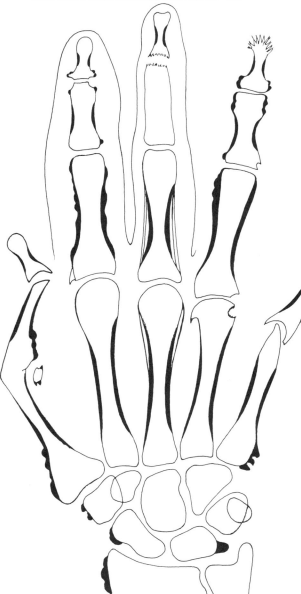

Fig. 106 **Synopsis of the possible roentgen findings in the hand during the course of psoriatic arthritis.**

Thumb (1st digit) = Concomitant occurrence of bony ankylosis and arthritic mutilation. Malposition of the joint. Periosteal reaction. New bone formation in the sesamoid bone of the MCP joint.

Index finger (2nd digit) = Erosive lesions and protuberances in the DIP joint, protuberance in the PIP joint. In the MCP joint, partial ossification of the joint capsule, starting from its insertion on the base of the proximal phalanx. *Undulating* metaphyseal and diaphyseal reaction on the part of the periosteum in the proximal phalanx. Sausage finger (compare the soft-tissue swelling of the entire finger with the normal contours of the 3rd finger).

Middle finger (3rd digit) = Small defect in the terminal tuft of the distal phalanx. Widened ("gaping") DIP joint space from extensive marginal resorption of bone with *denticulate* contours. *Lamellar* periosteal reaction, predominantly in the metaphysis and diaphysis of the proximal phalanx and the metacarpal. In the slightly coarsened middle phalanx—contrary to the other tubular bones of this digit—the cortex cannot be differentiated from the cancellous bone.

Ring finger (4th digit) = "Aspergillus aspect" due to osteolytic processes in the terminal tuft of the phalanx. Extensive fused protuberances in the DIP joint have led to coarsening of the articulating parts of the phalanx. In addition, the joint space is narrowed. Protuberance and erosion in the PIP joint. Erosions and narrowing of joint space in the MCP joint. Remodeling of the proximal phalanx into a so-called *bulbous phalanx*. The deformation develops when the periosteal new bone formation follows such protracted course that it at once fuses with the compacta and cannot be demarcated from the latter. A bulbous phalanx also occurs in gout, for instance.

Little finger (5th digit) = Bony ankylosis of the DIP joint. Erosions and narrowed joint space in the PIP joint. Mutilation and malposition of the MCP joint. Periosteal reactions and ossifying processes at the insertions of capsule, ligaments, and tendons on the base of the 5th metacarpal.

Carpus and its surroundings: Only ossifications of the insertions of capsule, ligaments, and tendons have been illustrated. The typical direct signs of arthritis (see Fig. 20), which can occur here as in any joint of the hand, have been omitted for the sake of clarity.

Note: In the present synopsis, the *predominance of the DIP joints* (so-called transverse type of manual involvement) and the *concordance of the DIP-PIP-MCP joint involvement* (so-called axial type of manual involvement) are not emphasized (compare Fig. 91) in order to present as nearly complete a picture as possible of the manifold roentgenographic findings in psoriatic arthritis.

Clinical Characteristics of Psoriatic Arthritis

Females and males are affected with about the same frequency. The rheumatoid factors in the serum are not encountered more frequently than among the average population (see p. 87); subcutaneous rheumatoid nodules are absent.

Psoriasis usually precedes the arthropathy; less frequently both diseases set in concomitantly. Even more infrequently, arthritis may be demonstrable prior to the affection of the skin *(prepsoriatic arthritis, psoriatic arthritis without psoriasis).* About every second patient reports an *acute* or *subacute* onset of the arthritis, not infrequently accompanied by local erythema and slight fever. Since, in addition, the initial attack of psoriatic arthritis is more frequently monoarticular or oligoarticular than polyarticular, the acute clinical symptomatology in small joints can be mistaken for a gouty attack or a felon.

Polyarticular joint manifestations of psoriatic arthritis are often not as symmetrical as in rheumatoid arthritis. Episodes of psoriasis and exacerbations of arthritis occur concomitantly in about 50 percent of patients. Sufferers from psoriatic arthritis frequently present a dermatologic aspect that differs from ordinary psoriasis (Braun-Falco and Rassner, 1969): involvement of the fingernails and toenails (pitting, "oil stains," subungual hyperkeratosis, crumbled nails, partial onycholysis, splinter hemorrhages) is observed with greater frequency. The morphology of psoriatic onychopathy evidently depends on the localization of the nail lesions (damage to the matrix, the nail bed, and/or the subungual layer). This accounts for the occasional difficulty in visually differentiating the nail involvement in psoriasis, in Reiter's syndrome and in onychomycosis. Nail lesions are encountered primarily in nails and toes whose interphalangeal joints are afflicted with arthritis *(vide infra).* The location and nature of the psoriatic effluorescences sometimes are atypical (palms, soles, skin folds, anogenital region; they often are pustular and pruritic, show little scaling and extend to erythroderma).

Radiographic Findings in Psoriatic Arthritis (Figs. 105 and 106)

1. Preferential involvement of the distal interphalangeal joints (DIP), including those of the thumb and the great toe at the onset or during the course of the disease *(DIP predominance,* also termed by this author the *transverse type* of psoriatic arthritis).
2. Concomitant involvement of the distal interphalangeal joints *and* the proximal interphalangeal joints (PIP) *and* the metacarpophalangeal (MCP) as well as the metatarsophalangeal joints (MTP) of one or more digits at the onset or during the course of the disease *(DIP-PIP-MCP-[MTP] concordance),* also termed by the author the *axial type* of psoriatic arthritis. From

the items 1 and 2 it can be inferred that psoriatic arthritis has a specific pattern of joint involvement (see Fig. 91).
3. Characteristically concomitant occurrence of osteodestructive *and* osteoproliferative joint lesions. The *resorption of cartilage and bone,* and thereby the destruction of the joint, evidently manifests itself by the direct signs of arthritis (narrowing of the radiographic joint space, alterations of the marginal subchondral lamella, erosions, arthritic geodes, etc.). Apart from this, extensive marginal resorption of bone in small joints sometimes leads to "widening of the joint space." The prognosis of psoriatic arthritis is unfavorable if mutilation and ankylosis, often in immediately contiguous joints, already occur within a few years, that is, early for a chronic arthritis (Moll and Wright, 1973). The concomitant occurrence of mutilation and ankylosis gives rise to the *irregular malposition* of the fingers that is frequently encountered in psoriatic arthritis. The *osteoproliferative processes* are demonstrable at the insertion of the joint capsule and its accessory ligaments as well as in the periosteum near the joint in the form of small new bone formations (Figs. 105 and 106). These have been termed in the literature protuberances (Schacherl and Schilling, 1967), spines, spicules, or spikes (Harvie et al., 1976).
4. *Psoriatic dactylitis* (Roberts et al., 1976). This term is meant to emphasize that not only are the joints of the hands and feet and their immediate neighborhood involved in psoriatic arthritis, but the disease is capable of producing lesions *remote from the joints.* Among the extraarticular findings are:

- "Sausage" fingers (sausage toes); i.e., a pronounced soft tissue swelling of the finger or toe with involvement of the tendon sheaths of the flexor muscles and accompanied by extraarticular edema
- *Extraarticular mutilation* (osteolysis) of the terminal tufts of the distal phalanx and/or (very infrequently) the metaphysis and diaphysis of the phalanx in cases where the epiphysis is preserved
- *Periosteal reactions in the metaphysis and diaphysis* (lamellae, undulations, bulbous appositions, club-shaped phalanx) and roentgenologically similar new bone formations at the anchorages of the tendon sheaths (Bywaters, 1979)
- *Dedifferentiation of cortical and cancellous bone* (Fig. 106, middle phalanx of third finger).

5. Juxtaarticular decalcification (see Collateral Phenomena of Arthritis) develops less frequently in psoriatic arthritis than, for example, in the subchondral layer of joints affected by rheumatoid arthritis. Even more infrequently, the phalanges present the very opposite of decalcification; namely, increased density *(ivory phalanx,* [Fig. 505]; Resnick and Broderick, 1977).

The foregoing roentgenologic differences between psoriatic and rheumatoid arthritis in the hands and feet are also demonstrable by light and electron microscope study (Rohe, et al., 1980). In addition, histologic findings in the extraarticular lesions of psoriatic arthritis in the hands and feet (Fassbender, 1979), as well as the results of nuclear medicine studies (Thiers et al., 1980), have supported the view that the extraarticular lesions in psoriasis evidence an involvement of bone that may occur with or without concomitant affection of the joints.

6. *Fibroosteitis* (see p. 73 ff; Fig. 79).
7. *Sacroiliitis of the "variegated picture" type* (see p. 490 ff), at the initial radiologic examination more frequently unilateral than bilateral. Depending on the duration of the disease, up to one third of the patients become affected.
8. Involvement of the axial skeleton *either* with the typical roentgenogram of ankylosing spondylitis (that is, bilateral sacroiliitis of the "variegated picture" type, syndesmophytes, box-shaped vertebrae etc. [p. 490 ff; 508]) *or* with the development of *psoriatic spondylitis*. This vertebral affection occurs either in association with a sacroiliitis of the "variegated picture" type or else without pathologic findings in the sacroiliac joints. The distinctive radiographic feature of this disease is the development of *parasyndesmophytes* (Dihlmann, 1968). These paravertebral and paradiscal new bone formations (Bywaters and Dixon, 1965) are visible in anteroposterior roentgenograms of the thoracicolumbar junction and the lumbar spine as well as in lateral roentgenograms of the cervical spine. The histocompatibility antigen HLA-B$_{27}$ (see under this heading), in patients with psoriatic arthritis, has proved to be a risk factor for the sacroiliac joints and the spine taking part in the disease process.

The description of the roentgen findings in psoriatic arthritis should be completed by the statement that the affection by this disease of *middle-sized* and *large* joints cannot, as a rule, be differentiated from the roentgen findings in rheumatoid arthritis. At most, juxtaarticular periosteal reactions and fibroosteitis occur with considerably greater frequency in psoriatic arthritis than in rheumatoid arthritis of adulthood.

Finally, the similarity or even identity of certain clinical and radiomorphologic findings in both psoriatic arthritis and Reiter's syndrome should be mentioned. This applies to the onychopathy and the psoriasiform skin lesions in Reiter's syndrome, the tendency of both diseases to induce periosteal reactions, and to fibroosteitis, to sacroiliitis of the "variegated picture" type (psoriatic spondylitis or spondylitis associated with Reiter's syndrome). The protuberances (spiculae, *vide supra*) of psoriatic arthritis also occur in Reiter's syndrome, though less frequently. Spiculae in the sense employed here also develop occasionally in gout.

Under the heading of *mucocutaneous syndromes* are grouped diseases whose principal manifestations are lesions of the skin and the mucous membranes. Officially, they also include Reiter's syndrome, but most important are **Stevens-Johnson syndrome** (the Stevens-Johnson type of erythema

multiforme with involvement of the skin and the mucous membranes) and **Behçet's disease** ("cutaneo-oculo-synovial syndrome") with painful ulcers of (1) the buccal mucosa, (2) the external genitals, and (3) ocular inflammations of which the most important pathologic lesions are anterior uvetis, iritis with hypopyon, and retinal vasculitis *(Behçet's triad)*. Among the various attendant manifestations of Behçet's disease—which, however, occur at most in every second patient—are to be mentioned the arthropathies, which range from arthralgia (possibly affecting numerous joints) to mono-, oligo-, or polyarthritis. Most frequently affected are the knee, the talocrural joints, and the joints of the hand (Mason and Barnes, 1969). The attendant arthritis in Behçet's disease usually runs its course without producing roentenologically demonstrable damage. (for exceptions see Vernon-Roberts et al., 1978).

Reiter's syndrome (Reiter's disease) occurs mainly in adult males and is characterized by the **classic triad:**

1. Nonbacterial urethritis (or inflammation of the urogenital organs),
2. Mucopurulent conjunctivitis, and
3. Seronegative mono-, oligo-, or polyarthritis.

This triad, which includes the most frequent symptoms and findings, has been termed classic because during the course of the (chronic, recurrent) Reiter's syndrome virtually any organ or tissue can be affected in addition. When certain skin manifestations (balanitis circinata, gonorrheal keratoderma, lesions of the oral mucosa, onychopathy) are superimposed on the main symptoms, one speaks of *Reiter's tetrad*. The disease sometimes follows an intestinal infection; it may develop within a few days or weeks after a bacillary dysentery, or an infection with *Salmonella* or *Yersinia*,[4] or it may occur subsequent to a gonorrheal or nongonorrheal urethritis. In such cases Reiter's syndrome has the character of a secondary disease. Sometimes it also occurs without a preceding disease. Arthritis of Reiter's syndrome affects primarily the joints of the *lower* extremities. In principle, however, any joint may be involved, including the joints of the hand. Direct signs of arthritis are to be expected primarily when the disease passes into a chronic stage (chronic recurrent course in about 50 percent of cases). It has already been mentioned that in both the peripheral joints and the axial skeleton there exist similarities or even identity between the roentgen findings in Reiter's syndrome and in psoriatic arthritis (see above). They also include the tendency to induce periosteal reactions (Fig. 107). See

---

[4] *Note: On the one hand,* an intestinal infection with *Yersinia enterocolitica* may be followed by Reiter's syndrome. *On the other,* there exists an acute (or subacute) oligo- or polyarthritis that immediately follows the *Yersinia*-induced diarrhea or occurs only a few days or weeks after the infection *(reactive* Yersinia *arthritis)* and which presupposes a genetic predisposition. In such patients the HLA-B$_{27}$ antigen is significantly elevated as compared with the "normal population" (Schilling, 1976). *Yersinia*-induced arthritis leads to serous joint effusions and is self limited, causing no permanent damage. The knee and the talocrural joint are frequently involved (Korting and Tröscher, 1978).

Fig. 107 **Reiter's syndrome in the hand.**
Subacute stage (for the past 3 weeks) = spotty demineralization in the vicinity of the diseased 2nd MCP joint, *lamellar* periosteal reaction of the 2nd proximal phalanx. Soft-tissue swelling.

Chronic stage (recurrences for a year) = erosions in the PIP joint of the 4th finger, juxtaarticular demineralization, soft-tissue swelling. Irregular periosteal reaction at the 4th proximal phalanx, erosions in the distal radioulnar joint and the styloid process of the ulna.

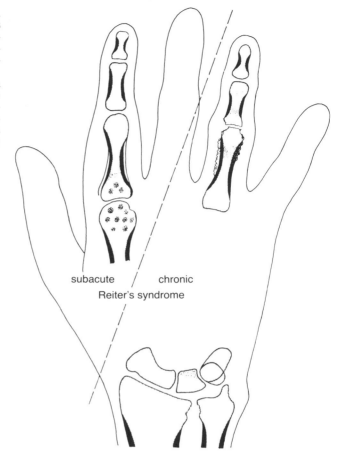

subacute / chronic
Reiter's syndrome

also under the headings of Fibroosteitis, Sacroiliitis, Spondylitis Associated with Reiter's Syndrome, and Ankylosing Spondylitis. Reiter's syndrome is a disease associated with HLA-B$_{27}$ (see under this heading).

A number of *chronic* intestinal diseases can be associated with joint manifestations. Among them are *ulcerative colitis, regional enteritis (Crohn's disease),* and *intestinal lipodystrophy (Whipple's disease).*[5] Since rheumatoid factors are not demonstrable and rheumatoid nodules do not occur in these concomitant joint diseases, they are not classified as instances of rheumatoid arthritis that accompany the intestinal diseases listed above. Rather, they are considered to be idiopathic clinical pictures (**"intestinal arthritis"**). *As a rule* there exist close temporal re-

lationships between the exacerbation or remission of regional enteritis or ulcerative colitis and the joint complaints, which sometimes improve or even regress following an intestinal resection.

Clinically, articular involvement manifests itself by arthralgia in a few or many joints, or a subacute migratory—sometimes even febrile—mono-, oligo-, or polyarthritis occurs, usually subsiding within a few weeks or months. In such cases, soft-tissue signs of arthritis (see under this heading) are to be expected. With a recurrent course or chronic manifestations, such an arthritis, especially one affecting the small joints of the extremities, collateral arthritic phenomena (see under this heading) or even direct roentgenologic signs of arthritis (see under this heading, Fig. 108) may be seen. This is also true of Whipple's disease (Staeffen et al., 1978).

In regional enteritis, noncaseating epithelioid cell granulomas are sometimes demonstrable in the synovial membrane of inflamed joints (Lindström et al., 1972). Another known characteristic of skeletal involvement in Crohn's disease is the tendency to induce periosteal reactions (Fig. 108). These occasionally have the aspect of hypertrophic osteoarthropathy

---

[5] Diarrheas with indistinct abdominal complaints, weakness and weight loss (as the results of malabsorption and steatorrhea), a dirty-gray complexion (pigment deposition), iron deficiency anemia, more or less extensive lymph node swelling, and joint discomfort are presumptive clinical evidence of the presence of Whipple's disease. The diagnosis is settled by the histologic demonstration of PAS-positive macrophages in the small intestinal mucosa, synovial cells, the bone marrow, the liver, and other organs.

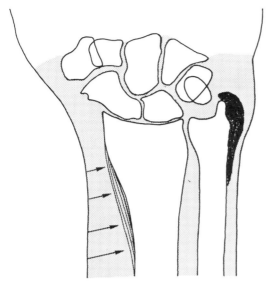

Fig. 108   Chronic intestinal arthritis in regional enteritis (Crohn's disease) (developing insidiously after the onset of the intestinal disorder. Rheumatoid factors not demonstrable).

Roentgen findings: In the radiocarpal joint, the joint space is narrowed and nearly absent, without causing any reaction. Erosions in the scaphoid and also in the styloid process of the ulna, due there to tenosynovitis of the extensor carpi ulnaris muscle *(particularly set off in the figure* but also *recognizable in the roentgenogram as a soft-tissue shadow).* Arrows = lamellar periosteal reaction, sometimes also occurring without arthritis of the neighboring joints. The periosteal new bone formation may fuse with the cortex. The cortex then seems to be more or less thickened.

(Marie-Bamberger syndrome; see under this heading), and in these cases they are accompanied by clubbing of the fingers and increased curvature of the nails. One of the peculiarities of the three types of intestinal arthritis listed is the occurrence of the "variegated picture" of sacroiliitis (p. 490 ff) which sometimes can develop into the full-blown picture of ankylosing spondylitis. Wright and Watkinson (1965) encountered inflammatory lesions of the sacroiliac joints in approximately every fifth patient with ulcerative colitis. In Crohn's disease, sacroiliitis is a less frequent event (observed by Mueller et al., 1974, in 10 percent of their cases). By and large the prognosis of sacroiliitis in the types of intestinal arthritis mentioned is favorable because the full-blown picture of ankylosing spondylitis develops much less frequently with these disorders than in ankylosing spondylitis *not* associated with intestinal disease (see under HLA-B$_{27}$).

Among the intestinal types of arthritis should also be mentioned the so-called *bypass arthritis* (Shagrin et al., 1971) and *arthralgia* or *arthritis* accompany-

ing the *carcinoid syndrome* (Solnica, 1976). Following intestinal (jejunoileal, jejunocolic) bypass surgery for the treatment of extreme obesity, polyarticular discomfort and even polyarthritis without demonstrable rheumatoid factors have been observed as complications. These disorders are accompanied by pain, more or less symmetrical swelling of joints, sometimes also by decalcification of the articulating bones or delicate erosions of the joint contours. In addition to this, a jejunoileal bypass can give rise to osteomalacia and secondary hyperparathyroidism (Compston et al., 1978). Joint symptoms and roentgen signs of arthritis can occur with carcinomas of the intestinal tract; these are probably precipitated by tumor metabolites.

Chronic arthritis of the small joints of the extremities in ankylosing spondylitis, occurring more frequently in the feet than in the hands, can present as a monarthritis, an asymmetrical oligoarthritis, or a seronegative polyarthritis. The following rule holds good: When the radiographic signs of chronic arthritis are encountered in one, two, or three *metacarpophalangeal* and/or *metatarsophalangeal joints,* while all the other joints of the extremities present a normal appearance, involvement of peripheral joints in an already known or not yet diagnosed ankylosing spondylitis should enter into the differential diagnosis (Fig. 109; compare p. 485), especially when male adolescents or young men are concerned.

Rheumatic fever (acute articular rheumatism) occurs as a delayed sequel of a throat infection with β-hemolytic group A streptococci, hence as a secondary disease. Among the classic findings is also an acute polyarthritis. *Clinically,* the latter manifests itself by a febrile, painful inflammatory infection that shifts from one joint to the other. *Serologically,* the significant rise in antistreptolysin O titer, which is demonstrable early in the disease, points to the pathogenetic importance of the preceding streptococcal infection. In recent years and decades, rheumatic fever not only has occurred less frequently but often also has pursued a modified clinical course. For example, it attacks only a few joints (oligoarticular instead of polyarticular involvement), or it assumes an attenuated form with fleeting joint discomfort (hence, minor exudative inflammatory manifestations). Thus, the physician is confronted with increasing difficulty in diagnosis. In rheumatic fever, radiologic study of diseased joints has no diagnostic importance because it would at most indicate an effusion into the joint. In rare cases, however, the acute episode or repeated recurrences are followed by a chronic disease picture in which radiologic studies are of definite value. Formerly, this evolution of the disease was termed "secondary chronic polyarthritis." At present, other eponyms are in use, such as **chronic streptococcal rheumatism, chronic rheumatic fever, chronic postrheumatic polyarthritis, Jaccoud's arthritis** or **Jaccoud's fibrotic rheumatism.** The diagnosis of this chronic type requires the following anamnesis and findings (Bywaters, 1950): rheumatic fever in the

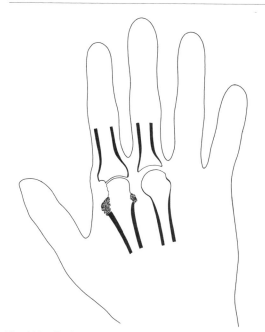

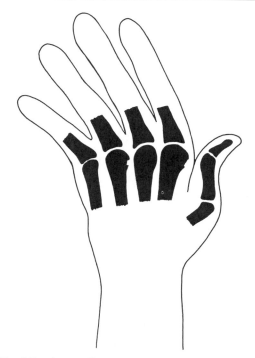

Fig. 109 **Patient with ankylosing spondylitis.** In the last few years pain and swelling in the metacarpophalangeal joint of the index finger and in several metarsophalangeal joints of both feet.

Roentgen finding in the right hand: Chronic arthritis of the 2nd metacarpophalangeal joint. Among other anomalies, there is a conspicuous, extensive, irregular periosteal reaction in the junction between metaphysis and diaphysis of the 2nd metacarpal.

Fig. 110 **Jaccoud's arthritis.** There is a striking discrepancy between *delicate* erosions in the metacarpal heads II and IV, as well as a slight narrowing of the joint space in the 5th metacarpophalangeal joint and the *pronounced* malpositions at these joints (ulnar deviation in the joints II to V, flexion and hyperextension at the joints of the thumb).

Characteristic radiographic features of Jaccoud's arthritis in small joints are, quite generally, the slight or absent destruction of the articulating bones *and* the striking malpositions of joints, which may even cause dislocations; they reflect the laxity of the fibrotic capsuloligamentous apparatus. Similar roentgen findings, however, may also be encountered in chronic involvement of joints accompanying disseminated lupus erythematosus (Fig. 111).

history, rheumatic endocarditis, elevated antistreptolysin titer.

Recurrent joint attacks develop into a chronic arthropathy that manifests itself primarily in the hand and less frequently also in the forefoot (Murphy and Staple, 1973). It causes little discomfort. The antistreptolysin titer shows marked elevation, particularly during a recurrence. An (acquired) valvular disease is clinically demonstrable. Jaccoud's arthritis is characterized by the discrepancy between the obvious physical findings (slight flexion and marked ulnar deviation at the metacarpophalangeal joints, more or less pronounced hyperextension at the proximal and distal interphalangeal joints, and even carpometacarpal and carpal malpositions, periarticular swellings) and the discrete pathologic roentgen findings in the subchondral bone (juxtaarticular decalcification and possibly delicate erosions in the metacarpal heads; see Fig. 110). Fibrotic capsular and periarticular processes (Girgis et al., 1978) outweigh a slight synovitis. For reasons of the roentgenologic differentiation, however, it should be mentioned that marked malpositions at small joints in the absence of destructive joint lesions may also occur in disseminated lupus erythematosus (Bywaters 1966; Russell et al., 1974) (Fig. 111).

The **classic collagen diseases** are disseminated (systemic) lupus erythematosus, polyarteritis (nodosa), progressive systemic sclerosis, and dermatomyositis (polymyositis). These diseases have been grouped together by Klemperer et al. (1942) under the name of "collagen diseases" because they reveal histologically a fibrinoid degeneration (fibrinoid necrosis) in the connectival intercellular substance (fibrils, ground substance). Considering the ubiquitous occurrence of the connectival intercellular substance and its limited reactivity, it might be expected that their common *staining* property would have caused very heterogeneous *clinical* entities to be grouped together. However, the classic collagen diseases present similarities between their clinical pictures and the serological findings as well as overlaps in their organic manifestations. Involvement of joints is an appropriate example.

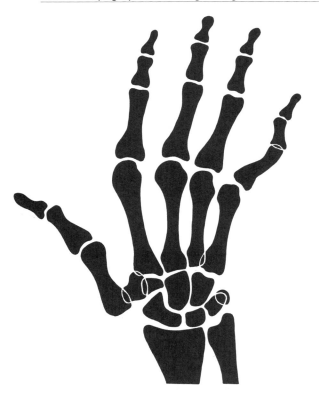

Fig. 111 **Disseminated lupus erythematosus** with malposition of joints of the hand but *without* erosive contour defects in the diseased joints.

Note: such predominance of severe malpositions of joints (in the hand and the foot), in contrast to normal or slightly eroded joint contours, occurs in disseminated lupus erythematosus and in Jaccoud's arthritis (Fig. 110). The Ehlers-Danlos syndrome also presents severe malpositions of joints, subcutaneous calcifications in necroses of adipose tissue, and roentgen signs of osteoarthrosis; for example, in the dislocated carpometacarpal joint of the thumb. Joint loosenings and the sequelae of attrition may (infrequently) be so marked that they give the impression of a neuropathic disintegration of joints—particularly in large joints of patients with the Ehlers-Danlos syndrome.

In **systemic lupus erythematosus,** predominantly a disease of women, the tolerance of the body to its own building elements, namely the protein of the cell nucleus, is impaired. Therefore, antinuclear autoantibodies against the native (double-stranded) deoxyribonucleic acid are demonstrable in this disease. About 90 percent of the patients complain of joint discomfort (Dubois and Tuffanelli, 1964) which appears as an initial symptom *or* concomitantly with other early manifestations of the disease *or* are reported by the patient at any time during the course of the disorder. The involvement of joints manifests itself either as clinically and roentgenologically nonobjectifiable arthralgia (polyarthralgia) or—in the majority of cases—as (poly-) arthritis. The arthritis primarily involves the joints of the hand and the knee. Even if the disease pursues a chronic course, it rarely produces erosive lesions in the joint contours. In this case the roentgen findings are similar to those obtained in rheumatoid arthritis (see under this heading). The following pathologic roentgen findings are encountered *in decreasing order of frequency* in the hands of patients with systemic lupus erythematosus: juxtaarticular decalcification, (peri-) articular swelling of soft tissues, acrosclerosis of the terminal tufts of the phalanges, (Weissmann et al. 1978), malposition of joints *without* erosive lesions (Fig. 111), calcifications of soft tissue (calcinosis), osteolysis of the terminal phalangeal tufts (concomitant clinical oc-

currence of Raynaud's phenomena such as intolerance to cold, episodes of painful disorders of circulation in the fingers with discoloration of the skin, avascular epiphyseal osteonecrosis with and without steroid therapy (Fig. 112), articular erosions, and narrowing of joint spaces.

Drug-induced (hence iatrogenic) systemic lupus erythematosis occurs with protracted (high-dose) administration of certain remedies; *for example* certain antihypertensive agents; antibiotics; chemotherapeutic substances; antiinflammatory, anticonvulsive, and anticonceptive agents; and following serotherapy (Rassner, 1966). Characteristically, the clinical symptomatology and the formation of autoantibodies gradually subside when the medication is discontinued. When, in rare cases, systemic lupus erythematosus persists, it is a matter of debate whether the previously latent disease has become activated by a certain drug.

Finally, *pseudolupus erythematosus* has been recognized. In this autoimmune disease, *antimitochondral* autoantibodies have been demonstrated. The disorder probably is due to the ingestion of certain drugs which in the meantime have been withdrawn (Flenker and Ricken, 1977).

Polyarteritis (nodosa) is a particular type of vasculitis that affects primarily middle-sized arteries and thereby impairs the function of the involved organ. These organs are, in decreasing order of frequency: kidneys, heart, intestinal tract, peripheral nervous system, *joints,* central nervous system, liver, lungs, pancreas, and skin. About every second patient complains of (poly-) articular discomfort or even

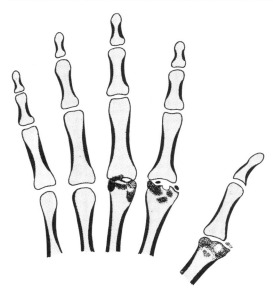

Fig. 112 Avascular epiphyseal necroses in the metacarpal heads I to III in disseminated lupus erythematosus.

During the course of this disease, one observes additional avascular necroses in the hand, particularly in the lunate and the triquetrum.

Radiographic characteristics: Deformation, disintegration, fragmentation, cystic translucences, increased density of bones.

(poly-) arthritis during the evolution of the disease. When polyarthritis develops, its radiographic manifestations are similar to those of rheumatoid arthritis. Further to be mentioned are painful periosteal reactions. Among the classic collagen diseases, such periosteal reactions occur most frequently in polyarteritis (see footnote on p. 34 and Fig. 514). Joint symptoms and/or roentgenologically identifiable joint lesions also occur in other types of vasculitis. Among these are *Wegener's granulomatosis* (granulomatous vascular necroses, primarily in the respiratory tract), *Schönlein-Henoch purpura* (most frequently involving the knee and the talocrural joints), *thrombotic thrombocytopenic purpura*, and *giant cell arteritis*.

Progressive systemic sclerosis (scleroderma) develops as an aftermath of inflammatory, fibrotic, and degenerative changes of the connective tissue and vascular lesions (frequently manifested by Raynaud's phenomena) in the skin and the subcutaneous tissues, the synovial membrane, various internal organs (esophagus and the remaining intestinal tract, lungs, heart, and kidneys), in the striated muscles, and in bones.

The *hand of the scleroderma patient* (Fig. 113) presents the following *classic* roentgen signs which, however, are *not* present *at the same time in every patient: Atrophy of soft tissues, osteolysis, osteoporosis, calcification of soft tissues,* and—in about one quarter of (temporarily hospitalized) patients—the roentgen signs of *seronegative or seropositive po-*

lyarthritis (Schacherl and Holzmann, 1967). Periosteal reactions also have been observed in progressive scleroderma.

Atrophy of the finger skin ("aclerodactyly") not only leads to obliteration of the physiologic folds but also contributes to stiffening of the fingers in pathologic flexion *(claw hand)*. The soft-tissue cover of the fingers has become, so to speak, too "tight." The atrophy of the soft tissues can be objectified *early* in the fingertips by using Yune's soft-tissue index (Fig. 114). In the advanced stage the involved finger has the shape of a sugar loaf (Fig. 114).

Nonreactive osteolysis occurs in the acral parts (terminal tufts of the fingers, styloid process of ulna and radius). In addition, apart from the hand, osteolyses occur in the acromion, the ribs (see Figs. 61 and 248), and the mandible. The periodontal cleft may be widened (see Fig. 587). Such nonreactive osteolyses also can originate in the subchondral layer of the joints (Fig. 113). In the initial stage it is difficult or impossible to differentiate such nonreactive osteolyses *in the roentgenogram* from early arthritic changes (Fig. 113). The same is true of the differential diagnosis by radiology between the nonreactive osteolysis sketched in Figure 113 (involving the interphalangeal joint of the thumb) and arthritic mutilation.

Decalcification of the hand skeleton manifests itself by diffuse or (less frequently) juxtaarticular increase in radiolucency.

Among the soft-tissue calcifications, localized (circumscribed) interstitial calcinosis predominates. Subcutaneous calcifications most frequently become apparent in the fingertips; i.e., an acral part. However, they are equally encountered in a periarticular location, less frequently, in an intraarticular location (Resnick et al., 1977), and over skeletal prominences. The calcium spots usually appear in clusters; sometimes they form larger conglomerates (Fig. 113) or extend into universal interstitial calcinosis.

The association of progressive scleroderma with soft-tissue calcifications is termed *Thibierge-Weissenbach syndrome*. The term *CRST syndrome* is applied to the combination of *C*alcinosis, *R*aynaud's phenomena (paroxysmal vasospasms), *S*clerodactyly, and *T*elangiectasias (Winterbauer, 1964). This syndrome, however, has also been observed in disseminated lupus erythematosus (Saporta et al., 1978). *CREST syndrome* corresponds to CRST syndrome plus additional esophageal involvement.

Joint discomfort in patients with progressive scleroderma can be produced by nonobjectifiable (poly-) arthralgias. Roentgen signs of chronic polyarthritis are depicted in Figure 113. Such polyarthritis is said to correspond histologically to a synovitis without pannus formation which gradually develops into a massive synovial fibrosis (Rodnan, 1962; Schumacher Jr., 1973). This synovial fibrosis is in part responsible for the impairment of motion and the stiffening of the joints in the hand of the scleroderma patient *(vide supra)*. Occasional difficulty in differentiating *roentgenologically* incipient subchrondral

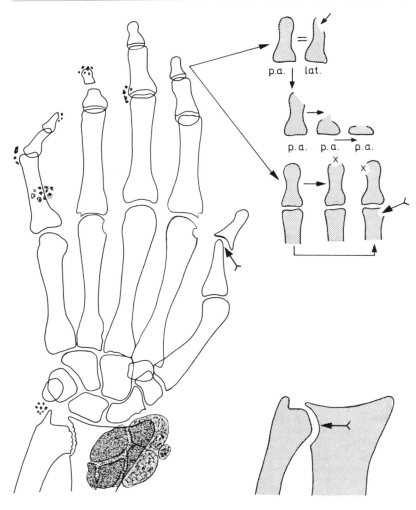

Fig. 113 **Hand in scleroderma.** Nonreactive osteolyses and acroosteolyses. At x small "rat-bite defects"; i.e., very incipient acroosteolyses. Localized interstitial calcinosis (partly crumbly, partly lumpy). Flexion contractures of the fingers and roentgen signs of chronic polyarthritis (metacarpophalangeal joints II and IV, carpometacarpal joint III, intercarpal joints, radioulnar joint).

The *Tailed arrows* point to contour defects which, without additional soft-tissue signs and/or collateral phenomena of arthritis, cannot be differentiated *in the roentgenogram* from nonreactive osteolyses!

Note: Acroosteolysis of the terminal phalanges usually begins on the *volar* side of the terminal phalangeal tuft (see above right). The detail *above right* also shows the different stages of acroosteolysis in the terminal phalanges. About one third of the patients with progressive scleroderma present pathologic roentgen findings in the hand (erosive contour lesions and/or soft-tissue calcifications) as early as the first 6 months of the disease (Yune et al., 1971).

nonreactive osteolysis from erosive arthritic contour defects has already been mentioned (Fig. 113). The *clinical* differentiation in the initial stage sometimes is fraught with similar possibilities of error because in rheumatoid arthritis "pseudosclerodermal" skin manifestations are apt to occur.

Progressive scleroderma starting *in childhood* sometimes interferes locally—in the immediate vicinity of the skin lesions—with the longitudinal growth of tubular bones and can give rise to the development of hypoplastic bones (e.g., the clavicle or the acromion) (Wolf et al., 1970).

Dermatomyositis (polymyositis) also belongs to the classic collagen diseases. In the forefront of the *clinical* picture is muscular weakness which in some cases is accompanied by spontaneous muscular pain or stiffness of the symmetrically involved muscles. Muscular atrophy and contractures also occur.

The disease most frequently affects the proximal muscles of the upper and lower extremities, hence those near the pelvic and shoulder girdle. The nuchal and the pharyngeal muscles (dysphagia, dysphonia) are also involved. The inflammatory disintegration of striated muscle fibers can be evidenced chemically (by enzyme tests), histologically, and by electromyographic examination. In the majority of cases the muscular phenomena are accompanied by skin manifestations; e.g., periorbital edema, erythema, and dark red discoloration (over the elbows, the knuckles, the knee joints, and the medical malleoli). These skin lesions are usually slightly elevated and may be scaly; the condition then is termed *dermatomyositis*. In polymyositis, the skin manifestations are absent. It is extremely infrequent for the characteristic skin lesions to occur *without* muscular signs and symptoms.

Among the possible attendant manifestations of

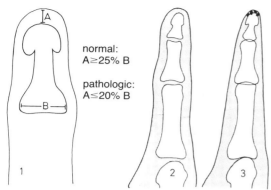

Fig. 114   1 = **Yune's soft-tissue index** for the early evidence of soft-tissue atrophy in the fingertips of patients with progressive scleroderma (Yune et al., 1971).

2 = **Normal** soft tissue contours of a finger.

3 = **"Sugarloaf" configuration** of the soft tissues of a finger in progressive scleroderma. (In addition, slight flexion contracture of the finger joints; see text). Soft-tissue atrophies in the fingertips are encountered in progressive scleroderma as well as in Raynaud's syndrome. The combined occurrence of soft-tissue atrophy of the fingertips plus calcium deposits in the soft tissues of the fingertips, however, is characteristic of scleroderma!

dermatomyositis (polymyositis) are vascular disorders (which may be accompanied by Raynaud's phenomena), pulmonary fibrosis, myocardial and pericardial involvement, hypomotility and hypotonicity of the esophagus and the small intestine, (poly-) arthralgia, and even (poly-) arthritis, calcinosis, and osteoporosis which may be diffuse or only juxtaarticular (Fig. 115). Periosteal reactions and acroostelolyses in the fingers are infrequent events. (Poly-) arthritis is mostly fugitive and manifests itself in the roentgenogram by the soft-tissue signs of arthritis. When the arthritis pursues a chronic course, collateral phenomena, soft-tissue signs, and direct signs of arthritis are observed. Circumscribed interstitial calcinoses occur in the hypoderm and even in deeper tissue planes. Therefore, they often present a crumbly, reticular or striated radiologic picture and may extend to universal interstitial calcinosis.

Calcinoses are seen in *juvenile* dermatomyositis (starting before the age of 16) with considerably greater frequency than when the disease begins in adulthood. Spontaneous regression of such soft-tissue calcifications has occasionally been observed (Sewell et al., 1978). In juvenile dermatomyositis, *local* disturbances of growth and development occur in bones and joints. These disturbances result from local muscular contractures (hence: immobilization joint, see the legend accompanying Figure 398; Ozonoff and Flynn Jr., 1973). In extreme cases, dermatomyositis-induced dwarfism may ensue (Canigiani and Zweymüller, 1972, see p. 93). About 15 percent of all

patients with dermatomyositis (polymyositis) acquire a malignant tumor during the course of the disease (Williams Jr., 1959). In patients beyond the age of 40, the incidence of tumors increases. It is rare for dermatomyositis (polymyositis) to develop in the presence of a preexisting tumor. The tumors gener-

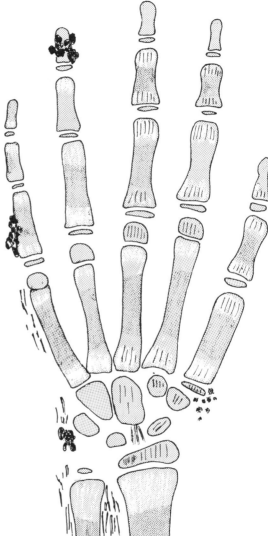

Fig. 115   **Dermatomyositis** (of 4 years' duration) in a child.

Pathologic roentgen findings: Demineralization *(osteoporosis)* primarily of cancellous bone (therefore giving the impression of being "joint-related") presenting a *fibrillar* character (so-called *hypertrophic atrophy of bone;* see the legend accompanying Fig. 13). The demineralization, however, may also be *uniform* and "joint-related" (see the two ulnar digits). Localized interstitial calcinosis in the hypoderm and the deeper soft-tissue planes (striated arrangement).

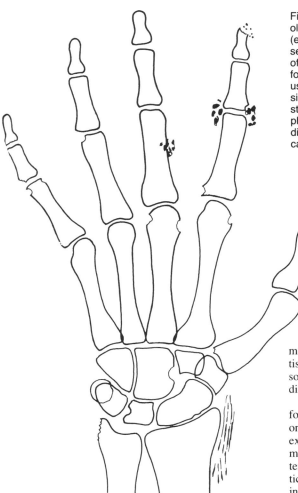

Fig. 116 **Sharp's syndrome** (diagnosis assured serologically). The demonstrable chronic polyarthritis (erosions, joint space narrowing, malpositions) presents the pattern of manual involvement characteristic of rheumatoid arthritis (compare Fig. 91). However, the following pathologic roentgen findings, which are unusual for rheumatoid arthritis, invite attention: Malpositions at joints without erosive lesions, localized interstitial calcinosis, acroosteolysis of the terminal phalangeal tuft of the index finger. Therefore the radiologist inquired of the referring physician whether the case might be one of mixed connective tissue disease.

ally occur in organs (bronchi, male and female genitalia, breast, colon, etc.). Sometimes the secondary disease is a malignant lymphoma or a leukemic blood disorder.

The preceding description of the *clinical* signs and symptoms as well as the roentgenologic changes reveals that "overlaps" are apt to occur in the classic collagen diseases; i.e. that individual or even several manifestations may occur in different diseases. However, the term **"mixed connective tissue disease (MCTD, Sharp's syndrome)** has been employed only since Sharp and his colleagues (1972) have described a *serologically defined* mixed picture of different classic collagen diseases (consisting principally of the manifestations of disseminated lupus erythematosus, progressive scleroderma, and polymyositis, associated with joint discomfort, Fig. 116). The Sharp syndrome is characterized by an elevated titer of specific antinuclear autoantibodies directed, among other substances, against ribonuclease-sensitive extractable antigens of the cell nucleus. The joint discomfort

manifests itself by (poly-) arthralgia or (poly-) arthritis. When the polyarthritis runs a chronic course associated with erosions, it cannot be radiologically differentiated from rheumatoid arthritis.

Concerning the classic collagen diseases, the following summary will be useful: The diagnosis of one of these diseases should be contemplated by the examiner when a roentgenologically demonstrable mono-, oligo-, or polyarticular arthritis is encountered in a patient who presents the following extraarticular manifestations or who reports their occurrence in the recent past: pleuritis, pericarditis, skin changes, soft-tissue calcifications, neurologic deficits, leukopenia, leukocytosis, eosinophilia, proteinuria, hematuria.

Primary biliary cirrhosis of the liver is a disease that preferentially attacks females and reveals the presence of antimitochondral antibodies. It is frequently associated with autoimmune diseases, such as Sjögren's syndrome or rheumatoid arthritis. The *suggestive clinical constellation* is therefore: *female patient, chronic pruritus, elevated alkaline phosphatase in the serum, antimitochondral antibodies and/or increased IgM immunoglobulin level*. Roentgenologically recognizable joint lesions have been observed primarily in the hand and the knee joint (O'Connell and Marx, 1978). The distal and the proximal interphalangeal joints—less frequently the metacarpophalangeal joints, the carpal region and the styloid process of the ulna—present soft-tissue swelling, marginal erosions, and narrowing of the joint space, generally in asymmetrical distribution. Roentgenologic differentiation from (seropositive) rheumatoid arthritis is not possible without the following *additional finding:* In addition to the radiologic findings described, osteoporosis (not related to the joints) has been observed, as well as osteomalacia, which may present the typical roentgenologic characteristics of malabsorptive secondary hyperparathyroidism (see under this heading). Hypercholesterolemia belongs to the clinical spectrum of primary biliary cirrhosis of the liver. This may be in relation to soft-tissue xanthomas and intraosseous cholesterol deposits which lead to flat-arched erosions on and inside the diaphyses of tubular bones, and to osteolyses in the spongiosa (see p. 141 f).

Recurrent polychondritis is a systemic disease of cartilage that often runs an episodic febrile course. Clinically, it is manifested by an inflammatory process in cartilaginous structures (gelling, hyalinization, asbestoslike degeneration, amounting to cartilage necrosis). Fiber-forming granulation tissue penetrating from the inflamed, infiltrated perichondrium replaces the destroyed cartilage (Jensen and Jensen, 1967; Johnson et al., 1973, Bachmann et al., 1976). During the evolution of the disease, noncartilaginous tissues (organs) also are involved; for example the eye (inflammation of the conjunctiva, cornea, sclera, iris, ciliary body, uvea), the audiovestibular apparatus (impaired hearing increasing to deafness, labyrinthine vertigo), and the heart (endocarditis, myocardial infarction, pericarditis). Among the leading symptoms and clinical stigmata of recurrent polychondritis are bilateral painful inflammation of the pinna (resulting in "cauliflower ears," "washcloth ears," possibly with *calcifications*. Etiologic differential diagnosis of calcifications of the pinna: trauma, repetitive trauma in boxers, frostbite, Addison's disease, gout, pseudogout [chondrocalcinosis], ochronosis, acromegaly, diabetes mellitus, hyperparathryroidism [Chune-Woo Yeh and Chan, 1979]). In addition, the following important diagnostic characteristics are known: nasal chondritis ("saddle nose"), involvement of the respiratory tract (e.g., hoarseness in affection of the larynx) as well as signs and symptoms suggesting a manifestation of polychondritis in the articular cartilage, the epiphsyeal cartilages, and the intervertebral disks (Thould et al., 1965, Spritzer et al., 1969). Such manifestations are low back pain, reduced respiratory excursions of the thorax, and increasing stiffness (requiring differentiation from ankylosing spondylitis). Articular involvement manifests itself clinically by arthralgia or seronegative oligoarthritis or polyarthritis, less frequently by monoarthritis. The arthritis attacks larger and smaller joints. It lasts from a few days to a number of weeks; its course is generally intermittent and, infrequently, chronic.

The arthritis manifests itself *roentgenologically* by the corresponding soft tissue signs (see under this heading) and by the collateral inflammatory phenomena (juxtaarticular osteoporosis). It is less likely that the disease give rise to narrowing of the radiographic joint space and erosions (Gordon et al., 1948; Harders, 1954; Johnson et al., 1973).

An important point to remember is that about one third of the polychondritis patients suffer *concomitantly* from inflammatory rheumatic affections or an autoimmune disease (McAdam et al., 1976). It must be emphasized again that it is not the (radiographic) findings in the joints but primarily the inflammation of the pinna and the nasal chondritis that are the decisive hallmarks of the disease.

The infrequent disease picture of **palindromic arthritis** (palindromic rheumatism, Hench and Rosenberg, 1944) (*palin* = again; *dromos* = course) in about 90 percent of the cases follows a monarticular course. This illness sets in acutely and recurs at irregular intervals. Each episode lasts only a few hours or a number of days. Frequent seats of the disorder are the knee joints, the finger joints, and the joints of the hands. However, any other joint of the extremities, the temporomandibular and the sternoclavicular joints, and the cervical spine may be affected. The radiologist should be familiar with this entity because—for example, in the finger joints—the (peri-) articular swelling of the soft tissues can also be recognized in the roentgenogram and because, on the other hand, a supposed palindromic rheumatism not infrequently turns out during the further course to be a (seropositive) rheumatoid arthritis of atypical onset

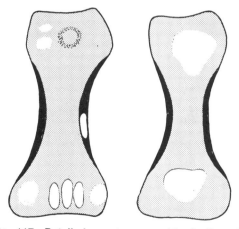

Fig. 117 Detailed roentgenographic findings in sarcoidosis of small tubular bones.
Circular, oval, and *heart shaped* osteolyses with and without marginal sclerosis, located chiefly in the epiphysis and metaphysis.

Note: Even in the patient with sarcoidosis, a single cystic osteolysis of the type illustrated does not prove skeletal sarcoidosis. In view of the systemic character of the disease, the findings sketched may be expected in the *majority* of patients with skeletal sarcoidosis. For the radiologic differential diagnosis see for example Lagier (1975). This writer illustrates remodeling processes in individual phalanges which correspond to the roentgen findings sketched here and in Figure 118. The radiologic differential diagnosis must also be made from enchondroma, fibrous dysplasia, advanced hyperparathyroidism, and tuberous sclerosis. (In tuberous sclerosis, not only cystic translucences but also trabecular, latticed, or honeycomb changes of structure are encountered in the small tubular bones, see Fig. 118 [Psenner and Schönbauer, 1958]).

(Mattingly, 1969). Apart from this, the condition has to be differentiated from disseminated lupus erythematosus, gout, and pseudogout (its so-called distant type, see Fig. 68).

The **reactive types of arthritis** are, as the term indicates, the expression of a mono-, oligo-, or polyarticular affection of joints. Frequently the symptoms are only fleeting; they are the result of an *allergic* or *toxic* reaction that may be systemic or limited to the synovial membrane. The causative offenders can be viruses, bacteria, protozoa, or parasites, but also endogenous tissues (for example of neoplasms, particularly of the pancreas) or foreign substances (drugs, chemical additives, etc.) *The pathogens are not demonstrable in the joint.* Postenteritic and post urogenital infection reactive arthritis is indicated by a high incidence of HLA-B_{27} and carries the risk to develop into sacroiliitis and ankylosing spondylitis respectively. In cases of HLA-B_{27} negative reactive arthritis, one should not expect in these cases to encounter pronounced pathologic findings; when the proximal or distal interphalangeal joints are involved, one notices a fusiform swelling that is demonstrable in the roentgenogram as well as on inspection and palpation. The same is true of other effusions in joints.

For **sympathetic arthritis** see p. 161 ff.

Skeletal sarcoidosis reflects the involvement of the supporting and gliding tissues in this systemic granulomatous affection of mesenchymal tissues. Histologically it is characterized by a noncaseating epitheloid cell granulomatosis. Particularly in the literature of the German-speaking countries, the disorder is also termed *"Boeck's disease,"* and skeletal sarcoidosis (of the small tubular bones) is named *"Jüngling's disease.* The epitheloid cell granulomas originate in the synovial membrane. In the bone marrow they may give rise to an acute, subacute, or chronic inflammation (synovitis, arthritis). In some cases of sarcoidosis-dependent arthritis, however, histologic study does not demonstrate synovial granulomas but only a nonspecific inflammatory synovitis. Occasionally, the joint involvement in sarcoidosis manifests itself only by a nonobjectifiable (poly-) arthralgia. When the sarcoid granulomas of the bone marrow expand, they give rise to osteolyses and (less frequently) to reactive osteoplastic changes. The skeleton is involved in about 15 percent of the sarcoidosis patients, there are also statistical reports on higher or lower incidences (Bouvier et al., 1972; Uehlinger and Wurm, 1976). Most reports on skeletal sarcoidosis so far have referred to the small tubular bones with the adjacent joints of the hands and feet. Less frequently, reports have been given on sarcoidosis of the carpal and tarsal bones, the long tubular bones, and the vertebrae.

Acute (subacute) sarcoidosis—Löfgren's syndrome—frequently starts with a rise in temperature and joint discomfort consisting of either polyarthralgia or a transient polyarthritis, often flitting from joint to joint. The arthritis frequently affects first and symmetrically the talocrural and knee joints and then also spreads to other joints; e.g., those of the hands and feet. A (tender) erythema nodosum (preferentially in the lower leg) precedes or follows the joint complaints. A roentgenogram of the thorax should be ob-

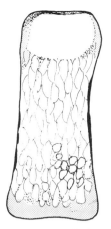 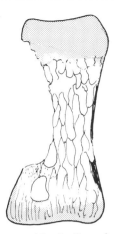

Fig. 118 Detailed roentgenographic findings in sarcoidosis of small tubular bones (continued). Remodeling of shape and structure (coarsening, expansion, wasting of the compacta; reticular, latticed, and honeycombed structures; marginal contour defects).

tained in every case of erythema nodosum. When the clinical symptoms described are accompanied by bilateral enlargement of the hilar lymph nodes, the presence of sarcoidosis is almost certainly established and the (most frequent) erroneous diagnosis of rheumatic fever is proved incorrect.

Joint complaints in *chronic sarcoidosis* also may be characterized by fleeting polyarthralgia, oligoarthritis, or polyarthritis; acute involvement of a single joint can mimic a gouty attack. Infrequently, an insidious or episodic seronegative chronic arthritis develops which, in the hands and feet, may present the radiologic picture of rheumatoid arthritis.

Involvement of bones becomes clinically the more manifest by localized swelling and redness, the younger the patient is. In early childhood, for instance, the diaphyses of the small tubular bones are not yet equipped with a marrow cavity but, instead, with coarse-meshed cancellous bone that impedes the expansion of the epitheloid cell granulomas less than cortical bone. The same is true of syphilitic and tuberculous osteomyelitis—(tuberculous) spina ven-

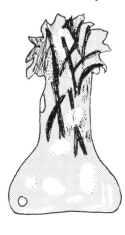

Fig. 119 Detailed roentgenographic findings in sarcoidosis of small tubular bones (continued). *Incipient* acroosteolysis in the terminal phalangeal tuft, trabecular remodeling of structure, small cystic osteolyses.

tosa—and the lesions of the small tubular bones in certain hemoglobinopathies, such as sickle cell anemia and thalassemia major (Cooley's anemia).

Most of the roentgen findings in sarcoidosis of the small tubular bones have already been described by Jüngling (1919–21, 1928) as ostitis (tuberculosa) multiplex cystica (cystoides). They are depicted in the Figures 117 through 120. The cystoid osteolyses, especially, are potentially reversible.

The lodging of bacteria in the gliding tissue of the hand gives rise to infection of the joint **(infectious arthritis)**. This condition may be hematogenous, propagated by extension from the surrounding soft tissues or bone, or it may develop after opening of the joint. The more acute the onset and the more pronounced the systemic manifestations, the more

probable is an infection of the joint by pyogenic pathogens **(pyogenic arthritis)**.

Rule I: The radiologic progression of a pyogenic infection is assessed at intervals of days and weeks. The more insidious the onset and the evolution, the greater the suspicion of tuberculosis of the joint.

Rule II: The progression of a tuberculous infection of the joint is assessed at intervals of months and years. On the other hand, the acute clinical picture of pyogenic arthritis can be obscured when a bacterial infection is superimposed on an inflammatory rheumatic arthropathy that is being treated locally or systemically with corticosteroids.

In the hand, pathogens most frequently become lodged in the carpal region and in the immediately contiguous joints (Fig. 121). In the finger joints, py-

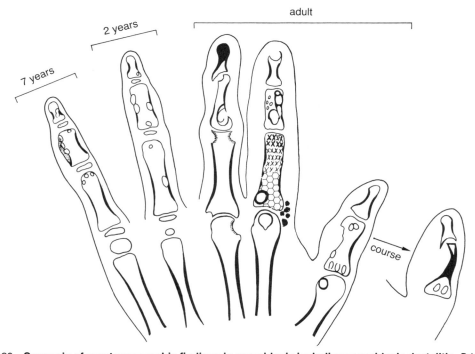

Fig. 120   **Synopsis of roentgenographic findings in sarcoidosis including sarcoidosis dactylitis.** *Primarily osseous* and *Primarily synovial* lesions are illustrated here side by side although the *concomitant* occurrence of these signs of sarcoidosis is the exception rather than the rule. Roentgen signs of the (infrequent) chronic sarcoid polyarthritis are illustrated in the metacarpophalangeal and proximal interphalangeal joints of the 3rd finger.

Osseous roentgen signs: Cystlike, heart-shaped, or oval, sharply demarcated translucences, prevalently in the juxtaarticular segments of bone, possibly also in the diaphysis (in children more frequently than in adults). Cystic osteolyses may invade the joint and give rise to articular destruction (see distal interphalangeal joint of 3rd finger). Larger epitheloid cell granulomas may also lead to (acro-) osteolyses of the terminal phalangeal tuft (see 2nd finger). Acroosteosclerosis of the distal phalanges (see 3rd finger) is said to occur with greater frequency in sarcoidosis patients than in the average population (compare Fig. 93; McBrine and Fisher, 1975). Marginal, initially cystic osteolyses may lead to extensive defects (mutilations; see proximal phalanx of thumb) or, in children, also to a periosteal reaction (middle phalanx of little finger). With diffuse involvement (proximal and middle phalanges of index finger), the shaft becomes expanded, the cortex thinned, and the bone sometimes undergoes reticular, latticed, honeycombed, or trabecular remodeling (proximal phalanx of index finger). The soft-tissue swelling then surrounds the shaft or spreads to the entire finger ("sausage finger"; see index finger, dactylitis). Symptomatic calcifications of soft tissues, which are liable to occur in sarcoidosis, have been sketched in the metacarpophalangeal joint of the index finger.

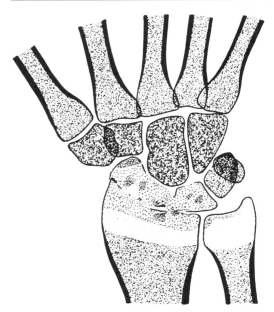

Fig. 121 **Metastatic pyogenic joint infection** follow-ing acute purulent tonsillitis. Initially, the condition was treated as a reactive arthritis. Only about 3 weeks later did the radiologically demonstrable arthritis of the ra-diocarpal joint provide a clue to the correct diagnosis.
Radiographic finding: Joint space between ra-dius, scaphoid, and lunate has largely disappeared. The partial wasting of the marginal subchondral lamella of the scaphoid and the lunate in the mediocarpal joint indicates that this joint, too, has already become af-fected by the infective arthritis. Diffuse decalcification of the metaphyseal bone, partly spotty and band-shaped in the radius (collateral phenomenon of arthritis). The distal ulna participates in the decalcification.

ogenic infections usually occur only after opening of the joint or as an extension of suppurative processes in the neighboring soft tissues and bones (Fig. 122). Figure 123 illustrates a *rule* for the radiologic differ-entiation between a bacterial infection of the carpus and an inflammatory rheumatic arthritis of the carpus that starts unilaterally (hence atypically).

In (acute) pyogenic arthritis, the soft-tissue signs *predominate initially* (Fig. 124). Tuberculosis of the joint presents considerable subchondral decalcifica-tion *early in the disease* (see p. 11 f); swelling of the soft tissues is less conspicuous. As a matter of prin-ciple, however, in both pyogenic (nontuberculous) and tuberculous infections of the joint the *extent to which the joint and the bone are destroyed* depends on when the diagnosis is established and adequate therapy is instituted.

In **gonorrhea,** various joint complications are known to occur. The pathogens migrate to the joint by way of the bloodstream (prevalently monarticular involvement). The arthritis sets in three or more weeks after the venereal infection. The joints of the wrist are among the preferred sites of gonorrheal arthritis.

If gonococci are not demonstrable in the syn-ovial fluid of the diseased joint, one is dealing either with a para- or postinfectious reactive arthritis (see p. 106) *or* an incipient postgonorrheal Reiter's syn-drome! Besides this, there also exists a gonococcal septicemia with polyarticular manifestations.

Primary synovial and **primary osseous tuber-culosis of joints** (Figs. 125–127) in the wrist, the metacarpus, and the fingers are outright types of adult tuberculosis. Primary synovial tuberculosis of joints usually follows a more insidious course, sparing the contours and structures to a greater extent than pri-mary osseous tuberculosis, which progresses more rapidly (Kastert and Uehlinger, 1964). This type is frequently accompanied by tuberculosis of the tendon sheaths in this area.

A differential diagnostic clue to the tuberculous etiology of an arthritis can be provided by the pa-tient's anamnesis; for example, a history of exudative pleurisy or extraskeletal tuberculosis (of the urogen-ital tract, for instance). One should in every case aim at settling the tentative diagnosis of tuberculous arthritis by histologic or microbiologic studies. **Synovial** or **osseous (gummatous) arthritis of late syphilis** should be ruled out by serological tests. The same rules apply to the infrequent articular, mostly endemic, **fungal infections;** e.g. coccidioidomyco-sis, sporotrichosis, histoplasmosis, mycetoma (mad-uromycosis), cryptococcosis (torulosis), and asper-

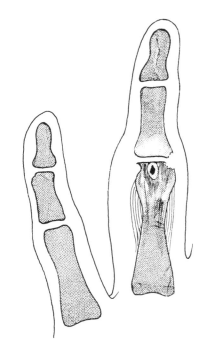

Fig. 122 **Pyogenic arthritis of the proximal inter-phalangeal joint** propagated by extension from a se-questrating osteomyelitis and periostitis of the proximal phalanx of the 4th finger.

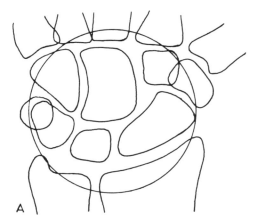

A

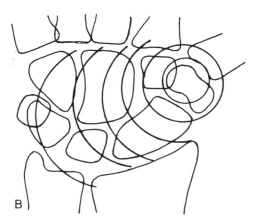

B

Fig. 123 **Radiologic differential diagnosis be-tween (unilateral) inflammatory rheumatic carpal arthritis and bacterial infection of the carpus** (compare Fig. 163). A = The inflammatory rheumatic process involves all carpal joints more or less simultaneously from the outset. B = In the early and intermediate stages of bacterial infection, a "center of destruction" that spreads successively is demonstrable.

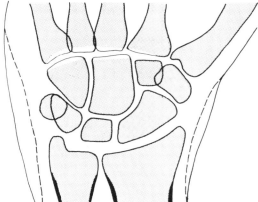

Fig. 124 **Pyogenic carpal arthritis** of 10 days' standing. Three radiologic findings suggest that the arthritis is pyogenic and neither tuberculous nor inflammatory rheumatic: (1) *Marked* soft-tissue swelling *(normal contours dashed).* (2) Slight band-shaped subchondral decalcification that (3) occurs "focally" (capitate, hamate, metacarpals II to V; also note the narrowing of the marginal subchondral lamella in these bones and the corresponding joints).

gillosis. These fungal infections of joints develop, as a rule, either by direct extension from a subchondral osseous lesion or by metastatic involvement of the synovial membrane.

In addition, prior to diagnosing a primary osseous tuberculous arthritis of the wrist, avascular osteonecrosis of the lunate and the scaphoid must be differentiated, as the possible disuse atrophy of the surrounding bones may be misinterpreted as a collateral arthritic phenomenon. **Viral infections** give rise, on the one hand, to a *reactive (symptomatic) arthritis* (see p. 106) and, on the other, to a *viral arthritis* in which the offenders are demonstrable in the joint effusion. The self-limited *arthritis of rubella,* for instance, occurs in connection with rubella infection or immunization. It primarily affects the joints of the

hand. In contrast, *arthritis from mumps*—likewise a self-limited condition—usually affects larger joints but occasionally also the joints of the hands and feet. The viral arthritis that accompanies or follows smallpox (it also may occur after vaccination) is the result of *smallpox-induced osteomyelitis* (p. 161). It can give rise to growth disturbances of the joint-bearing epiphyses (destruction, premature closure). Bacterial superinfection, as an additional complication of smallpox, destroys the joints and the articulating bones. Finally, there also exists a *reactive smallpox arthritis.*

Osteoarthrosis

Osteoarthrotic lesions of the hand are usually *polyarticular* and *bilaterally symmetrical*. It has been established that this polyosteoarthrotic condition, which affects climacteric and menopausal females with much greater frequency than males, is a heritable disease.[6] In the region of the hand, it manifests itself chiefly in the distal interphalangeal (DIP) joints (Figs. 128, 129, and 131), often concomitantly in the carpometacarpal joint of the thumb (Figs. 128 and 131), the proximal interphalangeal (PIP) joints (Figs. 129 and 131), and, less frequently, the metacarpophalangeal (MCP) joints (Figs. 130 and 131). Occasionally, roentgen signs of osteoarthrosis are also demonstrable in the articulat-

[6] Strictly speaking, this is true only for osteoarthritis of the *distal* interphalangeal joints.

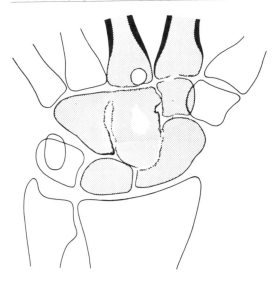

Fig. 125 **Primary osseous tuberculosis of the joints of the wrist and its surroundings.** The hematogenous focus was probably located in the capitate (the *diseased parts of bones and joints are shaded*). The condition must be differentiated from bacterial nontuberculous arthritis and from original carpal osteomyelitis (biopsy!).

Fig. 126 **Tuberculosis of the wrist.** Because of the advanced stage, one cannot determine whether the process is primarily synovial or primarily osseous. The marked inhomogeneous demineralization is striking. Few persisting differences in blackening between the soft tissues and the demineralized bone. Individual carpal bones can still be demarcated by the partly preserved (noncalcified or resorbed) marginal subchondral lamella (for example, the triquetrum). Other bones, among them the scaphoid, show little demineralization and therefore are recognizable. (The *darker the hue in the sketch, the more calcium the bone contains*).

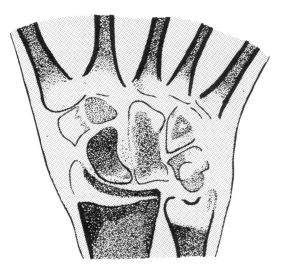

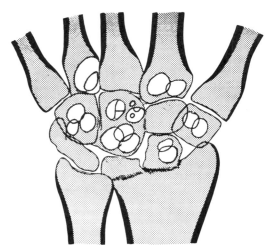

Fig. 127 **So-called cystic (cystoid) tuberculosis of the wrist** produced by a productive, nonfistulating tuberculous inflammation in the cancellous bone. The designation is merely descriptive, because the cystic translucences are a frequent but not a necessary manifestation. In addition, the sequelae of joint destruction (narrowing of joint space, destruction of bone, bony ankylosis) are demonstrable. The radiologic differential diagnosis from rheumatoid arthritis may be difficult so long as this disorder manifests itself (atypically) as a "monotopic" affection of the wrist.

Note: There are virtually no cancellous bones, cancellous (epiphyseal) parts of bone, or metaphyseal areas of a (long) tubular bone in which an isolated cystic destruction or a number of contiguous cystic osteolyses have not been produced by tuberculous granulation tissue. The same is true of sarcoidosis.

ing surfaces of the trapezium and trapezoid and the scaphoid (Figs. 128 and 131), as well as in the joint between the pisiform and the triquetrum (Fig. 131).

The appearance of the fingers and the roentgenogram in osteoarthrosis of the distal and proximal interphalangeal joints are quite typical because characteristic nodes (Heberden's nodes) or Bouchard's osteophytes develop in this arthropathy (Figs. 128, 129, and 131). These are spur-shaped marginal osteophytes whose prominence is increased, *on the one hand*, by cystlike regressive and metaplastic processes in the corresponding area of the capsule and in the subcutaneous connective tissue. (This, however, applies only to Heberden's nodes). *On the other hand*, these cystic soft-tissue structures in the interphalangeal joints often precede the development of osteophytes. They can therefore be conspicuous on mere inspection of the hand; they can alter the silhouette of the fingers and give rise to complaints, although the roentgenogram of the distal interphalangeal joints does not yet show any anomaly. Heberden's nodes develop principally at the *dorsal* and *lateral* contours of the DIP joints. Application of the term *''Bouchard's* osteophytes'' to the marginal osteophytes in osteoarthrosis of the PIP joints is historically incorrect.

Polyosteoarthrosis of the MCP joints occurs less frequently than osteoarthrosis of the interphalangeal joints and the carpo-metacarpal joint of the thumb. In pronounced form it has been observed particularly in persons who have done heavy manual work for a prolonged period of time.

The radiologic morphology of osteoarthrosis of the hand is depicted in Figs. 128 to 131 and is described in the accompanying legends.

A special type of osteoarthritis of the hand, **erosive osteoarthrosis** of the distal and proximal interphalangeal joints (and, less frequently, the carpo-metacarpal joint of the thumb) has been discussed on page 38 and illustrated in Fig. 46. The destruction of articulating bones, which is unusual for osteoarthrosis, is frequently initiated by extensive cystoid undermining of the articular surfaces (Fig. 46, PIP joint of index finger).

So-called **superimposed arthritis**—i.e., the advent of rheumatoid arthritis in patients with

Fig. 128 **Heberden's polyosteoarthrosis in the distal interphalangeal (DIP) joints** with characteristic secondary findings ("rhizarthrosis" = osteoarthrosis of the carpometacarpal joint of the thumb and osteoarthrosis of the joint between trapezium and scaphoid).

Typical "deformed picture" of osteoarthrosis (narrowed radiologic joint space, expanding enlargement and straightening of the articular surfaces, marginal osteophytes, band-shaped increased density of the subchondral cancellous bone, small debris cysts, possibly deviation or even subluxation of the articulating bones). Note the radial displacement and the considerable deformation of the articulating bones at the carpometacarpal joint of the thumb. The first metacarpal also seems to be "shortened," owing to the enlargement of its base. In osteoarthrosis of the carpometacarpal joint of the thumb, *capsular osteomas* are observed with particular frequency. However, such osteomas also occur as small *ossicles* in osteoarthrosis of the finger joints (e.g., DIP V). Delicate hook-shaped capsular ossification in DIP III.

Note: The so-called *Heberden's node* is initially a paraarticular, dorsolaterally located, cystic soft-tissue structure *(tailed arrow)* that only develops a roentgenpositive "nucleus" (osteophyte, *arrow*) with time!

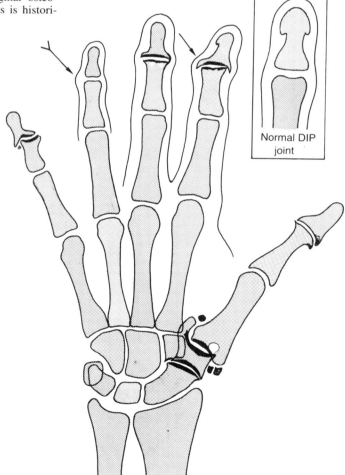

Normal DIP joint

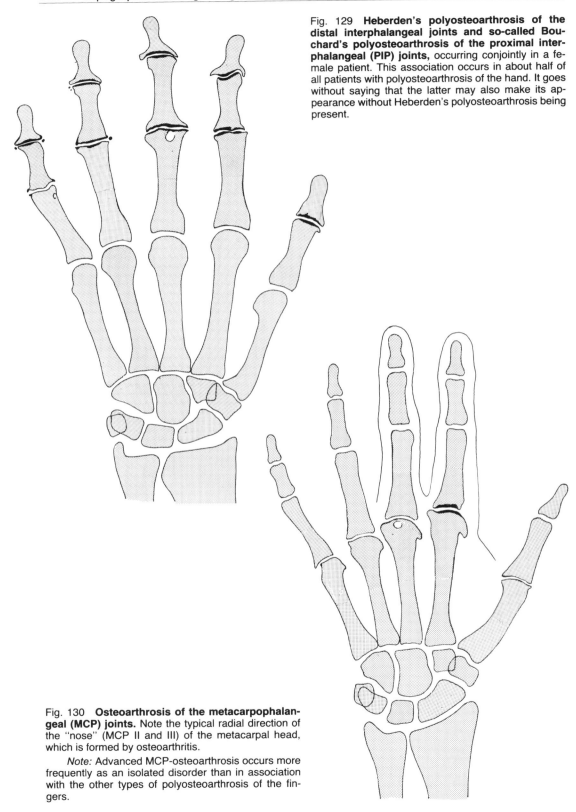

Fig. 129 **Heberden's polyosteoarthrosis of the distal interphalangeal joints and so-called Bouchard's polyosteoarthrosis of the proximal interphalangeal (PIP) joints,** occurring conjointly in a female patient. This association occurs in about half of all patients with polyosteoarthrosis of the hand. It goes without saying that the latter may also make its appearance without Heberden's polyosteoarthrosis being present.

Fig. 130 **Osteoarthrosis of the metacarpophalangeal (MCP) joints.** Note the typical radial direction of the "nose" (MCP II and III) of the metacarpal head, which is formed by osteoarthritis.

Note: Advanced MCP-osteoarthrosis occurs more frequently as an isolated disorder than in association with the other types of polyosteoarthrosis of the fingers.

Fig. 131 **Synoptic radiologic morphology of polyosteoarthrosis of the hand.** The illustration shows polyosteoarthrosis of the DIP, PIP, and MCP joints, osteoarthrosis of the carpometacarpal joint of the thumb, the joint between trapezium and scaphoid (see also Figs. 128, 129, and 130), and between pisiform and triquetrum (also recognizable in the volodorsal roentgenogram with the hand in semisupination, see p. 86).

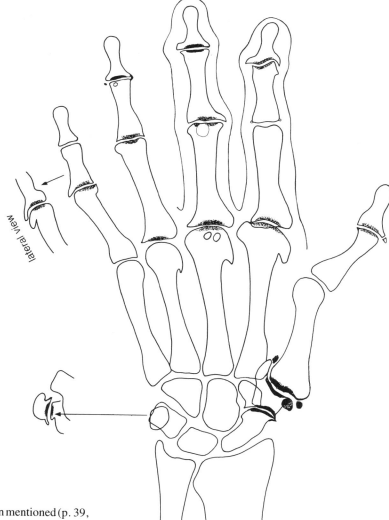

lateral view

polyosteoarthrosis, has already been mentioned (p. 39, Fig. 132). Monoarticular or oligoarticular-asymmetrical types of osteoarthrosis in the interphalangeal and metacarpophalangeal regions give rise to suspicion of secondary osteoarthrosis (as a posttraumatic event,[7] following or accompanying [poly-] arthritis, as an aftermath of avascular necrosis of bone, etc.). In such cases it is often possible to demonstrate the preosteoarthrotic deformities which have led to incongruity of the articular surfaces; for example the signs of a healed Bennett fracture, or Thiemann's disease, Dieterich's disease, osteomalacia of the lunate or pseudoarthrosis of the scaphoid, osteochondrodysplasia, or a mucopolysaccharidosis. In other cases the history provides a clue; for example, to frostbite of

the (distal) interphalangeal joints[8] (particularly when fishermen, hunters, soldiers or vagrants are concerned). Excessive occupational strain, especially on the carpometacarpal joint of the thumb, is known to produce localized osteoarthrosis; for example, in hatmakers, basket weavers and other trades requiring

[7] There also exist roentgenologically demonstrable traumatic Heberden's nodes. They develop and persist without other roentgen manifestations of osteoarthrosis of the DIP joint involved. Apart from this, an old avulsion of an extensor tendon can mimic a (dorsal) Heberden's node.

[8] Cold injuries to the fingers suffered during the growth period can also damage the epiphysis so that subsequent linear growth becomes impaired (Dreyfuss and Glimcher, 1955). The roentgenogram then reveals a conspicuous absence of the epiphyseal plate in the involved phalanges; there is no physiologic separation between the epiphysis and the diaphysis. The first signs of frostbite of the finger joints are mostly rounded subchondral translucences which sometimes communicate with the joint space. They may, over a period of months, lead to destruction of the articulating parts of the phalanx. Frostbite becomes roentgenologically demonstrable at the earliest between 5th and 12th months after the cold injury. Osteoarthrosis appears in the roentgenogram only years or decades later.

continued prehensile movement of that joint. Severe carpal and carporadial osteoarthrosis has sometimes been observed in professional boxers and in blacksmiths (Liebeskind, 1970). Osteoarthrosis of the distal radioulnar joint has been described as an aftermath of vibratory damage in power saw workers (Horváth and Kákosy, 1979).

Kashin-Beck disease (Fig. 134) is a generalized bilateral-symmetrical osteoarthrosis (Chu Chang-Jen and Tsui Te-Yu, 1978) of the peripheral joints (particularly the fingers, wrist, talocrural joint, knee, hip) and the axial skeleton. It develops on the basis of disordered endochondral ossification. The deficient maturation of the epiphyses, the disturbed growth and the avascular-necrotic processes have an adverse effect on the shape and stability of the epiphyses and metaphyses and also lead to shortening of the tubular bones. The disease occurs endemically in Eastern Siberia, Northern China, and North Korea. It usually starts in school-age children. The disease *probably* owes its origin to prolonged increased ingestion of iron salts in drinking water (Twersky, 1975).

Fabry's disease (angiokeratoma corporis diffusum) is a rare hereditary enzyme deficiency with deposition of lip-

ids. It sometimes leads to osteoarthrosis of the distal interphalangeal joints of the fingers (Wise et al., 1962).

The systemic preosteoarthrotic conditions also include the **Mseleni joint syndrome** (Lockitch et al., 1973). This snydrome has been observed among the native black population of Southern Africa. A hereditary systemic developmental disorder of the articulating bones (in the peripheral parts and in the axial skeleton) leads to the early development of osteoarthrosis.

The differential diagnosis between polyosteoarthrosis and rheumatoid arthritis is made from various points of view. Of *roentgenologic importance* are the search for roentgen manifestations of *osteoarthrosis* (p. 37 ff) and soft-tissue signs (Fig. 92), collateral phenomena (Fig. 13), and direct signs of arthritis (Fig. 20), as well as the consideration of the different patterns of involvement in the joints of the hand (Fig. 91). Finally, the osteoarthropathies (see under this heading) must also be ruled out. Although (in the advanced stage) the appearance of osteoarthrotic deformation of the fingers is definitely *characteristic*, it may be difficult to classify the pain, the intolerance

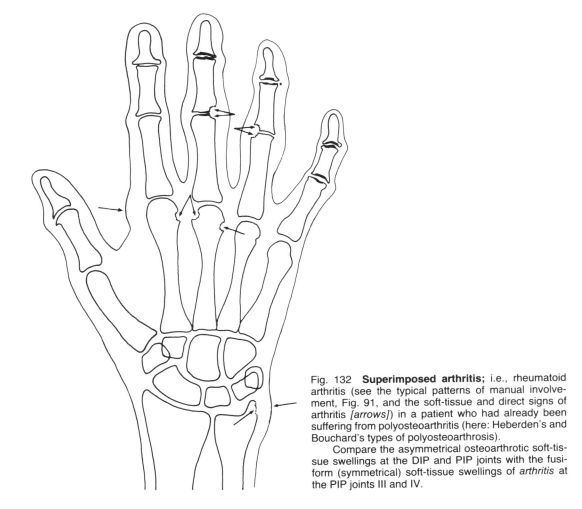

Fig. 132 **Superimposed arthritis;** i.e., rheumatoid arthritis (see the typical patterns of manual involvement, Fig. 91, and the soft-tissue and direct signs of arthritis *[arrows]*) in a patient who had already been suffering from polyosteoarthritis (here: Heberden's and Bouchard's types of polyosteoarthrosis).
Compare the asymmetrical osteoarthrotic soft-tissue swellings at the DIP and PIP joints with the fusiform (symmetrical) soft-tissue swellings of *arthritis* at the PIP joints III and IV.

Fig. 133 **Typical preosteoarthrotic conditions (p. 226 ff) in the joints of the hand.**

HP = *Incomplete supernumerary phalanx of the thumb.* The more incomplete (smaller) the third phalanx of the thumb is, the more difficult the differential diagnosis from a detached Heberden's node becomes (Fig. 131).

OD = Slight and moderately severe deformation of the articulating parts of bone in osteochondrodysplasias and mucopolysaccharidoses (illustrated here only in individual ends of bone).

Note: In the osteochondrodysplasias and the mucopolysaccharidoses one can observe contractures, arthralgias and, infrequently, the ankylosing arthritis of osteochondrodysplasia (Dihlmann and Cen, 1969). These symptoms and findings must not be misinterpreted as a superimposed inflammatory rheumatic arthropathy. Similar epiphyseal and metaphyseal deformations predisposing to osteoarthrosis have been observed in Turner's syndrome (gonadal dysgenesis).

TH = *Thiemann's disease* (epiphyseal acrodysplasia inherited as an autosomal dominant disorder that manifests itself in puberty; Kozlowski and Rupprecht, 1972). At the DIP joint, florid findings persist (phalanges forced into one another, epiphyseal debris squeezed out); at the PIP joint one sees stabilized findings (adaptive growth demonstrable in the head of the proximal phalanx, slight axial deviation).

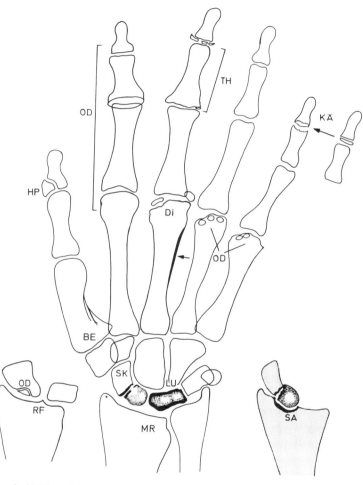

KA = Severe cold injury in the growth period (*right* = finding according to age; *left* = 9 months after cold injury). Cold injuries sometimes lead to premature closure of the epiphysis; in consequence, the finger remains shortened.

BE = *Bennett's fracture* combined with deformation.

DI = Revascularized aseptic necrosis of the epiphysis in the metacarpal head *(Dieterich's disease).*
→ = sometimes recognizable thickening of diaphysis or only periosteal lamella.

SK = Old *fracture of scaphoid* (pseudoarthrosis, ischemic osseous reaction in the proximal fragment which cannot participate in the decalcification of disuse and therefore seems to display increased density). *Note:* So-called congenital duplication of the scaphoid also occurs unilaterally (asymmetrically) and predisposes—especially in the dominant hand—to osteoarthrosis between the two parts. A congenitally duplicated scaphoid is liable to fracture and then must be differentiated from a tripartite scaphoid.

OD *(below left)* = osteochondrosis dissecans in dysplasia of the scaphoid (Baumann and Ilse, 1978).

LU = Repair stage of *subchondral necrosis of the lunate bone* in adults (Kienböck's disease). Minus variant of the ulna (relative shortness of the ulna, not illustrated here) probably predisposes to that disorder.

RF = *Anomalous shape of the radius* at the distal articular surface.

MR = *Minus variant of the radius,* (Mau, 1958) = forme fruste of Madelung's deformity (Fig. 88) with incongruity of the distal radioulnar joint and "neoarthrosis" between the styloid process of the ulna and the triquetrum. The neoarthrosis may also be the result of an isolated increase in size of the styloid process of the ulna.

SA = *"Attritional osteoarthrosis,"* here in pseudoarthrosis of the scaphoid.

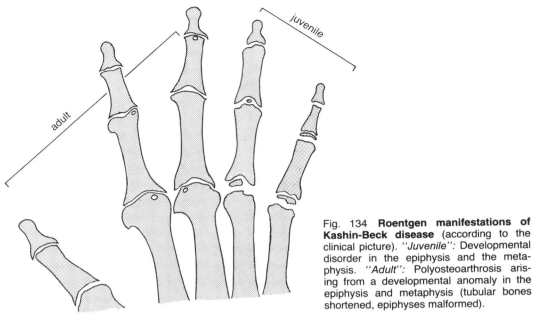

Fig. 134 **Roentgen manifestations of Kashin-Beck disease** (according to the clinical picture). *"Juvenile"*: Developmental disorder in the epiphysis and the metaphysis. *"Adult"*: Polyosteoarthrosis arising from a developmental anomaly in the epiphysis and metaphysis (tubular bones shortened, epiphyses malformed).

to cold, the paresthesias, and the sensation of stiffness as an incipient, still roentgen-negative, polyosteoarthrosis or a rheumatoid polyarthritis. In such cases the pattern of articular involvement in the hand is often a decisive diagnostic criterion, also from the *clinical* point of view.

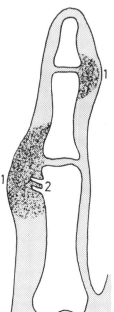

Fig. 135 **Detailed roentgen manifestations of gouty osteoarthropathy.**

1 = Owing to their sodium content, tophi in the soft tissues of the fingers and toes, display greater density than inflammatory or neoplastic swellings (see legend to Fig. 137).

2 = Periosteal tophaceous spines project into the soft-tissue tophus.

Osteoarthropathies

In about 25 percent of *gouty patients* (p. 41 ff), pathologic roentgen manifestations are to be expected during the course of the disease in the hand, more frequently in the finger joints than in the region of the wrist. When the disease manifests itself as a chronic polyarthritis (see quantity-time ratio of urate precipitation, Fig. 47), it may be difficult to differentiate the disorder from rheumatoid arthritis. One should then observe the following rules: When (1) the roentgenogram in chronic polyarthritis of the *hand* shows no conspicuous subchrondral demineralization; (2) the juxtaarticular cystic osteolyses have a diameter of more than 5 mm, and (3) the number of arthritic erosions is inferior to that of cystic osteolyses, the uric acid concentration in serum should be determined.

In addition, the cystic translucences should be differentiated from skeletal sarcoidosis and cystic tuberculosis of bone (Figs. 117, 118, 120, and 127). In contrast, gout must not be mistaken for *hereditary enchondromatosis* or *enchondromatosis associated with hemangiomas* (Mafucci's syndrome, in which phleboliths are visible in the soft tissues, Fig. 139; but compare Fig. 138, no. 14). Enchondromatosis becomes conspicuous, as a rule, in childhood by the disfiguring expansion of bones—or at least the small tubular bones as fingers and toes are uneven and lumpy to the touch. The enchondromas are predominantly located in the metaphysis and diaphysis, whereas intraosseous gouty tophi are found in the epiphysis, the metaphysis, and the diaphysis but rarely extend to the center of the diaphysis. The association of subchondral cysts and marginal osteophytes encountered in

Fig. 136 **Detailed roentgen manifestations of gouty osteoarthropathy** (continued).

3 = So-called punched-out defect (tophaceous osteolysis) with or without increased marginal density, multiple; diameter in small bones>5 mm.

4 = Longitudinal - ovoid tophaceous osteolysis extending to the epiphysis, metaphysis, and diaphysis (see p. 42).

5 = Overhanging osseous border from subperiosteal urate precipitation.

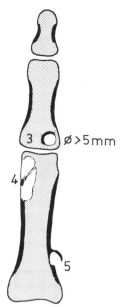

gout *as well as* in polyosteoarthrosis and in erosive osteoarthritis of the hand (see p. 38) can also, in individual cases, present a problem of radiologic differential diagnosis. It should be a rule to determine the uric acid level in every *male* with the typical roentgen manifestations of polyosteoarthrosis! (See Fig. 47.) Figures 135 to 138 present detailed roentgen findings in gouty osteoarthropathy of the hand (soft tissues, bones, joints). Figure 139 shows a synopsis of the roentgen findings in gout.

Among the congenital **coagulopathic osteoarthropathies** (p. 44 ff) it is primarily the hemophilic joint *(hemophilic osteoarthropathy)* that, also in the hand, engages radiologic diagnostic interest. Here also the pathologic roentgenogram is formed by recurrent

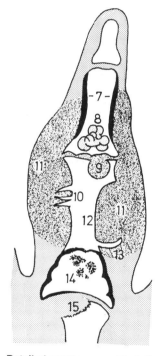

Fig. 137 **Detailed roentgen manifestations of gouty osteoarthropathy** (continued).

6 = Severe tophaceous destruction of joint and bone in a distal interphalangeal joint. The tophus also is recognizable in the periarticular tissues.

Note: The tophus in the soft tissues (of fingers and toes) reveals greater density than an effusion because the sodium component of the precipitated urate attenuates roentgen beam to a greater extent than the "water-equivalent" joint effusion (see p. 1) or synovial proliferations.

Exception: Pigmented villonodular synovitis. In this disorder, the proliferated synovial membrane contains iron and therefore attenuates the roentgen rays to a greater extent than a nonhemorrhagic effusion or synovial proliferation of a different nature.

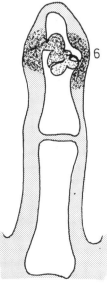

Fig. 138 **Detailed roentgen manifestations of gouty osteoarthropathy** (continued).

7 = Bulbous phalanx due to *protracted* periosteal apposition which instantly "fuses" with the compacta.

8 = Multiple punched-out defects communicating with one another.

9 = Destruction of a proximal interphalangeal joint with remodeling of the articulating bone.

10 = Tophaceous spine (see Fig. 135).

11 = Soft-tissue tophi.

12 = Pressure erosion produced by soft-tissue tophus (no. 11).

13 = Overhanging osseous border (see Fig. 136).

14 = Expansion of an osseous tophus with bulging of the involved part of bone, calcium urate deposition. Differential diagnosis from enchondroma!

15 = Narrowing of the radiographic joint space and erosion of the metacarpal head (direct sign of arthritis).

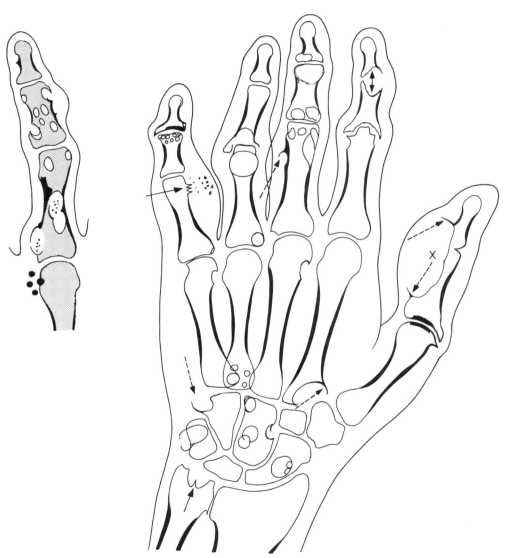

Fig. 139   *Right:* **Gouty hand** *(synopsis)*. Characteristic features of gout are the *tophaceous spine (arrow)*, the *overhanging osseous border (dashed arrow)*, and the *cup-shaped articular mutilation (two-pointed arrow)*. The so-called *punched-out defects* are suggestive of gout when they extend from the epiphysis through the metaphysis to the diaphysis (of small tubular bones) and/or when their diameter (in the regions of the hand and foot) exceeds 5 mm. The other roentgen manifestations of gout illustrated also occur in rheumatoid arthritis—e.g., erosions, joint space narrowing, bony ankylosis—or they may be encountered in osteoarthrosis (marginal osteophytes, band-shaped increased density of the subchondral bone). x = Pressure erosion produced by a soft-tissue tophus *or* starting from a subperiosteal tophus.

Left: **Finger with enchondromatosis** (see text). The rounded translucences frequently lie in the center of the diaphysis. Note the phleboliths adjacent to the metacarpal head (= *Mafucci's syndrome;* see text).

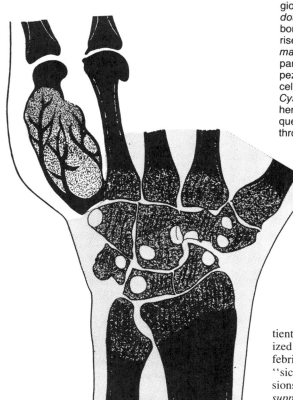

Fig. 140 **Osteoarthropathy of hemophilia** (early stage in the proximal segment of the hand). In the region of the 5th metacarpal, extensive *hemophilic pseudotumor* (see Fig. 52). *Deformations* of several carpal bones and at the distal ends of radius and ulna, giving rise to incongruities of individual joints and *radiologic manifestations of osteoarthrosis.* In addition, acquired partial *bony ankylosis* between the trapezium, the trapezoid, and the capitate. Slight *fibrillar* atrophy of cancellous bone in the carpal region and its surroundings. *Cystic translucences* in the carpal bones (see text). In hemophiliacs, the metacarpophalangeal joints frequently present the radiologic appearance of osteoarthrosis (Pavlov et al., 1979).

tient survives, the disease pursues a course characterized by alternating exacerbations (painful, frequently febrile, crises of vascular occlusion caused by sudden "sickling" of circulating erythrocytes) and remissions. The radiologically recognizable *lesions of the supporting and gliding tissues* can be traced to the following basic histologic processes (Fig. 141):

hemorrhages into the joint cavity, the synovial membrane, the fibrous joint capsule, and the periarticular soft tissues, as well as by the sequelae of subperiosteal and intraosseous hematomas. In Figure 140, hemorrhages into the bone marrow have given rise to rounded osteolyses in the carpal bones. In addition, a *hemophilic pseudotumor* has developed in the fifth metacarpal (see also Fig. 52). The cystic-trabecular structure of the pseudotumor and the expansion of the small tubular bones involved as well as the surrounding tissues are, together with the clinical history of hemophilia, quite characteristic. Hemophilic pseudotumors in the hand occur preferentially in the phalanges of the thumb and in the metacarpals (Brant and Jordan, 1972). Anomalies in the shape and growth of bones as well as roentgen signs of damage and even destruction of the articular cartilage as the result of recurrent hemorrhages into joints and bones have also been illustrated in Figure 140.

Congenital hereditary hemoglobinopathies— e.g., sickle cell anemia, thalassemia major (Cooley's anemia), and thalassemia minor—can be associated with skeletal lesions. Homozygous sickle cell anemia and its genetic variants manifest themselves in blacks *clinically* as early as the first year of life. If the pa-

1. *Erythroblastic hyperplasia of the bone marrow.* Roentgenologically demonstrable consequences: Resorption of the cancellous trabeculae. Coarsening of the preserved strands of cancellous bone. Apparent thinning of the cortical bone. Expansion of the marrow cavities of the diaphyses.

2. *Thrombosis of nutrient vessels of the bone and the synovial membrane (?).* Roentgenologically demonstrable consequences: Epiphyseal avascular necrosis of bone; e.g., head of femur (giving rise, in children, to a "Legg-Perthes picture"), and head of humerus. Infarcts in the metaphysis and diaphysis of long and small tubular bones; e.g., the metacarpals, metatarsals, and phalanges. These infarctions manifest themselves by areas of diminished and increased bone density *(hand-foot syndrome of infants and small children).* Noninflammatory, aseptic joint effusion. Osteoarthrotic destruction of joints due to subchondral infarcts (in weightbearing joints).

3. *Hematogenous osteomyelitis and arthritis* (frequently caused by staphylococci and *Salmonella*). Apart from these, there are reports of an *aseptic (?)* type of chronic arthritis which presents the picture of chronic arthritis in the roentgenogram and which is liable to terminate in bony ankylosis (Schumacher et al., 1977).

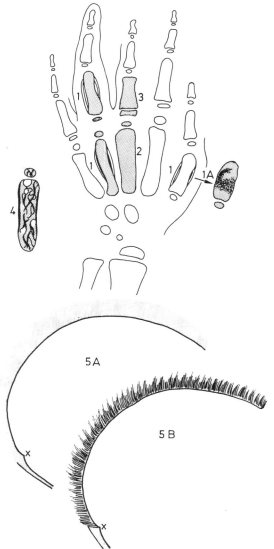

Fig. 142 Radiologic morphology of the polyetio-logic (acro-) osteolysis syndrome in the fingers (compare also Figs. 53 and 102 B). *Arrow* indicates the direction of the nonreactive osteolysis (e.g., in leprosy). The *double-pointed arrow* indicates the spread of the osteolysis; e.g., in progressive scleroderma (Fig. 113). X = band-shaped diaphyseal osteolysis (occurring, for example, in osteomalacia and in vinyl chloride disease). *Not illustrated* are *posttraumatic (acro-) osteolysis* of the *styloid process of the ulna* and of parts of individual carpal bones following isolated fracture of the distal radius (Fischer 1970), other (for example, hyperparathyroid) acroosteolyses of the styloid process (Fig. 150), hereditary carpal osteolyses (see Figs. 58 and 102 B), and massive osteolysis of Gorham-Stout (p. 59) in hemangiomatosis, which has also been observed in the skeleton of the hand.

Fig. 141 Congenital hereditary hemoglobinopa-thies. Synoptic picture of the hand in the child (1 to 3 = sickle cell anemia ; 4 = thalassemia major).

1 = Soft-tissue swelling and periosteal reaction (sometimes advancing to the "bone in bone" appearance) in "dactylitis" (hand-foot syndrome) following infarction of the small tubular bones *and/or* hematogenous bacterial osteomyelitis (in infarcted areas of bone?). Radiologic differential diagnosis between the two etiologies is usually impossible. Conversely, if sickle cell anemia is not diagnosed, the condition must also be differentiated from Caffey's *infantile cortical hyperostosis* (metacarpals, metatarsals), from tuberculosis (spina ventosa), and from hypervitaminosis A.

1A = Changes in shape and structure of the 1st metacarpal shown here also may be sequelae of infarction or infection. Therefore, when a bone infarct in sickle cell anemia is suspected clinically, even experienced workers (Sennara and Gorry, 1978) prescribe antibiotics "as a prophylactic measure."

2 = "Rectangular" remodeling of a metacarpal (metatarsal) as the result of "dactylitis."

3 = Growth disturbance following "dactylitis."

4 = *Reversible* remodeling of the trabecular structure in a metacarpal (metatarsal) in thalassemia major (see text).

5 = Remodeling of the calvarium—i.e., homogenously, loosened or even "foamy" enlargement of its structure (5A, however, not crossing the internal occipital protuberance)—and the so-called "hair-on-end" appearance of the flat bones of the skull (5B) in sickle cell anemia, thalassemia, and other congenital anemias; congenital hemolytic anemias; iron deficiency anemia; congenital cyanotic valvular diseases; primary polycythemia of childhood; or metastatic neuroblastoma.

Roentgenologic differentiation of 5A from Paget's disease and fibrous dysplasia: In the two last-named diseases, the calvarium is also thickened below the internal occipital protuberance (x).

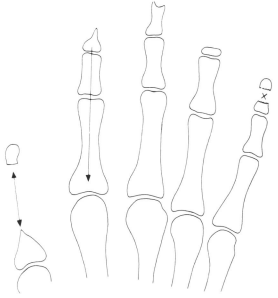

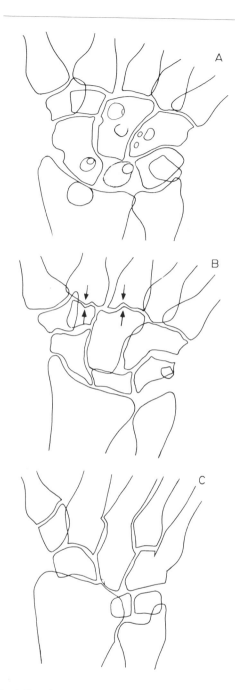

4. *Local disturbances of development and growth in the epiphyses and diaphyses.*

5. *Hyperuricemia amounting to (secondary) gout.*

Thalassemia is a hemolytic anemia that chiefly occurs among peoples originating in the Mediterranean basin; it indicates a defect of hemoglobin synthesis. The homozygous form of the disease is called *thalassemia major,* and the heterozygous manifestation is termed *thalassemia minor.* The roentgenogram reveals thickening of the calvarium; the flat bones of the skull may present a "hair-on-end" appearance (Fig. 141, no. 5 B). The remaining parts of the skeleton, also, shows the consequences of erythroblastic hyperplasia of the red bone marrow *(vide supra).* In childhood, the shafts of the small tubular bones contain red marrow. When the red marrow becomes physiologically transformed into fatty marrow, the trabecular structures undergo regressive changes caused by medullary hyperplasia (Fig. 141, no. 4). In thalassemia minor, a chronic recurrent mono- or oligoarthritis is known to occur. Roentgenologically, it runs a "non-erosive" course and preferentially involves middle-sized and large joints (Schlumpf et al., 1977).

In the **neurogenic osteoarthropathies** of the hand (p. 47 ff), non-reaching acroosteolytic or osteolytic processes are usually the principal features (Fig. 142). In the early stages, though, the *proximal segment of the hand* may present an indistinct radiologic appearance. Its detailed study (Fig. 143 A) can, however, offer the first clue to its neurogenic origin. In syringomyelia, a *generalized edema of the hand* (which, of course, by itself is equivocal) may be an early roentgen manifestation. In the dorsovolar roentgenogram, the edema manifests itself, among other signs,

thritic osteophytes arouses the suspicion of "trophic" narrowing of the articular cartilage.

Roentgenologic diagnosis in conjunction with anamnesis and physical findings: Chondroosteonecrosis in the *early stage of a neurogenic osteoarthropathy (syringomelia?).*

B: *Roentgen manifestations* = Atypical shape of the visible bones. Joint space in part of normal width, in part narrowed, and in part widened. Adaptive growth (adjusting itself to the contours; *arrows*). Absence of bony ankyloses.

Roentgenologic diagnosis: Disorder belonging among the groups of the *osteochondrodysplasias, mucopolysaccharidoses, mucolipidoses,* or *lipidoses* (see p. 238 ff).

C: Not all carpal bones are identifiable; some of them present an atypical shape. Carpometacarpal ankyloses. Slimming and shortening of the 4th and 5th metacarpal *(not illustrated).* No erosions, no collateral phenomena of arthritis.

Roentgenologic diagnosis: Status after arthritis of the growth period. (Clinically: Cured juvenile chronic arthritis 40 years previously at the age of 9. See Fig. 103).

Fig. 143 "Roentgenologic diagnosis at a glance" without exact analysis of *all* abnormal findings (hence not only those which are immediately conspicuous) can be misleading. The patients (A to C) were radiologically examined for "rheumatic" complaints in the wrist.

A: *Roentgen manifestations* = the shape of the visible bones gives a disharmonious, angular impression. Signs of osseous ischemia (increased density of the lunate, cystic osteolysis). Narrowing of the joint space between individual bones without other direct signs or collateral phenomena of arthritis and without osteoar-

Fig. 144 **Early stage of syringomelia.** A striking feature of the roentgenogram is the diffuse, hence not joint-related, edema of the soft tissues. It is demonstrable particularly beside the styloid process of the radius and the ulna *(marked)* and gives rise to convexity of the interdigital folds *(arrows)*. The normal appearance of these folds is shown above right; *tailed arrow*).

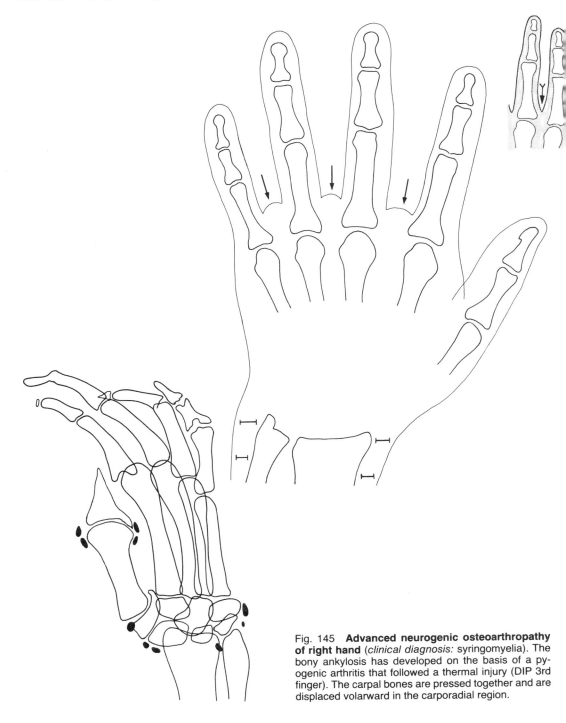

Fig. 145 **Advanced neurogenic osteoarthropathy of right hand** (*clinical diagnosis:* syringomyelia). The bony ankylosis has developed on the basis of a pyogenic arthritis that followed a thermal injury (DIP 3rd finger). The carpal bones are pressed together and are displaced volarward in the carporadial region.

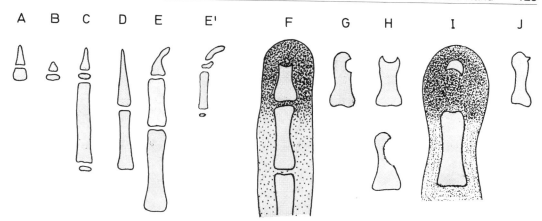

Fig. 146 **Roentgenologic differential diagnosis of the acro-osteolysis syndrome.**
A = Conical and bipartite distal phalanx in cleidocranial dysplasia. B = Brachytelephalangia in pyknodysostosis (acroosteolytic osteopetrosis) (child). C = Apert's syndrome (acrocephalosyndactyly, type 1) (child). D = Synphalangia. E = Kirner's deformity of the distal phalanx of the little finger.
E' = Kirner's deformity, radiographic aspect in the child (palmar and radial curvature of the distal phalanx of the little finger.). F = Osteomyelitis of the distal phalanx of the little finger with soft-tissue swelling of the entire finger ("sausage finger"). G = glomus tumor.
H = Pressure erosions from traumatic epithelial cyst or epithelial nodule. A similar appearance is also produced by benign tumors of soft tissues. I = osteolytic metastatic carcinoma (similar roentgen finding in carcinoma of the nail bed and in subungual sarcoma). J = No incipient osteolysis in the terminal phalangeal tuft but small *subungual* exostosis (lateral roentgenogram as in G and H [lower part of picture]).

by convexity of the interdigital folds (Fig. 144). The diagnosis can be established only by considering the anamnesis and the clinical findings. Figure 145 shows an advanced osteoarthropathy. For the manifold causes of nonreactive osteolysis, see p. 52 ff. Figure 146 illustrates the radiologic differentiation of osteolyses in the fingers.

Osteoarthropathy of amyloidosis (p. 60) is an infrequent finding. In the hand, it sometimes presents a certain *clinical* constellation of features, namely: bilaterally symmetrical, polyarticular, fusiform swelling of the proximal (possibly also the distal) interphalangeal and metacarpophalangeal joints (particularly noticeable in the first, second, and fifth me-

Fig. 147 **Amyloid osteoarthropathy in multiple myeloma (plasmacytoma).** About 10 percent of plasmacytoma patients acquire amyloidosis (Hannon et al., 1975).
Roentgen findings: Fusiform bulging of the proximal interphalangeal joints III to V and the metacarpophalangeal joints II and V. *No* joint space narrowing. Marginal erosions are apt to develop but are absent in the illustrated case. Irregularly rounded or oval larger osteolyses (without marginal sclerosis) in the distal radius, the distal ulna, the scaphoid, the base of the 5th metacarpal, and the proximal phalanx of the 4th finger. *Marginal* osteolyses, giving the impression of extraarticular *(juxtaarticular)* erosions, in the distal radius and the proximal phalanx of the 3rd finger. With consideration of the clinical diagnosis (multiple myeloma), the roentgen findings allow the diagnosis of amyloid osteoarthropathy.

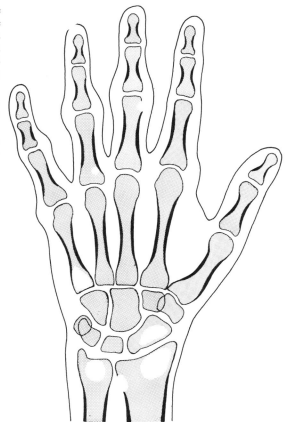

tacarpophalangeal joints), sensation of stiffness, limitation of motion, and more or less pronounced pain. Subcutaneous nodules are palpable over the diseased joints, and symptoms of a bilateral carpal tunnel syndrome are demonstrable (Hamilton and Bywaters, 1961).

In the presence of these findings, differential diagnosis should consider rheumatoid arthritis, secon-dary amyloidosis in rheumatoid arthritis, and amy-loid osteoarthropathy (most frequently as primary amyloidosis and as amyloidosis accompanying the paraproteinemias [see p. 60]). On the other hand, the roentgen findings sketched in Figure 147 should at least arouse the suspicion of a disease associated with the deposition of metabolic products (*"deposition disease," metabolic osteoarthropathy*).

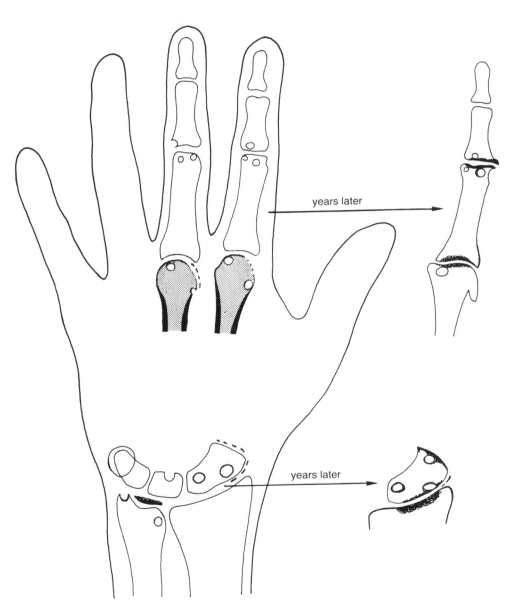

Fig. 148 Osteoarthropathy of hemochromatosis.
  Roentgen findings: Subchondral cysts with delicate sclerotic border, partly marginal (see text). Partial wasting of the marginal subchondral lamella (in the head of the 3rd metacarpal), producing a "nibbled" contour of the head of the 2nd metacarpal. Chondrocalcinosis of the distal radioulnar disk and the articular cartilage of the scaphoid.
  Roentgen findings (right): Appearance of osteoarthrosis (compare Fig. 131).

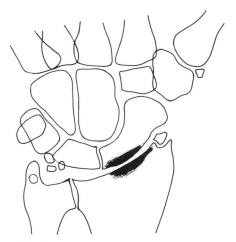

Fig. 149 **Osteoarthropathy in Wilson's disease.** Fragmentation of bone or bony metaplasia of soft tissues (five small loose bodies with marginal cortical seam; the "bed of a joint mouse" recognizable in the styloid process of the radius). Osteoarthrosis in the region of the carpus and forearm and in the distal radioulnar region. Cyst in the distal ulna.

Osteoarthropathy of hemochromatosis (p. 61 ff) generally shows, in the hand, a combination of polyosteoarthrosis, chondrocalcinosis and osteoporosis not related to the joints. In early and intermediate stages, analysis of the roentgenogram of the hand presents the following additional detailed findings (Fig. 148):

1. Preferential involvement of the metacarpophalangeal joints of the second and third fingers (see Fig. 91). The first pathologic roentgen findings in these and other joints (for example, the remaining metacarpophalangeal joints, the proximal interphalangeal, and the carpal joints) are subchondral cysts (geodes) measuring a few millimeters in diameter. They often have a delicate sclerotic seam. Marginal cysts with collapsed walls mimic erosions. The marginal subchondral lamella can be resorbed ("opened"); this sometimes gives the articular contour a "nibbled" appearance.
2. In the hand, chondrocalcinosis is most frequently encountered in the (distal) radioulnar disk.

In **osteoarthropathy of Wilson's disease** (p. 62, Fig. 149), the following roentgen manifestations have been observed in the hand (Feller and Schumacher, 1972):

1. The sequelae of damage to the articular cartilage, demonstrable already in the third and fourth decades of life (*premature* osteoarthrosis); subchondral cysts without other signs of osteoarthrosis.
2. Loose bodies from fragmentation of bone (similar to osteochondrosis dissecans) or from osseous metaplasia of soft tissues, therefore with or without "mouse bed."

3. Chondrocalcinosis.
4. Generalized osteoporosis without preference for the juxtaarticular parts of bone.
5. Roentgen manifestations of rickets or osteomalacia.

In the different types of autonomous (primary, tertiary[9]) and regulative (renal and intestinal, secondary) **hyperparathyroidism**, *subchondral* dissecting fibroosteoclasia can lead to breaks of the joint-bearing parts of bone and thereby to destruction of the articular cartilage. In the roentgenogram one then sees thinning or even absence of the marginal subchondral lamella (Fig. 96) as well as erosions and narrowing of the joint space (Figs. 150, 151, and 152); sometimes, however, the joint space appears to be widened (Figs. 365 and 366). Later on, signs of osteoarthrosis are demonstrable (in weightbearing joints). Since breakage of bone is followed by reactive inflammation of the synovial membrane and, frequently, by an effusion into the joint, the erroneous diagnosis of rheumatoid polyarthritis suggests itself, although the pattern of manual involvement typical of this disease is lacking (additional involvement of the distal interphalangeal joints). A similar finding is sometimes observed in **osteomalacia** (Bywaters et al., 1963). Contrary to these nondescript *articular* roentgen findings in hyperparathyroidism and osteomalacia are the characteristic *osseous* roentgen manifestations. Typical of osteomalacia are the frequently bilaterally symmetrical Looser's zones (Milkman's syndrome).[10]

Hyperparathyroidism presents a broad spectrum of pathologic roentgen manifestations in the skeleton:

1. *Intracortical resorption* in tubular bones. This finding in *small* tubular bones is illustrated by Figure 14. In *large* tubular bones, intracortical resorption of bone is caused by the cortex being "split off" or "scaled off." In addition, the roentgenogram often gives the impression of blurring of the osseous structure like that in osteomalacia, because this disorder (and also frequently hyperparathyroidism) is charac-

[9] The autonomous *tertiary* hyperparathyroidism develops from a regulative secondary hyperparathyroidism when a "hyperplasiogenic" adenoma arises in the reactive (regulative) hyperplastic parathyroid glands (Jesserer, 1979). For the regulative quaternary and the autonomous quinternary hyperparathyroidism, see Kuhlencordt and Kracht, 1968.

[10] In the hereditary and sporadic (acquired) *renotubular syndromes (renal tubulopathies)*, one or more functions of the renal tubules are disturbed. Experience has shown that initially the consequences of such tubular dysfunction are often more clearly manifest remote from the kidneys; for example in the skeleton, than in the kidneys themselves. Thus, in the adult, the association of osteomalacia with nephrocalcinosis is almost pathognomonic of *renal tubular acidosis*, provided that therapeutic hypervitaminosis D can be ruled out (Courey and Pfister, 1972). Among the causes of *acquired renal acidosis* are various congenital disorders of metabolism; e.g., Wilson's disease (see p. 62), cystinosis, Sjögren's syndrome, and the hypergammaglobulinemias. Wilson's disease sometimes also gives rise to the Toni-Debré-Fanconi syndrome (a complex renotubular defect consisting of glycosuria, phosphaturia, and aminoaciduria). This syndrome also is accompanied by rickets or osteomalacia.

terized by deficient mineralization of the newly formed bony matrix. This deficient mineralization, associated with osteoporosis *(vide infra)* and possible pathologic fractures, is responsible for the deformation of bones in advanced hyperparathyroidism (spinal deformities, increased kyphosis of the thoracic spine, bell-shaped thorax, heart-shaped pelvis, secondary basilar impression).

2. *Subperiosteal resorption of bone* (Figs. 14, 150, 151, 152, 365, and 366). Experience has shown that subperiosteal resorption of the cortex manifests itself *first* in the *radial aspect* of the middle phalanges of the fingers (Figs. 150 and 151). During the further course of the disease, the roentgenogram also shows involvement of the other tubular bones of the hand. In hyperparathyroidism, *endosteal* resorption in the

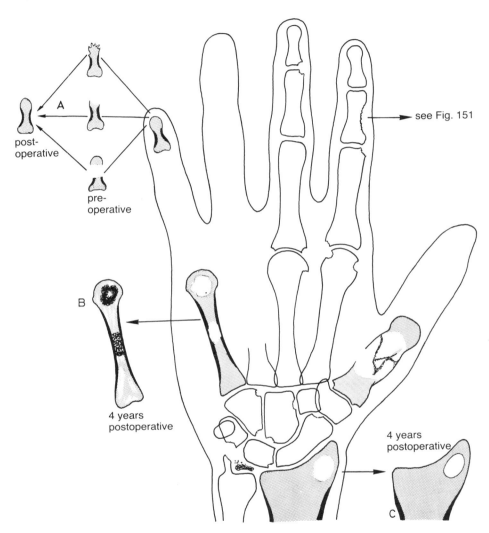

Fig. 150   Changes in the skeleton of the hand in hyperparathyroidism or renal osteopathy.
Subperiosteal resorption of bone (see radial aspect of the middle phalanx of index finger) is an *almost certain* sign of hyperparathyroidism (Kolb and Steinach, 1962). *Erosions* in various interphalangeal, metacarpophalangeal, carpometacarpal, and carpal joints as well as in the styloid process of the ulna; *narrowing of the radiographic interosseous space of several joints.* These findings require differentiation from rheumatoid arthritis (in the latter disease, however, chondrocalcinosis of the radioulnar disk and acroosteolysis in the distal phalanx would be atypical manifestations). *Cysts* (necrotic liquefied brown tumors) persist after operative removal of the parathyroid tumor. However, they usually present sharper contours; see C). *Brown tumors* are apt to enlarge and to expand the bone (1st metacarpal). Postoperatively, they present increased density (B). *Acro-osteolysis* also is reversible after surgery (see A).

Note: in secondary hyperparathyroidism or in the setting of renal osteopathy, brown tumors occur much less frequently than in primary hyperparathyroidism.

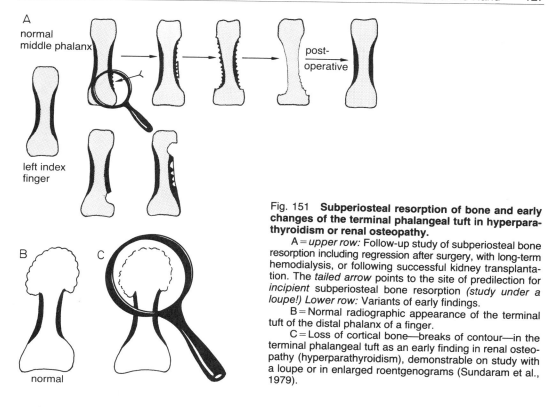

A = normal middle phalanx

left index finger

post-operative

B   C

normal

Fig. 151   **Subperiosteal resorption of bone and early changes of the terminal phalangeal tuft in hyperparathyroidism or renal osteopathy.**
A = *upper row:* Follow-up study of subperiosteal bone resorption including regression after surgery, with long-term hemodialysis, or following successful kidney transplantation. The *tailed arrow* points to the site of predilection for *incipient* subperiosteal bone resorption *(study under a loupe!) Lower row:* Variants of early findings.
B = Normal radiographic appearance of the terminal tuft of the distal phalanx of a finger.
C = Loss of cortical bone—breaks of contour—in the terminal phalangeal tuft as an early finding in renal osteopathy (hyperparathyroidism), demonstrable on study with a loupe or in enlarged roentgenograms (Sundaram et al., 1979).

tubular bones is much less striking than subperiosteal resorption (see Fig. 14). The radiographic appearance of *subchondral* resorption of bone in hyperparathyroidism has been described above. Finally, hyperparathyroidism is associated with a *subtendinous* type of bone resorption at the insertions of tendons and ligaments; for example, in the calcaneus (see Fig. 549), the ischia, the trochanters (Fig. 366), and the iliac wings. This agrees with the experience that, in hyperparathyroidism, increased remodeling (resorption) of bone becomes particularly manifest in the roentgenogram of those parts of the skeleton that are exposed to heavy mechanical strain; for example, in the acromio-clavicular joint (Fig. 269), the sacroiliac joint and the symphysis pubis (Fig. 366, Table 2).
3. *Osteolysis* (Fig. 150). *Circumscribed* extraarticular processes of bone resorption in hyperparathyroidism are acroosteolysis; for example, in the distal phalanges (early manifestation, see Fig. 151 C), in the ulnar and less frequently the radial styloid process, and the so-called "brown tumors." These resorptive giant cell granulomas are classical roentgen signs of advanced hyperparathyroidism *(vide infra);* they can give rise to pathologic fractures.

Table 2   **Minimal program of roentgenologic study in hyperparathyroidism**

Dorsovolar roentgenogram of both hands (mammography film)

Acromioclavicular joints (humerus abducted 90°, rotated dorsally, elbow flexed 90°)

Lateral roentgenogram of skull

Survey film of pelvis

Lateral roentgenogram of lumbar spine

Anterioposterior roentgenograms of both knees

Dorsoplantar roentgenogram of both forefeet

Upper and lower jaw (tooth sockets) only in children and adolescents

Comments: In the *skull* of the patient with hyperparathyroidism one observes a granular type of osteoporosis, the groundglass phenomenon, and disappearance of the three layers of the calvarium or thinning or thickening of the calvarium. In contrast to children and adolescents, complete resorption of the lamina dura dentium is a rare sign of adult hyperparathyroidism because it also occurs in a number of other local and systemic disorders, among them as an aftermath of periodontosis; in severe osteoporosis, rickets, osteomalacia, plasmacytoma, and leukemia; with diffuse skeletal metastases; in Cushing's disease and in Paget's disease. In addition, complete disappearance of the lamina dura is a late roentgen manifestation of hyperparathyroidism. In this stage, changes in the fingers are usually already demonstrable (Figs. 150 and 151; Prager et al., 1958).

4. *Osteoporosis.* Advanced hyperparathyroidism typically shows a generalized reduction of the mineralized mass of bone per unit of volume (= osteoporosis).

5. *Hyperostosis.* In hyperparathyroidism, new bone formation occurs as periosteal apposition of bone (Fig. 152). In addition, it is observed as increased bone density in the vertebral bodies (Fig. 660), in the bones of the skull, the ribs, and the pelvic region, and other cancellous parts of the skeleton (Fig. 152). In the newborn, the infant, and the small child, periosteal reactions are encountered more frequently than in the adult. Furthermore, at this age subperiosteal resorption of bone is more often demonstrable in the proximal humerus and the neck of the femur than in the phalanges (Nguyen et al., 1974).

6. *Ossification of soft tissues* (Figs. 150 and 152). Deposition of calcium in hyperparathyroidism is encountered as chondrocalcinosis in fibrous and hyaline cartilage. In addition to this, during the course of hyperparathyroidism one observes periarticular as well as cutaneous and subcutaneous calcifications at some distance from the joints. Calcifications of bursae and of the arterial tunica media also occur (more frequently in the lower than in the upper extremities).

7. *Disorders of the epiphyseal plates.* In hyperparathyroidism, cartilage and bone are resorbed in the

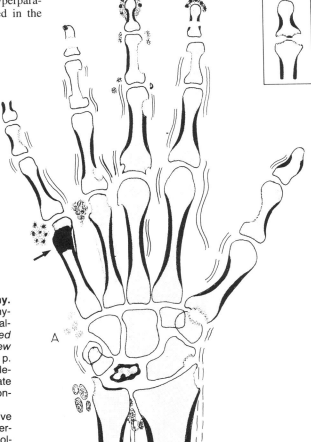

Fig. 152 Advanced renal osteopathy.
A = Arguments against primary hyperparathyroidism (see text) are the striking soft-tissue calcifications, the periosteal reactions, the *marked* calcifications of the arterial tunica media, the *few* cystic osteolyses (brown tumors or cysts; see p. 129 ff). *Arrow* points to a hyperostosis (sclerosis of cancellous bone; see text). The lunate has undergone avascular necrosis (osteochondritis of the lunate; Dihlmann, 1974).

B = Roentgen manifestation of extensive *subchondral* bone resorption in a distal interphalangeal joint (the roentgenologic morphology is identical to that of an arthritic erosion).

epiphyseal plate and the adjoining metaphysis. They are replaced by fibrous tissue and demineralized fibrocartilage (Krempien et al., 1973; Krempien, 1974). The chondrocytes lose their typical arrangement. The roentgenogram shows the following results of these processes of remodeling: General disturbance of linear growth (stunted growth; Ritz et al., 1975); broadening of the epiphyseal plates; narrowing of the breadth of the epiphyseal plates prior to (premature) closure of the epiphyses; epiphysiolysis which either follows fractures of the epiphysis and/or the metaphysis (Kirkwood et al., 1972) or is the result of remodeling processes that led to lateral displacement of the epiphysis due to shearing strain produced by muscle pull or gravity (Krempien et al., 1973; Fig. 365).

Advanced *primary* hyperparathyroidism is known as *von Recklinghausen's osteitis (osteodystrophia)— fibrosa cystica generalisata*. Primary hyperparathyroidism develops in primary diseases of the parathyroid gland; for example, in primary hyperplasia, in solitary or multiple adenomas, and (infrequently) in carcinoma of these endocrine glands. Familiarity with the roentgen manifestations described under items 1 to 7 allows the clinician to diagnose hyperparathyroidism in its early stages or, at least, to suspect the presence of this disorder. The skeletal roentgen manifestations of primary hyperparathyroidism, however, are potentially but in no way universally features of this disease. They occur in at most 50 percent of the patients (Pugh, 1951). Formally, this can be explained as follows: Hyperparathyroidism is associated with increased remodeling of bone; hence the disorder involves the osteoblasts *and* the osteoclasts. When increased osteoclastic resorption is compensated for by osteoblastic formation of new bone, the roentgenogram of the skeleton is normal, supposing that the newly formed osteoid becomes regularly mineralized. In the event of delayed mineralization or pronounced demineralization of the newly formed bony matrix, the bone structures appear ill-defined, "vague" *(vide supra)*. Excessive compensation of osteoclastic resorption leads to hyperostosis (periosteal reaction, increased density of cancellous bone).

The seven roentgen findings listed above are not only potential features of hyperparathyroidism but also vary among patients with skeletal changes. For example, subperiosteal resorption of bone in the middle phalanges of the fingers is an early skeletal manifestation. On the other hand, a brown tumor may infrequently occur without concomitant subperiosteal resorption (of the phalangeal cortex). Being familiar with the clinical signs and symptoms of primary hyperthyroidism and giving them due attention is therefore also important to the radiologic examiner. These manifestations include urolithiasis (in about 50 percent of the patients; Genant et al., 1973), nephrocalcinosis, polyuria, polydipsia, gastrointestinal complaints (anorexia, nausea, constipation, ulcer disease, pancreatic dysfunction, and mental symptoms (depressive mood, peevishness, irritability, lack of psy-

chomotor activity). The skeletal manifestations give rise to "rheumatic" complaints.

Finally, it should be pointed out that determination of the serum levels of alkaline phosphatase, calcium, and phosphate is of great diagnostic and differential diagnostic importance.[11] Primary hyperparathyroidism is a rare disease, but our knowledge of the skeletal changes involved has improved since it has become possible to analyze the skeletal findings in *secondary* hyperparathyroidism more exactly. Secondary hyperparathyroidism occurs with global (glomerular and tubular) renal insufficiency; i.e., in the setting of **renal (uremic) osteopathy** (osteodystrophy). Secondary hyperparathyroidism develops consistently as a result of hypocalcemia produced by a disorder of intestinal calcium absorption *plus* the accumulation of phosphate in the blood; such an accumulation indicates a disparity between the supply of phosphate and the capacity of the kidneys to excrete it. Renal osteopathy, however, is followed not only by (secondary) hyperparathyroidism but also by (renal) osteomalacia (or, in the growth period, by rickets). Typical cases of renal osteopathy then present a clinical picture of mixed hyperparathyroidism and osteomalacia. Today, renal osteopathy is observed with much greater frequency than previously because the life expectancy of patients with chronic uremia has considerably increased since the advent of long-term dialysis. In other words, in the past, the great majority of patients with global renal insufficiency died before the roentgen signs of renal osteopathy could become manifest. Long-term hemodialysis, however, modifies the clinical picture of the original renal osteopathy (Ritz et al., 1973). *For example,* the degree of medial calcification in the middle-sized and small arteries correlates with the duration of the dialysis, and the extraosseous soft-tissue calcifications are influenced by the calcium: phosphate ratio. When this ratio (measured in mg/dL) exceeds 70 to 80, soft-tissue calcifications—which frequently are very painful—occur in the majority of adult patients (Fig. 152). With a Ca^{++} to HPO_4^{--} ratio below 80, such calcifications are encountered in less than one third of the patients subjected to maintenance dialysis (Ritz et al., 1973).

Considering renal osteopathy and the influence of long-term dialysis on its manifestations, it should

---

[11] Particular clinical courses of hyperparathyroidism are *normocalcemic hyperparathyroidism* (Wills et al., 1969) and so-called *pseudohypo-hyperparathyroidism*, i.e., the combination of symptoms and findings (including roentgen signs) of pseudohypoparathyroidism (see pp. 143) and hyperparathryroidism (Kolb et al., 1962; Schwille et al., 1972). Besides these, *pseudohyperparathyroidism* with hypercalcemia and hypophosphatemia in nonendocrine malignant tumors (without skeletal metastases) has been described (Lafferty, 1966). These tumors—for example, renal adenocarcinoma or bronchial carcinoma—evidently produce a polypeptide resembling parathormone, which gives rise to a histologically demonstrable dissecting fibroosteoclasia. The skeletal roentgenogram is normal because the fatal progression of the tumor probably precedes the manifestation of the typical skeletal changes.

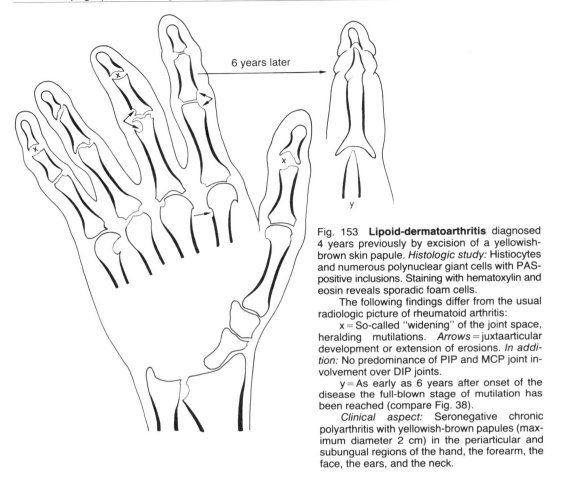

6 years later

y

Fig. 153 **Lipoid-dermatoarthritis** diagnosed 4 years previously by excision of a yellowish-brown skin papule. *Histologic study:* Histiocytes and numerous polynuclear giant cells with PAS-positive inclusions. Staining with hematoxylin and eosin reveals sporadic foam cells.

The following findings differ from the usual radiologic picture of rheumatoid arthritis:

x = So-called "widening" of the joint space, heralding mutilations. *Arrows* = juxtaarticular development or extension of erosions. *In addition:* No predominance of PIP and MCP joint involvement over DIP joints.

y = As early as 6 years after onset of the disease the full-blown stage of mutilation has been reached (compare Fig. 38).

Clinical aspect: Seronegative chronic polyarthritis with yellowish-brown papules (maximum diameter 2 cm) in the periarticular and subungual regions of the hand, the forearm, the face, the ears, and the neck.

be pointed out that the roentgen manifestations of primary and secondary hyperparathyroidism are qualitatively identical but differ quantitatively. Soft-tissue calcifications develop more frequently in secondary than in primary hyperparathyroidism (Irnell et al., 1970). Their incidence amounts to 50 percent in the former disorder and to between 5 and 10 percent in the latter. Periosteal reactions and increased density of cancellous bone are most often observed in patients with renal osteopathy. Brown tumors occur much less frequently in secondary than in primary hyperparathyroidism (Lindenfelser et al., 1974). In the roentgenologic differential diagnosis between brown tumors and genuine cysts (Fig. 150), which sometimes are the result of cystic transformation of brown tumors (produced by necrosis and subsequent liquefaction), angiography has proved helpful; brown tumors present a sharp contrast that is absent in cysts (Lindenfelser et al., 1974).

In cases where hyperparathyroidism has not yet been diagnosed, the roentgenologic differentiation between brown tumor and osteoclastoma, fibrous dysplasia, benign chondroblastoma, localized plas-

macytoma, an aneurysmatic bone cyst, and metastases (particularly of thyroid and renal malignancies) is based on the following considerations: Brown tumors are most frequently encountered in the metaphysis and diaphysis of the tubular bones. They are projected into the marrow cavity and erode the cortex on both sides of it. They also may expand the bone or are located eccentrically underneath the periosteum. Cystic lesions in the facial bones (including the mandible) and in the small tubular bones of the hands and feet are much more likely to be brown tumors than osteoclastomas. Finally, determination of the serum levels of alkaline phosphatase, calcium, and phosphate will be a decisive aid in making the differential diagnosis.

Surgical removal of the parathyroid tumor or successful kidney transplantation is usually followed by regression of the subperiosteal bone resorption, the acroosteolyses, and the soft-tissue calcifications. It is much less frequent for calcification of the arterial walls to recede (Meema et al., 1976). Long-term dialysis also can lead to regression of the subperiosteal bone resorption (Doyle, 1972). In secondary hyperparathyroidism, soft-tissue calcifications are often resorbed as soon as the blood concentration of phosphate is lowered by therapeutic measures. Brown tumors also tend to regress postoperatively or following transplantation. They then usually present calcifications which correspond to primitive bone substance (Fig. 150). In these areas of increased density, lamellar bone is apt to develop only some years later, if at all, which means that the bone again shows normal density and structure in the roentgenogram. Genuine cysts, in contrast, persist postoperatively more or less unchanged (Jesserer, 1979).

Lipoid-dermatoarthritis (synonym: **multicentric reticulohistiocytosis**) is a rare disorder in which lipids accumulate *principally* in the skin and the subcutaneous tissues, in the mucosa and the synovial membrane of joints, in the tendon sheaths, and in the tendinous insertions, giving rise to a tissue reaction. Therefore it is probably a storage disease. The joint manifestations frequently occur prior to the appearance of the nodules in the skin. The latter preferentially present a periarticular or subungual location. They are yellowish-brown or reddish-brown, copper-colored or purplish. Less frequently the lesions in the skin and in the joints develop concomitantly or the manifestations in the skin antedate those in the joints (Barrow and Holubar, 1969).

The radiologic appearance (Fig. 153) is that of a bilaterally symmetrical polyarthritis *without* its typical pattern of manual involvement. The condition runs a rapidly progressive course and can, after but a few years, reach the stage of mutilation. Sometimes, however, lipoid-dermatoarthritis becomes spontaneously inactive before that time; secondary osteoarthrosis then develops, particularly in the larger joints. In lipoid-dermatoarthritis, granulation tissue containing giant cells and possibly foam cells forms in the involved joint; this tissue coats the articular cartilage and erodes it, together with the bone. The joint space becomes narrowed. Marginal erosions appear, soon extending to the entire contour of the joint. On the other hand, massive resorption of subchondral bone can lead to ''widening'' of the joint space (in the finger joints). *Juxtaarticular* erosions, hence contour defects outside the insertion of the joint capsule, also form part of the roentgenologic features of lipoid-dermatoarthritis (Fig. 153). Despite extensive destruction of the joint, juxtaarticular osteoporosis is slight or absent. Equally remarkable is a *clinical* disproportion between the severe articular destructions and the relatively insignificant complaints. In the axial skeleton, destructive lesions occur primarily in the atlantoaxial region, in the intervertebral and costoverberal joints (Warren et al., 1957), and in the pelvis (sacroiliac joints and symphysis pubis; Martel et al., 1961). Deposits of lipids give rise to reactions on the part of the tendinous insertions, which can lead to contour defects; for example in the great tuberosity of the humerus, the ischial tuberosity, or the greater trochanter (Warin et al., 1957).

The *differential diagnosis* of lipoid-dermatoar-

thritis is facilitated by noting the characteristically colored skin papules. When these conspicuous efflorescences are (still) absent, it is necessary (in the hand) to rule out psoriatic arthritis, gout, and destructive polyosteoarthrosis. The following findings argue against rheumatoid arthritis: Absence of the rheumatoid factors; concomitant involvement of *all* levels of the finger joints, hence no predominance of the MCP and PIP joints over the DIP joints; mutilations occurring already only a few years' evolution.

Acromegaly of adult individuals is the result of increased or prolonged synthesis of the somatic anterior pituitary hormone. It manifests itself *externally* only in certain portions of the body, particularly the acral parts. When this hormonal overproduction occurs prior to the completion of growth, it results in *general* stimulation of endochondral growth leading to *giantism*. The acromegalic has a characteristic facial appearance (Fig. 154). No less conspicuous in the majority of patients are the changes in the hands, which manifest themselves equally in the soft tissues, the cartilages and the bones (Figs. 155 and 156). The *enlargement* of soft tissues in the fingers concerns not only the juxtaarticular parts (capsular thickening) but the entire finger. The adipose tissue in the subcutis is replaced by ''water-equivalent'' connective tissue (see

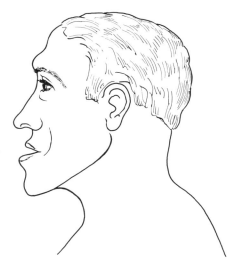

Fig. 154 **Characteristic facial appearance of an acromegalic** (facial skeleton elongated, protruding chin, teeth spaced as a result of mandibular enlargement, thick lips, bulging supraorbital arches). The roentgenogram reveals, in addition, widening of the angle between the body and the ramus of the mandible (see Fig. 584), increased volume of the paranasal sinuses (in the majority of cases), enlargement and erosion of the sella (produced by an eosinophilic adenoma of the anterior pituitary, which in most cases is responsible for the condition), and frequently a generalized thickening of the calvarium and/or circumscribed thickening of the external occipital protuberance.

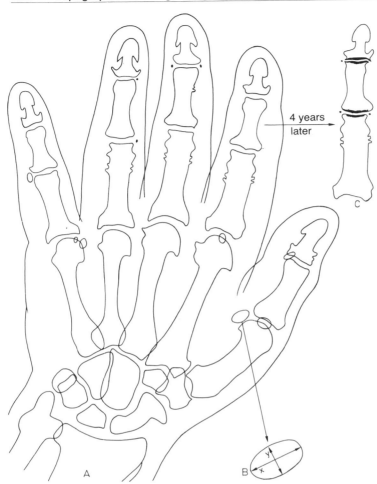

4 years later →

Fig. 155 Hand of an acromegalic. The picture is characterized by concomitant thickening of the soft tissues and the articular cartilage and by remodeling of bone.

A = Dorsovolar view of the hand. Roentgenologic appearance of "osteoarthrosis with widening of the joint space"; i.e., "outgrowing borders of the bones." Also note the spade- or anchor-shaped terminal tufts of the distal phalanges.

B = In acromegaly, the sesamoid bones are often enlarged and/or occur in atypical places (Wagner and Schaaf, 1963; see A). In addition, the *sesamoid bone index* (Kleinberg et al., 1966) should be a diagnostic adjunct in acromegaly (in this disease the product of *x* times *y* mm in the medial sesamoid bone of the thumb >30, Erbe et al., 1975).

C = Four years after the initial examination (see A) and hypophysectomy, polyosteoarthrosis of the *distal* interphalangeal joints (see text) is demonstrable (illustrated only in the index finger). In the *proximal* interphalangeal joint (of the index finger), the early stage of osteoarthrosis is manifested by slight narrowing of the joint space, a delicate increase in density of the subchondral cancellous bone, and small calcifications (ossifications) in the joint capsule.

Table 1). The soft tissues of the fingers appear in the roentgenogram to be "homogenized."

Proliferation of the articular cartilage leads to "widening" of the radiographic joint space. The proliferated articular cartilage can ossify and then sits as a cap over the previously subchondral bone (Fisher, 1978). On the one hand, the *acromegalic remodeling of bone* manifests itself by thickening of the metacarpal and phalangeal shafts without increase in bone length. On the other hand, the terminal tufts of the distal phalanges become typically deformed, assuming the shape of a spade or an anchor (Erbe et al., 1975). In addition, the capsular and ligamental insertions present bony protuberances, giving the impression of an *"osteoarthrosis with a widened joint space."* In the individual case, the bony deformations are variable (compare Fig. 155 with Fig. 156).

About 50 percent of the patients with acromegaly complain of joint discomfort in the extremities and/or pain in the spine ("low back pain"). When the joint discomfort cannot be objectified, one speaks of arthralgia. The picture of *acromegalic osteoarthropathy* also includes morning stiffness, joint pain, limitation of motion, and recurrent effusions into the joints. Moreover it should be mentioned that the proliferated articular cartilage—"widening of the joint space"—tends to premature abrasion so that, in addition, the *typical* radiologic appearance of osteoarthrosis (of the fingers) frequently develops during the evolution of the disease (see Fig. 155). Even *before*, circumscribed calcifications and ossifications of the joint capsule are demonstrable. Thickening of the tendons and tendon sheaths can give rise to the carpal tunnel syndrome (see under this heading) (Bluestone et al., 1971).

To assess the skeletal changes in an acromegaly patient, it is advisable to obtain—besides roentgenograms of the hands—especially dorsoplantar views of the forefoot and lateral views of the hindfoot (calcaneus; see Fig. 550), the skull, and the lumbar spine.

Fig. 156 **Hand of an acromegalic.** Striking features are increased density of the soft tissues in the fingers, widening of the joint spaces, and a partly bulbous, partly irregular enlargement of the shafts of the proximal phalanges, some of the middle phalanges, and the metacarpals. (No outgrowth of the "borders of the bones"; compare Fig. 155).

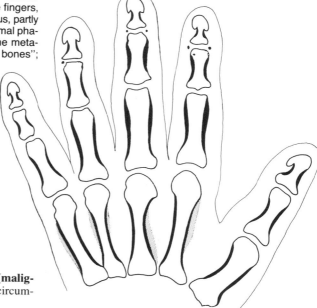

Joint complaints in conjunction with (malignant) tumors can occur under the following circumstances:

1. A benign or malignant neoplasm of the joint is present; e.g., a malignant synovialoma.
2. A carcinoma metastasizes to the synovial membrane (Goldenberg et al., 1975).
3. A paraneoplastic (febrile, acute, or subacute), mono-oligo- or polyarticular arthritis is present (Brunner, 1967).
4. In patients with leukemia and other malignancies, who are under treatment with antimetabolites, corticosteroids, etc., an *infectious* mono- or oligoarticular arthritis (caused, for example, by blood-borne intestinal bacteria) may be disguised by "rheumatic" complaints (Douglas et al., 1964).
5. Joint discomfort can be related to dermatomyositis (see p. 102 ff).
6. Arthralgia or arthritis (synovitis) develops in the setting of **hypertrophic osteoarthropathy (symptomatic pachydermoperiostosis, Marie-Bamberger syndrome,** Fig. 157).
7. Rickets or osteomalacia, as a paraneoplastic reaction, is apt to occur with benign or malignant tumors of bone and soft tissues as well as with tumorlike bone lesions. The condition can regress following surgical removal of the etiologic growth (Linovitz et al., 1976; Yoshikawa et al., 1977).

The disease picture listed under item 6 presents the following basic clinical and roentgenologic features: Generally bilateral, more or less symmetrical, periosteal reaction of bone in the diaphysis of large and small tubular bones (particularly, in decreasing order of frequency, the radius, ulna, tibia, fibula, humerus, and femur, the metacarpals, metatarsals, and the proximal and the middle phalanges); clubbing of fingers and toes with increased curvature of the nails; hyperhidrosis of the palms and soles; arthralgia amounting to arthritis (morning stiffness, limitation of motion, effusion with swelling, painful joints).

When attention is focused on the foregoing basic features, there evidently are *two causes* for this constellation of findings:

1. The clinical picture is due to a disease of the intrathoracic organs, the gastrointestinal tract, or the liver. In malignant tumors of the pleura, hypertrophic osteoarthropathy occurs more frequently than in bronchial cancer (von Wichert, 1967). Pulmonary metastases of extrathoracic tumors sometimes also give rise to hypertrophic osteoarthropathy, just as do chronic suppurative processes in the lungs and the pleura; for example, pleural empyema, lung abscesses, or bronchiectasis. Hypertrophic osteoarthropathy also occurs in cyanotic valvular diseases and in cancer of the esophagus (Peyman, 1959). *Unilateral* occurrence of the disease picture has been observed in aneurysms (Calabro 1967), of the aorta for instance, or with Pancoast tumor. Regional enteritis, ulcerative colitis (Farman et al., 1976), cirrhosis of the liver (Hansoti and Shah, 1966), and hepatocellular carcinoma (Morgan et al., 1972) are to be listed among the extrathoracic causes of hypertrophic osteoarthropathy. The signs and symptoms of the disease are reversible if the cause is removed by therapeutic measures.

2. **Idiopathic pachydermoperiostosis** presents—in addition to the periosteal reactions, arthralgia or synovitis, clubbed fingers and toes with increased curvature of the nails, and local dysfunction of the au-

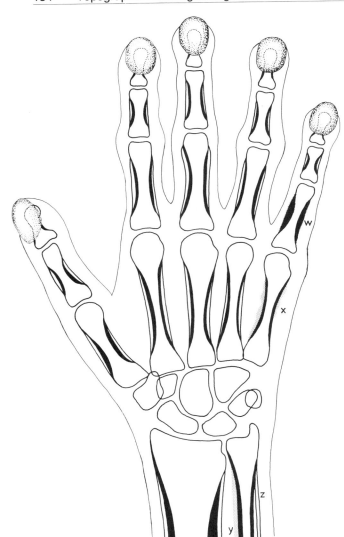

Fig. 157 Hypertrophic osteoarthropathy (symptomatic pachydermoperiostosis) in a patient with congenital bronchiectases.

1.   In digits I to IV and in the radius, the *classical* periosteal reaction is sketched = delicate lamella which is demarcated from the shaft of the tubular bone by a radiolucent area.

w to z are periosteal reactions that are less frequently observed in hypertrophic osteoarthropathy (sketched only in the 5th digit); namely:

w = The periosteal reaction fuses completely with the cortex, giving the latter a thickened appearance.

x = Solid periosteal reaction with wavy contour, sitting directly on the cortex.

y = Solid periosteal reaction (as in x) but with smooth contour.

z = stratified lamellar reaction.

2.   Clubbed fingers with increased curvature of nails.

3.   (Fusiform) swelling of the proximal interphalangeal joints II and IV due to synovitis, effusion into the metacarpophalangeal joint of the little finger (see Fig. 92, soft-tissue signs of arthritis).

Note: In hypertrophic osteoarthropathy the distal phalanges do not usually present periosteal reaction. Moreover, the periosteal reactions are not always recognizable in all the visible tubular bones. One or the other tubular bone may be free from them.

tonomic nervous system (hyperhidrosis of the palms and soles)—the following pathologic peculiarities: It is a hereditary disease with preference for the male sex, which usually begins in adolescence. Changes in the skin and the subcutis lead to pawlike enlargement of the hands and feet, column-shaped (cylindrical) forearms and legs, and thickening and furrowing of the facial skin and the scalp (cutis verticis gyrata, Fig. 158). Acro-osteolyses occur in the distal phalanges (see p. 57). Idiopathic pachydermoperiostosis pursues an insidious, progressive course and can, after years or decades, come to a spontaneous arrest. It can, however, also expand into generalized hyperostosis of the skeleton (generalized hyperostosis; Uehlinger, 1942). The bones of the extremities and the trunk become enlarged by periosteal apposition but do not increase in length. The ossification spreads to

the ligaments, joint capsules, and interosseous membranes and also involves cartilaginous structures, among them the menisci and the disks. Synostoses—for example, of the carpal, tarsal, carpometacarpal, tarsometatarsal, phalangeal, costovertebral, and sacroiliac joints and symphysis—as well as ossifications of the spinal ligaments can supervene. Besides the *complete* form of the clinical picture, which either is arrested spontaneously or expands into generalized hyperostosis, the disease can also run an *incomplete* course (forme fruste), presenting only individual signs and symptoms; for instance, hereditary clubbing of the fingers, isolated cutis verticis gyrata, or idiopathic pachydermoperiostosis without pachyderma.

The ''dualistic'' view—classification of acquired hypertrophic osteoarthropathy and idiopathic

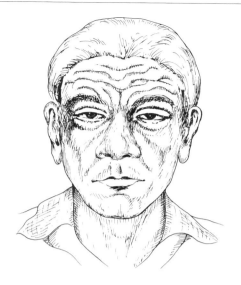

Fig. 158 **Facial appearance in pachydermoperiostosis.** Marked furrowing of the skin and coarsening of the facial structures give the face a worried expression. Slight ptosis due to thickening of the upper eyelid. Frequently also "oily face" from increased secretion of the sebaceous glands.

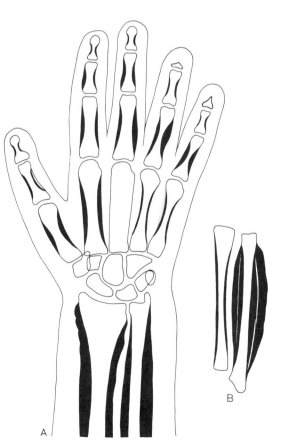

Fig. 159 **Spectrum of the hand in idiopathic pachydermoperiostosis** (A). The picture may vary, depending on the inherited individual mode of reaction and the clinical course (slowly progressive phase of evolution, spontaneous arrest, progression to generalized skeletal hyperostosis).

Soft tissues: Pawlike shape of the hand (with clubbed fingers and increased curvature of the nails) and columnar (cylindrical) transformation of the forearms.

Distal phalanges: Acroosteolyses in the 4th and 5th fingers.

Middle and proximal phalanges: Initially, often delicate periosteal lamella demarcated from the compacta (proximal phalanx I). Much more frequently, however, thickened compacta—the periosteal apposition has fused with the cortex. In addition, the waist of the phalanx may be completely lost (= *box-shaped phalanx;* see proximal phalanx II), or the phalanx may present a convex shape (see proximal phalanges III and IV, middle phalanx II). The marrow cavity of the diaphysis may be of a normal width (see proximal phalanx II) or maybe widened (see proximal phlanx III) or narrowed (see proxima phalanges IV and V).

Metacarpals: Thickening of the compacta (metacarpal I), box-shaped metacarpals II and III (in III, the compacta has become cancellous); the periosteal apposition may be demarcated from the original diaphyseal compacta (metacarapals IV and V).

Radius, ulna: The periosteal apposition has originated in the diaphysis, metaphysis, and epiphysis and has fused with the cortex. Portions of the periosteal appositions show an irregular surface contour (see distal radius). B = Roentgenologic aspect of Caffey's **infantile cortical hyperostosis** (the children are rarely older than 5 months!). Clinical onset in most cases with fever, elevated ESR, and a painful deep swelling that is located underneath the subcutaneous adipose tissue. Most frequent localizations are the ulna (with exception of the epiphyses), the mandible, and the clavicle. Unequivocal involvement of the phalanges and the vertebrae has so far not been observed. Differential diagnosis primarily from overdosage with vitamin A in small children, from trauma, and from osteomyelitis.

(hereditary) pachydermoperiostosis as two different entities—is opposed by the "unitary" view which is based on the following arguments:

Occasionally, hypertrophic osteoarthropathy is accompanied by an increase of the subcutaneous connective tissue, which leads to similar deformations of the forearms, hands, and feet to those in idiopathic pachydermoperiostosis. The latter disease, as well as hypertrophic osteoarthropathy can occur in the same family. In the *initial phase* of pachydermoperiostosis, the shelflike periosteal appositions in the roentgenogram are often indistinguishable from the findings in hypertrophic osteoarthropathy (Fig. 159, proximal phalanx I; Fig. 160). In this latter disease, the manifestations either regress after successful therapy or the patient dies from the underlying disease; e.g., bronchial cancer. Therefore, the stage in which the newly formed periosteal bone fuses completely with the cortex of the tubular bones (Fig. 157 W, X, and Y; Fig. 160) is seldom or never reached. In addition, hypertrophic osteoarthropathy is very rare in comparison with its underlying diseases. Therefore it is natural to assume that it also develops on the basis of a genetic predisposition, such as is an established fact in idiopathic pachydermoperiostosis. There exists, then, an *idiopathic (primary) pachydermoperiostosis* and a *symptomatic (secondary) pachydermoperiostosis* (= hypertrophic osteoarthropathy) (Vogl and Goldfischer, 1962).

Thyroid acropachy can occur in hyperthyroid patients in whom therapy has led to a euthyroid or hypothyroid disorder of metabolism. They present, besides pretibial edema and (malignant) exophthalmos, clubbing of fingers (and toes) and coarsening of the distal segments of the extremities. The roentgenogram shows periosteal changes of the nature illustrated in Figure 160. Differentiation from idiopathic and symptomatic pachydermoperiostosis is facilitated by the patient's clinical history. In addition, there exists an **idiopathic periosteal hyperostosis with dysproteinemia.** According to Goldbloom et al. (1966), this disorder is related to febrile infections of the respiratory tract.

About every tenth case of the carpal tunnel syndrome can be traced to hypothyroidism (Frymover and Bland, 1973). **Arthropathy of myxedema** also

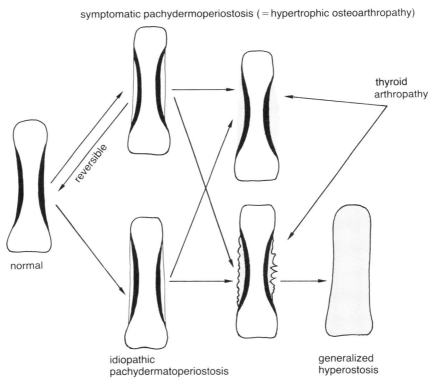

symptomatic pachydermoperiostosis (= hypertrophic osteoarthropathy)

thyroid arthropathy

reversible

normal

idiopathic pachydermatoperiostosis

generalized hyperostosis

Fig. 160 **Phase pattern of the periosteal reactions in symptomatic pachydermatoperiostosis (hypertrophic osteoarthropathy), in idiopathic pachydermatoperiostosis and in thyroid acropachy.** Thickening of soft tissues and clubbing of fingers (and toes) with increased curvature of the nails also belong among the characteristics of these disorders (see text). The *clinical history* is the most important criterion in making the differential diagnosis (see text)!

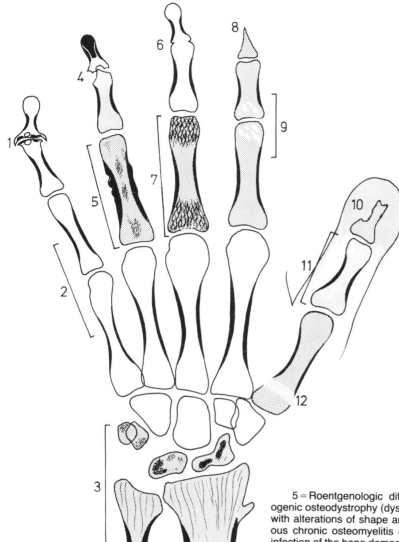

Fig. 161 **Synoptic roentgenogram of the hand in osteoarthropathy from ionizing rays.**

1 = Radiogenic osteoarthrosis of the distal interphalangeal joints (occupational radiation injury in a surgeon).

2 = Hypoplasia following damage to the epiphyseal plates of the proximal phalanx and the metacarpal of the little finger (roentgen irradiation of warts in childhood).

3 = Severe developmental disturbance of the distal parts of radius and ulna as well as the proximal carpal bones following repeated roentgen irradiation of a cutaneous cavernous hemangioma in this area in infancy and early childhood. In addition, a cartilaginous exostosis had developed as the result of irradiation (Kolář and Vrabec, 1976).

4 = Radiogenic arthritis, probably associated with an infection by bacteria that have invaded the joint by way of an irradiation dermatitis. Radiogenic damage of the articular cartilage.

5 = Roentgenologic differentiation between radiogenic osteodystrophy (dystrophic remodeling of bone with alterations of shape and structure) and an insidious chronic osteomyelitis developing after additional infection of the bone damaged by radiation. (A sequestrum, which would be an important differential diagnostic criterion, is not demonstrable in this case).

6 = Bony ankylosis following radiogenic arthritis (see no. 4).

7 = Fibrillar-cystoid remodeling of cancellous bone (similar to hypertrophic atrophy of bone; see Fig. 13) 9 years after roentgen therapy of chronic eczema.

8 = Radiogenic, noninflammatory and nonneoplastic acroosteolysis in a nurse working in a radiological department.

9 = Spotty decalcification several years after repeated roentgen irradiation for eczema.

10 = Invasion of the distal phalanx by a squamous cell carcinoma arising from an irradiation ulcer. Osteosarcomas, fibrosarcomas, and chondrosarcomas likewise are an infrequent result of therapy with ionizing rays.

11 = Diffuse, potentially reversible, osteoporosis of a bone situated in the cone of roentgen rays.

12 = Looser's zone following roentgen irradiation of the skin for a cavernous hemangioma.

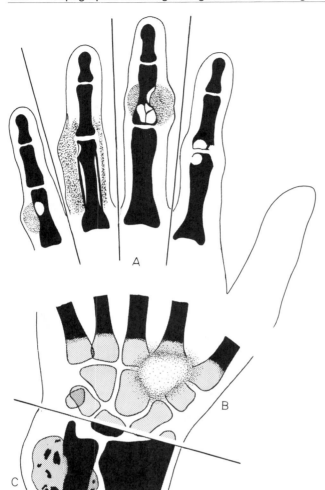

Fig. 162 **Pigmented villonodular synovitis (A) and malignant synovialoma (B, C) in the hand**(synopsis). A = Pigmented villonodular synovitis of the flexor tendon sheaths 3 to 5 = Circumscribed, unusually dense swelling of soft tissues (due to iron-containing pigment) with erosion of bone. En face = rounded, partly trabeculated osteolysis. In profile = radiographic aspect of the flat-arched pressure erosion. Diffuse involvement of the 4th flexor tendon sheath with lamellar periosteal reaction in the proximal phalanx.

The synovial membrane in the proximal interphalangeal joint of the index finger is diseased. Roentgen findings: Not very characteristic (slight swelling of joint; cystoid osteolyses on both sides of the joint space, which shows no narrowing; absence of subchondral osteoporosis). In any event, in the presence of such roentgen findings in a single joint and accompanied only by slight discomfort, pigmented villonodular synovitis also should enter into the differential diagnosis.

B = Osteolytic process with circumscribed swelling of soft tissues, which has completely dissolved the trapezoid and also has invaded the neighboring bones. Demineralization of the surrounding bones. If, in addition, local pleomorphic calcium shadows were visible, the roentgen finding alone would justify the suspicion of malignant synovialoma. In the present case, the diagnosis was settled by biopsy.

C = Swelling with increased density of soft tissues, irregularly shaped calcifications, and flat-arched erosion of the distal ulna. This radiologic finding suggests malignant synovialoma (see text).

is an infrequent finding. Arthralgia, sensation of stiffness, and joint effusion are the indistinct features of this hypothyroid arthropathy, which can manifest itself in the carpal region, in the metacarpophalangeal joints, in the knee, and in the talocrural joint. Histologically, one encounters a noninflammatory or slightly inflammatory synovitis accompanied by effusion into the joint (Golding, 1971). Calcification of articular cartilages (chondrocalcinosis) has also been observed in arthropathy of myxedema. Cretinism and juvenile myxedema can lead to delayed development, retardation of growth, and disordered epiphyseal ossification. Numerous ossification centers develop in the large epiphyses, which—roentgenologically—give the impression of fragmented epiphyseal nuclei. Adult hypothyroidism can give rise to avascular necrosis of bone; for example, in the lunate (Rubinstein and Brooks, 1977).

Osteoarthropathy from ionizing rays (Fig. 161) develops in the hand either following therapeutic irradiations or as occupational radiation damage. Depending primarily though not exclusively on the individual and total dosage, the intervals between radiation exposures and the nature of the rays, there arise (years later) regressive changes and necroses in the supporting and gliding tissues, which may become infected by irradiation ulcers. Lesions of the finger joints are to be expected, particularly in cases of occupational overexposure; they are associated with chronic irradiation damage to the skin. Growth disturbances in the hand and the distal forearm have been described; for example, as the result of inexpert irradiation of hemangiomas in infants and small children.

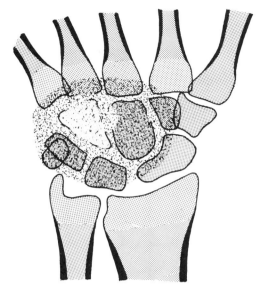

Fig. 163 **Carcinomatous metastasis in the wrist** (osteolysis, osteoporosis). Compare Figure 162. The condition must also be differentiated from arthritis of the wrist (Figs. 125 and 126). Arguments *against inflammation* are the absence of joint space narrowing and a dense soft-tissue shadow projected on the destroyed or decalcified carpal bones, which reflects the three-dimensional, unrestrained growth of the tumor. Tuberculosis (for instance) would spread in a rather "two-dimensional" manner; i.e., with limitation to the skeletal and articular structures. A tuberculous abscess would be fluctuating on palpation and possibly would be accompanied by fistulation. The expanding tumor masses are hard to the touch.

Neoplasms of Joints

This section deals with *space-occupying processes* that originate either in the glide tissues (synovial membrane of joints, bursae, and tendon sheaths), in the surrounding tissues, or in juxtaarticular bone, and which impair the glide tissue to varying degrees. The concept "space-occupying process" is conceived in a broad sense, so accumulations of metabolites will also be discussed (insofar as they have already been mentioned in other portions of this text).

Discussion regarding the nosological classification of **pigmented villonodular synovitis** of joints, tendon sheaths, and bursae has not yet ended. Jaffe et al. (1941) consider this disorder to be an inflammatory process, whereas Uehlinger (1977) classifies it as a semimalignant neoplasm. There are two types of the disease: the *diffuse* type, in which the entire synovial membrane is involved, and the *nodular* type, which occurs as a circumscribed affection of the synovial membrane. The nodular type is encountered especially often in the tendon sheaths of the flexor mus-

cles of the hand. Pigmented villonodular synovitis is much more likely to occur in a single site than in several sites. In the hand, the disorder prevalently affects the tendon sheaths and is characterized by the following, rather typical, roentgen manifestations (Fig. 162):

1. Circumscribed swelling of soft tissues without calcium shadows
2. Defects with smooth borders that may be classified as juxtaarticular pressure erosions (see p. 29).
3. Cystic osteolyses with smooth contours and a marginal seam, or without delicate increased thickness of the borders.
4. A lamellar periosteal reaction in the shaft of the phalanx develops, but infrequently. It occurs when pigmented villonodular synovitis involves the entire extent or at least larger segments of the flexor tendon sheath (Stern and Gauger, 1977). In such cases, growth may be disturbed (the finger increases in size).

When pigmented villonodular synovitis develops in the synovial membrane of a joint, the following pathologic roentgen manifestations are to be expected:

1. Joint-related swelling of soft tissues, which is more conspicuous the nearer to the surface the joint is situated.
2. There is no narrowing of the radiographic joint space.
3. Cystic osteolyses, either without a marginal seam or with a delicate increase in density of their marginal contours, situated *on both sides* of the joint space. Involvement of bone, however, is a late finding in pigmented villonodular synovitis. It reflects invasion of the proliferating tissue either through the nutrient channels or by way of the capsular insertion. Pressure erosions of the articulating bones in diseased joints occur less frequently than with involvement of the tendon sheaths and the bursae.
4. Juxtaarticular osteoporosis is usually absent.

The synovialoma originates in the synovial cells of the joints, the tendon sheaths, the bursae, and—less frequently—from the fasciae. Skeletal synovialomas are even less common. The histologic picture presents villous proliferations, clefts, and cysts that are coated with a cellular cover. The majority of synovialomas show the characteristics of a malignant tumor; hence the terms **malignant synovialoma** or **synovial sarcoma.** Figure 162 illustrates the roentgen findings in malignant synovialoma of the wrist and the distal forearm. In Figure 162 C one will find the characteristic roentgen manifestations of malignant synovialoma; namely, increased density of the soft tissues, calcifications in the soft tissues, and erosion of bone from pressure or from the invading tumor cells. These radiographic characteristics, however, occur *conjointly* only in a minority of the malignant synovialomas (Horowitz et al., 1973). Emphasis is to be placed on the diffuse demineralization of the remaining parts of the hand skeleton.

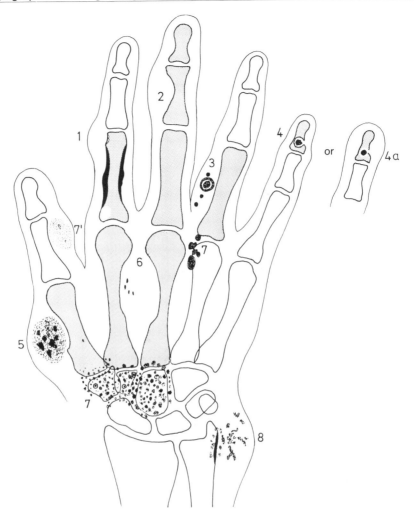

Fig. 164 **Visible and/or palpable space-occupying processes in the hand.** Diagnostic classification can be furthered decisively by roentgen examination.

1 = *Fibroma* with pressure erosion in the proximal phalanx in tuberous sclerosis. Identification on the basis of periosteal and endosteal new bone formation, including the cystic translucences of the osseous structure.

2 = Von Recklingausen's *neurofibromatosis,* identified by increase in size of the phalanges (growth disturbance). Pressure erosion by a neurofibroma.

3 = *Hemangioma* (pressure erosion possible but not illustrated). Identification by calcium shadows, which have the typical aspect of phleboliths.

4 = Painful *osteoid osteoma* with *calcified nidus* (characteristic, though not consistent, finding in osteoid osteoma of *cancellous* bone; compare Fig. 557). Fusiform bulging of the distal interphalangeal joint by an effusion of sympathetic arthritis (4, see p. 161 ff) or diffuse parosteal swelling of soft tissues (4a). In the growth period, osteoid osteoma may give rise to local growth disturbances; e.g., premature epiphyseal closure (Rosborough, 1966).

5 = *Soft-tissue chondroma* (originating in the synovial membrane of joints, in bursae, in tendon sheaths, or in parosteal connective tissue) with pressure erosion in the metacarpal of the thumb (the inhomogeneous calcification points to the cartilaginous matrix of the neoplasm).

6 = *Intermetacarpal lipoma* (compare Fig. 557) with extensive pressure erosions (delicate striated calcifications are possible).

7 = *Neoplastic synovial chondromatosis (Reichel's disease).* Identification by the (numerous) calcium shadows varying in size from dots to a few millimeters. Erosions may occur in small bones (Goutaillier et al., 1978).

8 = Neoplastic synovial chondromatosis of the flexor tendon sheath of the thumb (De Benedetti and Schwinn, 1979).

9 = *Peripheral chondrosarcoma* (early stage). A soft-tissue mass with bizarre, in part striated, calcium shadows appears to be attached to the bone. At the "site of attachment," the cortex is sometimes thickened. During its further course, the neoplasm destroys the contiguous bone. Roentgenologic differentiation from malignant synovialoma (compare Fig. 162 C).

This finding, in conjunction with slow growth and swelling of soft tissues, can lead to the erroneous diagnosis "tuberculosis of the joint." On the other hand, skeletal metastases of other malignant tumors sometimes present a similar radiographic appearance (Fig. 163).

In the fingers, and also in the remaining region of the hand, space-occupying processes starting from the joints, the extraarticular soft tissues, or the bones manifest themselves early in the disease, owing to their thin soft-tissue cover (Figs. 164 and 165). This applies to inspection and palpation on physical examination as well as to the roentgenograms (in two planes). In **lipomas** (growing, for example, entrapped between the metacarpals), in **fibromas** (isolated or in the setting of von Recklinghausen's neurofibromatosis), in **soft-tissue chondromas,** and in neoplastic synovial chondromatosis (see p. 66 ff), the roentgenogram can provide decisive additional information (Fig. 164). The same is applicable to the diagnosis of **hemangiomas** (isolated synovial hemangioma in joints and tendon sheaths or as part of a syndrome, for example the Klippel-Trenaunay syndrome [angioosteohypertrophic syndrome; see also p. 29], the Kasabach-Merritt syndrome [hemangioma-thrombocytopenia syndrome], of Mafucci's syndrome (see p. 116; Fig. 164).

In the *primary* hyperlipoproteinemias, **xanthomas** develop in the skin and subcutis, in the tendons—including the extensor tendons of the hands and feet—and in the bones. They can manifest themselves as space-occupying processes (Fig. 166). In addition, arthralgias and "migratory" kinds of arthritis with pain, swelling, limitation of motion, and even erythema over the involved joints have been observed in familial type II hyperlipoproteinemia (after Fredrickson and Lees, 1965) and in type IV hyperlipoproteinemia. Therefore, in these patients the radiologic suspicion of xanthoma or at least the hint of the presence of a storage disease is of diagnostic importance; for example, in differentiating the condition from rheumatic fever. Intraosseous xanthomas—i.e., primary involvement of bone in contrast to secondary involvement from pressure erosions—also occur in

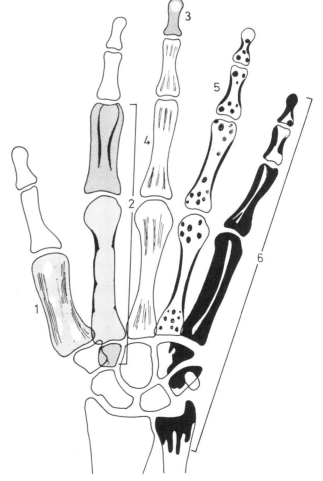

Fig. 165 Characteristic chance roentgenologic findings in patients whose hands are radiologically examined for joint discomfort of any kind.

1 = *Paget's disease of bone (osteitis deformans):* enlargement of bone, fibrillar structures, translucences.

2 = *Fibrous dysplasia:* polymorphic roentgenogram; for instance, sclerosis of cancellous bone in the trapezoid, slight expansion of the 2nd metacarpal with thinning of the cortex, "ground glass shadow," considerable thickening of the cortex (periosteal constriction) of the proximal phalanx of the index finger, part of whose original osseous shape is still visible.

3 = *Epithelial cyst* (following perforating injury to soft tissues and bone), often accompanied by blueish discoloration of the nailbed (compare Fig. 146 G and H).

4 = *Osteopathia striata* (Voorhoeve's disease). (Note the typical *metaphyseal* striation.)

5 = *Osteopoikilosis.*

6 = *Melorheostosis* (in the ulna, typical aspect of "melting wax flowing down the side of a burning candle"). The spread of melorheostosis probably follows the areas that are supplied by the sensory nerves (Murray and McCredie, 1979).

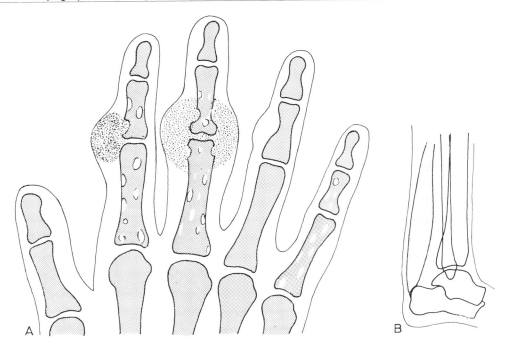

Fig. 166   **Hyperlipoproteinemia.**

A: *2nd and 3rd fingers* = soft-tissue xanthomas with pressure erosions, intraosseous cholesterol deposits (rounded or oval small osteolyses, in part with delicate increase in marginal thickness, frequently bilaterally-symmetrical in both hands).

4th finger = Soft-tissue xanthoma with pressure erosion. *Little finger* = intraosseous cholesterol deposits, sketched here as small osteolyses but sometimes also producing honeycomb remodeling of cancellous bone, *no* soft-tissue xanthomas. The soft-tissue swellings also should be radiologically differentiated from subcutaneous rheumatoid nodules in rheumatoid arthritis.

B: The finding that settles the roentgenologic diagnosis in the hyperlipoproteinemias is the bilateral fusiform swelling of the Achilles tendon produced by xanthomas of the tendon. (Deposition of calcium can take place in the xanthomas.)

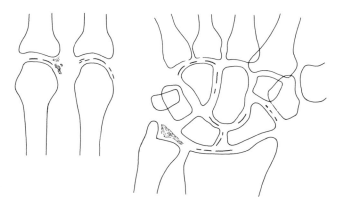

Fig. 167   **Radiographic morphology of chondrocalcinosis** in the region of the hand. (One of the metacarpophalangeal joints shows concomitant calcifications of the periarticular soft tissues; compare Figs. 68, 148, and 150).

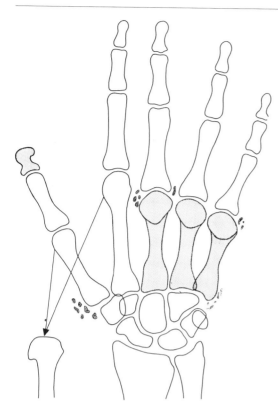

Fig. 168   Shortness of metacarpals and calcifications of soft tissues are the leading roentgenologic manifestations of pseudohypoparathyroidism and pseudopseudohypoparathyroidism (= short stature associated with short metacarpals and/or metatarsals; compare Fig. 561). The *metacarpals* IV, V, I, III, and II are involved in descending order of frequency (Spech and Olah, 1974). Epiphyseal deformations (even without shortening) also occur in the hand *(arrow)*, the feet, and other bones.

type III hyperlipoproteinemia (Kovac et al., 1976; Yaghmai, 1978). Similar findings, likewise caused by massive accumulation of cholesterol-laden foam cells, occur in *secondary* hyperlipoproteinemia; for example, in primary bilary cirrhosis of the liver (see p. 104) (Ansell and Bywaters, 1957).

Articular chondrocalcinosis occurs in a hereditary, sporadic, and symptomatic form (see p. 62 ff). Roentgenograms of chondrocalcinosis in the hand are reproduced in Figures 68, 148, 150, and 167.

Calcifications of Soft Tissues

The nosology of the periarticular calcifications has been discussed on p. 68 ff. Their roentgenologic aspect in the hand is reproduced in Figures 113, 115, 116, and 120.

Calcifications of soft tissues also occur in the

majority of patients with **pseudohypoparathyroidism** (PHP) (Albright et al., 1942), and those with **pseudo-pseudohypoparathyroidism** (PPHP). The former presents typical *constitutional characteristics* (short stature, round face, short neck, *shortness of metacarpals* more pronounced than shortness of metatarsals [particularly III to V, but also I], shortening of the distal phalanx of the thumb, disorders of epiphyseal ossification [deformations], exostoses, delayed eruption of teeth, enamel hypoplasias). Conspicuous *clinical* features are familial occurrence, mental deficiency, tetany and epilepsy, cataract, symmetrical calcifications of the basal ganglia, *calcifications of soft tissues,* osteoporosis, and hyperostosis. Important laboratory data are hypocalcemia, hyperphosphatemia, and a normal or *increased* serum concentration of parathyroid hormone. The result of the parathyroid hormone loading test can indicate resistance of the target organs to biologically active parathyroid hormone.

Pseudopseudohypoparathyroidism is a variant of pseudohypoparathyroidism. This is also suggested by the occurrence of both entities in a single family (Stögmann and Oser, 1974; Poznanski et al., 1977). In this disease, one does not observe the alterations of serum values that are characteristic of pseudohypoparathyroidism and their clinical consequences (tetanic seizures, for instance, do not occur). However, the constitutional characteristics described are identical in both diseases. In classifying the anomalies described, one can differentiate:

1. Constitutional anomalies (PHP, PPHP). These, however, whether congenital or acquired, also may occur as solitary findings and in various hereditary syndromes (see metacarpal sign, p. 79, Fig. 89).
2. Anomalous biochemical findings in blood (PHP) in (idiopathic) hypoparathyroidism and their consequences; for example, calcifications in the basal ganglia, deficient dentition, tetany, epilepsy (tetany-induced epilepsy; i.e., cerebral convulsions in tetany).
3. Calcifications (ossifications) of soft tissues, occurring about the joints, in the tendons, in the subcutis, and in muscles. Since they are encountered in pseudohypoparathyroidism as well as in pseudopseudohypoparathyroidism, they cannot be ascribed exclusively to the hypoparathyroid disorder of calcium metabolism.
4. The hypocalcemia and the increased serum level of parathyroid hormone (PHP) might lead one to expect that, histologically, the skeleton would reveal a dissecting fibroosteoclasia—hence the morphologic substrate of hyperparathyroidism. Such is indeed the case in pseudohypoparathyroidism. It also can be confirmed roentgenologically in a small percentage of patients (subperiosteal bone resorption, see p. 126 ff) (= pseudohypohyperparathyroidism, Kolb and Steinbach, 1962; Bronsky, 1970).

The *practical significance* of the disease pictures described can be summarized as follows: In convulsive disorders (tetany, epilepsy), the calcium-

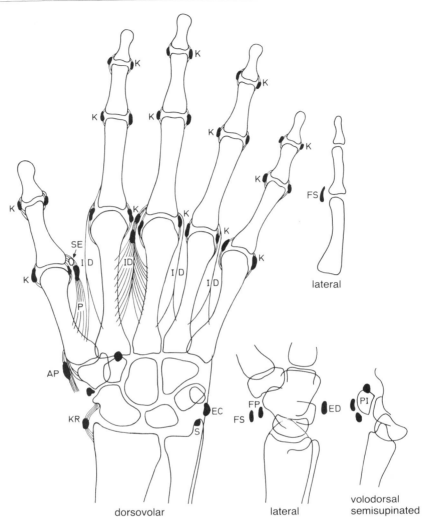

Fig. 169   Sites of predilection for so-called calcareous tendinitis (peritendinitis) in the hand.
    Clinically: Painless latent *or* chronic pain *or* acute inflammatory symptoms.
    Roentgenologic findings: Polymorphic soft-tissue calcifications (in tendons, ligaments, fibrous joint capsules).
    Topography: K = Fibrous joint capsule and collateral ligaments.
    ID = Dorsal interosseous muscles (Cooper, 1942). P = Flexor pollicis brevis muscle. SE = Sesamoid bone. AP = Abductor pollicis longus muscle.
    KR = Radial collateral ligament of carpus. S = Bursa of styloid process (Kessler and Silberman, 1961). EC = Extensor carpi ulnaris muscle. FS, FP = Flexor digitorum superficialis and profundus muscles (with acute onset often recognizable in the roentgenogram as edema [soft-tissue swelling]). ED = Extensor digitorum muscle.
    PI = Pisiform; calcium deposits in its surroundings point to involvement of the tendon of the flexor carpi ulnaris muscle. Calcium deposits are nonstructured. Supernumerary ossicles, traumatic avulsions (from the triquetrum, for instance), and osteoarthritic capsular ossicles have a structured cancellous bone and a cortex that is preserved entirely or in part (study under a loupe!). Neoplastic synovial chondromatosis not only occurs infrequently in the carpal region but also differs from the calcium deposits discussed here by the multiplicity of calcified synovial chondromas which are arranged in circular fashion around the carpus and the carpometacarpal joints (Fig. 164).

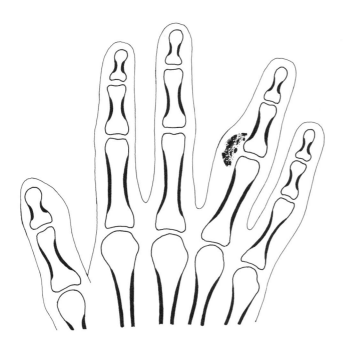

Fig. 170 Acute so-called calcareous tendinitis of the ring finger.

Clinically: Intense pain. Preferentially lateral swelling and reddening of the skin in the vincinity of the proximal interphalangeal joint of the ring finger of the right hand.

Roentgenologically: Radial to the proximal interphalangeal joint of the fourth finger, a crescent-shaped soft-tissue calcification is visible. Considerable edema of the immediately surrounding tissue. Slight swelling on the ulnar side of the joint.

Note: Calcareous tendinitis (peritendinitis) in the vicinity of the metacarpophalangeal joints manifests itself clinically by a more or less extensive swelling in the dorsum of the hand.

phosphate metabolism should always be checked by biochemical studies. On the other hand, in certain cases (in PHP and in PPHP), roentgenologic examination of the hands and feet (short metacarpals, short metatarsals [Fig. 561]; shortness of the distal phalanx of the thumb, calcifications of soft tissue [Fig. 168]) can provide decisive diagnostic information.

Calcium deposits in tendons, ligaments, and the fibrous portion of the capsule occur also in the hand (Figs. 169 and 170). Much like their best known counterpart, calcification of the rotator cuff in the shoulder, they sometimes remain clinically *latent*. However, they also may give rise to *chronic* pain on motion and even to *acute* signs of inflammation (intense pain, increased heat and reddening of the skin, limitation of motion and, infrequently, even fever and an elevated sedimentation rate). The condition then may be mistaken for an acute arthritis, a gouty attack, cellulitis, or acute osteomyelitis. Roentgenologic demonstration of soft-tissue calcification in the painful or evidently inflamed area leads to the correct diagnosis. The complaints often follow athletic activities that are associated with strong motion of the wrist; for example, playing golf.

It has already been mentioned (p. 73 ff) that a number of synonyms exists for such hydroxyl apatite deposits and their consequences, including *tendinitis, peritendinitis, myotendinitis, periarthritis, periarthropathy,* and *calcareous tendinosis.* The nomenclature depends on the clinical picture and the supposed site of the calcium deposits. It would therefore be appropriate to use the attribute "so-called" in connection with these denominations. The calcifications discussed here are, in principal, reversible. They are apt to be resorbed but can, after an interval, recur in the same place or elsewhere. This is true not only for the hand but equally for calcifications of tendons and ligaments that occur in many places synchronously or successively (see p. 74); *for example,* in the fingers, the wrist, the knee and, the shoulder regions.

Trauma to Joints

In **dislocations at the interphalageal and metacarpophalangeal joints,** the distal bone is usually dislocated dorsally because these injuries generally follow hyperextension (Fig. 171). Dorsal dislocation may be associated with a lateral displacement. Small breaks of bone, entrapment of sesamoid bones, and avulsion of tendons may complicate the dislocation. Tears or avulsions of the tendons of the extensors of the fingers without dislocation are illustrated in Figure 172. Interposition of parts of the collateral ligaments and of the sesamoid bones in the metacarpophalangeal joints II to V sometimes gives rise to an *irreducible* dislocation. In the metacarpophalangeal joint of the thumb, the dislocation becomes irreducible when, for example, the head of the first metacarpal is displaced

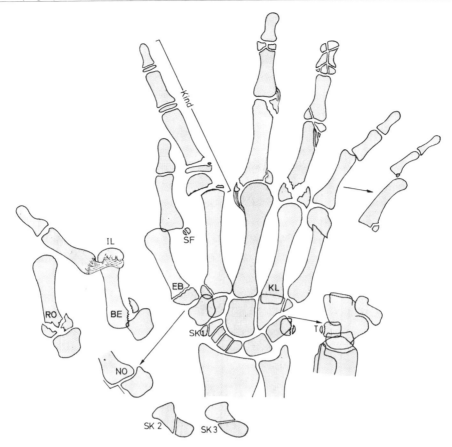

Fig. 171 **Synopsis of injuries to the hand with regular or potential involvement of joints** (part of the joint capsule and the ligaments illustrated).

Special indications: RO = Rolando's fracture (see text). BE = Bennett's fracture-dislocation (see text). IL = Irreducible dislocation at the metacarpophalangeal joint of the thumb (the head of the metacarpal being displaced volarward through a capsular tear; see text). EB = Extraarticular fracture of the base of the 1st metacarpal. SF = Fracture of sesamoid bone. Compare with the uninjured side because bipartite sesamoid bones are apt to occur. NO = Radial step in the 1st carpometacarpal joint is a normal finding (effect of projection) and *not* a subluxation. SK 1 = The most frequent fracture line in the scaphoid at a short distance from the center of the bone and running transversely.

SK 2 = Fracture line running an oblique perpendicular course.

SK 3 = Fracture line running an oblique horizontal course.

KL = Carpometacarpal dislocation, typical aspect in the dorsovolar roentgenogram. T = Characteristic dorsal avulsion of the triquetrum.

volarward in a buttonhole fashion through a capsular tear and cannot slip back.

Dislocations at the carpometacarpal joints II to V can be diagnosed in the dorsovolar roentgenogram. The articulating bones are then projected one above the other (Fig. 171). The direction of the dislocation—dorsal more often than volar—is indicated by the frontal roentgenogram or, in the ulnar carpometacarpal joints, by the dorsovolar roentgenogram in semisupination.

Intraarticular fractures of the fingers, the metacarpal, and the carpal bones also are illus-

trated in Figure 171. In the base of the first metacarpal, the following injuries occur (Fig. 171): *Extraarticular fracture of the base*, intraarticular *Bennet's fracture-dislocation*, and *Rolando's fracture* (intraarticular Y-shaped fracture). Bennet's fracture is the typical fracture-dislocation of skiers and boxers. The characteristic dislocation comes about by the pull of the abductor pollicis longus muscle, which inserts in the base of the first metacarpal.

There are various types of **dislocation of the hand,** among them volar rotary dislocation of the lunate bone. The conventional terminology of the

Fig. 172 **So-called mallet finger.** The dorsal extensor apparatus of the finger (E) has been ruptured by a trauma in extreme flexion; e.g. while playing a ball game. Thereby a flexion of about 30° is produced at the distal interphalangeal joint (due to pull of the flexor digitorum profundus—F). *Active* extension at the distal interphalangeal joint is impossible.

    Top = Tendon rupture.

    Center = Avulsion of extensor tendon from the bone with a small intraarticular fragment.

    Bottom = chondroepiphysiolysis; see Fig. 581. The dislocation is produced by pull of the extensor as well as the flexor muscles.

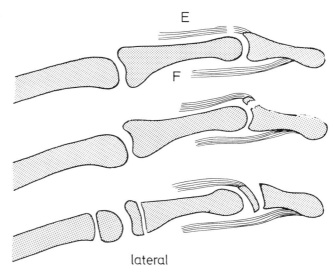

lateral

dislocations is based on the faulty position of the distal articulating bones. Therefore, some writers (Schneck, 1931; Jungbluth, 1973; Machan, 1979, and others) either refer to the latter injury as a dorsal perilunar dislocation or do not differentiate between the very rare pure dislocation of the lunate and the more frequent perilunar dislocation. Their approach is based on the following notions: the trauma dislocates *primarily* the capitate, together with the other carpal bones. The lunate, which is steadied by its volar and dorsal ligaments, at first remains in its normal place. The plane of the dislocation therefore surrounds the lunate. Only *secondarily,* following rupture of its dorsal ligaments, can the lunate be forced out toward the volar side by the dislocated capitate that has sunk back, comparably to the pit being squeezed from a cherry. It is uncommon for the carpal bones to become dislocated volarward around the lunate (volar perilunar dislocation). The plane of the dislocation—the dislocation line in the posteroanterior roentgenogram—does not always pass exclusively around the lunate; sometimes it is accompanied by fractures and dislocations of neighboring bones. This factor has led to the terminology of these *manifold* intercarpal dislocations and fracture-dislocations (Fig. 173). In addition, under the effect of gross direct violence to the wrist one, also sees dislocations of individual carpal bones as well as volar, dorsal, and lateral (mostly radial) dislocations at the radiocarpal joint with fracture of the styloid processes, or else dislocations in a number of directions (radial plus volar plus proximal, etc.). Owing to the strength of the ligaments in the carpal region, fracture-dislocations there occur more frequently than do pure dislocations, the accompanying fractures being very variable.

Among **isolated fractures of the carpal bones,** fracture of the scaphoid is a particularly frequent injury. Failure to recognize its presence involves the danger of pseudoarthrosis of the scaphoid with necrosis of the proximal fragment and the subsequent development of osteoarthrosis. The development of a pseudoarthrosis in the fractured scaphoid is favored both by the devascularization of the fragments and by their anatomically inadequate *reduction* and *adaptation,* as well as by deficient *compression* of the fractured parts. Suspicion of fracture of the scaphoid [12] calls for specific radiologic studies: By ulnar abduction of the hand and flexion of the fingers with dorsal semiflexion at the radiocarpal joint, the oblique position of the scaphoid in the wrist is corrected so that its longitudinal axis approximately parallels the plane of the film. Fracture clefts running in the dorsovolar direction then are met by the x-rays tangentially and can be identified in the roentgenogram. It is advisable to repeat the roentgen examination after one or two weeks because a previously invisible fracture line sometimes becomes demonstrable after the border of the fracture has been resorbed. It should be mentioned here that *osteochondrosis dissecans of the scaphoid* is an extremely infrequent event and that its occurrence has even been doubted (Meves and Schneider-Sickert, 1975). It should be differentiated from traumatic avulsion or detachment of a necrotic portion of the scaphoid.

Avascular necrosis of the lunate bone is apt to develop as the result of undiagnosed or inadequately treated injuries to this bone. Therefore, patients with this disorder sometimes give a history of major trauma. Apart from this, experience has shown that patients without a previous major trauma often have a rela-

---

[12] When the metacarpophalangeal joints II to V and the proxial interphalangeal joints II to V are flexed, the axes of the apposed fingers run toward the scaphoid. Tenderness on pressure elicited over the proximal thenar in the prolonged longitudinal axis therefore suggests injury to the scaphoid.

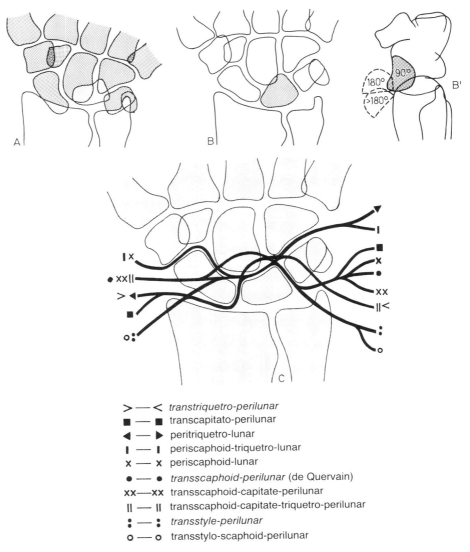

Fig. 173 **Intercarpal dislocations and fracture-dislocations.**
A = *Pure* perilunar dorsal dislocation of the carpus with slight proximal displacement of the dislocated carpal bones. The lunate lies in its normal location!
B, B' = perilunar dorsal dislocation of the carpus with additional volar dislocation of the lunate (so-called rotary volar dislocation of the lunate). (In *A* and *B*, the informative carpal bones are stippled; in *C*, the most frequent injuries are underlined).
C = Examples of combined perilunar dislocations and fracture-dislocations.

tively short ulna (Hultén) and/or work with pneumatic drills. Finally, it should be mentioned that a supposed refractory sprain of the wrist actually may be caused by a dorsally located, flat, generally shelf-like avulsion of the triquetrum (Fig. 171 I)—to be differentiated from the epitriquetrum (De Cuveland, 1955) and from avulsion of the posterior extremity of the lunate!—or by an undiagnosed fracture of the pis-iform, the body of the triquetrum, and the capitate, as well as by the infrequent fractures of the other carpal bones (not described here).

Injuries and, possibly, inflammatory processes (rheumatoid arthritis, Meythaler and Bach, 1979) are sometimes the stimulus for the ossification of a previously cartilaginous accessory ossicle which therefore is not visible in the roentgenogram (Brauer, 1959). Awareness of this possibility

Fig. 174 **Fracture of distal radius at its typical site, depending on age and the mechanism of trauma (see text).** Fractures extending into the radiocarpal joint and thereby producing the formation of steps in the contour of the distal radial joint are not illustrated (see Fig. 175, *right,* and compare Fig. 581).

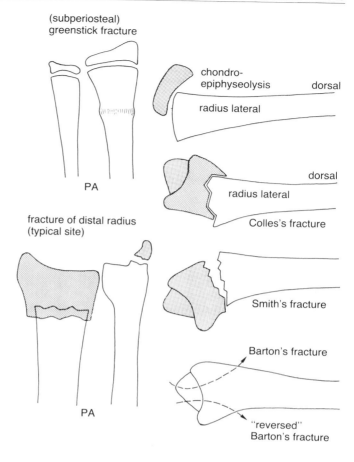

(subperiosteal) greensteck fracture

chondro-epiphyseolysis   dorsal

radius lateral

PA

dorsal

radius lateral

Colles's fracture

fracture of distal radius (typical site)

Smith's fracture

Barton's fracture

PA

"reversed" Barton's fracture

protects against the general assumption of a posttraumatic capsuloligamentous ossification or an osteogenic avulsion of periosteum in places where accessory ossicles are known to occur. It should therefore be taken into consideration in giving expert opinion. Finally, apophyses or epiphyses (for example, the styloid process of the ulna) which had broken off in the growth period can unite again and increase in size; i.e., undergo postraumatic hypertrophy. If bony consolidation fails to take place and a pseudoarthrosis develops, the broken-off part of bone often continues growing and becomes smooth and rounded. In this way, for example, a "posttraumatic os triangulare" (Pöschl, 1957) can develop.

Distal fracture of the radius at the typical site, following closure of the distal radial epiphysis, is a paraepiphyseal fracture. The fracture line courses between 1 and 3 cm proximal to the carpal articular facet of the radius. About 50 percent of the patients suffer concomitant avulsion of the ulnar styloid process (Engeloch and Stirnemann, 1978). Much more infrequent *concomitant injuries* are fractures of the head of the ulna, the scaphoid, the triquetrum, and/or the pisiform.

The following fracture types are known (Fig. 174): *Colles's fracture* from hyper*extension* and compression, *Smith's fracture* from hyper*flexion* and

compression, *Barton's fracture,* a fracture of the dorsal border of the radius from hyperflexion and compression, *"reversed" Barton's fracture* of the volar border of the radius from hyperflexion and compression, and *comminuted fracture of the distal radius.* The classification is based on the roentgenologic aspect and indicates the therapeutic modality. *Late complications* of these fractures are to be expected in the first place when the fracture has united with shortening, malposition, and/or loosening in the distal radioulnar joint (Fig. 175):

1. When the fracture heals in a position that is not conformable to the function of the joint—i.e., when the dorsoradial or volar angulation or displacement has not been completely corrected, the result is limitation of motion and a predisposition to osteoarthrosis of the radiocarpal joint. The same is true of fracture-dislocations.

2. In addition to the transverse and oblique fracture clefts, there exist fractures of the distal radius with T-, V- or Y-shaped fracture lines. In the latter cases, and also in comminuted fractures, the joint is frequenty involved. When such intraarticular fractures unite with incongruity of the articular surfaces (when,

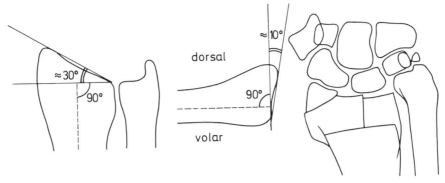

Fig. 175 **Causes of limitation of motion and development of osteoarthrosis in the radiocarpal and distal radioulnar joints** following deformed healed intraarticular fracture of the distal radius at its typical site.
Right: Instances of preosteoarthrotic deformities (recognizable in the dorsovolar roentgenogram) (see text).
Center and left: Normal angular measurements between the shaft of the radius and the carpal articular facet of the radius, ≈10° *(center)*, ≈30° *(left)*.

for example, a step remains in the articular surface of the radius) the result is a preosteoarthrotic deformity of the radiocarpal joint. When a pseudoarthrosis develops in the avulsed styloid process of the ulna, the patient may *occasionally* be left with refractory pain. 3. With major compression of the fragments, the radius may become shorter. The result is relative lengthening of the ulna, which likewise furthers the development of orteoarthrosis. In addition, with major compression of the radius, dislocation at the distal radioulnar joint is to be expected. The capsuloligamentous apparatus of this joint can rupture, and "springy ulna" (p. 80 ff) then makes its appearance as a postraumatic event. Fracture of the distal radius with concomitant damage to the periarticular radioulnar soft tissues leads, as a rule, more frequently to osteoarthrosis than isolated fracture of the distal radius. A fracture between the distal and the middle

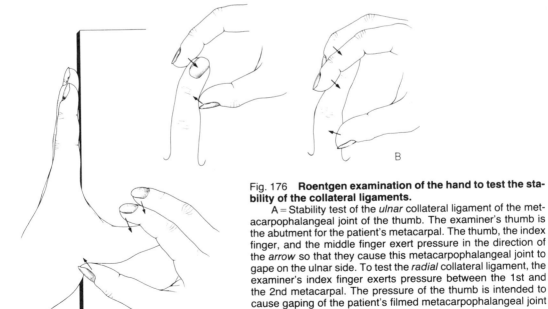

Fig. 176 **Roentgen examination of the hand to test the stability of the collateral ligaments.**
A = Stability test of the *ulnar* collateral ligament of the metacarpophalangeal joint of the thumb. The examiner's thumb is the abutment for the patient's metacarpal. The thumb, the index finger, and the middle finger exert pressure in the direction of the *arrow* so that they cause this metacarpophalangeal joint to gape on the ulnar side. To test the *radial* collateral ligament, the examiner's index finger exerts pressure between the 1st and the 2nd metacarpal. The pressure of the thumb is intended to cause gaping of the patient's filmed metacarpophalangeal joint on its *radial* side.
B = Technique of stability testing of the *ulnar* collateral ligament at the distal *(left)* and the proximal *(right)* interphalangeal joints. To test the stability of the *radial ligaments,* the procedure is modified accordingly. In these tests the patient can assume the examiner's role, using the sound hand, if the provocation of pain is prevented by local anesthesia!

third of the radial shaft, associated with dislocation at the distal radioulnar joint and possibly with avulsion of the ulnar styloid process, is termed *Galeazzi's fracture.*

Fractures of the distal forearm in the growth period should be regarded and treated not only from the viewpoint of epiphysiolysis—chondro- and osteoepiphyseolysis (epiphyseal fracture), see Figure 581 —or epiphyseal damage (compare p. 78: pseudo-Madelung's deformity) but also with respect to potential stimulation of local growth, which may occur in connection with healing of the fracture (hyperemia?), and which can give rise to faulty growth in the forearm region (*vide supra:* posttraumatic hypertrophy of the ulnar styloid process). The stability of the finger joints is assessed by *roentgenologic stability tests* (p. 4). The technique for the "separation" of these joints is illustrated in Fig. 176.

The **pronatus quadratus sign** (Fig. 177) is a useful aid in the diagnosis of certain pathologic changes in the distal forearm. The pronatus quadratus muscle passes from the distal anterior aspect of the ulna to the anterior aspect of the radius. It is covered by a layer of adipose connective tissue that separates it from the flexor digitorum profundus. Since adipose tissue attenuates the x-rays less than the other soft structures (Table 1), this separating adipose layer appears in the strictly lateral roentgenogram as a narrow "black" stripe ("pronator quadratus sign") situated between the pronator quadratus and the flexor tendons. With injuries to the distal forearm—for example, fractures, volar infractions, epiphyseal separations, but also sprains that are accompanied by a deep hematoma—the volar soft tissues frequently thicken and thereby cause the adipose layer described to become displaced and deformed. The edema of inflammatory processes in the radiocarpal region is apt to infiltrate the adipose layer which, similarly to the other soft structures, in this way becomes equivalent to water, thereby completely or partly obliterated or deformed. In addition to this, the increase in volume leads to enlargement of the entire volar soft structures. The morbid changes mentioned frequently leave a deformation of the blackened stripe. It should, however, be mentioned that the pronator quadratus sign is of diagnostic value only when compared with the (sound) contralateral side.

The **scaphoid fat stripe** (Terry, Jr. and Ramin, 1975) is an indicator of trauma, particularly fractures of the carpal bones, the styloid process of the radius, and the base of the first metacarpal. In the great majority of adult individuals—less frequently in children and juveniles—a striated or triangular blackened

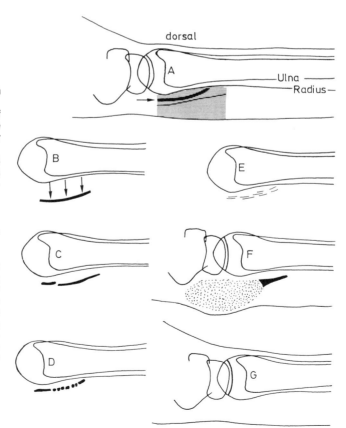

Fig. 177 Pronator quadratus sign (PQS)

A = Normal aspect of the layer of adipose connective tissue that covers the pronator quadratus muscle (= pronator quadratus sign = "black stripe" = *arrow*).

B to G = Modifications of the PQS with injuries (hematoma) and in diseases of the distal forearm and the carpal region.

B = Displacement of the PQS.

C = Step formation in the PQS.

D = Ill-defined, blurred middle segment of the PQS.

E = Fraying (splintering) of the PQS.

F = Inflammation of the common tendon sheath of the flexores digitorum (so-called ulnar bursa; Weston, 1973); for example, during the course of rheumatoid arthritis. The inflamed, edematous tendon sheath (*dotted*) manifests itself in the roentgenogram by increased thickness and density of the soft tissues. In this way the PQS may be shortened or enlarged and may, in its distal part, become concave.

G = Complete (or only partial) obliteration of the PQS following infiltration with edematous or sanguineous fluid.

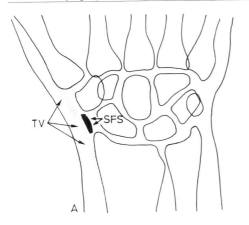

Fig. 178 **Scaphoid fat stripe (SFS)**
A = Adipose layer *(blackened area)* extending from the scaphoid toward the thumb. It is situated between the radial collateral ligament and the common tendon sheath (TV) of the abductor pollicis longus and the extensor pollicis brevis *(arrows)*.

B = The distention of the capsule that accompanies an effusion into the radiocarpal joint deforms (displaces) the SFS.

area extends toward the thumb, parallel to the scaphoid (Fig. 178). Its morphologic substrate is a layer of adipose tissue situated between the radial collateral ligament and the common tendon sheath of the abductor pollicis longus and the extensor pollicis brevis. The scaphoid fat stripe is particularly demonstrable in roentgenograms taken without use of a foil and in industrial roentgen films (mammography films). The fat stripe becomes invisible when it becomes impregnated with blood or an edema of the soft tissues (*vide supra* under pronator quadratus sign). An effusion into the radiocarpal joint can displace the scaphoid fat stripe (Fig. 178 B).

The **turret-shaped exostosis** (Wissinger et al., 1966) develops as the result of a minor *open* injury to the *dorsal* aspect of the proximal or middle phalanx of a finger that has healed by primary intention, but on condition that the periosteum was perforated with formation of a subperiosteal hematoma. Such a periosteal hematoma ossifies in a number of places, and after approximately 6 months the solid "ripened" turret-shaped exostosis is visible in the roentgenogram (Fig. 179).

The **carpometacarpal protuberance** (Artz and Posch, 1973) is recognizable on inspection of the dorsum of the hand as a prominence over the bases of the second and/or third metacarpals. On palpation, this painful or asymptomatic prominence proves to be "as hard as bone"; i.e., its consistency differs from that of the so-called ganglia. The carpometacarpal protuberance can develop posttraumatically or in the absence of a major injury. It is likely that an excessive (occupational) strain on the strong dorsal lig-

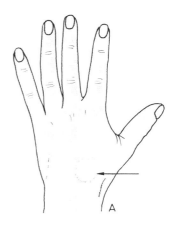

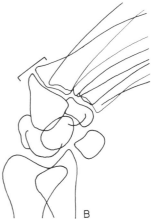

Fig. 180 **Carpometacarpal protuberance.**
A = Visual appearance of the carpometacarpal protuberance *(arrow)* on the base of the 2nd or 3rd metacarpal.

B = Radiographic appearance of the carpometacarpal protuberance *(marked)* in the *lateral ulnoradial* roentgenogram with volar flexion of the hand. The bony prominence has developed in the base of the 3rd metacarpal and in the capitate. A small ossicle is sometimes visible in the cleft between the two bony prominences *(not illustrated)*.

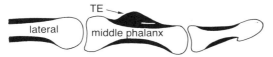

Fig. 179 **"Ripened" turret-shaped exostosis (TE);** see text.

Fig. 181 **Graphic depiction of the (right) carpal tunnel** after Hart and Gaynor (1941). (For the focusing technique see Fig. 182.)

Tinted black = Accessory bony element observed by Diller and Lamoth (1966). Fracture (pseudoarthrosis) of the hook of the hamate gives rise to compression of the median nerve in the carpal tunnel, not only through displacement of the broken-off hook but also as the result of an increase in volume as the fracture hematoma organizes into connective tissue.

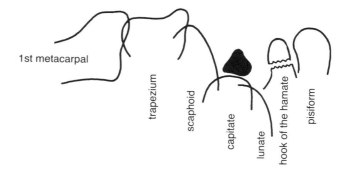

aments between the carpal and metacarpal bones leads to ossification, which can also be identified in the roentgenogram (Fig. 180).

The **carpal tunnel syndrome** manifests a disproportion between the volume of the carpal canal (closed dorsally by the carpal bones and bridged anteriorly by the tight retinaculum of the flexor muscles) and the space required by its soft structures. A sensitive indicator of lack of space in this osteofibrous tunnel is the median nerve that traverses it. Impingement on the nerve becomes manifest subjectively and objectively. A well-known early symptom, for example, is the statement by the patient that he has difficulty in clasping and holding a bottle. Other symptoms of the carpal tunnel syndrome are tingling and/or numbness in the area supplied by the median nerve (second and third finger, medial half of the fourth finger, less frequently the thumb) which are often worse at night. Paresis of motor portions of the median nerve leads to atrophy of the thenar. "Trophic" ulcerations of the skin with osteolyses in the distal phalanges (Bouvier et al., 1979) are a rare complication. The *acute* carpal tunnel syndrome sets in within hours or days (sometimes even later) after an *injury to the wrist or the distal forearm.* It also accompanies purulent inflammations; for example, a suppurative tenosynovitis, or an inflammatory, edematous swelling of the paratenon.

Pseudogout (chondrocalcinosis) also can give rise to the carpal tunnel syndrome. It can be identified roentgenolologically by deposits of calcium pyrophosphate in the carpal canal (Spiegel et al., 1976). *Glass splinters* that have penetrated the canal are likewise visible in the roetgenogram. In *traumatic volar dislocation of the lunate,* the carpal tunnel syndrome becomes clincally manifest only after a few weeks (p. 147).

The *chronic* carpal tunnel syndrome develops without a preceding acute event that could be responsible for the condition. When a chronic unilateral or bilateral carpal tunnel syndrome is supposed to be present, the following diseases and abnormalities should enter into the differential diagnosis: rheumatoid arthritis (tenosynovitis, radial rotation of the car-

pus as a result of weakness of the radial extensors, Schilling, 1974), psoriatic arthritis, disseminated lupus erythematosus, gouty tophus, sarcoidosis, *carpal osteoarthrosis,* hypothyroidism, acromegaly, amyloidosis, *tumors of the distal radius* (Wessinghage, 1972), tumors of the soft tissues in the carpal canal—for example, lipomas and hemangiomas, but also so-called ganglia—and mucopolysaccharidosis I–S (Scheie's disease, previously called mucopolysaccharidosis V). The latter has also been observed as a familial, hence hereditary, disorder (Gray et al., 1979). Finally, it should be mentioned that the carpal tunnel syndrome has been described as an accompaniment of anatomic variants; namely, anomalous proximal

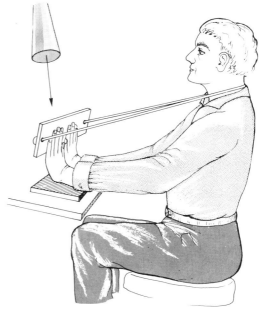

Fig. 182 **Focusing technique for demonstrating the carpal tunnel after Hart and Gaynor (1941).** The so-called central beam should pass in front of and parallel to the 3rd metacarpal.

origin of a lumbrical muscle (Eriksen, 1973) and *accessory carpal ossicles*. It also has been seen in pregnancy. The enumeration of these diverse etiologies should impress the reader with the necessity of studying the carpal canal of *both hands* radiologically in every case of carpal tunnel syndrome, although the roentgenogram will clarify the diagnosis in only a small proportion of patients (see the italicized etiologies). In addition, an anteroposterior roetgenogram of the elbow should be taken in every case of the carpal tunnel syndrome! Compression of the median nerve can also be produced by a *supracondylar process* and Struthers' ligament, which passes from its tip to the medial epicondyle of the humerus. The supracondylar process is a phylogenetically conditioned (atavistic) bone spur on the medial border of the distal humerus. The spur and the ligament form an osteofibrous ring that is traversed by the median nerve which is liable to be compressed at this site (Fig. 183, no. 14).

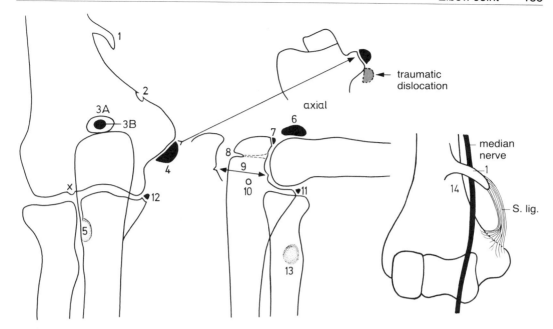

Fig. 183   **Variants of normal in the elbow joint.**

1 = Supracondylar process (atavism?).

2 = Sulcus or foramen.

3A = supratrochlear foramen (the bony septum between the coronoid fossa and the olecranon fossa is absent). Intermediate between the supratrochlear foramen and the normally developed bony septum is the so-called free supratrochlear septum (3B). Some writers also speak of an os supratrochleare (Canigiani et al., 1972) or of osteochondrosis dissecans of the supratrochlear septum. The latter eponym is based on the observation that the centrally ossified part of the septum may become detached from the peripheral fibrous portion and then becomes a loose body (Viehweger, 1968).

4 = Bony structure or structures distal to the medial epicondyle; persistent unicentrically or multicentrically ossified apophysis which, by its shape and position, completes the normal outline of the epicondyle. This condition must be differentiated from (A) disorders of traumatic origin (fracture or detachment of the apophysis, wrenching away of the metaphysis with the apophysis appendant, avulsion of the epicondyle). In these cases, the axial roentgenogram of the olecranon *(see above right)* usually reveals a distal and slightly medial dislocation *(arrow)*. (B) Circumscribed metaplastic ossification and calcium deposits in the flexor tendons and/or the collateral ligament in lesions due to excessive strain; e.g., in competitive athletes (throwing sports) or following an injury to the soft tissues (also calcified hematomas and localized myositis ossificans; p. 68). In these cases, however, the medial epicondyle retains its typical normal shape. The same considerations are applicable to the lateral condyle

5 = Radiolucence from a groove (instead of protuberance) of the annular ligament of the radius (Höffken, 1952).

6 = Patella cubiti (sesamoid bone in the triceps muscle or the result of trauma; i.e., avulsion with continued independent growth; Ishikawa et al., 1976). To be differentiated from old fracture of the olecranon or epiphysiolysis; in this case, the olecranon is "too short." A calcified bursa has a lumpy appearance; cortical seam and structured cancellous bone are absent.

7 = Persistent ossification center in the tip of the olecranon (to be differentiated from a posttraumatic condition).

8 = Partial persistence of the proximal epiphyseal plate in the ulna *(dashed = total persistence)*.

9 = Crest or groove in the trochlear incisura.

10 = Nutrient canal on the radial side.

11 = (Persistent) apophysis of the coronoid process or os cubiti anterius (both are infrequently present at the same time).

13 = Translucence due to orthograde view of the radial tuberosity (see also Fig. 31). x = Radial border of trochlea.

14 = Potential compression of the median nerve by the supracondylar process and/or Struthers' ligament *(S. lig.)*, which originates in this process. See p. 153 ff = carpal tunnel syndrome. *Tinted black:* Parts of bone in surrounding soft tissue and median nerve.

Elbow Joint

Variants from Normal and Malformations

Knowledge of the variants from normal protects against misdiagnosing pathologic changes (Fig. 183). Among the malformations, *aplasia of the joint* (congenital synostosis) can involve all three articulating bones or only two of them; for example, the humerus and the ulna. The upper arm and the forearm then form an angle. Congenital synostosis of the elbow is mostly associated with other malformations of the upper extremities. Familial and nonhereditary synostosis of the proximal ulna and radius—aplasia of the proximal radioular joint (Fig. 184)—occurs more frequently than synostosis between the humerus and the bones of the forearm. Bilateral occurrence of proximal radioulnar synostosis has been reported more frequently than its unilateral occurence (Walter, 1978). Rotary motion of the forearm is prevented by this malformation; the hand is in the pronated position. *Distal* radioulnar synostosis, in contrast, is a very uncommon malformation. In later childhood the synostosis is apt to become distended. In some cases, the opposing cortices of the two bones can, initially, still be delineated; in others, even in small children,

the bones are firmly united. The association of malformations of the elbow, among them radioular synostosis, with certain malformations of the bones of the lower leg and the foot, has been termed *Nievergelt's syndrome* (hereditary systemic malformation of the skeleton of the extremities).

Congenital impairment of supination of the forearm (Fig. 185) results from a developmental disorder of the capitellum of the humerus and a valgus deformity of the head and neck of the radius; it leads to the pathologic valgus position of the elbow. The physiologic cubitus valgus owes its origin to the fact that the distal epiphyseal plate of the humerus does not run parallel to the longitudinal axis of the upper arm. When the elbow is extended and the hand is supinated, the axes of the upper and lower arm consequently form a radially open angle of 160 to 170 degrees. Major variations from these normal values—pathologic *cubitus valgus* and *cubitus varus*—occur with diverse malformations of the elbow and also as an aftermath of juxtaarticular fractures. Bilateral cubitus valgus is, next to dissociated infantilism and bilateral pterygium colli, one of the prominent diagnostic features of *Turner's syndrome* (gonadal dysgenesis).

The shape of the *tarsoid and gonoid malformation of the upper* extremities (Andrén and Theander, 1975) suggests a disturbance of morphologic differentiation between the upper and lower extremities,

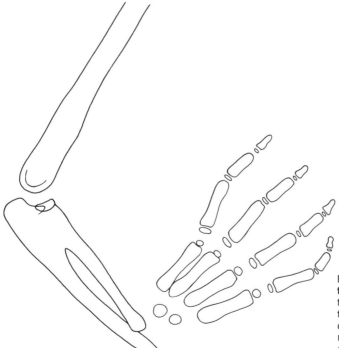

Fig. 184 **Proximal radioulnar synostosis—aplasia of the radioulnar joint**—in the setting of complex malformations of the upper extremity (age 4, male), hence *combined malformation* in this case. It may, however, occur as a *solitary malformation.*

which manifests itself by a knee-shaped structure of the wrist (Fig. 186).

The following **congenital dislocations at the elbow joint** are known:

The (very infrequent) *dislocation of both radius and ulna* (congenital and recurrent)[13] presupposes severe malformations and a slack capsuloligamentous apparatus, particularly in the humero-ulnar segment of the joint.

Congenital and recurrent dislocation of the radial head posteriorly, anteriorly, or laterally (in descending order of frequency) accompanies malformations of the elbow joint. The latter, however, do not necessarily involve only the head and the neck of the radius. A major disturbance of longitudinal growth of the ulna—for example, Ollier's enchondromatosis—can lead to dislocation of the radial head just as the dislocation can be caused by a disorder of the articular mechanics resulting from a paralysis that has been acquired in early childhood. A posterior or anterior dislocation (or subluxation) is demonstrable in the lateral roentgenogram of the elbow because, with (rectangular) flexion of the elbow, the axis of the radial head and neck no longer points to the ossification centers of the capitellum and the trochlea of the humerus, which are projected one above the other (Fig. 187). Dislocation of the radial head is often observed in conjunction with a malformation of the knee (the patella) and also in various malformation syndromes, for example the nail-patella syndrome (osteoonychodysostosis with pelvic protuberances; Valdueza, 1973).

Habitual dislocation of the ulna on a congenital basis—that is, as the result of a deformity of the humeroulnar segment of the joint—is a rare event; more frequently this condition follows an injury.

A *preliminary condition* for the development of a congenital dislocation of the elbow is, as has been mentioned above, the presence of deformities of the articulating bones.

[13] As a matter of routine, any *recurrent* dislocation should radiologically examined to determine whether it has developed in response to a malformation or whether the proneness to dislocation has been acquired; for example, as a sequel to trauma.

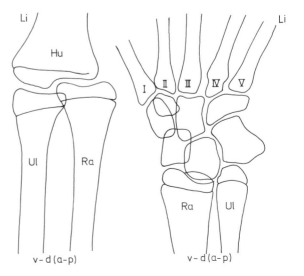

Fig. 185 **Dysplasia of the humeroradial portion of the joint** with congenital impairment of supination (and extension) of the left forearm (in the presence of pathologic cubitus valgus of less than 160°; see text). Differential diagnosis from *acquired* impairment of rotation, particularly postraumatic, or due to rachitic bending.

Fig. 186 **Main radiographic features of the tarsoid and gonoid malformation in the upper extremities (Andrén-Theander syndrome).**

Ra = Radius presenting similarities to the tibia. Ul = Ulna with similarities to the fibula. Hu = Humerus. I to V = metacarpals. The elbow joint shows a resemblance to the knee joint; the connection between the carpus and the forearm resembles the talocrural joint. The pisiform is absent.

(The concomitant giantism of the *tarsal bones* has not been illustrated.)

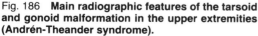

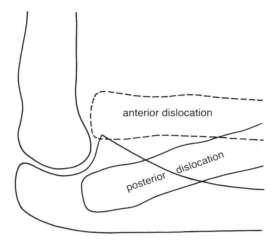

Fig. 187 Congenital dislocation of the radial head in malformation of the elbow. Typical deformity of the head and elongation of the neck of the radius (adult patients).

As the *result* of such deformities, the contact between the articulating bones is disturbed so that even normal movement or a trivial injury leads to dislocation or subluxation. Deformities can become visible in any place in the articulating bones (the head and the neck of the radius, the olecranon with its trochlear or radial incisura, the coronoid process, the capitellum and the trochlea of the humerus, etc.). When a deformity, with or without faulty position of the articulating bones, leads to incongruity of these bones, it becomes a preosteoarthrotic lesion. Finally, the deformity can limit the range of motion. However, deformities of the articulating bones are not in every case the result of hereditary damage or external agents. The latter are only effective in a definite period of fetal development— in the present instance at the time when the elbow becomes differentiated. Deformities can also develop on the basis of hereditary disorders of metabolism which lead to skeletal deformation by producing an anomaly of the gliding and supporting tissues in the mesenchymal stage, or even later in the cartilaginous stage (Schmid, 1967). Among such disorders are the mucopolysaccharidoses, the mucolipidoses, and the lipidoses. These hereditary diseases are the result of enzyme deficiencies in the breakdown of complex carbohydrates. They are accompanied by anomalous storage, and frequently increased renal elimination, of these substances. They present the radiographic appearance of *dysostosis multiplex* (see under this heading) (Fig. 188). Finally, inflammation of juxtaarticular parts of bone and the synovial membrane (compare arthritis of the growth period), as well as insufficient use or disuse (e.g., with paresis in the growth period), play a part in the deformation of articulating bones and likewise give rise to the disorders of articular function listed above; i.e., dislocation, preosteoarthrotic deformities, and limitation of motion.

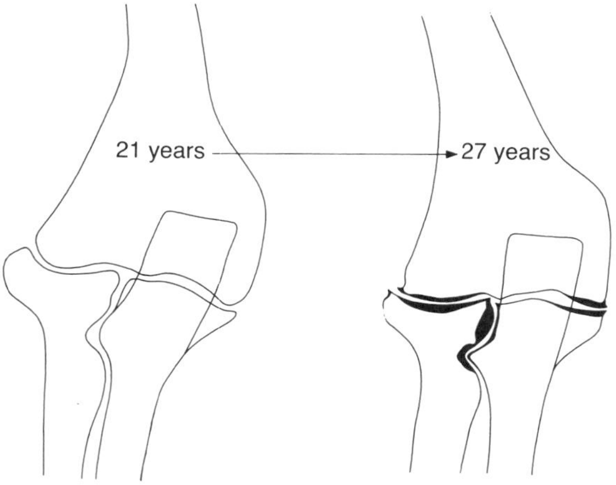

Fig. 188 Radiographic approach of dysostosis multiplex in the elbow accompanying mucopolysaccharidosis.
Left: Deformity of the articulating bones of the right elbow joint.
Right: Six years later, signs of osteoarthrosis of the elbow. The deformity has proved to be a preosteoarthrotic condition.
Note: The deformation of the articulating bones (see 21 years) could also be the result of an arthritis experienced in the (early) growth period (p. 90 ff).

Arthritis

The arthritic joint effusion and the inflammatory proliferation of the synovium lead to an *intraarticular* increase in volume. An identical increase in volume may also be expected as the result of a traumatic effusion into the joint, an intraarticular hematoma, and tumorous proliferation of the synovium. Owing to the anatomic pecularities of the elbow joint, an intraarticular increase in volume of only 5 mL can be identified roentgenologically (Norell, 1954; Bledsoe and Izenstark, 1959). A layer of adipose tissue that is interposed between the synovial membrane and the fibrous capsule forms the morphologic substrate of the anterior and the posterior **cubital fat pad sign** in the lateral radioulnar roentgenogram of the elbow when the joint is flexed at a right angle. The *anterior* fat pad is recognizable in the healthy joint at the level of the coronoid fossa and immediately in front of it as a drop-shaped area of increased blackening measuring about 5 mm in width (Fig. 189). The *posterior* fat pad is projected into the olecranon fossa and is therefore not visible under normal circumstances. An intraarticular increase in volume of at least 5 mL lifts the anterior fat pad from the deep structures; the fat pad thus becomes separated from the contour of the humerus (positive fat pad sign, Fig. 189). When the posterior fat pad is lifted from the olecranon fossa, it

Fig. 189 Cubital fat pad sign (CFS) and supinator fat line (SFL).

A = Negative CFS (normal finding), normal SFL.

B to D = Positive CFS indicates intraarticular increase in volume. Pathologic alteration of the SFL (*arrow;* see text).

E = *Paradoxical* positive posterior CFS (see text).

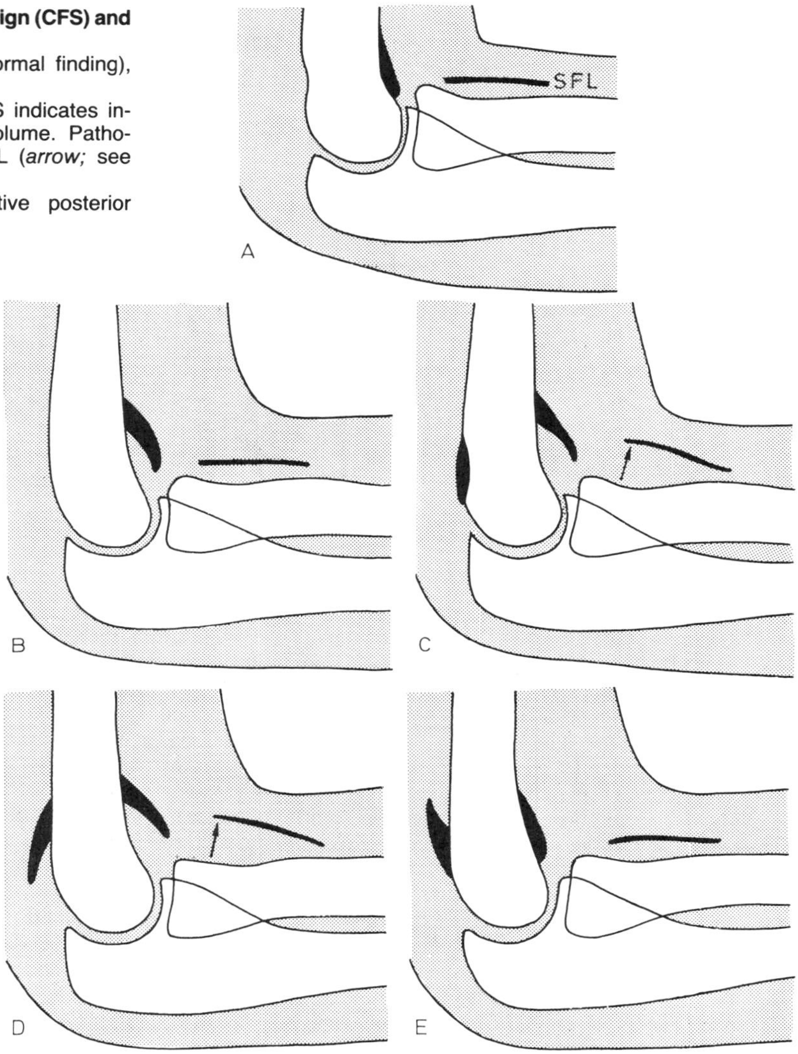

becomes visible. This always constitutes a pathologic roentgen finding. With a joint effusion accompanying a capsular tear, the fat pad sign usually remains negative. A positive paradoxical posterior fat pad sign (Fig. 189) is produced by a subperiosteal hematoma or a neoplastic reaction on the part of the periosteum (Murphy and Siegel, 1977).

The **supinator fat line** (Fig. 189) runs above the supinator muscle, parallel to the proximal part of the radius (Rogers and Mac Ewan, 1969). It is from 3 to 4 cm long and from 2 to 3 mm broad. An arthritis of the elbow joint, an anterior synovial cyst in the joint, a traumatic effusion, or a fracture of the proximal radius (the radial head or neck, for instance) *can* modify the shape and course of the supinator fat line; i.e., it can displace it toward the surface, deform it, enlarge it, and/or cause its contour to become indis-

tinct (see also Fig. 212). The positive fat pad sign *plus* concomitant juxtaarticular demineralization (see collateral phenomena of arthritis, p. 12, Fig. 13) indicates arthritis of the elbow joint, provided a preceding trauma or an operation of the joint with several weeks' immobilization (disuse decalcification) has been ruled out. The same is applicable to the concomitant evidence of direct signs of arthritis (p. 17 ff, Fig. 20). *Nosological classification* of an arthritis of the elbow joint that has been identified radiographically is generally impossible without knowledge of the history, the clinical findings, and the radiologic aspect of other joints (Figs. 190 through 193). The following points should, however, be heeded when the roentgen finding is indicative of "cubital arthritis":

In monoarthritis of the elbow joint, it is more

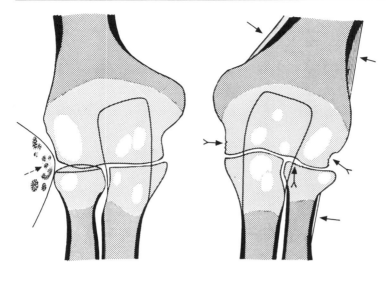

Fig. 190 **Relatively early cubital arthritis** in rheumatoid arthritis *(right)* and in tuberculous infection *(left)*. Nearly identical roentgen findings (conspicuous juxtaarticular cystoid osteolyses without marginal sclerosis, joint space narrowing, juxtaarticular demineralization). The right side of the figure illustrates, in addition, the sites of predilection for arthritic erosions *(tailed arrows)* as well as the shape and seat of lamellar periosteal new bone formations, also in arthritis *(arrows)*. This supplementary information (set off by a *curved line*) can be of aid in narrowing the diagnostic possibilities: calcified (tuberculous) pus, calcified (intraarticular) gouty tophi, arthritis with attendant calcinosis (primarily collagen diseases). The dashed arrow points toward shady calcifications.

justifiable to presume a bacterial infection than to diagnose a rheumatoid arthritis starting atypically there, or another type of inflammatory rheumatic arthritis. Nor does the bilateral occurrence of a cubital arthritis exclude its being tuberculous. Sequestra and intraarticular or juxtaarticular amorphous calcifications (calcified pus) are encountered most frequently in tuberculous infections (Fig. 194). However, an arthritis with attendant calcinosis and calcified gouty tophi should enter into the differential diagnosis.

When an oligoarthritis or polyarthritis affects the elbow *together with other joints,* the findings in the elbow do not as a rule allow of it to be accurately classified. In these instances one should first of all make an attempt to classify the disorder on the basis of the roentgenologic pattern of manual involvement (compare Fig. 91). In addition, it should be remembered that in every case of roentgenologically evidenced arthritis (whether it be a mono-, oligo-, or polyarthritis), the serological tests for syphilis should be *routine,* so as not to overlook an occult syphilitic arthropathy, although this is a diagnosis of remote likelihood.

Conspicuous periosteal reactions in a cubital arthritis, particularly one affecting a single joint or a few joints, occur most frequently in Reiter's syndrome and in psoriatic arthritis. In childhood, however, they can accompany any kind of arthritis.

The bacterial and the inflammatory rheumatic types of arthritis, but also lipoid-dermatoarthritis (multicentric reticulohistiocytosis) of the elbow joint, often present—in adults as well as in growing individuals—larger, cystic juxtaarticular osteolyses. Erosions and joint space narrowing are usually less striking initially. The arthritic genesis, or at least the development of these cystoid osteolyses on the basis of an arthropathy, is very probable when these findings are present in all three articulating bones. A

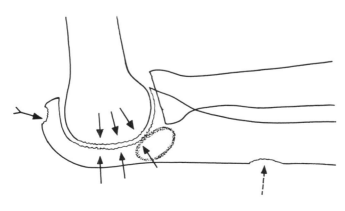

Fig. 191 **Advanced cubital arthritis in the lateral roentgenogram** (in the present case: rheumatoid arthritis). The destroyed trochlear incisura "engulfs" the eroded trochlea humeri. The *dashed arrow* points to a nonreactive erosion in the ulna by a palpable subcutaneous rheumatoid nodule. The *tailed arrow* points to a defect in the olecranon bursa (a frequent finding in inflammatory rheumatic polyarthritis, but occasionally also encountered in tuberculous arthritis and in gout; Fig. 200). These findings provide important additional information. *Arrows* point to the areas of predilection for arthritic erosions in the convex and concave parts of the joints.

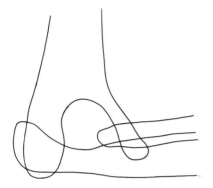

Fig. 192 **"Burned-out" stage of mutilation in cubital arthritis** in rheumatoid arthritis of many years' standing. Similar osteolyses in the elbow (occurring, however, *already in childhood*) have been observed in a hereditary disorder of metabolism that is closely related to the mucopolysaccharidoses (Winchester's syndrome); see also Fig. 206. If, in addition, conspicuous periarticular bone shadows are demonstrable, the identical roentgenologic finding suggests a neurogenic osteoarthropathy (see Fig. 206).

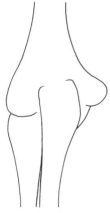

Fig. 193 **Arthritic bony ankylosis of the elbow of many years's standing.** The ossifying process, which followed destruction of the articular cartilage and erosive lesions of the subchondral bone, not only has united the three articulating bones but also has smoothed out the erosions, etc. The present roentgenogam, however, may also suggest that no major erosive changes of the contours have occurred but that bony ankylosis has immediately followed the arthritic resorption of the articular cartilage (*example:* juvenile chronic arthritis).

rounded juxtaarticular osteolysis in a single bone in conjunction with conspicuous demineralization of the articulating bones and/or sequestration can suggest the hematogenous origin of an osseous tuberculosis of the joint. *Focally* arranged destructions in two or all three articulating bones in the presence of roentgenologic signs of arthritis also suggest a tuberculous infection (Fig. 194). Without subchondral demineralization, however, cystic juxtaarticular osteolyses limited to a single bone are an ambiguous radiographic finding (p. 20 ff). The spottier the attendant collateral demineralization is, (see Collateral Phenomena of Arthritis, p. 12) and the hazier the juxtaarticular cancellous structures are, the fresher and more acute is a cubital arthritis.

Arthritis of the elbow in the growth period and its differential diagnosis have been discussed on page 90 ff (compare Fig. 188). The distal metaphysis of the humerus is partly covered by the joint capsule. Therefore, osteomyelitis of the distal humerus in children often produces a pyogenic infection of the joint without spreading necessarily by way of the epiphysis. Osteomyelitis of the distal humerus thus can give rise to disorders of growth and, later on, to deformation of the elbow joint.

The elbow very frequently is the seat of acute **osteomyelitis of variola** (p. 109), which often occurs bilaterally and symmetrically (Lentz and Noyes, 1979). Small children are its principal victims. Disorders of development and growth, therefore, are potential sequelae of this viral infection that may also affect the elbow *joint*. An early roentgenologic manifestation of smallpox osteomyelitis is a very extensive periosteal reaction. Destructive foci in the metaphysis may supervene. The epiphyseal centers of ossification are affected only later in the disease. The arthritic destructions can thereby become intensified.

Sympathetic arthritis is a sterile, nonsuppurative inflammation of the joint that commonly occurs as the result of a morbid process in the bone (marrow). It is indicative of involvement of the synovial membrane in a primary affection of bone (Greek *sympathēs* = affected by like suffering). Sympathetic arthritis is commonly precipitated by an inflammatory condition (nonspecific osteomyelitis, tuberculosis of bone, and, infrequently, even nonspecific bacterial arthritis of a neighboring joint; Baker and Robinson, 1978). Sympathetic arthritis has also been described in osteoid osteoma, osteoblastoma, aneurysmatic bone cyst, osteoclastoma, osteosarcoma, and fibrosarcoma. Sherman (1947), Marcove and Freiberger (1966), Simon et al. (1972), and Snarr et al. (1973) have reported the occurrence of sympathetic arthritis in intraarticular osteoid osteoma of the elbow (Fig. 195). Histologically, sympathetic arthritis presents the features of a chronic nonspecific synovitis or a lymphoid-follicular synovitis with and without germ centers (Snarr et al., 1973; Dihlmann and Fernholz, 1978). Sympathetic arthritis manifests itself as a serous arthritis (painful effusion into the joint with osteoarthrosis as a possible late sequel) and, very in-

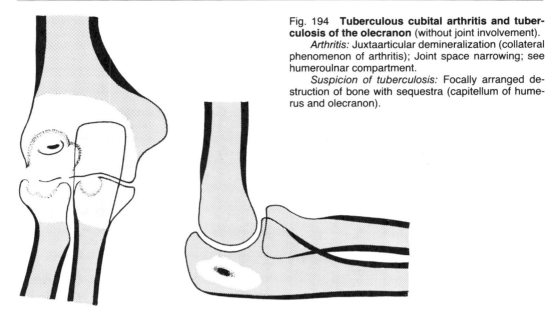

Fig. 194 **Tuberculous cubital arthritis and tuberculosis of the olecranon** (without joint involvement).
Arthritis: Juxtaarticular demineralization (collateral phenomenon of arthritis); Joint space narrowing; see humeroulnar compartment.
Suspicion of tuberculosis: Focally arranged destruction of bone with sequestra (capitellum of humerus and olecranon).

frequently, as a chronic erosive arthritis and polyarthritis with direct arthritic signs (Christoph et al., 1977; Dihlmann and Fernholz, 1978).

The closely contiguous bursae of the elbow (subcutaneous olecranon bursa, intratendinous olecranon bursa, subtendinous bursa of the triceps muscle) are frequently involved in rheumatoid arthritis and other inflammatory rheumatic types of arthritis, in gout, and in tuberculosis. These diseases should be taken into consideration when a swelling of the soft tissues occurs dorsally to the olecranon and a pathologic roentgen finding the elbow is concomitantly demonstrable. When the roentgenogram of the elbow is normal, a soft-tissue swelling behind the

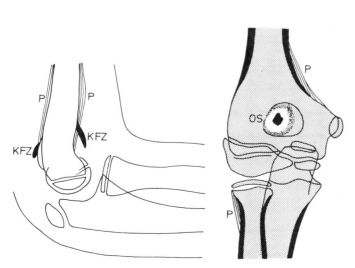

Fig. 195 **Osteoid osteoma in the olecranon fossa with sympathetic cubital arthritis.**
Roentgen findings: Osteoid osteoma (OS) with central calcified nidus and partial marginal sclerosis presenting ill-defined contours. Lamellar periosteal reaction (P) in humerus and radius. Soft-tissue swelling. Positive cubital fat pad sign (KFZ, see Fig. 189) evidences the effusion of sympathetic arthritis.
Radiographic differential diagnosis in the present case from osteochondrosis of the supratrochlear septum: Osteochondrosis dissecans is not accompanied by periosteal reaction.
Note: In *cancellous* bone, the nidus of osteoid osteoma is often demonstrable as an area of increased density with or without surrounding radiolucency, whereas in *cortical* bone it manifests itself generally by an area of radiolucency. (Nonmalignant) osteoblastoma frequently differs roentgenologically and histologically from osteoid osteoma only by a nidus the diameter of which may reach 1, 2, or more cm. Therefore, the synonym "giant osteoid osteoma" is used (instead of osteoblastoma).

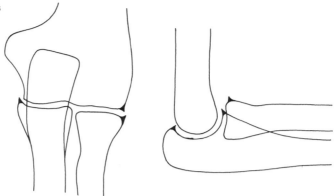

Fig. 196 **Early marginal osteophytes in osteoarthrosis of the elbow joint.**

olecranon suggests, generally speaking, a bursal affection (compare Fig. 200 with Fig. 213).

Osteoarthrosis

In the average population, complaints referable to osteoarthrosis of the elbow are of minimal significance. Osteophytes commonly appear first in the head of the ulna and the capitellum of the humerus. In addition, osteophytic outgrowths are observed in the coronoid process and the proximal border of the trochlear notch (Fig. 196). The increasing size of the osteophytes leads to elongation of the ulnar hook that grasps the trochlea, with consequent impairment of flexion and extension. Subsequently, the head of the radius becomes mushroomed and the other bones also assume a plumper shape. Osteophytes in the sulcus of the ulnar nerve sometimes damage this nerve by compression (indication for a so-called axial roentgenogram of the elbow joint; compare Fig. 183). "Joint mice" *regularly* are observed in osteoarthrosis of the elbow. On the one hand, they suggest concomitant involvement of the synovial membrane. When, on the other hand, they are a primary affection, they predispose to the development of osteoarthrosis. This is particularly true of neoplastic synovial chondromatosis (Fig. 197) which may occur as a multifocal disorder but usually occurs at a single site. In somewhat more than 25 percent of cases the elbow is the seat of the disease, which is a typical preosteoarthrotic condition. This also applies to *osteochondrosis dissecans* of the elbow joint, which can give rise to the development of "joint mice" (compare p. 299). This disease, which has a preference for the male sex, affects principally the right joint. In the majority of cases—generally concerning patients in the second decade of life—the detached fragment is derived from the capitellum of the humerus (Fig. 198) and much less frequently from the head of the radius or the trochlea of the humerus. Initially, the bed of the joint mouse is demonstrable in the roent-

genogram as a hollow. With time it flattens out so that later on it is frequently recognizable only as a depression or as a flattening of the capitellum humeri. The radiologic differential diagnosis of osteochondrosis dissecans of the supratrochlear septum has been reviewed briefly in the captions to Figures 183 and 195.

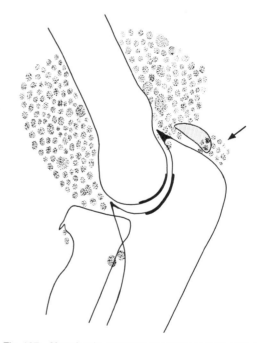

Fig. 197 **Neoplastic synovial chondromatosis of the elbow.** The olecranon bursa is concomitantly involved *(arrow).* Minor roentgen manifestations of secondary osteoarthrosis (see osteophytes in head of radius). Elongation of the coronoid process and the proximal end of the trochlear notch, sclerosis of the subchondral cancellous bone, capsular osteoma with cortical bone in the vicinity of the olecranon (compare the absence of cortical bone in the numerous calcified capsular chondromas).

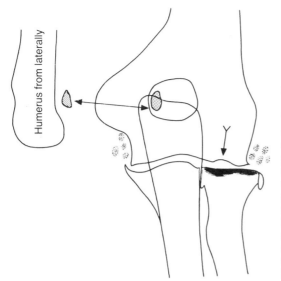

Fig. 198 **Secondary osteoarthrosis of the elbow** (marginal osteophytes, calcified capsular chondromas, subchondral sclerosis in head of radius) **following osteochondrosis dissecans of the humeral capitellum.** Bed of loose body *(tailed arrow)* is almost leveled (recognizable only as a flat depression of the capitellum humeri; see text). The loose body lies in front of the coronoid fossa *(arrow)*.

result of injuries to the joint that have been described on page 175 ff. For the deformations and faulty positions of joints, which gave rise to osteoarthrosis, see page 157 ff and Figure 188.

Osteoarthropathies

The elbow joint rarely is involved during the course of **chronic gout** (p. 41 ff). Osteoarthrosis, especially osteophytes and narrowing of the joint, are usually prominent features of the roentgen picture. Subchondral cystic osteolyses can reflect debris cysts as well as tophi. In any case, the radiographic finding in gout of the elbow can become relatively characteristic by association of osteoarthrosis with gouty olecranon bursitis. This bursal affection may be anticipated in about 20 percent of patients with chronic gout. This disorder gives rise to a *dense* soft-tissue swelling dorsally to the olecranon, in which calcium shadows are frequently demonstrable (Fig. 200). Gouty (tophaceous) bursitis sometimes leads to a pressure erosion in the olecranon. The possible affection of the elbow in **ochronosis** (p. 43) manifests itself in the roentgenogram as osteoarthrosis. Involvement of the elbow joint is a common event in *hemophilia*. The elbow and the knee joint are therefore the test joints for **osteoarthropathy of hemophilia.** The processes described on page 44 ff gradually lead to considerable

Juxtaarticular bone infarcts are of frequent occurrence in *congenital hereditary hemoglobinopathies associated with sickling.* During the repair stage, artifacts that resemble osteochondrosis dissecans develop, subsequently terminating in osteoarthrotic deformations.

Juvenile avascular necrosis of the capitellum humeri, and the still more infrequent avascular necrosis of the ossification centers of the trochlea and the head of the radius, become preosteoarthrotic conditions only when they heal with deformations. Hemophilia, also, is one of the manifold (known) causes of avascular necrosis of bone (compare p. 254 ff) in the elbow joint, particularly in the head of the radius.

Compressed air damage to the elbow joint (which is more pronounced in the work arm than in the contralateral arm) presents a polymorphous though rather characteristic radiographic appearance, especially when certain findings in the wrist and in the acromioclavicular joint are taken into consideration. (Principal among the former are subchondral necrosis of the lunate bone, pseudoarthrosis of the scaphoid, cysts in the lunate and the scaphoid, and signs of necrosis in both styloid processes). The roentgen manifestations in the elbow are (1) signs of osteoarthrosis, (2) loose bodies as the result of osteochondrosis dissecans, detached portions of the metaplastic capsule, broken-off osteophytes, and (3) fibroostoses (Fig. 199). Posttraumatic preosteoarthrotic deformities are the

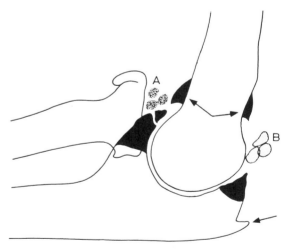

Fig. 199 **Compressed air damage of the elbow joint.** Increased size of the hook of the olecranon through considerable coarsening of the coronoid process, the tip of which has become detached, and through widening of the trochlear notch whose proximal margin is elongated and deformed. Marginal lipping in the head of the radius. Loose bodies (A = cartilaginous type [calcified]; B = osseous type [with cortical bone]). Fibroostosis *(arrow)* of the capsular insertions in the humerus and the olecranon (insertion of the triceps muscle). *(The most important sites from the diagnostic point of view are tinted black).*

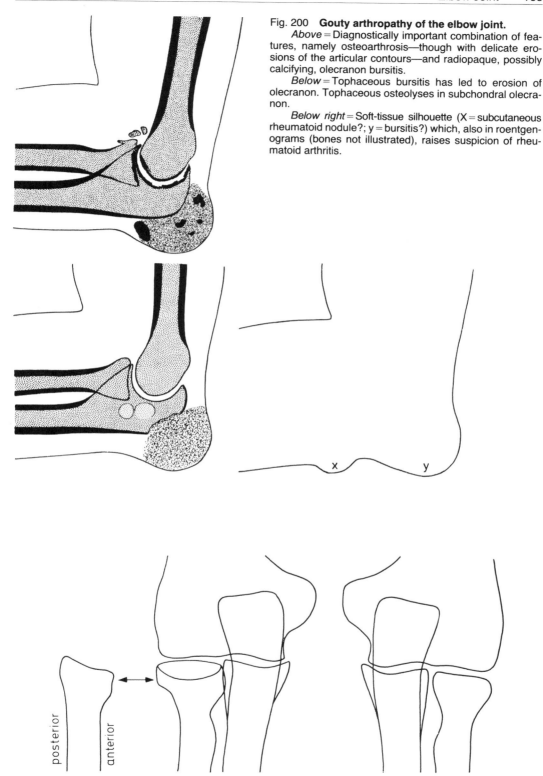

Fig. 200   **Gouty arthropathy of the elbow joint.**

Above = Diagnostically important combination of features, namely osteoarthrosis—though with delicate erosions of the articular contours—and radiopaque, possibly calcifying, olecranon bursitis.

Below = Tophaceous bursitis has led to erosion of olecranon. Tophaceous osteolyses in subchondral olecranon.

Below right = Soft-tissue silhouette (X = subcutaneous rheumatoid nodule?; y = bursitis?) which, also in roentgenograms (bones not illustrated), raises suspicion of rheumatoid arthritis.

Fig. 201   **Hemophilia A** (age 21, male). *Right:* Normal left elbow joint. *Left:* Early stage of hemophiliac joint. Head of radius increased in size and beveled anteriorly.

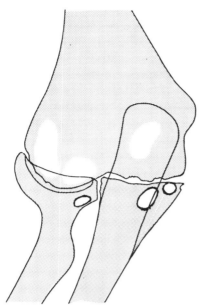

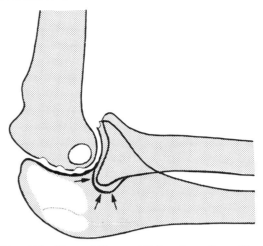

Fig. 203 **Hemophiliac cubital osteoarthropathy** (deformation of the articulating bones, joint space narrowing, delicate erosions of the trochlear notch and the distal humerus, cystic osteolyses). *Arrows* point to an erosion of the radial notch of the ulna (Perri, 1978).

Fig. 202 **Advanced cubital osteoarthropathy in hemophilia.** Deformation of the articulating bones, cubitus valgus, eroded articular surfaces, joint space narrowing, subchondral cystic osteolyses (result of intramedullary hemorrhages? This assumption is justifiable because such cystic osteolyses, with or without increased density of the marginal contours, can develop into hemophiliac pseudotumors).

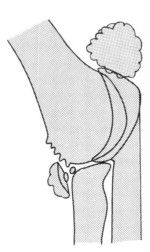

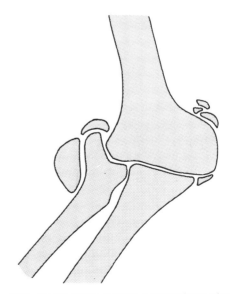

Fig. 204 **Neurogenic osteoarthropathy of the elbow in syringomyelia.**
Typical features: Nonreactive osteolyses leading to "simplification of shape." Ossifications of the periarticular soft tissues. Faulty position of the articulating bones.

Fig. 205 **Neurogenic cubital osteoarthropathy in syringomyelia.**
Typical features: "Simplification of shape" of the ends of the articulating bones, faulty positions, ossifications of the periarticular soft tissues.

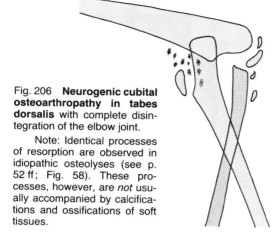

Fig. 206 Neurogenic cubital osteoarthropathy in tabes dorsalis with complete disintegration of the elbow joint.

Note: Identical processes of resorption are observed in idiopathic osteolyses (see p. 52 ff; Fig. 58). These processes, however, are *not* usually accompanied by calcifications and ossifications of soft tissues.

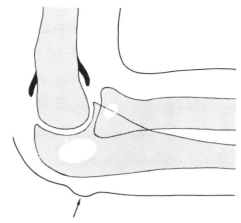

Fig. 208 Amyloid osteoarthropathy must be included in the differential diagnostic considerations when this roentgenogram is obtained (positive fat pad sign, see Fig. 189; nonreactive spherical or ovoid osteolyses; circumscribed bulging of the soft-tissue contour *[arrow]* due to a palpable periosteal (amyloid) nodule [Goldberg et al., 1964]), particularly when these findings are bilaterally symmetrical and polyarticular, when rheumatoid factors are not demonstrable in the serum, and/or when a disease is present that sometimes leads to amyloidosis (see p. 60).

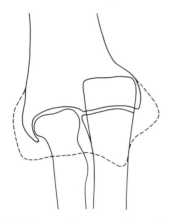

Fig. 207 Posttraumatic resorption (osteolysis, abrasion) in the humeral condyle following dislocation of the elbow in adolescence (more than 20 years previously). The contour of the distal humerus on the sound contralateral side is *dashed.*

Neurogenic osteoarthropathies (p. 47 ff) of the elbow occur chiefly in syringomyelia. Tabes dorsalis and other diseases (p. 49 ff) are much less frequently the cause of a neurogenic osteoarthropathy of the elbow or a nonreactive osteolysis of the cubital parts of the ulna, the radius, and the humerus. Early in the disease they can offer difficulties in diagnosis because the frequent ossifications and calcifications[14] of the periarticular soft tissues and the increased size of the olecranon hook are associated with the pictures of both neurogenic osteoarthropathy and cubital osteoarthrosis. Eventually, the pronounced osteolyses in the three articulating bones (see, however, also Fig. 192), in conjunction with the more or less pronounced soft-tissue ossifications—hence the typical anarchic remodeling of the joint and its disintegration (Figs. 204, 205, and 206; p. 47)—enable the correct diagnosis.

Posttraumatic osteolyses are known to occur also in the humerus (Fig. 207).

Amyloid osteoarthropathy (p. 60) is commonly a bilaterally symmetric, polyarticular disorder. The findings to be expected in the elbow are illustrated in Fig. 208.

Idiopathic hemochromatosis (p. 62) in the elbow shows an osteoarthritic roentgen picture and dotted

damage of the elbow joint, which impairs the function of the joint and can be identified in the roentgenogram. Repeated hemorrahages into the joint and the sunchrondral layer, which are to be expected as early as in childhood and early adolescence, not only damage the gliding tissue and the bone but also accelerate maturation and interfere with the growth of the ossification centers in the vicinity of the elbow. The head of the radius (Figs. 201, 202, and 203), and also the condyle of the humerus and the olecranon then present an atypical shape; cubitus valgus is frequently observed (Fig. 202). The hemophilic pseudotumor, also, has been described in the elbow. As the term suggests, the roentgenogram in this condition is governed by severe cystic destruction of bone resulting from repeated intramedullary and subperiosteal hemorrhages; the bone is expanded concomitantly.

---

[14] Cubital osteoarthrosis and compressed-air damage of the elbow joint show, as a rule, a far greater number of calcified capsular chondromas than capsular osteomas. The reverse is true of neurogenic osteoarthropathies, which chiefly present ossifications in the soft tissues and only few calcifications of cartilage and soft tissues.

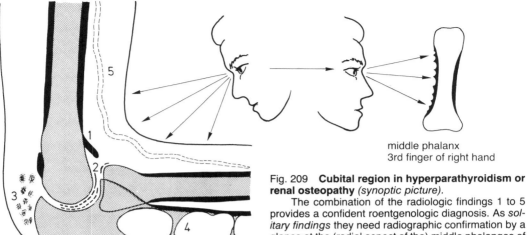

middle phalanx
3rd finger of right hand

Fig. 209 Cubital region in hyperparathyroidism or renal osteopathy (synoptic picture).
The combination of the radiologic findings 1 to 5 provides a confident roentgenologic diagnosis. As *solitary findings* they need radiographic confirmation by a glance at the (radial aspect of the) middle phalanges of the fingers. There, hyperparathyroid subperiosteal resorption of bone becomes manifest early in the course of the disease (see Fig. 151).
     1 = Positive fat pad sign, see Fig. 189; erosions not demonstrable.
     2 = Chondrocalcinosis of the hyaline articular cartilage.
     3 = Calcifications of the periarticular soft tissues.
     4 = Expanding osteolyses.
     5 = Calcifications of the arterial tunica media.

or broken calcifications of the articular cartilage (chondrocalcinosis).
     Osteoarthropathy of Wilson's disease (p. 62) also manifests itself in the elbow as osteoarthrosis. Loose bodies likewise form part of the radiographic appearance. They develop as the result of either synovial changes or detachment of bone due to osteochondrosis, which are known to occur in Wilson's disease. Roentgen manifestations of chondrocalcinosis also can be recognizable. Looser's zones (e.g., in the neck of the radius) as additional diagnostic information, are indicative of renal rickets or osteomalacia, which frequently accompany Wilson's disease.
     As with the other joints, the roentgenogram of the elbow can reveal subchondral resorption of bone and microfractures as manifestations of **hyperparathyroidism** or **renal osteopathy** (p. 125 ff), which may give the impression of arthritic erosions. The hyaline cartilage over these more or less extensive breaks disappears so that the radiographic joint space appears to be narrowed and even a reactive effusion into the joint is apt to occur (positive fat pad sign, Fig. 189). Finally, when subchondral cysts are formed in addition, the roentgenogram of the elbow joint also mimics a chronic arthritis. Such a misinterpretation is obviated if concomitant roentgen manifestations of chondrocalcinosis, soft tissues, and arterial walls in the vicinity of the joint, or even a brown tumor (Fig. 209) is demonstrable. In addition to this, the patients

complain of discomfort in one or several joints, so that the signs of extraarticular hyperparathyroid subperiosteal bone resorption can be searched for in other joints; for example, in the hand (see Figs. 150, 151, and 152). With hyperparathyroidism and with osteomalacia, the resorption of bone in the areas of heavy compressive and tensile stress (for example, near the tendon insertions) is particularly conspicuous and runs a precipitous course (compare Fig. 279). Thus, (acro-) osteolysis occasionally develops in the olecranon (Fig. 210).

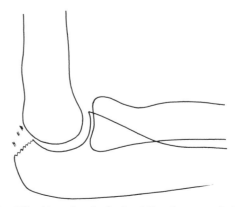

Fig. 210 (Acro-) osteolysis of the olecranon in hyperpathyroidism or osteomalacia (see text).

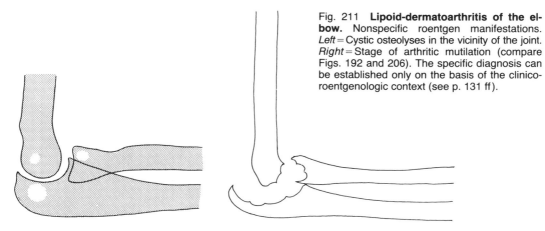

Fig. 211 **Lipoid-dermatoarthritis of the elbow.** Nonspecific roentgen manifestations. *Left* = Cystic osteolyses in the vicinity of the joint. *Right* = Stage of arthritic mutilation (compare Figs. 192 and 206). The specific diagnosis can be established only on the basis of the clinico-roentgenologic context (see p. 131 ff).

In **lipoid-dermatoarthritis** (p. 131 f), hardly any tissue, organ, or joint is spared the storage of lipids, according to the cases published so far. In the elbow joint, this polyarticular, bilaterally symmetrical disorder shows the radiographic characteristics of chronic arthritis which, often within a few years, reaches the stage of mutilation (Fig. 211).

Neoplasia of the Joint

Suspicion of a neoplasm developing from the periarticular soft tissues or the connective tissue in the vicinity of the joint is aroused in the presence of a dense soft-tissue swelling, that is also demonstrable in the roentgenogram. In addition, **malignant synovialoma** (p. 139 ff) is often accompanied by deposition of calcium so that, also in the elbow and its immediate surroundings, the roentgen finding of "circumscribed juxtaarticular resorption of bone and irregularly lobulated or homogeneous increase of soft tissue with calcifications" should raise suspicion of malignant synovialoma. Occasionally, a trivial trauma (to the elbow) gives rise to pain. One then often thinks of a calcifying hematoma (erosion of bone not being a necessary characteristic of malignant synovialoma) until a biopsy, performed because of the refractory nature of the condition, leads to the correct diagnosis.

In **pigmented villonodular synovitis** (p. 139 ff), a roentgen finding similar to that in malignant synovialoma is to be expected (Fig. 212). However, this disorder, which as a result of its abundant content in hemosiderin, produces a dense, frequently lobulated or nodular, soft-tissue shadow, generally does not show calcifications of soft tissues. Demineralization of the juxtaarticular bones is absent or extremely infrequent. This circumstance facilitates differentiation from tuberculosis of the elbow joint. Apart from this, the radiographic joint space—at least in the physiologically non-weightbearing elbow joint—is not usually narrowed in pigmented villondular synovitis. The bone is not involved until late in the disease!

For **neoplastic synovial chondromatosis (Reichel's disease)** (p. 66 f) in the elbow joint see Figure 197.

In rheumatoid arthritis, cystic fluctuating struc-

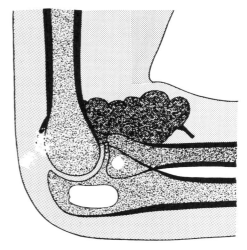

Fig. 212 **Pigmented villonodular synovitis in the elbow joint.**
Suggestive roentgen manifestations: Osteolytic area *(here)* in the olecranon and the head of the radius, lobular and nodular swelling and increased density of soft tissues in the antecubital fossa, positive (posterior) fat pad sign (see Fig. 189), and pathologic modification of the supinator fat line (see Fig. 189). No calcifications within the increased density of soft tissues.

tures that originate in the synovial membrane of the joint occur also in the elbow (**cubital cysts, cubital synovial cysts**). They must be differentiated from tumors (palpation, consistency!) and acquire clinical importance only when they rupture, limit the motion of the joint, become infected, or lead to compression of the nerves that pass in the vicinity of the joint (Ehrlich, 1972).

Xanthomas of soft tissues (p. 141 ff) also should enter into the differential diagnosis of increased soft-tissue densities at the elbow. The same applies to bursitis and cubital synovial cysts (Figs. 200 and 213).

Articular and Periarticular Calcifications and Ossifications of the Soft Tissues

The roentgenologic morphology of hereditary, sporadic, and symptomatic **chondrocalcinosis** (p. 62 ff) of the elbow is illustrated in Figures 209 and 214. Severe, painful, destructive osteoarthropathies during the course of chondrocalcinosis also occur in the elbow (Cosendai et al., 1976).

For **capsular calcifications** and **ossifications** see page 66 ff, Figures 197, 198, and 199.

The most frequent causes of so-called **localized myositis ossificans** (p. 68) in the elbow are traumas [15] and organic nervous diseases. The disorder can give rise to extraarticular ankylosis of the joint. *Posttraumatic* myositis ossificans has no relation to **progressive myositis ossificans,** which has a poor prognosis (p. 70). Neurogenic paraarticular formations of new bone can occur without a concomitant arthropathy. Paraarticular ossifications in the elbow have been observed following burns and tetanus infection. Figure 215 shows the typical picture of localized myositis ossificans of the elbow. A connection with trauma may be presumed either when residuals of trauma are visible in the articulating bones or when the clinical findings leave no doubt as to a preceding major injury to the soft tissues.

Figure 216 reproduces the pictures of **localized, universal,** and **pseudotumorous interstitial calcinosis** (p. 69 ff).

Among the **pathologic findings in the fibroosseous junction** (see p. 72 ff) is the *olecranon spur* (Fig. 199). When it gives rise to pain, an attendant inflammation of a neighboring bursa should be diagnosed—similarly to other tendon spurs.

The so-called *tennis elbow* (Schneider, 1972) also belongs to the fibroosseous disorders. The pain is triggered in the lateral epicondyle of the humerus where

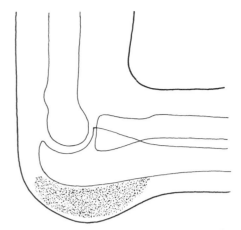

Fig. 213   **Tendon xanthoma in the elbow.** *Differential diagnosis* by differences in consistency on palpation from chronic bursitis and synovial cysts, which have developed from the olecranon bursae and are apt to spread toward the forearm, by differences in consistency on palpation (Palmer, 1969).

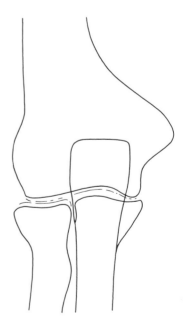

Fig. 214   **Chondrocalcinosis of the elbow joint.** Only the calcification of the articular cartilage is illustrated. However, calcifications in the synovial membrane, in the fibrous joint capsule, in ligaments, and in tendons may be observed concomitantly (McCarthy Jr. and Silcox, 1973).

---

[15] Posttraumatic myositis ossificans of the brachialis muscle—visible in the antecubital fossa—frequently follows dislocation of the elbow. It is, however, still a matter of debate whether the condition is an (often inevitable) sequel to trauma or is due to incompetent therapy.

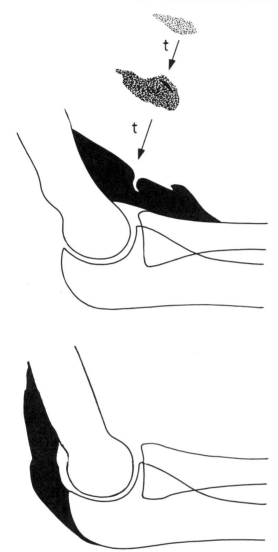

Fig. 215 Localized myositis ossificans in the elbow (typical site).

Above = Development of localized myositis ossificans in the antecubital fossa (t = time)

Below = posterior ossification of tendon and muscle. "Above" and "below" may occur concomitantly.

the extensor muscles of the hand and the fingers originate. Therefore, this condition, which is the result of excessive strain or an injury, and which can be accompanied by reactive inflammatory lesions, has been termed "humeral epicondylitis." The medial epicondyle is less frequently the seat of the complaints; these are due to pathologic changes in the origin of the flexor muscles (so-called *pitcher's elbow;* Heiss 1972). On the one hand, a normal roentgen finding does not

rule out a humeral epicondylitis, but, on the other, there are reports on spurs in the tendinous attachments *(fibroosteoses)* as well as cloudy, rounded calcium deposits at a few millimeters' distance from the insertions, and sometimes demineralization of the epicondyle and its surroundings (Fig. 217). These roentgen findings show no qualitative relation to the clinical picture. The latter can be silent, or there may be pain on exercise (particularly on prehension) as well as persistent pain. In chronic sports injuries to the tendinous insertions mentioned, additional osteoarthrotic lesions in the elbow joint (particularly in its humeroulnar compartment) and damages to the collateral ligaments are frequently demonstrable (Lehmann and Saxer, 1976).

Fibroosteitis has been discussed on page 73 (see Fig. 79). Figure 217 E shows this finding in the elbow.

Metaplastic ossifications in the ulnar and radial collateral ligaments and their insertions are also known to occur. They can follow a trauma or be the result of excessive strain (Fig. 217). Ossification of the attachment of the interosseous membrane and its diagnostic significance are shown in Fig. 218.

Affections of the bursae in the immediate neighborhood of the elbow sometimes manifest themselves by calcifications (Figs. 197 and 200).

It can be seen from the preceding remarks and the caption to Figure 183 (no. 4) that *periarticular* calcifications and ossifications of the soft tissues occur in a large variety of anatomic structures. Therefore, despite the considerations presented above and the accompanying figures, it is—in an individual case—not always possible to determine the *anatomic seat* of the calcium deposit or the newly formed bone. To the physician referring a patient to the radiologist, however, it is of the highest importance to obtain detailed information concerning the *position* of the calcification or ossification with regard to palpable reference points in the elbow so as to be able to differentiate a painful morbid condition from a painless chance finding by palpation.

Injuries to the Joint

Among the **pure dislocations,** posterior dislocation of the forearm takes first place (Fig. 219). Concomitant injury to the collateral ligament frequently produces an additional lateral displacement (radial dislocation). The latter injury, however, also occurs without dorsal dislocation. Anterior and ulnar dislocations usually are accompanied by fractures or avulsions. Divergent dislocation of the elbow is spoken of when the humerus is pushed between the anteriorly dislocated radius and the posteriorly dislocated ulna. Isolated anterior dislocation of the radial head is the result of a tear in the annular ligament of the radius. The radial head also can dislocate posteriorly or laterally.

Subluxation of the radial head in infancy and

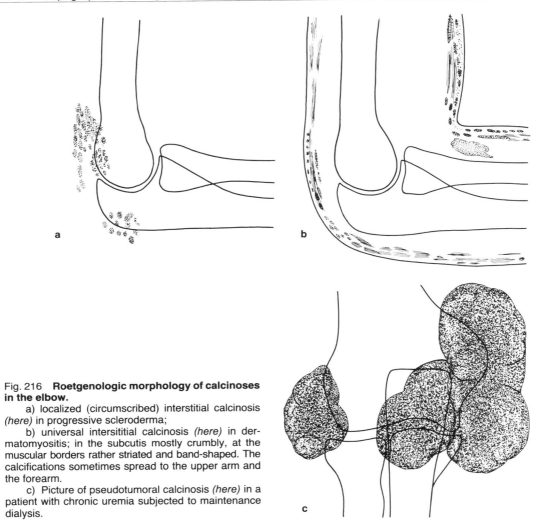

Fig. 216 **Roetgenologic morphology of calcinoses in the elbow.**
   a) localized (circumscribed) interstitial calcinosis *(here)* in progressive scleroderma;
   b) universal intersititial calcinosis *(here)* in dermatomyositis; in the subcutis mostly crumbly, at the muscular borders rather striated and band-shaped. The calcifications sometimes spread to the upper arm and the forearm.
   c) Picture of pseudotumoral calcinosis *(here)* in a patient with chronic uremia subjected to maintenance dialysis.

childhood is termed **pulled elbow (Chassaignac's painful pseudoparalysis).** This dislocation comes about in a typical manner: the toddler usually stumbles and the parent prevents him from falling by jerking him up. By so doing, the radial head is caused to slip out of the annular ligament and comes to lie partly or entirely in the cul-de-sac of the joint. The arm hangs down flaccid, as if paralyzed; the hand is pronated, and supination is blocked. The primary cause of this subluxation of the radius is longitudinal traction on the arm. The injury also occurs, even after the toddler stage, in predisposed individuals (for example, when dressing and undressing, or when hanging from a horizontal bar). "Predisposed" here means that *absence* of the conical shape of the radial head and neck that is physiologic in infancy and childhood

(their transverse diameters hence being equal) persists in later life. The faulty position of the radial head is recognizable in the lateral roentgenogram of the elbow when the axis of the radius (the radial neck) does not pass in the direction of the ossification center of the capitellum, which usually ossifies as early as the end of the first year of life (Fig. 220).

   In **dislocations of the elbow when the bone is wrenched away,** it is primarily the two epicondyles, the capitellum of the humerus, the tip of the olecranon, the coronoid process, the head of the radius, and the insertions of ligaments that, frequently in combination, are broken off, sheared off, or avulsed. The respective centers of ossification likewise can be detached (Fig. 221).

   A rupture of the ulnar collateral ligament can

Fig. 217 **Roentgen findings in so-called epicondylitis humeri** (A to E)

A = Rounded, cloudy calcium deposits at a few millimeters' distance from the origin of the extensor muscles. Conspicuous demineralization of the lateral epicondyle and the contiguous portion of the condyle (not illustrated) sometimes occurs.

B = Osseous tendon spur (Fibroostosis).

C = Epicondylitis may present a normal roentgen finding. Local tenderness, however, is a necessary accompaniment.

NV = typical radiographic morphology of calcification of peripheral nerves (solid, cylindrical calcium shadows); e.g., in leprosy.

D = Calcium deposits or ossifications in the illustrated collateral ligaments (due to excessive strain or posttraumatic) or—when situated near the bone—traumatic avulsions of epicondylar bone. For the differential diagnosis compare Fig. 183, no. 4; only the medial epicondyle is sketched there. Fibroostosis (tendon spur) at the insertion of the biceps muscle in the tuberosity of the radius.

E = Productive fibroosteitis in the tendon insertions on the lateral epicondyle (here in ankylosing spondylitis).

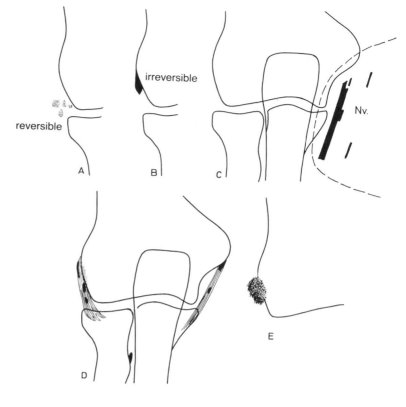

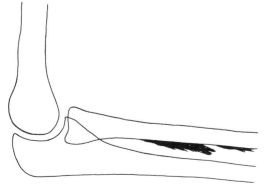

Fig. 218 **Ossification of the insertion of the interosseous membrane in the radius** is a characteristic roentgen finding in **fluorosis of bone.**

Chronic endemic (drinking water!) and industrial fluorine poisoning does not develop in all exposed individuals. It manifests itself roentgenologically by a diffuse alteration of the bone structure (hyperostosis of cancellous bone, periosteal and endosteal formation of new bone—"white" bone in the film), and ossification of the insertions (large fibroostoses) or complete ossification of tendons, ligaments, fasciae, interosseous membranes, and fibrous joint capsules. Partial regression of these alterations, which are more pronounced in the axial than in the peripheral skeleton, is possible after discontinuation of the exposure to fluorine (Dominok, 1975).

Differential diagnosis from osteomyelosclerosis in which myeloid metaplasia is to be expected and which is absent in chronic fluorosis.

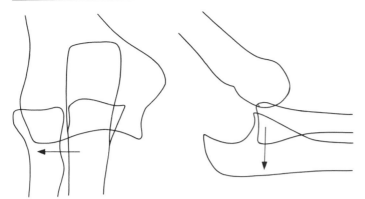

Fig. 219 **Posterior dislocation of the forearm with slight additional lateral displacement.** *Arrows* indicate direction of dislocation.

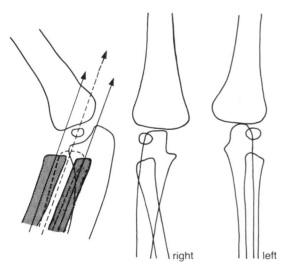

Fig. 220 **Chassaignac's painful pseudoparalysis of the right arm in early childhood** (see text).

Roentgen findings: In the lateral view, the longitudinal axis of the radial neck does not pass through the middle of the ossification center of the capitellum *(normal position dashed)* but deviates either anteriorly or posteriorly *(unbroken arrows;* Frank, 1967). In the anteroposterior view, the generally obstructed supination of the forearm is demonstrable by the strongly pronated position of the radius *(see:* right forearm).

Note: The roentgen finding is not pathologic in every case of clinically suspected Chassaignac's subluxation. In this instance, the radiologic examination serves to identify or exclude secondary injuries of bone. The pain-dependent unrest and crying of the child do not always allow normal focusing to obtain a lateral roentgenogram with an as nearly rectangular flexion as possible.

best be identified in *roentgenograms with the arm held in a certain position:* After donning radioprotective gloves, the examiner fixes the humerus above the condyles. With his other hand he flexes the forearm as far as possible to the side of the radius (following administration of a local anesthetic!). The humeroulnar interspace can normally be separated by a maximum of 5 mm. A comparative roentgenogram of the uninjured side is indispensable.

Among the **fracture-dislocations of the elbow** (Fig. 222) are:

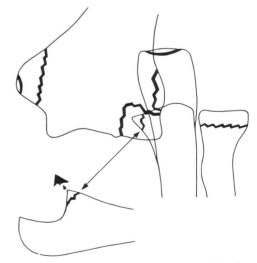

Fig. 221 **Left-sided radial dislocation of the forearm.** The additional breaks, shearings, and avulsions that most frequently accompany a dislocation are shown schematically (without the dislocation). (See text.) *Double-pointed arrow* indicates the broken-off coronoid process in the *two standard planes of exposure* and its displacement into the antecubital fossa *(small arrow).*

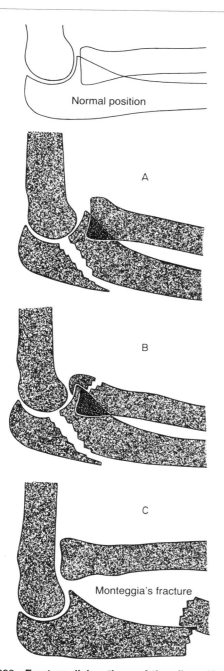

Normal position

A

B

C

Monteggia's fracture

Fig. 222 Fracture-dislocations of the elbow (A to C; see text).

1.   Proximal fracture of the ulna with anterior dislocation of the forearm (Fig. 222 A)
2.   Fracture of the proximal ulna and the radial head with anterior (Fig. 222 B) or posterior dislocation of the forearm

3.   Monteggia's fracture in the proximal or middle third of the ulna, associated with anterior (Fig. 222 C) or, less frequently, posterior dislocation of the radial head

Included among **complications in dislocations of the elbow** are:

1.   Localized (traumatic) myositis ossificans (p. 68, Fig. 215).
2.   In fracture-dislocations, the median nerve is most likely to be injured. If, with a Monteggia fracture (Fig. 222 C), the dislocation of the radial head is not reduced, a shelflike—sometimes reversible—capsular calcification often develops, contrasting sharply with the biconcave radial head. This finding should not be mistaken for an avulsed part of bone (Schmitt, 1967).
3.   Limitation of motion due to shrinking of the capsule and the muscles or to myositis ossificans (see item 1).
4.   The capsule of the elbow joint encloses not only the region that is covered by cartilage but also areas that are devoid of cartilage. Broken-off or sheared-off parts of bone (for example, as secondary injuries in dislocations) may therefore be displaced within the joint and may become loose bodies.

The capsule inserts in the neck of the radius about 1.5 cm distal to the radial head. In the humerus, the insertion of the capsule runs about 2 cm proximal to the border of the cartilage of the capitellum and the trochlea. The epicondyles lie outside the capsular insertion, but they are more or less bound to the joint capsule by the insertion of the collateral ligaments. The coronoid fossa lies in the joint cavity. One half of the olecranon fossa lies inside and the other half outside the joint cavity.

The **anterior humeral line** (AHL) (Rogers et al., 1978, Fig. 223) is a radiographic aid in identifying a **supracondylar fracture of the humerus** in children. With the humerus in an exactly lateral position, a tangent to the anterior contour of the humeral shaft is erected in the roentgenogram. This anterior humeral line passes distally as a secant to the projection of the capitellum humeri. The tangent to the distal contour of the capitellum humeri (TC) runs vertically to this secant. TC is divided into three parts according to the extension of the capitellum. Normally, AHL intersects the *middle* third of TC. With supracondylar fractures of the humerus, including greenstick fractures, AHL passes through the anterior third of TC. In addition, a positive fat pad sign (see Fig. 189) may be expected, *provided the joint capsule is not torn.* The latter reservation applies on principle to the development of the cubital fat pad sign in traumatic joint effusions!

Flexion types of supracondylar fractures sometimes present T-, Y- or V-shaped fracture clefts that extend into the joint (Fig. 224). They often heal with the formation of steps in the articulating surface and also can be followed by malalignment (valgus or varus deformity).

Among the *extraarticular supracondylar frac-*

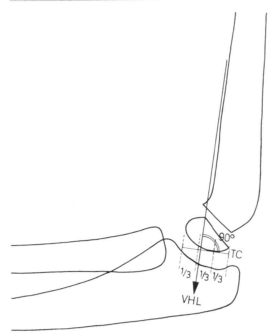

Fig. 223. Anterior humeral line (VHL) to facilitate the roentgenologic diagnosis of a supracondylar fracture in children. (Normal finding illustrated; see text.)

TC = distal tangent to the capitellum humeri, which runs perpendicular to the VHL, divided into three parts.

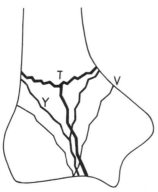

Fig. 224 Supracondylar fractures with T-, Y-, and V-shaped fracture cleft *(diagrammatic).*

Note: It is not the course of the fracture lines but the incomplete adaptation of the (displaced) fragments that leads to the formation of steps in the articular surface (preosteoarthrotic deformity) and to malalignments in the elbow region.

tures of the humerus, the **extension types of fractures** (fractures with dorsal and proximal displacement of the fragments) can interfere with the function of the elbow joint. The proximal fragment, which lies to it anteriorly, sometimes consolidates with the formation of a step and shortening so that flexion is impaired (Fig. 225). Since this fracture mostly occurs in the growth period, the offending step grows, as a rule, away from the elbow joint (in the direction of the shoulder), and normal flexibility is gradually restored.

Following reduction of a supracondylar fracture of the humerus in childhood, the orienting line of Baumann (1960)—**Baumann's line**—indicates the course of the axis of the distal fragment. When the reduction has achieved correct alignment, the angle between Baumann's line and the longitudinal axis of the humerus is between 75 and 80 degrees (Fig. 226).

Volkmann's ischemic contracture of the arm and the hand (''claw hand'') is a dreaded complication following particularly, though not exclusively, supracondylar fractures of the humerus in children. The condition is diagnosed clinically. It should, however, be remembered that the exact site and the extension of traumatic damage to the blood vessels can be determined only by angiography. On the other hand, the clinical concept of Volkmann's contracture, with regard to its etiology and pathogenesis, is at present understood in a broader sense than it was originally. Not only arterial ischemia but also the sequelae of venous stasis and toxic damage, as well as nerve injuries and reflex influences of the vegetative nervous system, are suggested etiologic factors (Makoski and Löhr, 1972).

In **diacondylar fractures,** the cleft extends more or less transversely through the condyle of the humerus, the greatest part of the fracture cleft occupying an extraarticular position. **Condylar fractures** occur more frequently laterally than medially. The fracture cleft, which usually follows an oblique course, extends into the joint. The more peripheral the course of the fracture cleft, the more shelflike the appearance of the fragment (Fig. 227). Shearing fractures of the lateral condyle of the humerus are related to a typical mechanism of accident: with a fall on the hand, the radius transmits the blow proximally in its longitudinal direction and thus gives rise to a shearing fracture of the lateral condyle of the humerus. The same process can cause the radial head to break off.

Finally, **avulsion of the epicondyles** is a well-known injury that mostly concerns children and adolescents. In most cases the medial epicondyle is injured; the fragment can be impacted in the joint (see the legend to Fig. 227).

Breaks of the capitellum and the trochlea of the humerus are only rarely associated. Individual fractures, however, occur quite frequently, ranging from shelflike breaks to total separation, particularly of the capitellum (Fig. 228). They are not always limited to the anatomic boundaries between the trochlea and capitellum. Persons with a constitutionally

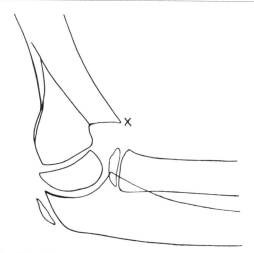

Fig. 225 **Extension type of supracondylar fracture healed with deformation and impairment of flexion at the elbow** (X = site of impact).

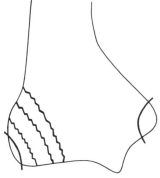

Fig. 227 **Courses of the fracture clefts in fracture of the lateral condyle** (fracture of the *medial* condyle is very rare). If a proximal displacement of the sheared-off portion ot the lateral condyle is not corrected, a pathologic cubitus valgus is likely to develop. Among epicondylar avulsions (marked by *curved lines*), fracture of the medial epicondyle occurs most frequently. This injury is incurred primarily in the growth period (Fig. 183, no. 4). In dislocations, the concomitantly broken-off epicondyle may be displaced into the joint and may give rise to manifestations of locking.

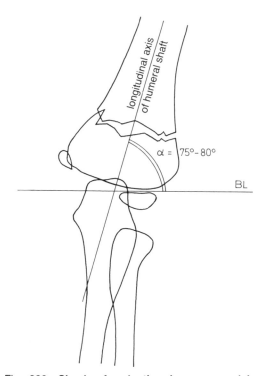

Fig. 226 **Check of reduction in supracondylar fracture of the humerus in children by measuring the angle between Baumann's line (BL) and the longitudinal axis of the humeral shaft.** Normally, the angle $\alpha = 75$–$80°$. Baumann's line is the straight line drawn through the epiphyseal plate of the capitellum humeri.

marked cubitus valgus are susceptible to these kinds of fractures. Böhler (1953) therefore has referred to them as injuries of typical anatomic-constitutional origin. Since both of these parts of the humerus have their own centers of ossification, young individuals are more likely to suffer an epiphysiolysis than a fracture. In childhood, detachment of the ossification center of the capitellum can be mistakenly diagnosed unless one remembers that the opposing contours of the condyle and the capitellum form, as a rule, a dorsally open angle (Matzen, 1959, Fig. 229). A comparative roentgenogram of the other elbow joint will prevent this erroneous diagnosis.

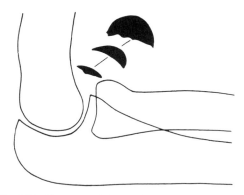

Fig. 228 **Fracture of the capitellum humeri,** ranging from shelflike break to total separation *(synopsis).* The smallest shelflike part of the capitellum indicates the most frequent site of dislocation in the lateral roentgenogram of the elbow.

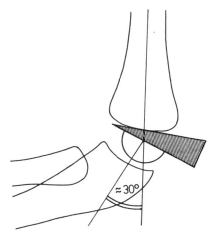

Fig. 229 **Two tangents drawn to the opposing humeral condyle and capitellum** form, in early childhood (age 4 in the present case), a posteriorly open angle. *Caution:* Beware of misinterpreting this finding as traumatic epiphysiolysis. Normal epiphysis: shaft angle of the humerus (about 30°).

Fractures of the proximal part of the radius (Fig. 230) range from a so-called chisel fracture to total separation and to comminution of the radial head. The neck of the radius may be involved in comminuted fractures, but it also may break off without an injury to the radial head. Epiphysiolysis occurs in the growth period, after the ossification center of the radial head has appeared between the fourth and seventh years of life.

Comparison with a dissected specimen of the elbow shows that anteroposterior radiograph with supination of the hand demonstrates the head of the radius in about the same way as does a lateral radiograph with the hand *pronated* (the palm resting on a table). Consequently, for the second plane, a lateral film with supination of the hand (its ulnar border resting on the table) should be taken as a matter of principle.

In the proximal end of the ulna, **fractures of the olecranon and the coronoid process** are of interest (Fig. 231). The pull of the triceps muscle may lead to con-

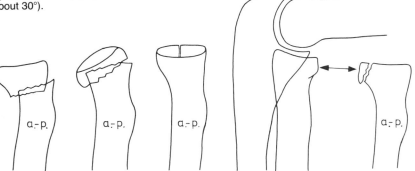

Fig. 230 **Fractures of the proximal part of the radius.** *From right to left:* Chisel fracture with slightly lateral course of the fracture cleft (difficult to identify in the lateral roentgenogram). Chisel fracture in the center of the radial head (compressed fracture of the radial head with lateral and volar angulation). Fracture of the radial neck (slightly displaced).

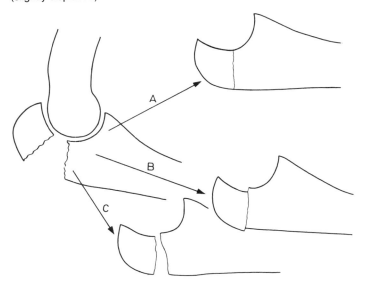

Fig. 231 **Fracture of the olecranon with distraction of fragments.** A = Desirable union. B (union with step formation) and C (pseudoarthrosis) are preosteoarthrotic deformities.

siderable diastasis of the olecranon fragments. Unless this condition is corrected, there is a threat of pseudoarthrosis with impairment or loss of extension at the elbow joint. Consolidation with formation of a step in the articular surface results in a preosteoarthrotic deformity, just as does a pseudoarthrosis. The coronoid process usually breaks off with severe fractures of the elbow and as a complication of dislocation (Fig. 221).

Apart from the characteristic fractures of the elbow discussed in the foregoing, there occur **comminuted fractures** in which, depending on the intensity of the blow, the articulating bones are more or less completely and irregularly shattered.

The involvement of the elbow joint in fractures of the articulating bones can manifest itself by the positive fat pad sign (intraarticular hematoma, traumatic joint effusion, Fig. 189). The escape of (fatty) bone marrow through the fracture cleft into the elbow joint is demonstrable roentgenologically as **lipohemarthrosis** (Yousefzadeh and Jackson Jr., 1978) (Fig. 232).

In *summarizing the undesirable sequelae of elbow fractures, mention should first be made of impairment* or even *loss of function,* which can develop in a variety of ways (as the result of intra- and extraarticular ankylosis, of a flail joint, etc.), and in posttraumatic *osteoarthrosis* of the elbow joint. In this connection it should be remembered that limitation of flexion and extension at the elbow joint cannot be counterbalanced by other joints! Moreover, there

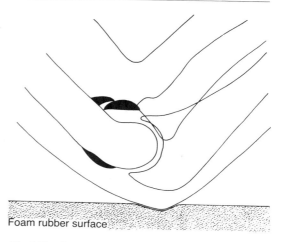

Foam rubber surface

Fig. 232 Cubital lipohemarthrosis in the roentgenogram. Lateral roentgenogram of the elbow with *horizontal* incidence of rays reveals, in addition to the positive fat pad sign, intraarticular fat level formation.

is the threat of *injuries to nerves and arteries* that, apart from accurate reduction, require additional therapeutic measures. Late nerve damage, particularly of the ulnar nerve, may develop as the result of posttraumatic osteoarthrosis and also of inadequate adaptation of the fragments in the region of the medial olecranon groove.

Joints of the Shoulder Girdle

Variants and Malformations

Typical variants and modifications of density are shown in Figure 233. The radiologic examiner is interested primarily in those deformities of the joints of the shoulder girdle that manifest themselves unilaterally or bilaterally in the *immediately* articulating parts of the bones. Figure 234 presents malformations in the scapulohumeral joint (shoulder joint). The acromioclavicular joint and/or the sternoclavicular joint are involved in aplasia of the acromion, frequently also in cleidocranial dysplasia (generally bilateral hy-

poplasia or aplasia of the clavicle, sometimes only absence of its middle portion) and in cleidofacial dysostosis, which is a very rare disorder. Occasionally, such embryologic errors are chance findings without clinical importance. At times they may interfere with motion or may promote attrition of the articular cartilage; in the latter instance they are preosteoarthritic deformities. Deformation of joints can also be the result of an arthritis in the growth period (p. 93 ff), a pyogenic septicemia in infancy with localization in the proximal end of the humerus, or an injury incurred in the growth period. Prior to diagnosing a congenital malformation, those etiologies must be ruled out by the history.

Arthritis

Demonstrations of the soft-tissue signs of arthritis in the shoulder joint depend on the patient's age, the stage of the arthritis, and its etiology. In infancy, an effusion into the joint manifests itself by distention plus (sub-) luxation plus lateralization of the proximal end of the humerus (Fig. 235). **Nonspecific bacterial arthritis of the shoulder joint** can, at any age, lead to periarticular edema, which causes the juxtaarticular soft tissue to become swollen and "homogeneous" (Figs. 235 and 236). **Tuberculosis of the shoulder joint** has its origin either in a subchondral focus in the bone marrow or in the infected synovial membrane. The "synovial type" of tuberculosis (Fig.

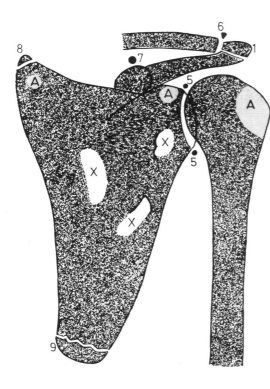

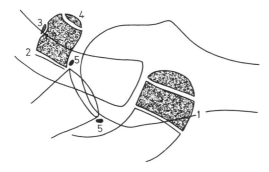

Fig. 233 **Variants in the shoulder region** (1 to 9). Multiple pleomorphic circumscribed *ossification defects* (X; Cigtay and Mascatello, 1979) and typically located circumscribed **areas of increased radiolucency** without pathologic significance (A).

1 = OS acromiale, possibly bipartite. Roentgenological differential diagnosis between os acromiale and acromial pseudoarthrosis with a history of trauma sometimes is difficult.

2 = Os coracoideum.

3 = Persistent apophysis of the coracoid process.

4 = Persistent epiphysis of the coracoid process.

5 = Bones or ossification centers that become detached during development of glenoid fossa and are apt to persist at any point on the glenoid (nomenclature nonuniform).

6 = Accessory acromioclavicular bone?

7 = Sesamoid bone in the coracoclavicular ligament (posttraumatic ligamentous ossifications are not as harmoniously rounded).

8 = Persistent apophysis at the superior angle of the scapula.

9 = Persistent apophysis at the inferior angle of the scapula.

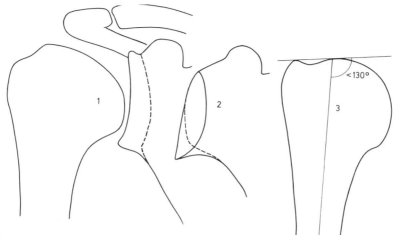

Fig. 234   **Malformations of the shoulder joint.**
1 = Congenital malformation of the humeral head and embryologic error of the glenoid (flat glenoid, neck of scapula shortened). *Dashed line* indicates contour of the glenoid in aplasia.

Note: As with the acetabulum, embryologic errors are more frequent in the region of the glenoid than in the head of the humerus. Embryologic errors may lead to *congenital* or *recurrent* dislocation (subluxation) of the shoulder joint.

2 = "Shovel-shaped" glenoid *(normal contours of glenoid dashed)*.

3 = Humerus varus (angle between neck and shaft of humerus smaller, normal values ranging from 130° to 140°). Humerus varus may be congenital or symptomatic (e.g., in achondroplasia, in the osteochondrodysplasias and mucopolysacharidoses, in cretinism and hemophilia, following osteomyelitis, following arthritis in the growth period [see Fig. 242], or posttraumatic).

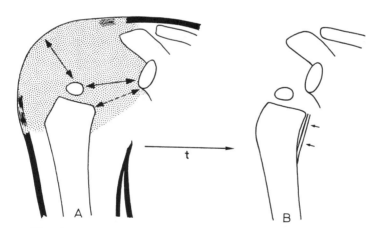

Fig. 235   **Empyema of the shoulder joint,** in the present case as the result of acute osteomyelitis of the proximal metaphysis of the humerus (patient over 1 year old, onset of the disease one week previously).

A = *Lateralization of the ossification center in the humeral head (approximately horizontal double arrow)* is a sign of capsular distention (effusion; pus was aspirated). When, depending on the patient's age, the ossification center is still absent, distention of the joint capsule by the effusion is recognizable by the lateralization of the proximal diaphysis of the humerus *(dashed double arrow)*, in comparison with the contralateral side. A traumatic (hemorrhagic) effusion may also give rise to lateralization; for example, one following obstetric epiphyseolysis (p. 203 ff). Swelling of soft tissues *(approximately vertical double arrow)* due to periarticular inflammatory edema, which impregnates the subcutaneous fat stripe *(black)* and renders it roentgenologically equivalent to water. It then can no longer be radiologically differentiated from the surrounding soft tissues.

B = Regression of the suppurative arthritis under antibiotic treatment. Six weeks after onset of the disease, only a delicate lamellar periosteal reaction in the proximal humerus *(arrows)* indicates the past osteomyelitis (t = time; follow-up study).

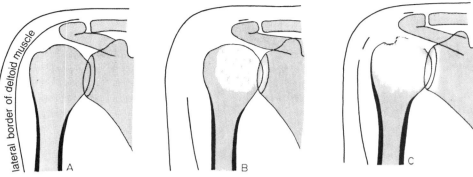

Fig. 236 Evolution of a case of pyogenic arthritis of the shoulder joint.
A = Normal roentgen finding on the day of local injection of a corticosteroid for clinically diagnosed periarthritis of the shoulder.
B = Fifteen days after A. Strong periarticular, homogenizing swelling of soft tissues, spotty demineralization of the articulating bones. Antibiotic treatment these last 3 days.
C = Thirty days after A. The periarticular soft-tissue swelling tends to regress. Uniform decalcification of the articulating bones. Delicate erosion in the upper region of the capsular insertion and partial obliteration of the marginal subchondral lamella of the humeral head. The clinical and serological data indicate subsiding of the process. Histologic repair and removal of the debris may, however, persist for months; only then does the total extent of the destruction manifest.

237) manifests itself, *as a rule*, by periarticular swelling of the soft tissues and marked decalcification of the articulating bones. In synovial tuberculosis, erosive changes become demonstrable in the roentgen picture only after a prolonged period; they start in the area exposed to least mechanical strain,

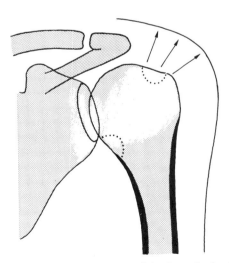

Fig. 237 Suspicion of synovial tuberculosis of the shoulder joint is aroused when the roentgenogram reveals a (insidiously developing) periarticular soft-tissue swelling *(arrows) plus* decalcification in the juxtaarticular parts of bone, particularly the head of the humerus. Areas where the arthritic erosions (not only in synovial tuberculosis) first become manifest are *dotted* (see Figs. 236 and 240).

and at the greatest possible physiologic distance from the humerus and the glenoid fossa of the scapula (Ganguli, 1963). In the "osseous type" of tuberculosis one observes atrophy of the periarticular soft tissues (compare both sides) and irregularly shaped osteolysis, usually in the head of the humerus. Initially, these lesions are sometimes accompanied by a hazy contour and later by erosions of the articular surface (Fig. 238). When the tuberculous destruction of bone takes place in the *metaphysis,* it is commonly associated with a delicate periosteal reaction. Tuberculous (calcified) pus is seen in the synovial as well as in the osseous type of tuberculosis of the shoulder joint. Sequestra and detached fragments of bone develop during the course of tuberculous breakdown of bone. Cutaneous fistulas may also occur. A very infrequent complication is necrosis of the humeral head related to tuberculous destruction of nutrient vessels (Ganguli, 1963).

Sometimes, tuberculosis of the shoulder joint starts from an infection of the *subdeltoid bursa.* This bursa is also known to be an infrequent primary site of rheumatoid arthritis in the region of the shoulder girdle, or it may be a secondary finding in various types of arthritis of the shoulder joint. Finally, this bursa can be involved in neurogenic osteoarthropathies (see Fig. 262) and in affections of the rotator cuff (see Figs. 70 and 277). The lesion can also be demonstrated roentgenologically. In the anteroposterior roentgenogram (with the humerus externally rotated) an *inconstant* ("black") fat stripe measuring 1 or 2 mm in width indicates the location of the normal bursa (Fig. 239). The swollen subdeltoid bursa is often demarcated from its surroundings by a lateral, caudal, and medial ("black") fat stripe which

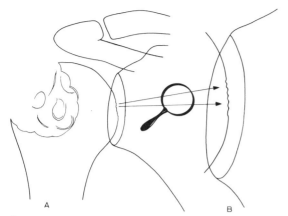

A   B

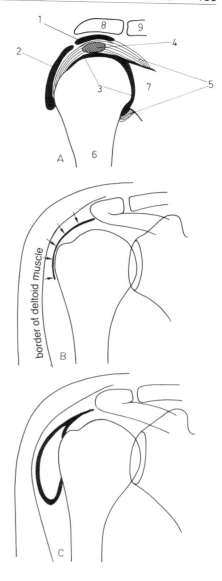

Fig. 238 Centrolateral osteolysis of the humeral head, in part trabeculated (A). *Only under a magnifying glass* can a definite, though flat, erosion be identified in the articulating region of the humeral head (B).

Radiographic diagnosis: Arthritic process (tuberculosis?); no tumor; see Figs. 22 and 23.

Radiographic differential diagnosis: Pigmented villonodular synovitis, osteoarthropathy of amyloidosis.

Result of biopsy: Caseating tuberculosis **(osseous type of articular tuberculosis).**

Fig. 239 Subdeltoid bursa.

A: anatomy. 1 = Subacromial bursa, often communicating with the *subdeltoid bursa* (2). 3 = Joint cavity. 4 = Tendon of supraspinatus muscle. Communication between 3 and 1 only with perforation or with rupture of 4. 5 = Joint capsule. 6 = Humerus. 7 = cavity of shoulder joint, neck of scapula. 8 = Acromion. 9 = Clavicle.

B = *Inconstant* fat stripe *(arrows)* which indicates the *normal* subdeltoid bursa (Weston and Palmer, 1978).

C = *Enlarged* subdeltoid bursa which is marked laterally, caudally, and in part also medially by the subsynovial layer of adipose tissue *and/or* which displaces the border of the deltoid muscle (compare Fig. 236).

Note: In rheumatoid arthritis, larger or smaller fluctuating cysts may develop from the diseased subacromial and subdeltoid bursa (Palmer, 1969; compare Fig. 244).

also reflects the subsynovial position of the adipose layer, and/or it displaces the border of the deltoid muscle (Fig. 239; Weston and Palmer, 1978). The enlarged bursa has the appearance of a big "tear."

Inflammatory rheumatic diseases, for example, rheumatoid arthritis, psoriatic arthritis, and involvement of peripheral joints in ankylosing spondylitis, present the picture of chronic arthritis in the shoulder joint. Destructive phenomena—direct signs of arthritis—are in the forefront of the radiographic picture. Erosions start, as a rule, from the capsular insertion and therefore become manifest in the upper and lower borders of the anatomic neck of the humerus. Erosions and destructions developing in the anterior and posterior aspects of the capsular inser-

tion in the humerus become manifest in the anteroposterior roentgenogram as equivocal "cystic" translucencies of the bone structure. Only the axial view of the shoulder identifies these lesions as erosions of the capsular insertion (Figs. 240 and 241). In the inflammatory rheumatic diseases mentioned above—excepting ankylosing spondylitis—the shoulder joint is not usually the initial articular manifestation. Thus, their roentgenologic differentiation—for example, from tuberculosis of the shoulder joint—hardly ever meets with difficulties. On the other hand, ankylosing spondylitis as the initial manifestation of *peripheral* joint involvement *can* lead to chronic arthritis of the shoulder joint. In these cases, however, the primary disease has usually been known for years.

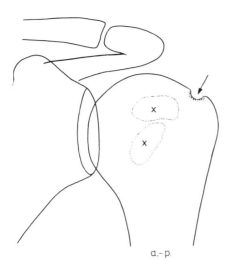

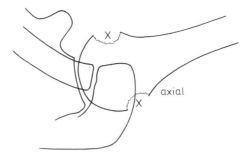

a.-p.

axial

Fig. 240 Early erosion in arthritis of the shoulder joint *(arrow)* in the upper contour of the anatomic neck of the humerus. Depressions—but also affections—of the rotator cuff occur in this place (see Fig. 277)! X = Larger erosions of the capsular insertion in the anterior and posterior aspect of the humeral head appear in the anteroposterior roentgenogram as equivocal "cystic" translucent areas in the humeral head.

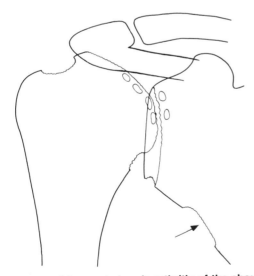

Fig. 241 Advanced chronic arthritis of the shoulder joint (in the present case rheumatoid arthritis) with narrowing of the interosseous space, erosions, destructions, and attendant arthritic cysts. The elevation of the humeral head in the glenoid fossa indicates damage of the rotator cuff (see Fig. 277, no. 12), which in this patient is probably caused by the arthritic processes. *Arrow* points to an erosion of the lateral border of the scapula, which can be observed in rheumatoid arthritis.

Arthritis of the growth period (see p. 93 ff) and *deformation of the joint due to immobilization* (see the legend to Fig. 398) are shown in Figure 242.

Chronic arthritis of the joints of the shoulder girdle in teritiary syphilis can be diagnosed from the radiographic appearance only in connection with the positive result of serological tests. It should be remembered that congential as well as acquired syphilis attacks not only the knee joints but also the sternoclavicular, sternocostal, and temporomandibular joints with particular frequency (Sundt, 1948).

Fungal infections of the joints of the shoulder girdle also present the roentgen findings of chronic arthritis. Inflammatory rheumatic and bacterial types of arthritis *may* be followed by bony ankylosis. The reduced mobility is compensated in part by the associated movement of the scapula.

Roentgen findings in acromioclavicular arthritis are shown in Figure 243.

Chronic sternoclavicular arthritis is known to occur in inflammatory rheumatic diseases (see also Fig. 244) or may, for example, be transmitted from a juxtaarticular osteomyelitis of the clavicle (Fig. 245). Tomographs are essential to the early and confident diagnosis of sternoclavicular arthritis.

Painful, inflammatory swelling of the sternoclavicular and/or acromioclavicular joint is known to occur as an early—though roentgenologically negative—symptom of *polymyalgia rheumatica*.

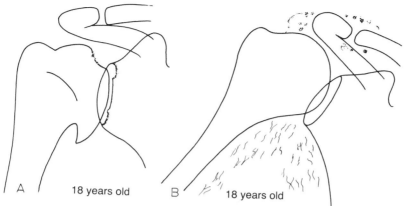

Fig. 242 Scapulohumeral arthritis of the growth period (A) and **deformation of the joint due to immobilization** (B).

A = Deformity of the humeral head and humerus varus (Fig. 234) *plus* arthritic erosions in the humeral head and the glenoid fossa suggest an arthritis of the shoulder joint that started in childhood (according to the history, juvenile rheumatoid arthritis is present since the age of 7; the patient is now 30).

B = Crumbly, and reticular calcification of soft tissues. The disordered growth of the proximal humerus (disproportion between the humeral head and the thickness of the humeral shaft) *without* roentgen manifestations of arthritis and the atypical radiologic attitude in the shoulder joint raise suspicion of dermatomyositis starting in youth (see pages 93 and 102).

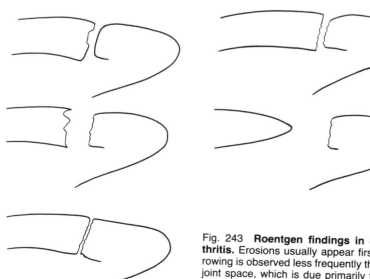

Fig. 243 Roentgen findings in (chronic) acromioclavicular arthritis. Erosions usually appear first in the clavicle. Joint space narrowing is observed less frequently than "widening" of the radiographic joint space, which is due primarily to resorption of the lateral (distal) end of the clavicle *(middle row)*. For the differential diagnosis of this osteolysis of the clavicle see pp. 58 and 195.

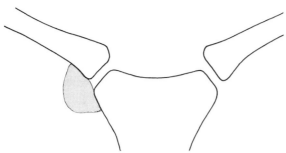

Fig. 244   Synovial cyst of the right sternoclavicular joint in rheumatoid arthritis (Grelier and Hardin, 1975) that has spread posteriorly into the upper mediastinum and gives the impression there of a space-occupying process with cyclic borders. (Detail from a posteroanterior roentgenogram of the thorax.) To be differentiated from other space-occupying processes in the mediastinum!

The (radiographic) differential diagnosis of **sclerosing (hyperostotic) clavicular processes** is shown in Figure 246.

Pathologic (osteolytic) findings in the ribs in rheumatoid arthritis and other diseases, among them progressive scleroderma (ribs, acromion) can be observed in Figures 247 and 248.

Osteoarthrosis

The typical picture of *osteoarthrosis of the shoulder joint* and the acromioclavicular joint is shown in Figures 45, 249, 250, and 251 (marginal osteophytes, narrowing of the radiographic joint space, increased density of the subchondral layer and "cystic" translucencies of the bone structure, remodeling of the articulating parts of bone leading to deformation). Advanced osteoarthrosis of the shoulder joint is an infrequent finding. In certain cases, the patient's history and/or the radiographic appearance provides a clue concerning the etiology of the cartilage attrition. It may be possible, for instance, to identify the residues of an injury to the shoulder, the repair stage of

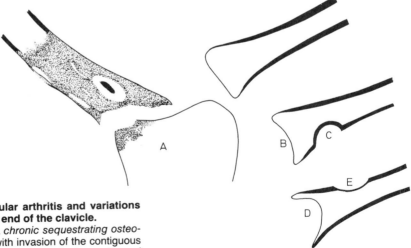

Fig. 245   Sternoclavicular arthritis and variations of shape of the sternal end of the clavicle.

A = Tomograph of a *chronic sequestrating osteomyelitis of the clavicle* with invasion of the contiguous sternoclavicular joint (destructions, faulty position of joint).

B = *Cupping* of the sternal clavicle, generally bilateral, sometimes as a transient phenomenon in the growth period.

C = *Sulcus* of the costoclavicular ligament, unilateral or bilateral (variant of normal).

D = *"Fishmouth"* shape of the sternal end of the clavicle, generally bilateral, sometimes as a transient phenomenon in the growth period.

E = *Sulcus at the origin of the sternocleidomastoid muscle* (variant of normal).

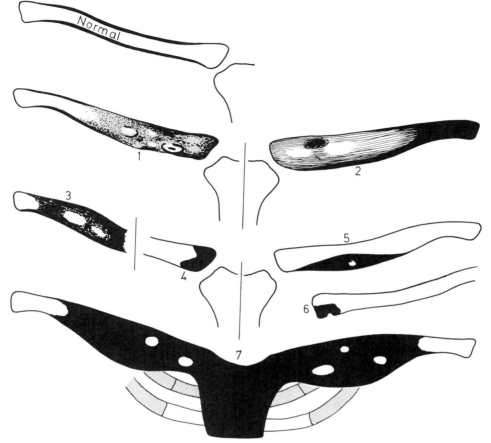

Fig. 246   Radiographic differential diagnosis of adult sclerosing (hyperostotic) clavicular processes.
1 = Chronic sequestrating pyogenic osteomyelitis.
2 = Paget's disease of bone.
3 = Suspicion of tertiary syphilitic (gummatous) osteomyelitis. To be differentiated from no. 1 (tests for syphilis?).
4 = So-called ostitis condensans claviculae (Brower et al., 1974), often painful, unilateral. Sternoclavicular joint roentgenologically normal, no histologic or clinical signs of inflammation. Reaction to mechanical stress?
5 = Osteoid osteoma.
6 = Friedrich's disease (avascular necrosis of the sternal end of the clavicle). *Clinical findings:* Pain on weight-bearing, swelling of soft tissues over the diseased portion of the clavicle. *Roentgen findings:* Increased density of cancellous bone asociated with areas of radiolucency from resorptive processes within the osteonecrosis. The disease exclusively attacks the *caudal* portion of the sternal end of the clavicle (Lingg and Heinemeier, 1981); sometimes demarcation (perisclerotic seam of increased translucence) and delicate irregularities of contour, increasing coarsening of shape, termination in osteoarthrosis of the sternoclavicular joint.
7 = Painful sternoclavicular hyperostosis—late finding (Köhler et al., 1975, 1977). Insidious development bilaterally, initially also destructive phenomena in the sternoclavicular joints and the ribs (Heimstädt, 1978). Sternoclavicular joints ankylosed, cartilage of the first or additional pairs of ribs ossified. Unilateral or bilateral occlusion of the subclavian vein possible; sometimes elevated sedimentation rate. To be differentiated from Garré's sclerosing osteomyelitis and from nos. 1, 2, 3, and 5 (see also Keipert and Campbell, 1970).

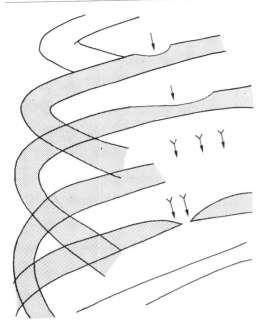

Fig. 247 **Pathologic findings in the ribs in rheumatoid arthritis** *(arrows)* (Sargent et al., 1969). The *upper borders* of the posterior segments of the 2nd to 5th ribs are affected, often in bilaterally symmetrical fashion. Identical or similar findings are encountered in progressive scleroderma *(arrows; tailed arrows,* Fig. 61), disseminated lupus erythematosus, Sjögren's syndrome, hyperparathyroidism, polymyelitic paresis, and tetraplegia (Woodlief, 1978). Pressure erosions with a similar radiographic aspect are known to occur in neurofibromatosis and in cardiovascular malformations; for example coarctation of the aorta (defects of the upper and/or lower borders of the ribs), as well as in multiple cartilaginous exostoses and in thoracic neuroblastoma. Circumscribed alterations of contour occur in osteogenesis imperfecta, in Marfan's syndrome, in progeria (Greenfield, 1969), and following irradiation.

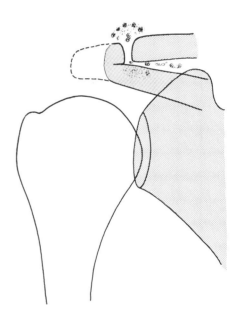

Fig. 248 **Acromial osteolysis in progressive scleroderma** (see also localized crumbly intersitital calcinosis). *(Initial contour of acromion dashed.)*

necrosis of the humeral head[16] (Fig. 252), osteochondrosis dissecans, synovial chondromatosis (Fig. 253), or deformations in epiphyseal osteochrondro-

dysplasias and mucopolysaccharidoses (p. 239 ff). In rheumatoid arthritis, the secondary osteoarthrosis sometimes overshadows the roentgenologic signs of arthritis (Fig. 254) to such a degree that, on the one hand, anamnestic statements and the results of physical examination are needed to establish the correct (roentgenologic) diagnosis. On the other hand, the development of osteoarthrosis secondary to arthritis suggests little activity of the inflammatory process or a healed arthritis, because a secondary osteoarthrosis develops exclusively in a joint that is being moved; i.e., one that is not too painful.

---

[16] The (infrequent) *necrosis of the acromial apophysis* and the *avascular necrosis of the sternal end of the clavicle (Friedrich's disease)* or of the *acromial end of the clavicle* can also induce repair processes that alter the shape of the bones and thus give rise to a preosteoarthrotic deformity. In the florid stage, these conditions must be differentiated clinically and roentgenologically from inflammatory diseases of bone!

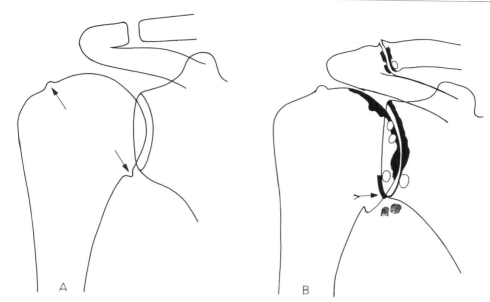

Fig. 249 **Osteoarthrosis of the shoulder joint and the acromioclavicular joint.** A = Early marginal osteo-phytes in the head of the humerus *(arrows)*. B = Remodeling with deformation, marginal osteophytes, sclerosis of subchondral cancellous bone, solitary detritus cysts, joint space narrowing. In the axillary capsular cul de sac, two calcified loose bodies (detached capsular chondromas?). *Tailed arrow* points to a partial calcification (ossifi-cation) fo the glenoidal lip.

Note: Ossifications of the glenoidal lip also occur without roentgen signs of osteoarthrosis. Traumatic avul-sions of the glenoidal lip can be identified in the roentgenogram when the lip is calcified.

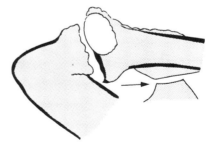

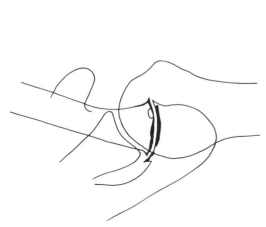

Fig. 250 **Acromioclavicular osteoarthrosis** (axial view of the shoulder).

Fig. 251 **Severe osteoarthrotic remodeling of the acromioclavicular joint** 25 years after amputation of the right thigh. The patient has never worn a prosthesis but has used exclusively forearm types of crutches. (Uric acid concentration in serum normal, no local or hu-moral signs of inflammation.)

→ = The so-called coracoclavicular joint is in all probability an anatomic variant (Heitzeberg and Reiner-Theisen, 1978; Cockshott, 1979). Its *posttraumatic* de-velopment becomes more likely the more the shape of coracoclavicular ossification and the joint formation varies from the picture sketched; i.e., the more irregu-lar the shape becomes (Fig. 286).

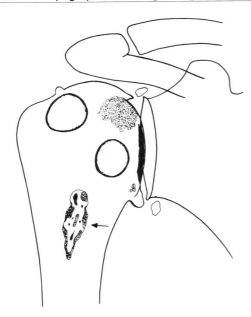

Fig. 252 **Repair stage of necrosis of the humeral head with secondary osteoarthrosis of the shoulder joint.** Regarding the multiple causes of epiphyseal osteonecrosis, see p. 254 ff). *Roentgenologic morphology* of the *revascularized* necrosis: Top part depressed, marginal parts raised, areas of increased density, small irregular fragments of bone (detached fragments), larger resorptive cysts in regions of the humeral head that are more distant from the joint. Concomitant clues to a prior *infarct of the metaphyseal bone marrow (arrow)* suggest that it was *not a localized* but a systemic process (e.g., the decompression syndrome) that has led to the circumscribed devitalization of bone.

Note: Malignant tumors developing in the cicatricious area of the infarct have been described as a complication of infarcts of the bone marrow (McCarthy et al., 1979).

Additional information in osteoarthrosis of the shoulder joint is provided by the following roentgen findings: changes of contour and structure in the greater tubercle and the acromion; elevation of the head of the humerus in the glenoid fossa; formation of a pseudoarthrosis between the head of the humerus and the inferior surface of the acromion (Fig. 255). These roentgen signs suggest with a high degree of probability a concomitant perforation or rupture of the degenerated or injured rotator cuff. This tendinous sheet, which is formed by the supraspinatus, infraspinatus, and teres minor muscles, increases the size of the

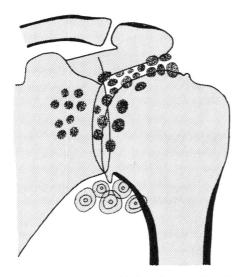

Fig. 253 **Neoplastic synovial chondromatosis of the shoulder joint and the juxtaarticular bursae** with roentgen signs of osteoarthrosis. Capsular chondromas with stratified calcification are demonstrable in the axillary cul de sac of the joint.

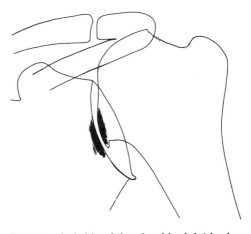

Fig. 254 **Arthritis of the shoulder joint in rheumatoid arthritis.** The prominent features of the radiologic finding are the inflammatory secondary osteoarthrosis and the clue to (inflammatory?) damage of the rotator cuff (elevation of the humeral head in the glenoid fossa; see text).

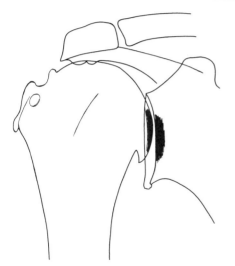

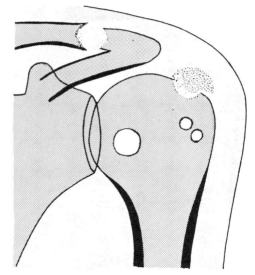

Fig. 255 Advanced osteoarthrosis of the shoulder joint with additional roentgen manifestations of severe damage to the rotator cuff (elevation of the humeral head in the glenoid fossa. Deformation of the greater tubercle. Osteophytosis of the inferior surface of the acromion). (See Fig. 277, no. 11.)

Fig. 257 Chronic gout in the scapulohumeral and the acromioclavicular joint. Erosion in the cranial cartilage: bone interface of the humeral head with increased density of the surrounding soft tissues (soft-tissue tophus). This area of cloudy condensation is recognizable in the roentgenogram only when it contains calcium urate in addition to sodium urate. However, it does *not* present the dense shadow of a calcium deposit in the rotator cuff. Urate deposits in the bone marrow manifest themselves as "cysts" with increased density of the marginal seam in the humeral head. Widening of the acromioclavicular joint space produced by the tophus as a nonspecific mode of reaction in this joint; see Fig. 243.

articulating abutment of the humeral head, since the glenoid fossa is too small in proportion to the circumference of the humeral head. When the soft-tissue abutment is injured, the resting tonus of the deltoid muscle or its voluntary contraction cause the head of the humerus to rise, and the normal adaptation of the

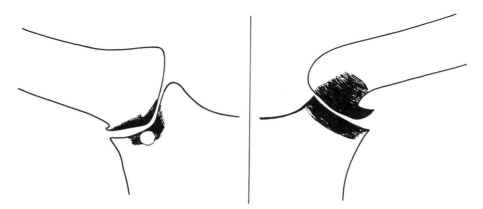

Fig. 256 Osteoarthrosis of the sternoclavicular joint (in tomographs). Less advanced *on the left* than *on the right*. (Joint space narrowing, increased density of subchondral bone, debris cysts, deformation of the sternal end of the clavicle.)

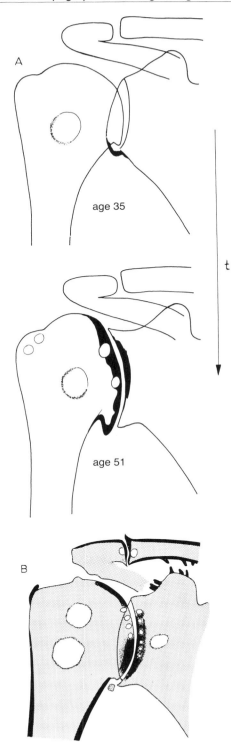

articular surfaces is disrupted. This favors attrition of the cartilage and thus leads to the development of osteoarthrosis in the shoulder joint. Perforation and rupture of the rotator cuff can be verified and localized by arthrography. The air or the water-soluble contrast medium injected into the joint then enters the subacromial bursa (compare Fig. 239).

Compressed-air damage to the joints of the shoulder girdle manifests itself as osteoarthrosis —more frequently in the acromioclavicular than in the scapulohumeral joint—but it does not usually reach the same extent as, for example, in the elbow. In addition, osteolyses occur in the acromial end of the clavicle.

Pathologic studies have revealed that *osteoarthrosis of the sternoclavicular joint* as well as of the *acromioclavicular joint* is a frequent finding. In the sternoclavicular joint, however, the condition is hardly of clinical importance. Figure 256 shows the radiographic features of two sternoclavicular joints with degenerative changes.

Osteoarthropathies

Gout (p. 41 ff) affects the distal joints of the extremities with greater frequency than those near the trunk. Therefore, the manifestation of gout in the joints of the shoulder girdle is not only one of its less frequent localizations, but in this stage of chronic gout the diagnosis usually has already been established. Urate deposits in the acromioclavicular joint cause the radiographic joint space to widen (Fig. 257). It is also true of the shoulder joint that erosive, destructive, or even mutilating lesions in the articulating bones, par-

Fig. 258 Ochronotic osteoarthropathy in the shoulder region.
A = Follow-up study. Initially (age 35), insignificant roentgen manifestations of osteoarthrosis of the shoulder joint (small osteophyte in the lower part of the humeral head, slight lipping in the caudal rim of the glenoid fossa). Equivocal cystic radiolucency with irregular marginal seam in the humeral head. *Sixteen years later:* Advanced osteoarthrosis of the shoulder joint. Considering the patient's age, the condition is unusually severe, and considering the time interval, the progression is very rapid. (The ochronosis, which has been diagnosed in the meantime, accounts for the unfavorable evolution.)
B = Osteoarthrosis of the humeroscapular and the acromioclavicular joint with atypical secondary findings (numerous *fibroosteoses).* The three larger, irregularly rounded translucences with sclerotic margins in the head and neck of the humerus and the neck of the scapula are not debris cysts but ochronotic foci in bones remote from the joints like those described by Bauer and Kienböck (1929). Roentgenologic differentiation from similar translucences in osteoarthropathy of hemophilia is by roentgenograms of the lumbar spine, the disks of which are the test joints for ochronosis (see Fig. 50).

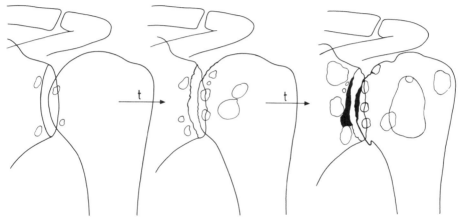

Fig. 259 **Follow-up study of an osteoarthropathy of the left shoulder joint in hemophilia** (from *left* to *right*; 32, 35, and 41 years old). Onset with small, irregularly rounded translucences in the cancellous bone, which increase in number and size, occur also outside the subchondral bone, and do not present the appearance of osteoarthrotic debris cysts. Increasing signs of cartilage destruction and erosion of subchondral bone, minor signs of secondary osteoarthrosis (t = time).

ticularly in the head of the humerus, associated with a *circumscribed increase in thickness of the soft* tissues (which reflects the invasion of these tissues by the tophi), should raise suspicion of gout (Fig. 257).

Ochronotic osteoarthropathy (p. 44 ff) manifests itself in the joints of the shoulder girdle either as typical osteoarthrosis or as osteoarthrosis with atypical secondary findings. Atypical in this connection are the often numerous fibroosteoses and spher-

ical translucences in the cancellous bone. The latter are encountered at some distance from the joints and should not be labeled as osteoarthrotic debris cysts (Fig. 258).

Osteoarthropathy of hemophilia in the region of the shoulder girdle involves primarily the shoulder joint. The processes in the hemophiliac joint described on page 44 ff characterize the radiographic picture. The picture reflects the destruction of the joint,

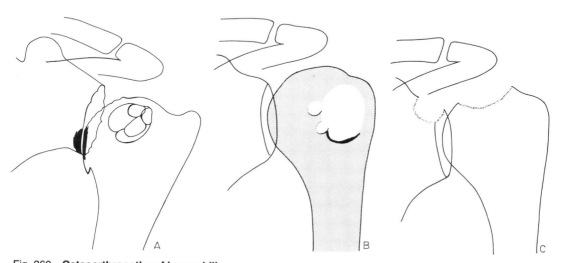

Fig. 260 **Osteoarthropathy of hemophilia.**

A = Roentgen manifestations suggesting onset in the growth period are humerus varus and elongation of the neck of the scapula. Adduction contracture (due to eccentric shrinking of the capsule).

B = Intraosseous hematomas have led to cystoid osteolyses. Also in the hemophiliac, the condition must be differentiated (for example) from tuberculosis of bone and a cystic bone tumor!

C = Erosive changes of contour which can occur in hemophilia as well as in inflammatory or tumorous proliferations of the synovial membrane.

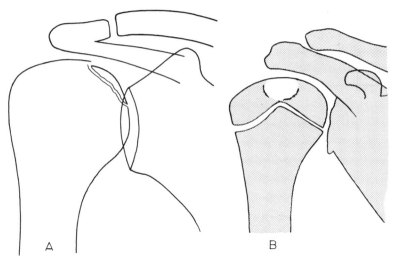

Fig. 261 **Florid damage of the shoulder joint in hereditary hemoglobinopathies with sickled erythrocytes.**

A = Avascular osteonecrosis in the head of the humerus following thrombosis of nutrient arteries. The atraumatic fracture of the top part with depression of the fragment, *without* sclerosis of the cancellous bone or roentgen signs of bone resorption, suggests a *fresh* event.

B = Nonspecific hematogenous bacterial abscess in the proximal epiphysis of the humerus of a child. The *slight* increase in density of the marginal seam indicates a *fresh* breakdown of bone.

cystoid resorption of the cancellous bone—even at some distance from the joint—possibly secondary osteoarthrotic reactions and, when the arthropathy begins in childhood, also disorders of growth (Figs. 259 and 260).

Congenital hereditary hemoglobinopathies with sickled erythrocytes (p. 119 and 121 ff) damage the joints of the shoulder girdle *primarily* in two ways. *First* by thrombosis of nutrient vessels (of the humeral head) and *second* by promoting the hematogenous lodgment of bacteria in the subchondral bone or the synovial membrane (Fig. 261).

Involvement of the shoulder joint in *syringomyelia* is the prototype of the **neurogenic osteoarthropathies** (p. 47 ff) in the region of the shoulder girdle (Figs. 262 and 263). Figure 262 shows a follow-up observation. In differential diagnosis *at the onset of the disease,* an arthritic process, especially tuberculosis or an osteolytic tumor, must be ruled out.

This is true of any manifestation of the osteolytic syndrome. In *the advanced stage,* when the roentgenologic diagnosis is unequivocal, the various other causes of neurogenic osteoarthropathies[17] or of the osteolytic syndrome must be differentiated from syringomyelia. These causes have been listed on page 48 ff.

Osteolyses of the *acromial end of the clavicle*—i.e., its lateral (distal) part—and, less frequently, of the *acromion* have a variety of causes. Their inflammatory (arthritic) genesis has already been mentioned

---

[17] In exceptional cases, the mutilating stage of rheumatoid arthritis also leads to complete resorption of the humeral head and the glenoid fossa. However, the concomitant pain and the roentgen manifestations of arthritis in other joints distinguishes this condition from neurogenic osteoarthropathy. Osteolyses of the proximal humerus (head and neck) occur, rather infrequently, as side reactions to corticosteroid therapy.

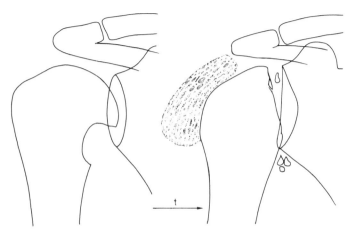

Fig. 262 **Neurogenic osteoarthropathy of the right shoulder joint** (observation over 3 months, hence *rapid* progression; t = time).

Left: In this stage, the roentgen finding (nonreactive contour defect) suggests primarily neoplasm, tuberculosis, or neurogenic osteoarthropathy. *Clinically:* Dissociation of sensation (syringomyelia).

Right: The *roentgenologic diagnosis* of "neurogenic osteopathy" is now certain. The nonreactive osteolysis has involved both the humeral head and the glenoid fossa; solitary fragments of bone lie in the joint cavity; a large amount of bone debris has invaded the subdeltoid bursa, which functions as a "mud trap" (see Figs. 70 and 239).

(see Fig. 243). In addition, the following etiologies are to be listed: lipoid-dermatoarthritis (see Fig. 270), progressive scleroderma (see Fig. 248), osteoarthropathy of amyloidosis, gout, hyperparathyroidism, osteomalacia, posttraumatic osteolysis—very infrequently even in the humeral head with periarticular calcifications or remnants of bone (see Fig. 62)—and progeria.

Posttraumatic osteolysis of the clavicle can also follow a blunt injury to the shoulder. The ensuing loss in length of the clavicle is 2 or 3 cm at most. Osteolysis can be accompanied by periclavicular calcifications, sometimes after a few weeks. In other cases, months or even years may elapse before the osteolysis becomes manifest (Levine et al., 1976). Repeated microtraumas (in compressed-air workers and athletes, see p. 58) as well as gas embolisms in divers (Feindt, 1974) also are liable to cause osteolyses in the clavicle (see Fig. 264).

Osteolysis in the (lateral) clavicle following fracture of a radiation osteonecrosis and *late radiation damage of the shoulder joint* presenting the appearance of erosive arthritis have been reported (Kolář and Vrabec, 1959).

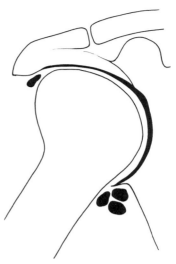

Fig. 263 **Neurogenic osteoarthropathy** (in syringomyelia). The bone has been completely remodeled (phase of stabilization after Fried (p. 48).

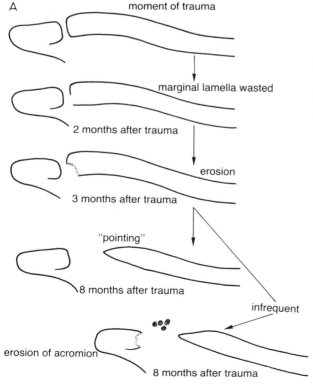

A   moment of trauma

marginal lamella wasted

2 months after trauma

erosion

3 months after trauma

"pointing"

8 months after trauma

infrequent

erosion of acromion

8 months after trauma

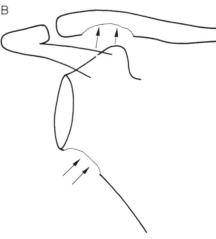

B

Fig. 264 **Development of lateral (distal) posttraumatic osteolysis in the clavicle** (A). Partial or complete reconstruction (reossification) is possible. Flat contour defects *(arrows in B)* in *nonfamilial acroosteolysis with cortical defects* (Gilula et al., 1976; see p. 55).

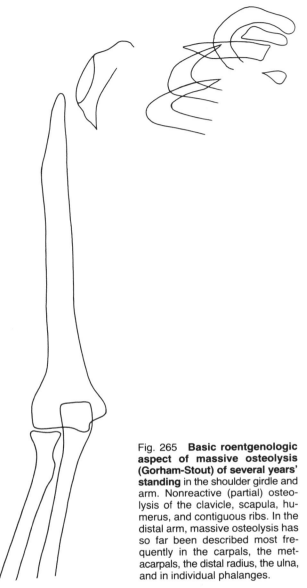

Fig. 265 Basic roentgenologic aspect of massive osteolysis (Gorham-Stout) of several years' standing in the shoulder girdle and arm. Nonreactive (partial) osteolysis of the clavicle, scapula, humerus, and contiguous ribs. In the distal arm, massive osteolysis has so far been described most frequently in the carpals, the metacarpals, the distal radius, the ulna, and in individual phalanges.

In *pyknodysostosis,* the hypoplasia of the acromial end of the clavicle sometimes mimics an osteolysis.

The association of osteolysis in the clavicle with dissolution of contiguous ribs occurs in progeria and, more frequently, in *massive osteolysis (Gorham-Stout),* see p. 59. This disease is a tumorous affection of bone with a predilection for the shoulder girdle and the pelvic ring. It is regarded to be the consequence of an osseous hemangiomatosis or lymphangiomatosis. The disorder is fittingly defined as "massive"

because it is not confined to the original bone and leads, after a time, to disintegration of contiguous, even large, bones (Fig. 265). It also can spread to the soft tissue. It is common for the disease to become spontaneously arrested and to burn out.

Periarticular ossifications are a typical finding in the neurogenic osteoarthropathies, but they also occur without remodeling of the articulating bones **(neurogenic paraosteoarthropathies)** (Figs. 57, 266, and 267).

Osteoarthropathy of amyloidosis (Fig. 65, p. 60) gives the visual impression (shoulder pad sign) and presents the radiographic appearance of articular, periarticular, and osseous deposits of amyloid. The deposition of amyloid can erode the lateral end of the clavicle and thus lead to widening of the acromioclavicular joint space.

Osteoarthropathy of hemochromatosis (p. 89) presents the appearance of osteoarthrosis. However, particularly in the early stages, this can vary from the typical picture of osteoarthrosis (Fig. 268). In addition, articular chondrocalcinosis has also been described in hemochromatosis.

In **osteoarthropathy developing during the course of Wilson's disease** (p. 62) the region of the shoulder girdle will show a *premature* osteoarthrosis, loose bodies, chondrocalcinosis, generalized demineralization of bone (not related to the joints), and the roentgen manifestations of rickets (osteomalacia). Looser's zones are demonstrable in roentgenograms of the shoulder joint, particularly in the scapular neck, and in the spine.

The minimal program of roentgenologic diagnosis in **hyperparathyroidism** (p. 160 ff) presented in Table 2 (p. 127) also includes the acromioclavicular joints. In these joints, hyperparathyroidism frequently gives rise to disappearance of the marginal subchondral lamella, erosions, and, eventually, widening of the joint space (compare Fig. 243). However, widening of the acromioclavicular joint space alone is an equivocal reaction of this joint or the articulating lateral (distal) end of the clavicle (see p. 195). In addition, roentgenograms of the shoulder in patients with hyperparathyroidism occasionally reveal resorption of bone in the acromion, in the proximal humerus, and the ribs, as well as chondrocalcinosis, "brown tumors," and calcification of soft tissues (Fig. 269).

Lipoid-dermatoarthritis (p. 131 ff) can give rise to a variety of articular and extraarticular destructions in the shoulder region (Fig. 270).

In **acromegaly,** (p. 131 ff) the articular cartilage also proliferates; this can lead to "widening of the joint space." In addition, the articular cartilage of acromegalic patients evidently is more prone to attrition than that in individuals with normal levels of somatotrophin. The degeneration of the articular cartilage in the shoulder joint sometimes gives rise to the remodeling of bone that, in the advanced stage, presents neurogenic "features" (Campbell and Feldman, 1975; Fig. 271).

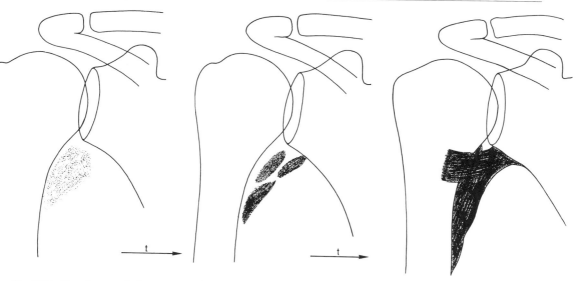

Fig. 266 **Development of a neurogenic paraosteoarthropathy** within 5 months (in the present case following a severe craniocerebral injury). The roentgenogram is consistent with so-called localized myositis ossificans (see p. 68). (t = time; follow-up study).

Note: After improvement of the neurologic symptomatology, ossifications that are not too extensive may (partially) regress.

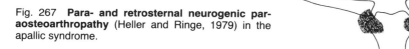

Fig. 267 **Para- and retrosternal neurogenic paraosteoarthropathy** (Heller and Ringe, 1979) in the apallic syndrome.

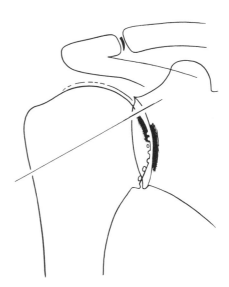

Fig. 268 **Early stage of hematochromatosis-dependent osteoarthropathy of the shoulder joint.**

Roentgen manifestations of a not very marked osteoarthrosis of the shoulder joint with delicate marginal osteophytes, small subchondral cysts, and band-shaped areas of increased density in the subchondral cancellous bone. The cyst walls have collapsed to some extent, so that in these places the contour of the humeral head has a "nibbled" appearance *(lower part of the humeral head)*. Chondrocalcinosis *(upper part of the humeral head and acromioclavicular joint)*.

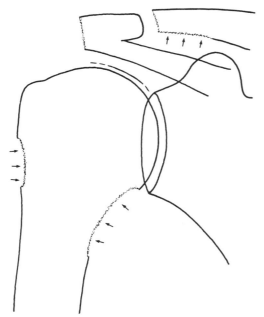

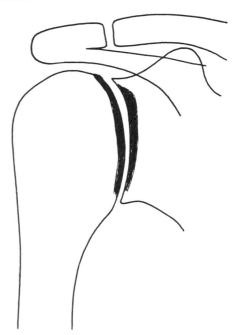

Fig. 269 **Roentgen manifestations of hyperpara-thyroidism in roentgenograms of the shoulder.**
Among the diverse findings (see text), the following have been illustrated: Widening of the acromioclavicular joint space due to resorption of the lateral end of the clavicle; partial osteolysis in the acromion; subperiosteal resorption of bone in the medial and the lateral contour of the proximal metaphysis of the humerus and the inferior border of the clavicle *(arrows);* chondrocalcinosis of the shoulder joint.

Fig. 271 **Advanced osteoarthropathy of the shoulder joint in acromegaly.** The roentgenologic aspect of the osteoarthrotic remodeling *resembles* a neurogenic osteoarthropathy (compare Figs. 262 and 263).

Neoplasms of the Joints of the Shoulder Girdle

Pigmented villonodular synovitis (p. 139 f) can lead to an (lobulated) increase in density of the juxtaarticular soft tissues, though without calcifications. This disease should also be taken into consideration when destructions of bone starting from the capsular insertion are visible on both sides of the joint space. These lesions give the impression of marginal erosions and destructions; in viewing the joint from above, they appear to be "cystic" osteolyses (see Fig. 240). However, neither narrowing of the joint space nor subchondral demineralization is demonstrable. Oc-

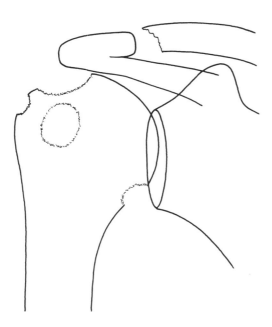

Fig. 270 **Lipoid-dermatoarthritis.** The following *pathologic roentgen findings* are conspicuous: Erosions in the humeral head and the lateral end of the clavicle (widening of the acromioclavicular joint space). Elevation of the humeral head in the glenoid fossa. Erosion in the great tuberosity. Cystic osteolysis in the humeral head. *Roentgenologic diagnosis:* chronic arthritis of the shoulder joint and the acromioclavicular joint, severe lesion of the rotator cuff, erosion at the capsular insertion (rarefying fibroosteitis?). The larger osteolysis in the humeral head remote from the joint could suggest a storage disease, including lipoid-dermatoarthritis.

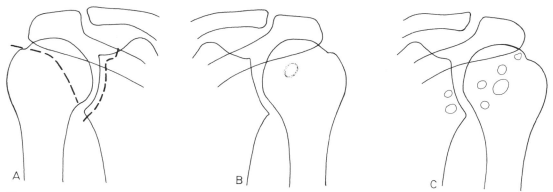

Fig. 272   A = **Course of the capsular insertion in the shoulder joint** *(dashed)*.
   B = **Cystoid osteolysis** starting from the capsular insertion in the proximal humerus. In the present case this osteolysis indicates invasion of the humerus by **pigmented villonodular synovitis.**
   C = **Pigmented villonodular synovitis** with cystoid osteolyses reaching the size of a cherry on both sides of the joint space, which presents a normal width. In addition, marked swelling of the periarticular soft tissues *(not illustrated)*. No juxtaarticular decalcification.

casionally, a solitary, and therefore *equivocal,* cystic osteolysis, which is not demonstrable as a marginal erosion in the roentgenogram, points to invasion of the capsular insertion by pigmented villondular synovitis. It is therefore of diagnostic importance to the radiologist to be familiar with the course of the capsular insertion in the shoulder joint (Fig. 272).

A roentgenogram of **neoplastic synovial chondromatosis** (Fig. 66 f) in the shoulder joints is shown in Figure 253.

The radiologic picture of **malignant synovialoma** is characterized by the triad: increased density of the juxtaarticular soft tissues, calcification of soft tissues, and erosion of bone. This association of signs indicates extraarticular growth and regressive changes in the tumor. However, the pleomorphic, sometimes shelflike, calcifications are demonstrable in only about

one third of malignant synovialomas. If the increased density of the soft tissues appears lobulated, the diagnosis of tumor is more likely. The more extensive the destruction of bone, the less certain becomes the specific diagnosis of malignant synovialoma or any other malignant soft-tissue tumor (for example, rhabdomyosarcoma), but the more justifiable is the suspicion of a malignant growth in general.

Calcifications of the Soft Tissues and Enthesopathies

The possible locations of **chondrocalcinosis** (p. 62) in the region of the shoulder girdle are depicted in Figure 273. Also in the shoulder joint, chondrocalcinosis sometimes gives rise to severe destruction (see

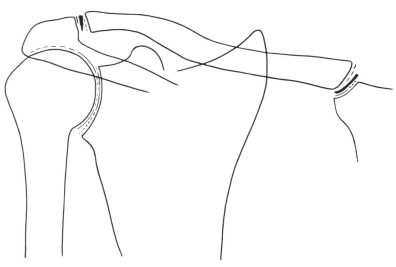

Fig. 273   **Chondrocalcinosis of the joints of the shoulder girdle** (calcification of the articular cartilage and the disks).

p. 64 ff). Its development can be described by the following formula: chondrocalcinosis → osteoarthrosis + avascular necrosis = chondrocalcinosis-induced destructive osteoarthropathy resembling Charcot's joint (Fig. 274). The chiefly descriptive significance of the **calcinosis** concept and the manifold causes of periarticular calcium deposits have been discussed on page 69 ff. In Figure 275, three different forms of calcifications have, for didactic reasons, been illustrated next to each other. The periarticular calcifications in a uremic patient subjected to long-term dialysis (1) are consistent with the picture of pseudotumorous calcinosis. The calcium deposits in dermatomyositis sketched under (2) are instances of localized interstitial calcinosis. They lie in the subcutis and present a netlike appearance. The crumbly calcifications in a scleroderma patient (3) also have to be classified as localized interstitial calcinosis. The radiographic morphology of the **fibroosteoses** in the shoulder region (p. 72 ff) have already been depicted in Figure 258 B. These bony spurs have been sketched as secondary manifestations in the tendon and ligament insertions occurring in osteoarthropathy of ochronosis. Examples of **productive** and **rarefying fibroosteitis** (p. 73) are shown in Figure 276 as typical findings at the origin of the long head of the triceps muscle and at the origin and insertion of the coracoclavicular ligament.

The diagnosis of so-called **periarthritis of the shoulder (Duplay's disease;** p. 73 ff) rests on the clinical findings. The term denotes a painful limitation of motion in the shoulder joint due to an affection of the periarticular tissues—to be specific, pathologic changes in the vault of the shoulder. The vault of the shoulder enlarges and completes the glenoid and adapts it to the size of the humeral head. The coracoacromial ligament, which extends from the coracoid process to the acromion, forms the roof of the glenoid fossa. Underneath it passes the rotator cuff, which is made up of the tendons of the supraspinatus, infraspinatus, and teres minor muscles. In addition, these rotators and the subscapularis muscle fix the head of the humerus against the glenoid fossa so that other muscles, e.g., the deltoid muscle, can fulfil their function.

Underneath the rotator cuff lies the capsule of the shoulder joint. It is additionally strengthened in this region by the coracohumeral ligament. The tendons of the subscapularis muscle and the long head of the biceps complete the vault of the shoulder anterolaterally. The long tendon of the biceps passes initially inside the shoulder joint and then through the intertubercular sulcus. It prevents the humeral head from dislocating anteriorly and superiorly. During motion of the shoulder joint, the gliding of the tendon between the structures mentioned above is furthered by various bursae, primarily the subacromial bursa and the subdeltoid bursa, which often communicates with it. Lesions from excessive strain, which in a joint would lead to osteoarthrosis, cause the gliding structures in the shoulder region to suffer degenerative changes. Initially, osteoarthrosis is only a potential disease; it does not acquire the subjective characteristics of a real disease until some irritative factor becomes operative (activated osteoarthrosis). This irritative condition is caused by an inflammatory reaction of the synovial membrane. Therefore, one may infer that degenerative changes of the rotator cuff, particularly the supraspinatus tendon, likewise assume the features of a disease as the result of reactive inflammatory processes in the bursal synovium. For example, this may occur when calcium deposits in the tendon invade the subacromial or the subdeltoid bursa and give rise there to a bursal synovitis (Fig. 70). An additional cause of discomfort in periarthritis of the shoulder is perforation or rupture of the supraspinatus tendon, leading to instability of the vault of the shoulder. Moreover, the developing cicatricious tissue leads to thickening of the tendon; it impairs the glide process in the subacromial space and increases friction. This also may be the cause of complaints. Calcium deposits in the rotator cuff do not give rise *there* to major acute inflammation. When, on the other hand, the calcium deposits lie in the junction between muscular and tendinous tissues, acute inflammatory changes are encountered in the musculature (Pedersen and Key, 1951). These processes also can be the cause of pain. The clinical picture of the "frozen shoulder" (fibrotic stiffness of the shoulder) is due to shrinking of the joint capsule, which can be demonstrated by arthrography. This shrinking is evidently the result of inflammatory changes in the

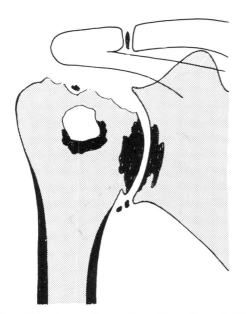

Fig. 274 **Destructive osteoarthropathy of the shoulder joint in (sporadic) chondrocalcinosis** (see text). In this sketch, the chondrocalcinosis can be recognized only by the calcified disk in the acromioclavicular joint.

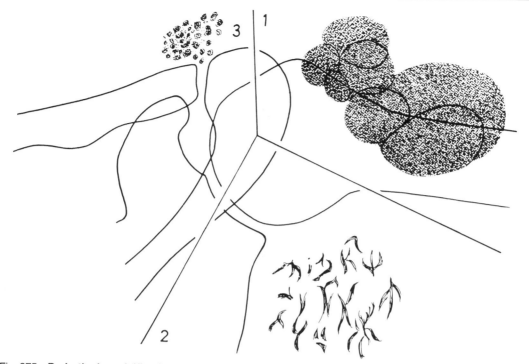

Fig. 275   **Periarticular calcifications in the shoulder** (anteroposterior roentgenogram of left shoulder joint with the humerus externally rotated and in 90° of abduction. Elbow flexed to a right angle).

1 = Larger homogeneous calcium deposits (pasty in consistency on biopsy) in a uremic patient subjected to long-term dialysis. Type of pseudotumorous calcinosis. 2 = Localized interstitial type of calcinosis located subcutaneously, netlike projection (observed in dermatomyositis). 3 = Crumbly and spotted type of localized interstitial calcinosis (observed in a case of progressive scleroderma).

Note: The projection sketched *(radiographic focusing technique)* is particularly suitable for assessing the acromioclavicular joint.

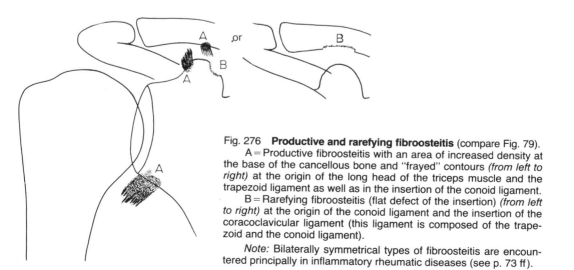

Fig. 276   **Productive and rarefying fibroosteitis** (compare Fig. 79).

A = Productive fibroosteitis with an area of increased density at the base of the cancellous bone and "frayed" contours *(from left to right)* at the origin of the long head of the triceps muscle and the trapezoid ligament as well as in the insertion of the conoid ligament.

B = Rarefying fibroosteitis (flat defect of the insertion) *(from left to right)* at the origin of the conoid ligament and the insertion of the coracoclavicular ligament (this ligament is composed of the trapezoid and the conoid ligament).

Note: Bilaterally symmetrical types of fibroosteitis are encountered principally in inflammatory rheumatic diseases (see p. 73 ff).

Fig. 277 Synopsis of possible roentgen findings in so-called periarthritis of the shoulder. When this disorder is suspected clinically (Fig. 278), as many as four roentgenograms of the shoulder joint are necessary: An anteroposterior film with the arm extended and externally rotated and the shoulder pulled actively in direction of the fingers (A); an anteroposterior film with strong internal rotation (B); an axial view (C) to demonstrate the soft tissues surrounding the lesser tuberosity; and (D) a tangential view of the intertubercular sulcus in which the long tendon of the biceps muscle, enclosed by the intertubercular tendon sheath, glides freely. When motion of the shoulder is impaired by severe pain, only roentgenogram A is taken, and two spot examinations with the fluoroscope are made (with variable rotation of the humerus).

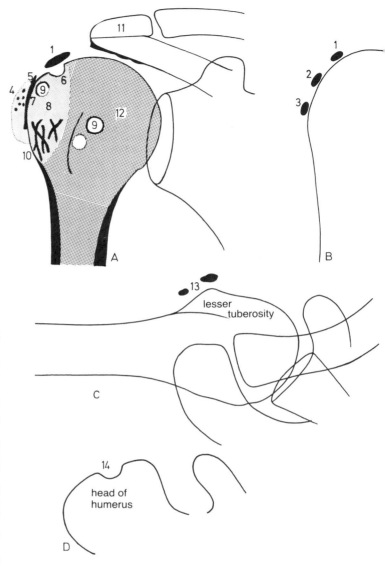

1 = Calcium deposit in the supraspinatus tendon. It differs, as a rule, by its oval (biconvex) or rounded shape from calcification of the subacromial bursa, which usually has a half-moon appearance.

2 = Calcification in the infraspinatus tendon (mostly visible only in a roentgenogram with internal rotation of the humeral head.)

3 = Calcification in the tendon of the teres minor muscle (with internal rotation of the humeral head).

4 = Invasion of the subdeltoid bursa by calcification in the tendon ("cast" or crumbly or lumpy appearance).

5 = Fibroosteosis in the greater tuberosity.

6 = Resorptive hollow in the greater tuberosity.

7 = Band-shaped or linear sclerotic area in the tendinous insertion on the greater tuberosity.

8 = Apophyseal osteoporosis (Otte, 1964). Differentiation from the physiologic, though variable, translucence in the tuberosity sketched in Fig. 233 by comparison with the sound side!

9 = Cystic translucences in the tuberosity with or without marginal seam.

10 = Irregularly arranged, thickened cancellous trabeculae in the region of the greater tuberosity *(schematic, magnified).*

11 = Osteophytes on the inferior surface of the acromion.

12 = Elevation of the humeral head in the glenoid fossa (compare with the opposite side!). *Etiology:* Rupture of the supraspinatus tendon (see Fig. 239 A) *or* reflex hypertonicity of the synergistic deltoid muscle to relieve the degenerated supraspinatus tendon from weight. (Differential diagnosis by arthrography of the shoulder joint.) **Rupture of the supraspinatus tendon can be recognized indirectly by the following radiologic examination:** Anteroposterior roentgenogram of the shoulder joint with the patient standing and his arm hanging down; anteroposterior roentgenogram with the arm in 45° of active abduction. A lesion of the supraspinatus tendon is present when the second roentgenogram shows an unequivocally greater elevation of the humeral head in the glenoid fossa than the first.

13 = Calcification in the subscapularis tendon or in the tendon of the long head of the biceps (see also no. 14).

14 = Normal appearance of the intertubercular sulcus (calcium shadows? osteophytes?).

outer segments of the capsule and the contiguous adipose tissue (Schallock, 1971). In periarthritis of the shoulder, both structures share in the inflammatory reaction. For the pathogenesis and etiology of the affection of the rotator cuff and its surroundings, compare p. 74.

The radiologist should draw the following conclusions from the processes described:

1. Calcifications of tendons and bursae in the region of the shoulder must first of all be localized (e.g., in the supraspinatus tendon, in the subdeltoid bursa, etc.).

2. Since the nomenclature of these findings is inconsistent (p. 73) and often problematic—this is particularly applicable to the suffixes *-itis* and *-osis* (periarthritis, periarthrosis, tendinitis, tendinosis, etc.)— these terms should only be used with the attribute "so-called" or should be replaced by "periarthropathy" (p. 73). These terms will then not mislead the

examiner into regarding the calcification in a tendon *generally* as a periarthritis—hence an inflammation—and treating it accordingly.

3. Although the calcium deposits are conspicuous, they often are not the only changes recognizable in the roentgenogram, which indicate an affection of the vault of the shoulder. This is the reason why all the possible roentgen findings in the disorder described here have been combined synoptically in Figure 277.

4. In the presence of the pertinent symptomatology, a negative roentgen finding does not rule out acute periarthritis of the shoulder.

Injuries to the Joints

The **upper arm type of obstetric brachial plexus paralysis (Erb's paralysis)** and of course also the infrequent **total paralysis of the arm** produce, among other manifestations, deficient fixation of the humeral head in the glenoid fossa. This leads to subluxation of the humeral head *downward and, to a lesser extent, laterally.* In the newborn, the ossification centers in the proximal end of the humerus have not yet developed. The faulty position of the joint on the paralyzed side can therefore be identified only by the increased distance between the proximal end of the humeral diaphysis and the glenoid fossa (Fig. 279).

The consequences of a permanent obstetric paralysis are delayed development of the ossification centers, disuse hypolasia of the humerus and the scapula and, less frequently, even deformation of the articulating bones. These findings, including faulty position of the joint, are also encountered in poliomyelitic paresis of the muscles of the upper arm and shoulder occurring in early childhood. In the differential diagnosis of the upper-arm type of brachial plexus paralysis that has become manifest *immediately after delivery,* the following findings must be taken into consideration:

1. **Dislocation of the shoulder joint in congenital malformations.** In the majority of cases, the head of the humerus dislocates posteriorly so that the malposition cannot be identified in the anteroposterior roentgenogram. In addition, only severe malformations of the scapular neck can be radiologically diagnosed in the newborn.

2. **Obstetric separation of the upper humeral epiphysis** also impairs active motion of the shoulder. In the newborn, an epiphysiolysis cannot be demonstrated directly on the roentgenogram because—as has already been mentioned—the ossification center in the epiphysis has not yet developed. However, on comparing both sides, a major secondary hematoma in the joint can be recognized by the conspicuous lateralization of the proximal humeral diaphysis (Fig. 235; compare the difficulty of roentgenologic diagnosis with Fig. 279). A fracture of the epiphysis can usually be diagnosed by radiographic examination. When the fracture cleft is not recognized in the initial roentgenogram, a follow-up study after about 10 or 15 days

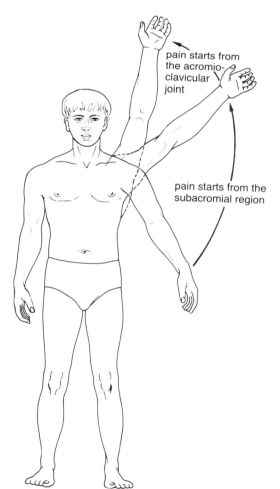

pain starts from the acromio-clavicular joint

pain starts from the subacromial region

Fig. 278 **Diagnosing the localization of pain in the shoulder region prior to radiologic examination— so-called painful arc.**

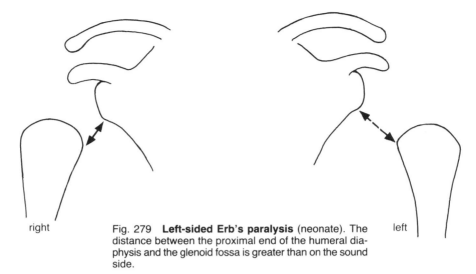

right   Fig. 279 **Left-sided Erb's paralysis** (neonate). The   left
distance between the proximal end of the humeral diaphysis and the glenoid fossa is greater than on the sound
side.

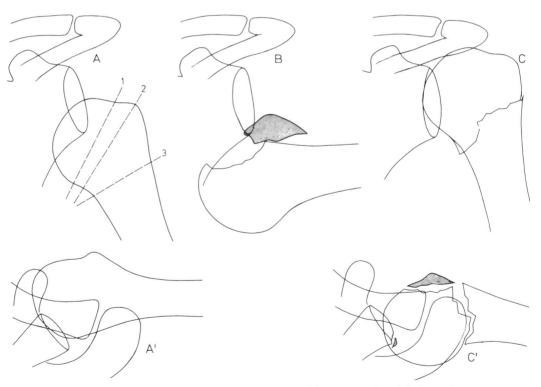

Fig. 280 **Traumatic dislocations of the shoulder with and without secondary injuries to bone.**
    A, A' = Preglenoidal subcoracoid dislocation of the humerus. Course of the fracture lines with additional
fracture of the anatomic neck (1), with pertubercular fracture (2), and with fracture of the surgical neck of the
humerus (3). B = Horizontal axillary dislocation of the humerus with avulsion of the greater tuberosity. C,
C' = Retroglenoidal subacromial dislocation of the humerus with secondary injuries (fracture of the surgical neck
of the humerus, avulsion of the lesser tuberosity, posterior rim of the glenoid sheared off). Only an axial roentgenogram reveals the full extent of the injuries.

is very likely to reveal the calcifying subperiosteal hematoma and/or the periosteal callus. A clavicle fractured by birth trauma can also mimic clinical aspects of Erb's paralysis. In addition, it should be mentioned that occasionally an ipsilateral paresis of the diaphragm (from radicular damage at the level of C_4) accompanies Erb's paralysis (radicular damage at the levels of C_5 and C_6). This paresis will then aid in making the differential diagnosis.

3. **Parrot's pseudoparalysis in congential syphilitic separation of the epiphysis** cannot usually be identified immediately post partum but develops after the first or second week, or even later. The condition is coupled with the characteristic, though not specific, roentgen manifestations of syphilitic osteochondritis (metaphyseal band-shaped translucences and even destructions). Congenital syphilis manifests itself at many sites, often symmetrically.

Altogether, *immediately after delivery* it is difficult to form an accurate view, clinically and roentgenologically, of the causes of impaired active mobility of the shoulder, particularly since paralysis and injuries to the bone can occur concomitantly.

In the majority of cases of **traumatic dislocation of the shoulder,** (Fig. 280) the head of the humerus leaves the glenoid fossa anteriorly. Since in all dislocations of the shoulder the humeral head approaches the midline of the trunk, it usually glides under the coracoid process *(preglenoidal subcoracoid dislocation of the humerus)* or, with major disruption of the capsule, it glides still further medialward *(preglenoidal subclavicular dislocation of the humerus)*. When the humerus dislocates posteriorly, it is encountered either under the acromion *(retroglenoidal subacromial dislocation of the humerus)* or under the scapular spine *(retroglenoidal infraspinous dislocation of the humerus)*. In the first-named case, the humeral head is, therefore, slightly dislocated in the anterosuperior direction, whereas in the latter case it is dislocated posteroinferiorly. The axial view is particularly suitable for identifying a dorsal dislocation. In the anteroposterior roentgenogram of the shoulder, the following findings can raise suspicion of the presence of a retroglenoidal (posterior) dislocation of the humeral head:

1. The posteriorly dislocated head of the humerus is fixed springily in *internal* rotation. If the patient is capable of positioning his humerus in external rotation for an anteroposterior roentgenogram, a retroglenoidal dislocation can be ruled out.
2. In a retroglenoidal dislocation of the humerus, the roentgenologic shoulder joint space—the space between the medial contour of the humeral head and the *anterior* rim of the glenoid fossa (Fig. 281)—is

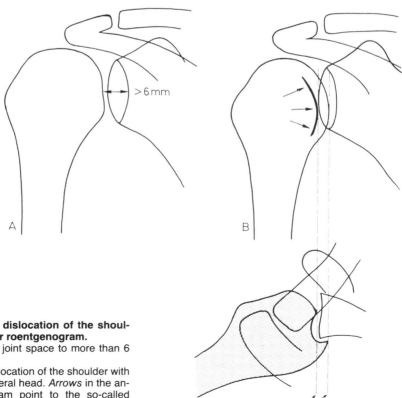

Fig. 281 **Retroglenoidal dislocation of the shoulder in the anteroposterior roentgenogram.**
   A = "Widening" of the joint space to more than 6 mm (see text).
   B = Retroglenoidal dislocation of the shoulder with depressed fracture of humeral head. *Arrows* in the anteroposterior roentgenogram point to the so-called *trough line* (see text).

"widened" to more than 6 mm (focal distance 1 m). This is true of patients with complete closure of the proximal humeral epiphysis, hence from the 18th year of life upward (Arndt and Sears, 1965). The condition has to be differentiated from a major intraarticular hematoma, from distraction-dislocation of the shoulder *(vide infra)*, and from flaccid paresis of the muscles of the shoulder girdle because these can also "widen" the shoulder joint space!

3. The *trough line* (Cisternino et al., 1978) indicates a posterior dislocation of the shoulder with concomitant depression of the humeral head through the dorsal rim of the glenoid fossa (Fig. 281).

Depending on the course of the longitudinal humeral axis of the springily fixed arm, axillary dislocation of the shoulder allows differentiating, in addition, between *erect axillary dislocation* and *horizontal axillary dislocation* of the humerus.

Finally, two more types are known: *central dislocation of the humerus,* in which at least the glenoid fossa has been shattered, and *supracoracoid dislocation of the humerus.* Shattering of the bony roof of the shoulder is a prerequisite for the latter injury. *Distraction-dislocation of the shoulder* is the result of sudden, excessive pull on the shoulder joint, which also leads to rupture of the rotator tendons. The roentgenogram shows an increased distance between the humeral head and the glenoid (compare with the contralateral side and *vide supra* under item 2).

In dislocations of the shoulder, the clinician dreads injuries to the vessels and nerves, whereas the radiologist is afraid of overlooking the presence of a dislocation or subluxation. Therefore, every injury to the shoulder requires that roentgenograms be taken in *at least* two planes, first an *anteroposterior roentgenogram* and second an *axial roentgenogram in dorsal decubitus,* or even better the transscapular so-called Y-radiograph (Rubin et al., 1974). However, roentgenograms in two planes, supplemented by *fluoroscopic spot examinations* if necessary, are needed not only to accurately assess the faulty position but also to recognize manifold secondary injuries to bones (fracture-dislocations). The head of the humerus and the glenoid fossa, the two tuberosities and the surgical neck, as well as the acromion and the coracoid process, must be most accurately examined for changes of contours and structures and the neighboring soft tissues for fragments of bone. To identify such avulsed fragments, *check radiographs following reduction* are sometimes more important then the initial films because the arm is then no longer in a posture of painful, springy fixation but can be cautiously brought into a position adequate for taking the roentgenogram!

Among the *secondary injuries to bone in dislocation of the shoulder* are fractures of the tuberosities, the head of the humerus and the anatomic neck, as well as pretubercular fractures and, (marginal) fractures of the glenoid fossa (Fig. 280). Also observed with some frequency without concomitant dislocation are fractures of the anatomic and the surgical neck of the scapula, fractures of the acromion, avulsions of the coracoid process, but primarily abduction fractures, adduction fractures, and impacted fractures of the surgical neck of the humerus. The same can be said of separations of the epiphyses and apophyses in the vicinity of the shoulder joint. Such losses in continuity—and also epiphyseal fractures in which the dividing line runs partly in the calcified cartilage and partly in the metaphysis—usually occur in children and juveniles after injuries that cause dislocation in the adult.

The finding of **lipohemarthrosis** in the roentgenogram (Fig. 282) indicates that fatty bone marrow has entered the joint cavity. The causes of a fat-blood level in the shoulder joint are usually fracture-dislocations, fractures, and sometimes also fissures that are not recognizable in the roentgenogram. When the injury has led to rupture of the rotator cuff or when rupture or perforation of this tendinous cuff has preexisted, the fat-blood level can be identified in both the joint cavity and the subacromial bursa.

Among the *posttraumatic sequelae in the soft tissues and the* articulating bones of the shoulder joint, the following findings are of interest to the radiologist: calcifications and ossifications in the soft tissues—for example, in a hematoma, in the injured capsular tissue, or in ligaments, tendons, and muscles. A separated periosteum is also capable of forming new bone. This occurs preferentially in the neck of the scapula and the humerus. Avulsed fragments of bone and persistent ossification centers (Fig. 233) must be differentiated from these findings. Other well-known pictures are traumatic rupture of the tendinous rotator cuff, especially the supraspinatus tendon (Fig. 277, no. 12), and posttraumatic periarthritis of the shoulder, diagnosed clinically and roentgenologically (Figs. 277 and 278). The inflammatory periarticular irritation probably develops as an immediate reaction to the formation of a hematoma and/or edema; hence it may even follow simple contusions and sprains. This consequence of trauma should be kept in mind when the complaints outlast the accident by 10 to 14 days with undiminished intensity even though an injury to bone has been ruled out (Bloch and Fischer, 1958). Partial or total necrosis of the humeral head (Fig. 252) and osteoarthritis of the shoulder (Fig. 249) are also possible posttraumatic events. A neoarthrosis developing after an undiagnosed or unreduced dislocation should be relegated to history.

Recurrent dislocation of the shoulder is usually the result of a traumatic dislocation in which injuries of the bones and soft tissues have paved the way for a habitual—i.e., constantly recurrent—dislocation. The development of this condition is favored primarily by a refractory rupture or wrenching away of the labrum in the anteroinferior rim of the glenoid fossa and by bony avulsion of the rotator tendons. In addition, malformations or developmental

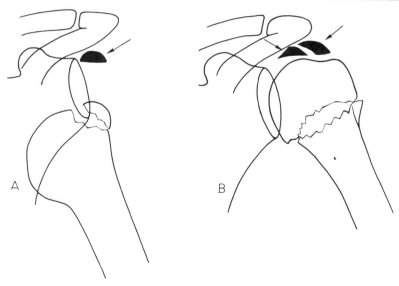

Fig. 282 **Lipohemarthrosis of the shoulder joint,** recognizable in the anteroposterior roentgenogram with the patient *sitting*. The fat from the bone marrow that has penetrated the joint cavity floats on the sanguineous effusion and attenuates the roentgen rays less than the blood (see Table 1). Thus it manifests itself in the roentgen film as an area of increased blackening *(arrows)*.

A = Preglenoidal dislocation of the shoulder with secondary injury to bone. This leads to lipohemarthrosis, unless the capsular tear allows the joint effusion to escape.

B = Fracture of the surgical neck of the humerus. A roentgenologically invisible fracture line must have extended as far as the intraarticular surface of the humerus. Fat-blood level in both the joint cavity and the subacromial bursa (see text). The cuff of the rotator tendons passes between the two.

disorders of the glenoid fossa can facilitate the initial dislocation and its recurrence. The "typical defect of the humeral head," i.e. the Hill-Sachs Lesion, in dislocation of the shoulder is a depressed fracture (indentation) of the posterolateral part of the articular surface of the humeral head (Fig. 283), dorsal and medial to the greater tuberosity. Avulsion of the tuberosity is a rare event. The "defect" develops by the anteriorly dislocated part of the humeral head being pressed against the inferior rim of the glenoid fossa. This defect, depending on its depth and dimension, contributes to the development of recurrent dislocation of the shoulder and probably is one of the reasons why the humerus commonly dislocates anteriorly (subcoracoid dislocation). The typical defect of the humeral head can be demonstrated best in spot

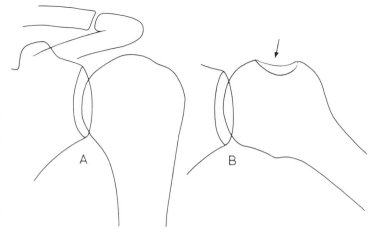

Fig. 283 **Reduced preglenoidal dislocation of the shoulder.**

A = Physiologic contours of the humeral head in the anteroposterior roentgenogram.

B = **Typical defect of the humeral head** *(arrow; see text),* recognizable only on a spot radiograph with internal rotation, slight abduction, and retroflexion.

radiographs of the internally rotated, slightly abducted, and retroflexed upper arm. In a retroglenoidal dislocation of the shoulder, the defect will be encountered closer to the anterior aspect of the humerus (see Fig. 281).

In **dislocation of the acromioclavicular joint** (Fig. 284), the clavicle is displaced mostly superiorly *(supraacromial acromioclavicular dislocation or subluxation)*. When the lateral (distal) end of the clavicle surmounts the acromion by a distance equal to or even greater than the total breadth of its shaft, *all* ligamental connections of the acromioclavicular joint are ruptured (Fig. 285). When the clavicle is demonstrable underneath the acromion, a *subacromial* or *subcoracoid dislocation* at the coracoacromioclavicular joint is present. When the longitudinal axis of the clavicle passes dorsally to the acromion, the injury is termed *supraspinous acromioclavicular dislocation*. A recurrent type of acromioclavicular dislocation is also known.

Secondary injuries accompanying these dislocations cannot be identified in the plain roentgenogram because they involve nerves and vessels.

Osteoarthrosis (Figs. 249 and 250), posttraumatic osteolysis of the clavicle (Fig. 264), and reparative calcification of the capsule and ligaments (Fig. 286) are *delayed sequelas. Roentgenograms in a strained posture* give information about the maximal possible dislocation as an indicator of the extent of a capsuloligamentous rupture. It is advisable to make such roentgenograms at the outset, when acromioclavicular dislocation is suspected upon physical examination. To this end, the patient lowers his shoulders as far as possible anteriorly with internal rotation of the upper arms and extension of the cervical spine. The stability of a reduced and healed acromioclavicular dislocation is also tested by *weight-bearing radiographs:* The downward extended arms of the standing patient are each loaded with a weight (e.g., a sandbag) of 3 to 4 kg. In this way, strong traction is applied to the acromioclavicular joints. When the joint is unstable—including undiagnosed dislocations undergoing spontaneous reduction and ruptures of the capsule and ligaments without dislocation—the load causes the joint space to gape, and the lateral end of the clavicle lies higher than the acromion (for com-

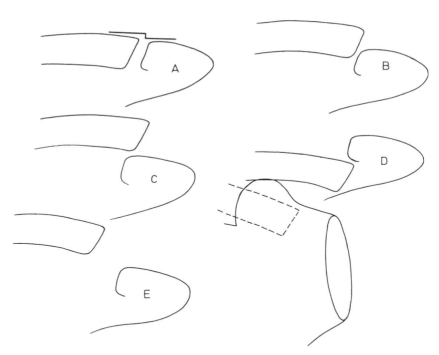

Fig. 284 Examples of dislocations of the acromioclavicular joint (see p. 4 ff, roentgenogram under weight-bearing).

A = Normal finding; the lateral end of the clavicle slightly surmounts the acromion.

B = Incomplete supraacromial acromioclavicular dislocation.

C = Supraacromial acromioclavicular dislocation. The articulating bones are somewhat displaced relative to each other.

D = Subacromial and subcoracoid *(dashed)* acromioclavicular dislocation.

E = C, except for diastasis of the articulating bones.

Note: Palpation sometimes gives more useful information than an axial view about anterior and posterior dislocations of the clavicle (for example, supraspinous acromioclavicular dislocation), because in these injuries the typical focusing technique for an axial roentgenogram of the shoulder joint is impracticable.

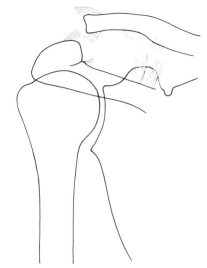

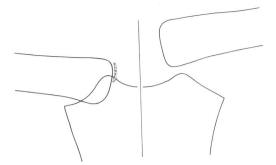

Fig. 287 **Sternoclavicular dislocation;** *right* suprasternal; *left:* pre- or retrosternal. The simplest way of differentiating these two types of dislocation is by palpation. **Secondary finding:** Persistent ossification center (often bilateral), no avulsion.

Fig. 285 **Supraacromial acromioclavicular dislocation.** A prerequisite for displacement of the clavicle by at least the breadth of its shaft is complete disruption of the acromioclavicular ligament and both parts of the coracoclavicular ligament (illustrated in the sketch).

parison with the uninjured side, picture both joints in a single film).

The terminology of the **sternoclavicular dislocations** (Fig. 287) also depends on the direction in which the clavicle has dislocated, hence *pre-, retro-* and *suprasternal dislocation.* In addition, all three directions of dislocation are usually accompanied by

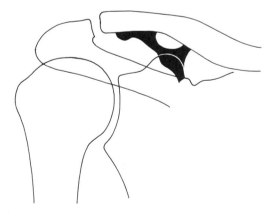

Fig. 286 **Posttraumatic ossification of the coracoclavicular ligament** following (reduced) supraacromial dislocation at the acromioclavicular joint 4 months previously.

medial displacement of the clavicle. Whether a dislocation identified in a survey film is presternal or retrosternal can be determined by computed tomographs or, more simply, by palpation. Compared with the uninjured side, one palpates a bony prominence in presternal dislocation and a depression at the sternal end of the clavicle in retrosternal dislocation.

Secondary injuries accompanying *retrosternal* dislocation manifest themselves in the trachea, the esophagus, the lungs, the pleura, the great vessels of the mediastinum, the phrenic nerve (singultus) and the vagus nerve (e.g., hoarseness, dysphagia). *Suprasternal* dislocation can damage the larynx (dyspnea). Osteoarthrosis (Fig. 256) can occur as a late sequel of sternoclavicular dislocation. Recurrence of this dislocation is, among other factors, also favored by severe disruptions of the capsule and the ligaments.

Ipsilateral subluxation of the clavicle at the sternoclavicular joint is sometimes observed following radical neck dissection. The most frequent event is displacement of the medial end of the clavicle superiorly and anteriorly, less often posteriorly. In addition, the clavicle rotates to a greater or lesser extent around its longitudinal axis (Gorman et al., 1971).

Subluxation of the sternoclavicular joints as the result of excessive strain is known to occur in *weight lifters:* on transmitting the weight above the clavicles, the sternoclavicular joints are subjected to considerable strain. The developing force pushes the clavicles medially and anteriorly so that a presternal subluxation can occur with time. If this sport is started in childhood, local growth disorders (flattening and broadening of the sternal articular surface) can ensue (Korkusuz et al., 1972).

Hip Joint

In judging the anteroposterior projection of the hip joint we make use of a survey film of the pelvis (in doing this, the feet are internally rotated about 20° to compensate for the anteversion of the femoral neck). If the patient is adjusted and positioned accurately, such a film not only outlines both hip joints under the same roentgenographic conditions but it also furnishes additional diagnostic information. For example, pathologic changes of the sacroiliac joints, the symphysis pubis, and the origins of the tendons in the ischium can, in certain inflammatory rheumatic conditions, facilitate the nosological classification of pathologic findings in the hip joints.

To appraise the proportions of the pelvis and its joints and synchondroses properly, one should bear in mind that a survey film of the pelvis magnifies the diameters of the femoral heads by approximately 1 cm and that the actual distance between the femoral heads is about 5 cm less than in the survey film of the pelvis (Fassbender et al., 1969). An anteroposterior roentgenogram of one hip joint only is reserved for postoperative, post-traumatic and similar *check radiographs*. The focusing technique for roentgenograms in the second plane depends on the clinical problem or on the disorder that is either diagnosed or suspected in studying the survey film of the pelvis (pages 3, 247 ff, and 271 ff).

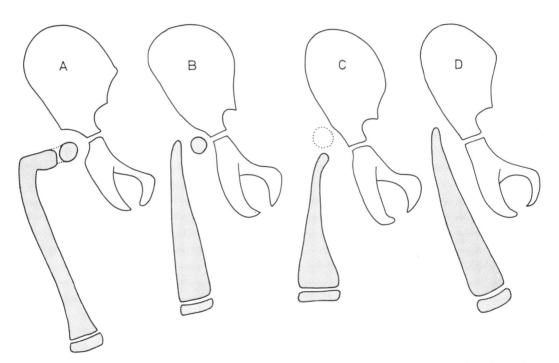

Fig. 288 **Basic radiomorphologic pattern of the different degrees of congenital defect of the femur** (Levinson et al., 1977).

A = Femur shortened; continuity of femur preserved after completion of growth *(dotted);* femoral head concentrically seated within the acetabulum; neck-shaft angle in varus position.

B = Femur shortened; continuity of femur has failed to develop, even after completion of growth; shape of acetabulum adequate for the femoral head to be concentrically seated.

C = Femur shortened; if the *dislocated* rudiment of the femoral head is at all recognizable after the completion of growth *(dotted),* the continuity of the femur fails to develop; malformed, flat acetabulum.

D = Femur shortened; even after completion of growth, acetabulum is absent and femoral head is not visible in the roentgenogram.

Concerning C and D the following rule holds true: The stronger the malformation of the acetabulum, the rounder the obturator foramen.

Note: Classification of congenital defects of the femur in early childhood does not necessarily correlate with that obtaining after the completion of growth! In infants or small children, arthrography of the hip joint usually reveals delayed ossification of the center in the femoral head when a congenital defect of the femur is present. This technique may therefore assist in the classification because its result answers the question of whether a cartilaginous center of ossification exists in the femoral head.

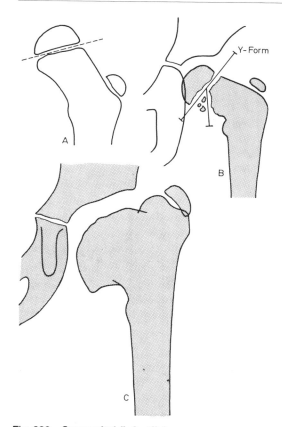

Fig. 289   **Congenital (infantile) coxa vara.**
A = Normal finding in a 5-year-old child (proximal epiphyseal line coursing approximately horizontally; *dashed line*).
B = Congenital coxa vara in 5-year-old child. Neck-shaft angle less than 120°. Steeply coursing epiphyseal line with irregular contours and y-shaped projection; metaphysis fragmented; femoral neck shortened and coarsened; greater trochanter hypoplastic and elevated.
C = Congenital coxa vara in 8-year old child. Typical shepherd's staff deformity (see Fig. 336) already suggested. Premature bony closure of the epiphyseal line in the proximal femur. Adaptation of acetabulum to shape of femoral head.

Malformations

The so-called **congenital defect of the femur** is a unilateral or, less frequently, bilateral malformation of the *proximal* segment of the femur. *Aplasia of the femur* is therefore not included in the group of developmental anomalies of the skeleton, but belongs, rather, among the *phocomelia* group, in which the extremity involved is shortened through the absence of long tubular bones and the distal segments of the limb are closely approximated to the trunk. Conversely, in *peromelia,* the peripheral end of the limb

is absent, whereas the proximal stump is preserved. *Hypermelia* occurs in the femur and the humerus, usually in the form of an incomplete double malformation. In this instance, the socket may also present a rudimentary duplication.

The *indispensable hallmark* of the different manifestations of a congenitally defective femur, the complete extent of which is often recognizable only after the completion of growth, consists in the shortened and "stunted" proximal segment of the femur. The acetabulum may embrace the head of the femur; in other instances it may be very flat or not at all laid down as a socket. The proximal end of the femur is connected to the shaft by bone or by cartilage; the continuity of the femur is then preserved from the beginning or becomes established with increasing maturation of the skeleton. At times, however, the fusion of the femoral shaft with the proximal end of the femur fails to take place, or the proximal end is entirely absent in the roentgenogram, which reveals only the "stunted" proximal portion of the femoral shaft. This outline will make it clear that the congenital defect of the femur may be present in different degrees of severity (Fig. 288).

The radiologic similarity between **congenital (infantile) coxa vara** and type A of a congenitally defective femur (see Fig. 288) is evident. The former therefore is spoken of in the literature as the slightest degree of a congenitally defective femur. In addition, the *primary* type of congenital coxa vara can be classified as dysostosis—i.e., a malformation of a solitary skeletal segment (Lindemann, 1949)—even if such a malformation, as frequently happens, is associated with ipsilateral aplasia of the fibula. Conversely, the *secondary* type of congenital coxa vara occurs in connection with systemic malformations of the skeleton; i.e., one of the osteochondrodysplasias (Walker, 1973). "Congenital" (infantile) coxa vara following osteomyelitis of the femur in early infancy or fracture of the femoral neck is discussed on page 242 and 243.

Indispensable and potential radiographic signs of congenital coxa vara in the anteroposterior roentgenogram (Fig. 289) are:

1. Reduced neck/shaft angle
2. Approximately vertical course of the epiphyseal line of the femur
3. Y-shaped projection of the proximal epiphyseal line of the femur, caused by the fragmented metaphysis
4. Shortened and coarsened femoral neck
5. Elevation of the greater trochanter
6. Delayed ossification of the center in the femoral head; the center may be deformed.
7. Premature closure of the proximal epiphysis of the femur
8. Possible dysplasia of the acetabulum
9. Possible slipping of the femoral head
10. Possible aseptic necrosis of the femoral head (Johanning, 1951/52)

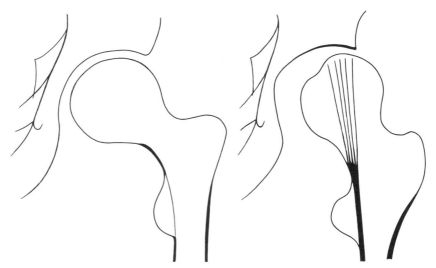

Fig. 290 Paralytic hip (left) in malformation of the lumbosacral cord and **paretic hip** undergoing subluxation *(right)* following poliomyelitis in the years of growth. Because of the partially preserved mobility of the left leg, the paretic hip shows trajectories and less marked thinning of the compacta than the paralytic hip, which leaves the patient incapable of walking. The preponderance of the iliopsoas muscle has produced (relative) hyperplasia of the lesser trochanter while the preserved activity of the adductor muscles has led to coxa valga *(right)*. A typical radiographic hallmark of the paralytic and the paretic hip is the normal-appearing size of the femoral head and the "thin" femoral shaft!

11. Possible attendant intertrochanteric and/or subtrochanteric pseudarthrosis

By the end of the growth period, items 1, 4, 5 and possibly 9 concur to produce the typical *shepherd's staff deformity* in the roentgenogram (see Fig. 336). Infrequently, congenital coxa vara can develop into valgus. A pseudarthrosis of the intertrochanteric or subtrochanteric region may develop and may even heal completely without therapy. As a rule, however, coxa vara deteriorates from early childhood up to puberty. Orthopedic treatment is therefore mandatory to prevent the condition from terminating in a preosteoarthrotic deformity of the hip joint (see p. 226 ff.) or at least to reduce this danger.

Teratologic dislocation of the hip is a malformation acquired in embryonic life. It is often associated with other skeletal anomalies (compare Fig. 288); e.g., in the setting of an alcoholic embryopathy (Leiber, 1978). However, the condition also is encountered in congenital disorders that do not primarily interfere with skeletal development (Rompe, 1968); for instance, *arthrogryposis multiplex congenita* (leading signs: absence of spontaneous motion and muscle wasting in the extremities). Of clinical importance, on the other hand, is the **anthropologic dislocation of the hip,** universally known under the designation of **congenital dislocation of the hip.** This disorder will be discussed with preosteoarthrotic conditions of the hip joint (p. 226 ff.).

Dislocations from imbalance develop in disorders of the muscular equilibrium about the hip joint; for instance, in meningomyelocele, which is associated with a functional preponderance of the flexors of the hip and the adductor muscles. This condition increases the *anteversion* of the proximal end of the femur and favors the tendency to dislocation (Rossak et al., 1970). Besides this, any flaccid or spastic paralysis of the hip muscles occurring during growth, as well as hereditary systemic diseases of the musculature, are apt to produce malpositions of the hip joint and deformations of the articulating bones (Fig. 290).

Arthritis

Coxarthritis (Inflammatory arthritis of the hip joint)

Roentgenographic diagnosis of **coxarthritis** (coxitis) requires:

1. Attention to the periarticular soft tissues (signs of arthritis in the soft tissues)
2. Estimation of the subchondral mineralization by comparison with the unaffected side (collateral phenomena of arthritis)
3. Roentgenographic evaluation of the width of the joint space as well as the contours and structures of the juxtaarticular bones (direct signs of arthritis)

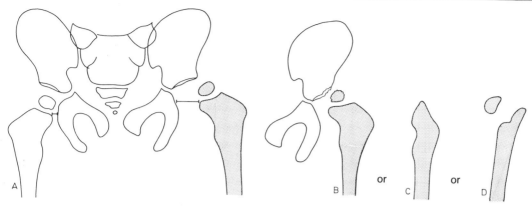

Fig. 291   A = **Dislocation of the left hip joint resulting from distention** by an effusion into the joint, in the present instance produced by coxarthritis (coxitis) in a small child, accompanied by high fever and marked swelling of the soft tissues in the region of the left hip. No evidence of acetabular dysplasia. Inflammatory bone changes not (yet) demonstrable.

B = **Dislocation from destruction** in coxarthritis (coxitis) of an infant. Delayed diagnosis and therefore inadequate therapy. The chief cause of the malposition is the inflammatory destruction of the acetabulum, whatever the etiology of the coxarthritis. The irregular ossification of the center in the femoral head indicates inflammatory damage.

C, D = Other possibilities of destruction of the proximal femur following bacterial coxarthritis in infants: C = destruction of the epiphyseal center of ossification. D = persistent epiphysiolysis and destructon of the metaphysis.

In **bacterial coxitis of infants and small children** (Fig. 291), the inflammatory edema often causes a striking periarticular swelling. In addition to this, the periarticular edema alters the **structures of the soft tissues about the hip joint** (Figs. 292 and 293) and thereby suggests the presence of an inflammatory edema, impregnation with pus, or an extensive hematoma in the vicinity of the hip joint, this is also indicative when an adult patient is concerned. We then have to decide in each individual case whether the edema and the other manifestations are due to a blood-borne bacterial arthritis of the hip joint, to a juxtaarticular osteomyelitis, to a traumatic hematoma, or to **fleeting coxitis (coxitis fugax, irritable hip).** The last-named disorder, which is mostly unilateral and much more infrequently bilateral, affects children between the ages of 1 and 14 years (Mills, 1964). It starts acutely or insidiously with pain and/or limping. Fleeting coxitis has differential diagnostic significance because it must be distinguished from the initial stage of juvenile rheumatoid arthritis and from bacterial coxarthritis. In addition, experience has shown that some of the children who have suffered a fleeting coxitis a few months later develop the clinical and roentgen signs of Legg-Calvé-Perthes disease (see under this disorder). Therefore, one should make it a rule to radiologically reexamine the hip of every patient about two months after an attack of supposed fleeting coxitis. The alteration of the physiologic periarticular soft structures—ie., their partial or complete obliteration—is a potential pathologic manifestation of fleeting coxitis in the roentgenogram. In small children, it is apt to produce a minor distention-dis-

location (see Figs. 291 and 339). The etiologic factors are still under debate; among them are mild infection, an allergic reaction of the synovial membrane, trauma, and aseptic necrosis of bone (Legg-Calvé-Perthes disease; *vide supra*). At times, an increase in size of the femoral head has been observed as a late sequel (Heine and Leitz, 1972). In these cases, fleeting coxitis as an **arthritis of the growth period** has accelerated and stimulated the development and growth of the femoral head.

In the hip joint, the general sequelae of arthritis of the growth period are completed by certain specific alterations of shape and structure, namely:

1. Bell-shaped deformity of the femoral head (Fig. 294)
2. Coxa valga (Fig. 295 A)
3. Developmental disorders and malpositions of the femoral head resembling the radiographic appearance of congenital dislocation of the hip (Streda and Bardfield, 1964; Fig. 295 B).
4. Fibrillar, so-called hypertrophic, atrophy of bone (Figs. 13 and 295 C)
5. In children with juvenile rheumatoid arthritis who are confined to bed permanently or for a prolonged period, the coxarthritic destructions in the articulating bones of the hip joints are much less marked than in children who have not been immobilized. In patients who are allowed to be up and about, the bone of the inflamed weight-bearing joints obviously may become necrotic. The necrotic bone is resorbed, and extremely severe mutilations develop (Fig. 296)
6. Following ankylosis of the hip (due to juvenile

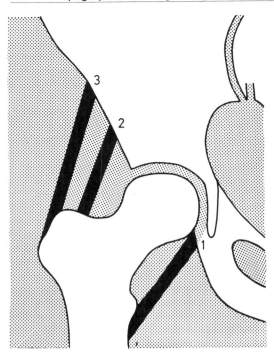

Fig. 292 **Pericoxal fat streaks** (see Reichmann, 1967). For intrapelvic soft-tissue shadows see Fig. 390.

1 = Fat streak medial to iliopsoas muscle

2 = Fat streak mainly medial to the gluteus minimus muscle

3 = Fat streak mainly between gluteus minimus and gluteus medius muscles (variably demonstrable)

Periarticular saturation with edema, pus, or blood renders the fat streaks equivalent to water (see Table 1) so that they can no longer be delimited radiologically. Inflammatory edema, pus, or a traumatic hematoma also homogenizes the soft structures in this fashion. The fat streaks may become interspersed by infiltrating soft-tissue tumors and thus be broken (compare Fig. 370) or displaced (Fig. 371).

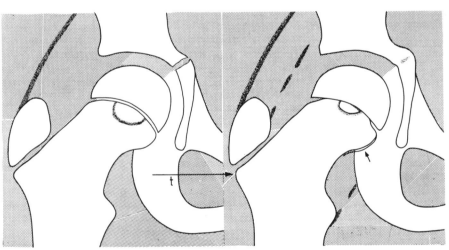

Fig. 293 **Development of an osteomyelitis of the femoral metaphysis with sympathetic coxarthritis in school age child.** *Left:* Poorly defined focus of destruction in the proximal metaphysis of the femur; pericoxal edema (the fat streaks 1 and 2—see Fig. 292—have been obliterated). Study of the aspirated effusion determines whether a purulent or sterile serous effusion (hence, either a pyogenic or a sympathetic coxarthritis) is present.

Right: *Three months* later—t stands for time—the infection has regressed. *Signs of repair:* Focus in the femur has decreased in size and presents marginal sclerosis, there is a periosteal reaction in the femoral neck *(arrow),* and the fat streaks 1 and 2 are visible again to some extent. Partial closure of the femoral and acetabular epiphysis indicates accelerated maturation induced by the inflammatory hyperemia.

Note: Sympathetic arthritis (see p. 161 ff) is accompanied by a sterile serous effusion. Destruction of joints does not usually occur, but accelerated maturation and disorders of growth in the articulating bones may be observed and are apt to result in a preosteoarthrotic deformity. With coxarthritic edema, the fat stripes 1 and 2 (at times also 3) generally are obliterated. With *unilateral* obliteration of the fat streaks—for instance either 1 or 2 and 3 (Fig. 292), one also should consider the presence of edema that has been triggered directly by an extra-articular process, such as osteitis or saturation with pus. Obliteration of the pericoxal fat stripes does *not* belong among the radiographic findings in rheumatoid arthritis. When it is observed in this disorder, it should arouse suspicion of an additional pyogenic infection of the hip joint (see p. 88).

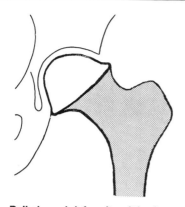

Fig. 294   Bell-shaped deformity of the femoral head (Dihlmann and Peter, 1965) as a general clue to an inflammation of the hip joint that started at or was experienced between the 10th and 12th year of life and prior to the age of 17 to 20. In this period of life the central portions of the proximal femoral epiphysis are already ossified; in its periphery, however, epiphyseal *cartilage* persists. Inflammatory damage ("irritation" but not "destruction") to the peripheral epiphyseal cartilage alters the normal direction of bone and cartilage growth, causing the borders to become raised and thus leading to the bell-shaped appearance of the femoral head. A double-sided bell-shaped appearance arouses suspicion of (past) inflammatory rheumatic coxarthritis, whereas a one-sided bell-shaped appearance is only a general clue to arthritis. The bell-shaped deformity should be considered as a preosteoarthrotic condition of the hip joint.

rheumatoid arthritis), "compensatory" pseudoarthroses in the cartilaginous epiphysis of the femur have been observed that are, in a sense, "false hip joints" (Stovell et al., 1975).

It is true that some of the findings listed under items 2 and 4 are related to the long-standing immobilization of the joint or the patient. However, these anomalies develop exclusively during growth and indeed—as is the case with most of the sequels of arthritis of the growth period—occur more frequently, the younger the patient is at the onset of disease. In the hip joint, just as in the vicinity of other joints, the fibrillar atrophy of bone persists throughout life and many decades later still evidences the arthritis and/or the long-term immobilization experienced in the years of growth!

The *collateral demineralization in arthritis* manifests itself in the neighborhood of the hip joint by an ill-defined bone structure (in acute or subacute arthritis) and by a patchy or homogeneous increase in translucence (in subacute or chronic processes) (see Fig. 13).

Prior to diagnosing collateral demineralization in arthritis (see Figs. 292 and 293) *without* concomitant evidence of soft-tissue signs of arthritis and/or direct signs of arthritis (Fig. 20), the following conditions must be considered in the differential diagnosis:

1. Demineralization of disuse; i.e., decalcification due to sparing of the joint

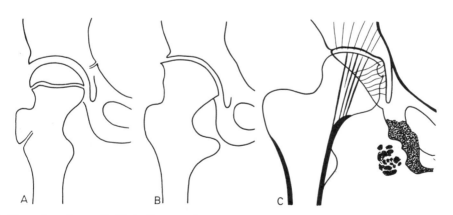

Fig. 295   Sequelae of coxarthritis in the growth period

A = Coxa valga as a consequence of juvenile rheumatoid arthritis (onset in 3rd year; present age 14). Only by the combined results of anamnesis, a general check-up, and arthritic radiologic findings (for instance, in the joints of the hands) may one determine the cause of the deformity.

B = Serious deformations and premature closure of the epiphyses as a consequence of juvenile rheumatoid arthritis (onset in 3rd year; present age 13). The illustrated deformities conform to the picture of congenital dislocation of the hip (see under this heading) and cannot be differentiated from this disorder without data from the anamnesis!

C = Tuberculosis of the hip joint and the ischium at the age of 10 (present age 35). Long-term treatment by immobilization. Hypertrophic atrophy of the cancellous bone; minor osteoarthrosis of the hip (delicate osteophytes on the borders of the fovea); sclerotic defect of the ischium with calcified tuberculous pus in the soft tissue.

Note: In general, major disorders of growth of the articulating bones are to be expected only when the arthritis started before the age of 10 and following injuries to the bone.

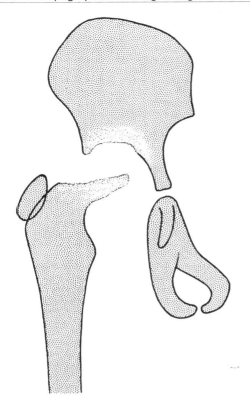

Fig. 296   Mutilation of the right hip joint in juvenile chronic arthritis (sequel to chronic arthritis *and* to arthritis-induced aseptic necrosis of bone?)

2. Transient osteoporosis of the hip joint (p. 14 ff, Fig. 16).

Figure 297 shows those areas of bone in which juxtaarticular demineralization manifests itself very early and unequivocally. Narrowing of the joint space in the hip joint furnishes important radiographic information (Fig. 298). In arthritis, the damage soon involves the entire extent of the articular cartilage. An even, *concentric* narrowing of the joint space develops. Osteoarthrosis, however, at first leads to *eccentric* narrowing of the joint space; for instance, in the pressure-absorbing zone of the joint (Fig. 298 B). The association of concentric narrowing of the joint space with *minor* formation of marginal osteophytes and an equally slight density of the subchondral cancellous bone is very suggestive of *chronic* coxitis (Fig. 299 A) that has not yet led to erosion of the subchondral bone. The articular cartilage is uniformly damaged (thinned and resorbed) by the arthritis and can no longer withstand the everyday stress; a paraarthritic osteoarthrosis of the hip develops with time, and marginal osteophytes make their appearance. Such paraarthritic or postarthritic osteoarthrosis (secondary inflammatory osteoarthrosis) can assume such proportions that they completely overshadow the roentgen manifestations of arthritis (Fig. 299 B). Only anamnesis and/or the radiographic signs of arthritis in other joints will indicate the damage to the articular cartilage. Finally, there exists the possibility that an arthritis of whatever etiology (Figs. 299 C and 300) does not make itself manifest at all in the roentgenogram. In any case, it will already have interfered with the nutrition of the articular cartilage—for instance, by producing a sterile serous effusion—to such an extent that an osteoarthrosis (secondary para- or post-arthritic osteoarthrosis) develops. Occasionally the so-called *lobster claw* (osteophytes on the acetabulum and the head of the femur atypical of osteoarthrosis, adapted to each other) will arouse suspicion of an arthritic origin of osteoarthrosis of the hip (Fig. 301).

Among the chronic arthritides of the hip joint are to be mentioned in the first place the inflammatory rheumatic and the tuberculous affections. **Adult rheumatoid arthritis** manifests itself in the hip joint the more frequently the longer the patient has suffered from this disease. Only in a few of the patients (about 3 percent according to Lenoch et al., 1966) is the hip joint the initial site. Apart from this, there exists an **isolated rheumatoid coxarthritis** that begins as a monoarticular or biarticular symmetrical in-

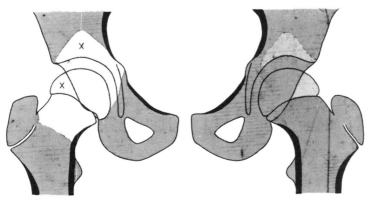

Fig. 297   Collateral arthritic phenomenon in the right hip joint. Typical localization. Without concomitant signs in the soft tissues and/or direct signs of arthritis, the condition must be differentiated from demineralization of disuse (p. 13) and transient osteoporosis (p. 14 ff). The areas marked with x display decalcification from inflammation or other causes very early since, for anatomic reasons, they are more translucent to the roentgen beam than their surroundings (compare with the sound *left* hip joint).

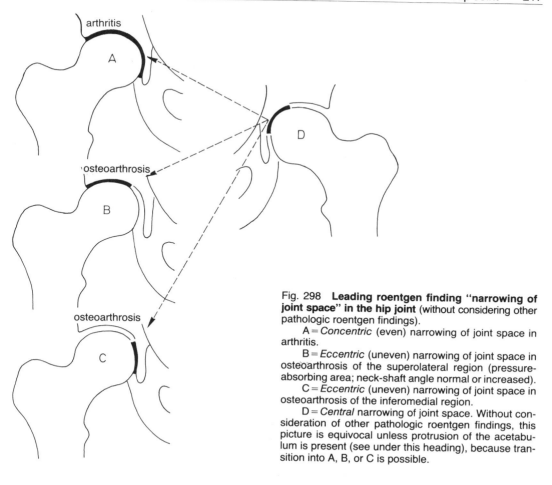

arthritis

A

osteoarthrosis

B

osteoarthrosis

C

D

Fig. 298 **Leading roentgen finding "narrowing of joint space" in the hip joint** (without considering other pathologic roentgen findings).

A = *Concentric* (even) narrowing of joint space in arthritis.

B = *Eccentric* (uneven) narrowing of joint space in osteoarthrosis of the superolateral region (pressure-absorbing area; neck-shaft angle normal or increased).

C = *Eccentric* (uneven) narrowing of joint space in osteoarthrosis of the inferomedial region.

D = *Central* narrowing of joint space. Without consideration of other pathologic roentgen findings, this picture is equivocal unless protrusion of the acetabulum is present (see under this heading), because transition into A, B, or C is possible.

flammation of the hip joint and runs its course as such; i.e., without terminating in the polyarticular stage (Arlet et al., 1971).

In rheumatoid arthritis, the roentgenogram of the hip joint principally reflects the destructive and metaplastic potentials of the pannus, which is an inflammatory fibrovascular resorptive tissue (Fig. 302). At times, centrally located "cystic" or crescent-shaped marginal osteolyses of typical roentgenographic appearance form in the junction of the femoral head with the femoral neck or directly in the latter (Fig. 303). This resorption of bone is initiated by the pannus, by focal rheumatoid necrosis of bone, or by rheumatoid nodules (see p. 18 f.).

The involvement of the hip joint in the course of **ankylosing spondylitis** shows variable clinical expressions (Fig. 304). Osteoarthrosis of the hip from excessive strain affords the best prognosis. It occurs as a consequence of seriously faulty posture of the stiffened spine. Chronic coxarthritis, which often is bilateral and also more or less affects the subchondral bone, is likewise depicted in Figure 304. The younger the patient is at the onset of the manifestation in the

hip, the more rapidly the disorder is likely to terminate in bony ankylosis. The coxarthritis may even be the first *clinical* manifestation of ankylosing spondylitis. The affection of the hip is then frequently initially misdiagnosed as tuberculosis because the involvement of the sacroiliac joints either occurs a little later or remains unnoticed in the survey film of the pelvis, and the coxarthritis is indeed in the forefront of the patient's complaints. This type of evolution generally starts between the ages of 15 and 20. Whether and to what extent secondary osteoarthrotic deformations are superimposed depends on the activity (progression) of the coxarthritis and the mobility of the patient (see p. 218). Finally, the characteristic inherent tendency of ankylosing spondylitis for pathologic ossification of the gliding tissue can, also in the hip joint, lead to ossification of the articular cartilage and the joint capsule. In this case, the joint already ankyloses *prior to* the inflammatory destruction of the articular cartilage. This process, also, can be inferred from the roentgenogram (Fig. 304 D).

In general, coxarthritis occurring during the evolution of **psoriatic arthritis** and in **Reiter's syn-**

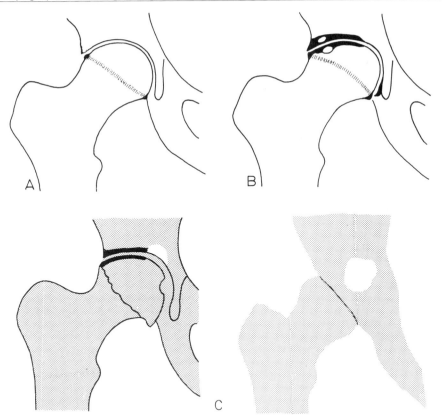

Fig. 299   A = **Coxarthritis running a protracted course** (in this instance in rheumatoid arthritis). The diagnosis is derived from the combination of "concentric narrowing of the joint space *and* minor formation of marginal osteophytes" (see text).

B = **Full-blown paraarthritic osteoarthrosis of the hip joint** in rheumatoid arthritis. The roentgen signs of arthritis are completely overshadowed. Only the anamnesis and the roentgen findings in the other joints allow correct diagnosis from the roentgenogram.

C = **Osteoarthrosis of the hip joint in a younger individual (aged 23 years) without recognizable preosteoarthrotic deformity.** This appearance is an indication for tomography. The tomograph reveals that the acetabular radiolucency, which is not very conspicuous in the survey film, corresponds to a large indolent cavitation in the ilium. *Diagnosis:* Sympathetic coxarthritis—radiographically, secondary osteoarthrosis—in juxta-articular tuberculosis of the ilium, or (less probably) nonspecific bacterial abscess in the ilium.

drome offers a better prognosis than involvement of the hip in rheumatoid arthritis and in ankylosing spondylitis. Severe destruction of the hip joint, including bony ankylosis, is seen but rarely—particularly in Reiter's syndrome. The radiologist should consider ankylosing spondylitis, psoriatic arthritis, and Reiter's syndrome when confronted with the following constellation of pathologic roetgen findings in the pelvic region:

1. Unilateral or symmetrical bilateral *coxarthritis*
2. Unilateral or bilateral *sacroiliitis* or the "variegated picture" type (see p. 490 ff)
3. *Fibroosteitis* at the sites of predilection in the pelvic region (see Figs. 79, 304, and 378)

Lipoid-dermatoarthritis can, from erosions through destruction and mutilations, lead to devastation of the hip joint (Fig. 305) that at times may extend to the femoral neck. Since these lesions are situated on both sides of the joint space, they indicate an (inflammatory) affection of the joint. However, further information concerning the etiology of this disease cannot be obtained from the roentgenogram.

The radiographic morphology of **bacterial coxarthritis** is governed primarily by the clinical course (from acute to chronic), the type of pathogens involved, and the patient's age at onset.

Nontuberculous bacterial coxarthritis develops most frequently by hematogenous lodgment of the bacteria in the synovial membrane or in the sub-

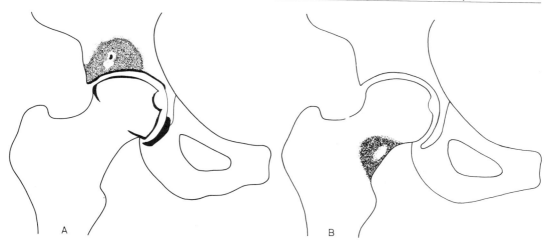

Fig. 300   A = **Osteomyelitis of the acetabular roof with bland sympathetic coxarthritis** manifested radiographically by the secondary osteoarthrosis. The *extensive* sclerotic area *(screened)* around the granulation cavity containing a sequestrum indicates an adequate local defense mechanism and/or little virulence of the invading organisms.

B = **Osteoid osteoma in the femoral neck. To be differentiated from A.**

The nidus of the osteoid osteoma in *cancellous* bone may undergo partial or complete calcification. It can then be recognized in plain roentgenograms either as a circumscribed density of bone with difficulty *or* not at all (tomography, angiography!). In the present case the nidus lies in the midst of compact bone (in the so-called Adam's arc) and therefore appears as a translucent area.

chondral bone marrow. Injury, aspiration of the joint, and surgical intervention are infrequent causes of bacterial invasion. In acute osteomyelitis, the close anatomic relationships between the proximal epiphysis or metaphysis of the femur and the hip joint often lead to concomitant involvement of this joint. The same pathway of infection is frequently respon-

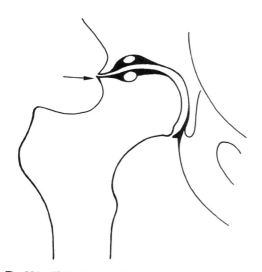

Fig. 301   **"Lobster claw" appearance** (*arrow;* see text) arouses the suspicion of osteoarthrosis of the hip induced by arthritis (see also Fig. 302 D and E).

sible for acute coxarthritis (coxitis) of infants and small children, in whom the intraarticular increase in volume produced by the effusion manifests itself as a faulty position of the articulating bones (Fig. 291), as distention-dislocation, and as destruction-dislocation of the hip joint. **Distention-dislocation** can occur with nonspecific bacterial, tuberculous, and fungous types of arthritis as well as with juvenile rheumatoid arthritis or as a complication of a traumatic effusion. It should be mentioned here that infections with opportunistic fungi depend on certain prerequisites; for instance, immunologic deficiency, cytostatic therapy, wasting diseases, broad-spectrum antibiotics, and also measures of intensive care (infusion catheters, etc.). **Obstetric femoral epiphysiolysis** initially also presents femoral distention as a consequence of intraarticular hemorrhage before, after an interval of 10 to 14 days. The calcifying hematoma and possibly a periosteal reaction furnish a clue to this injury (Figs. 291 and 314). The roentgenogram of distention-dislocation differs from that in congenital dislocation of the hip by the normal shape and the normal state of development of the articulating bones. In older children, a large effusion sometimes produces a slight widening of the joint space in the roentgenogram (compare Fig. 306 A). This finding may also occur in adults, although rarely.

The more *acute* the course a nontuberculous bacterial coxarthritis pursues, the *more distinctive* are the signs of arthritis in the soft tissues (p. 213), the *less sharp* are the contours and cancellous structures of the subchondral bone, and the *more strongly and*

Fig. 302 **Roentgen finding "chronic coxarthritis"** (here in rheumatoid arthritis).

A = *Early roentgen findings* (attendant arthritic cyst in acetabulum, delicate erosion of femoral head; partial wasting of the marginal subchondral lamella in the femoral head). Narrowing of joint space not yet demonstrable.

B = Concentric narrowing of joint space; flattening of femoral head through superficial erosion.

C = Secondary (inflammatory) protrusion of acetabulum with pathologic fracture, femoral head "cervicalized."

D to E = Follow-up study (t = time). After the hyaline cartilage has been destroyed by the pannus, the metaplastic potential of the inflammatory pannus may manifest itself by the formation of a fibrocartilage (fibrocartilaginous ankylosis, frequently with residual mobility). Since the fibrocartilage occupies a larger volume than the pannus, the joint space at times "widens" again. During the period of observation the attendant arthritic cysts assume sharp contours (evidence that the process has become stabilized).

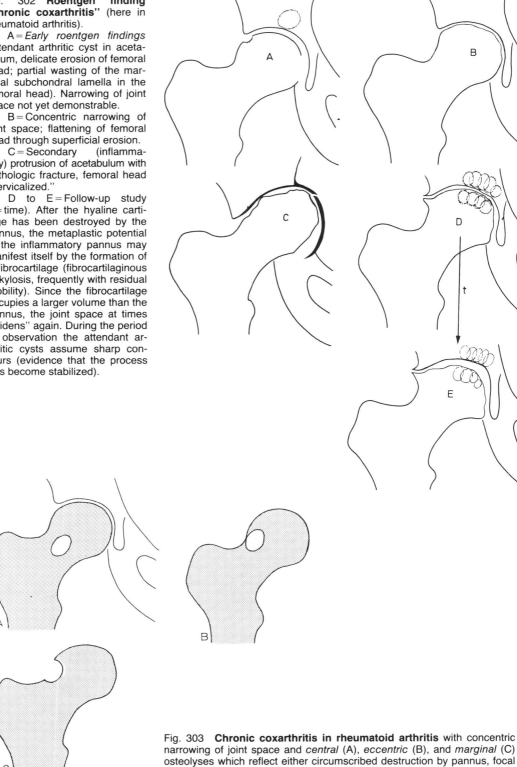

Fig. 303 **Chronic coxarthritis in rheumatoid arthritis** with concentric narrowing of joint space and *central* (A), *eccentric* (B), and *marginal* (C) osteolyses which reflect either circumscribed destruction by pannus, focal rheumatoid necroses of bone, or rheumatoid nodules (Hunder et al., 1965).

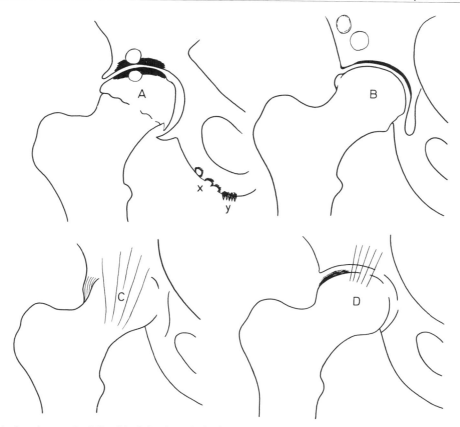

Fig. 304 **Involvement of the hip joint in ankylosing spondylitis.** A = *Osteoarthrosis of the hip joint from excessive strain* as a consequence of faulty posture of the spine (lumbar kyphosis, thereby elevation of the os pubis; x = rarefying and y = productive fibroosteitis at the sites of origin of the ischiocrural muscles (Fig. 79).

B = *chronic coxarthritis with little secondary paraarthritic osteoarthrosis.* The cystic radiolucencies are not osteoarthrotic debris cysts but osteolyses developing in direct connection with the coxarthritis during the course of ankylosing spondylitis. At times they have a diameter of several centimeters.

C = *Bony ankylosis* following arthritic destruction of the articular cartilage and the articulating bony areas. Capsular ossification. Hypertrophic trajectories course uninterrupted from the ilium to the femur.

D = *Bony ankylosis with false joint space.* The typical radiographic appearance arises either by ossification of the preserved articular cartilage (particular mode of reaction in ankylosing spondylitis!) or by osseous metaplasia of the inflammatory pannus *and* the more or less preserved marginal subchondral lamella.

Note: The coxarthritis in rheumatoid arthritis of the adult tends to fibrocartilaginous ankylosis (see legend accompanying Fig. 302), whereas the coxarthritis occurring during the course of ankylosing spondylitis is apt to develop bony ankylosis. These morphologic characteristics are also reflected in the roentgenogram.

readily the demolition of the articular cartilage (narrowing of the joint space) and the joint-bearing bones (erosion, destruction, mutilation) occurs.

Tuberculosis of the hip joint (tuberculous coxitis) develops by hematogenous lodgment of the pathogens in the synovial membrane or the subchondral bone marrow as well as by spreading from abscesses in other neighboring organs affected by tuberculosis. *Synovial* tuberculosis of the hip joint manifests itself by juxtaarticular decalcification (compare Fig. 297), which is demonstrable at the earliest between 2 and 3 months after onset of the

symptoms. This collateral phenomenon of inflammation will be recognized earlier, the more strictly the radiologist adheres to the rule that paired articulations should be subjected to paired roentgenologic examination (p. 4), i.e., evaluation of the painful hip joint by means of a survey film of the pelvis. In this connection it is well to remember that a juxtaarticular decalcification may be due to different individual causes or it may be occasioned by a combination of several factors (collateral inflammatory phenomenon, splinting or immobilization, damage to osteoblasts by bacterial toxins, p. 11). In the further course

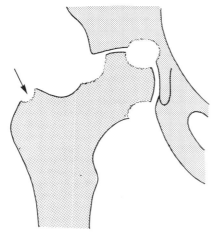

Fig. 305 **Lipoid-dermatoarthritis** *Roentgenogram:* Mutilating coxarthritis developed in the setting of a polyarthritis as evidenced by the findings in other joints. The defect in the tendinous insertion *(arrow)* into the greater trochanter is also in inflammatory rheumatic disorders and in hyperparathyroidism.

of synovial tuberculosis, erosions and narrowing of the joint space develop (Fig. 306 B). In contrast to this, sequestra and calcified pus from an abscess are late roentgen findings in tuberculosis of the hip joint. The primary lesion of *osseous* tuberculosis of the hip is an intraarticular skeletal focus in the head or neck of the femur in the acetabulum or, less frequently, an extraarticular bony focus; e.g., in the greater trochanter. In the beginning, this ill-defined "focus," presenting more or less marginal sclerosis, dominates over the roentgenologic signs of coxarthritis (narrowing of the joint space, etc.). The following rules will once again summarize and complete the roentgenologic differential diagnosis of the *painful hip* with regard to coxarthritis:

1. An insidious course of the disease accompanied by periarticular demineralization *without* narrowing of the joint space, *without* defective contours, and *without* juxtaarticular breakdown of bone arouses suspicion of the *early stage* of tuberculous coxitis. The next step in the roentgen diagnosis is tomography of the hip joint. Differential diagnosis must be made from transient osteoporosis (p. 14, Fig. 16),

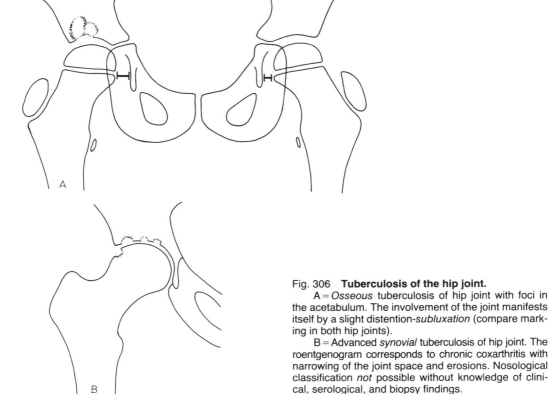

Fig. 306 **Tuberculosis of the hip joint.**
    A = *Osseous* tuberculosis of hip joint with foci in the acetabulum. The involvement of the joint manifests itself by a slight distention-*subluxation* (compare marking in both hip joints).
    B = Advanced *synovial* tuberculosis of hip joint. The roentgenogram corresponds to chronic coxarthritis with narrowing of the joint space and erosions. Nosological classification *not* possible without knowledge of clinical, serological, and biopsy findings.

posttraumatic demineralization, and other osteoporoses of disuse, in children also from Legg-Calvé-Perthes disease.

2. Periarticular demineralization occurs in connection with juxtaarticular breakdown of bone—with or without sequestrum formation or dissection—both in nontuberculous bacterial and in tuberculous infections. In children, the diagnostic differentiation of such cases from the initial stage of Legg-Calvé-Perthes disease sometimes presents considerable difficulty.

3. Periarticular demineralization, narrowing of the joint space, defective contours, and/or subchondral focal osteolyses are seen in nontuberculous bacterial, tuberculous, and inflammatory rheumatic affections of the hip joint. The *more rapidly* these changes develop—e.g., within the space of 1 or 2 months—and the *more ill-defined* (hazy) the structures appear because of the juxtaarticular demineralization, the greater the probability of a nontuberculous bacterial etiology in unilateral involvement of the hip.

4. Any osteoarthrosis of the hip in *younger* patients (between the third and fourth decade of life or so), *not* presenting a preosteoarthrotic deformity, may be an inflammatory secondary osteoarthrosis. One can then differentiate, for instance, a juxtaarticular breakdown of bone from bacterial inflammation in the survey film or only in tomographs (see Fig. 299 C), or the sacroiliac joints may reveal early signs of ankylosing spondylitis.

5. For the differentiation between inflammatory rheumatic and bacterial disorders of the hip joint, the radiologist also should resort to the available clinical and serological findings (compare p. 105). ''Gas'' manifests itself in the roentgenogram in two ways. First by the so-called *vacuum phenomenon* (Fig. 307 A) and secondly as *pneumarthrosis* (Fig. 307 B).

Osteoarthrosis

Ovid's saying *principiis obsta* (nip things in the bud) applies especially to osteoarthrosis of the hip. It is not only the most frequent pathologic finding in the hip but, in its active stage, is also the source of considerable discomfort (pain, uncomfortable muscle strain, a sense of weight in the leg, etc.) that torments the patient on standing and walking as well as in sitting and during recumbency. Osteoarthrosis of the hip heralds its presence in the roentgenogram by osteophytes on the margin of the fovea capitis (Fig. 308, no. 1), by flat appositions of bone on the anterior surface of the femur—*plaque sign* (Fig. 308, no. 2, compare Fig. 309) (Dihlmann and Frik, 1971)—and by the *supercilium of the acetabular roof* (Fig. 308, nos. 3 B and C). Osteophytes are sensitive indicators of excessive strain on the articular cartilage. Their size informs one about the nature and extent of damage to the articular cartilage (Dihlmann et al., 1979) but does not influence the course or prognosis of osteoarthrosis (Danielsson, 1964).

During the further evolution of osteoarthritis of the hip, marginal osteophytes also develop on the rims and in the depth of the acetabulum (Fig. 310). At times the acetabular rim displays marked bulging that manifests itself in the roentgenogram as a *pseudo-fracture line* (Fig. 311; Herzog, 1933, Dihlmann, 1964). With a normal or increased neck-shaft angle, increased density of the cancellous bone, cysts of osteoarthrotic disintegration and eccentric narrowing of the roentgenologic joint space are to be expected at first in the superolateral and superomedial regions of the joint; i.e., in the pressure-absorbing area (Fig. 310). In the normal adult hip, the thickness of the adult cartilage (equal to the width of the joint space

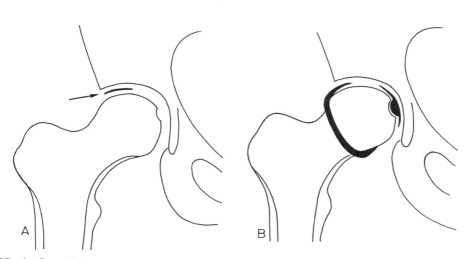

Fig. 307   A = **So-called vacuum phenomenon *(arrow).*** B = **Pneumarthrosis of hip joint** in anaerobic infection. (For additional causes of such accumulations of gas in the joint see p. 20).

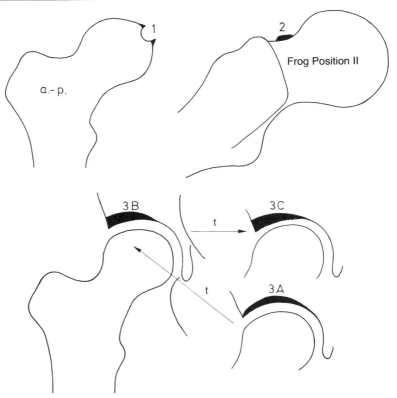

Fig. 308 Early radiographic signs of osteoarthrosis of the hip.

1 = *Osteophyte on the margin of the fovea capitis.*

2 = In the so-called frog position II roentgenogram (taken in dorsal decubitus, with the upper legs anteflexed, abducted but *not* externally rotated), the *plaque sign* "grows out" of the *concave* or *straight* contour of the anterior surface of the femur neck (compare Fig. 309). The plaques on the anterior surface of the femur (which are more infrequent than those on its posterior surface) are derived from a variable cartilage covering of the femoral neck or are circumscribed neoplastic cartilage formations. Being a regenerative tissue response to degenerative lesions of the articular cartilage, the cartilage in the area of these plaques undergoes proliferation. This process initiates its ossification. The cartilage then develops a base which in the roentgenogram (taken in the so-called frog position II) becomes visible as the plaque sign. (In the European literature the frog position roentgenogram is also known as the Lauenstein roentgenogram.)

3 = The "supercilium of the acetabular roof"—3B—(Pauwels, 1976) develops when the articular pressure is no longer evenly distributed over the bearing surface. Experience has shown that the "supercilia" appear preferentially with a wide neck-shaft angle (coxa valga, dysplasia of the hip) and then constitute the radiographic expression of excessive strain on the articular cartilage.

3A = Normal finding,

3B = Supercilium of the acetabular roof.

3C = Supercilium of the acetabular roof plus narrowing of the joint space in the pressure-absorbing zone *(schematic drawing; t = time course).*

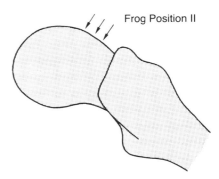

Fig. 309 Radiographic differential diagnosis of the plaque sign (compare Fig. 308, no. 2). *Arrows* point to the "eminentia articularis colli femoris" (Fick, 1904). This convex articular hump of the femoral neck commonly has a cartilaginous sheath and is a variant (Dihlmann and Frik, 1971).

Fig. 310 Roentgen signs in osteoarthrosis of the hip.

Note: The fovea capitis femoris may ossify completely, creating a knoblike bulge into the joint cavity (compare Fig. 311). *Arrow* points to an osseous metaplasia (capsular osteoma) in the fibrosed capsule of the osteoarthrotic joint. Likewise, solitary (calcified) synovial chondromas *(tailed arrow)* may develop in the synovium of the osteoarthrotic joint through cartilaginous metaplasia (compare Figs. 372 and 373). The osteoarthrotic narrowing of the joint space *begins* eccentrically, most often superiorly (superolaterally or superomedially). Less often it begins centrally; for instance in osteoarthrosis following idiopathic protrusion of the acetabulum, or inferiorly (inferomedially). Laterocaudally to Köhler's tear-shaped figure = calcification of the labrum acetabuli (see p. 267).

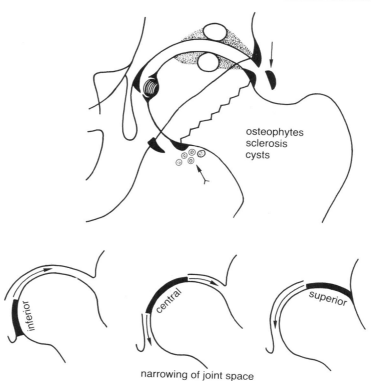

osteophytes
sclerosis
cysts

narrowing of joint space

in the roentgenogram) above the center of the femoral head is somewhat greater than 4 mm (Fredensborg and Nilsson, 1978). Only with time does the osteoarthrotic narrowing of the joint space extend to the entire circumference of the joint (Fig. 311). However, the location of the narrowing is influenced not only by the neck-shaft angle but also by the extent of anteversion or retroversion, the angle of inclination, and the depth of the acetabulum.

The roentgen findings listed are accompanied by processes of resorption and apposition that constitute the deforming character of the osteoarthrosis. These processes may also lead to decentralization of the hip joint. With decentralization, the virtual centers of the circles of the acetabulum and the femoral head are no longer congruent. There are three roentgen signs of decentralization: (1) *duplication of the acetabular floor*, (2) *subfoveal osteophytes*, and (3) *the Wiberg signs* (Dihlmann and Hopf, 1971). Not only do they indicate the decentralization of the hip, but the first two signs also evidence its irreversibility.

At times, osteoarthrosis of the hip follows an atypical course (Fig. 313). Instead of the slowly progressive roentgen signs of osteoarthrosis, a considerable aggravation sets in within a couple of months. A painful destruction, particularly of the femoral head,

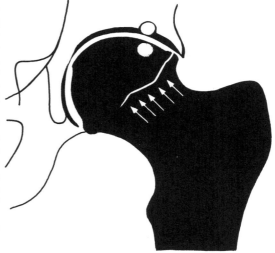

Fig. 311 Pseudofracture line in osteoarthrosis of the hip. This line develops through a Mach effect in the osteoarthrotic bulge of the anterior and/or posterior rim of the acetabulum *(arrows)* and may mimic a fracture line. (In the optical illusion named after *Ernst Mach,* the subjectively experienced contrast is greater than the actual, photometrically demonstrable contrast).

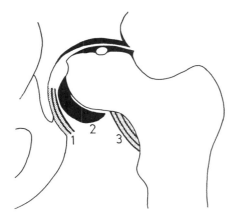

Fig. 312 **Signs of decentralization in osteoarthrosis of the hip** (see text).
1 = Duplication of acetabular floor.
2 = Subfoveal osteophyte.
3 = Wiberg sign ("hammock").

Note: It is rare for all three signs of decentralization to coexist. Usually only one or two of these signs are present; the Wiberg sign is the most sensitive, and therefore most frequent, indicator of decentralization.

without major formation of osteophyes occurs in about 10 percent of cases. (Abelanet et al., 1974). This is the picture of **(rapidly) destructive osteoarthrosis of the hip.** It is still a matter of debate whether the histologic cause of such rapid destruction is not an inflammatory chondroosteolysis (Abelanet et al., 1974) but a local disorder of circulation with strong reactive synovitis (Puls, 1974).

Classic Preosteoarthrotic Conditions of the Hip Joint

The articular cartilage multiplies in its upper layers near the joint cavity (Otte, 1965). Its loss of substance, which manifests itself in the roentgenogram by narrowing of the joint space, likewise begins at the surface of the cartilage. This accounts for the lack of regenerative capacity of the damaged, abraded hyaline articular cartilage in osteoarthrosis and other pathologic conditions. This piece of insight was the starting point of the formulation and justification of the *doctrine of the* preosteoarthrotic conditions (Hackenbroch, 1943). The same may be said of the wish to supplement the roentgenologic diagnosis of

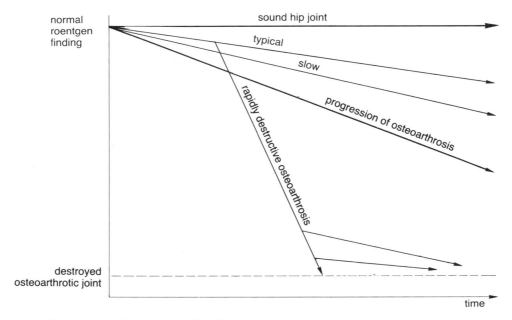

Fig. 313 **Time relationships in osteoarthrosis** (see text).

osteoarthrosis by clues to an etiology that might be demonstrable roentgenographically and so to fully exploit the information furnished by the film.

Furthermore, the doctrine of the preosteoarthrotic conditions brought new realizations concerning the etiology, pathogenesis, prophylaxis, and therapy of osteoarthrosis. Although it was founded in the hip joint, it claims heuristic interest. The doctrine originated with the observation that incongruities of the articular surfaces due to congenital or acquired deformity, malposition or malalignment, and also the disturbed coordination of the hip muscles, are factors that predispose to osteoarthrosis because they interfere with the physiologic equilibrium between articular pressure and resistance of the articular cartilage. The mechanically active incongruities displace and increase the articular pressure so that the cartilage cover is no longer able to cope with the strain: it is abraded and worn away. In addition, the resistance of the articular cartilage can be lowered by an arthritic effusion and by the arthritic pannus, by chondrotrophic disorders of metabolism, by inherited inferiority of the cartilage, and so on. In these instances, early degeneration of the cartilage will ensue, even in the presence of congruent articular surfaces. Preosteoarthrotic conditions are therefore, quite generally, all those conditions and processes that are *very likely* to lead to osteoarthrosis either by disturbing the mechanics of the joint or by damaging the biologic milieu; such interference can take place either directly or indirectly via damage to the articular cartilage. The following classic preosteoarthrotic conditions of the hip joint are known.

Congenital dislocation of the hip—a disorder that has special predilection for females—is commonly subdivided into *three degrees,* namely: (1) *dysplasia of the hip,* (2) *subluxation,* and (3) *dislocation.*

For reasons of therapy, an intermediary form is sometimes distinguished from dislocation. Such differentiation, however, is only possible by means of arthrography of the hip joint. Nevertheless, the following findings in the anteroposterior survey film of the pelvis are highly suggestive of the intermediary form (Dörr, 1971): The epiphyseal nucleus of the femoral head is situated laterally (Fig. 318). The femoral head is displaced laterocranially without, however, completely crossing the superiorosseus margin of the acetabulum. In the intermediary form, arthrography additionally reveals craniomedial flattening of the femoral head without narrowing of the capsular hood. From the viewpoint of articular mechanics, the intermediary form therefore behaves like a subluxation and not like a dislocation; among other features, the latter would display narrowing of the capsular hood by the so-called isthmus.

Congenital dislocation of the hip is also designated "anthropological dislocation of the hip," as contrasted with the teratological variety (see p. 212). It is the most frequent preosteoarthrotic deformity of the hip joint and, if untreated, often leads to osteoarthrosis of the hip as early as the third decade of life. "Congenital" means that in this disorder of the hip joint the proneness to dislocation as a consequence

of inadequate preservation of the articular shape is already present at birth.

There is still a divergence of opinion as to the morphologic cause of dislocation proneness. In particular, changes in shape and disturbed ossification of the acetabulum, but also irregularities in shape of the proximal end of the femur and hormonal loosening of the capsuloligamentous apparatus in utero have, with variable emphasis, been listed as decisive causes of the dislocation proneness. The etiology of the disorder is apparently complex. Hereditary factors, however, play a definite role (Wynne-Davies, 1970).

It is primarily muscular forces and the mechanical (static and dynamic) load that *in extrauterine life* add to the defective preservation of shape and thus are apt to induce the faulty position of the articulating bones in a superolateral and posterior direction. The objective of therapy is to obtain a complete preservation of the shape of the hip joint. The successful therapeutic result depends on the earliest possible establishment of the diagnosis and thereby on the commencement of therapy. The method of treatment is selected according to the degree of dislocation and also to the patient's age. Ortolani's sign (Ortolani 1951; Dörr, 1969, 1970) is commonly the earliest *physical* finding, enabling diagnosis to be made in the first 4 weeks of life. It demonstrates the possibility of displacing the femoral head out of the acetabulum or vice versa into the primary acetabulum.

The *roentgenologic diagnosis* is based on recognizing a disordered shape of the acetabulum and the proximal end of the femur as well as the faulty position of the proximal end. In subluxation and dislocation it is as a rule possible, during the first weeks of life, to provoke the faulty position of the articulating bones by applying the roentgenographic technique of Andrén and von Rosen (1958) and to visualize it in the roentgenogram (Fig. 314). After the first 3-month period, the roentgenogram gains more and more importance in demonstrating *all* degrees of dislocation because the ossification of the primarily cartilaginous portions of the joint has assumed increasing proportions, at least on the sound side. Numerous angles and subsidiary lines have been devised to facilitate the roentgen diagnosis of congenital dislocation of the hip, especially during the first years of life. Moreover, the success of the therapeutic measures can be checked in this way.

Kopits' rectangle (Kopits, 1939) can be constructed even before the ossification of the nucleus in the femoral head has started (Fig. 315 A). If a rhomboid results instead of a rectangle, congenital dislocation of the hip is present (Fig. 315 B).

The earlier and the more confidently the roentgen diagnosis of congenital dislocation is to be established, the stricter are the criteria to be followed in correctly adjusting the survey film of the pelvis and in positioning the child (Melzer, 1977):

1. The iliac wings and the obtruator foramina of both sides should be filmed as symmetrically as possible to avoid any *torsion* (to the left or the right). Any

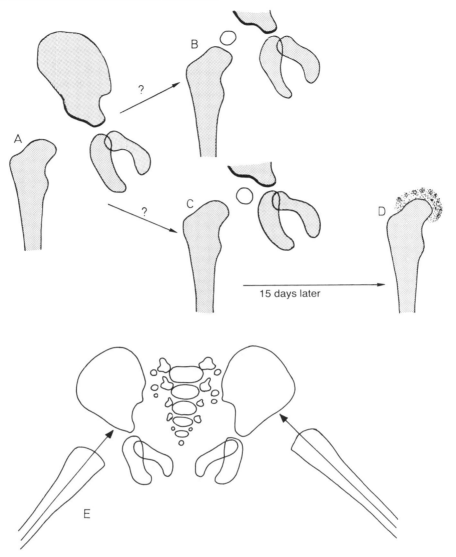

Fig. 314 **Roentgenologic differential diagnosis between congenital dislocation of the hip and obstetric separation of the femoral epiphysis in the newborn.**

A = Dislocation of the proximal end of the femur.

B, C = The problem is one of distinguishing between congenital dislocation of the hip (B) and obstetric epiphysioloysis (C). The proximal femoral epiphysis is not yet ossified and therefore not visible in the roentgenogram.

D = Obstetric epiphysiolysis is accompanied by an intraarticular hematoma and therefore leads to the development of a distention-dislocation (A, C, Fig. 291). The early calcification of the hematoma in the newborn allows differential diagnosis between B and C (Dihlmann, 1972) after only 2 weeks.

E = Roentgenographic technique after Andrén and von Rosen (1958): Patient in dorsal decubitus. The upper legs are abducted 45° (so that their longitudinal axes enclose an angle of about 90°) and are strongly rotated internally to compensate for the greater anteversion in the newborn. Normally (*left*) the axis of the femoral shaft points to the superolateral corner of the already ossified portion of the acetabulum. By contrast, in congenital dislocation of the hip, beginning from the stage of subluxation, the axis of the femoral shaft meets the pelvis above the acetabulum (*at the right* in the figure).

Fig. 315 **Kopits' rectangle**
A = *Normally,* the tangent to the acetabular roof and the tangent to the proximal metaphysis of the femur run parallel.
If their end points are connected, a *rectangle* (a *rectangular parallelogram*) results.

B = In congenital dislocation of the
hip, the tangents to the acetabulum and
the femoral metaphysis do not run parallel. They form a *rhomboid* (an unequal,
oblique-angled parallelogram).

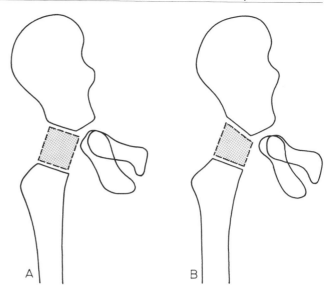

A

B

torsion of the pelvis with respect to the longitudinal
axis of the body (so that the buttocks fail to lie parallel to the cassette) will, for instance, alter the measurable angle of the acetabular roof (see Fig. 318). A
torsion of the body to the other side will increase this
angle to a certain extent, while a rotation to the same
side will decrease it.
2. On a survey film of the pelvis made in dorsal decubitus, the symphysis pubis presents caudally to the
promontory. This is due to the *physiologic inclination of the pelvis* (in the erect position, the linea terminalis forms an angle of between 50 and 70 degrees
with the horizontal). For instance, *tilting of the pelvis*
(i.e., increased inclination with caudal "displacement" of the symphysis pubis) produces diminution
of the measurable acetabular roof angle and an alteration in shape of the Kopits' rectangle. In contrast,
elevation of the pelvis (i.e., diminished inclination
with cranial "displacement" of the symphysis pubis)
increases the measurable acetabular roof angle. Pelvic tilting and inclination are recognized or ruled out
in the anteroposterior roentgenogram by paying attention to the anatomic relationships of the cranial
ends of the pubis and the ischium (Fig. 316).
3. Roentgenograms of the pelvis should be taken with
the legs in intermediate rotary position. This is accomplished if the lower legs, with the knees flexed at
right angles, depend vertically across the edge of the
Bucky table.
4. Adduction and abduction of the upper legs falsify
certain results of measurement; for instance, the Beta
angle.

The Z line and the Beta angle (Zsernaviczky and Türk,
1974, 1975) are also suitable for the roentgen diagnosis of congenital dislocation of the hip (Fig. 317).
The Beta angle can, under favorable conditions, be

measured even prior to the ossification of the center
in the femoral head. To determine the *acetabular roof
angle* (Hilgenreiner, 1925; Fig. 318), a connecting
line is drawn, close to the acetabular epiphysis, between those points in the two ilia that project farthest
caudally, and a straight line is carried on either side
of these points to that edge of the acetabular roof that
projects farthest *laterally.* Values of maximally 29
angular degrees (boys) and 32 angular degrees (girls)
are normal for infants. The corresponding values for
6-month-old children are about 26° (boys) and 28°
(girls). For children aged 1 year the values are about
24° (boys) and 26° (girls). The acetabular roof angle
decreases still further with advancing age and in the
7-year-old child reaches values of maximally 18°
(boys) and 19° (girls). (Tönnis and Brunken, 1968).

The center-corner angle (*Wi angle of Wiberg;*
1939) cannot be measured before the femoral capital
center of ossification has made its appearance (Fig.
318). In the small child, this angle varies according
to the externally rotated position of the upper leg because at that age the femoral head is apt to undergo
slight lateral deviation. Therefore, in positioning the
child care must be taken to see that both patellae (of
the extended legs) are directed exactly forward (and
upward). The Wi angle is measured between the lines
running parallel through the center of the femoral head
to the longitudinal axis of the body and the line connecting the center of the femoral head with the lateral
corner of the acetabular roof. In the first and second
years of life, values below 10° are pathologic (Thomas
1969). From the third year up to puberty, the lower
limit of normal values is about 15°, and from the 14th
year upward, it is 20°. The degree of the Wi angle
depends on the breadth of the acetabular roof and the
topographic relationship between the femoral head and
the acetabulum. It is therefore a measure both of the

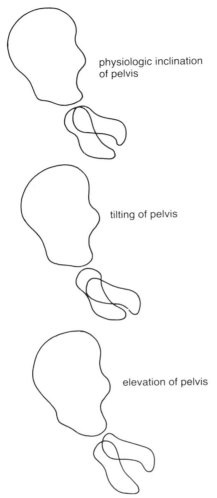

physiologic inclination
of pelvis

tilting of pelvis

elevation of pelvis

Fig. 316 Physiologic inclination of the pelvis, tilting of the pelvis, and elevation of the pelvis. Parameters are the topographic relationships between the cranial ends of the pubis and the ischium. Physiologic inclination of the pelvis, which proves the correct adjustment and positioning of the child, can also be recognized by the fact that the connecting line of Hilgenreiner (Fig. 318) runs approximately between the 4th and the 5th sacral vertebrae.

osseous development of the acetabular roof and the faulty position of the femoral head.

The *vertical line of Ombrédanne* (Fig. 318) gives information about the position and displacement of the ossification center of the femoral head. A plumb line is drawn from the lateral corner of the acetabular roof to the connecting line of Hilgenreiner to form four quadrants. Normally, the capital ossification center lies prevalently in the inner lower quadrant. The vertical line of Ombrédanne then intersects the proximal metaphysis of the femur so that approxi-

mately two thirds lie medially and one third lies laterally to this line.

The line of Shenton-Ménard: Normally, the medial contour of the femoral neck and the cranial contour of the obturator foramen form a smooth, harmonious arc (Fig. 318). This arc is disrupted by subluxation or dislocation of the hip joint *(vide supra).* The usefulness of this line again depends on positioning the child correctly in making a survey film of the pelvis. In the first place, the upper legs should be neither abducted nor adducted but must lie parallel to the longitudinal axis of the body. A glance at the survey film of the pelvis will show whether these conditions have been satisfied. *Lateralization of the cartilaginous femoral head* is present when the so-called diaphyseal spine (the tip of the medially directed femoral neck) lies outside the vertical line of Ombrédanne. *Cranialization of the cartilaginous femoral head* is to be assumed when the diaphyseal spine has crossed the top point of the obturator foramen (Fig. 318).

Finally, it should be pointed out that *in congenital dislocation of the hip the appearance of the ossification center is often delayed* (later than the eighth month) or *that its size lags behind that of the sound side.*

When a congenital dislocation of the hip has been treated for several months by orthopedic immobilization in the position of flexion and abduction, contractures are apt to develop that make it impossible to perform a roentgen examination in the normal position *(vide supra)* without major tilting of the pelvis. The child is then examined in the flexed and abducted position (Lorenz position) to evaluate the development and ossification of the acetabulum, particularly its posterior rim (Fig. 319).

Determination of the *vertical neck-shaft angle* (angle between the center of the femur, the collum femoris, and the diaphysis equals the CCD angle) and the *angle of anteversion* (AV angle) are additional information necessary in regard to children with congenital dislocation of the hip, and, particularly, to the treatment planning. Experience has shown that the AV angle and the CCD angle are the greater the steeper the anatomic acetabular roof is, and that the AV angle becomes the greater the flatter the anterior rim of the acetabulum is. (Gross et al., 1969). Increase of the CCD angle is termed *coxa valga;* when the angle is less than the normal values, *coxa vara* is present.

Coxa valga develops during the period of growth *or* it can be caused by reduction of the work load on the leg through shortening, amputation, or *many years'* confinement in bed. Other etiologies are flaccid and spastic paralysis (absolute or relative weakness of the abductors of the hip in comparison with the adductors) and local disorders of the proximal femoral epiphysis (fracture of the femoral neck, operation, inflammation, tumor). It is also possible that a congenital type of coxa valga exists which is unrelated to the different degrees of dislocation encountered in the common type. *During the growth period,* differences

Fig. 317   **Z line (A) and β angle (B) for the roentgen diagnosis of congenital dislocation of the hip** (Zsernaviczky and Türk, 1974, 1975).

Normal findings: The projecting rim of the acetabulum, the ossification center of the femoral head, and the spine of the femoral diaphysis (see *dashed arrow* in Fig. 318) lie on the Z line. The Z line and the tangent to the proximal femoral metaphysis enclose the β angle. In the first year of life, a β angle of more than 56° is pathologic; the present β angle of less than 50° is definitely normal.

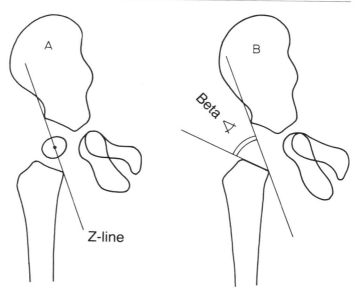

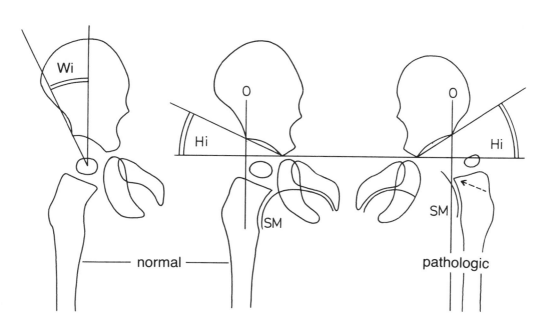

Fig. 318   **Angles and subsidiary lines for the early diagnosis of congenital dislocation of the hip.**
Hi = Acetabular roof angle (Hilgenreiner, 1925).

Wi = Angle of Wiberg (1939), O = Ombrédanne's vertical line. SM = Line of Shenton-Ménard. Besides the other features, the figure on the right presents the following "signs of dislocation": Retarded ossification of the femoral head: primordium of the ossification center in the femoral head lies laterally. Cranial and lateral displacement of the femoral head. The diaphyseal spine *(dashed arrow)* lies above the highest contour of the obturator foramen and outside Ombrédanne's vertical line. The illustrated hypoplasia of the iliac wings (in high congenital dislocation) is due to insufficiency of the gluteal muscles. Such weakness of contraction occurs when origins and insertions of the glutei are greatly approximated.

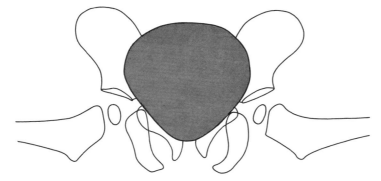

Fig. 319 **Check radiograph with protective screen for the ovaries** following several months' orthopedic immobilization for the treatment of congenital dislocation of the hip. The acetabular roof angle is measurable; the ossification of the posterior rim of the acetabulum can be evaluated.

in leg length accompanied by a compensatory contralateral scoliosis of the lumbar spine and the oblique position of the pelvis therefore can produce a steep, flat acetabulum and sometimes can lead to subluxation of the femoral head—hence to deformities which, in the roentgenogram, cannot be differentiated from congenital dislocation of the hip (Bierkreim, 1974). **Measuring techniques for determining the neck-shaft angle:** The normal CCD angle varies between 120° and 140°, depending on the age of the individual. In the adult, values between 120° and 130° are normal. In infants and small children, one encounters values decreasing from 140° to 130°. The question of whether a normal CCD angle, a coxa valga, or a coxa vara is present can be answered in the following way:

1. In the presence of a normal CCD angle after puberty, the vertical constructed in the longitudinal axis of the femur as a tangent to the greater trochanter runs approximately level with the center of the femoral head (Bessler and Müller, 1963). In coxa valga, it runs below the reference point, and in coxa vara, above it (Fig. 320). This relationship between the tip of the trochanter and the center of the femoral head is largely independent of external rotation of the leg;

i.e., the protective posture of the hip joint (Otte and Seybold, 1974).
2. After puberty, the lesser trochanter has a definite relationship to the femoral head that depends upon the CCD angle (Lange, 1921; Fig. 321).
3. Measurement of the CCD angle following the establishment of the center of the femoral head, the longitudinal axis of the femoral neck and the longitudinal axis of the femoral shaft (Fig. 322). Since the projection of the CCD angle is influenced by anteversion, the legs are positioned in slight internal rotation (of about 20°) for taking the survey film of the pelvis.

Measurement of the angle of anteversion: In the roentgenogram of the hip joint, the AV angle (Fig. 323) can be estimated in so-called false profile ("faux profil," Lequesne 1967). Figure 324 portrays the roentgen findings with normal and with pathologically increased anteversion. In the adult, the normal angle of anteversion varies between 10° and 15°. From infancy through early childhood to puberty, the AV angle decreases from about 35° to adult values. For the purpose of routine diagnosis, the false profile roentgenogram suffices.

For the *preoperative determination* of the AV

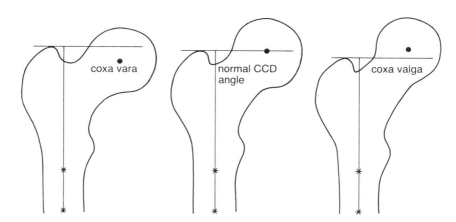

Fig. 320 **Estimation of the neck-shaft angle (CCD angle);** see text.

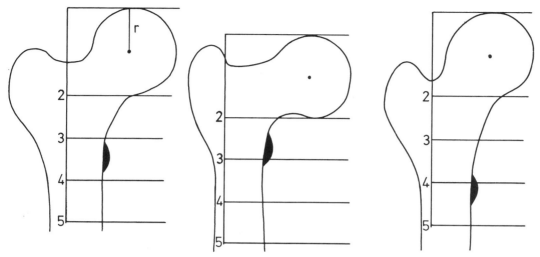

Fig. 321   Determination of coxa vara and coxa valga (method of Lange, 1921). Lines running parallel to the horizontal tangent at the upper border of the femoral head are drawn at distances amounting to 2, 3, 4, and 5 times the radius of the femoral head. (The horizontal tangent is vertical to the axis of the femoral shaft or one of its parallels. Normally, the bulk of the lesser trochanter is found between parallels 3 and 4; in coxa vara it is between 2 and 3, and in coxa valga between 4 and 5.

angle, one makes use primarily of the radiographic techniques of Dunlap, et al. (1953), Ryder and Crane (1953), and Rippstein (1955). To this end, two roentgenograms are needed:

1. A survey film of the pelvis is made in midposition between internal and external rotation (with the patient recumbent, the patellae are directed precisely upward), or the patient is examined in recumbency with his legs dangling across the edge of the Bucky table. In this position, the CCD angle is measured.

2. A roentgenogram is taken in the abducted position. To this end one uses an adjustable leg-holding device which, employing the Rippstein technique, abducts each upper leg about 20°. Both the hip and knee joints of the recumbent patient are flexed 90°; the lower legs are placed in the rests of the holding device, parallel to the longitudinal axis of the body. The transverse bar of the holding device is included in the roentgenogram; it corresponds with the posterior transverse tangent to the femoral condyles or the bicondylar axis of the femur. The so-called central

Fig. 322   Measuring points to determine the CCD angle.

1. Mark out the *center of the femoral head.*

2. Sketch in the *longitudinal axis of the femur:* The circular arc around the center of the femoral head (C) intersects the medial and lateral contours of the femoral neck. A straight line is drawn through the intersections and is then bisected. The connecting line between the center of the femoral head and the point of bisection may be continued as the longitudinal axis of the femur.

3. *Ascertain the longitudinal axis of the femur* (supposing that the femoral shaft is straight and not deformed by rickets or otherwise) = the line connecting the points of bisection of two transverse diameters of the subtrochanteric femoral shaft.

Note: In congenital coxa vara the medial contour of the femoral neck often appears to be absent. In place of the medial point of intersection of the circular arch, one then uses the point where a vertical constructed upon the longitudinal axis of the femoral shaft intersects the highest point of the inferomedial contour of the femoral neck to define its midportion (see Fig. 336).

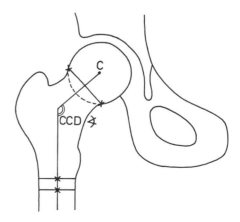

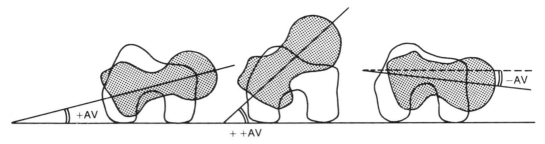

Fig. 323 **The angle of anteversion** is formed by the posterior transverse tangent to the femoral condyles—or else the bicondylar axis—and the axis of the femoral neck. *Left:* Normal anteversion *(viewed from above in the direction of axis of the left femoral shaft). Center:* Increased angle of anteversion (pathologic). *Right:* Negative anteversion (= retroversion). Measurement of the angle by parallel displacement of the condylar tangent of the bicondylar axis.

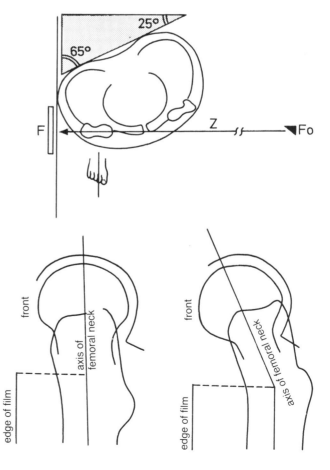

Fig. 324 **False-profile roentgeno-gram** *(faux profil;* Lequesne, 1967) for the identification of increased or diminished anteversion and maldevelopment of the anterior acetabular roof.

Above: Focusing technique with the patient standing, pelvis rotated 25° backward. The foot near the film remains parallel to the latter (F). The so-called central ray (Z) is aimed at the inguinal region of the leg near the focus (Fo). With marked contracture in external rotation (more than 25°), the false-profile focusing technique is no longer applicable because it would mimic an increased anteversion.

Bottom left: With normal anteversion, the parallel drawn through the femoral shaft to the edge of the film and the axis of the femoral neck would form an *approximately* straight line.

Bottom right: With a pathologic increase in anteversion, the axis of the femoral neck is plainly inclined anteriorly, and with retroversion posteriorly.

Table 3   Corrective table of Rippstein (1955) for determination of real CCD angle and AV angle from the angles ascertained roentgenometrically. The real values of the angles sought are found in the square of two intersecting columns. The upper (smaller) figure in the square shows the respective real AV angle. The lower (greater) figure corresponds to the real CCD angle.

		\ Roentgenometric angle of anteversion															
		5	10	15	20	25	30	35	40	45	50	55	60	65	70	75	80
	100	4/101	9/100	15/100	20/100	25/100	30/98	35/99	40/98	45/97	50/96	55/96	60/94	65/94	70/93	75/92	80/91
	105	4/105	10/105	15/104	20/104	25/103	30/103	36/102	41/101	46/100	51/99	56/99	60/97	65/96	70/95	75/94	80/92
	110	5/110	10/110	16/109	21/108	26/108	31/107	37/106	42/105	47/104	52/103	57/101	61/100	66/98	71/97	76/95	80/93
	115	5/115	11/115	16/114	21/112	27/112	32/111	37/110	43/109	48/107	52/105	57/104	62/102	67/101	71/99	76/96	81/94
	120	6/120	11/119	17/118	22/117	28/116	33/115	38/114	44/112	49/110	53/108	58/106	62/104	68/103	72/101	77/98	81/95
Roentgenometric, neck-shaft angle	125	6/125	12/124	17/123	23/121	28/120	34/119	39/118	44/116	50/114	54/112	59/109	63/106	68/105	73/103	77/100	82/96
	130	6/130	12/129	18/127	24/126	29/125	35/124	40/122	46/120	51/117	55/115	60/112	64/109	69/107	73/104	78/101	82/97
	135	6/134	13/133	19/132	25/131	31/130	37/129	42/126	47/123	52/120	57/118	61/114	66/112	70/109	74/105	78/102	83/98
	140	7/139	13/138	20/137	26/135	32/134	38/132	44/130	49/127	53/124	58/120	62/116	67/115	71/111	75/107	79/103	83/100
	145	7/144	14/143	21/142	27/139	33/138	40/136	45/134	51/131	55/128	59/124	63/119	68/117	72/114	76/110	79/104	83/101
	150	8/149	15/147	22/146	29/144	35/143	41/141	47/138	52/135	57/133	61/129	65/124	69/120	73/116	77/112	80/106	84/102
	155	9/154	17/153	25/151	31/149	38/148	44/146	50/142	55/139	59/136	63/132	67/128	71/124	75/119	78/115	81/108	85/103
	160	10/159	19/158	28/157	34/154	41/153	47/151	52/147	57/144	62/140	66/136	69/132	73/128	76/122	79/117	82/111	85/105
	165	12/164	23/164	32/161	40/159	47/158	53/156	58/153	63/149	65/144	69/140	72/135	75/130	78/126	81/119	83/113	86/106
	170	15/169	27/168	37/166	46/164	53/162	58/159	63/157	67/154	71/150	73/145	76/141	78/134	81/129	83/122	85/116	87/109

beam traverses the symphysis pubis. Figure 326 shows the measuring lines designed to ascertain the "measured" *(roentgenometric)* angle of anteversion. As abduction at the hips is bound to produce a standardized error, the *real* angle of anteversion must be calculated trigonometrically and be read on Table 3. By analogy, the *real* CCD angle has to be taken from this table. These, however, are only mathematical approximations which have been corrected in the meantime by Elsasser and Walker (1973; Table 4).

For the management of displaced fractures of the femur in children between the ages of 2 and 12, vertical extension by the procedure of Weber has been recommended (Saxer, 1978). A special traction device (Weber, 1963) enforces the positioning of the child with the hips and knees in 90 degrees of flexion and the upper legs in 20 degrees of abduction (Rippstein position). The pelvic roentgenogram made in this position serves to ascertain the roentgenometric ("measured") angle of anteversion. Angles of anteversion that are equal on both sides rule out any malrotation of the proximal fragment of the femur.

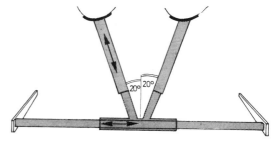

Fig. 325   Leg-holding device for measuring the angle of anteversion after Rippstein (principal structure; commercialy available).

The angle of anteversion can also be measured by computed tomography (Peterson et al., 1981; Grote et al., 1980). The different degrees of congenital dislocation of the hip are shown in the Figures 327 through 329. Specific preoperative roentgenograms are depicted in Figure 330.

Table 4 Corrective table of Elsasser and Walker (1973) for determination of real CCD angle and AV angle (see text). Table also allows measuring the CCD angle in congenital coxa vara.

Roentgenometric, neck-shaft angle	Roentgenometric angle of anteversion															
	5	10	15	20	25	30	35	40	45	50	55	60	65	70	75	80
45	3/45	7/45	10/45	13/46	17/46	21/47	25/47	29/48	33/49	38/50	43/52	49/54	54/57	61/61	68/65	75/71
50	4/50	7/50	11/50	14/51	18/51	22/52	26/52	30/53	35/54	40/56	45/57	50/59	56/62	63/65	69/69	76/74
55	4/55	7/55	11/55	15/56	19/56	23/57	27/57	32/58	37/59	41/61	47/62	52/64	58/66	64/69	70/72	77/76
60	4/60	8/60	12/60	16/61	20/61	24/62	29/62	33/63	38/64	43/65	48/66	53/68	59/70	65/72	71/75	77/78
65	4/65	8/65	12/65	17/66	21/66	25/66	30/67	34/67	39/68	44/69	49/70	55/72	60/73	66/75	72/77	78/79
70	4/70	9/70	13/70	17/70	22/71	26/71	31/71	35/72	40/72	45/73	50/74	56/75	61/76	67/77	72/79	78/81
75	4/75	9/75	13/75	18/75	22/75	27/76	32/76	36/76	41/76	46/77	51/77	57/78	62/79	68/80	73/81	79/82
80	5/80	9/80	14/80	18/80	23/80	28/80	32/80	37/80	42/80	47/80	52/81	58/81	63/81	68/82	74/82	79/83
85	5/85	9/85	14/85	19/85	24/85	28/84	33/84	38/84	43/84	48/84	53/84	58/83	64/83	69/84	74/84	79/84
90	5/90	10/90	15/90	19/89	24/89	29/89	34/88	39/88	44/87	49/87	54/86	59/86	64/86	69/85	75/85	80/85
95	5/95	10/95	15/94	20/94	25/94	30/93	35/92	40/92	45/91	50/90	55/89	60/88	65/88	70/87	75/86	80/86
100	5/100	10/100	15/99	21/99	26/98	31/97	36/96	41/95	46/94	51/93	56/92	61/91	66/90	71/89	75/87	80/86
105	5/105	11/105	16/104	21/103	26/102	32/101	37/100	42/99	47/98	52/96	57/95	62/93	66/92	71/90	76/89	81/87
110	5/110	11/109	16/109	22/108	27/107	32/106	38/104	43/103	48/101	53/99	58/97	62/95	67/94	72/92	76/90	81/88
115	6/115	11/114	17/114	22/113	28/111	33/110	39/108	44/106	49/104	54/102	58/100	63/98	68/96	72/93	77/91	81/89
120	6/120	12/119	18/118	23/117	29/116	34/114	40/112	45/110	50/108	55/105	59/103	64/100	68/97	73/95	77/92	81/90
125	6/125	12/124	18/123	24/122	30/120	35/118	41/116	46/114	51/111	56/108	60/105	65/102	69/99	73/96	78/93	82/90
130	6/130	13/129	19/128	25/127	31/125	37/123	42/120	47/118	52/115	57/111	61/108	66/105	70/102	74/98	78/95	82/91
135	7/135	13/134	20/133	26/131	32/129	38/127	43/124	49/121	53/118	58/115	63/111	67/107	71/104	75/100	79/96	83/92
140	7/140	14/139	21/138	27/136	34/134	40/131	45/129	50/125	55/122	60/118	64/114	68/110	72/106	76/102	79/97	83/93
145	8/145	15/144	22/143	29/141	36/138	41/136	47/133	52/129	57/126	61/122	65/117	69/113	73/108	77/104	80/99	83/94
150	8/150	16/149	24/147	31/145	38/143	44/140	50/137	55/133	59/129	63/125	67/120	71/116	74/111	78/106	81/100	84/95
155	9/155	18/154	27/152	34/150	41/148	47/145	53/141	58/137	62/133	66/129	70/124	73/119	76/113	79/108	82/102	85/96
160	11/160	21/159	31/157	39/155	46/152	52/149	57/145	62/141	66/136	69/132	72/127	75/121	78/115	81/109	83/103	85/97
165	14/165	27/163	38/161	46/158	53/155	59/152	64/148	68/143	71/139	74/134	76/128	79/123	81/117	83/111	85/104	86/98
170	23/169	41/167	52/164	60/160	66/156	70/151	74/147	76/142	78/137	80/131	82/126	83/120	85/114	86/108	87/102	88/96

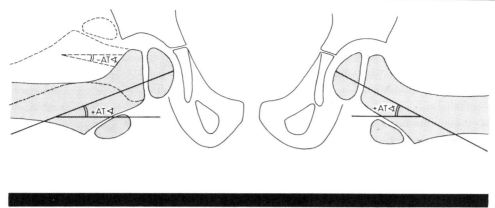

metal bar and its parallels = posterior transverse tangent to the femorfal condyles = bicondylar axis of femur

Fig. 326 Roentgenometric angle of anteversion (+AV angle) determined by the Rippstein technique. The roentgenometric angle of anteversion is formed by the axis of the femoral neck and the parallels to the metal bar. −AV angle = retroversion.

Children with congenital dislocation of the hip develop more often than average an avascular necrosis of the femoral head (**"dislocation-induced Legg-Perthes disease"**). It is still a matter of debate whether the ischemia of the capital center of ossification appears as a sequel to manipulative reposition or to the attitude of retention enforced for months to maintain the result of reposition. (The disorder may also develop on the unaffected side.) In addition, the abduction treatment is said to be capable of producing defects at the lateral junction between the head and neck of the femur (Papadopulos, 1972).

So-called **duplication of the femoral head** (Fig. 331) is apt to follow a (pressure-induced?) damage to the femoral head such as can occur in the treatment of congenital dislocation of the hip, or it may be due to an inflammatory process and also to defective healing of Legg-Perthes disease. Duplication can occur in the sagittal as well as in the frontal plane.

The term **cretin's hip,** which is too limited from the nosological point of view, points to disorders of skeletal maturation and growth in congenital, infantile, or juvenile athyreosis and hypothyroidism. These disorders are demonstrable in the entire skeleton; for

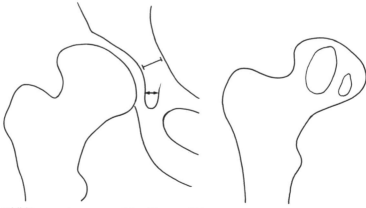

Fig. 327 Dysplasia of the hip in the adult. *Roentgen characteristics:* Steep, flat acetabulum with hypoplasia of the acetabular roof (underdeveloped superior margin of the acetabulum and thickened acetabular floor; decreased roundness of the femoral head. Coxa valga; increased antetorsion. These roentgen signs are encountered in varying degree.

Notes: 1. Dysplasia of the hip exhibits a regular course of the Shenton-Ménard line. In congenital subluxation of the hip, this line is already disrupted. 2. The distance between the two sides of Köhler's tear-shaped figure *(arrow with double point)* corresponds to the thickness of the acetabular floor. Normally, the tear-shaped figure is visible from the 6th month of life onward (Peic, 1971). Thickening of the acetabular floor is also recognizable by the enlargement of this structure opposite the fovea of the femoral head *(marking)*. 3. The larger cystic translucences (sketched at the *right*) are not cysts of osteoarthrotic disintegration, particularly because other roentgen signs of osteoarthrosis are absent. These cysts are apt to regress after a corrective osteotomy; they probably reflect the inadequate adaptability of the femoral head to the unphysiologic strain.

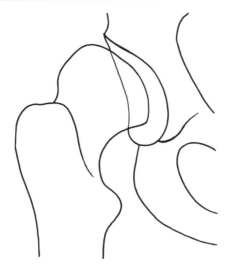

Fig. 328 **Congenital subluxation of the hip in the adult.** *Roentgen characteristics:* Signs of dysplasia of the hip (Fig. 327) with additional disruption of the Shenton-Ménard line. Hence, the femoral head is situated too far superolaterally and is not embraced (not "covered") by the steep, flat, oval acetabulum.

instance, delayed ossification of the epiphyses and retarded epiphyseal closure. They are, however, particularly striking in the hip and produce a preosteoarthrotic deformity there. The delayed ossification of the femoral head has its origin in numerous small, irregular centers which, in typical cases, coalesce to form a broad, flat epiphysis of irregular thickness (Fig. 332) that adapts itself to the femoral neck and thus

appears enlarged and shortened in the roentgenogram. This description shows the similarity between this picture and the stage of fragmentation and remodeling in Legg-Perthes disease (see under this heading). However, the clinical signs of this entity are missing. Besides this, in case of doubt the radiologist can search for other signs of hypothyroidism in the skeleton, such as multicentric ossification in other epiphyses, "stenosis" of the femoral marrow cavity through endosteal thickening of the compacta, pseudoepiphyses in the metacarpals, and so on. The subsequent development of osteoarthrosis is favored not only by the anomalous mushroomlike or rollerlike shape of the femoral head, which may be associated with coxa vara, but frequently also by *deficient ossification* of the femoral head, which manifests itself as largish, rounded, central or marginal translucences.

The survey film of the pelvis revealing the radiographic morphology of the hip joint plays an important part in the diagnosis of certain congenital, mostly inherited, systemic disorders of growth and development of the cartilage and bone tissues. The pathogenesis of these **osteochondrodysplasias** is either not known or has been investigated only fragmentarily. At times these disorders are already present at birth. In other instances, they appear phenotypically in the first years of life or even later. To recognize and classify these diseases, the clinician searches in the first place for parameters such as body height, body proportions, and mobility of joints as well as lesions of skin and nails, dental anomalies, and opacities of the cornea. The *minimum program of roentgen diagnosis* in this group of disorders includes (apart from a survey film of the pelvis) lateral roentgeno-

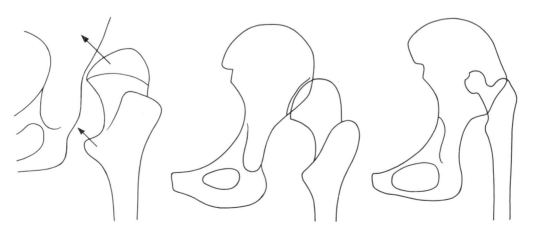

Fig. 329 **Congenital dislocation of the hip.** *Left:* Findings in 14-year-old girl. During the further evolution of the disorder the femoral head, if untreated, probably would become displaced behind the ilium and find a support there (formation of a secondary acetabulum). The lesser trochanter than could give rise to a so-called pelvitrochanteric neoarthrosis *(arrows). Center:* The displaced femoral head has hollowed out for itself a flat secondary acetabulum in the posterior surface of the ilium. In the adult, severe osteoarthrotic lesions and processes of remodeling *(not sketched in)* are always to be anticipated in these cases. *Right:* High posterior dislocation. The femoral head is supported by the gluteal muscles and has no contact with bone. Therefore, neither a secondary osteoarthrosis nor a major remodeling of the underdeveloped femoral head is to be expected.

Fig. 330 **Preoperative roentgenograms with abduction and adduction at the hip joint.** In dysplasia and in subluxation of the hip *(above)* with or without secondary osteoarthrosis, a displacement osteotomy (abduction or adduction osteotomy) often can correct the roofing of the femoral head and/or obtain congruity of the joint. To judge the problem of improved roofing of the femoral head (particularly in children and adolescents), an abduction roentgenogram *(below left)* is needed. Evaluation of the congruity of the joint (in secondary osteoarthrosis) requires *both* an abduction and an adduction roentgenogram *(below left and right).*

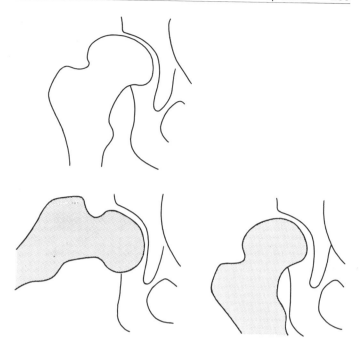

grams of the spine and roentgenograms of the hands, the knee joints, and the lateral skull.

Osteochondrodysplasias with particular involvement of the epiphyses of the long bones—for instance, multiple epiphysial dysplasia (Ribbing disease, Fairbank disease) or dysplasia spondyloepiphysial tarda (Fig. 333)—lead in adult age to severe osteoarthroses, among them, and with special frequency, early osteoarthrosis of the hip. The association of disproportionate ''stunted growth with bilateral osteoarthrosis of the hip'' therefore should always arouse suspicion of an osteochondrodysplasia.

The **mucopolysaccharidoses** and **mucolipidoses** are genetically determined diseases of metabolism and therefore belong to the hereditary systemic disorders of skeletal growth and development of *recognized* pathogenesis. They reflect inborn enzyme defects, namely the insufficient breakdown of complex carbohydrate compounds, the fragments of which are stored in body cells. In the mucopolysaccharidoses, an increased proportion of these fragments is also eliminated by the kidneys. The nosological classification of these disorders depends on the specific enzyme deficiencies and thus on the qualitative and

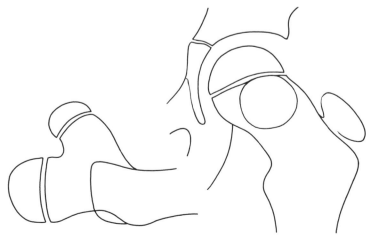

Fig. 331 **Roentgenogram of the femoral head duplicated in the sagittal plane** (see text). *Right:* anteroposterior roentgenogram. *Left:* Frog position roentgenogram. With duplication in the frontal plane, the anteroposterior roentgenogram *(not illustrated)* reveals the more or less bipartite cap of the femoral head.

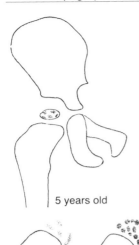

5 years old

7 years old

20 years old

Fig. 332 **Instances of the so-called cretin's hip.**
Five years old: Small proximal epiphysis of femur with stippled areas of increased density. No ossification center yet visible in greater trochanter.
Seven years old: Eccentric center of epiphyseal ossification or mulberry-shaped ossification of the capital epiphysis of the femur.
Twenty years old: Epiphyseal closure still incomplete. Flattened upper femoral epiphysis with structure of irregular density. Irregular contour of acetabulum. Femoral neck shortened and enlarged.

quantitative differences in the occurrence and distribution of the stored products, as well as on genetic points of view and clinical criteria. The mucopolysaccharidoses and mucolipidoses are typified by Roman numerals (I to VII) and by adding proper names. The most frequent mucopolysaccharidosis (I–H, the Hurler-Pfaundler syndrome, also known as dysostosis multiplex) is characterized by skeletal anomalies which, in varying degrees of severity, are also demonstrable in the other mucopolysaccharidoses and mucolipidoses, in mannosidosis, fucosidosis, the gangliosidoses, and similar disorders. The roentgen diagnosis "dysostosis multiplex," therefore, should prompt the referring physician to differentiate *the individual* mucopolysaccharidoses and mucolipidoses on the basis of clinical, genetic, biochemical and other points of view!

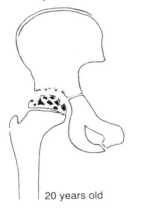

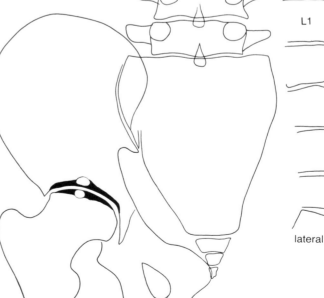

L1

lateral

Fig. 333 **Dysplasia spondyloe-piphysaria tarda.** Usual manifestation between the 6th and 12th years of life. In adulthood, early osteoarthrosis, especially in the hip joint (as illustrated) and in the shoulder joint.

Fig. 334 **Roentgen appearance of the hip in mucopolysaccharidosis and mucolipidosis** (*upper row:* growth period; *lower row:* adulthood). The deformities are demonstrable in *both* hip joints. In the differential diagnosis, other skeletal roentgen findings of dysostosis multiplex (gargoylism; Fig. 335) should be searched for. Athyreosis and hypothyroidism (Fig. 332) as well as the sequelae of a polyarthritis in early childhood and septicopyemia in infancy must be ruled out.

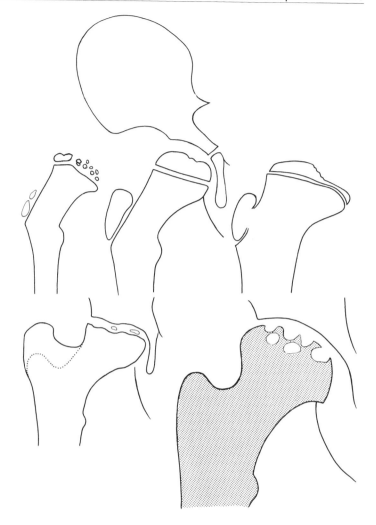

From the second year of life on, the roentgen characteristics of dysostosis multiplex are (Figs. 334 and 335; Kozlowski and Rupprecht, 1972; Spranger et al., 1974):

• *Cranium:* Macrocephaly, dyscephaly, atypical profil of the sella (Fig. 335), thickened cap
• *Thorax:* Lateral and anterior costal segments resembling oar blades, clavicles short and stubby, scapulae deformed
• *Spine:* Vertebral bodies ovoid, in the thoracolumbar junction resembling fishhooks on lateral roentgenograms; vertebrae flat
• *Pelvis:* Iliac wings resembling "mouse ears" (Fig. 334); acetabulum deformed, disordered development and ossification of the proximal femoral epiphysis, coxa valga
• *Long tubular bones:* Short and coarsened irregular contours of diaphyses, beveled distal radius and ulna
• *Short tubular bones:* Shortening, metaphyses enlarged, epiphyseal dysplasia (malformation), proximal ends of the metacarpals II to V conical, phalanges resembling sugar loaves
• *Bone structure:* Osteoporosis, coarse strains of cancellous bone

Besides this, the following *characteristic* combination of roentgen signs is demonstrable in mucopolysaccharidosis IV Morqio: Generalized flatness of vertebrae is apparent. The vertebral bodies in the thoracolumbar region have hooklike (tonguelike) anterior extensions. The odontoid process of the axis is hypoplastic, and there is atlantoaxial instability (an indispensable sign also in mucolipidosis III). Bilateral dysplasia of the hip (malformation of the acetabular roof, disordered ossification and shape of the femoral head), bilateral coxa valga. Bilateral genu valgum due to lateral hypoplasia of the proximal portions of the tibiae and the lateral condyles of the femur. Conical shape of the proximal ends of the metacarpals II to V.

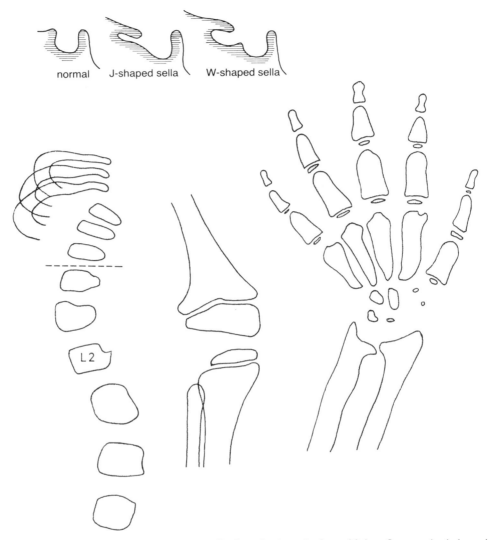

normal   J-shaped sella   W-shaped sella

Fig. 335 **Characteristic extrapelvic roentgen findings in dysostosis multiplex.** *Cue words:* J-shaped sella turcica; W-shaped sella; oar-blade shape of the ribs; persistence of ovoid infantile shape of the vertebral bodies; flat vertebrae; fishhook dysplasia of the vertebrae in the thoracolumbar junction, also beyond infancy (see Fig. 609). Genu valgum; distal slope of ulna and radius; proximal metacarpals conical; phalanges resembling sugar-loaves.

In the Mseleni district of North Zululand (South Africa), a hereditary generalized malformation of the epiphyses with or without involvement of the spine has been observed among the native population—Mseleni joint syndrome—which leads to early osteoarthrotic lesions.

The radiographic morphology of **congenital (infan-tile) coxa vara** was described on page 211. The un-derlying cause for the deformity is a disorder of the proximal metaphysis of the femur that must become operative during the second year of life. It gives rise to the **shepherd's staff deformity** of the proximal femur. This deformity is a preosteoarthrosis of the hip joint (Fig. 336). On the other hand, the term "shepherd's staff deformity" is also applied to the malformation of the femur in fibrous dysplasia (Fig. 337). Furthermore, **symptomatic coxa vara** must be differentiated, also roentgenographically, from con-genital coxa vara. Symptomatic coxa vara is in some cases a partial manifestation of a *generalized* de-crease in skeletal strength, for instance in rickets—*rachitic coxa vara* (Fig. 338)—in osteomalacia, in the skeletal manifestations of hyperparathyroidism,

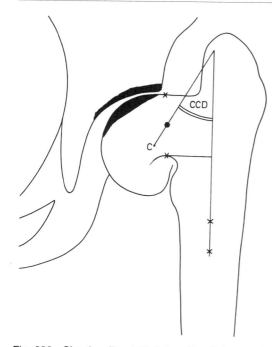

and so on. Symptomatic coxa vara can also develop as a result of *local* damage to the neck-shaft junction; e.g., following trauma or owing to inflammatory processes localized there. A symptomatic decrease of the neck-shaft angle is accompanied by deformation in the region of the femoral head and neck only when the underlying process has a damaging effect on the proximal femoral epiphysis or on the metaphysis. For instance, an osteomyelitis in the metaphysis of the femoral neck or a fracture of the femoral neck (infrequent in early childhood) can give rise to a malformation that resembles congenital coxa vara but differs from its primary and secondary type by *additional* changes in bone structure (scars) in the region of the femoral head and neck (compare p. 211 ff).

Epiphyseal separation of the upper end of the femur is still sometimes called adolescent or epiphyseal coxa vara. This term, however, should no longer be used because other disorders that likewise can present a decreased neck-shaft angle (Legg-Perthes disease, for instance) would then also have to be included in the coxa vara group.

Legg-Calvé-Perthes (-Waldenström) disease is an avascular (aseptic) necrosis of the femoral head occurring between the ages of 3 and 10 (occasionally 15) years; it is found much more commonly in boys than in girls. The disease occurs about ten times less frequently in Negroes than in other races (Golding et al., 1959). This circumstance speaks in favor of a genetic predisposition, as does the experience that in some of these patients disorders of skeletal maturation—generally retardation and rarely acceleration—are found (Katz and Siffert, 1977). Bilateral involvement does occur; in such instances, the femoral heads

Fig. 336 Shepherd's staff deformity of the proximal femur in congenital coxa vara with secondary osteoarthrosis of the hip. The measuring points and lines to ascertain the neck-shaft angle (CCD angle) are sketched in (see legend accompanying Fig. 322). Secondary osteoarthrosis of the hip following congenital coxa vara cannot, as a rule, be expected to develop before the second half of life.

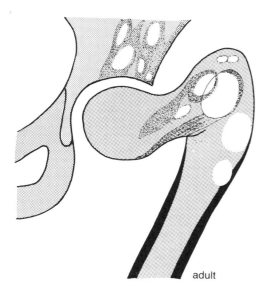
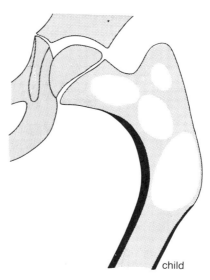

Fig. 337 Shepherd's staff deformity of the proximal femur in fibrous dysplasia. The typical curving develops as a consequence of the normal cancellous and cortical bone being replaced by statically insufficient fibrous bone and the endosteal cortical bone being resorbed.

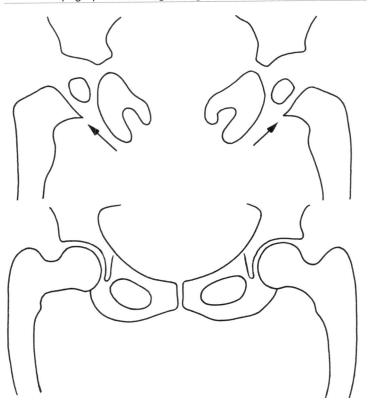

Fig. 338 **Rachitic coxa vara,** *above* in a 6-month-old child, *below* in an adult. The *pointed* so-called diaphyseal spine *(arrows)* is a sign of rickets; coxa vara is recognizable by the steep course of the epiphysis and the equally steep contour of the metaphysis.

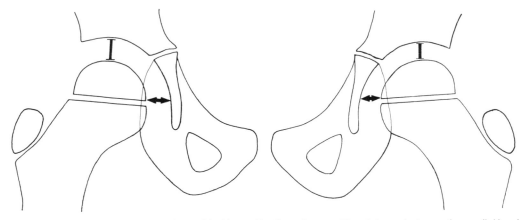

Fig. 339   **Early roentgen signs of right-sided Legg-Perthes disease.** The distance between the medial border of the upper femoral epiphysis and the lateral contour of Köhler's tear-shaped figure is increased in comparison with the unaffected side *(arrows)*. The same is true of the distance between the upper femoral epiphysis and the acetabular roof *(markings)*.

Note: In fleeting childhood coxitis (pp. 213 and 214), the distance between the upper femoral epiphysis and the acetabulum is sometimes also increased (distention-[sub-]luxation) (Anderson and Stewart, 1970) so that this finding, without modifications of contours (different on the two sides) and/or structural lesions in the femoral head can only be considered as suggestive evidence of Legg-Perthes disease.

Fig. 340   **Roentgen signs of early Legg-Perthes disease** (continued). The roentgenogram in dorsal decubitus (A) shows flattening of the femoral head with hazy contours *(arrow)*. In comparison with the unaffected side, the height of the femoral head, in addition, appears to be diminished in its entirety *(not illustrated)*. In the Frog position roentgenogram (B), an additional *subchondral marginal fracture,* is visible which *in this instance,* as frequently happens, is not demonstrable in the roentgenogram A.

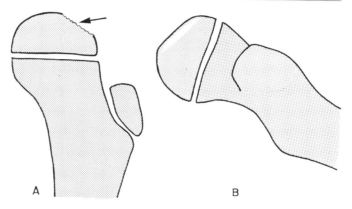

A   B

are affected with great regularity, *one following the other,* mostly at an interval of a few months. This observation is of importance in the differential diagnosis because *synchronous* involvement speaks against Legg-Perthes disease and, rather, suggests an epiphyseal disorder of different (hormonal, hereditary) genesis (compare Figs. 332 and 334 that present a roentgenographic morphology similar or even identical to the fragmentation stage in Legg-Perthes disease; see Fig. 341). Legg-Perthes disease of the femoral head tends to recur very rarely (Kemp et al., 1971). Only on rare occasions is injury to the hip (contusion, dislocation) occurring at the age typical of Legg-Perthes disease followed by this illness (Hofer, 1973). For that matter, it is a matter of debate whether Legg-Perthes disease is not primarily a necrosis of the femoral head due to arterial ischemia but rather the sequel to a chronic trauma that causes the femoral head to be compressed by the acetabular roof (Caffey, 1968).

In undertaking the clinical differential diagnosis of Legg-Perthes disease, one must pay attention to the limitation of hip mobility. A tentative bedside diagnosis is based on the limitation of abduction (adduction contracture). Limitation of movement on all sides suggests coxarthritis. In adolescence, an inhibition of internal rotation from a resting position of external rotation arouses suspicion of epiphysiolysis.

The *early roentgenographic signs* of the disorder take a number of months to become manifest. Therefore, follow-up checks must be made when the roentgen findings are normal but Legg-Perthes disease is suspected clinically. The most frequent roentgen signs are as follows:

1.   *Widening of the medial portion of the joint space* as compared with the unaffected side (Fig. 339). Histologic studies have shown that this roentgen finding is due to thickening of the cartilage in the femoral head (Larsen and Reimann 1973; Robichon et al., 1974). Since the difference between the two sides is only a few millimeters, any asymmetry in positioning must be avoided and ruled out. Asymmetries are recognized by the different projection of the obturator foramen and the iliac wing; the "smaller" obturator foramen then indicates the direction in which the pel-

vis (i.e., the patient) has rotated. In contrast, the width of the gap between the femoral head and the acetabular roof is independent of the rotation of the pelvis; therefore it also has been recommended for the comparison between the two sides (Papadopulos and Malahias, 1973; Fig. 339).
2.   *Subchondral marginal fracture of* the upper epiphyseal nucleus of the femur, which usually is slightly flattened (has lost its roundness) and which in the flattened area often displays hazy contours (Fig. 340). The site of most severe involvement is the superoanterolateral segment of the head. This is why the pathologic roentgen findings listed are most distinctly (or even exclusively) demonstrable in the frog position roentgenogram.

Occasionally, a vacuum phenomenon may develop at the site of the fracture and in the anatomical joint space. The vacuum phenomenon then will be detectable on the roentgenogram taken in the frog position.
3.   Sparing of the painful hip can, after a few months, manifest itself by *disuse osteoporosis* in the vicinity of the acetabulum and in the femoral neck (compare with the unaffected side).

The *typical* further evolution of Legg-Perthes disease during a number of years can be surmised from Figure 341, which chiefly shows:

·   Diffuse increased density of the femoral head
·   So-called fragmentation of the femoral head
·   Metaphyseal defects
·   Typical deformity of the femoral head (in the shape of a roller or mushroom)
·   Shortening and enlargement of the femoral neck
·   Coxa vara
·   Elevation of the greater trochanter

The fragmentation is caused mechanically by the compressive strain on the necrotic femoral head and by the pressure of the growing cartilage cover of the capital epiphysis of the femur (Otte, 1968) as well as by repair processes. These processes are associated with the proliferation of noncalcified cartilagenous cells between the necrotic trabeculae of the spongiosa, such as occur in enchondral ossification (Larsen and Rein-

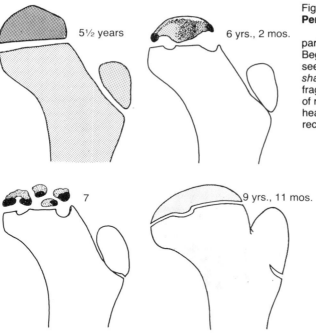

5½ years

6 yrs., 2 mos.

7

9 yrs., 11 mos.

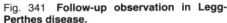

Fig. 341 Follow-up observation in Legg-Perthes disease.
Above left: Slightly increased density and partial flattening of femoral head. *Above right:* Beginning of repair process (revascularization; see text). Marginal subchondral fracture *(non-shaded area). Below left:* Full-blown stage of fragmentation (see text). *Below right:* Process of repair and remodeling of the femoral neck and head area (small metaphyseal translucence still recognizable).

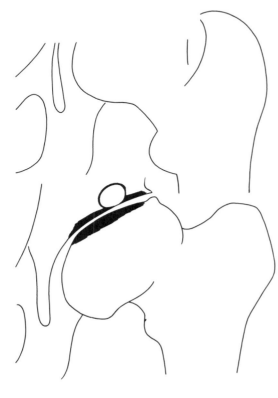

mann, 1973). The ingrowth of vascular and connective tissue leads to the resorption of devitalized bony trabeculae and to the formation of new bone, which may originate from various centers ("fragments") mostly lying medial and lateral to the necrotic remainder of the epiphysis (Bergstrand and Norman, 1961). These histologic processes are visible in the roentgenogram as circumscribed "translucences" and circumscribed areas of "increased density" in the femoral head, which present, or at least accentuate, the appearance of a fragmentation.

Metaphyseal defects in the femoral neck point to a disorder of enchondral ossification in the proximal epiphysis of the femur. These defects are produced by tonguelike expansions of cartilage invading the femoral neck and by islets of noncalcified and proliferating ephiphyseal cartilage (Ponsetti, 1956; Caffey, 1968). Because of these defects it may become difficult, in a given case, to differentiate Legg-Perthes disease from osteomyelitis of the femoral neck

Fig. 342 Status after healed Legg-Perthes disease
Above: 21-year-old individual. Roller-shaped head to which the acetabulum has adjusted itself. Femoral neck shortened. Coxa vara. *Below:* 59-year-old individual. Secondary osteoarthrosis as a sequel to Legg-Perthes disease.

with a subsequent disturbance of the blood supply to the upper epiphyseal nucleus of the femur. In such instances it is advisable to search for delicate periosteal lamellae at the medial contour of the femoral neck (Fig. 293), the roentgen signs of an effusion into the hip joint (Fig. 291), and pericoxal edema (Fig. 292). All these signs are lacking in Legg-Perthes disease. The shortness of the femoral neck also reflects the disorder of enchondral longitudinal growth of the proximal epiphysis. Since the progression of the periosteal growth of the femoral neck parallels the development of the greater trochanter, the femoral neck enlarges, and coxa vara and elevation of the trochanter ensue. With increasing revascularization, the growing bony fragments "fuse," and the head enlarges until finally it assumes the shape of a mushroom or a roller (Figs. 341 and 342). The acetabulum adjusts itself to the remodeling of the femoral head. This preosteoarthrotic deformity is followed, generally after several decades (commonly after the 50th year of life) by osteoarthrosis of the hip (Fig. 342). The treatment should interrupt this evolution of avascular necrosis of the femoral head into the preosteoarthrotic deformity. Therapy is the more promising the earlier the disease is radiographically diagnosed.

A vascular necrosis of the femoral head, for instance in Gaucher's disease or in sickle cell anemia, presents itself in the roentgenogram under the guise of Legg-Perthes disease.

Slipping of the capital femoral epiphysis—juvenile separation of the femoral head—commonly manifests itself clinically between the 12th and 15th years of life, hence in puberty. On the average, girls become affected somewhat earlier than boys. Slipping of the capital femoral ephiphysis has been observed prior to that age; for instance, following radiotherapy of a malignant tumor when the epiphyseal zone had been exposed to the cone of rays (Wolf et al., 1977).

Uremic epiphysiolysis (which occurs in the aetting of renal osteopathy) is not linked to a definite age but owes its development exclusively to the failure of epiphyseal closure (Kirkwood et al., 1972). Certain constitutional types, such as adiposogenital dystrophy, eunuchoidism, and giantism, occur with particular frequency among patients with slipping of the capital femoral epiphysis (Taillard, et al., 1964) and may suggest the (etiologic) hormonal dysregulation. Slipping of the femoral head is typically preceded by a complete break in continuity of the epiphyseal cartilage. The break, however, leaves the actual zone of cartilage proliferation completely intact. This zone lies proximal to the gap so that growth as a rule continues after the epiphysiolysis has come to a halt either spontaneously or in response to therapy. Hence, shortening of the concerned leg does not belong among the clinical findings following slipping of the capital femoral epiphysis.

In epiphysiolysis, the roentgenogram not only settles the diagnosis but also indicates the direction and the degree of the displacement of the femoral head.

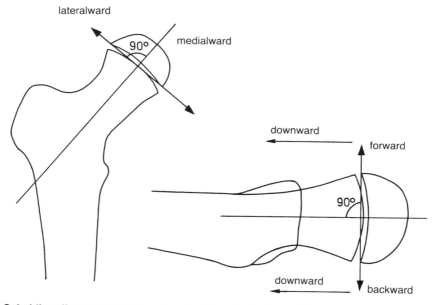

Fig. 343 **Subsidiary lines to determine the direction of slipping of the femoral head in slipping of the capital femoral epiphysis.** Normally, in the anteroposterior roentgenogram the projection of the femoral head is approximately bisected by the longitudinal axis of the femoral neck. The base line of the cap and the longitudinal axis of the femoral neck form an angle of 90°. Also in the Lauenstein roentgenogram (frog position; for focusing technique, see text), the base line of the cap normally is vertical to the longitudinal axis of the femoral neck.

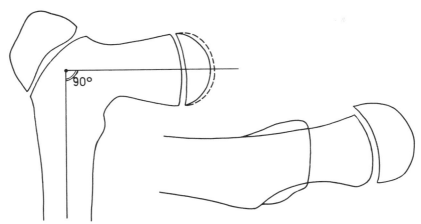

Fig. 344 **With a neck-shaft angle of 90°,** the separated femoral epiphysis is tilted *anteroinferiorly* (compare Fig. 343; see text).

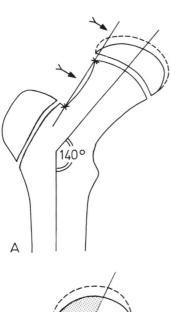

A

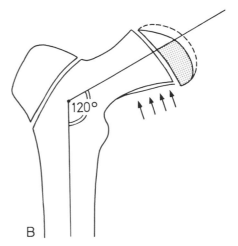

B

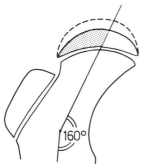

Fig. 345 **The direction of slipping of the femoral head depends on the degree of the neck-shaft angle.** (compare Fig. 344).

A: With 140°, the slipping proceeds *postero*inferiorly. The original projection of the femoral head is *dashed* (compare with the sound side). As a result of the slipping, the height of the femoral head in the roentgenogram is diminished (*roentgen sign:* "setting sun"). (See also B and C).

Tailed arrows: With displacement of the femoral head, the tangent to the superior contour of the femoral neck intersects a smaller segment of the femoral head than on the sound side or does not cross the femoral head at all (see B).

B: Direction of posteroinferior and *medial* displacement with a neck-shaft angle of about 120°. The longitudinal axis of the femoral neck intersects the femoral head eccentrically. *Arrows:* Bone-forming periosteal lamella lifted at the medial contour of the femoral neck. (Lifting triggered by the slipping.)

C: With a neck-shaft angle of about 160°, the femoral head slips posteroinferiorly and *laterally.*

In undertaking the radiographic examination, a standardized focusing technique is advisable, especially with regard to surgical therapy (Imhäuser, 1969). For the anteroposterior roentgenogram, the anterior surface of the patella should lie exactly parallel to the plane of the Bucky table. To this end, it may be necessary to lift the pelvis on the affected side (with the aid of pillows). In this way the anteroposterior roentgenogram may also reveal whether or not the gliding process takes place medialward or lateralward (Fig. 343). The Frog position I roentgenogram (taken with flexion, abduction, and external rotation at the hip joint) shows the posteroinferior or anteroinferior displacement of the head cap. To this end, the leg is rotated externally to such a degree that the lower leg, flexed at the knee joint, lies parallel to the Bucky table. With this focusing technique, the line connecting the two corners of the femoral heads (the base line of the cap) normally is perpendicular to the longitudinal axis of the femoral neck (Fig. 343).

The direction of displacement of the femoral head depends on the neck-shaft angle (CCD angle) (Imhäuser, 1969)! With a CCD angle of about 90°, the femoral head slips *antero*inferiorly (Fig. 344); with a CCD angle of about 120°, it slips posteroinferiorly and *medially* (Fig. 345B); with a CCD angle of about 140°, it slips *postero*inferiorly (Fig. 345 A), and with a CCD angle of 160°, it slips posteroinferiorly and *laterally* (Fig. 345 C). Posteroinferior displacement is the one most frequently observed (in more than four fifths of the cases) so that it can be said that epiphysiolysis occurs chiefly with a steep neck-shaft angle.

Since in the majority of cases juvenile separation of the femoral head occurs bilaterally (mostly successively), the roentgenographic morphology of **premobile loosening of the epiphysis** is likewise known. In comparison with the sound side (and with the epiphysis of the greater trochanter), the loosened epiphyseal cartilage appears enlarged and, moreover, the metaphyseal contour of the epiphysis is indefinite in outline (Fig. 346). The metaphyseal bone structure is loosened and slightly decalcified. However, the axial relationships are normal (Fig. 343). The temporal and spatial relationships *(vide supra)* of the displacement of the femoral head reveal certain regular features which are reflected by the nonmenclature proposed by *Imhäuser*. "Softening" of the metaphysis (occurring dorsally when the displacement is directed posteroinferiorly) causes the femoral head to tilt *slowly* in a posteroinferior direction without the spatial displacement manifesting itself by the formation of a step between the contour of the femoral neck and the base of the femoral head *(tilting stage; Fig. 347 top)*. In the *shearing stage* (tilting plus slipping), the Frog position I roentgenogram reveals a step between the head and the neck of the femur (Fig. 347, center). *Acute slipping* (Fig. 347, bottom) in the direction predetermined by the neck-shaft angle presupposes a complete break in continuity of the epiphyseal cartilage and produces acute symptoms resembling a fracture of the femoral neck. In the roentgenogram, one sees a gaping cleft between the femoral head and neck,

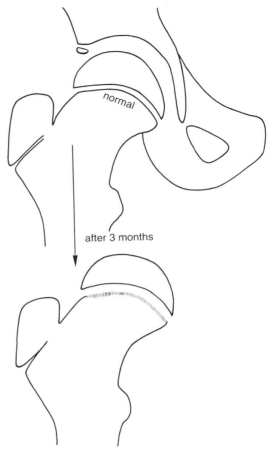

Fig. 346 **Premobile slipping of the capital femoral epiphysis.** *Roentgen signs:* Slight enlargement of the epiphysis; haziness of its metaphyseal contour; slight reduction of epiphyseal height possibly already demonstrable (compare with sound side).

with the femoral head "riding" more or less distinctly on the border of the metaphysis.

In addition, the following roentgen signs suggest separation of the epiphysis: The femoral head on the affected side is lower than that on the sound side (roentgen sign of the "setting sun," Fig. 345). The tangent to the superior contour of the femoral neck either intersects a smaller segment of the head than on the unaffected side, or, even, becomes a tangent to the cap, or no longer meets the femoral head (Fig. 345). A delicate periosteal lamella is recognizable on the medial side of the femoral neck (Fig. 345 B). The juvenile epiphysiolysis comes to a halt with the age-related ossification of the proximal epiphyseal cartilage. Figure 348 shows a case in which either the slipping was not diagnosed and therefore not treated or the treatment was inadequate. The typical hump developing on the femoral neck (Fig. 348, *arrow)* can restrict the movements at the hip joint considerably. Furthermore, every hip joint with an epiphysi-

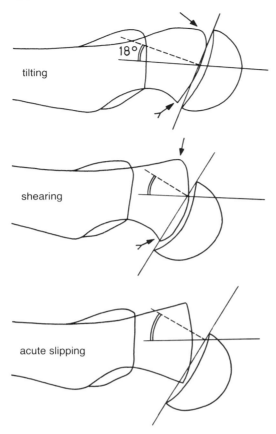

Fig. 347   Data on juvenile slipping of the capital femoral epiphysis obtained from the Frog position roentgenogram.
Above and center: Femoral head and neck remain in contact, but axial relationships are disturbed (measurable tilting angle above = 18°). Therefore *slow* slipping in a *posteroinferior* direction is occurring. No step is demonstrable between the contour of the femoral neck and the base of the femoral head (= *tilting* stage). By contrast, the drawing in the *center* does show a step (= *shearing stage*). Arrows point to metaphyseal areas in which slow slipping is accompanied by adaptive processes of remodeling (*arrow* = area of bone resorption; *tailed arrow* = area of bone formation).
Below: Gaping cleft between the neck and head of femur as well as femoral head riding on posterior border of femoral neck are indicative of *acute slipping* in posteroinferior direction.
Note: Acute slipping may follow both the stage of premobile loosening (Fig. 346) and the other stages.

olysis whose tilting angle exceeds 40–45° is threatened by osteoarthrosis of the hip.

A complication of untreated or (surgically) treated—hence diagnosed—slipped proximal femoral epiphysis must be considered when the pain increases without an exterior cause or when an impairment of joint mobility is demonstrable. Such complications are:

- Further displacement of the femoral head
- Avascular (aseptic) necrosis of the femoral head (Mickelson et al., 1979; for roentgen signs see pp. 251–252)
- Necrosis of the articular cartilage (so-called chondrolysis)
- Postoperative infection (leukocytosis, increased sedimentation rate, etc.)

So-called **chondrolysis of the hip joint** occurs as a complication of juvenile epiphysiolysis as well as on the sound contralateral side and, very infrequently, even *without* epiphysiolysis (El-Khoury and Mickelson, 1977; see also p. 254). *Histological* findings in such cases are dead chondrocytes, loss of the upper layers of the acetabular cartilage, and an inflammatory reaction of the synovial membrane (Goldman et al., 1978).

The following roentgen findings are indicative of chondrolysis:

- Extensive concentric narrowing of the roentgenologic cartilage space (to at least 50 percent of that on the sound side)
- Flat erosions of the femoral head and/or the acetabulum may be seen.
- Osteoporosis (of disuse?) in the vicinity of the joint

Chondrolysis is reversible with the cartilage space regaining its normal width (compare with the sound side). Bony ankylosis ensues infrequently, but the condition may terminate in osteoarthrosis of the hip (Maurer and Larsen, 1970).

Intrapelvic protrusion of the acetabulum may be either unilateral or bilateral. A slight intrapelvic bulge of the acetabulum between the seventh year of life and puberty (*physiologic prominence of the acetabular floor,* Imhäuser, 1952) is a normal event related to adolescence (Fig. 349). In this case, the acetabulum thickens, but the head of the femur shows no displacement into the acetabulum such as in actual protrusion of the acetabulum. In the adult, however, the condition must always be regarded as a pathologic finding, whether it be primary or secondary in origin (Fig. 350).

Primary (idiopathic) protrusion of the acetabulum is a deformity that is found more often in females than in males. Various causes are debated; e.g., coxa vara with retroversion of the femoral neck that generally coexists, or premature closure of the Y-shaped acetabular epiphysis so that in this instance the regression of the physiologic prominence of the acetabulum fails to take place. Apart from the still debatable cause of idiopathic intrapelvic protrusion of the acetabulum, it is an established fact that this acetabular deformity originates at adolescence.

Secondary protrusion of the acetabulum occurs at any age, principally with inflammatory destruction of the acetabulum (Fig. 350), in Paget's disease, as a result of osteoporotic or osteomalacic lesions of the skeleton, in osteoradionecrosis following radiotherapy of the pelvic organs (Hasselbacher and Schu-

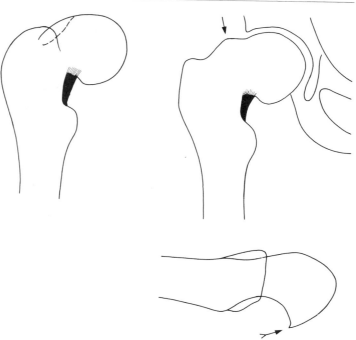

Fig. 348 **Posteroinferior juvenile slipping of the capital femoral epiphysis stabilized with deformation.** *Arrow* points to typical hump on femoral neck. *Tailed arrow* points to equally typical spur (Lauenstein roentgenogram: frog position). Appearance of the hump on the femoral neck depends on the degree of slipping and is thus *not* an indispensable roentgen finding *(left)*. Adam's arc—the medial cortex of the femoral neck—follows a steep course. In contrast to the reformation in Legg-Perthes disease, the acetabulum retains its normal shape! The normal superior contour of the femoral neck in the presence of a femoral head that has not slipped and has not been remodeled by osteoarthrosis is indicated by *dashed lines*.

macher, 1977), and as an aftermath of trauma. Paget's disease of the proximal femur leads to coxa vara.

Among the causes of **osteochondrosis dissecans** (Fig. 351) affecting the femoral head and, less frequently, the acetabulum are segmental avascular (aseptic) necrosis of bone, ossification centers that remain isolated, fatigue fractures (compare p. 299 ff), and also osteochondrodysplasias and mucopolysaccharidoses (see Fig. 334). Finally, in the repairing

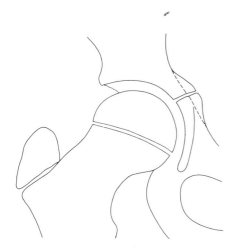

Fig. 349 **Physiologic prominence of the acetabular floor at prepuberty.** (*Dashed* line continues the course of the linea terminalis that would have been anticipated).

stages of Legg-Perthes disease, individual centers of ossification may fail to fuse with the bulk of the remodeled femoral head and then may also appear to be dissected. Osteochondrosis dissecans may occur bilaterally (Guilleminet and Barbier, 1957). It is readily diagnosed in the roentgenogram, but the radiographic appearance offers no more than conjectures regarding the etiology.

Devitalization of the bone of the proximal end of the femur in adult life—**adult avascular necrosis of the femoral head**—is recognizable in the roentgenogram, but its pathogenesis and etiology are widely debated. *Idiopathic* necrosis of the femoral head (i.e., a disorder of unknown origin) commonly occurs between the ages of 30 and 50. In nearly 50 percent of such cases, the disease becomes bilateral after a number of months or years. Its counterpart is *symptomatic* necrosis of the femoral head. The literature of the past decades shows that the group of idiopathic necroses has been decreasing in number as compared with the symptomatic necroses. It should be mentioned, however, that particularly casuistic publications do not always make a clear distinction between coincidence—i.e., fortuitous concurrence—and causality. *For instance,* it is quite possible in gout that demonstrable deposits of urate crystals in a necrosis of the femoral head have led to a devitalization of bone. On the other hand, this finding may be evidence of a dystrophic elimination of urates into necrotic tissue (of different origin?), analogous to dystrophic tissue calcification (Doerr, 1974).

Roentgen signs of adult necrosis of the femoral head:

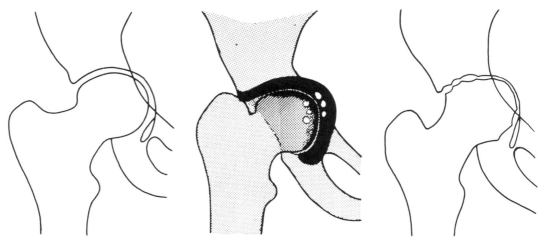

Fig. 350 **Intrapelvic protrusion of the acetabulum.** *Left* and *center: Primary* (idiopathic) type. *Right: Secondary,* inflammatory protrusion of the acetabulum, in the present instance accompanying rheumatoid arthritis. The sketch in the *center* illustrates the marked sclerosis of the acetabulum, narrowing of the joint space, and detritus cysts (secondary osteoarthrosis).

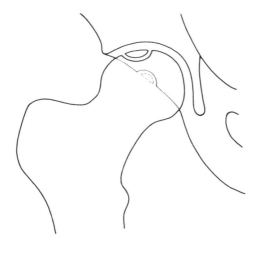

Fig. 351 **Osteochondrosis dissecans of the femoral head.** The "joint mouse" has not (yet) left its "bed." Osteochondrosis dissecans is much less frequent in the acetabulum than in the femoral head.

Prior to diagnosing osteochondrosis dissecans of the acetabulum, the following conditions must be differentiated: fracture of the acetabular rim; accessory bones of the acetabular rim (Heidenblut, 1963; indicated by *dashed* line); osteomyelitic dissection of the acetabular rim; circumscribed ossification of the acetabular lip; metaplastic ossification close to the origin of the iliofemoral ligament; osteochondropathy of the anteroinferior iliac spine (De Cuveland and Heuck, 1951); avulsion fracture or a persistent epiphyseal nucleus of the anteroinferior iliac spine (compare Fig. 389), and the radiologic os acetabuli. This osseous element increases in frequency with advancing age (Schmidt and Braun, 1961) so that circumscribed metaplasias of the capsule of the hip joint are debated as being its morphologic substrate. In addition, this element could be derived from the persisting apophysis of the acetabular rim or from the persisting, often polynuclear, os coxae quartum (anatomic os acetabuli) so that these two elements also have to be differentiated from osteochondrosis dissecans of the acetabulum.

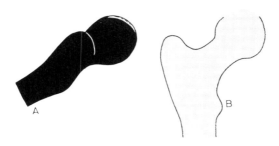

Fig. 352 **Early roentgen signs of adult necrosis of the femoral head.**

A = Accurate subchondral fracture line reflecting a fatigue fracture. It is seen with particular frequency in the superoanterolateral region of the femoral head and therefore is best or exclusively visible in the Frog position roentgenogram.

B = Circumscribed resorption (decalcification) of the marginal subchondral lamella in the superolateral region of the femoral head. *Clinically,* no signs of inflammation. The patient gives a history of a fall while skiing downhill 9 months previously, with fracture of both malleoli.

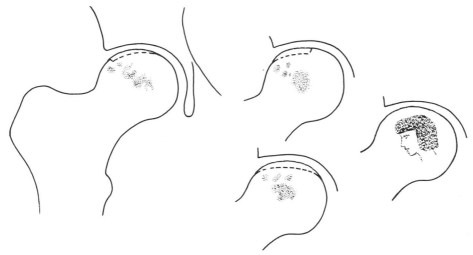

Fig. 353 Early roentgen signs of adult necrosis of the femoral head (continued). Delicate, irregularly shaped and irregularly distributed foci of increased density, sometimes resembling a ski cap (right) and sagging or mere flattening of the cranial head segment. Normal contour *dashed*.

1. *Fracture, dissection, fragmentation, collapse of the femoral head* (Figs. 352, 353, and 354). In the beginning, necrotic bone tissue differs biologically from living bone tissue with adequate blood supply only by its diminished weight-bearing capacity.

2. *Bone resorption, increased density of bone* (Figs. 353 and 354).

The repair process occurs by means of revascularization. As this takes place, the dead bone is at times resorbed, and cystlike osteolyses, concentric osteolyses, (Fig. 354 B) and radiotranslucent marginal seams make their appearance. Regenerated bony trabeculae can refill the areas of resorption or are apposed to dead trabeculae. In the latter instance, the bone reveals greater radiologic density than its surroundings. Moreover, dystrophic deposits of calcium in the necrotic bone marrow add to attenuation of the films. This is particularly known of metaphyseal and diaphyseal bone infarcts. Finally, the impaired mo-

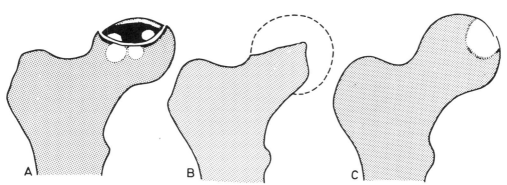

Fig. 354 Roentgen signs of advanced ischemic reaction of the femoral head (the roentgen signs of secondary osteoarthrosis to be expected in this stage are not illustrated).

A = Necrotic collapse, demarcating repair process (revascularization). In the *dark* area, prevalent apposition of bone to the devitalized trabeculae. The translucences indicate processes of revascularization with prevalent resorption of the necrotic parts. In the remainder of the femoral head the osteonecrosis has not yet been revascularized; there one sees a marginal subchondral fracture line.

B = Revascularization has led to concentric resorption of bone (*original* contour *dashed*).

C = Small necrotic area has been resorbed (cystic appearance of the avascular necrosis).

In epiphyses exposed to static load, this process is observed less frequently than in non-weightbearing bones; e.g., the head of the humerus.

bility of the adjacent joint leads to disuse demineralization of the live bone tissue in which the devitalized cancellous trabeculae do not (cannot) partake. This explains why the radiologic density of the area of dead bone is greater than that of its surroundings. Moreover, in weight-bearing portions of bone the devitalized cancellous trabeculae become sintered and compressed and thus increase the bone mass per unit of volume. This event also contributes to the increased density of dead bone. Hence, the attenuation of the roentgen beam in devitalized areas of bone can be traced to different histologic processes in which, as a matter of experience, revascularization and its consequences play a prominent part.

The most frequent (late) sequela of necrosis of the femoral head is *osteoarthrosis of the hip* (Fig. 355). *Necrosis of the articular cartilage*—so-called chondrolysis (Lequensne, 1972; see p. 250 ff)—is a much less frequent complication: In a case of previously diagnosed necrosis of the femoral head, the radiologic cartilage space becomes narrowed within a few months without the appearance of major marginal osteophytes (Fig. 355 B). The process is accompanied by an increase in discomfort.

Pathogenesis of adult necrosis of the femoral head: Adult necrosis of the femoral head, like other *epiphyseal or apophyseal* osteonecroses, is basically a *subchondral* fatigue fracture in a pathologically altered portion of the skeleton, or the fatigue fracture occurs in the setting of a generalized skeletal disease. The segmental blood supply to the femoral head in the absence of efficient interconnections and possibilities of collateral pathways (Trueta and Harrison, 1953) constitutes the most important morphological prerequisite for adult necrosis of the femoral head and one that occurs more frequently there than in other bones. The blood supply to the femoral head can be interrupted by (1) thrombosis and embolism, (i.e., fat emboli in the bone marrow; Fisher 1978), (2) an affection of the vessel wall, (3) the compressive effect of abundant pathologic cells invading the marrow cavity, and (4) traumatic rupture of blood vessels, and (5) necrosis of bone due to corticosteroid therapy. In the latter, apart from stenosis by intraosseous inflammatory lesions of arteries (Jansen, 1967; see also p. 59), the compression of blood vessels by perivascular edema (Uehlinger, 1964) is a subject of debate.

Etiology of adult necrosis of the femoral head: posttraumatic necrosis of the femoral head, (item (4) of the foregoing) can develop following fractures of the medial or lateral neck of the femur, following pertrochanteric fractures and isolated fractures of the trochanter, as well as following an intertrochanteric osteotomy. It also occurs after dislocation of the hip. *Early posttraumatic necrosis* occurring within a few weeks or months after an accident is distinguished from *late necrosis* occurring after one, two, or more years.

Symptomatic necrosis of the femoral head is also seen in the *decompression syndrome* (caisson disease, diver's disease), as a consequence of gas embolism. The characteristic roentgen picture of the *meta- and diaphyseal* bone infarct has been studied particularly in the decompression syndrome (Horváth, 1978). Calcification of the bone marrow is most marked in the marginal portions (compare Fig. 252). Periosteal thickening can occur at the level of the infarct. The inner contour of the compacta in tubular bones does not become altered; therefore it is possible in the roentgenogram to differentiate the condition from enchondroma and central chondrosarcoma. Calcified syphilitic gummas also must be considered in the differential diagnosis of an infarct in the diaphysis, metaphysis, or epiphysis of long tubular bones (Jakob, 1951). Perform serologic tests for syphilis in oligoosteal infarction!

Diseases of the blood can also produce necrosis of the femoral head; for instance, hemoglobinopathies with formation of sickle cells (item 1 of the foregoing), hemophilia and primary polycythemia.

During the course of *Gaucher's disease* (a disorder due to an enzyme deficiency), the femur is as a rule the *first* bone to be affected; moreover, it also reveals the *most frequent* pathologic alterations visible in the roentgenogram (Amstutz and Carey, 1966). Among them are necrosis of the femoral head (item 3 of the foregoing), pathologic fracture of the femoral neck, and a flasklike deformity of the distal third of the femur *(Erlenmeyer flask deformity*, Fig. 355).

Avascular necrosis of bone—for instance, the neck of the femur—is known to be a side effect of oral, parenteral, or intraarticular corticosteroid therapy (Compare p. 59). The steroid genesis of such necroses of bone cannot be doubted in diseases that otherwise run their course without involving the skeletal system (Klümper et al., 1967). On the other hand, it is difficult to prove the side effect of steroids when aseptic necroses of bone develop during the course of steroid-treated diseases in which avascular necroses of bone are also apt to occur *without* the administration of steroid therapy. This applies primarily to rheumatoid arthritis but equally to disseminated lupus erythematosus (infarction of bones by antigen-antibody complexes?) and to osteoarthrosis of the hip. Finally, there are reports on adult necrosis of bone in osteomyelitis of the femoral neck; in endocarditis; in Cushing's disease (Sharon et al., 1977); in *adult* myxedema (Rubinstein and Brooks, 1977); in inflammatory and degenerative vascular diseases; in sarcoidosis (Edeiken et al. 1967); in progressive scleroderma, even without corticosteroid treatment (Wilde et al., 1977); in pancreatitis; following burns; in gout and in hyperuricemia (see p. 251); in connection with pregnancy (Storey, 1968); in amyloidosis; in histiocytosis X; in inflammatory and degenerative vascular diseases; in sarcoidosis (instance of foregoing pathogenesis no. 3; Edeiken et al., 1967); and following the administration of the plasma substitute polyvinylpyrrolidone (Mazière et al., 1980). Especially in the opinion of French writers (compare Simon et al., 1975), chronic alcoholic abuse is the most frequent cause of adult avascular necrosis of the femoral head. Ethylic hyperlipidemia is thought to produce mi-

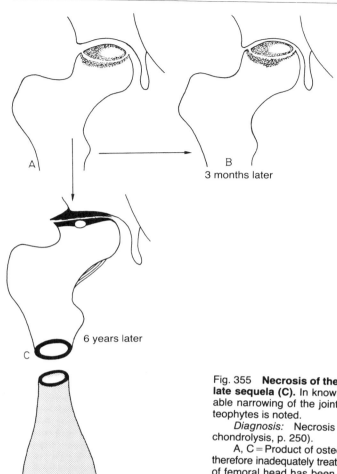

A

B
3 months later

6 years later

C

Fig. 355 Necrosis of the femoral head (A) complication (B) and late sequela (C). In known necrosis of the femoral head, considerable narrowing of the joint space without formation of marginal osteophytes is noted.

Diagnosis: Necrosis of the articular cartilage (so-called chondrolysis, p. 250).

A, C = Product of osteoarthrotic destruction in undiagnosed and therefore inadequately treated necrosis of femoral head. Necrotic area of femoral head has been resorbed; decentralization of the femoral head (see Fig. 312, no. 3). Without knowledge of roentgen finding A, the necrosis of the femoral head can no longer be identified unless a roentgenogram of the distal femur is available! *In this case* the roentgenogram shows the so-called *Erlenmeyer flask deformity* (C). This deformity, in connection with necrosis of the femoral head and its sequelae, is found only in Gaucher's disease (see text).

croembolisms of fatty particles and thus to trigger the devitalization of the femoral head. This theory can be compared with the view that necrosis of the femoral head is also apt to develop in hyperlipoproteinemia (Eichler, 1975; Hackenbroch, Jr., et al., 1978, and other writers).

Necrosis of the femoral head following radiotherapy of the pelvic organs—compare similar reports on necrosis of the head of the humerus following radiotherapy of breast cancer (Sengupta and Prathap, 1973)—leads to necrosis of the femoral head in *generalized* skeletal diseases; for instance, during the course of osteomalacia (Laurent et al., 1973; Strauss et al., 1979). In these instances, the subchondral fatigue fracture in the proximal femur *(vide supra* under "Pathogenesis of adult necrosis of the femoral head")* occurs after *direct* damage to the bone substance by ionizing rays. In CT of the head of the femur, a star-shaped structure, that Dihlmann (1982) refers to as the *asterisk sign,* can be seen. The asterisk is formed by thickened weight-bearing bone trabeculae. It can be shown by CT that the asterisk exhibits a characteristic change in avascular bone necrosis of the femoral head, even when the disease is in an early stage. CT of the hip joint is therefore an important examination for the early diagnosis of ischemic disease of the femoral head. The same is true of imaging the capsule and effusion of the hip joint by CT (Dihlmann and Nebel 1983).

Osteoarthropathies

In the radiologic differential diagnosis of **gouty osteoarthropathy** of the hip joint (see p. 41), the following two points of view must be taken into consideration:

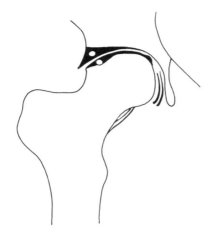

Fig. 356 **Gouty osteoarthropathy of the hip joint masquerading radiographically as "nonspecific" osteoarthrosis of the hip joint.** (see text).

1. Gouty arthritis shares the tendency to preferential involvement of the lower extremities with two other diseases—namely, Reiter's syndrome and ankylosing spondylitis—*and* it affects mostly males.
2. The (radiologic) morphology of gouty arthropathy is determined not only by the quantity-time quotient in the precipitation of urates (p. 41) but also by the surface relationship between the articular cartilage and the capsule of the affected joint (Uehlinger, 1975). With a relative preponderance of the surface of the articular cartilage, the osteoarthrotic phenomena are in the forefront, for instance in the hip joint (Fig. 356), the knee joint and the talocrural joint.

Ochronotic osteoarthropathy (p. 44 ff.) manifests itself in the hip joint as osteoarthrosis of the hip. Other striking features in the vicinity of the hip are often very pronounced fibroosteoses and/or rounded bony foci (Bauer and Kienböck, 1929); for instance, in the ischium or in the vicinity of other tendinous insertions (Fig. 357).

Hemophilic osteoarthropathy manifests itself in the hip joint and its vicinity principally as arthropathy and as pseudotumor. The recurrent hemorrhages into the joint and the bone marrow give rise to the reactions and alterations described on p. 46 ff. These result in roentgen signs indicating variable degrees of cartilage destruction and osseous proliferation (Figs. 358 and 359). The growth of the juxtaarticular bone may be disturbed (coxa valga) and the juxtaarticular cancellous bone may be remodeled with consequent hypertrophic atrophy. These findings are also well known to occur in arthritis of the growth period (p. 93 ff). Hemorrhages into the bone marrow lead, on the one hand to cystic translucences of bone at a distance from the joint and, on the other, to recurrent intraosseous and subperiosteal hematomas that form the cystic *hemophilic pseudotumor* (Fig. 358 A), which is frequently loculated. In the vicinity of the hip joint, the tumor is most often found in the ilium (for the differential roentgen diagnosis, see p. 46). When the acetabulum is concomitantly involved, the hip joint undergoes central dislocation. Hemorrhages into the soft tissues of the pelvis can give rise to ossification of these structures (Fig. 360; Hutcheson, 1973). At times, hematomas in the iliac muscle produce an injury of the femoral nerve with paresis of the quadriceps femoris muscle (Grauthoff et al., 1978).

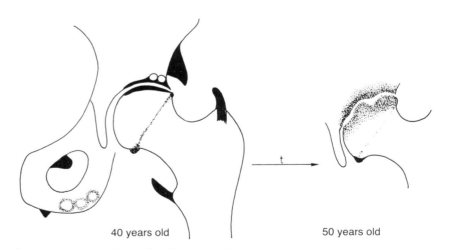

40 years old   50 years old

Fig. 357 **Ochronotic osteoarthropathy of the hip joint.**
    1. Premature **osteoarthrosis of the hip joint** (see "40 years old") which not only reveals rapid progression but in this instance also shows the roentgen signs of avascular osteonecrosis of the femoral head (see "50 years old").
    2. Comparatively oversized fibroosteoses.
    3. Bauer-Kienböck osseus foci (p. 44 ff.) have developed (t = time of evolution).

Fig. 358 **Hemophilic osteoarthropathy of the hip joint and its surroundings.**

A = Extensive hemophilic pseudotumor in the ilium.

B = Osteoarthropathy of the hip with osteoarthrotic and arthritic (destructive) roentgen signs.

C = Intraosseous translucences remote from the joint with marginal sclerosis, which gives the impression of cystic translucences with marginal sclerosis (The dividing lines are intended to emphasize that the roentgen findings A, B, and C also can occur singly).

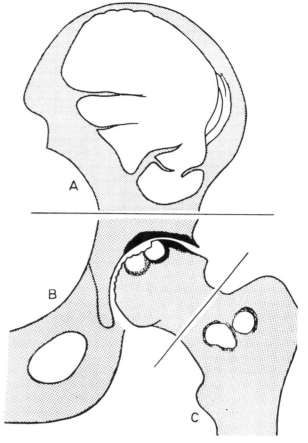

The **hereditary congenital hemoglobinopathies** (pp. 117 and 119 ff)—e.g., sickle cell disease—manifest themselves in the hip joint *principally* by necrosis of the femoral head. In children the "Legg-Perthes picture" then develops (Figs. 340 and 341), whereas in adults the typical appearance of osteonecrosis is found (Figs. 352 to 355). If not treated or inadequately treated, this condition leads later to osteoarthrotic destruction of the joint.

Neurogenic osteoarthropathies (p. 47 ff.) of the hip joint occur most frequently in the tabes dorsalis. Initially, the head and neck of the femur as well as the acetabular region show nondescript cystic translucences and/or erosions and/or narrowing of the cartilage space, as in arthritis or osteoarthrosis (Fig. 298). In other instances, the clinical picture begins with a spontaneous fracture of the femoral neck. Much more characteristic, however, is the finally dominating, nonreactive, more or less concentric osteolysis. With time it leads to complete resorption (disappearance) of the head and neck of the femur with widening of the roentgenologic joint space. In the surroundings, one sees many grumous or lumpy bone fragments or ossifications of soft tissues. The acetabulum widens through resorption of bone; this can lead to the development of a flail joint or to dislocation. The corresponding reontgenogram (Fig. 361) in all likelihood evidences a neurogenic osteoarthropathy of the hip so that only its etiology has to be determined. As mentioned above, a postsyphilitic affection of the spinal cord must be considered first; secondly, one must consider the diseases listed on p. 49 ff. In the presence of nonreactive osteolyses near the hip joint, particularly in the femoral head and neck, the following disorders have to be ruled out in addition: osteoradionecrosis and necroses of other etiology (p. 254 ff; Fig. 354 B), in which progressive resorption sometimes occurs instead of the repair of dead bone (reparative formation of new bone). It is very rare for the stage of mutilation in rheumatoid arthritis, the same as for lipoid-dermatoarthritis or for a neglected tuberculosis, to disintegrate the head and neck of the femur. As for *juvenile* chronic arthritis, see page 213 and Figure 196. With advanced osteolytic sarcomas and metastatic malignancies, the region of the femoral head and neck may at times be resorbed to a large extent. However, paraarticular bone shadows are absent in these cases, as in inflammatory

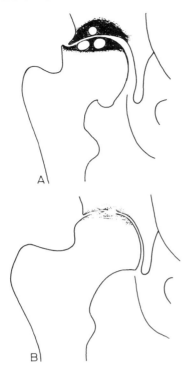

Fig. 359   Osteoarthropathy related to a coagulation defect
    A = Hemophilia A; unequivocal *osteoarthrotic* roentgen appearance. The strongly projecting lesser trochanter indicates a contracture in external rotation.
    B = Congenital hypoproconvertinemia. This observation shows a preponderance of *arthritic* roentgen signs (concentric narrowing of the joint space, erosions in the femoral head and the acetabulum).

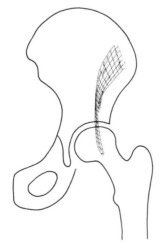

Fig. 360   Hemophilic sequelae in the surroundings of the hip joint.
    1. Coxa valga (see text).
    2. Ossification (for instance) of the iliac muscle (see text).

joint diseases. Severe avascular disorganization of the hip joint, as well as other joints, has been observed, especially as an aftermath of repetitive intraarticular injections of corticosteroids so that, in analogy with tabetic osteoarthropathy, the term *"pseudo-Charcot's joint* (see p. 59) has been applied to these cases (Chandler et al., 1959).

Finally, for reasons of differential diagnosis, mention must be made of *massive osteolysis (Gorham-Stout)* (p. 59). This disorder has been repeatedly reported in the region of the pelvic girdle and the hip. The spreading of massive osteolysis to ilial segments remote from the hip and to the regions of the ischium and pubis argues against neurogenic osteoarthropathy (Figs. 63 and 362). Neurogenic osteoarthropathies following severe (e.g., traumatic) damage to the central nervous system are characterized primarily by processes of ossification in the immediate vicinity of the hip. They have therefore been classified as **neurogenic paraosteoarthropathies** (p. 52 ff, Fig. 363). Bony hooks developing in the muscles, tendons, ligaments, and joint capsule increasingly impair the mobility of the hip joint. Figure 57, moreover, shows that severe damage to the central nervous system (e.g., traumatic paraplegia) can lead to extensive osteolyses in the hip and pelvis.

The proximal end of the femur is one of the sites of predilection for **amyloid osteoarthropathy** (p. 60). This disorder manifests itself by osteolyses appearing as large cysts that frequently are bilaterally symmetrical or sometimes marginal, and by erosions in the area of the capsular insertion. The radiographic joint space remains unaltered (Fig. 364).

Osteoarthropathy of the hip joint related to hemochromatosis should be considered in the differential diagnosis when the roentgen findings of "osteoarthrosis of the hip" are associated with those of "chondrocalcinosis of the hip joint and the symphysis pubis" (demonstrable in the survey film of the pelvis).

Kashin-Beck disease (p. 114) leads to generalized deformation of the epiphyses (see Fig. 134) which also affects the hip joint, producing a preosteoarthrotic deformity. The disorder must be differentiated clinically *and* roentgenologically from the osteochondrodysplasias, the mucopolysaccharidoses, and the mucolipidoses.

Osteoarthropathy in Wilson's disease (hereditary hepatolenticular degeneration) (p. 62) manifests itself as a *premature* osteoarthrosis (1). In the joints, there is a tendency toward the development of marginal fragmentations of bone (similar to osteochondrosis dissecans) and to osseous metaplasias in the soft structures of the joints (2). In addition, it is likely that chondrocalcinosis appears in these patients with above average frequency (3). As a result of renal rickets or osteomalacia (4), whose occurrence in Wilson's disease is well known though not inevitable, one finds generalized skeletal osteoporosis, Looser's pseudofractures, and/or the Milkman syndrome (p. 125). In children, the epiphyses are wid-

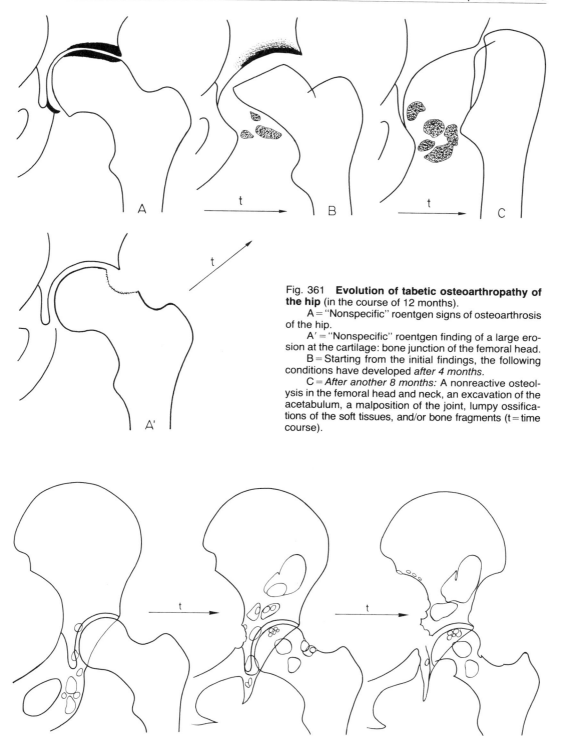

Fig. 361 **Evolution of tabetic osteoarthropathy of the hip** (in the course of 12 months).

A = "Nonspecific" roentgen signs of osteoarthrosis of the hip.

A' = "Nonspecific" roentgen finding of a large erosion at the cartilage: bone junction of the femoral head.

B = Starting from the initial findings, the following conditions have developed *after 4 months.*

C = *After another 8 months:* A nonreactive osteolysis in the femoral head and neck, an excavation of the acetabulum, a malposition of the joint, lumpy ossifications of the soft tissues, and/or bone fragments (t = time course).

Fig. 362 **Follow-up observation over 2 years of a massive Graham-Stout osteolysis** in an adult.

Principal features of roentgenologic morphology: Nonreactive osteolysis with a tendency to skip joints, beginning with nondescript rounded translucences. *Complications:* Pathologic fracture; dislocation. In the initial stage, the condition cannot be differentiated *in the roentgenogram* from osteolytic metastases (compare Fig. 63). (t = time course).

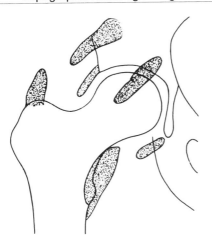

Fig. 363 **Neurogenic paraosteoarthropathy** *(schematic drawing)* with ossification of soft tissues (capsule, ligaments, tendons, muscles) in traumatic paraplegia (19 months after accident). Condition started 3 months after accident.

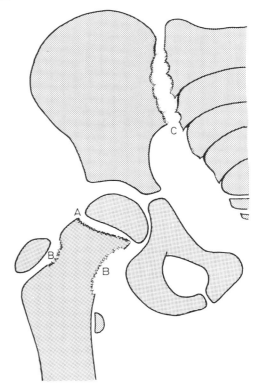

Fig. 365 **Roentgen signs of hyperparathyroidism in a child** (selection).
A = Epiphysiolysis (see p. 127).
B = Subperiosteal resorption of bone (see p. 126 ff).
C = Garland-shaped pseudodilatation of the sacroiliac joint space through subchondral resorption of bone (see p. 488 ff.).

ened. The roentgen signs mentioned under (4) are particularly marked in the pelvic girdle.

In cases of suspected **hyperparathyroidism** or **renal (uremic) osteopathy** (p. 125 ff), the minimum program of roentgen diagnosis (Table 2, p. 127 ff) includes a survey film of the pelvis. Figures 365 and 366 show pathologic roentgen findings which *may* be encountered in this group of diseases.

Insofar as **acromegaly** (p. 131 ff) manifests itself at all in the hip joint, it shows at first the radiographic appearance of "osteoarthrosis with widened

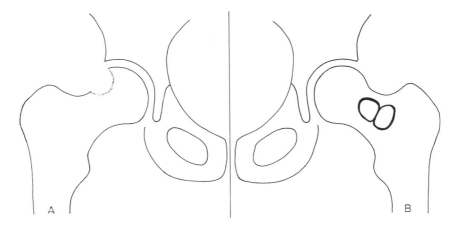

Fig. 364 **Amyloid osteoarthropathy of the hip joint.**
A = Subchondral deposit of amyloid lies eccentrically in the junction between head and neck of femur. (compare Fig. 303).
B = Osteolysis through deposition of amyloid in the area of the capsular insertion. It is possible to make the differential diagnosis between this condition and pigmented villonodular synovitis (Fig. 371) only by the clinical identification of amyloidoisis.

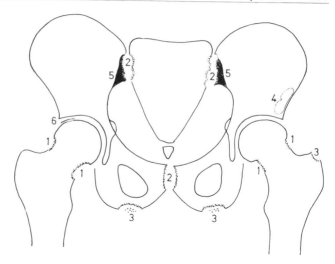

Fig. 366 **Roentgen signs of hyper-parathyroidism in the adult** (selection; compare Fig. 728).

1 = Subpoeriosteal resorption of bone.

2 = Subchondral resorption of bone (pseudodilatation of the sacroiliac joints and the symphysis pubic).

3 = Subtendinous resorption of bone, partly with stippled ossifications of soft tissues (see p. 126).

4 = Brown tumor (see p. 125 ff.).

5 = Subchondral hyperostosis of ilium presenting a triangular appearance (see p. 505).

6 = Chondrocalcinosis (see p. 69 ff.).

joint space'' (Fig. 367). At a later stage, however, the characteristic findings of osteoarthrosis of the hip develop, including the (initially) eccentric narrowing of the joint space.

Late **radiation injury** to the articulating bones of the hip joint appears primarily following radiotherapy of female genital carcinoma. The interval between the period of irradiation and the commencement of the complaints varies from 6 months to several years. Figure 368 also depicts the *early roentgen signs* of osteoradionecrosis in the region of the femoral head and neck (Fries, 1967). They become manifest at the marginal subchondral lamella, particularly in the central region of the femoral head and in the head-neck junction. During the further course, spontaneous fracture of the medial neck of the femur supervenes. It can heal by impaction of the fragments without active therapeutic measures, but it involves the danger of pseudoarthrosis, necrosis of the femoral head, and osteoarthrosis of the hip, (and thereby functional incapacity of the hip joint). Necrosis of the femoral head occurs either directly—i.e., without preceding fracture of the femoral neck—or following such a radiogenic fracture treated by internal fixation or by conservative means. The necrosis can be revascularized with a preosteoarthrotic deformity, or it can be resorbed with formation of a defect. Lesions of the acetabulum following radiation develop, on the one hand, in the setting of a postnecrotic osteoarthrosis of the hip. On the other hand, the resorption and insufficient weight-bearing capacity of necrotic portions of the acetabulum lead, infrequently, to a spontaneous fracture or, here also, to osteodystrophic processes of remodeling. In unfavorable cases, these processes extend to the entire field of irradiation and can reach as far as the sacroiliac region (Fig. 369). The cancellous structures undergo *irregular* consolidation, and calcification of the bone marrow develops. Apart from this, translucences are visible. Regarding its structure, this picture resembles Paget's disease but differs from this entity by its abrupt borders and the possible event of an acetabular fracture due to the radiogenic brittleness of the supporting tissues. Moreover, Paget's disease displays an increase in volume and deformation of the affected bones, which can lead to protrusion of the acetabulum and—when the femur is affected—also to coxa vara. On the other hand, protrusion of the acetabulum has also been observed as an aftermath of a radiation injury.

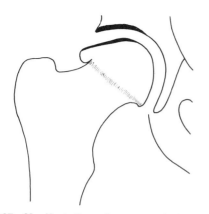

Fig. 367 **Manifestation of acromegaly in the hip joint.** Roentgen appearance of osteoarthrisis of the hip with "wide" joint space.

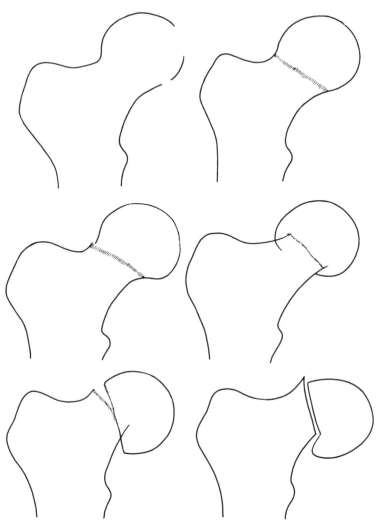

Fig. 368 **Manifestations and stages of radiogenic fracture of the femoral neck.** Possible early roentgen signs *(above)* are the disruption—(partial) obliteration—and haziness of the marginal subchondral lamella and an intraosseous callus.

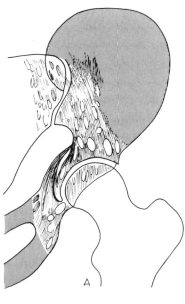

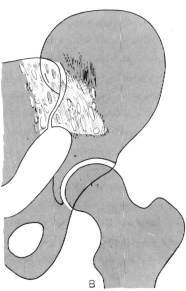

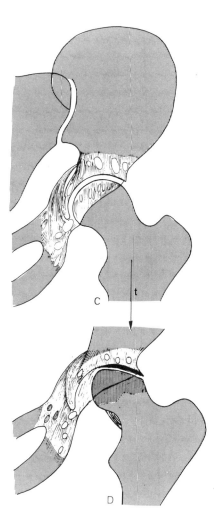

Fig. 369 **Pelvifemoral osteoradionecrosis following gynecologic radiotherapy.**

A = Sacroiliac and periacetabular osteoradionecrosis (fibrillar structures of cancellous bone; areas of increased density alternating with translucences; pathologic fracture of acetabular floor).

B = Sacroiliac osteoradionecrosis limited to the upper parts of the field of irradiation.

C = Radiation damage to acetabulum with pathologic fracture of the acetabular floor.

D = Four years later (t = time), advanced osteoarthrosis of the hip joint. The increased density of the entire femoral head justifies the supposition of additional radiogenic necrosis of the femoral head.

Note: The radiogenic lesions, which frequently are bilateral and symmetrical, should not be confused with Paget's disease or with a mixed osteolytic-osteoplastic metastasis. The same is true of late radiogenic damages, which must not be interpreted as sequelae of an osteolytic metastasis of the irradiated tumor.

Neoplasia of the Joint

In the hip joint also, the roentgen diagnosis of **malignant synovialoma** can in all probability be made when pleomorphic calcifications are recognizable within a closely periarticular, often lobulated, consolidation of the soft tissues, and when erosions of bone are present. When attention is paid to the three periarticular strips of fat illustrated in Figure 292, not only an inflammatory periarticular edema but also the infiltrating growth of a tumor in the soft tissues can be diagnosed relatively quickly.

Important points are comparison of the pericoxal soft-tissue structures on both sides of the body in a survey film of the pelvis and the pattern of the soft tissues in the Frog position roentgenogram (Fig. 370). Even without any erosion of bone, a lobulated, irregularly shaped consolidation of the soft tissues—with or without deposition of calcium—should always arouse suspicion of a malignant tumor of the soft tissues and should prompt a biopsy of the palpable mass. Also in the hip joint, cystlike osteolyses appearing on one or both sides of the normally wide joint space and the concomitant, normal mineralization of the subchondral layer are recognized as the principal roentgen signs of **pigmented villonodular synovitis** (p. 139 ff). After the knee joint, the hip joint is the most frequent localization of this disease, which commonly manifests itself in early adulthood by discomfort of insidious onset in one joint, and less frequently in two joints. Bone lesions visible in the roentgenogram are not to be expected before a late stage, hence after several years' evolution; they then reflect the extension of the pathologic tissue to the capsular insertions and/or via vascular channels. The cystic, or even polycystic, roentgen appearance (Fig. 371) develops when large fossae of erosion are met *en face* by the roentgen beam. The border of the cyst is marked off sharply or indistinctly, with or without a marginal seam. When a very great number of cystic osteolyses is present in the femoral head, its cap is liable to collapse. At times the pericoxal soft tissues appear to be consolidated. The pericoxal strips of fat may become displaced (Fig. 371 E). Calcifications are not among the roentgen findings in pigmented villonodular synovitis.

Capsular or *bursal cysts* developing in rheumatoid arthritis (Palmer, 1969), if of sufficient size, appear in the roentgenogram as a consolidated, space-occupying soft-tissue process in the *extra-* and *intrapelvic* surroundings of the hip joint.

Neoplastic synovial chondromatosis (p. 66 ff) also starts from the synovial membrane of the hip joint or from a juxtaarticular bursa. The synovial chondromas, which frequently are very numerous, become recognizable in a plain roentgenogram only when they undergo calcification (Fig. 372). They are capable of producing pressure erosions in the articulating bones (Fig. 373). Postoperatively—hence following removal of the synovial chondromas—the pressure erosions sometimes regress. Neoplastic synovial chondromatosis in time leads to osteoarthrosis. It is therefore a preosteoarthrotic condition. On the other hand, synovial chondromas can also develop through cartilaginous metaplasia in the synovial membrane of osteoarthrotic joints. These metaplastic synovial chondromas (see Fig. 310), however, do not occur in such great numbers as do the cartilaginous proliferations in neoplastic synovial chondromatosis.

Cystic skeletal angiomatosis (compare the legend accompanying Fig. 25) is a more or less generalized condition. Histologically, hemagiomas or lymphangiomas are demonstrable, usually manifesting themselves by the pathologic fracture of a long bone (Singh et al., 1974). Alternatively, the condition may be detected as an incidental finding; for in-

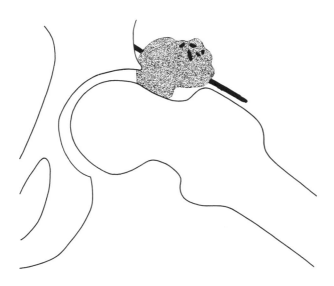

Fig. 370 *Biopsy:* **Malignant synovialoma.** Anteroposterior roentgenogram of the hip joint *(not illustrated)*; fat stripes, partially disrupted medial to the gluteus minimus muscle. Pleomorphic calcium shadows in this area. In the Frog position II roentgenogram, the increased density of the soft tissues with irregular calcifications between the greater trochanter and the acetabulum is shown more distinctly than in the anteroposterior roentgenogram. No erosion of bone.

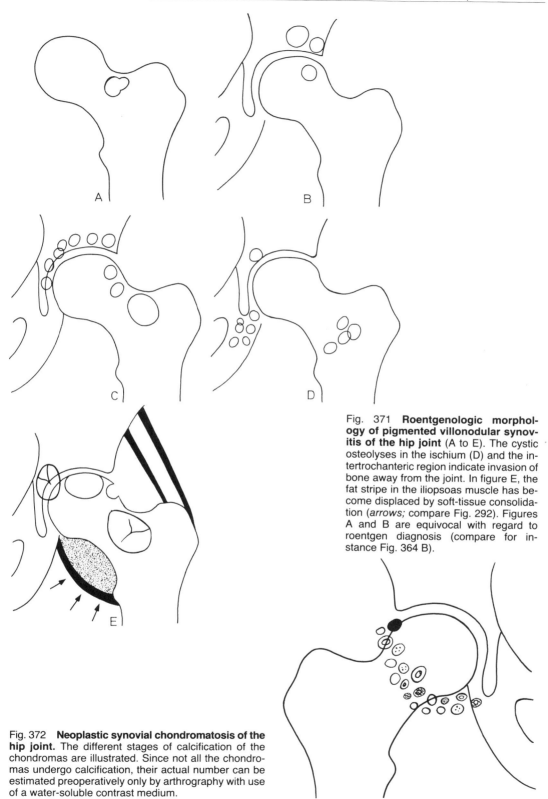

Fig. 371 **Roentgenologic morphology of pigmented villonodular synovitis of the hip joint** (A to E). The cystic osteolyses in the ischium (D) and the intertrochanteric region indicate invasion of bone away from the joint. In figure E, the fat stripe in the iliopsoas muscle has become displaced by soft-tissue consolidation (*arrows;* compare Fig. 292). Figures A and B are equivocal with regard to roentgen diagnosis (compare for instance Fig. 364 B).

Fig. 372 **Neoplastic synovial chondromatosis of the hip joint.** The different stages of calcification of the chondromas are illustrated. Since not all the chondromas undergo calcification, their actual number can be estimated preoperatively only by arthrography with use of a water-soluble contrast medium.

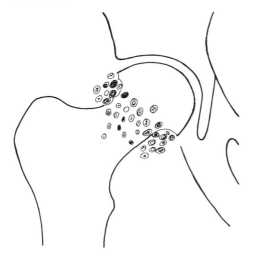

Fig. 373 **Neoplastic synovial chondromatosis** with pressure erosions recognizable in the superior and inferior junction between femoral head and neck.

stance, when performing intravenous urography (Fig. 374). The lesions may enlarge (hazard of a pathologic fracture), may remain unchanged, or may regress and thereby undergo reossification. Skeletal lymphangiomatosis is sometimes accompained by a chylous effusion into the pleura. Cystic skeletal hemangiomatosis may be associated with hemangiomas of the skin and the deeper soft structures (phleboliths). The differential diagnosis should consider different polyostotic disorders; *for instance,* histiocytosis X, fibrous dysplasia, incipient massive osteolysis of Gorham-Stout (see Fig. 63) and skeletal metastases (see also the legend accompanying Fig. 25).

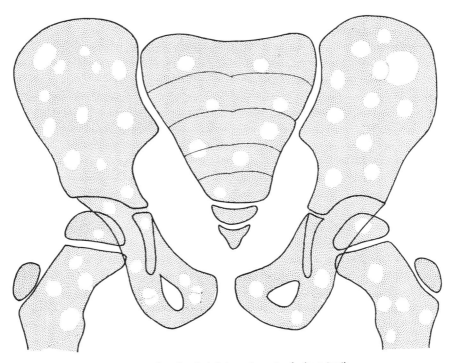

Fig. 374 **Cystic skeletal angiomatosis** (see text).

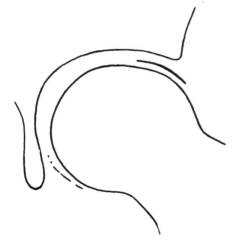

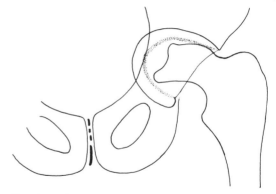

Fig. 375 **Chondrocalcinosis in the hip joint.** *Markings* indicate locations where superficial calcifications of the articular cartilage are most frequently recognizable in the roentgenogram.

Fig. 376 **Severe destructive chondrocalcinosis-induced osteoarthropathy of the left hip joint with secondary protrusion of the acetabulum.** Since the articular cartilage has been completely destroyed, the only sign indicating chondrocalcinosis is calcification of the symphyseal cartilage.

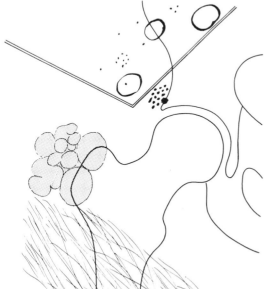

Articular and Periarticular Calicifications and Ossifications of Soft Tissues

The delicate linear or punctiform calcifications of the superficial articular cartilage in **chondrocalcinosis** (p. 62 ff) are visible particularly at the superior (lateral) and inferior (medial) circumference of the femoral head (Fig. 375). The occurrence of severe destructive osteoarthropathy during the course of chondrocalcinosis has been pointed out on page 64 ff (Fig. 376). Calcifications or ossifications of the acetabular fibrocartilage are encountered in elderly individuals, in osteoarthritis of the hip, and also in ankylosing spondylitis (Fig. 310). Circumscribed, slab-shaped, capsular ossifications (capsular osteomas) are a frequent finding in advanced osteoarthrosis of the hip (Fig. 310). Extensive capsular ossifications have sometimes been observed in ankylosing spondylitis. Figure 377 shows the different forms in which the *calcinoses* in the vicinity of the hip joint are projected. Regarding the terminology, the site, and the cause of these calcium depositions, see p. 69 ff.

Fig. 377 **Calcinoses about the hip joint** (here in dermatomyositis; reproduced synoptically). The separate part of the drawing shows, at the typical site, non absorbed remnants of the intramuscular injection of a medication containing metal salts. Furthermore, one sees ring-shaped calcium shadows (parietal calcifications of a local necrosis of adipose tissue or a hematoma resulting from inadvertent subcutaneous injection of a drug destined for intramuscular administration).

Among the *sequelae of hemophilia,* we have mentioned muscle ossifications in the vicinity of the hip joint (Fig. 360).

Neurogenic paraosteoarthropathies are depicted in Figure 363. The ossifications of soft tissues sketched in Figures 360 and 363 have also been grouped together under the term of **localized myositis ossificans** (p. 68).

Affections of the Fibroosseous Junction (Enthesopathy)

In this group of diseases, fibroosteoses, fibroosteitis, and so-called periarthritis coxae are of particular significance in roentgen diagnosis. In the vicinity of the hip joint, fibroosteoses occur prevalently in the tro-

chanters, the iliac crests, and the tendinous insertions on the ischium (Fig. 378). They appear in the roentgenogram as sharply delimited pin-shaped or lumpy bulgings of the contour. We have already pointed out on page 72 ff that particularly pronounced fibro-osteoses develop in certain diseases such as hyperostotic spondylitis, fluorosis, ochronosis (Fig. 357), and acromegaly. Besides this, excessive occupational strain upon circumscribed muscle groups, and also traumas, are apt to induce the development of more or less striking fibroosteoses.

Productive and **rarefying fibroosteitis** (Fig. 378) occurs with particular frequency in the tendinous insertions on the anterior pelvic ring. It is, as a rule, an accompaniment of inflammatory rheumatic arthropathies (p. 73 ff). The associated findings of "bilat-

Fibroostosis   **Fibroosteitis**

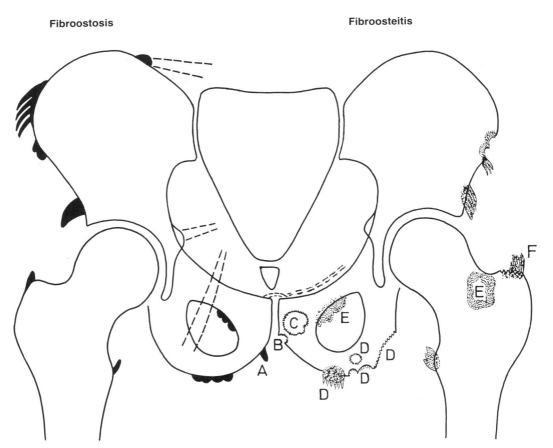

Fig. 378   **Sites of predilection for fibroosteoses** *(left, shaded black, sharply delimited)* and **Fibroosteitis** *(right, shaded gray, often with increased density of surrounding tissues)* **in the region of pelvis and hip. Ligamentous ossifications** *(from above downward* = iliolumbar, sacrospinal, tuberosacral, pectineal ligament [Nebel and Dihlmann, 1979] and ligamentum superius pubis) indicated by *dashed* lines.
Peculiarities: A = fibroosteosis of Muscularis gracilis. B = rarefying fibroosteitis of the arcuated pubic ligament. C = rarefying fibroosteitis *(top view)* at the origin of the adductor longus and brevis muscles. D = productive and rarefying types of fibroosteitis (partly *top view* and partly *in profile*) in the ischium. E = fibroosteitis at the origin and insertion of the obturator externus muscle (Birkner and Consentius, 1977). F = rarefying and productive fibroosteitis at the insertion of the gluteus medius.

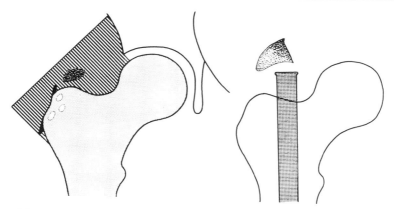

Fig. 379 **Reversible non structured calcium deposits,** which may occur in any part of the iliotrochanteric region *(hatches)* are among the inconstant roentgen findings in clinically diagnosable so-called **periarthritis coxae.** Fibroosteosis of the trochanters, structural loosening in the greater trochanter, and slight decalcification of the trochanters *(not set off in the figure)* are occasional additional manifestations. *On the right* one sees "Küntscher's cap" after intramedullary nailing of the femur; this pattern enters into the differential diagnosis.

eral sacroiliac pseudodilatation and rarefying (and/or productive) fibroosteitis of the ischial bones'' are an important diagnostic clue to ankylosing spondylitis, especially when no roentgen signs of this disease are yet visible in the spine. Similar findings, however, namely bilateral pseudodilatation of the sacroiliac joints and excavated defects at the muscle origins in the convex portion of the ischium, also occur in hyperparathyroidism and in renal osteopathy (Fig. 366, nos. 2 and 3). Though, in hyperparathyroidism and in renal osteopathy—contrary to rarefying fibroosteitis—stippled or lumpy calcium shadows are visible in the defects of the ischium and sometimes in the region of the pseudodilatation. In hyperparathyroidism, the lesions in the ischium are due to precipitate remodeling of bone with prevalent resorption in the areas of strong mechanical strain.

The terminological problems concerning the concept of periarthritis, the associated ideas regarding its pathogenesis, and the clinical symptomatology of the disorder have already been discussed under the heading of Humeroscapular Periarthritis (p. 200 ff). So-called **periarthritis coxae** shows an acute, subacute, or chronic recurrent symptomatology and variable roentgen findings reflecting morbid lesions of tendons, bursae, and fasciae in the vicinity of the hip joint, particularly near the greater trochanter. Reversible *structured* and *nonstructured* calcium deposits may become visible in the soft-tissue compartment between the greater trochanter and the superolateral margin of the acetabulum (Figs. 81 and 379).

Possible additional roentgen findings in so-called periarthritis coxae are structural loosenings and minor decalcifications identifiable only on comparison with the opposite side, as well as fibroosteoses in the greater trochanter. The roentgen findings support the presumptive clinical diagnosis. They may, however,

be present *without* any complaints and then will prompt the referring physician to search for the local symptoms of the affection. It should be remembered that local overexertion and excessive strain, for instance, in pelvic obliquity as a consequence of leg length discrepancy, and trivial local traumas are, as experience shows, the most frequent causes of so-called periarthritis coxae.

Injuries to the Joint

In **traumatic dislocation of the hip,** the head of the femur is levered out completely from the acetabulum and comes to lie in the pericoxal soft structures (Fig. 380).

1. In iliac dislocation, the head displaces *postero*superiorly (most frequent type of dislocation).
2. In sciatic dislocation, it displaces *postero*inferiorly.
3. In pubic dislocation, it displaces *antero*superiorly.
4. In obturator dislocation, it displaces *antero*inferiorly.

Infrequent types are perineal and scrotal dislocation.

Avulsion of bone from the acetabulum occurs as an additional trauma (fracture-dislocation). So-called **central dislocation of the hip** (Fig. 381) is always a fracture-dislocation. The head of the femur is driven through the acetabulum into the pelvis and also forces the fracture of portions of the acetabulum into the interior of the pelvis.

Anterior dislocations of the hip are liable to compress the femoral artery, whereas posterior dislocations can injure the sciatic nerve. As a general rule, the most probable late sequela of anterior and posterior dislocation is necrosis of the femoral head

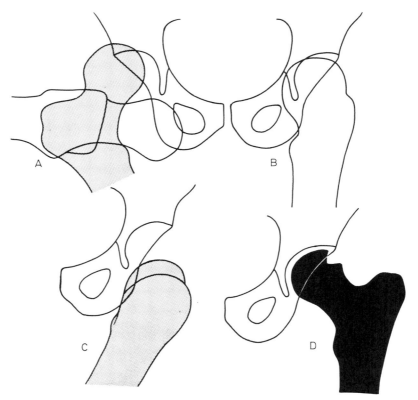

Fig. 380 **Classic traumatic dislocations of the hip joint.** (Possible fractures of the acetabulum are not illustrated.)

A = Iiac dislocation *(screened);* obturator dislocation.

B = Pubic dislocation.

C = Sciatic dislocation.

D = Status following reduction of an obturator dislocation of the hip with depressed fracture of typical localization (at times also shearing injury, *not illustrated*). These injuries *may* come about by violent impingement of the femoral head against the junction between the acetabulum and the superior ramus of the os pubis.

Note: In anterior dislocations, the leg is externally rotated (the lesser trochanter becomes more prominent); in posterior dislocations *(stippled),* the leg is internally rotated.

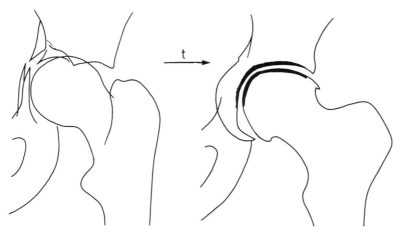

Fig. 381 **Central traumatic dislocation of the hip joint.** *Left* Roentgenogram immediately after accident. *Right:* Four years after accident (posttraumatic osteoarthrosis of the hip); t = time course.

(p. 251 ff), whereas in central dislocation the most threatening complication is (posttraumatic) osteoarthrosis of the hip. It is rare for dislocation of the hip and fracture of the pelvis to be followed by heterotropic formation of bone in the soft tissues (so-called *traumatic myositis ossificans*).

Fractures of the acetabulum (acetabular floor, roof, or rim) can occur as additional injuries to bone in dislocations *(vide supra)*, without presenting a faulty position of the proximal end of the femur. The identification of fractures of the acetabular rim is relevant to prognosis and therapy because with small avulsions the hip joint remains stable, whereas with major ones it becomes unstable. Small fractures of the acetabular rim must be differentiated from the *radiologic os acetabuli*, from osteochondrosis dissecans *of the acetabulum,* from persistent portions of the *anatomic os acetabuli (os coxae quartum),* and from accessory bones and the apophysis of the acetabular rim (compare the legend accompanying Fig. 351).

To evaluate a fresh injury in the region of the hip joint, the following roentgenograms are made *routinely:*

1.   An anteroposterior survey film of the pelvis
2.   An oblique roentgenogram in dorsal decubitus with the injured half of the pelvis lifted 60° (Urist roentgenogram). Taken in the second plane, the oblique roentgenogram yields valuable information concerning the position of the femoral head and possible injuries to the acetabular rim.

If, however, the circumstances require and admit it, the following roentgenograms are advisable in the presence of an injury to the hip joint:

1.   An anteroposterior survey film of the pelvis (as indicated above)
2.   An oblique roentgenogram with the *noninjured* half of the pelvis lifted 45° (so-called Ala roentgenogram)
3.   An oblique roentgenogram with the *injured* half of the pelvis lifted 45° (so-called obturator picture).

In addition, the Göb technique (roentgenogram taken in the squatting position: Wilhelm 1973; Fig. 382) and, ideally, computed tomography can be useful in the demonstration and evaluation of the *posterior area of the acetabulum.*

Following reduction of a traumatic dislocation of the hip, a survey film of the pelvis is obtained. The study of *this* roentgenogram should answer four questions:

1.   Has the reduction been successful?
2.   Does this roentgenogram reveal any additional injuries to bone that were not demonstrable in the roentgenogram(s) taken immediately after the accident?
3.   Is an intraarticular *osteochondral* fragment plainly visible?
4.   Is the *medial* portion of the roentgenographic cartilage space on the reduced side wider (more than 2 mm difference as compared with the sound side;

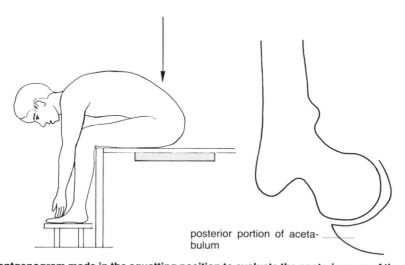

posterior portion of acetabulum

Fig. 382   **Roentgenogram made in the squatting position to evaluate the posterior area of the acetabulum** (if a computed tomograph is not available).
Left: Position for filming the patient, who should be capable of flexing the hip joints by at least 90 to 100° because the angular degrees (40°) remaining until extreme anteflexion is obtained can, in this instance, still be compensated for by tilting the roentgen beam emitter. In the figure, the patient's hip joints can be anteflexed to the maximum. The so-called central beam *(arrow)* is then directed at the sacrum at the level of the greater trochanter, perpendicular to the board of the Bucky table.
Right: Detail from the roentgenogram taken in the squatting position. Only the left side of the roentgenogram with its *most important* contours is reproduced.

Smith and Loop, 1976) than in the nontraumatized hip joint? In this case, tomography of the reduced joint must be resorted to in search of an intraarticular osteochondral fragment. If no such fragment can be identified although the difference in width of the cartilage space between the two sides persists and the patient complains of discomfort when weight is borne by the hip joint, the suspicion of an intraarticular *cartilage* fragment is justified!

Isolated fractures of the femoral head are a rare event. They generally come about by shearing or longitudinal compression. Apart from this, it should be recalled that the concomitant faulty position of the femoral head may have corrected itself spontaneously so that the subluxation or dislocation component of the initial fracture-dislocation has escaped attention.

Traumatic epiphysiolysis of the proximal end of the femur is to be mentioned here as an infrequent sequel to trauma during the growth period (compare Fig. 314—obstetric epiphysiolysis).

In **fractures of the femoral neck** (Fig. 383), the break is either medial (intracapsular) or lateral (extracapsular). For considerations of prognosis and therapy, a distinction is made in *medial fractures* on radiologic grounds between the unstable adduction or varus fracture (Fig. 384), which occurs more frequently and is less favorable, and the (commonly impacted) abduction or valgus fracture (Fig. 385). The *medial* fractures of the femoral neck are apt to trigger a partial or total *necrosis of the femoral head,* and involve the danger of *pseudoarthrosis of the femoral neck.* (Fig. 386). Both complications can lead to considerable impairment of function in the hip joint. Moreover, a medial fracture of the femoral neck can be followed by secondary *osteoarthrosis of the hip.* The accident endangers, for topographic reasons, the

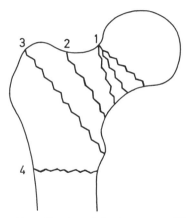

Fig. 383   Classification of the fractures of the femoral neck near the hip joint.
1 = Medial fracture of the femoral neck. The steeper the course of the fracture line, the graver the prognosis for healing of the fracture and frequency of complications (pseudoarthrosis, necrosis of the femoral head, osteoarthrosis of the hip). Accordingly, experience has shown that fractures of the femoral neck in which the fragment of the femoral head has rotated laterally unite more readily than those in which the fragment has rotated medially. The primary prognosis of fractures of the femoral neck is therefore the more favorable the more the fragments are subjected to compressive load; the more shearing force develops between the fragments the less favorable the prognosis (Pauwels, 1935).
2 = Lateral fracture of the femoral neck.
3 = Pertrochanteric fracture of the femur
4 = Subtrochanteric fracture of the femur.

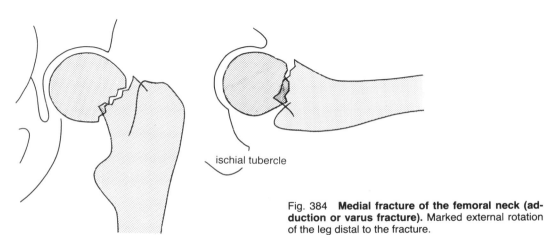

ischial tubercle

Fig. 384   Medial fracture of the femoral neck (adduction or varus fracture). Marked external rotation of the leg distal to the fracture.

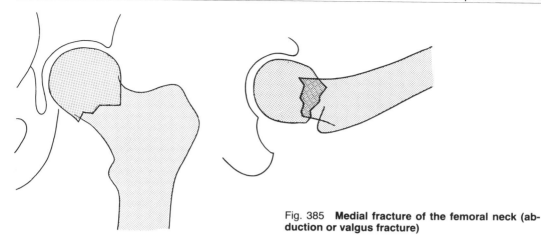

Fig. 385 **Medial fracture of the femoral neck (abduction or valgus fracture)**

nutrient vessels of the femoral head, principally the so-called lateral epiphyseal arteries, which are derived from the—equally endangered—deep branch of the medial circumflex artery of the femur, which courses behind the femoral neck. In the adult, the lateral epiphyseal vessels supply nearly four fifths of the epiphyseal area of the femoral head. These vessels enter the bone at the posterolateral circumference of the head, commonly 0.5 cm distally to the border of the articular cartilage. In medial fractures of the femoral neck, the plane of the fracture often traverses this area, so that these vessels are apt to be torn. However, direct damage to the articular cartilage and the subchondral cancellous bone, as well as capsular tears produced by the accident, also pave the way for

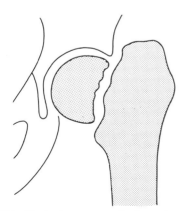

Fig. 386 **Typical roentgen findings in pseudoarthrosis of the femoral neck;** i.e., fracture cleft coursing steeply, cranial displacement of femoral shaft (elevation of trochanter), shortening amounting to resorption of the stump of the femoral neck. Besides these features, attention should always be paid to signs of necrosis of the femoral head (Figs. 352, 353, and 354).

the three undesirable consequences of medial fractures of the femoral neck listed above.

In elderly individuals, the brittle osteoporotic bone favors the occurrence of fractures of the femoral neck, which sometimes accompany a minor, even trivial, injury. Still, in such cases a pathologic fracture should also be taken into account, for instance one due to a metastatic tumor of the femoral neck or to an osteoradionecrosis (p. 261).

Lateral fractures of the femoral neck occur closely proximal to the trochanter mass. In the majority of cases, the fragments show a nonimpacted varus position. The extracapsular situation of the break generally does not compromise the vascular supply to the femoral head.

Pertrochanteric fractures of the femur always lie outside the capsule of the hip joint and therefore hardly ever involve the hazard of injury to the deep branch of the medial circumflex femoral artery.

Fatigue fractures of the femoral neck (Fig. 387) extend vertically to the compact bone of the medial femoral neck—Adam's arc. They occur, for instance, in osteomalacia due to malnutrition or renal osteopathy, and are known as *Looser's zones of remodeling* or, if bilateral and symmetric, as the milkman syndrome. Only rarely do these fractures produce a break in continuity of the region of the femoral neck (Hauer et al., 1977).

In the region of the pelvis and femur (Fig. 388), **deformations of the apophyses**[18] owe their origin to various causes:

1. Multicentric ossification and persistence as *developmental variants*
2. *Apophyseal osteochondropathy* (avascular disorder of ossification)

---

[18] Apophyses are projections of bone for the insertion of tendons and ligaments. They develop, either constantly or inconstantly, their own centers of ossification.

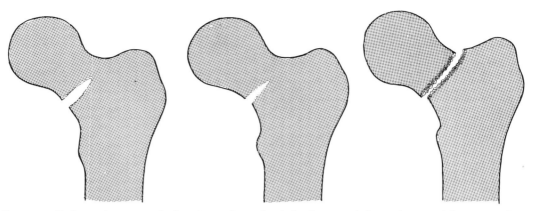

Fig. 387 **Fatigue fracture of the femoral neck.** *Left* = Aspect of Looser's pseudofractures. *Center* = "Infraction." *Right* = Fracture (with increased density of the marginal seam).

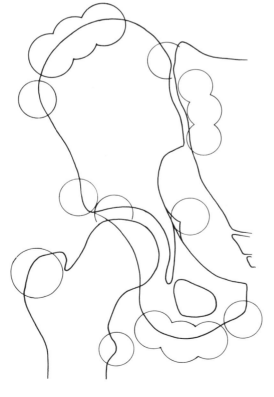

3. *Avulsion of the apophysis* (frequently as a sports accident)

The developmental variants are incidental roentgen findings, whereas the etiologies named under (2) and (3), in their fresh or florid stage, are accompanied by pain. Additional distinctive features are the youth of the patients—the femoropelvic apophyses fuse at the end of the second or the beginning of the third decade of life—and athletic activities in the history. The roentgenographic differential diagnosis between (2) and (3) is shown in Figure 389. Besides this, the condition must be differentiated from traumatic or non-traumatic localized myositis ossificans.

Physiologic soft-tissue shadows in the pelvis are noticeable in the roentgenogram only if the subjacent structures are covered with sufficiently thick layers of adipose tissue. It is true that on this premise they become inconstant elements of the survey film of the pelvis. In a given case, however, they can furnish certain information; for instance, about the sequelae of trauma to the soft tissues of the pelvis (Fig. 390).

Fig. 388 **Location of the apophyses in the femoropelvic region.** Concerning the basic pathology of the apophyses, see Fig. 389.

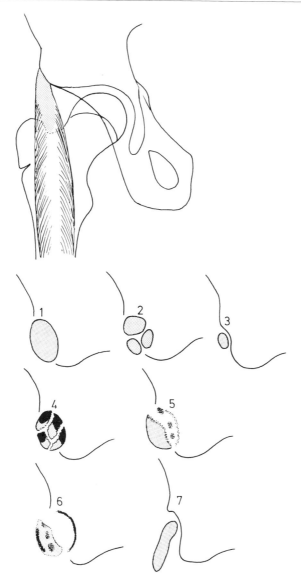

Fig. 389 **Apophysis of the anteroinferior iliac spine.**
(The findings illustrated are also valid in respect to other
apophyses.)

1 = Normal finding. Appearance between the 13th
and 15th year of life; fusion approximately between the
16th and 17th year.

2 = Multicentric apophyseal ossification (variant).

3 = Persistent apophysis (variant).

4 = Apophyseal osteochondropathy (fragmented,
inhomogeneous, dense roentgen appearance).

5 = Fresh avulsion of apophysis (displacement;
bowl-shaped, cloudy and lumpy, fragmented roentgen
appearance).

6 = Apophyseal avulsion about 6 weeks old with
signs of repair (increased densifications of bone).

7 = "Old" apophyseal avulsion, healed with deformation and persistence.

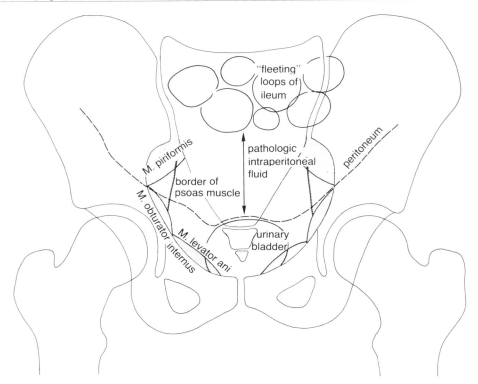

Fig. 390 **Pelvic soft-tissue shadows potentially distinguishable in the roentgenogram** (Kalman, 1978, and others). Most frequently recognizable are the bladder filled with urine and the obturator internus muscle (obliteration by hematomas and in [purulent] coxarthritis).

Knee Joint and Tibiofibular Joint[19]

The anteroposterior and the tibiofibular (lateral) roentgenograms are used routinely in examining the knee joint. The anteroposterior roentgenogram *with the patient standing* furnishes more accurate information on the extent of narrowing of the cartilage space and faulty positions in varus or valgus as a consequence of soft tissue lesions than does the anteroposterior roentgenogram *with the patient lying down* (Ahlbäck, 1968). In taking an anteroposterior roentgenogram one *may* equalize the slight, physiologic inclination of the tibial articular surface from anterosuperiorly to posteroinferiorly by tilting the x-ray tube (about 5° to 10° in direction of the feet) or by placing pillows under the popliteal space, thereby obtaining a position of 170° flexion. This is not absolutely essential, however. Rather, the separate projection of the anterior and posterior border of the head of the tibia can yield additional localizing information.

When an affection of the patella is suspected, a posteroanterior roentgenogram should be taken (p. 4). In positioning the patient for a lateral roentgenogram, a small pillow is placed underneath the heel to obtain a partial view of the tibiofibular joint, and the knee joint is flexed 30° from the extended position.[20]

Apart from tomography, certain situations require the addition of two types of roentgenograms:

First, the Frik roentgenogram (intercondylar roentgenogram) is used to obtain a clear view of the intercondylar eminence in injuries and for the better identification of osteochondrosis dissecans and loose bodies. With the patient in dorsal decubitus, a commercially available saddle-shaped cassette padded with foam rubber is placed underneath the knee joint. By doing so, a flexion of 45° is accomplished, and the so-called central beam is directed at the cartilage space and deflected about 40° toward the head.

The *second* additional roentgenogram, recommended for the evaluation of the shape of the patella and—conditionally—the glide surfaces of the femoropatellar joint, is the so-called *axial roentgenogram.* For instance, with the patient in dorsal decubitus and the knee flexed 45° from the extended position, the central beam coming from below is adjusted parallel to the articular surface of the patella. It then meets the cassette placed above the knee joint vertically. As

for "défilé roentgenograms," see Figures 395 and 396.

Concerning roentgenograms with the lower leg bent toward the intact side, see Figures 462 and 464. For level roentgenograms see Figure 479.

Malformations and Deformities

Ossification of the patella starts from a number of small centers and begins at about the third year of life. Failure of these ossification centers to fuse completely produces a bipartite patella *(patella bipartita, tripartita, multipartita,* Fig. 391). This diagnosis, however, can be made only after the completion of growth because individual ossification centers that initially have remained isolated sometimes fuse belatedly and call for the following differential diagnostic considerations:

A bipartite patella must be differentiated not only from fracture, but especially from pseudoarthrosis. It also must be borne in mind that this deformity may be the aftermath of trauma. Following avascular necrosis of the patella *(juvenile patellar osteopathy,* Larsen-Johansson), a revascularized portion of the tip or base of the patella may remain isolated. This finding must be distinguished from bipartite patella, as must inflammatory dissections. Generally, however, the revascularized, previously necrotic portion of the tip or base of the patella fuses again and thus often leads to deformation of its superior or inferior border (Fig. 391, no. 9). As a clue to differential diagnosis, it should further be mentioned that bilateral occurrence of bipartite patella is the rule, whereas with trauma it is the exception. In addition, the shape and size of the broken-off portion of the patella correspond with the "defect" in the patella. By contrast, in bipartite patella the persistent center of ossification usually is smaller or larger or shaped differently and therefore does not "fit" exactly into the adjacent patella area. Unilateral duplication of the patella—*patella duplex*—is an infrequent finding. Its differentiation from traumatic avulsion of an ossification center dating back for years may be difficult or impossible because the functional remodeling of the avulsed (smaller) portion also, with time, reestablishes the typical shape of the patella. This is why some writers (Jonasch, 1964) have questioned the occurrence of congenital duplication of the patella.

Aplasia, hypoplasia (Fig. 392), and *dysplasia of the patella* have been observed unilaterally and bilaterally, often as part of a hereditary malformation syndrome, for instance, osteoonychodysostosis (nail-patella syndrome, onychoosteodysplasia; Valdueza,

---

[19] The popliteal bursa overlies the femoral condyle dorsally and *always* has direct communication with the knee joint. (The anatomic nomenclature therefore speaks of the subpopliteal recess.) The popliteal bursa *frequently* communicates with the tibiofibular joint (Fick, 1904). Both joints can thus be interconnected and will be discussed conjointly.

[20] When it is proposed to specifically investigate the tibiofibular joint, the roentgenogram is made with the heel lifted about 45°.

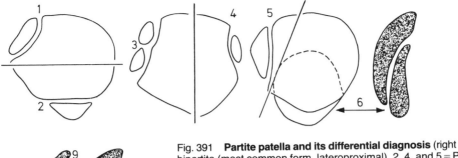

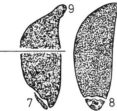

Fig. 391   **Partite patella and its differential diagnosis** (right leg). 1 = Patella bipartita (most common form, lateroproximal). 2, 4, and 5 = Patella bipartita. 3 = Patella tripartita. 6 = Patella bipartita with frontal cleft. 7 = Differential diagnosis of the sketched roentgen finding ("older" juvenile osteopathy of the patella [Larsen-Johansson]? Delayed appearance or delayed fusion of the ossification center?) can often be made only on clinical grounds (local tenderness in osteopathy). 8 = Florid juvenile osteopathy of patella. Weeks or months after onset of pain, circumscribed structural disturbances (translucences and increased densities) are recognizable in tip of patella. 9 = (Revascularized) juvenile osteopathy of patella in the base of the bone, healed with deformation.

1973). The weight-bearing capacity of knee joints with these malformations is less than that of those with a normally shaped patella. The malformations constitute a preosteoarthrotic condition and, besides, they further the instability of the knee. Hypoplastic patellae, for instance, have a tendency to dislocate laterally.

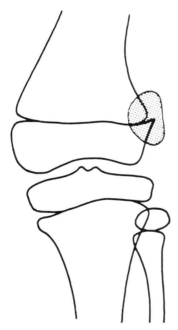

Fig. 392.   **Congenital hypoplasia and ectopia** (fibular subluxation) **of the patella** *(stippled),* associated with a slight degree of genu valgum.

Deformities of the femoropatellar glide way can, on the one hand, be identified in the axial roentgenogram of the patella *(vide infra)* and, on the other hand, favor the development of *chondromalacia of the patella.* The *causative factors* of this disorder are excessive strain on the hyaline cartilage of the posterior surface of the patella and the cartilage of its opposite femoral condyle and/or disturbed nutrition of these structures (Bandi, 1976). The process is initiated by circumscribed necroses (softenings) and ulcerations of the cartilage and eventually terminates in osteoarthrosis of the femoropatellar joint.

The *clinical* symptomatology of chondromalacia of the patella includes circumscribed tenderness of the medial border of the patella and retropatellar pain that increases upon rising from the squatting position and upon climbing stairs, ladders, etc., because the pressure with which the patella is forced against the condyles correlates with the bending angle of the knee. The greatest compression load is to be expected with approximately 90° flexion of the knee. The retropatellar pressure can reach values of 600 to 800 kp (1 kp = 9.81 N(ewton) = SI unit of force) (Bandi, 1972).

As a result of chondromalacia of the patella, cartilage detritus passes into the cavity of the knee joint and frequently causes a painful reaction of the synovial membrane with swelling of the capsule and an effusion into the joint that is also recognizable in the roentgenogram. During the evolution of this inflammatory synovial reaction, demineralization of the patella (Fig. 393) and, less frequently, juxtaarticular decalcification of the other two articulating bones *may* develop after a few weeks or months. The end result of this subacute or chronic, insidious process, if not treated or inadequately treated, is osteoarthrosis. It will be seen from the description of the clinical pic-

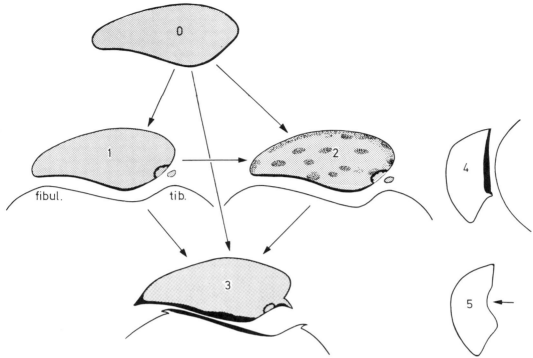

Fig. 393 **Right-sided chondromalacia of the patella and its sequelae.**
0 = Clinically diagnosed chondromalacia of the patella with great tenderness of the medial border of the patella and effusion into the joint. The plain axial roentgenogram shows type III of patellar shape (see Fig. 394). No other radiographic anomalies.

1 = Status following past chondromalacia of the patella. (Small crater with sclerotic borders near the medial facet; part of the focus in the patella has become a loose osteochondral body and may give rise to symptoms of locking. Frequently such a loose body can be identified only in the axial roentgenogram of the patella).

2 = Recurrent chondromalacia (renewed appearance of spotty demineralization, often following an effusion into the joint).

3 = Roentgen signs of osteoarthrosis of the femoropatellar joint. The lateral displacement of the patella toward the fibula arouses suspicion about the etiologic role of chondromalacia of the patella. (This disorder gives rise to atrophy of the vastus medialis so that the pull of the quadriceps displaces the patella lateralward.) With progressive osteoarthrosis of the femoropatellar joint, the direct residua of chondromalacia of the patella are increasingly less recognizable in the roentgenogram.

4 = "Old" chondromalacia of the patella (irregular subchondral sclerosis of the cancellous bone in the glide surface of the patella). Discrete marginal osteophytes.

5 = Haglund depression in the patella (variant of shape *unrelated* to trauma or chondromalacia).

ture and the roentgen morphology (effusion, demineralization) that primary inflammatory affections of the joint enter into the differential diagnosis of *florid* chondromalacia of the patella. Microscopic and bacteriologic study of the joint aspirate is therefore often indispensable.

For morphological reasons, chondromalacia of the patella develops *primarily when the femoropatellar glide way is disturbed,* e.g., in dysplasia of the patella or the (medial) femoral condyle, and also with recurrent dislocation or subluxation of the patella. The

tendency for the patella to assume a faulty position can be tested by two roentgenograms:

• *Roentgenogram 1:* Anteroposterior position of the knee joint with the quadriceps femoris muscle *relaxed*

• *Roentgenogram 2:* Anteroposterior position with the quadriceps femoris muscle *tensed*

• *Normally,* the patella lies higher (more proximal) in roentgenogram 2 than in roentgenogram 1. A proximal *and* lateral (fibular) displacement of the pa-

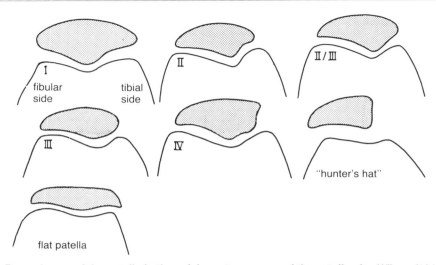

Fig. 394 **Bony shapes of the patella in the axial roentgenogram of the patella** after Wiberg (1941), Baumgartl (1964), Rau et al. (1979). (Right leg.)

Note: Studies on cadaver patellae (Nebel and Lingg, 1981) have supported the classification of patellar shapes in axial roentgenograms suggested by Wiberg and Baumgartl. However, Nebel and Lingg obtained completely different results concerning the frequency of their occurrence! The shape types II/III and III—hence dysplasia of the patella in the sense of Wiberg and Baumgartl—outnumbered the shape types I and II, hence the "normal shapes." In addition, the patellar types I to IV revealed *no differences* regarding the frequency of degenerative cartilage lesions and osteoarthrotic osteophytes. Therefore it may be stated that the bony patellar shapes I to IV are variants of the normal and that none of them is a preosteoarthrotic deformity.

tella is pathologic, indicating a tendency for subluxation

The *second* morphologic cause of chondromalacia of the patella is a *disturbance of the femoropatellar glide surface;* for instance, (post) traumatically or symptomatically in chronic arthritis (of whatever etiology) or in advanced osteoporosis.

The different bony shapes of the patella in plain axial roentgenograms are shown in Figure 394. A disadvantage of the plain axial roentgenogram has been pointed out particularly by Rau, et al. (1979): In comparative studies on cadaver knee joints, the shape of the *bony* posterior surface of the patella often diverges from the shape of the *cartilage cover.* Moreover, cartilage tears and cartilage ulcers are not, of course, directly recognizable in the plain axial roentgenogram. Finally, the contact surfaces of the patella and the femoral condyles change as a result of the variable flexion of the knee joint. Hence, the plain axial roentgenogram of the patella only reproduces the *bony shape* of the patella with a given degree of flexion. More accurate information concerning the condition and shape of the *cartilage cover* of the patella is obtained from the so-called *défilé roentgenograms* (Ficat, 1970; Figs. 395 and 396). With this technique, the roentgen examination is undertaken following intraarticular injection of a water-soluble contrast medium or by double-contrast study (Rau et al., 1979). Three roentgenograms are taken at 40,

70, and 100 degrees of *real* flexion from the extended position of the knee joint. However, to meet the patellofemoral articular surface tangentially, the central beam must be deflected about 10° from the longitudinal axis of the lower leg (compare Fig. 395 E). Thus, the diffraction angle between the longitudinal axis of the femur and the central beam in the défilé roentgenogram is 30, 60, and 90 degrees respectively (Fig. 395; Kölbel et al., 1979).

Dystopias of the patella are divided into upward positioning *(high patella),* downward positioning *(low patella)* and lateral positioning *(lateral patella).* The faulty position may be permanent, habitual, or recurrent. *Habitual dystopia* (dislocation) has morphological causes, among them underdevelopment of the lateral condyle, giving rise to genu valgum, a flat glide groove, small, rounded shape of the patella, and soft-tissue alterations (overstretching of the medial patellar retinaculum, underdevelopment of the vastus medialis muscle). Habitual lateral dislocation mostly occurs in the flexed position and becomes reduced when the knee joint is being extended. On the one hand, both habitual and recurrent dislocations are promoted by a preceding trauma, and on the other, a traumatic dislocation can be favored by the deformities mentioned.

High or low positioning of the patella is recognized by the method of Insall and Salvati (1971) (Fig. 397). Individuals with osteoarthrosis of the femoropatellar joint more often have a high patella than those

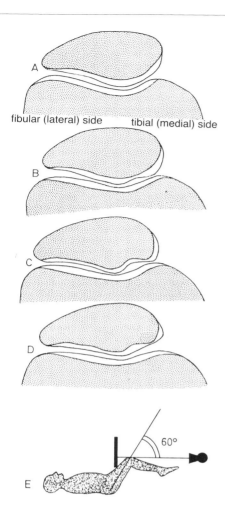

fibular (lateral) side   tibial (medial) side

Fig. 395 **Défilé roentgenograms of the right patella.** (See text and Figs. 394 and 396. Contrast media *not* illustrated, excepting Fig. 396 B).

A = Identical shape of the posterior surface of the patella composed of bone and articular cartilage (type III).

B = Plain axial roentgenogram suggests patellar type III, whereas the shape of the articular cartilage of the patella in the défilé roentgenogram suggests type IV.

C = Patellar type IV according to both the bony and the cartilaginous shapes of the posterior surface of the patella.

D = In the plain axial roentgenogram, patellar type IV; in the défilé roentgenogram, type II/III (compare Fig. 394).

E = Principal focusing technique for défilé roentgenograms (Kölbel et al., 1979).

Note: It is only the défilé roentgenogram of the patella that furnishes information about the actual conditions of the transfer of pressure in the femoropatellar joint. Arthrography with single or double contrast study has the same importance as the three serial roentgenograms. The ridge of the articular cartilage at the medial (tibial) facet of the patella (see B and C) is not only a frequent variant of shape but is also much less often premodeled in bony than in cartilaginous form (Rau et al., 1979). When chondromalacia of the patella is suspected clinically, défilé roentgenograms are therefore indispensable! Rau and Kauffmann (1978) have indicated a simple device for taking standardized défilé roentgenograms.

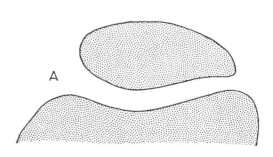

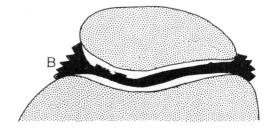

Fig. 396 **Comparison between the information from a plain axial roentgenogram of the left patella (A) and a défilé roentgenogram (B; contrast medium illustrated) in the same patient.** Only the défilé roentgenogram (B) reveals cartilage ulcers at the medial (tibial) patellar facet, whereas displacements of the patella—for instance, laterally (toward the fibula)—and the bony shapes of the patella (see Fig. 394) are recognizable in both A and B.

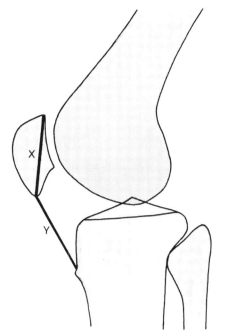

Fig. 397 Roentgenometry of patellar dystopias by the method of Insall and Salvati (1971).
With the knee joint flexed between 20 and 70° $\frac{y}{x}$ = normally 0.8–1.2; y = line drawn from the tip of the patella to the upper border of the tuberosity of the tibia; x = line drawn from the posterosuperior corner of the patella to the tip of the patella. $\frac{y}{x}>1.2$ = high patella; $\frac{y}{x}<0.8$ = low patella.

with a normal femoropatellar joint. High patella is found more frequently in females than in males; it often occurs bilaterally (Ahlbäck and Mattsson, 1978). Bilateral occurrence of high patella has also been observed in Little's disease, whereas unilateral high patella predominates following rupture of the patellar ligament or osteomyelitis of the femur, in paralysis related to poliomyelitis, in avascular necrosis of the tibial apophysis (Osgood-Schlatter disease), et cetera. Low positioning of the patella also may be congenital or acquired; e.g. in quadriceps paresis due to poliomyelitis or as a sequel of rupture of the rectus femoris tendon. Sideward (medial or lateral) displacements reveal themselves by the fact that the patella "rides" on one of the femoral condyles (Fig. 392); that is, has given up its normal, slightly eccentric position between the two condyles.

Congenital malformations of the femoral and tibial condyles often give rise to faulty positions and impaired mobility of the knee joint. There exist three degrees of *congenital dislocation of the knee joint:* Congenital genu recurvatum, congenital subluxation, and complete congenital dislocation of the knee. As a rule, both tibiae are displaced anteriorly. Lateral and rotary displacements also occur.

Discoid meniscus is a malformation that prevalently involves the lateral semilunar cartilage. Discoid meniscus impairs the function of the joint because it occupies excessive space and therefore acts as a "foreign body." In standing and walking, it is exposed to increased compressive, rotary, and shearing forces and thereby tends to premature attrition, so that frequently even children and juveniles complain of discomfort and present an effusion into the joint as well as discreet signs of osteoarthrosis. An

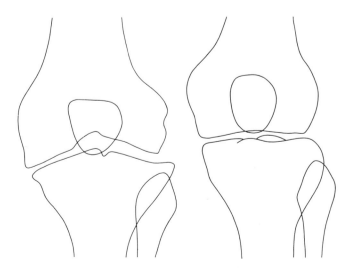

Fig. 398 Disorders of modeling and growth in the knee joint following past poliomyelitis with extensive residual pareses (paretic joint). *Left:* Present age 37, poliomyelitis at age 3. *Right:* Present age 32, poliomyelitis at age 7.

Note: The concepts "paretic joint" and "paralytic joint" should be superordinated by the concept *"immobilization joint,"* because the disordered shape ("smoothing") of the articulating portions of bone is not brought about by the paralysis of muscles but by the permanent or long-continued incomplete or complete immobilization of a joint in (early) childhood, undertaken for whatever reason; see text.

unequivocal roentgen diagnosis can be made only by use of arthrography. In contrast, widening of the lateral portion of the joint space, flattening of the lateral edge of the head of the tibia, hypoplasia of the lateral femoral condyle, and the consequent relative elevation of the head of the fibula (with lateral discoid meniscus) are no more than unreliable, suspicious signs.

Congenital contractures of the knee joint permit only rocking movements. These deformities of the soft-tissue cover (capsule, ligaments, tendons, muscles) are often associated with other malformations.

Acquired flaccid paralyses of the muscles acting on the knee joint, for instance those due to poliomyelitis, can—depending on the age of occurrence, the extent of the paralysis and the kind of treatment—lead to malpositions (e.g., paralytic genu recurvatum) but also to deformities of the articulating bones and to fibrillar remodeling of the structure of the cancellous bone. Figure 398 illustrates the examples of *paralytic knee joints*. An immobilizing therapy in childhood that has been prolonged for many years (which today is hardly any longer necessary)—for instance, a plaster cast including the leg and pelvis for tuberculosis of the hip joint—may not only bring on a fibrillar alteration of the structure of the cancellous bone in the concomitantly immobilized *unaffected* joint but also changes in shape (incongruities) that later on act as a preosteoarthritic deformity. Besides this, immobilization of a healthy joint also leads to muscular atrophy, impaired mobility related to shrinking of the capsule, and drying of the joint cavity (Spranger, 1974). These factors pave the way for malnutrition of the articular cartilage; regressive changes of the cartilage are the consequence. Later on, when the joint is moved again, osteoarthrosis supervenes.

Arthritis

Arthritis of the knee joint *(gonarthritis)* manifests itself *radiologically* by:

- Soft-tissue signs
- Collateral arthritic phenomena
- Direct arthritic signs.

The soft-tissue signs indicate an increase in volume within the cavity of the knee joint that can be brought about by an inflammatory or traumatic effusion, by intracavitary accumulation of blood, or by tumorous proliferation of the synovial membrane. The anatomic structure of the knee joint facilitates the radiographic demonstration of an intracavitary increase in volume which becomes visible especially in the lateral roentgenogram and, less reliably, in the anteroposterior view (Figs. 399 and 400). A preliminary condition for radiographically identifying an intracavitary increase in volume—e.g., an effusion into the joint—is the accurate knowledge of the normal soft-tissue structures of the knee joint (Fig. 399 A and B). Moreover, the position of the fabella ("little

bean") in the lateral head of the gastrocnemius can evidence an intracavitary increase in volume.

Between 10 and 20 per cent of adult individuals possess a lateral fabella, which in about three quarters of the cases occurs bilaterally. Much more infrequent are the *medial* fabella in the tibial head of the gastrocnemius (Freyer, 1960) and the distal fabella of the popliteus muscle (Slanina, 1956), dorsally and medially to the head of the fibula (Fig. 400 G). With increasing flexion of the knee joint, the fabella even normally moves away from the femoral condyle and approaches the tibia. This must be taken into consideration when comparing both sides (see legend accompanying Fig. 400 G).

In the class of *pathologic synovial structures* at the knee belongs *Baker's cyst* (synovial cyst, popliteal cyst, arthrocele, hygroma; Fig. 400 E). It is derived from communicating and noncommunicating bursae, primarily the gastrocnemius-semimembranosus bursa (Doppman, 1965) and from synovial diverticula protruding through the fibrous membrane of the knee joint. In children, malformations of the capsule as a causative factor are a matter of debate (Crasselt, 1968). A check-valve mechanism between the cavity of the knee joint and the communicating gastrocnemius-semimembranosus bursa probably contributes to the development of Baker's cyst. This check-valve mechanism allows synovia to pass from the joint cavity into the bursa, but not in the opposite direction. The mechanism promotes the development of a "pressure balance chamber" which becomes the palpable Baker's cyst in the *medial* area of the popliteal space; it is apt to extend far into the lower leg. Baker's cyst either remains asymptomatic and/or displays an alternate increase and decrease in size, or it gives rise to pain and impairment of motion. Rupture of Baker's cyst presents the clinical picture of acute thrombophlebitis of the lower leg (differential diagnosis). Baker's cyst has also been observed after trauma, in intestinal lipodystrophy (Whipple's disease) (Kelly and Weisiger, 1963), in gout (Peavy and Franco, 1974), and in hypothyroidisms (myxedema; Dorwart and Schumacher, 1975). Apart from this, hypothyroidism also is known to cause effusions, particularly into the knee joint, the talocrural joint, and the joints of the hand (pp. 136 and 138). The dimensions of Baker's cyst and its contents can be determined by arthrography (single and double contrast) and by sonography. The condition must be differentiated from lipoma, fibroma, ganglion of the knee joint, aneurysm of the popliteal artery, thrombophlebitis, popliteal varicosities, and cold (tuberculous) abscess.

Ventral and lateral cysts of the knee joint (Reinhardt, 1972) rank as very infrequent findings. They also give rise to a rubbery swelling. The more acute the evolution of arthritis of the knee joint, the earlier and more striking are the *collateral arthritic phenomena* (for the differential diagnosis, particularly from transient osteoporosis, see p. 12 ff and Fig. 17). Initially, the lateral roentgenogram usually shows *spotty*

Fig. 399 **Roentgen signs of increased volume in the cavity of the knee joint** (effusion, synovial proliferation).

A = *Normal orienting structures: Fatty layers* near the rectus femoris muscle (1), the vastus intermedius muscle (2), the border of the gastrocnemius muscle (7).

Suprapatellar (4), anterior (3), and posterior (5) *fat pad* at the femoral metaphysis (more marked in the child than in the adult). (6) indicates *physiologic layers of fat* (pursuing a course like the figure 3; often *not* visible without an intraarticular increase in volume). Fabella (8).

B = A sharp posterior contour of the rectus femoris tendon (1, *dashed*) and the *distance 2* of less than 5 mm (base of the suprapatellar recess [bursa]) very likely rule out an effusion into the knee joint (Hall, 1975), Accordingly, recognized roentgenographic clues to the presence of an effusion into the knee joint—in the most favorable case measuring between 1 and 2 mm—are beginning haziness of the tendon contour (1, *dashed*) and an increase of the *distance 2* to more than 5 mm. A technical prerequisite is that the femoral condyles should *not* be projected one upon the other—For the lateral roentgenogram, tilt the roentgen tube 5° cranially—and that the knee joint should not be flexed more than 45°. Haziness or (partial) obliteration of the *contour 3* (dashed) raises the suspicion of *bacterial* infection or superinfection of the knee joint (e.g., in rheumatoid arthritis), in which

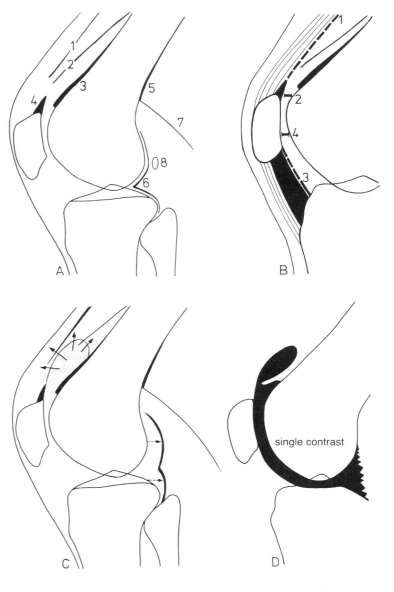

the edema renders the infrapatellar fat pad more or less equivalent to water (see p. 1; Gelman and Ward, 1977).

An increase of more than 5 mm in the distance between the patella and the femoral condyle is also considered a roentgen sign of effusion.

C = Major effusion and/or synovial proliferation recognizable by the ovoid ballooning of the suprapatellar recess. *Arrows* sketched there indicate its further potential expansion. Possible displacement of the "3" sign (Weston, 1971) by an effusion and/or synovial proliferation *(dashed arrows)*.

D = The suprapatellar bursa almost always communicates with the joint cavity (= suprapatellar recess). There are numerous variations between a wide communication and a slit delimited by a band-shaped plication (suprapatellar plica). The plica is apt to become fibrotic, hyalinized, and *calcified* (Pipkin, 1950). These processes interfere mechanically with the mobility of the knee joint; pain and a chronic effusion into the joint may ensue — plica syndrome.

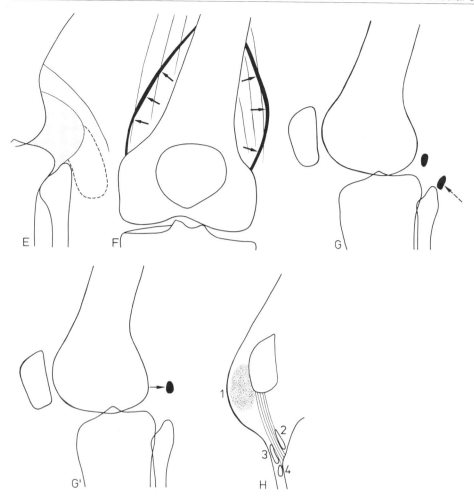

Fig. 400 Roentgen signs of increased volume in the cavity of the knee joint and its immediate vicinity (continued from Fig. 399).

E = Mostly inhomogeneous, dorsal densification of soft tissues as a consequence of effusion and/or synovial proliferation. When such a densification extends in the direction of the calf *(dashed line)*, it raises the suspicion of an arthrocele (Baker's cyst).

F = The suprapatellar bursa *(recess),* which has been ballooned by a major effusion, appears in the antero-posterior roentgenogram as a medial and/or lateral convex line (fatty layer, *arrows;* Harris and Hecht, 1970) which overlies the vastus strips without obliterating them. G, G' = The dorsal displacement of the fabella (G'; *arrow*) in the (approximately) extended position of the knee joint (see text) is a roentgenographic sign of intracavitary increase in volume (G = comparison with the unaffected side). The same is true of the dorsal displacement of a popliteal artery, which has a calcified wall. The *dashed arrow* points to a distal fabella (see text).

H = Juxtaarticular bursae. 1 = Prepatellar bursitis, possibly with calcium shadows. As a rule, one cannot discern from the roentgenogram whether a subcutaneous, subfascial, or subtendinous bursa is involved. 2 = Deep infrapatellar bursa. 3 = Subcutaneous infrapatellar bursa. 4 = Subcutaneous bursa on the tuberosity of the tibia. (2 to 4 = Location of the bursae not increased in size.)

decalcification of the patella. In the anteroposterior roentgenogram, a band-shaped demineralization is recognizable immediately in the subchondral area of the femur (Figs. 401 and 402). Finally, the decalcification spreads more or less evenly to involve the juxtaarticular portions of the femur and the tibia. In acute arthritis or during acute episodes of chronic arthritis, the structure of the cancellous bone becomes hazy, assuming a blurred appearance. With a chronic evolution of the arthritis, the haziness of the demineralized bone is less obvious or not at all apparent.

In **pyogenic gonarthritis,** the *direct signs* of ar-

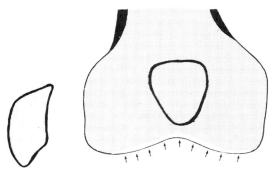

Fig. 401 **Early localizations of collateral arthritic phenomena and local demineralization of varying genesis in the knee joint** (p. 12 ff.) Spotty patella (lateral view), subchondral band in femur (anteroposterior roentgenogram; *arrows*). Additionally, a transverse band-shaped zone of demineralization is to be expected in the metaphysis of femur and tibia (*not illustrated in the figure;* see Fig. 403). Compare Fig. 13.

Note: Knee pain *plus* spotty decalcification of patella *plus* effusion = arthritis *or*—though less probably—transient osteoporosis (see p. 14). Knee pain *plus* spotty patella *without* effusion = (very probably) transient osteoporosis (see p. 15 ff.), provided demineralization of disuse (trauma or operation in the anamnesis with prolonged immobilization of the knee joint) can be ruled out by the history and the physical findings.

of arthritis—for instance, disappearance of the marginal subchondral lamella—are sometimes "skipped" in acute pyogenic gonarthritis. Among adult individuals, pyogenic gonarthritis occurs with particular frequency in patients under corticosteroid therapy and in those suffering from diabetes mellitus or rheumatoid arthritis (Kelly et al., 1970; Baum, 1971). This group of people definitely is afflicted more often with pyogenic arthritis than the average population. The suspicion of a local pyogenic complication becoming superimposed upon a known inflammation of the knee in a patient with rheumatoid arthritis should be aroused when the effusion (without additional trauma) increases notably and rapidly despite antirheumatoid therapy and/or when a rapid deterioration is observed in comparison with other diseased joints; for example, partial sequestration of bone or subluxation of the femur in the weight-bearing knee joint (see p. 88).

Among the **blood-borne gonorrheal infections of joints,** the knee joint occupies a preferential position. In this connection, one may be dealing with a suppurative arthritis similar to an infection with pyogenic pathogens, or there may be only a reactive para- or postinfectious arthritis without demonstrable offenders in the joint and offering a more favorable prognosis. In the latter instances, the onset of a postgonorrheal Reiter's syndrome must also be borne in mind! It should be mentioned here that Reiter's syn-

thritis sometimes appear after only a few weeks. Particularly striking are the narrowing of the joint space and the *hazy* boundaries of the defects in the contours (erosions, destructions). These findings are accompanied by soft-tissue signs of arthritis and juxtaarticular decalcification (Fig. 403). Discrete direct signs

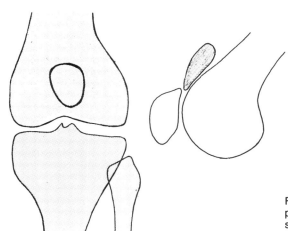

Fig. 402 **Subacute arthritis of the knee joint,** recognizable in the roentgenogram by ovoid densification and ballooning of the suprapatellar recess (bursa) *and* the narrow, band-shaped supratubercular zone of demineralization in the femur.

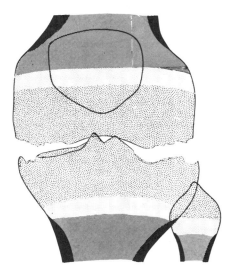

Fig. 403 **Pyogenic arthritis of the knee joint** (empyema following perforating injury). Pronounced destruction of cartilage and bone; collateral phenomena (see Fig. 13). When the suppurative inflammation is as far advanced as sketched here, fibrotic or bony ankylosis is threatening. (*The lighter the shading, the more advanced is the decalcification of bone;* compare also the band-shaped zone of demineralization in the metaphysis of femur, tibia, and fibula.)

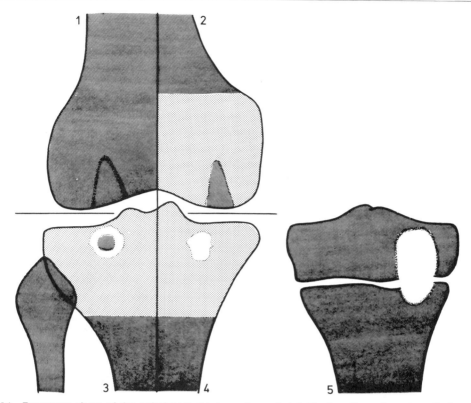

Fig. 404   Roentgen signs of the subchondral tuberculous skeletal lesion. Normal roentgen findings (plain roentgenogram, tomogram) do not rule out a *fresh* tuberculous necrosis of bone and bone marrow, because the shape and arrangement of necrotic trabeculae initially remain intact, and caseous bone marrow attenuates the roentgen beam the same way as living marrow tissue. *This is the reason why a tuberculous skeletal lesion frequently is more extensive than would be expected from the roentgenographic findings.*

1 = Demarcation of a wedge-shaped tuberculous necrosis of bone by perifocal apposition of bone (increased density of the marginal seam).

2 = Apparent area of increased density within pronounced perifocal demineralization (the tuberculous necrosis of bone does not take part in the perifocal decalcification).

3 = Partial resorption of the tuberculous necrosis of bone. (In the *center* one recognizes the sequestrum that does not take part in the perifocal demineralization or the resorption of bone; this roentgen finding is also known to occur in *sarcoidosis!* [Bjarnason et al., 1973].)

4 = So-called cavernous lesion of bone (the necrotic bone being resorbed). Extensive cavitation with a sharply delimited, *narrow* marginal sclerosis has also been termed "cystic tuberculosis" (see legend accompanying Fig. 127).

5 = Cystlike tuberculous focus in the epiphysis and metaphysis with obliteration of the cancellous structure and delicate marginal density (see Fig. 519). *(Principle of the drawing; the darker the stippling the greater the calcium content of the bone.)*

Note: In the growing skeleton, tuberculous and pyogenic infections occur in the same segments of bone (epiphysis, metaphysis, diaphysis) and frequently give rise to identical roentgen findings (resorption of bone, apposition of bone, formation of sequestra). Finally, (in the years of growth) even maligant tumors, particularly Ewing's sarcoma, may be very similar to the "inflammatory" roentgen picture. Moreover, certain bone tumors—for instance, osteoid osteoma (Bussière et al., 1976)—sometimes produce a sympathetic arthritis of the knee joint (see p. 161 ff). This knowledge underlines the great responsibility of the radiologic examiner in interpreting *findings in the juxtaarticular bones!*

drome presenting as arthritis of the extremities most frequently affects the knee joint. Gonorrheal involvement of joints follows the venereal infection after an interval of several weeks. Bacterial arthritis, including gonarthritis, has been reported as a complication of long-term dialysis in patients with chronic uremia (Massry et al., 1975). In these individuals, bacterial arthritis must be differentiated from symptomatic chondrocalcinosis (p. 62) and also from painful periarticular precipitations of calcium which are known to occur in chronic uremia, sometimes accompanied by edematous swelling and erythema (p. 69).

Hematogenous fungus infections (compare p. 108), **tuberculosis,** and **tertiary syphilis** also run a *chronic* course in the knee joint. Among the skeletal manifestations of tuberculosis, gonarthritis ranks second to spondylitis in frequency (p. 108, Fig. 404). In addition, experience has shown that the ipsilateral talotibial joint is often concomitantly involved. This fact should be considered in the differential diagnosis. Similarly to tuberculosis (p. 108), arthritis in tertiary syphilis occurs as a synovial and as an osseous form. Therefore, syphilitic arthritis is apt to be confused with tuberculosis of the joint. For this reason it should be the rule for any chronic arthritis running an insidious course, and *particularly* with *symmetrical* involvement of the knee joints, to obtain serological tests for syphilis. Besides this, young males toward the end of the second and third decades of life suffering from subacute or chronic gonarthritis should be subjected to a roentgenologic study of the sacroiliac joints because in this age group gonarthritis is one of the *early clinical manifestations of ankylosing spondylitis!* This matter of experience applies especially to the industrialized countries. Finally, in rheumatoid arthritis the knee joint is second only to the joints of the hand in the frequency of initial involvement.

On page 93 ff, **disseminated lipogranulomatosis (Farber's disease)** has been differentiated from juvenile rheumatoid arthritis. In this storage disease, juxtaarticular, bilaterally-symmetrical erosions of bone on the medial side of the proximal shaft of the tibia are known to occur (Fig. 405 A). Viewed as an *isolated* finding, these tibial lesions resemble Wimberger's roentgen sign of congenital syphilis (Dihlmann, 1972). Prior to diagnosing Farber's disease, syphilis must therefore be ruled out clinically and serologically (compare the legend accompanying Fig. 405 A).

As a complication of intracutaneous BCG vaccination, hematogenous lodgment of Bacillus Calmette-Guérin leads to **BCG osteomyelitis and arthritis** (Mortensson et al., 1976; Bachmann et al., 1977). Especially in the long tubular bones—more infrequently in flat or short bones—monoostotic or oligoostotic destructions develop in the metaphysis (Fig. 495 B) and are apt to spread to the neighboring joint or, less often, to the diaphysis. Striking features are the *slight* or *absent* tendency to periosteal reaction and sequestration, as well as the bland clinical symptomatology; for instance, the afebrile or subfebrile course. Differential diagnosis from infection with human or bovine tubercle bacilli is not possible without cultural examination. Arguments against infantile osteomyelitis (which frequently is polyostotic) are the negative response to customary antibiotic therapy, the discrete clinical symptomatology, and the slight or absent periosteal reaction.

A case of **sympathetic gonarthritis** (p. 161 ff) in plasma cell osteomyelitis is shown in Figure 406.

Chronic gonarthritis of whatever etiology (Fig. 407) can lead to considerable narrowing of the joint space (not accompanied by subchondral sclerosis),

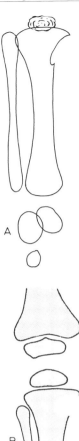

Fig. 405   **A = juxtaepiphyseal marginal defect** on the medial side of the proximal tibia *(right side illustrated; corresponding finding also on the left side).* This finding—**Wimberger's sign**—is known to occur in **congenital syphilis.** Congenital syphilis shows lesions in the diaphyses and metaphyses but not in the epiphyses. In the present instance, additional epiphyseal lesions (irregular ossifications of the proximal tibial epiphysis) are recognizable. Here, the marginal defect has occurred in **Farber's disease** (p. 93 ff). During the course of this disease of neonates and infants, marginal defects are found in the tibia, ulna, femur, humerus, acromion, clavicles, and vertebrae. Flexion contractures of the joints and nodular joint swellings also have been observed. However, very similar juxtaepiphyseal marginal defects are known to occur in (polyostotic) **infantile osteomyelitis** (to be differentiated by the clinical features).

B = BCG-induced osteomyelitis and arthritis of the tibial metaphysis and the knee joint (effusion into the joint, demonstrable physically and roentgenologically, *not illustrated*). Differential diagnosis from infantile osteomyelitis and human as well as bovine skeletal tuberculosis; see text.

even with no, or insignificant, defects in the contour (Fig. 408). In the majority of cases, however, contour defects or circumscribed areas of decalcification (Fig. 409) are recognizable prior to narrowing of the joint space or concomitantly with this direct sign of arthritis. They should be sought in the edges of the tibia—especially laterally but also dorsally and medially—and in addition, on lateral roentgenograms, in the femoral condyle, approximately at the level of the inferior border of the patella or closely underneath it, as well as at the level of the superior border of the patella (Fig. 409). There, one also encounters a conspicuous narrowing or obliteration of the marginal subchondral lamella. During the further course of gonarthritis, breakdown of the joint (narrowing of the joint space, erosions, destructions, attendant cysts) come increasingly to the fore and can involve all portions of the joint (Fig. 410). The condition rarely progresses to the stage of mutilation (Fig. 411) but rather to bony ankylosis. Advanced chronic gonar-

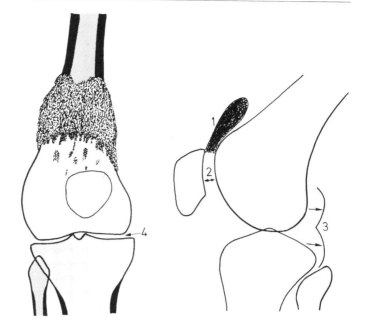

Fig. 406 **Roentgenogram in chronic plasma cell osteomyelitis and periostitis of the femur, accompanied by sympathetic (sterile) gonarthritis.** Roentgen signs 1 to 3 = Effusion or synovial proliferation (compare Fig. 399). 4 = Narrowing of joint space by destruction of the articular cartilage, because a **chronic** sympathetic arthritis *may* be associated with synovial proliferation and consequent erosion of cartilage. The bacterial process in the femur shows marked periosteal reaction in the metaphysis and diaphysis as well as extreme demineralization of the condyles. In the border zone between these findings, foci of cancellous sclerosis are interspersed (Dihlmann and Fernholz, 1978).

thritis hence gives a typical roentgen picture. When similar lesions are also encountered in other joints, the presence of an inflammatory-rheumatic, polyarticular arthropathy, principally rheumatoid arthritis, must be suspected. Figure 407 once more should demonstrate the difficulty or impossibility of drawing conclusions regarding the etiology of a given arthritis without knowing the history and the clinical findings. The roentgenogram as such only allows making the diagnosis of "chronic gonarthritis." In the *present* figure, tuberculosis and rheumatoid arthritis show a largely identical radiographic picture.

However, the following *additional information concerning the differential diagnosis* can at times be obtained from the radiographic picture of chronic gonarthritis: In contrast to adult rheumatoid arthritis, **psoriatic arthritis, Reiter's syndrome** (see p. 96 ff), and **arthritis of the extremities in ankylosing spondylitis** are characterized by their particular tendency to periosteal reactions and fibroosteitis. This tendency frequently also manifests itself in the knee joint (Figs. 412 and 413). As for periosteal reactions in **Crohn's regional enteritis,** see Fig. 412, p. 33 and p. 134).

Lipoid-dermatoarthritis (multicentric reticulohistiocytosis, p. 131 ff) can lead to erosions in the knee joint and destruction of the articulating bones; it therefore presents the radiographic appearance of

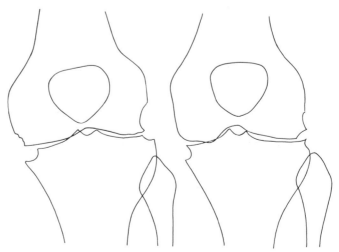

Fig. 407 **Approximately identical roentgen findings in rheumatoid arthritis** *(left)* **and synovial tuberculosis of the knee joint** *(right).*

Note: The suspicion of tuberculosis was raised because the affection of the knee developed 2 years after an exudative pleuritis and appeared as a chronic monarthritis of insidious onset. The sacroiliac joints presented a normal radiologic picture (see text). The findings on the *left* developed during the course of a rheumatoid arthritis that had been known for years.

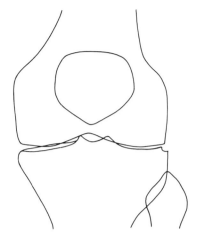

Fig. 408 Chronic gonarthritis with nonreactive narrowing of the joint space without major destruction of bone (only a delicate erosion in the fibular edge of the tibia) during the course of rheumatoid arthritis.

chronic (poly-) arthritis. Rather atypical are the juxtaarticular marginal defects of bone, which have been described for the hand (p. 131 ff) and which occasionally also are observed in the knee joint.

The less active a (chronic) gonarthritis is, the more the patient will move and burden the knee joint. Thus, a secondary (inflammatory) osteoarthrosis develops with time (Fig. 413) because the articular car-

tilage damaged by the arthritis can no longer cope with its normal load. During the course of this process, the osteoarthrotic lesions can completely overshadow the arthritic roentgen signs, so that the latter become almost or entirely unrecognizable. On the other hand, it is possible for the less aggressive serous-inflammatory effusion, which is not accompanied by any direct signs of arthritis, to damage the articular cartilage to such an extent that it paves the way for the development of an osteoarthrosis.

Arthritis of the growth period (p. 93 ff) leads also in the knee joint to deformations, shortening or lengthening of the articulating bones (Fig. 414), and sometimes to a fibrillar alteration of the bone structure (Fig. 13, compare also Fig. 436) that persists throughout life. In small children, an inflammatory (arthritic or osteomyelitic) acceleration of growth is often reflected by the *shape of the distal femoral epiphysis, resembling an aspergillum* (Fig. 415). This deformity, though less obvious, is also seen in the other two bones. It is rare for inflammatory processes in the knee joint or its immediate vicinity to cause a perichondral ossification in the growing skeleton, hence bone shadows which are separated from the epiphyseal nucleus by a translucence (cartilage). Figure 51 shows a so-called widening of the intercondylar fossa which is apt to develop not only in hemophilia—as in Figure 51—but also in juvenile rheumatoid arthritis and other types of chronic arthritis, including tuberculosis of the knee joint (compare Fig. 414 A). A likewise varied etiology is attributed

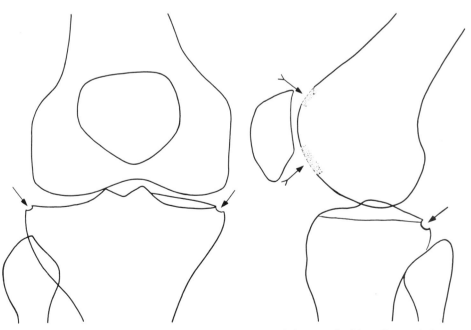

Fig. 409 Most frequent sites of erosions *(arrows).* **Lesions of the marginal lamellae and circumscribed zones of decalcification** (tailed arrows) which occur as **early** direct arthritic signs in rheumatoid arthritis but also in arthritis of different etiology.

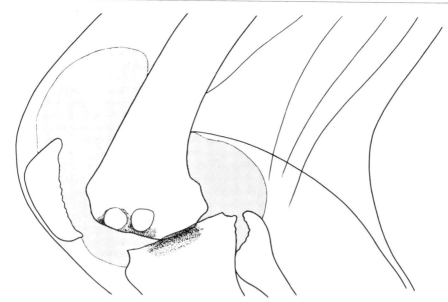

Fig. 410 **Chronic arthritis of many years' standing affecting the knee joint and the tibiofibular joint in rheumatoid arthritis.** Marked effusion and/or inflammatory synovial proliferation *(screened light gray).*

Note: In tight joints (here in the tibiofibular joint) erosions often lead to "widening" of the roentgenologic joint space.

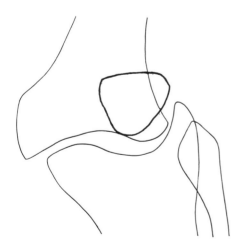

Fig. 411 **Stage of mutilation** (with flail joint and genu valgum) in rheumatoid arthritis of about 30 years' standing. If the history were not known, a neurogenic osteoarthropathy also would have to be considered.

Note: Even in not very far advanced chronic gonarthritis, lateral subluxation of the tibia is a frequent finding that points to destruction of the capsuloligamentous apparatus.

to the *so-called acquired rectangular patella,* whose diameter in depth has increased at the expense of its diameter in height (Figs. 416, 435, and 437).

In **juvenile chronic arthritis,** the joints most frequently affected are those of the knee, the hand, and the ankle joint (compare p. 88). This disease, the onset of which may be monoarticular, oligoarticular, or polyarticular, is associated relatively soon with posterior subluxation of the tibia (Fig. 415). To be sure, this roentgen sign is not evidence of juvenile chronic arthritis but, in children, it should be regarded as a clue to chronic gonarthritis.

The differential diagnosis of rounded translucences ("cystic" structures) in the subchondral bone of the knee joint will be discussed now for two reasons:

1. Given the small size of the patella and its close topographic relation to the knee joint, a variety of pathologic processes—whose *chief characteristic* is a circumscribed translucence in the patella—can cause discomfort in the knee joint. Therefore, a great number of gonarthritic signal cysts visible in the roentgenogram (Fig. 20), which naturally also may occur in the patella, must be differentiated. They will be summarized as follows (compare Reinhardt, 1969):

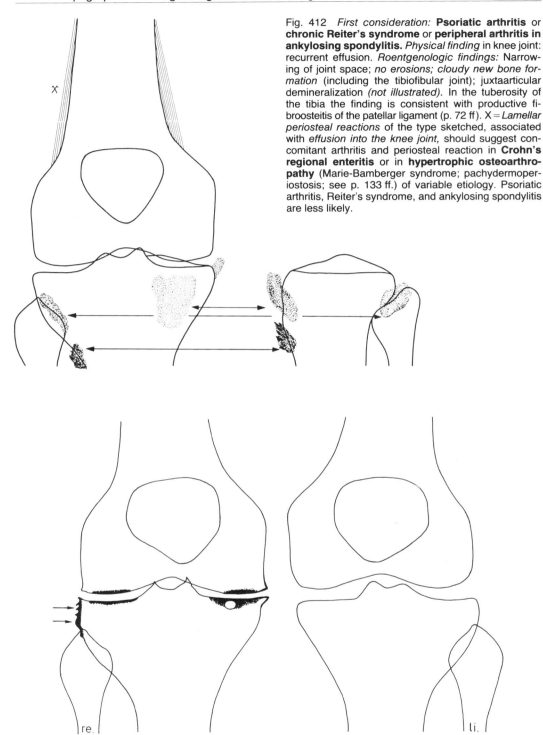

Fig. 412 *First consideration:* **Psoriatic arthritis** or **chronic Reiter's syndrome** or **peripheral arthritis in ankylosing spondylitis.** *Physical finding* in knee joint: recurrent effusion. *Roentgenologic findings:* Narrowing of joint space; *no erosions; cloudy new bone formation* (including the tibiofibular joint); juxtaarticular demineralization *(not illustrated).* In the tuberosity of the tibia the finding is consistent with productive fibroosteitis of the patellar ligament (p. 72 ff). X = *Lamellar periosteal reactions* of the type sketched, associated with *effusion into the knee joint,* should suggest concomitant arthritis and periosteal reaction in **Crohn's regional enteritis** or in **hypertrophic osteoarthropathy** (Marie-Bamberger syndrome; pachydermoperiostosis; see p. 133 ff.) of variable etiology. Psoriatic arthritis, Reiter's syndrome, and ankylosing spondylitis are less likely.

Fig. 413 **Osteoarthritis of right knee with periosteal reaction atypical of osteoarthrosis on the lateral border of the head of the tibia** *(arrows).*

Even without knowing the history and the physical findings, such a periosteal reaction raises the suspicion of secondary osteoarthrosis following (chronic) serous or serofibrinous gonarthritis in psoriatic arthritis, Reiter's syndrome, or ankylosing spondylitis.

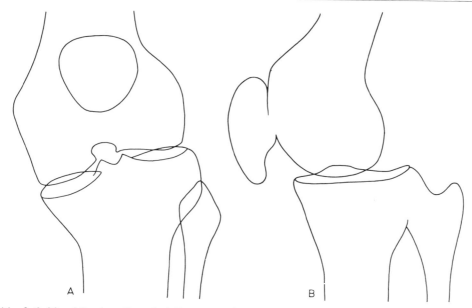

Fig. 414 Arthritis of the growth period. Roentgen signs in the knee joint.

A = 20-year-old patient, male. Ankylosing spondylitis that began as gonarthritis (recurrent serous effusion into the joint) at age 15. This led to deformation of the articulating parts of femur and tibia and to fibrillar structure of the bone *(not illustrated)*. There were, however, no erosions or other direct signs of arthritis.

B = 21-year-old patient, male. Juvenile chronic arthritis since age 9. Deformation of the articulating bones; bony ankylosis in the region of the femoropatellar and the tibiofibular joint.

Concerning the **roentgenologic differential diagnosis** between sequelae of arthritis of the growth period and a joint damaged by immobilization, compare Fig. 414 with Fig. 398.

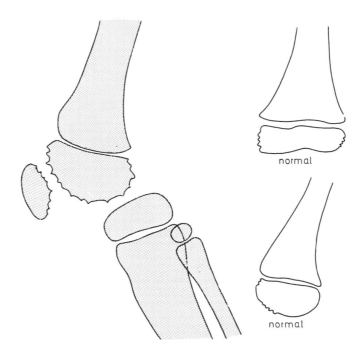

Fig. 415 **Inflammatory (arthritic) acceleration of growth of the ossification centers in small children.** *Left:* Age 5, female, suffering for about a year from rheumatoid arthritis. Accelerated growth of the ossification centers in the distal femoral epiphysis and the patella ("aspergillum"; see text). In addition, dorsal subluxation of tibia. *Right:* Irregularities of contour to be observed *normally* at the distal femoral epiphysis of small children.

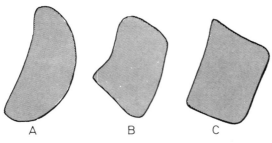

Fig. 416 **Typical acquired deformations of patella (B, C) due to arthritis of the growth period or recurrent hemorrhages into the joint in hemophilia.**
A = Normal roentgen finding.
B, C = **Rectangular patella.**

Osteomyelitis including Brodie's abscess (with or without sequestrum; sequestra found also in tuberculosis); (cystic) tuberculosis of bone (possibly associated with prepatellar swelling of soft tissues, due to tuberculous bursitis); syphilitic gumma (sometimes with striking periosteal reaction in the anterior surface of the patella); mycetoma; gouty tophi (with or without deposits of calcium and prepatellar swelling of soft tissues due to bursitis); solitary bone cyst; eosinophilic granuloma; enchondroma; hemangioma;

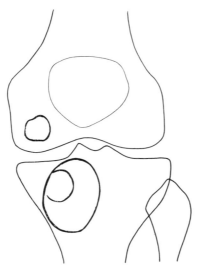

Fig. 417 **Rheumatoid arthritis persisting for 3 years;** since then treated orally with corticosteroids. In the *joints of the hand,* roentgen signs of chronic polyarthritis. In the *left knee joint,* minor effusion and thickening of the joint capsule demonstrable physically. In the roentgenogram, strikingly large, cystlike destruction of epiphyseal and metaphyseal bone with delicate, sharply delimited marginal sclerosis. A smaller cavity has developed in the subchondral bone of the femur (see text).

benign chondroblastoma (delicate calcium shadow in the area of osteolysis); osteoblastoma; osteoclastoma; sarcoma; plasmacytoma; metastatic tumor; focus of leukemia; fibrous dysplasia; Paget's disease; and hyperparathyroidism ("brown tumor," Fig. 445). Also, the so-called *dorsal* patellar defect, situated in the superolateral subchondral area of the patella, must be taken into consideration for the roentgenologic differential diagnosis of cystic structures in the patella of younger individuals. This infrequent finding, at times occurring bilaterally, is often detected incidentally by a roentgen examination undertaken for an accident. Histologically, dense fibrous tissue is encountered so that an atypical localization of a fibrous cortical defect possibly is involved (see p. 30) (Goergen et al., 1979).

2. In patients with rheumatoid arthritis to whom corticosteroids have been administered *orally* for years, cystic osteolyses with a very delicate sclerotic marginal seam are sometimes observed, particularly in the head of the tibia but also in the subchondral layer of other long bones (Fig. 417). They often expand as far as the metaphysis and contain necrotic tissue (Kindermann et al., 1969). These findings frequently occur in joints that are painful but which, in contrast to other of the patient's joints, reveal no erosion, narrowing of the joint space, or other lesions. In such instances, the roentgenographic differentiation from arthritic signal cysts (p. 23) or the infrequent focal necrosis in rheumatoid arthritis (p. 18; Uehlinger, 1971) is therefore difficult or impossible. On the other hand, the relationship of such juxtaarticular cystic osteolyses to cortisonoid therapy is manifest when they develop in disorders that do not involve the joints. In these cases, extensive avascular necrosis of bone has been demonstrated in the terminal bloodstream of intraosseous arteries, among other sites in the head of the tibia (Uehlinger, 1964). The further fate of these epiphyseal avascular necroses can consist in gelatinous pulpefaction of the devitalized tissue, delimited by a delicate osseous shell. At times part of the necrotic tissue calcifies and then presents the typical roentgenologic appearance of a bone infarct (Fig. 252, *arrow*) or manifests itself as osteochondrosis dissecans (Rudermann and McCarthy Jr., 1964). Finally, pictures can develop which go far beyond the characteristic appearance of avascular necrosis and indicate the complete disintegration of the supporting and gliding tissues involved. These severe joint destructions have already been described as *pseudo-Charcot's joints* elsewhere in this book (compare p. 59). These severe disintegrations of joints, which are encountered in arthritis and osteoarthrosis, especially as an aftermath of repeated intraarticular steroid injections, sometimes manifest themselves by certain noncystic alterations (bite sign; Fig. 418).

It should be emphasized here that an inflammatory reaction of the knee joint—the largest joint of the body—is a frequent, and even preferential, advent in various *intermittent* or *periodic diseases.* In this connection, intermittent means that the signs and

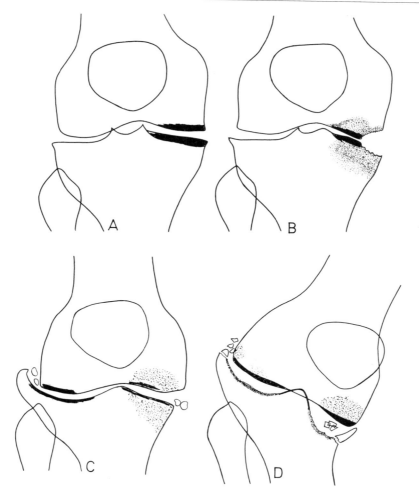

Fig. 418 Development of a pseudo-Charcot joint in osteoarthrosis of the knee following numerous intraarticular injections of corticosteroids (compare Fig. 64).

A = Osteoarthrosis of knee. Commencement of local injections.

B = Radiologic check after 15 injections (about 18 months later than A). So-called *bite sign* (Miller and Restifo, 1966).

C = Pseudo-Charcot joint (about 4 years after the first injection) with destruction of the articular cartilage. "Crumbling" of bony particles. Resorption and remodeling of the articulating bones. In addition, increased subchondral densities exceeding the degree commonly seen in osteoarthrosis.

D = During the further evolution, increasing joint disintegration, now associated with striking malalignment.

Note: Pseudo-Charcot joints have also been observed in weight-bearing joints with osteoarthrotic lesions (hip, knee) following treatment with nonsteroidal anti-inflamatory and analgesic agents. It has therefore been suggested that relief of pain with medications may favor excessive use of the diseased joint and thus precipitate osteochondral fractures which can lead to the appearance of Charcot joint.

symptoms appear at irregular intervals, whereas periodic diseases are characterized by regular intervals.

Intermittent hydrarthrosis (periodic course, hence a paradoxical term in the foregoing sense) occurs in form of more or less painful attacks lasting between 3 and 5 days and commonly is limited to a single joint, preferentially the knee. Onset is often as early as the growth period. Intervals of recurrence usually range between 2 and 4 weeks. Sometimes there occurs a transition to rheumatoid arthritis. Secondary osteoarthrosis (of the knee joint) can develop as a sequela to the periodic joint effusions.

Palindromic arthritis (palindromic rheumatism) (see p. 105): this disorder pursues an intermittent course.

Behçet's disease (p. 96): the Course is intermittent, presenting arthralgia and even arthritis; infrequently accompanied by erosions (Hamza et al., 1975).

Familial Mediterranean fever (intermittent course). It affects certain ethnic groups who inhabit or inhabited the countries bordering on the eastern Mediterranean; for instance, Sephardic Jews, Armenians, Turks, and Arabs. In addition, it is supposed that the disease occurs sporadically in other races (Brodey and Wolff, 1975). Familial Mediterranean fever usually makes its first appearance in childhood or adolescence. Its cardinal symptoms are febrile episodes frequently lasting for only a day or two, with temperatures rising as high as 40°C. These episodes are accompanied by other complaints, primarily intense abdominal (peritoneal) pain, pleural or pericardial discomfort, an erythema resembling erysipelas, and, in the majority of patients, also joint manifestations. The prognosis depends on the (frequent) development of secondary amyloidosis. In this case, renal amyloidosis often leads to death from renal insufficiency.

The episodic joint complaints—the second most frequent manifestation of the disease—occur in three forms:

1. Arthralgia and polyarthralgia, commonly in the lower extremities
2. (Febrile) oligoarthritis or polyarthritis running an acute or subacute course of several days, weeks or even months
3. Monoarticular involvement of large joints with effusion, swelling of soft tissues and collateral arthritic phenomena, which sometimes linger on for months

When the affection of the joints runs a chronic recurrent course, one may also encounter erosions, subchondral cysts, narrowing of the joint space, and even fibrous ankylosis (Sohar et al., 1967). In addition, a secondary osteoarthrosis can develop. In the majority of patients, however, the arthritis heals without permanent damage.

The knee joint, the talocrural joint, and the hip joint are the most frequent sites of articular involvement. Compared with other joints, the sacroiliac joints apparently are affected with above average frequency. Unilateral or bilateral sacroiliitis of the "variegated picture" type is encountered (Heller et al., 1966; Brodey and Wolff, 1975). In addition, there are reports on familial Mediterranean fever occurring in association with the full-blown (radiographic) picture of ankylosing spondylitis (Lejeune et al., 1975, and other writers).

Etiocholanolone fever, similar to familial Mediterranean fever, belongs in the group of diseases pursuing an intermittent course. The febrile episodes, which commonly endure no longer than a day or two, are accompanied mostly by monarthritis of one of the *larger* joints that may outlast the fever by weeks or months. Joint effusion, collateral arthritic phenomena, and (infrequently) erosions are apt to occur. During the attacks, an elevated plasma level of un-conjugated etiocholanolone is demonstrable. The disorder, therefore, is evidently a disease of metabolism.

Osteoarthrosis

When faced with a degenerative arthropathy, the principal interest of the radiologic examiner attaches to the early signs of the disorder and, in addition, to the question of whether the roentgenogram allows the drawing of conclusions concerning the causes and extent of cartilage attrition. In the knee joint, one distinguishes osteoarthrosis of the posterior surface of the patella and its glide layer—**femoropatellar** and **subpatellar osteoarthrosis**—from **osteoarthrosis of the entire joint.** In the medial femorotibial compartment, degenerative damage of the articular cartilage and its sequelae are demonstrable with much greater frequency than in the lateral femorotibial segment of the joint. This is particularly true of roentgenograms taken with the patient standing (Ahlbäck, 1968).

Variants of the anatomic shape of the patella occur more frequently than such variants in the articulating portion of the femur and tibia. However, the elevated load on the patella (p. 278) is tolerated in the long run only if the femoropatellar segments of the joint are congruent. Chondromalacia of the patella, as the consequence of excessive strain on the femoropatellar joint, has already been discussed on page 278 ff, and its significance in the development of femoropatellar osteoarthrosis has been emphasized. With time, femoropatellar osteoarthrosis can develop into osteoarthrosis of the entire knee joint. When a lateral roentgenogram of the knee joint taken because of joint pain and an effusion reveals delicate osteoarthrotic steophytes on the posterosuperior and posteroinferior borders of the patella (Fig. 419), whereas the other portions of the joint show *no anomaly*, the next steps in the radiologic diagnosis should be a plain axial roentgenogram and/or roentgenograms taken with the knee in 30, 60, and 90 degrees of flexion, which have still greater informative value (Figs. 395 and 396; p. 279 ff). These views will show whether the femoropatellar glide way presents any deformity; e.g., hypoplasia of the medial trochlea. In some of the cases a preosteoarthritic deformity will be ascertained and conclusions regarding therapy can be drawn. In other patients no primary deformity is demonstrable in the roentgenogram, despite osteoarthrosis of the femoropatellar joint. In such cases a careful search should be made for secondary, for instance posttraumatic, deformations and anomalous positions of the patella. Both can lead to the development of femoropatellar osteoarthrosis. When, on the other hand, the roentgen examination fails to detect neither a deformity of the patella and/or the patellar glide way nor an anomalous position, it could be that the patient gives, for example, a history of inflammatory gonarthritis or Sudeck's syndrome that might account for the development of femoropatellar

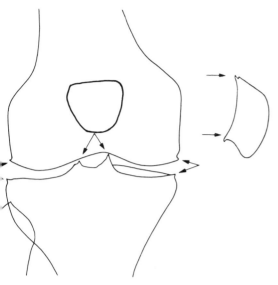

Fig. 419   **Localization** *(arrows)* **of early osteoarthritic osteophytes in the femoropatellar and femorotibial sections of the joint.**

osteoarthrosis. Finally, there remains the hypothetical assumption of constitutional inferiority of the cartilage. In this case, also, the patient should be advised to give up any activities or sports (for instance, football) that subject the knee joint to addition strain, thereby to slow down or prevent the progression of articular wear and tear.

A direct conclusion regarding the condition of the articular cartilage of the patella can be deduced from the size of the marginal osteoarthrotic osteophytes in lateral and axial roentgenograms of the patella (Dihlmann et al., 1979). If the size of the osteophytes exceeds 2 mm, retropatellar cartilage ulcers are present in the entirety of the cases. If the size of the osteophytes is about 2 mm or less, 80 percent of the patients have cartilage ulcers. These figures allow conclusions to be drawn about the activating potential of femoropatellar osteoarthrosis (as for activated osteoarthrosis, see p. 36 ff).

Osteoarthritic osteophytes in the region of the femorotibial joint develop—as elsewhere—upon the cartilage-bone interfaces (Fig. 419); i.e., likewise on the margin of the intercondylar fossa. Here, they usually are only demonstrable in the Frik view (intercondylar view). Delicate osteophytes (elongations) upon the two intercondylar tubercles attract attention before long. During the further course, the articular surfaces become realigned, the osteophytes develop into coarse marginal bulges, the intercondylar tubercles become rounded, and the subchondral layer consolidates (Fig. 420). At times, the detritus cysts develop (in the tibia). The joint space between the tibia and femur narrows (if unequally, this gives rise to **osteoarthrotic genu varum** [Fig. 421] or **osteoarthrotic genu valgum**)[21] until finally the osteoarthrotic remodeling into a largely nonfunctional knee

---

[21] These terms have a double meaning since the malalignment may be the primary condition or else an osteoarthritis exists which has produced a secondary malalignment.

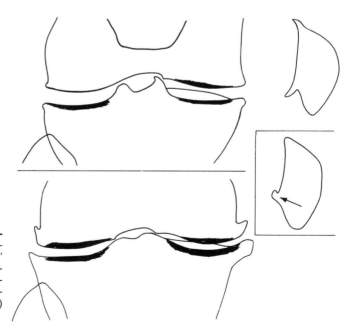

Fig. 420   **Advanced stages of osteoarthrosis of the knee** (see text). *Arrow* points to a *"patellar exostosis."* (Status after juvenile osteopathy of patella [compare Fig. 391, no. 9]?, but certainly not an osteophyte due to osteoarthrosis!) in an otherwise normal knee joint.) (Only patella illustrated.)

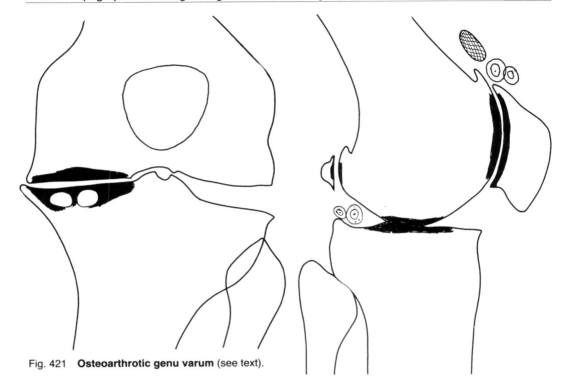

Fig. 421 **Osteoarthrotic genu varum** (see text).

Fig. 422 **Osteoarthrosis of the knee.** Among other features, abrasion of femoropatellar interfaces; calcified synovial chondromas; a synovial osteoma with cancellous structure; deformed fabella.

joint is completed. In the osteoarthrotic knee joint, calcified synovial chondromas and osteomas (Fig. 422)—i.e. fixed or detached loose bodies—are encountered with greater frequency than in osteoarthrosis of other joints (excepting cubital osteoarthrosis and carpometacarpal osteoarthrosis of the thumb, which shows a similar tendency for capsular metaplasia). The different ways in which loose bodies develop have been described on page 66. The fabella (the sesamoid bone in the lateral head of the gastrocnemius) often takes part in the osteoarthrotic deformation (Fig. 422).

The roentgen signs of the infrequent tibiofibular osteoarthrosis are depicted in Figure 423.

Figure 424 shows again the typical radiographic picture of osteoarthrosis of the knee joint. In this instance it has developed from a roentgenologically demonstrable chronic juxtaarticular osteomyelitis of the femur.

The movements of the knee joint are guided and restrained primarily by the capsule, the ligaments, the semilunar cartilages and the infrapatellar fat pad, but also by the muscular tone. Traumatic or other damage to these structures—for instance, **slack knee** (Fig. 425)—promote malalignments and faulty positions of the articulating bones (Fig. 426), and therefore are preosteoarthrotic conditions. Tears of the semilunar cartilages lead to *local* incongruities of the articulating surfaces. This is why excessive strain on the articular cartilage and its consequences are to be expected initially only in the compartment of the knee

where the tear has occurred. Besides this, the soft tissues of the joint listed play an auxiliary part in attrition of the joint and can intensify as well as accelerate the process. Disorders of muscular coordination—for instance, in the knee of spastic patients—and excessive strain following amputation of the contralateral lower leg are also preosteoarthrotic conditions. The same is true of arthritis-induced damage to the cartilage and traumatic lesions of cartilage and bone. Finally, among preosteroarthrotic conditions mention must be made of deformities accompanying the osteochondrodysplasias and other congenital systemic disorders as well as *local* acquired disorders of growth and ossification. Among the last-named acquired deformities, particular importance attaches to idiopathic, symptomatic (e.g., rachitic), and compensatory genu varum (occurring as a result of faulty static posture).

Tibia vara (Blount's disease, osteochondrosis deformans tibiae; Fig. 427) is a disorder of growth at the medial portion of the proximal end of the tibia, implying disturbed growth in the medial regions of the epiphyseal plate, epiphyseal line, and metaphysis (Bathfield and Beighton, 1978). In spite of straight growth of the tibial diaphysis, an increasing varus position of the proximal portion of the tibia develops.

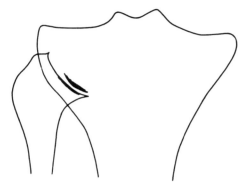

Fig. 423 **Typical appearance of tibiofibular osteoarthrosis** in the anteroposterior roentgenogram of the knee joint.

Whether bilateral or—as is usual—unilateral, the condition becomes manifest when the toddler starts walking (*infantile* type of Blount's disease). The less frequent *adolescent type* reveals the typical deformity only at the end of the first or the beginning of the second decade of life. Tibia vara (when not treated or inadequately treated)—similarly to **idiopathic, symptomatic,** and **compensatory genu valgum** as well as **genu recurvatum**—belongs to the class of preosteoarthrotic conditions. The osteopathic form of genu recurvatum, for instance, is apt to develop as an aftermath of inflammatory growth disturbances at the juxtaarticular epiphyseal plates.

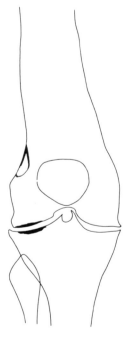

Fig. 424 **Long-term chronic osteomyelitis of femur, status after sequestrotomy.** Osteoarthrosis of the knee probably superimposed on a so-called sympathetic arthritis (compare p. 161 ff).

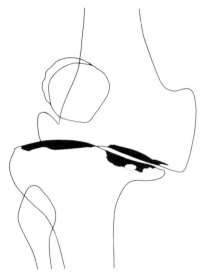

Fig. 425 **Osteoarthrotic slack knee.** About 40 years previously, severe fall from a bicycle with fracture of the patella and rupture of the collateral ligaments. Inadequate therapy. (Serological tests for syphilis repeatedly negative; normal findings on neurologic examination. A postsyphilitic [neurogenic] osteoarthropathy, which would show a more or less identical roentgenogram, can therefore be ruled out).

Osteochondrosis dissecans, spontaneous osteonecrosis, and neoplastic synovial chondromatosis are also to be classified as preosteoarthrotic conditions of the knee joint.

The knee joint is second only to the elbow joint in the incidence of **osteochondrosis dissecans** (Fig. 428). This disorder, which sometimes occurs bilaterally, affects primarily the medial and less frequently the lateral condyle of the femur. Osteochondrosis dissecans of the lateral condyle is often recognizable only in the intercondylar roentgenogram after Frik.

Formerly, the views on the pathogenesis of osteochondrosis dissecans were based on the assumption of an initial, focal, spontaneous ischemia with subsequent infarction and dissection. Other workers, for instance, Chiroff and Cooke III (1975), interpreted osteochondrosis dissecans as being a variant of epiphyseal development, which would lead to the formation of a separate center of ossification. The "self-healing tendency" of this ossification center, hence its fusion with the main portion of the epiphysis, was thought to be proved by the fact that osteochondrosis dissecans is observed principally in the years of growth. The theory of pathogenesis currently in favor is based on the following findings:

Histologic study of detached fragments removed surgically has shown that only parts of them are necrotic (Milgram, 1978). Surgeons are familiar with the fact that the articular cartilage over the roentgeno-

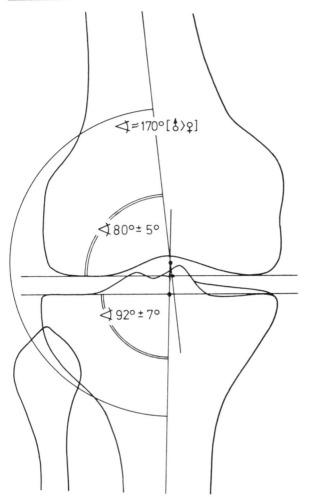

Fig. 426 **Axial relationships of femur and tibia in the anteroposterior roentgenogram** (taken to ascertain the extent of deformation or destruction of the supporting and gliding tissues in genu valgum or varum). In genu recurvatum the *lateral* roentgenogram, with the knee completely extended or hyperextended, is used to determine whether the hyperextensibility is related to flattening of the anterior tibial region. (Normally, the head of the tibia is found to lie at a somewhat higher level anteriorly than posteriorly). Additional causes of recurvature may be variations in shape of the femoral trochleae or deformities of the shaft of the tibia and lesions of the semilunar cartilages.

logically visible detached fragment is sometimes unchanged on gross inspection. The corresponding *biomechanical* considerations have identified osteochondrosis dissecans as a fatigue fracture that initially is subchondral and subsequently becomes osteochondral (Bandi, 1978).

Small, immediately subchondral, bone infarcts in hemoglobinopathies with sickle cell formation are sometimes resorbed. In such a case, the roentgen finding resembles the empty bed of a loose body in osteochondrosis dissecans. In hemoglobinopathies with sickle cell formation (for other causes see p. 254 ff), such a subchondral avascular necrosis of bone, depending on its extent, may also give rise to a preosteoarthrotic deformity in the knee joint. It should be mentioned that Gaucher's disease also leads to bone infarcts in the subchondral area. These infarcts at times become separated and, as additional roentgen information, then show the typical Erlenmeyer flask deformity of the distal end of the femur (Fig. 355 C).

This deformity is seen in the anteroposterior roentgenogram of the knee joint. Certainly, it is not a specific feature of Gaucher's disease (Greenfield, 1969, 1970) but it narrows the diagnostic possibilities to a small number of clinical pictures (compare, however, the legend accompanying Fig. 355).

Spontaneous osteonecrosis in the knee joint (Ahlbäck et al., 1968) also may lead to osteoarthrosis of the knee joint, and in severe cases to osteoarthrotic genu varum. This clinical picture must be differentiated from osteochondrosis dissecans (Fig. 428), circumscribed subchondral bacterial (tuberculous) inflammatory conditions, the early stage of a neurogenic osteoarthropathy of the knee joint, metastatic tumor, and, finally, from avascular osteonecrosis of known etiology (hemoglobinopathy with sickle cell formation, Gaucher's disease, etc., see p. 254 ff). Differentiation is possible with attention to the following characteristics of spontaneous osteonercrosis of the knee joint: The disease very frequently starts with

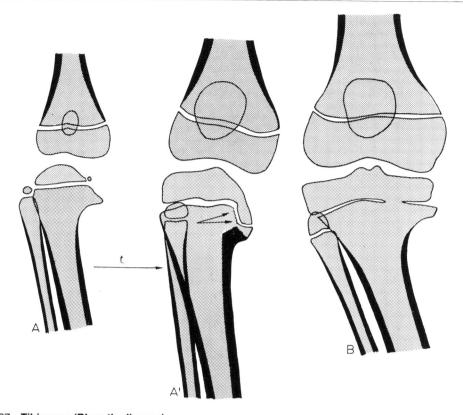

Fig. 427   **Tibia vara (Blount's disease).**
A, A′ = Infantile type (t = follow-up study).
B = Adolescent type (see text). In this type, there is comparatively little deformation of the proximal tibial epiphysis. In particular, no "step" is encountered in the epiphyseal line (see A′; *arrows*). In addition, note the bony bridge between the epiphysis and metaphysis in B (Langenskiöld and Riska, 1964).

acute intense pain in the knee, for which the patients (who generally are in the second half of life, usually beyond the age of 60) find no convincing explanation. The first pathologic roentgen sign to appear, 3 weeks after the onset of pain at the earliest, is a slight straightening (flattening) of the *medial* femoral condyle, which is recognizable in both the anteroposterior and the lateral roentgenograms (Fig. 429).

In general, the flattened area lies more medially, i.e., nearer the medial epicondyle of the femur, than does the typical site of osteochondrosis dissecans. At times, the cancellous bone in the immediate neighborhood of the flattened contour shows a slight increase in density, probably as the consequence of the homogenization of the devitalized trabeculae. About 2 months after the onset of pain, however, the subchondral area of the medial femoral condyle clears until one finally sees a flat defect of the bony contour which may encompass a characteristically even (flattened) bone shadow (Fig. 429 D). The radiolucency of the cancellous bone and the defect of the bony contour show a more or less extensive increase in density of the perifocal cancellous bone.

In some instances, there also develop alterations in the opposite medial condyle of the tibia; namely a circumscribed increase in density of the cancellous bone during the course of the disease. Less frequently, small fragments of bone become detached from the area of increased density. Occasionally, a periosteal aposition of bone is seen proximal to the medial femoral condyle (Fig. 429 D and E, *arrow*).

In **neoplastic synovial chondromatosis** (Fig. 430), the chondroma formation starts from the synovial membrane. Numerous clustered or rounded, frequently stratified, calcareous shadows are visible. The *calcified,* roentgenologically identifiable synovial chondromas, however, are present in only some of the cases. The *noncalcified* chondromas, sometimes the majority of cases, are not visible in the plain roentgenogram. At best, they can manifest themselves in the form of dense, homogeneous suprapatellar, infrapatellar, and popliteal soft-tissue shadows containing rounded calcium shadows.

In these instances, the disorder must be differentiated, also in the knee joint, from a synovial or capsular hemangioma with phleboliths. Malignant

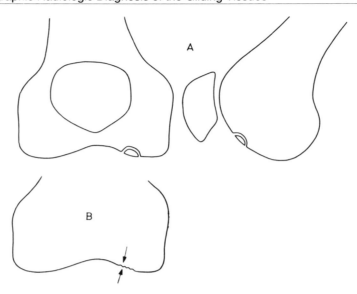

Fig. 428   **Osteochondrosis dissecans of the right knee joint.**
   A = Typical (most frequent) site. (Medial femoral condyle, nearer the intercondylar fossa, about the middle third of the circumference of the trochlea). The loose body is demarcated (but not yet "born").
   B = After the loose body became detached and was removed surgically because of locking, scar tissue formed in its former bed. Through (fibrous) cartilaginous and subsequent osseous transformation of the scar tissue, the defect has been largely filled *(arrows)* and is hardly or not at all recognizable in the film. (It is still best visible in the intercondylar roentgenogram after Frik.) Regarding the roentgenologic differential diagnosis of the "born" loose body not (yet) removed surgically, with its bed leveled, the infrequent **menisceal ossicles** (in the posterior extremity of the medial meniscus) are recalled (Glass et al. 1975, Kossoff et al. 1979). It is a matter of debate whether these structures constitute a posttraumatic metaplasia or an atavism (menisceal ossicles are frequently present in rodents). When the knee is flexed under the fluoroscope, the menisceal ossicles move together with the tibia (differential diagnosis from free loose bodies!).

degeneration into synovial chondrosarcomatosis is a very rare event. In advanced cases, the differentation between osteoarthrosis of the knee joint with synovial chondromas and synovial chondromatosis with secondary osteoarthrosis of the knee can be very difficult, since—as mentioned above—synovial chondromas occur with particular frequency in osteoarthrosis of the knee joint. In the early and intermediate stages, the diagnosis depends on the "majority conditions." (Many synovial chondromas but few signs of osteoarthrosis speak in favor of neoplastic synovial chondromatosis; in osteoarthrosis of the knee joint, accompanied by synovial chondromas, the relation is reversed and, in addition, synovial osteomas are observed together with the chondromas.)

There have been a number of reports on a **trough-shaped defect of the bone contour in the anterior surface of the distal femur** in which, with the knee extended, the patella finds space (Sutro, 1964; Fig. 431). Since this trough is found particularly in osteoarthrotic knee joints, relationships between that defect and femoropatellar osteoarthrosis have been suspected. The differential diagnosis by radiography must take into consideration a pressure erosion from

a soft-tissue tumor and, in general, a tumor-induced osteolysis.

Osteoarthropathies

In **gout** of the knee joint (p. 41 ff), the local reaction and, thereby, the roentgenologic morphology are materially influenced by the magnitude of the quantity to time quotient of the precipitation of urates. The great majority of gouty patients with involvement of the knee present the picture of osteoarthrosis of the knee. Osteophytes, straightening of the joint contours, narrowing of the joint space, and similar defects are striking features. In addition, discrete direct signs of arthritis as well as tophaceous deposits in bone sometimes give the osteoarthrosis an atypical appearance, and soft-tissue tophi become visible in the form of pleomorphic calcifications (Figs. 432 and 433). Under effective treatment, tophaceous osteolyses are apt to diminish in size with time or even to reossify. If gouty arthropathy takes the course of chronic gonarthritis, pronounced direct arthritic signs are encountered. Owing to the chronicity of the dis-

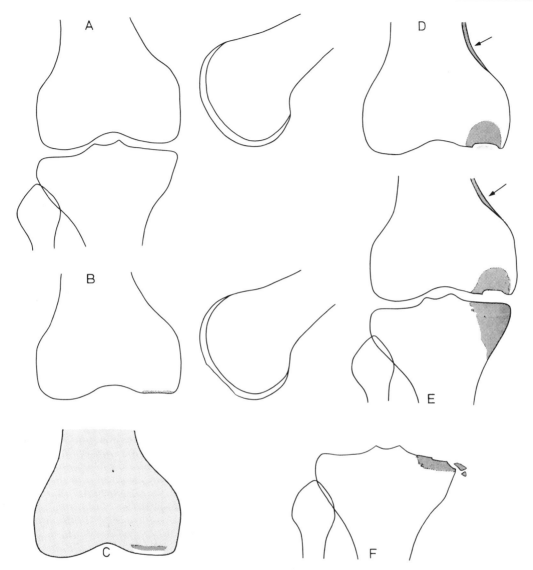

Fig. 429 **Manifestations of spontaneous osteonecrosis in the knee joint.**

A = Normal roentgen finding (at least 3 weeks after the onset of pain). Scintigraphy with bone-tracing radio-isotopes is positive (pathologic accumulation of tracers) sooner than the result of radiologic examination!

B = slight straightening (flattening) of the medial femoral condyle (early roentgen finding!), often accompanied by a very delicate subchondral area of increased density.

C = Two months after onset of the disease at the earliest, increased subchondral radiolucency with more or less pronounced increase in perifocal density of cancellous bone.

D = Oval, trough-shaped defect with increased perifocal density of cancellous bone. The *flattened* bone plate in the defective contour is a characteristic roentgen finding (compare the finding in osteochondrosis dissecans in Fig. 428). Contingent periosteal reaction *(arrow)*.

E = The necrotic plate-shaped portion of bone has been resorbed. In the opposite medial condyle of the tibia an increased density of the spongiosa has appeared which (by no means an indispensable sign) is often deeper and broader than the area of increased density in the femur. Contingent periosteal reaction *(arrow)*.

F = In addition to the changes depicted in E, gradual densification and fragmentation of bone occur in the tibia.

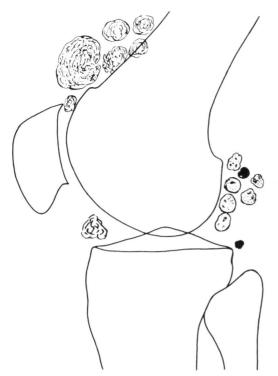

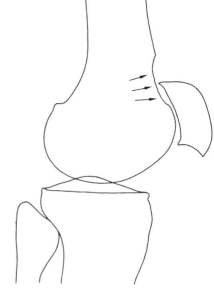

Fig. 431 **Trough-shaped defect in the contour of the distal anterior aspect of the femur,** *so-called anterior distal erosion of the femur (arrows).* In the extended position part of the patella glides into the defect. Osteoarthrosis of the knee (marginal osteophytes; narrowing of the femoropatellar joint space).

Fig. 430 **Neoplastic synovial chondromatosis of the knee joint.** Numerous calcified synovial chondromas, only minor secondary osteoarthrosis (see text).

order, however, these signs are often overshadowed by a secondary osteoarthritis. It should further be mentioned that, also in gout, the semilunar cartilages of the knee joint are apt to become calcified (p. 63, symptomatic chondrocalcinosis). For the gouty tophus in the patella and its radiologic differential diagnosis, see page 294. Dissection of the necrotic upper portion of the patella has also been observed (Seewald, 1971). The devitalization of bone demonstrated in this case has been attributed to a local vascular reaction demonstrated histologically.[22]

Of the large peripheral joints, the knee is the most frequently involved in **ochronotic osteoarthropathy** (p. 44 ff). The roentgenogram reveals osteoarthritis of the knee joint with (calcified) synovial chondromas and osteomas, and occasional calcification of the menisci (Fig. 434). In patients with ochronosis, however, the osteoarthrosis frequently appears as early as the third or fourth decade of life. The patients often report episodes of acute locking produced by loose bodies. These free loose bodies in ochronotic patients are either detached cartilaginous

or osseous synovial metaplasias or ("grown" and/or calcified) fragments of the brittle articular cartilage that have been split off. Since in anteroposterior roentgenograms of the knee joint not only the femoral condyles but usually also part of the femoral shaft can be evaluated, the ochronotic foci of Bauer and Kienböck (rounded translucences, Fig. 434 B; compare Fig. 258) sometimes attract attention as additional information. The nearer *and* farther bony surroundings of the knee joint are favorite sites for these findings.

The knee and the elbow are the test joints of **hemophilic osteoarthropathy.** However, these test joints also are subject to the rule that the development of this osteoarthropathy depends on the severity of the disorder, hence the genetically determined percentile of residual activity of the clotting factors. The pathologic processes in the hemophilic joint described on page 46 ff, with their serious morphologic and functional effects on the supporting and gliding tissues of the joint, have been studied preferentially in the knee. Figures 435 through 439 illustrate different degrees of severity of the alterations in the knee joint. Particular emphasis is to be laid on the usually asymmetrical increase in size of the distal femoral epiphysis with the consequent valgus—less frequently varus—of the knee, and also the pronounced (at times fibrillar) juxtaarticular demineralization (Fig. 436). It gives rise to a supracondylar fracture of the

---

[22] Proliferations of the vessel wall are regarded as a reaction to the proximity of a gouty tophus. Apart from this, compression of the blood vessels by a neighboring tophus can lead to impairment of circulation (Ganz, 1971).

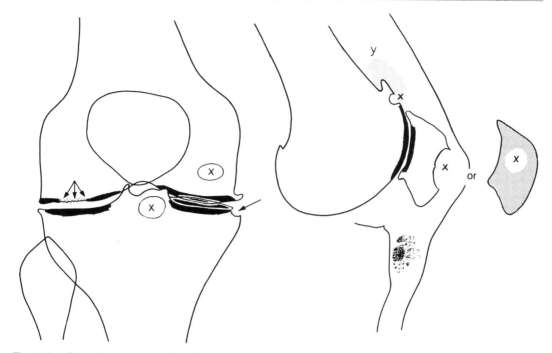

Fig. 432. **Chronic gout persisting for 10 years.** Principal roentgen findings are the characteristic osteoarthrosis deformations of the knee joint. *Atypical* of banal latent osteoarthrosis (see p. 36) are, however, *(synoptically):*

1. An (arthritic) marginal erosion and fine serration (breakage of the marginal lamella) *(arrows).* 2. Sharply delineated defects of bone (x), in part (see patella) with swelling of soft tissues. These are gouty tophi. 3. Pleomorphic calcifications above the tuberosity of the tibia (calcified tophus in the patellar ligament or in a bursa (compare Fig. 400 H). Effusion into the suprapatellar recess (bursa) = y. Calcium shadows are apt to occur in the cavity of the knee joint (calcium urate; *not illustrated*).

Fig. 433 **Infrequent roentgen findings in gout.**

A = Knee joint complaints in known gout with attacks of podagra. The roentgenogram shows discreet signs of osteoarthrosis of the knee joint (delicate osteophytes) and a cystlike osteolysis in the medial femoral condyle (compare legend of Fig. 49). The osteolytic area has a marginal seam of alternating density and contains pleomorphic calcium shadows. Biopsy reveals a calcified urate tophus. *Differential radiologic diagnosis:* Bone infarct; enchondroma; chondroblastoma.

B = Chronic effusion into the knee joint in known gout. Dorsally and caudally a bulging soft-tissue tumor is palpable which (possibly) contains pleomorphic calcium shadows. This is a Baker's cyst (p. 283 ff) in gouty arthropathy (Peavy and Franco, 1974) with precipitates of calcium urate.

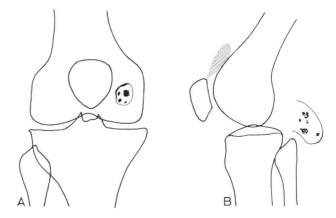

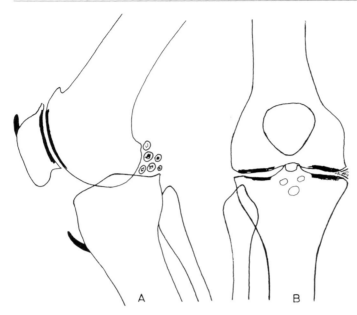

Fig. 434 **Ochronotic osteoarthro-pathy of the knee joint in a 50-year-old patient.** (Five years previously there were slight complaints, but the roentgen findings were still normal).
A = Typical roentgenogram of osteoarthrosis with metaplastic calcified synovial chondromas. Fibroosteoses at the patella and the tuberosity of the tiba (see p. 44).
B = Osteoarthrosis of the knee joint with "peculiarities" (chondrocalcinosis of the medial meniscus). The cystlike structural defects underneath the intercondylar eminence are, according to their location, not osteoarthrotic detritus cysts but (very probably) Bauer-Kienböck osseous foci (see p. 44 ff.).

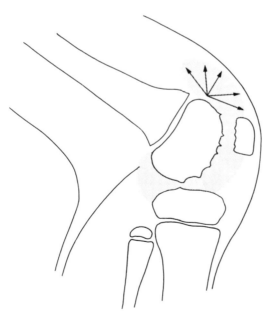

Fig. 435 **Hemophilia** (7-year-old child); recurrent hemorrhages into the knee joint. Disturbed growth; see distal femoral epiphysis and patella (rudimentary "aspergillum," Fig. 415; "rectangular" shape of patella, Fig. 416, instead of normal harmonious rounding). In the region of the joint cavity, distention and *increased density* from effusion of blood, reactive proliferations of the articular soft tissues, and *hemosiderin precipitates* are demonstrable (see the *arrows* in the ballooned suprapatellar recess of the joint).

femur, which is a typical event in hemophilia and frequently occurs even with a trivial trauma (Landbeck and Kurme, 1970). It has already been mentioned that widening of the intercondylar fossa (Figs. 51 and 437; pp. 46 ff and 290) is a general sign of disordered growth, which is encountered not only in hemophilia but also in arthritis of the growth period. With large effusions of blood, the resorptive processes are apt to produce dull contours of the joint, erosions, and haziness and blurring of the juxtaarticular cancellous structures. These pictures are reminiscent of arthritis and its collateral phenomena. Fixed high-grade flexion contracture with subluxation of the tibia, the most severe clinical manifestation of the hemophilic joint, nowadays is avoidable or at least correctable. With a serious clinical course, it is particularly the patella that is apt to undergo bony ankylosis with the femur. Fibrotic-bony ankylosis rarely, if ever, occurs between the femur and the tibia. The hemophilic pseudotumor (Fig. 439)—for its development see page 46—shows severe changes (remodeling with prevalent resorption of bone) *and* extensive circumscribed expansion of the soft tissues. Initially, the roentgenogram makes one suspect a malignant tumor. However, a previous history of hemophilia strongly suggests a hemophilic pseudotumor.

The distal femoral epiphysis is an area of particularly pronounced longitudinal growth, for it accounts for about two thirds of the increase in length of the femur. In the **congenital hereditary hemoglobinopathies**—for instance during the course of sickle cell anemia (pp. 117 and 119)—the distal femur is frequently the site of avascular bone infarcts and

Fig. 436 **Hemophilic osteoarthropathy of the right knee joint.** *Asymmetrical* acceleration of growth *(arrow)* at the distal femoral epiphysis has produced genu valgum (see text). Fibrillar juxtaarticular decalcification (Fig. 13). So-called lines of growth (arrest) are demonstrable in the tibia, the fibula, and the femur. Normal roentgen finding in the *left* knee joint (no joint hemorrhages in the history).

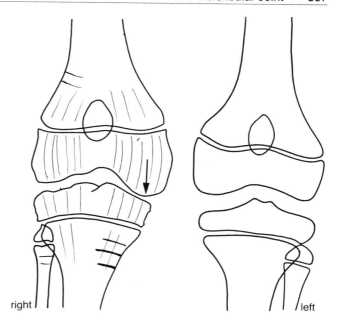

right   left

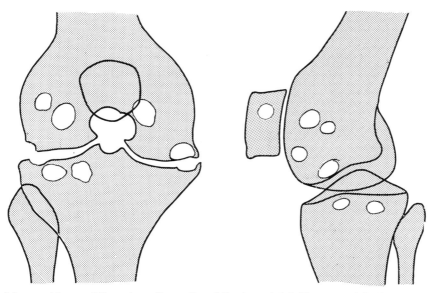

Fig. 437 **Advanced hemophilic osteoarthropathy of the knee joint.** Note especially the "widening" of the intercondylar fossa (compare Fig. 51) and the "rectangular patella." These signs of disordered growth occur frequently in hemophilia but also in other acquired growth disturbances; for instance, arthritis of the growth period. The rounded translucences in the subchondral area and at some distance from the joint are the consequences of hemorrhages into the bone marrow.

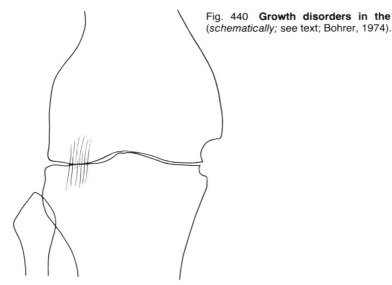

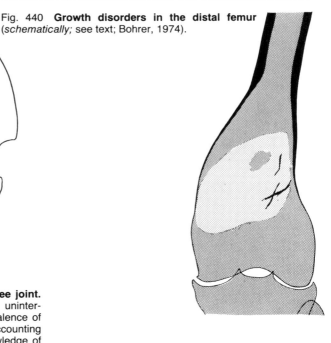

Fig. 440   **Growth disorders in the distal femur** (*schematically;* see text; Bohrer, 1974).

Fig. 438.   **Final stage of a hemophilic knee joint.** Partial bony ankylosis (trajectories coursing uninterrupted from the femur to the tibia) but prevalence of fibrotic ankylosis. Marked demineralization (accounting for the patella being invisible). Without knowledge of hemophilia in the history the roentgenogram would suggest a (past) arthritic process.

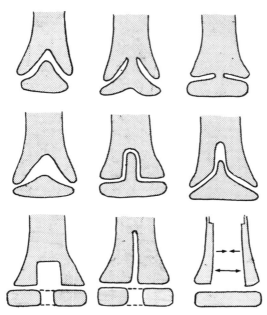

Fig. 439   **Hemophilic pseudotumor in the distal femur.**

hematogenous osteomyelitis (p. 119). In early childhood, depending on their localization (in the diaphysis, metaphysis, or epiphysis), these processes can lead to the disordered growth and development of the epiphysis and its cartilage. Such deformations (Fig. 440) also occur as a result of trauma or osteomyelitis without sickle cell anemia. Thus, the only decisive factors are the *early* growth period and the point where the damaging agent attacks.

Neurogenic osteoarthropathies (p. 47 ff) of the knee joint are to be expected primarily in tabes dorsalis. However, besides in *acquired* diseases (p. 49 ff), neurogenic osteoarthropathies and the so-called pseudo-Charcot's joints (p. 59; Figs. 64 and 418) also occur in the knee. Although certain neurogenic osteoarthropathies take years to develop, it has—though less frequently—been observed that a clinical course eventuates within weeks or months in the typical "anarchic rearrangement" of the joint (Norman et al., 1968). Instability, dissolution of smaller or larger portions of the articulating bones, and, finally, complete disorganization of the joint are the stages in the development of neurogenic osteoarthropathy of the knee (Figs. 441 and 442). The late stages present characteristic roentgen findings. The early stages—insofar as they are at all identifiable in the roentgen-

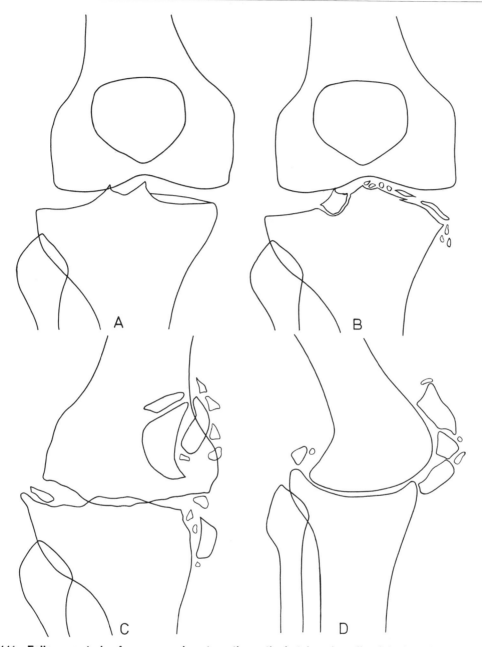

Fig. 441   **Follow-up study of a neurogenic osteoarthropathy in tabes dorsalis of the knee joint.**

A = Radiologic examination undertaken because of an effusion into the joint. Slight subluxation (instability); minor signs of osteoarthrosis not exceeding those to be expected at age 65 (extended intercondylar tubercle). In the absence of *clinical* signs suggestive of neurosyphilis or some other disease presenting neurogenic joint lesions, the diagnosis "early stage of a neurogenic osteoarthropathy" *cannot* be made from the roentgenogram.

B = Increasing instability (genu varum) and "melting away" (fragmentation) of the head of the tibia. Roentgen examination about 4 weeks later than A (hence considerable progression). The roentgen diagnosis "neurogenic osteoarthropathy" or pseudo-Charcot joint (see text) can now be established.

C and D = Roentgen examination 18 months later than B. Advanced neurogenic osteoarthropathy (among other features, complete fragmentation of patella).

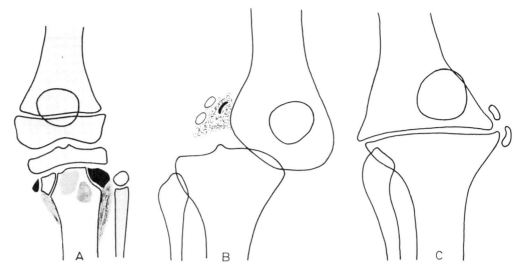

Fig. 442 **Neurogenic osteoarthropathies.**
    A = 12-year-old patient. Painless expansion in the region of the knee with congenital analgesia (p. 49). The pathologic reactions consist chiefly of metaphyseal fractures with excessive callus formation and increased densities of the cancellous bone. Slight widening of the cleft of the proximal epiphyseal cartilage of the tibia.
    B = Tabes dorsalis.
    C = Diabetes mellitus of several decades' standing. The severe deformity of the knee joint causes almost no disomfort!

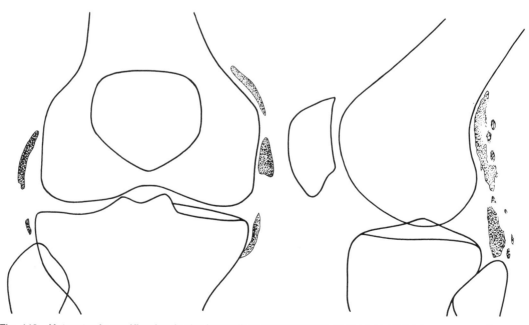

Fig. 443 **Heterotopic ossification in the immediate surroundings of the knee joint** (appearance of neurogenic paraosteoarthropathy) **following extensive burns of the body surface.** (The surroundings of the right knee joint in the case illustrated are, however, not directly involved in the burn).

ogram—may considerably hinder the roentgen diagnosis or may even go undiagnosed. This is because, on the one hand, a neurogenic osteoarthropathy may be the first manifestation of tabes dorsalis or another disease, and, on the other hand, a neurogenic (tabetic) osteoarthropathy (in a patient with late syphilis) is apt to develop subsequent to a capsuloligamentous injury. In this instance, a compensable sequel to trauma will be accepted under the following premises (Jonasch, 1964):

Prior to the accident, a neurogenic osteoarthropathy was *not* demonstrable in the part involved. The accident involved the joint in which the neurogenic osteoarthropathy subsequently manifested itself. Finally, no (or only minor) osteoarthropathies have developed in any other part of the body not directly affected by the accident (i.e., the difference in degree as compared to the injured joint must be striking).

Tabetics are liable to suffer spontaneous fractures in the vicinity of neurogenic osteoarthropathies. However, spontaneous fractures also occur in these patients in the absence of such an adjacent affection. A typical event is the *spontaneous supracondylar fracture of the femoral shaft,* which is often followed by excessive callus formation.

Heterotopic extracapsular neoformations of bone—as the expression of a neurogenic paraosteoarthropathy (p. 52 ff)—in patients with hemiplegia, paraplegia, and quadriplegia, but also in pareses due to poliomyelitis, occur exclusively in areas with a disturbed nerve supply (Wharton and Morgan, 1970). This disorder can give rise to extraarticular bony ankylosis, which, however, is much less common in the knee joint than in the joints of the hip, shoulder, and elbow. Heterotopic neoformations of bone also sometimes are observed in the knee joint following thermal injuries[23] (Fig. 443) and as a complication of tetanus infection. These neoformations cannot be differentiated radiographically from neurogenic extracapsular ossifications.

Massive osteolysis (Gorham-Stout) (p. 59) is also seen in the joint-bearing bones of the knee (Fig. 444). The adjective ''massive'' characterizes the typical, progressive, extensive, nonreactive dissolution of these bones.

In the region of the knee, **osteoarthropathy from amyloidosis** (p. 60) is an infrequent roentgen finding as compared with the manifestations of the disease; for instance, in the shoulder and hip joints. Cystlike osteolyses and cortical defects of the articulating bones are to be expected in this disorder (Gordon et al., 1973). Without awareness of the disease in the history, it is not possible to classify roentgenologically

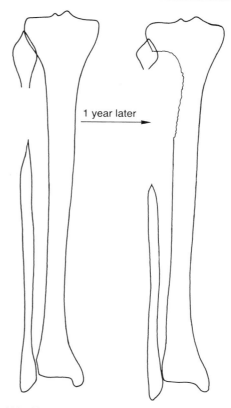

1 year later

Fig. 444   **Massive osteolysis (Gorham-Stout) in the lower leg.** A 32-year-old male developed an osteolysis of the fibula and tibia. No remaining bone shadows in the soft tissues. An extensive biopsy gave no clue to malignancy.

the osteolyses or erosions reflecting the masses of amyloid.

Osteoarthropathy from hemochromatosis (p. 61 ff) in the knee joint shows the roentgen signs of osteoarthrosis and chondrocalcinosis (of the hyaline cartilage and the menisci), hence an ambiguous combination of findings. The chondrocalcinosis can give rise to acute arthritic irritation (pseudogout, see p. 62 ff). The physician referring the patient for radiology usually is cognizant of the presence of idiopathic hemochromatosis. The nosological classification of the roentgen findings mentioned therefore hardly ever meets with difficulty if it is borne in mind that up to 50 percent of all patients with idiopathic hemochromatosis complain of discomfort in the joints, which commonly follows the other symptoms. In addition, it should be pointed out that, owing to chondrocalcinosis in the region of the carpus and the metacarpals, the metacarpophalangeal joints II and III are the test joints of arthropathy related to hematochromatosis (compare Fig. 148).

Kashin-Beck disease has been discussed in detail on page 114. In the knee joint, the disordered

---

[23] If, following an extensive thermal injury—for instance, to the lower leg or foot—an insidious destruction of the knee joint develops, one has to consider primarily an infection of the joint propagated by extension from the surrounding tissue or by way of the bloodstream or the lymphatics. It is very rare for extreme destruction of the joint to take place following a thermal injury. Such destructions can closely resemble neurogenic osteoarthropathies, even without infection of the joint!

endochondral ossification leads to deformation of the articulating epiphyses and thereby to early attrition of the joint (osteoarthrosis of the knee).

In the knee joint, **osteoarthropathy of Wilson's disease** (p. 62) manifests itself as a slight osteoarthritis of the knee that already appears in early adulthood and can be associated with chondrocalcinosis. Moreover, one frequently encounters small, free, loose bodies ("fragments") and the irregularities of contour in the condyles and the patella (lateral view), occasionally even the full-blown picture of osteochondrosis dissecans. It has already been pointed out on page 62 that *renal* rickets (*renal* osteomalacia) occurring in Wilson's disease manifests itself particularly in the pelvic girdle. In the vicinity of the knee joint, Looser's zones (which, *by definition* are repair stages of persistent fractures in the diseased skeleton) are to be expected in the metaphyseal regions of the articulating bones. They originate in the medial contour of these bones.

Hyperparathyroidism (p. 125 ff) also manifests itself in the knee joint and its immediate surroundings. The same applies to **renal (uremic) osteopathy** (p. 129 ff). In roentgenograms of the knee joint, signs of subperiosteal bone resorption are recognizable *primarily* in the medial contour of the proximal third of the tibia (Figs. 445 and 446). Less frequent are lesions of the joints (Fig. 446), particularly calcifications of the menisci and the hyaline articular cartilage (chondrocalcinosis). In addition, the fibroosseous destruction, which of course also involves the subchondral area, leads to breaks in the articulating bones. These have the radiographic ap-

pearance of (arthritic) erosions. In these cases, the clinical suspicion of chronic arthritis will be further strengthened if the synovial membrane reacts to such breaks with inflammation, and an effusion into the joint makes its appearance (Fig. 446). Since the patella is exposed to a great compressive load, its glide surface sometimes becomes depressed and resorbed in hyperparathyroidism. The patella then "envelops" the opposite femoral condyle (Bywaters et al., 1963; Fig. 446). Attention is called to the fact that in hyperparathyroidism the walls not only of the major but also of the minor arteries frequently calcify (Fig. 446).

Osteoarthropathy of the knee joint in acromegaly (Fig. 447) manifests itself as osteoarthrosis of the knee with a "wide" roentgenologic joint space (p. 131 ff). With time, however, this characteristic roentgen finding merges into the picture of typical osteoarthrosis because the articular cartilage, which has proliferated under the action of pathologic hormonal impulses, is subject to premature attrition (follow-up study in Fig. 447). Other conspicuous features of acromegaly, also visible in the knee joint, are the coarse shape of the articulating bones and (frequently) the fibrillar bone structure.

Osteoarthropathy due to ionizing rays occurs rarely in the knee joint. Its manifestations are (unilateral) osteoarthrosis of the knee, growth disturbance, circumscribed alteration of the normal structure of cancellous bone, and osteochondrosis dissecans, accompanied or not by metaplasia of the synovial membrane, into cartilage and bone. The concomitant radiation injury to the skin points to the causal connection. Radiation osteoarthropathy in the treatment

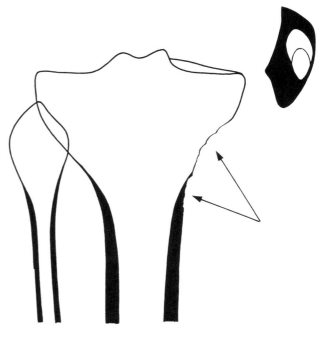

Fig. 445 **Extraarticular roentgen signs of hyperparathyroidism recognizable in radiographs of the knee joint.** *Arrows* point to a typical localization of subperiosteal bone resorption in the medial contour of the proximal third of the tibia; during the further course, subperiosteal resportion of bone also may become visible in the proximal fibula. "Brown tumor" in the patella (rare finding; more frequent in the pelvic bones, the ribs, and the long tubular bones). In about 3 percent of cases (Greenfield, 1969) a *solitary* brown tumor occurs in hyperparathyroidism (therefore, determine the serum calcium and serum phosphate in the presence of solitary bullous osteolyses).

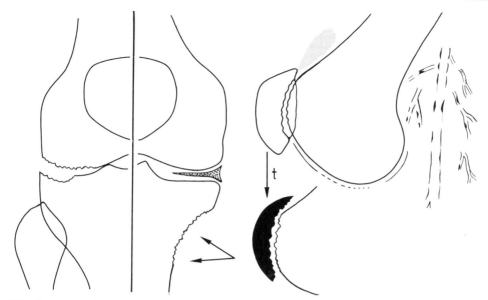

Fig. 446 **Roentgen signs of hyperparathyrodism** (continued). Effusion into the suprapatellar recess; erosions; narrowing of the joint space; depression of the patellar glide surface progressing to extensive resorption of the posterior surface of the patella. Course (t) illustrated: The patella "envelops" the femoral condyles; the menisci and the hyaline cartilage become calcified. Subperiosteal resporption of bone in the typical place (see *arrows* and Fig. 445) usually demonstrable earlier than subchondral erosions. In addition, calcified arterial vessels are sketched in the figure. Deposition of calcium even in *small* vessels is a typical feature. *Note:* In Wilson's Disease irregularity of the patellofemoral contours associated with narrowing of the joint space can also occur.

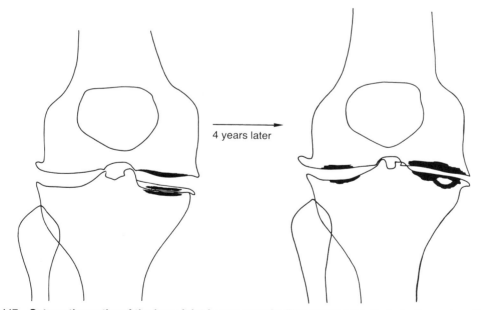

4 years later

Fig. 447 **Osteoarthropathy of the knee joint in acromegaly.** This disorder manifests itself as osteoarthrosis of the knee joint without narrowing of the joint space ("wide" roentgenologic joint space). With time it merges into the typical radiographic appearance of osteoarthrosis *(right part of the figure).*

of malignant tumors must be accepted on careful consideration of the benefits and risks. It should, however, by no means be the consequence of intraoperative fluoroscopy; for instance, in searching for bomb or shell splinters (Kolář et al., 1967).

Neoplasms of Joints

Establishment of the diagnosis of **malignant synovialoma** is reserved for histologic study. The gliding tissue of the knee joint is the most frequent site of this neoplasm, which starts there primarily from the bursae (Ebbinghaus, 1953). In the region of the knee joint, this tumor manifests itself roentgenographically as a rounded or lobulated increase in density and swelling of the soft tissues (Fig. 448). In about one third of the cases, pleomorphic calcium shadows appear within the area of increased density. This finding substantiates the suspected roentgenologic diagnosis (Lewis, 1947). The malignant synovialoma *may* invade the articulating bones as a cone-shaped structure. This process is revealed in the roentgenogram by rounded, more or less marginal, osteolyses (Fig. 449). Occasionally, the tumor also produces periosteal reactions. In contrast to **pigmented villonodular synovitis**[24] (p. 139 ff), which likewise manifests itself by rounded or lobulated increases in density of the soft tissues, malignant synovialoma is often characterized by the location of the increased density of the soft tissues. Roentgenologic study often succeeds in localizing the tumor entirely or partially outside the known borders of the joint capsule (see Figs. 399 and 400). Conversely, an increased density produced by pigmented villonodular synovitis lies inside the borders of the capsule. Moreover, in pigmented villonodular synovitis, no calcifications are seen in the proliferated tissue. Initially, direct signs of arthritis are lacking in pigmented villonodular synovitis of the knee joint; cystlike osteolyses on one or both sides of the joint space or marginal erosions from skeletal invasion are to be expected only *after many years* (Fig. 450).

It should be mentioned here that the knee joint is also the most frequent site of pigmented villonodular synovitis. This disease occurs in the knee joint, as in the other large joints, in its diffuse form (see p. 139). In addition, both malignant synovialoma and pigmented villonodular synovitis are seen with the highest frequency between the ages of 20 and 40.

Regarding the *differential diagnosis of malignant synovialoma*, the following examples will be listed:

Calcifications are occasionally observed in front of the *trough-shaped defect in the contour of the distal anterior aspect of the femur* (Fig. 431). These calcifications are situated in the synovial membrane (Doppman, 1964). However, the location of the trough-shaped femoral erosion is so characteristic that one should consider primarily the latter lesion and only secondarily a malignant synovialoma.

The infrapatellar fat pad, similarly to the infrequent **lipoma of the joint,** can become calcified. The calcium shadows occupy their typical place within the infrapatellar fat pad.

In hemangiomas of the knee joint—**synovial hemangiomas**—circumscribed increased densities of the soft tissues and, frequently, calcium shadows likewise are to be expected. However, the calcifications show the appearance of phleboliths (rounded calcifications, part of them stratified), and they are not as pleomorphic as in malignant synovialoma. The synovial hemangiomas occur either as solitary tumors or in association with hemangiomas of the skin; for instance, in the setting of the Klippel-Trenauny syndrome or the Kasabach-Merritt syndrome (hemangiomas associated with coagulation defects). The synovial hemangiomas frequently manifest themselves already in early childhood by pain, swelling, and impaired mobility. They give rise to recurrent hemorrhages into the joint; the reactive processes of resorption produce not only the roentgen signs of increased intraarticular volume (see Figs. 399 and 400) but also disturbances of the normal development of the articulating bones; e.g., deformation of the femoral epiphysis with widening of the intercondylar fossa or rectangular shape of the patella (Resnick and Oliphant, 1975).

Traumatic rupture of the quadriceps tendon (see p. 324 ff; Fig. 466) in adipose individuals presents a distinctive clinical finding; i.e., the inability actively to extend the leg. *Frequent* roentgenologic features, especially in ruptures of some standing, are effusion (hemorrhage into the joint), increased density of the suprapatellar soft tissues with *calcium shadows* (retracted tendon, dystrophic calcifications of the tendon) or calcifying hematoma (Newberg and Wales, 1977).

Swelling of soft tissues and increased densities in the immediate vicinity of the joint are also produced by **lipomas, neurofibromas, fibromas of the gliding tissues** (including the menisci), **arthroceles, bursal hygromas** (p. 283 ff), and **menisceal ganglia.** These ''ganglia'' will be taken up in greater detail (Fig. 451): Ganglia of the menisci and the joint capsule (which, outside the joints, can arise from tendons and their insertions, from peritendinous tissues, and from ligaments) owe their origin not to degenerative processes but possibly to dysontogenetic events. Rests of the arthrogenic mesenchyme (embryonal remnants) are thought to start proliferating for various reasons and differentiating into myxomatous or fibromatous tissue. The eventual cystic transformation is said to be an inherent property of

---

[24] The following constellation of findings will suggest the presence of pigmented villonodular synovitis: Chronic or recurrent, often blood-tinged effusion into the joint, which initially may have occurred after an injury to the soft tissues; palpable swelling of the capsule or striking increase of the soft tissues of the knee; and normal or slightly pathologic roentgen findings in the articulating bones.

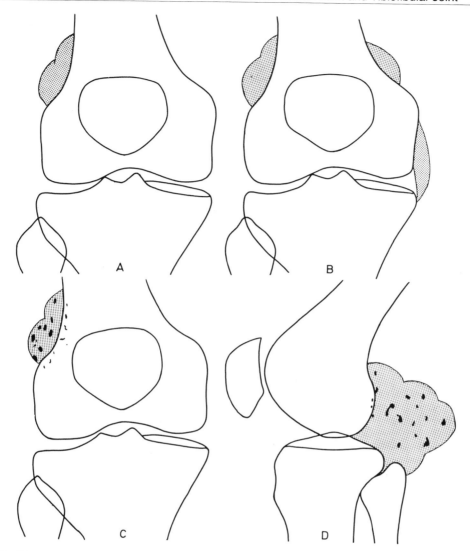

Fig. 448 Differential radiologic diagnosis of circumscribed increased densities of soft tissue near and inside the knee joint.

A = Circumscribed (lobulated) increased density of soft tissues, hence an ambiguous finding that may suggest hemangioma, lipoma (Pudlowsky et al., 1979), pigmented villonodular synovitis, malignant synovialoma.

B = Multicentric, circumscribed increased densities of soft tissues, initially suggesting pigmented villonodular synovitis or malignant synovialoma.

C = Circumscribed increased density of soft tissues with scattered calcifications. Strong suspicion of malignant synovialoma.

Note: Lipomas of the joints and hemangiomas (phleboliths) may also reveal calcium shadows. Synovial lipoma with a villous configuration is termed *lipoma arborescens.* It may occur bilaterally in the knee joint and, during its slowly progressive development, it gives the following findings: massive increase in soft-tissue density (tumor tissue and considerable effusion); calcified areas (mostly dorsal to the femoral condyles); lateral subluxation of the tibia; osteoarthrosis (Arzimanoglu, 1957). Lipoma arborescens also occurs in the carpal region and in the talocrural joint (Weitzman, 1965).

D = Lobulated increase in soft-tissue density very probably caused by a malignant synovialoma. (1. Scattered pleomorphic calcium shadows. 2. Partly extraarticular expansion of the area of increased density?)

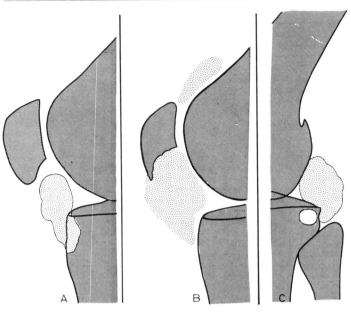

Fig. 449 **Difficult or impossible roentgenologic differentiation between pigmented villonodular synovitis (A) and malignant synovialoma (C).** (Pleomorphic calcifications are present only in one third of malignant synovialomas.) In either case, erosions of bone are apt to occur. In pigmented villonodular synovitis, however, this would take a number of years. The malignant synovialoma (C) had been neglected over a prolonged period because the soft-tissue shadow did not stand out and because the concomitant (independent) osteoarthrosis of the knee caused the cone-shaped expansion of the tumor into the posterior portion of the tibial plateau to be misdiagnosed as an osteoarthrotic detritus cyst. B shows a roentgen finding that justifies diagnosis of a malignant neoplasm of the joint.

the arthrogenic mesenchyme. Ganglia develop more frequently in the lateral than in the medial meniscus (Masshoff and Schultz-Ehrenberg, 1974). Menisci with ganglia often present congenital deformations; they may be discoid and frequently show (acquired) tears, or they are encountered in knee joints with disordered static conditions; for instance, axial deviations. With equal frequency, the patients give a history of excessive athletic strain and consequent stretching of the insertions of the menisci. This is a summary of the possible causes for proliferation of the mesenchymal remnants *(vide supra)*.

Clinically and radiographically, ganglia of the menisci reveal the characteristics of a (nonmalignant) tumor: They displace other structures as they grow, and they tend to recur. When their size and location are adequate, ganglia protrude lateralward from the joint space as a circumscribed increase in density of the soft tissues. On physical examination, nonmalignant and malignant meniscus tumors can mimic a minisceal ganglion. Every supposed menisceal ganglion therefore should be examined histologically.

Xanthomas accompany the hyperlipoproteinemias; they are found in the skin, the subcutaneous and tendinous tissue, and bone (p. 141). Xanthomas in the region of the knee are depicted in Figure 452.

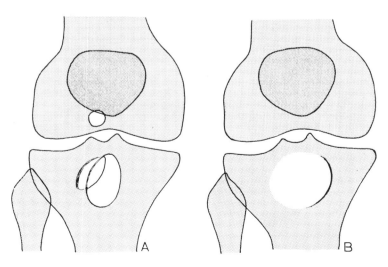

Fig. 450 **Patterns of pigmented villonodular synovitis with involvement of bone** (after many years' evolution).

A = Cystic osteolyses on both sides of the joint space suggest a disorder that originated in the knee joint.

B = The cystlike osteolysis in the tibial plateau, with or without increased density of the marginal seam, arouses suspicion of a malignant tumor. The diagnosis was only settled by biopsy.

Correct interpretation of the roentgen findings A and B would be facilitated if in either instance an effusion into the knee joint were demonstrable (see Fig. 399 C).

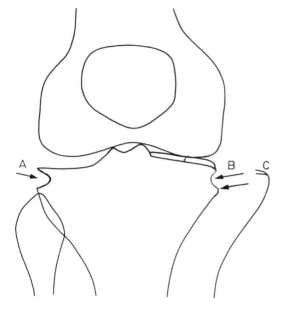

Fig. 451 **Signs of meniscus ganglion in the plain roentgenogram.** A = *Pressure erosion* (depression). It does *not* extend to the articular surface *(arrow);* thereby it generally can be differentiated from an arthritic erosion. In its florid stage, moreover, an arthritic erosion has ill-defined borders, whereas a pressure erosion has sharp contours. B = *Pressure erosion (upper arrow)* and small *exostosis (lower arrow)* due to traction on the insertions of the capsule and the ligaments. (Comparison with the sound side = C).

Note: The pressure erosion persists even after removal of the meniscus ganglion. The roentgen signs of meniscus ganglion appear within the first 3 years (Jonasch, 1964). The exostosis alone does not suffice to diagnose a meniscus ganglion in the plain roentgenogram (see Rauber's console and De Gerdy's tubercle; Fig. 457).

Figure 453 shows a large, monarticular, monotopic **intraarticular osteoma** in the typical site of the knee joint. Its edges are apt to develop contact scleroses.

For **neoplastic synovial chondromatosis** see Figure 430.

During the *growth period,* various "erosive" changes of contour are observed in close proximity to the knee joint (in the femur and, less frequently, in the tibia). Among those that play an important part in the differential diagnosis from osteosarcoma are:

- The **fibrous cortical defect** (p. 30, Fig. 35 A)
- The **cortical desmoid** (p. 31, Fig. 36)
- The **anterior distal defect of the femoral metaphysis** (Keats, 1974; Fig. 454).

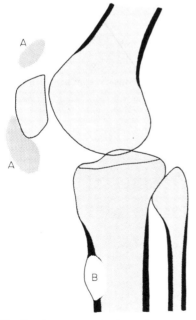

Fig. 452 **Xanthomas at the knee joint in hyperlipoproteinemia** (see Fig. 166).
A = Xanthomas in tendon and in ligament.
B = Intraosseous xanthoma with the roentgen appearance of an expansive, space-occupying tumor.

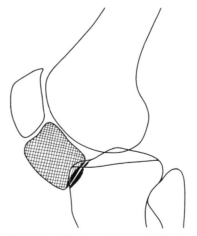

Fig. 453 **Intraarticular osteoma of the knee joint** in its typical location. Contact sclerosis at the tibial head.

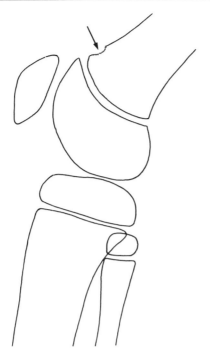

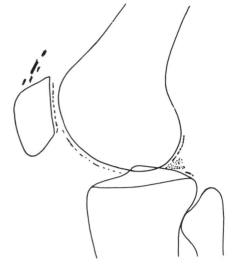

Fig. 454 **Defect of the anterior distal metaphysis of the femur** (Keats, 1974). *Arrow* points to the typical location—above the epiphyseal cartilage—of this developmental variant in adolescence.

Fig. 455 **Roentgenographic appearance of chondrocalcinosis in the lateral roentgenogram of the knee joint.** Note the calcifications in the quadriceps tendon. Calcification of tendons in chondrocalcinosis is known to occur primarily in the quadriceps and the Achilles tendon as well as in the plantar aponeurosis (Gerster et al., 1977). These linear tendon calcifications identifiable in the roentgenogram have diagnostic significance. When, for instance, an arthropathy due to chondrocalcinosis (resembling a Charcot's joint) has completely destroyed the articular cartilage and the menisci so that the *chondro*calcinosis is no longer visible, the calcifications in the tendons provide *the* clue to the etiolgy of the knee affection.

Articular and Periarticular Calcifications and Ossifications. Affections of the Fibroosseous Junction and the Bursae

The roentgen signs of **chondrocalcinosis** (p. 62 ff) of the knee joint are depicted in Figures 66 and 455. In Figure 66, the chondrocalcinosis accompanied hyperthryoidism *symptomatically*. The counterpart of symptomatic chondrocalcinosis is chondrocalcinosis of unknown etiology. In these cases, calcium pyrophosphate precipitates in the hyaline and fibrous cartilage, less frequently also in other structures (Fig. 455), with *no* underlying disease being clinically responsible for this metabolic disorder. At times, however, these patients present a *familial* predisposition. When *neither* an underlying *nor* a familial (hereditary) chondrocalcinosis is present, the condition is also referred to as "sporadic chondrocalcinosis." When chondrocalcinosis begins in old age, the mono- or oligoarticular type occurs more frequently than the polyarticular manifestation (Asshoff et al., 1967).

As for the destructive osteoarthropathy in chondrocalcinosis resembling Charcot's joint, see Figure 69 and p. 64 ff.

It has already been pointed out on page 301 ff that, on the one hand, (calcified) synovial chondromas are frequently observed in osteoarthrosis of the knee joint (Fig. 422) and, on the other, neoplastic synovial chondromatosis (Fig. 430) has, also in the knee joint, to be regarded as a preosteoarthrotic condition. Smaller synovial osteomas also belong to the picture of osteoarthrosis of the knee. Regarding the (monotopic) intraarticular osteoma of the knee joint, see Figure 453.

When confronted with roentgenologically demonstrable calcium deposits and ossifications of soft tissues in the region of the knee, the radiologist should ask:

1. Are these findings referable to a *local* condition or to a *generalized* process which can also be identified in the vicinity of other joints and in soft tissues remote from the joints (see, for instance, Fig. 456)?
2. Is it possible to locate the calcifications or ossifications (as, for instance, those depicted in Figs. 457 to 460) in identifiable *anatomic structures;* e.g., in bursae, ligaments, menisci, the joint cavity?
3. Are they situated in *pathologic substrates* (see malignant synovialoma, Fig. 448; see calcified tophi, Fig. 432), in tuberculous pus, etc.?

Fig. 456 **Roentgenographic appearance of interstitial universal calcinosis** (involving the entire upper leg, only the juxtaarticular region being illustrated) *(left)* and **interstitial localized calcinosis** *(right)*. Only the clinical examination revealed that the calcinosis *on the left* was referable to dermatomyositis, whereas the calcinosis *on the right* was due to progressive scleroderma. The calcinosis type sketched on the *left* must be differentiated from the (bilateral) **cuff-shaped,** flat, reticular **subcutaneous stasis ossification in the upper and lower leg** (Frössler and Osmers, 1976). In chronic venous insufficiency (thrombophlebitis, varices, arteriovenous fistula, congenital anomalies, vascular tumors), various sequelae can be observed, such as discoloration and ulceration of the skin; edema; calcification of thrombi, vein walls, and the perivenous connective and adipose tissues; as well as the subcutaneous stasis ossifications mentioned above (see also p. 33).

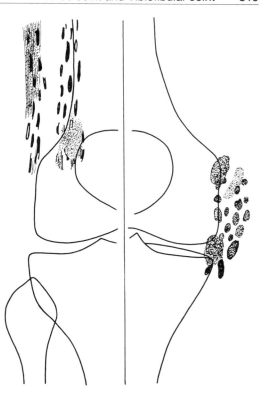

Fig. 457 **Special changes in the contours of the articulating bones as well as paraosteal calcium and bone shadows.**

1 = Fibroosteoses sketched at the origin of the fibular collateral ligament.

2 = Calcium deposit in the tendon of the popliteus muscle or in the fibular collateral ligament. *Clinical finding:* Painful swelling on the lateral aspect of the knee joint. Resorption within 6 weeks (hence so-called calcareous tendinitis; p. 74 ff).

3 = Posttraumatic **Stieda-Pellegrini shadows** (types I to III after Volkmann, 1949):

I = Fibroosteosis or ossified avulsion at the insertion of the adductor magnus muscle ("pronounced" adductor tubercle or else bone shadow standing out against the tubercle *[not illustrated]*).

II = Paraosteal metaplastic new formation of bone not related to the tibial collateral ligament (situated in tendon tissue; or hematoma firm contact with femur possible).

III = Ossified avulsion of collateral ligament (commonly associated with unstable knee). With major avulsions, the dislocated portion of bone "fits" into an adequately shaped bed in the femoral condyle.

4 = **Rauber's console** on the medial and/or lateral edge of the tibia. This sign appears only a few months after the tear of a meniscus and is of diagnostic aid exclusively in the absence of roentgen findings suggesting osteoarthrosis of the knee!

5 = **De Gerdy's tubercle** (variant of normal).

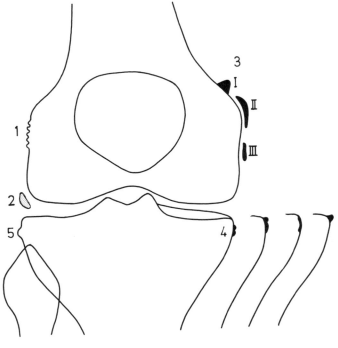

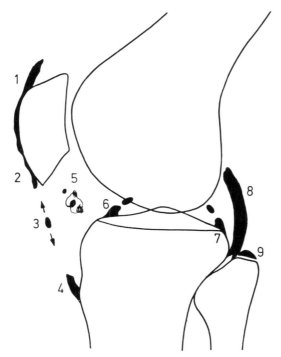

Fig. 458 **Special changes in the contours of the articulating bones as well as paraosteal calcium and bone shadows** (continued from Fig. 457).

1 = Superior patellar spur (fibroosteosis at the insertion of the rectus muscle).

2 = Inferior patellar spur (fibroosteosis of the origin of the patellar ligament [continuation of the rectus ten-

don]). Between 1 and 2—at times irregular appositions of bone on the patella, such as illustrated here.

3 = Osseous metaplasia in the patellar ligament; e.g., following trauma or Osgood-Schlatter disease. *Arrows* indicate course of patellar ligament and thus possible additional sites of osseous metaplasias or calcifications in this ligament.

4 = Fibroosteosis of the patellar ligament on the tibial tuberosity.

5 = Inhomogeneous (mostly posttraumatic) calcifications in the infrapatellar fat pad (differential diagnosis from free loose bodies of variable origin and calcifications of the deep infrapatellar bursa [compare Fig. 460]).

6 = **Third intercondylar tubercle**—very likely a fibroosteosis of the insertion of the anterior cruciate ligament, because this tubercle occurs in 51 percent of laborers, in 41 percent of football players, and in only 18 percent of the average population (Arndt, 1965). *Above 6 and 7:* (Posttraumatic) calcifications or ossifications in the cruciate ligaments. (These also occur without a tubercle; complete ossification of the cruciate ligaments is a very rare event.)

7 = **Fourth intercondylar tubercle,** very likely a fibroosteosis of the insertion of the posterior cruciate ligament.

8 = This (posttraumatic?) bone shadow may be an ossification of the oblique popliteal ligament (Jonasch, 1963) or the arcuate popliteal ligament (Seyss, 1958). *Differentiation in the anteroposterior roentgenogram:* the former ligament courses from inferiorly and medially to superiorly and laterally; the other ligament (bone shadow) courses from the fibular head superiorly and medially.

9 = Persistent portion of the proximal fibular epiphysis or persistent fibular apophysis (?). (Differential diagnosis from avulsion of the collateral ligament.)

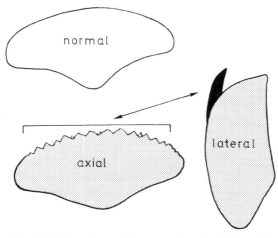

Fig. 459 **Superior patellar spur** (see Fig. 458, no 1) **in the axial and lateral roentgenogram of the patella.**

Osgood-Schlatter disease is caused by excessive strain on the apophysis of the tibial tuberosity. It occurs in adolescence and is accompanied by pain and local swelling. Figure 461 shows the roentgen signs in its florid stage, and its residuals, recognizable in adulthood.

Injuries to the Knee Joint

In the knee joint, one distinguishes between *injuries to the soft tissues* (contusion, distortion, rupture), *dislocations,* and *fractures of the articulating bones.*

The knee joint, like any other joint of the human body, requires an *intact* set of ligaments to perform its function. This applies to motion as well as to standing without muscular fixation. The collateral ligaments impede any lateral displacement of the lower leg relative to the upper leg and also any stronger rotary movement between one articulating bone and the other.

Fig. 460 **Examples of calcifying diseases of bursae** (see Fig. 400 H). 1 = Prepatellar bursa. This bursa may lie in the subcutaneous, subfascial, or subtendinous tissue. 2 = Calcifications in the subcutaneous infrapatellar and/or the deep infrapatellar bursa. 3 = Calcifications in a popliteal cyst (*synonyms:* Baker's cyst, arthrocele, popliteal hygroma; see Fig. 400 E).

Note:The illustrated calcifications (rarely are they ossifications; see Fig. 72) are also termed *calcereous bursitis* because they occur in chronically inflamed bursae. This inflammation most commonly sets in after an excessive mechanical stress (tile setters, houseworkers, etc.— nos. 1 and 2), though sometimes without a recognizable cause, or in connection with a tuberculous infection or rheumatoid arthritis (no. 3).

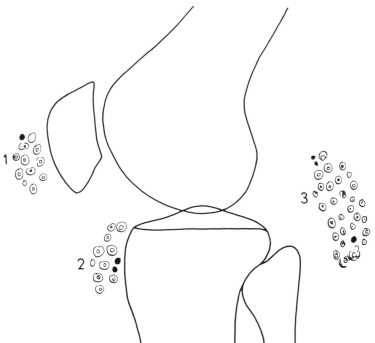

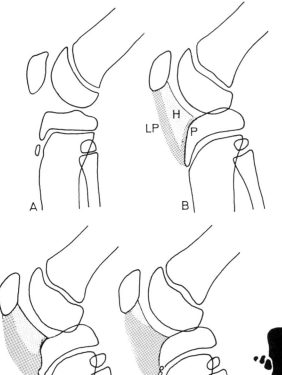

Fig. 461 **Osgood-Schlatter disease.**

A, B = Normal development of the beak-shaped proximal apophysis of the tibia. Smooth contours of the infrapatellar fat pad (H), which is sharply delimited from the patellar ligament (LP) and the prearticular connective tissue (P). In Osgood-Schlatter disease, an edema develops which extends cranially, involving the patellar ligament, the prearticular connective tissue, and the infrapatellar fat pad.

C, D = Fragmentation of the apophysis and edema with thickening of the patellar ligament and more or less extensive homogenization of P, H, and LP in Osgood-Schlatter disease. The "lower angle" of the infrapatellar fat pad (see C) is first affected by the edema; it loses its sharp contour or becomes obliterated (Scotti et al., 1979). The lesions are better recognizable in xeroradiographs than in roentgenograms; the latter should be read under a strong light. Since the differentiation between multiple centers of ossification in the apophysis (i.e., developmental variants) and fragmentation in Osgood-Schlatter disease offers difficulty, demonstration of the soft-tissue lesions described has particular importance in the differential diagnosis.

E = Status after Osgood-Schlatter disease in an adult.

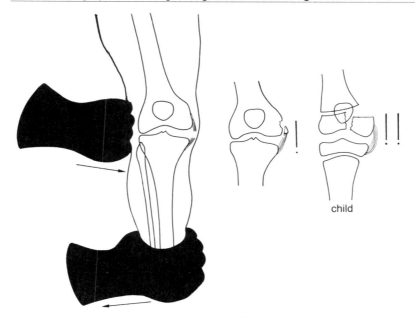

child

Fig. 462 **Rotational roentgenogram (see p. 4) of the (right) knee joint to demonstrate a rupture of a Valgus stress collateral ligament and to differentiate it from other lesions.** One hand (wearing a radioprotective glove) is applied laterally to the knee joint; it serves as an abutment to fix the leg. The other hand clasps the lower leg above the malleoli and pulls it in the direction of the *arrow* to separate the articular surfaces of the joint.

Note: A local anesthetic agent may be administered at the point where pain is greatest. A wedge-shaped bolster of foam rubber should be placed underneath the popliteal space to produce slight flexion of about 15°. Although the intact cruciate ligaments may—even in the presence of a rupture of the medial collateral ligament—impede the separation of the articular surfaces in complete extension, a rupture of the cruciate ligaments sometimes permits separation of the articular surfaces while the collateral ligaments are uninjured (Schobert, 1972). **Roentgenologic demonstration of an unstable knee joint is, in principle, no more than a basic topographic diagnosis and does not justify the assumption that the other soft tissues are intact.** Only the operative findings give an accurate picture of the real extent of damage suffered by the soft tissues! As an additional measure, roentgenograms of the uninjured side should always be taken for comparison, because the physiologic separability of the articular surfaces amounts to about 5 mm. Rupture of the external collateral ligament with or without avulsion of the fibular head involves risk of injury to the common peroneal nerve. The same applies to the broken-off head of the fibula.

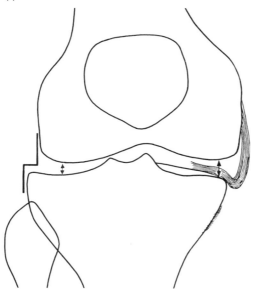

Fig. 463 **Roentgenologically suspected interposition of the avulsed portion of the medial collateral ligament.** *Reasons:* Physical examination and valgus stress roentgenogram suggest a rupture of the medial collateral ligament. In the position of rest (anteroposterior roentgenogram), lateral *subluxation* of the lower leg ("step") and "widening" of the medial joint space.

Note: With isolated injuries of the medial collateral ligament, the palpable point of greatest tenderness is found two fingerbreadths above the joint space; with isolated injuries of the medial meniscus it lies exactly at the joint space (Groh, 1972).

Fig. 464 **Stress examination of the cruciate ligaments by roentgenograms.**
The patient lies supine; the knee joint is flexed about 90°. The so-called central ray passes transversely through the joint. An assistant holds the film cassette lateral to the knee joint. With a fresh injury to the cruciate ligament, any major effusion of blood should be aspirated prior to the radiologic examination because the joint capsule, which has become greatly distended by the effusion, may impede the mobility of the tibia.

A = Roentgenogram in intermediate position (with 90° flexion). Both knee joints should be examined for comparison.

B = Rupture of the anterior cruciate ligament (the *anterior drawer sign* can be elicited). The examiner (radioprotective gloves!) clasps the patient's lower leg with both hands and *pulls* it continuously in the direction of the *arrow* while the film is being exposed.

C = Rupture of the posterior cruciate ligament (the *posterior drawer sign* can be elicited). The examiner clasps the patient's leg with both hands and *pushes* it continuously in the direction of the *arrow* while the film is being exposed.

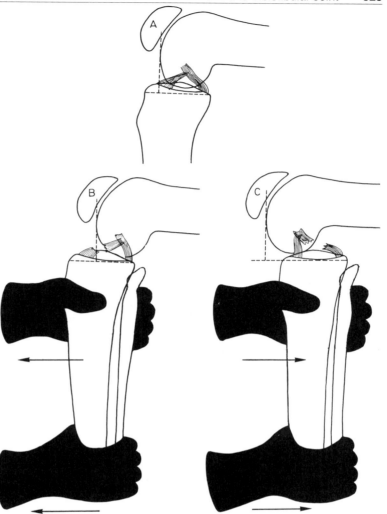

Note: Drawer signs of up to 5mm are still physiologic (comparison with the uninjured side is therefore mandatory). In testing of the drawer signs it is also true that demonstration of a lesion to the cruciate ligaments is only a basic diagnosis. With a positive posterior drawer sign, for instance, *both* the posterior cruciate ligament and the joint capsule may have been torn or at least overstretched. With an anterior drawer sign, additional rupture of the capsule is even necessarily present. Finally, the anterior drawer sign may also be elicited with an intact anterior cruciate ligament if a *bilateral* lesion of the collateral ligaments has occurred!

The cruciate ligaments do not permit any (major) sagittal displacement of the tibia relative to the femur. Finally, the incongruent contact surfaces of the femur and tibia are adapted by the menisci.

Roentgen examination is capable of revealing pathologic changes in the soft tissues. Thus it confirms, supplements, and documents the results of physical examination. In this connection, the **roentgenograms** play a special part (Figs. 462 through 464).

Stress roentgenograms should be made when the result of the physical examination of the knee joint suggests an injury of the collateral and/or cruciate ligaments, or when the standard films in two planes show alterations of bone that may be associated with avulsions of ligaments (e.g., Fig. 465). During the *growth period, any* clinically demonstrable injury of the collateral ligaments requires radiologic documentation of the finding, either by survey films in two planes or by stress roentgenograms. This is necessary because shortly before the complete closure of the distal femoral epiphysis, a trauma is liable to detach the still cartilaginous portion of the epiphysis and to

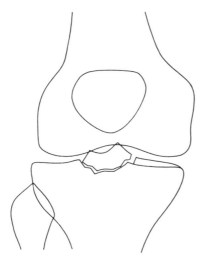

Fig. 465 **Avulsion of the cruciate ligament from the bone with dislocation** (also occurring without displacement). When only *one* intercondylar tubercle or its tip has broken off, only *one* cruciate ligament has usually been avulsed (Jonasch, 1964). This inference is also applicable to isolated avulsions from the anterior intercondylar area (anterior cruciate ligament) and the posterior intercondylar area (posterior cruciate ligament).

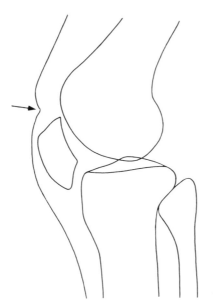

Fig. 466 **Rupture of the quadriceps tendon.** Low position of the patella (compare with the other side!) and typical depression above the patella *(arrow)*, which is visible and palpable in the skin.

Note: In elderly individuals, degenerative lesions in the tendon promote its rupture so that sometimes even minor traumas may precipitate this injury (compare p 314).

cause the already closed portion to collapse or to break off. Then, on clinical examination, the detached (broken-off) portion of the epiphysis can be separated from its base (Titze, 1956). This finding only mimics a lesion of the collateral ligament (see Fig. 462) which, *at the extreme right,* depicts the *principal* pathologic situation.

The precise evaluation of a meniscus injury is reserved for arthrography. Still, **Rauber's console** (Fig. 457, no. 4) is an indirect clue to a meniscus injury (of some standing), and various other roentgen findings in Figure 457 can indicate certain older soft-tissue injuries of the knee joint received several weeks, months, or years previously.

Rupture of the quadriceps tendon can be seen radiographically in the lateral roentgenogram of the knee joint (Fig. 466). The same applies to **rupture of the patellar ligament.** The tendon rupture produces a caudal position of the patella, and rupture of the ligament leads to cranial displacement of the patella (compare the two sides). The history of trauma and the attending clinical manifestations (effusion, swelling of soft tissues) allow the diagnostic differentiation from congenital low positioning of the patella or patella alta. The further differential diagnosis of a "neglected" rupture of the quadriceps tendon (rectus femoris tendon) is discussed on page 314. With flexion of the knee joint, a strong, abrupt contraction of the quadriceps muscle can produce an *avulsion fracture* of the tibial tuberosity or the beak-shaped apophysis of the tibia (Fig. 467).

Traumatic dislocation of the patella (Fig. 468) is the effect of considerable violence. The most common direction of dislocation is outward, but the patella also may be dislocated inward or may become twisted around a vertical axis (up to 180° rotation) and horizontal axis (*horizontal dislocation* following rupture of the tendon or the ligaments; see Fig. 468, no. 5). Immediately after reduction, an axial roentgenogram of the patella should be obtained in every case so as not to overlook any avulsions of bone or cartilage from the patella and/or the femoral condyles (Fig. 469). In **habitual dislocation of the patella,** a minor force such as a kink or twist of the leg may be sufficient to produce the dislocation. Chief causes include congenital or acquired deformities, as well as anomalous positions of the patella and the distal end of the femur. Finally, congenital weakness or acquired lesions of the capsuloligamentous apparatus or the extensor muscles of the knee joint (lateralization of the quadraceps femoris or atrophy of the vastus medialis) play a part in these dislocations of the patella.

In **traumatic dislocation of the knee joint** (dislocation of the tibia at the knee joint), the lower leg becomes dislocated relative to the upper leg at the knee joint. The direction of dislocation may be forward or backward, lateralward or medialward. Usually, the tibia becomes displaced in *at least* two directions, most commonly forward and lateralward. Additional cranial displacements and a rotation around

Fig. 467 **Traumatic avulsion of the tibial tuberosity** (14-year-old patient). *In a later stage,* difficulties may be encountered in the radiologic differential diagnosis of avulsion of the tuberosity versus the status after Osgood-Schlatter disease.

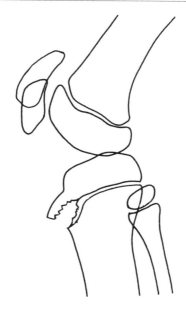

the longitudinal axis of the tibia result from analysis of the roentgen sketch in Figure 470. The dislocation may be closed or open. Secondary injuries to vessels and nerves are recognized by physical examination. The nature, site, and extent of an injury of the popliteal artery should be established by angiography, since these factors affect the therapy. Additional injuries of bone must be ascertained by roentgenograms taken prior to and following reduction. Strangulations of capsule, ligaments, and tendons come to the fore when reduction is attempted, and sometimes are suspected by the radiologist following successful reduction (compare Fig. 463).

Dislocation of the fibular head at the tibiofibular joint occurs more frequently with fractures of

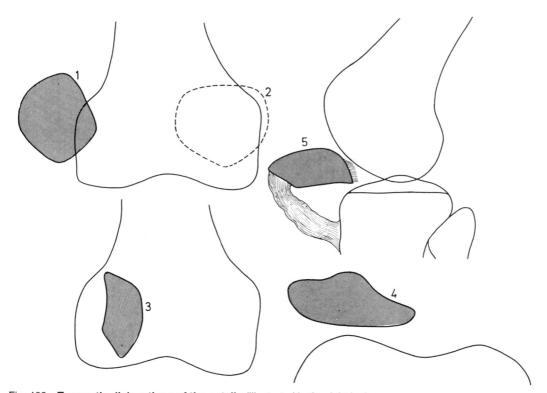

Fig. 468 **Traumatic dislocations of the patella** (illustrated in the right leg).
    1 = Lateral dislocation (plus slight deviation from the frontal plane).
    2 = Medial subluxation.
    3 = Rotary dislocation (90° around the longitudinal axis of the patella).
    4 = Lateral rotary dislocation (180° around the longitudinal axis of the patella; extensive rupture of the joint capsule to be expected as a preliminary condition). Axial view.
    5 = Horizontal dislocation (90° around the transverse axis of the patella), in the present case following rupture of the quadriceps tendon; may also occur following rupture of the patellar ligament.

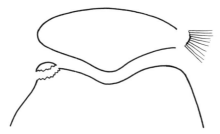

Fig. 469 **Typical additional injuries of bone following (lateral) disclocation of the patella,** detected on axial roentgenogram of the patella after reduction. Avulsion of the (medial) edge of the patella (roentgenologically invisible fibrous structures included in the sketch) and shearing of a cartilage-bone fragment from the (lateral) condyle of the femur.

the lower leg than as an isolated injury (Fig. 471). Depending on the nature and direction of the traumatic dislocation, one distinguishes (Ogden, 1974):

- Subluxation
- Anterolateral dislocation (most frequent)
- Posteromedial dislocation
- Cranial dislocation

Supracondylar fractures of the femur (Fig. 472) endanger the knee joint only when its superior recess

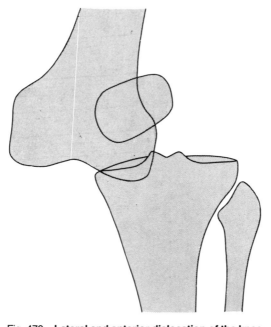

Fig. 470 **Lateral and anterior dislocation of the knee joint** (the latter direction of dislocation, recognizable in the lateral roentgenogram, not included in the sketch). There is also a cranial dislocation with a rotary component (see the position of the tibia and the projection of the tibiofibular joint).

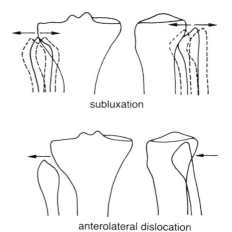

subluxation

anterolateral dislocation

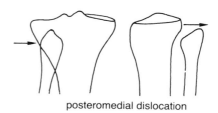

posteromedial dislocation

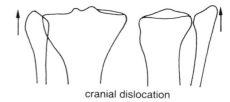

cranial dislocation

Fig. 471 **Subluxation and dislocation in the tibiofibular joint.**
Note: Any traumatically induced instability in the tibiofibular joint may injure the (common) peroneal nerve.

(infrequently) extends so far proximally that the joint is opened by the proximal fragment. This injury manifests itself by an effusion of blood into the knee joint. As a rule, however, the supracondylar fractures of the femur are classed among the **fractures in the vicinity of the knee** without involvement of the joint. This group also includes most of the traumatic epiphysiolyses in the distal femur and the proximal end of the tibia, infracondylar fractures of the tibia, and isolated fractures of the fibular head. When an effusion into the joint (infrequently) accompanies such fractures in the vicinity of the knee, it is generally not sanguinous (as for an exception: *vide supra*).

Among the **fractures of the knee joint** in which the fracture lines extend into the joint or which lead to the avulsion of ligaments inside the joint are the

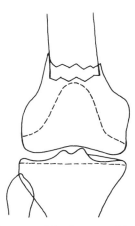

Fig. 472 **Supracondylar fracture of femur.** The usual course of the insertion of the joint capsule in the anterior aspect of the femur as well as the anterior and posterior insertions of the capsule in the tibia is indicated by *dashed lines.* The posterior insertion of the capsule in the femur *(not sketched in)* does not extend as far cranially as the anterior insertion. Specifically with a supracondylar fracture of the femur, and to a variable extent also with monocondylar and bicondylar fractures, the pull of the gastrocnemius muscle produces dorsal tilting of the condylar fragment.

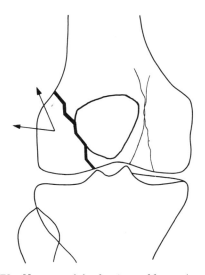

Fig. 473 **Monocondylar fracture of femur** (most frequent site of the lesion in the lateral condyle). *Arrows* indicate the main directions in which the fragments dislocate. If the fragment is markedly displaced sideward, the condition is spoken of as a *fissured fracture.* **Monocondylar fissures** in the medial condyle.

following types: *Isolated detachment of a femoral condyle* is a rare sequela to trauma. More frequent events are *fissures, monocondylar* or *bicondylar fractures with V-, Y-, or T-shaped clefts, comminuted fractures,* and *dorsal fractures of the trochleae* (Figs. 473, 474). The fracture clefts commonly extend into the knee joint (hence their classification as joint fractures); involvement of the joint manifests itself clinically by hemarthrosis. The articular cartilage suffers damage by the injury; the patient is at risk of subsequent posttraumatic osteoarthrosis of the knee. In addition, poor adaptation and healing of the fragments, which lead to the formation of a step in the joint surface, can result in a preosteoarthrotic deformity. Condylar fractures that have healed with deformation frequently interfere with the function of the joint and/or lead to a valgus or varus position. These malpositions of the knee joint are worsened by the concomitant traumatic damage to the capsuloligamentous apparatus. They also favor attrition of the cartilage related to the uneven load on the joint. Open condylar fractures are exposed to the additional hazard of pyogenic infection of the joint.

Fractures of the tibial head occur more frequently than fractures of the femoral condyles. These fractures involve one or both condyles (Figs. 475 and 476). In monocondylar fractures, the fibular portion of the tibial head is affected more frequently than is the tibial. Included among the monocondylar fractures are fissures, minor avulsions, or slight depressions (see the legend accompanying Fig. 475). However, it is also possible for the larger portions of the tibial head to become impressed or depressed in such a way that the step in the articular surface must be corrected by therapeutic measures. Lateral dislocation of the fragment produces a fissured fracture. At times, the fissured fracture is depressed concomitantly, and/or the additionally fragmented articular surface can be impressed distally into the gaping cleft. (Fig. 475 D).

In monocondylar fractures, the development of a posttraumatic osteoarthrosis of the knee joint depends not only on the formation of a residual step in the articular surface of the tibia but also on the nature and extent of secondary injuries to the capsuloligamentous apparatus and the menisci, as well as the degree to which they have healed.

Bicondylar fractures of the tibial head have V-, Y-, and T-shaped fracture clefts (Fig. 476) and can present recurvation or antecurvation, and a valgus or varus position. They are to be classed among the fissured or comminuted fractures.

In fractures of the tibial head, rupture of the popliteal artery and nerve damage occur as secondary injuries. These, however, can be of decisive importance to the function of the knee joint or even to the preservation and unimpaired function of the lower leg and the foot. With open injuries, osteomyelitis and pyogenic infection of the knee joint are dreaded complications. Fractures of the fibular head, the patella, and the femur also may occur as "secondary inju-

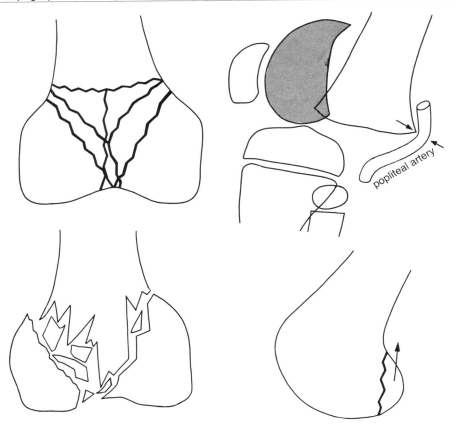

Fig. 474 **Traumas to the distal femur.** *Above left:* Principal course of the V-, Y-, and T-shaped fracture clefts in bicondylar fracture of the femur. *Below left:* Severe type (dislocation) of epiphysiolysis in the distal end of the femur. In these cases the proximal fragment, which is displaced toward the popliteal space, threatens to introduce complications from the side of the popliteal artery *(arrows). Below right:* Dorsal fracture of the femoral trochlea.

ries'' in fractures of the tibial head. The development of a posttraumatic osteoarthrosis of the knee joint—as in monocondylar fractures of the tibial head—depends on the firmness of the joint (the capsuloligamentous apparatus) achieved by the therapeutic measures. Furthermore, in judging the therapeutic result it is important that full extensibility be reestablished.

Fractures of the fibular head (fractures in the vicinity of the knee joint, *vide supra*), occurring either as a secondary injury in fractures of the tibial head or as an isolated event, are of importance because of their complications. Among these are to be mentioned injuries to the (common) peroneal nerve and loss of tension of the fibular collateral ligament, which leads to instability of the knee joint.

Before diagnosing **fracture of the fabella,** primordial duplication of the fabella must be ruled out. Such a duplicated fabella generally is larger than the fabella of the opposite side.

During the growth period, traumatic epiphyseolyses (chondroepiphyseolyses)—possibly also epiphyseal fractures (osteoepiphyseolyses)—of the femur (Fig. 474) and the tibia in the vicinity of the knee joint occur with greater frequency that the comparable fractures in adults. (For the classification of injuries to the open epiphyseal cartilage, see Fig. 581). Epiphyseal injuries rarely induce stimulation or inhibition of growth and thereby lead to bending, shortening, and/or deformation of the bone involved (Fig. 477).

Fractures of the patella involve the joint and occur as transverse, double transverse, oblique, longitudinal, star-shaped, and comminuted fractures (Fig. 478). Apart from these injuries, fissures, small avulsions, lacerations of the articular facets, and (infrequent) fractures in the frontal plane have been observed. When the physical examination suggests fracture of the patella, three radiographs are required: A posteroanterior and a lateral view of the knee joint and an axial roentgenogram of the patella. The therapeutic measures aim at establishing the normal shape of the patella by correcting a possible dehiscence of the fragments and by preventing the formation of a persisting step in the articular surface of the patella.

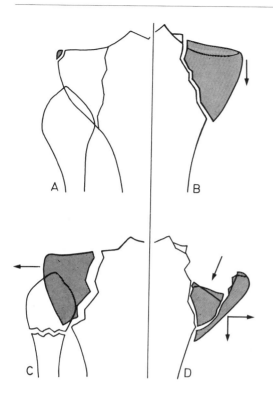

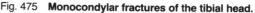

Fig. 475 **Monocondylar fractures of the tibial head.**
A = Monocondylar fissure and small avulsion.
B = Monocondylar fracture of the tibial head with slight distal displacement of the fragment *(depressed fracture)*.
C = Fissured fracture of the tibial head. Additional fracture of the fibular head.
D = Monocondylar fissured and depressed fracture with additional severe impression (see text).
E = *Impressed fracture.* Impressions of the (lateral) tibial plateau can be radiologically diagnosed only from a depth of about 5 mm upward (Niethard and Plaue, 1976). (*Arrows* indicate the direction of the dislocation. Combined fractures do occur; for instance, mixed types of fissured and depressed fractures).

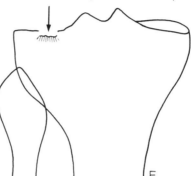

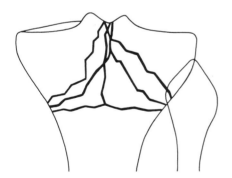

Fig. 476 **Bicondylar fractures of the tibial head** (principal course of the V-, Y-, and T-shaped fracture clefts). In the lateral view, care must be taken to see whether the proximal portion of the tibial head has been tilted anteriorly or posteriorly (bicondylar fractures of the tibial head with antecurvation or recurvation). When extensive splintering or shattering has occurred and the typical course of the fracture cleft is no longer recognizable, one speaks of a *splintered* or *comminuted* fracture of the tibial head, perhaps with the attribute "bicondylar" or "infracondylar," depending on the location and extent of the shattered bone.

In this way the development of a pseudoarthrosis and a postraumatic osteoarthrosis is obviated. An open fracture of the patella involves the danger of pyogenic infection of the joint and thereby favors the development of an ankylosis of the patella (with the femur). Extensive destructions sometimes require a partial or total patellectomy. Following an "untidy" operation, residual pieces of periosteum can lead to (painful) regeneration of tissue. Fractures of the tip of the patella are situated outside the joint.

Lipohemarthrosis (Fig. 479) in the knee joint indicates that either the infrapatellar fat pad or the fatty alar folds have been crushed by the injury *or* that fat from the bone marrow has invaded the joint. The latter event presupposes *at least* a traumatic fissure which may or may not be demonstrable in the roentgenogram (tomography).

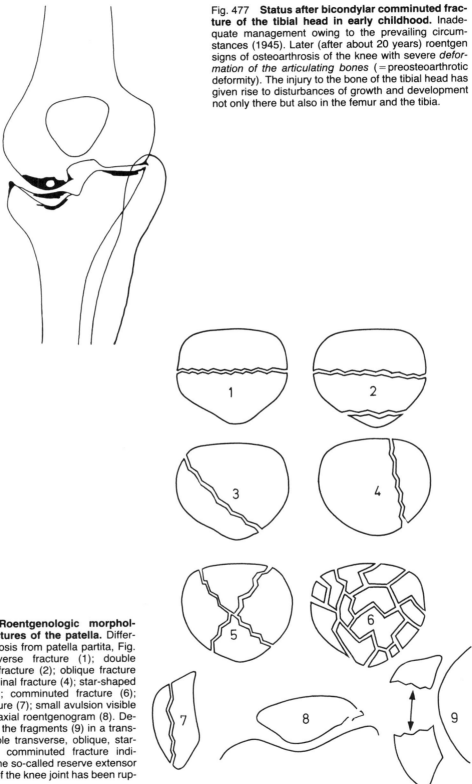

Fig. 477 **Status after bicondylar comminuted fracture of the tibial head in early childhood.** Inadequate management owing to the prevailing circumstances (1945). Later (after about 20 years) roentgen signs of osteoarthrosis of the knee with severe *deformation of the articulating bones* (= preosteoarthrotic deformity). The injury to the bone of the tibial head has given rise to disturbances of growth and development not only there but also in the femur and the tibia.

Fig. 478 **Roentgenologic morphology of fractures of the patella.** Differential diagnosis from patella partita, Fig. 391; transverse fracture (1); double transverse fracture (2); oblique fracture (3); longitudinal fracture (4); star-shaped fracture (5); comminuted fracture (6); frontal fracture (7); small avulsion visible only in the axial roentgenogram (8). Dehiscence of the fragments (9) in a transverse, double transverse, oblique, star-shaped, or comminuted fracture indicates that the so-called reserve extensor apparatus of the knee joint has been ruptured.

Fig. 479 A = **Level roentgenogram to demonstrate lipohemarthrosis in the knee joint** (Holmgren, 1942). The roentgenogram is made with the knee extended and in the horizontal view. In the presence of larger quantities of fat in the (sanguineous) effusion (see text), it is possible to identify not only the ballooned suprapatellar recess but also a stratification, because the fat floats on the sanguineous fluid and attenuates the roentgen beam less strongly than the other components of the fluid. This is why the roentgen film is darker there.

B = **The demonstration of lipohemarthrosis in the lateral roentgenogram of the knee joint (in the recumbent position) is successful only with a high concentration of fat in the sanguineous effusion.** The joint capsule, which exhibits decreased radiolucency in the soft-tissue roentgenogram, is then surrounded on the inside by a sanguineous effusion that contains a large quantity of fat from the bone marrow and on the outside by an extracapsular fatty layer of the suprapatellar bursa (recess) or the infrapatellar fat pad (C). Where the joint capsule is met tangentially by the beam, it stands out against the surrounding fat as an arched stripe of increased density (Sacks et al., 1977). (The "ideal case" has been illustrated.)

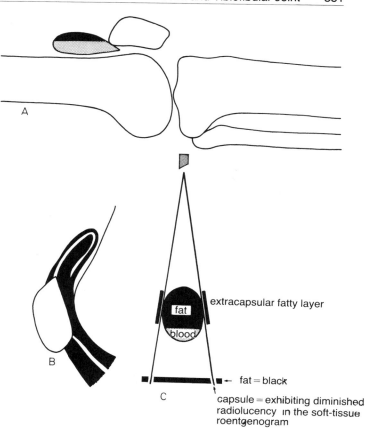

extracapsular fatty layer

fat

blood

fat = black

capsule = exhibiting diminished radiolucency in the soft-tissue roentgenogram

Joints of the Foot, Including the Ankle Joint

At least four different roentgenograms are needed to give an estimate of the joints to be discussed:

1. A dorsoplantar view of the forefoot
2. A plantar-dorsal oblique view of the foot[25]
3. A tibiofibular frontal view of the (lateral) hindfoot with the ankle joint
4. An anteroposterior view of the ankle joint (with the leg rotated internally by about 20° so that the distance between the posterior margins of *both* malleoli and the film cassette becomes identical as a preliminary condition for a "genuine" anteroposterior view of the ankle joint)

With lesions of the longitudinal plantar arch it may become necessary to obtain a tibiofibular frontal view of the entire foot, with the patient standing, as an *alternative roentgenogram* and thus to replace the roentgenogram number 3. For the so-called axial view of the calcaneus, which is an *additional roentgenogram,* see Figure 480.

---

[25] When a particularly accurate evaluation of the first and second ray is contemplated, it is advisable to make an oblique dorsoplantar roentgenogram. By positioning the foot on the inner aspect of the sole, the film to object distance of the two rays is diminished as compared with the plantardorsal roentgenogram (p. 4).

Embryologic Errors, Congenital and Acquired Malpositions of the Joints

Congenital synostosis between the middle and terminal phalanx of the fifth toe (Fig. 487) is a frequent, inconsequential finding. In the other toes, synostoses of the middle and terminal phalanges are much less common. Congenital *coalitions in the tarsal and metatarsal regions* (Fig. 481) develop on a fibrous, cartilaginous, or osseous basis. They may either remain asymptomatic or may give rise to discomfort (generally not before the second decade of life). The possible ossification of fibrous and cartilaginous bridges begins during this period. Chronic pains in the foot occur, often intensified or triggered by prolonged standing and walking, and stiffness is felt on motion. At times, a painful, peroneal spastic flatfoot is present (particularly with calcaneonavicular and talocalcaneal coalition—congenital synostosis between the body of the talus and the sustentaculum tali of the calcaneus). The oblique roentgenogram of the foot, the axial roentgenogram of the calcaneus, and (preferably) the lateral tomogram (Hessge, 1961) or computed tomography (Sarno et al. 1984) provide a

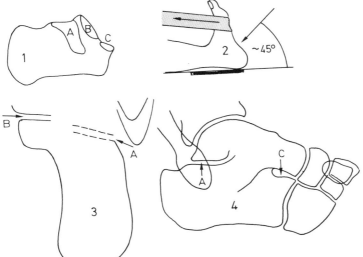

Fig. 480 **Normal anatomic relationships (1), roentgenologic technique (2), normal roentgenologic morphology (3, 4) in the region of the hindfoot.**

1 = Right calcaneus viewed laterally. A = Posterior articular surface. B = Medial articular surface—most frequent site of coalitions. C = Anterior articular surface of the corresponding joints.

2 = Positioning for taking an axial roentgenogram of the calcaneus.

3 = Axial projection of the right calcaneus.

4 = Oblique roentgenogram of the (hind part of the) foot.

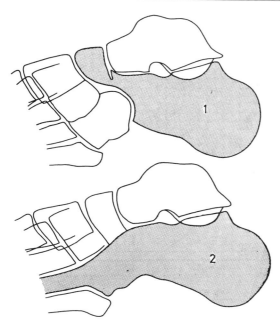

Fig. 481 **Examples of congenital coalitions.**
1 = Calcaneonavicular coalition. 2 = Coalition between the calcaneus, the cuboid, and the fourth metatarsal.

view of the anomalous bony connections and of the topographically analogous accessory bones (os calcaneum secundarium, [calcaneus secundarius], os sustentaculi). Indirect clues (suggestive signs) of diminished or absent mobility in the subtalar joint are depicted in Figure 482 B, C, and D.

Coalitions have been observed between most of the tarsal bones, between the tarsal and metatarsal bones, and between the bases of the metatarsals. These coalitions vary from monoarticular fusion to synostosis of all the joints of the tarsus and metatarsus. When coalition in the region of the hindfoot renders supination and pronation of the foot impossible (this can occur with talocalcaneal fusion as well as with talonavicular and calcaneocuboid coalition), the an-

kle joint is transformed into a ball and socket joint between the second and fourth years of life (Fig. 483). This morphologic transformation of the ankle joint (into a diarthrodial talus with reduction of the lateral malleolus) is the consequence of disturbed function (Imhäuser, 1970). However, the impairment of motion mentioned and the secondary transformation of the ankle joint occur not only with synostoses of the hindfoot but also as an aftermath of pareses from poliomyelitis. Moreover, in certain cases of diarthrosis, a *primary* malformation is also a matter of debate (Hensage, 1974). To facilitate the distinction between congenital and acquired synostoses it is well to remember that congenital synostoses of the carpus and tarsus are sometimes observed concomitantly. The occurrence of a (poly-) arthritic os tarsale (Fig. 499) as well as a (poly-) arthritic os carpale is generally recognized. The roentgen finding of polyarthritis in other (neighboring or remote) joints and/or the history of local arthritis settles the diagnosis. The same applies to osteolmyelitic or posttraumatic synostoses of the tarsus. However, difficulties of differential diagnosis are encountered if the arthritic process has occurred and healed in early childhood. This has already been mentioned under the heading of the carpal synostoses (p. 77 ff).

The congenital malpositions of the toes usually can be diagnosed without radiologic examination, but the roentgenogram serves to document the finding and suggests the therapeutic procedure. Among the congenital deformities of the toes are:

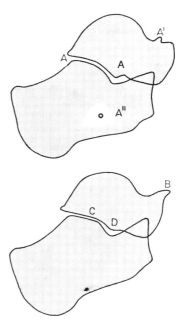

Fig. 482 **Indicators of impaired mobility in the subtalar region—hence signs suggestive of talocalcaneal coalition—in lateral roentgenograms of the hindfoot** (B to D; Conway and Cowell, 1969).
A = Normal roentgen finding (compare with B to D).
A' = Nose of talus, i.e., hypertrophied talar ridge (projection for the insertion of the talonavicular ligament and of the capsule of the ankle joint). Variant of normal; its origin and growth are probably favored by excessive athletic strain on the area of insertion; for instance, in hurdlers and football players (Keats and Harrison, 1979).
A" = solitary bone cyst of calcaneus or foramen nutricium, to be considered in the differential diagnosis. Both may be accompanied by a triangular translucence of bone structure, in which the foramen nutricium (A") is visible, whereas it is absent in a cyst (Keats and Harrison, 1979).
B = so-called talar beak (differential diagnosis from A').
C = Narrowing of the posterior talocalcaneal joint space.
D = Broadened and flattened processus lateralis tali.

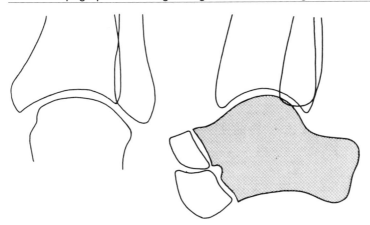

Fig. 483 **Talocalcaneal coalition** with secondary remodeling of the ankle joint into a ball-and-socket joint.

1. **Congenital claw toe**[26] with hyperextension at the metatarsophalangeal joint, angular flexion of the proximal interphalangeal joint, and slight hyperextension of the distal interphalangeal joint. The second toe is most frequently involved.
2. **Digitus superductus.** In this malformation there is strong adduction at the metacarpophalangeal joint so that the dorsoflexed and externally rotated toe overlaps the (medial) adjacent toe.
3. **Congenital varus of the distal phalanx (varus toe); congenital valgus of the distal phalanx (of the hallux).** Both types are probably due to a unilateral growth disturbance of the distal phalanx of the toe. The valgus deformity involves the great toe, whereas the varus deformity also occurs in the other toes. It is possible for the flexed distal phalanx to be overlapped by the adjacent toe.
4. **Congenital hallux valgus; congenital hallux varus.** Both malpositions are commonly associated with additional malformations of the foot.

Congenital pes adductus (congenital metatarsus varus) is an adducted malposition that is limited to the forefoot (Fig. 484). The roentgenogram reveals a medial angulation (varus position) of the metatarsals at the tarsometatarsal joints. It is most pronounced in the first metatarsal and decreases continuously from the second to the fifth metatarsal. The heel never stands in the varus position, but rather in slight valgus.

The deformations in **congenital clubfoot (talipes equinovarus)** can be subdivided into five individual components; the management depends on their variable extent:

1. Pes adductus (adduction of the forefoot)
2. Pes varus (supination of the heel)
3. Pes equinus (due to equinus position at the ankle joint)
4. Pes cavus (equinus position at Chopart's joint—the joint between talus and calcaneus on the one side and between cuboid and navicular on the other)
5. External rotation of the malleolar mortise

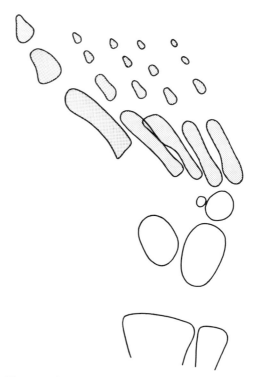

[26] Most of these (congenital) deformities of the toes may also be acquired, frequently as an accompaniment of foot deformities of varied origin. It should be pointed out that *claw toe* must be differentiated from *hammer toe*. In this deformity, there is more or less pronounced flexion at the distal interphalangeal joint; and for the hammer hallux at the corresponding interphalangeal joint.

Fig. 484 **Congenital pes adductus (congenital metatarsus adductovarus).** The faulty position in adduction involves only the forefoot.

Fig. 485 **Roentgenometry for the diagnosis of club-foot in infants.** *Lateral roentgenogram:* The longitudinal axis of the tibia intersects the talus in its posterior third *(in clubfoot the talus is situated in front of the longitudinal axis of the tibia).* The angle between the longitudinal axes of talus and calcaneus measures approximately 40° *(in clubfoot it measures considerably less than 40°).* In clubfoot, the sinus tarsi of the calcaneus is not visible.

Dorsoplantar roentgenogram: The longitudinal axis of the talus runs approximately toward the first metatarsal! *(In clubfoot it does not meet the 1st metatarsal.)* The longitudinal axis of the calcaneus meets the cuboid and runs approximately parallel to the 5th metatarsal *(in clubfoot it does not meet the cuboid; it runs strongly lateral and intersects the 5th metatarsal).* The angle between the longitudinal axes of talus and calcaneus measures between 30° and 40° *(in clubfoot it measures less than 30°).*

In addition: In clubfoot, the centers of ossification appear later and are smaller than on the sound side. On the lateral roentgenogram, the indentation of the sinus tarsi in the calcaneus becomes visible after the first few weeks of life; this is not the case in clubfoot. In clubfoot, the talus has slipped forward across the calcaneus.

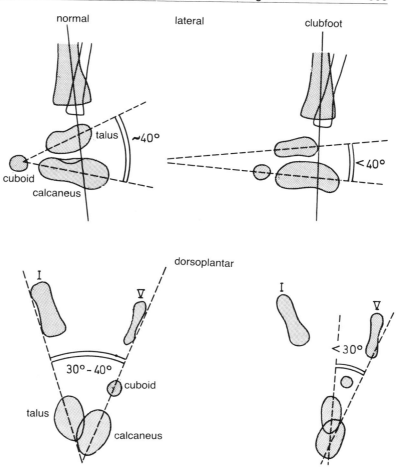

Figure 485 shows the most important lines and angles in the normal foot and in clubfoot of the *infant* on the lateral and the dorsoplantar roentgenogram with the leg held fixed in the corrected *position.* In the majority of cases, a clubfoot termed *genuine* is encountered. The skeletal parts show no embryonic error; the foot presents the clinical picture of a contracture. In *teratogenic clubfoot,* by contrast, there exist primary skeletal defects or congenital disorders of the central nervous system with spastic or flaccid paralyses. *Acquired* talipes equinovarus, pes equinus, and other deformities of the foot can develop as a result of flaccid or spastic paralyses, injuries, or habitual postures; for instance, uncorrected shortening of the leg.

In congenital **talipes calcaneus (talipes calca-**

neovalgus), the dorsum of the foot can be approximated to the anterior surface of the lower leg. In contrast, plantar flexion is limited significantly. This contracture distinguishes congenital talipes calcaneus from a foot that has been turned up during delivery (as a consequence of an anomalous position associated with general muscle weakness and delayed onset of muscular activity [Schlegel, 1972]). This condition in the newborn and infant can be as readily diagnosed as pes calcaneus acquired from paralysis or injury to the Achilles tendon (see also Pes calcaneocavus). Conversely, roentgenologic examination plays an important part in the diagnosis of **congenital pes planovalgus (congenital** vertical talus).[27]

Congenital pes planovalgus must be differentiated from **acquired pes planovalgus (acquired vertical talus).** This deformity has, for instance, been observed as a late complication of thermal burns in

---

[27] "Flatfoot" is a comprehensive term for changes of the longitudinal arch. Pes calcaneovalgus is characterized by sagging of the longitudinal arch, associated with valgus position of the heel. The valgus component is seen best on inspection of the weight-bearing foot (with the patient standing).

infancy and in childhood, which has led to a cicatricial contracture (clinical history and findings) (Jackson, 1978). Congenital as well as acquired pes planovalgus with vertical talus presents a typical picture in the lateral (tibiofibular) roentgenogram taken in recumbency (Fig. 486).

The real extent of acquired sagging of the longitudinal arch—acquired flatfoot—can only be estimated in the lateral roentgenogram with the patient standing; i.e., bearing weight. Acquired sagging of the arch can be the result of paralysis, fracture of the calcaneus, rickets, and various affections of the joints and bones of the foot. Constitutional weakness of the muscles and ligaments that preserve the plantar arch also leads to imbalance between the weight-bearing capacity and the actual strain on the arch, hence to the development of flatfoot. Overweight and continued (occupational) standing are additional factors that stimulate sagging of the plantar arch; they favor wear and tear of the articular cartilage, especially in the lowered navicular. In stiffened—hence contracted—flatfoot, an underlying calcaneonavicular coalition or an etiologic inflammatory condition of joints or bones can be identified in the roentgenogram. A ligamentous or muscular contracture is demostrable upon physical examination. The preceding classification of flatfoot takes into consideration partly morphological and partly functional points of view. Therefore, close cooperation between the referring physician and the radiologist is also, in this instance, indispensable.

Pes cavus is the counterpart to flatfoot. Clinically, pes cavus differs from ''foot with a high instep'' in that the heel is supinated[28] and the forefoot pronated. In either case, the vertical calcaneus is the prominent roentgen finding. The navicular may be projected in the form of a wedge.

Hollow clawfoot shows additional clawing of the toes. Paralyses are the most common cause of this deformity, which infrequently may be congenital. In severe hollow clawfoot, troublesome subtalar osteoarthrosis is liable to develop.

Pes calcaneocavus is a result of paresis of the triceps surae muscle. In this case, the patient walks on the tuberosity of the calcaneus.

In **splayfoot (pes transversoplanus,** Fig. 487), ''fanning'' (divergence) of the metatarsals through sagging of the anterior transverse arch of the foot is best recognizable in the dorsoplantar roentgenogram of the forefoot, with the patient standing (i.e., bearing weight). A particularly striking feature is the divergence between the first and second and between the fourth and fifth metatarsals.

Hallux rigidus (rigid great toe) is a flexion contracture of insidious onset in the tarsometatarsal joint of the great toe, which leads to the typical formation of marginal osteophytes (Fig. 488). The disorder af-

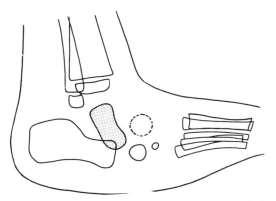

Fig. 486 **Congenital pes planovalgus** with typical vertical position of the longitudinal axis of the talus **(vertical talus).** In addition, the talus is displaced medially, and the calcaneus is tilted. The primordium of the navicular—which in the present case is not yet ossified (dotted ring)—lies dorsolaterally to the talus; hence, it has been "dislocated." This can be inferred indirectly by the position of the corresponding metatarsal.

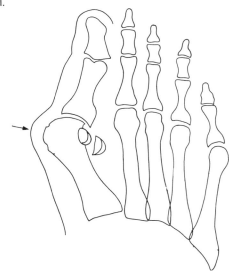

Fig. 487 **Splayfoot** associated with **hallux valgus** (and, as a frequent event, *minor* secondary osteoarthrosis) and slight **digitus quintus varus.** Note the divergence between the first and second and between the fourth and fifth metatarsals. In hallux valgus, the great toe deviates laterally at the tarsometatarsal joint and is *pronated.* The head of the first metatarsal projects medially. The base of the proximal phalanx still articulates only with the lateral portion of the metatarsal head. As a result of the valgus position, the muscles of the hallux modify their topographic relations to their fulcrum in the tarsometatarsal joint of the great toe. This causes the sesamoid bones to become displaced toward the little toe. Hallux valgus is a preosteoarthritic deformity. However, the medial extraarticular soft-tissue callosity (bursitis, etc.; *arrow*) causes the principal discomfort.

Accessory finding: Aplasia of the distal interphalangeal joint of the little toe.

---

[28] The stronger the supination of the heel, the better the view of the joint space of the *anterior* talocalcaneal joint (compare Fig. 480, 1 C).

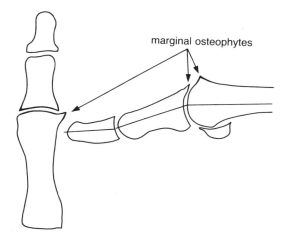

marginal osteophytes

Fig. 488 **Osteoarthrosis due to hallux rigidus.** Typical spiny marginal osteophytes *(arrows)*. In addition, a sesamoid bone deformed by osteoarthrosis and the axial relationships are sketched in the lateral roentgenogram.

fects not only adult individuals but also juveniles, sometimes even children.

Exostosis of the cuneiform is the term applied to a visible and palpable bony projection on the dorsal aspect of the first (more infrequently, the second) cuneiform. A bulge of less marked proportions also commonly is found on the adjacent base of the first metatarsal. These deformities, which are recognizable in a lateral roentgenogram, occur in patients with a fallen arch, but also in those with cavus foot, and, finally, in individuals not presenting any of these deformities. Exostosis of the cuneiform can give rise to complaints due principally to counterpressure exerted

by the footwear. Besides this, it is a matter of debate whether shoes that are too narrow or too hard (e.g., clogs) are the actual cause of these new growths of bone that are supposed to originate as a periosteal reaction. Apart from this, exostosis of the cuneiform undoubtedly can be due to other causes: (1) It may be an extreme variant of the normal shape of the first cuneiform and the first metatarsal. (2) It may result from a second ossification center of the first cuneiform. (3) It may be the expression of a permanently isolated or synostosed accessory ossicle. (4) It may be the consequence of osteoarthrotic changes in the joint between the first cuneiform and the first metatarsal (Bauer, 1968).

Arthritis

In the region of the foot, as elsewhere, the soft-tissue signs of arthritis are the expression of an increase in intraarticular volume. In arthritis, such an increase is produced by inflammatory effusion and inflammatory proliferation of the synovium. On the other hand, these roentgen signs also may be the consequences of a neoplastic intracavitary increase of soft tissues or a traumatic (sanguineous) effusion.

An increase in volume in the ankle joint manifests itself on the lateral roentgenogram (Fig. 490) and, less frequently, also on the anteroposterior roentgenogram. A sanguineous effusion (hemarthrosis), owing to its content of iron, is more conspicuous than a serous, serofibrinous, or purulent effusion. Consequently, synovial proliferations are more demonstrable (in the form of increased densities) in pigmented villonodular synovitis than, for instance, in rheumatoid arthritis.

An intraarticular increase in volume of the toe joints produces a fusiform distention of these joints

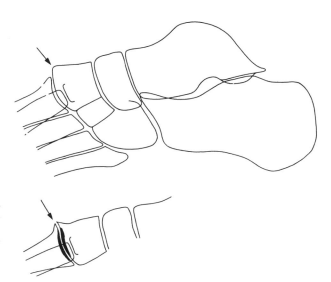

Fig. 489 **Exostosis of the cuneiform** *(arrow)*. In the lower part of the figure, an osteoarthrosis of the joint between the medial cuneiform and the first metatarsal is the cause of this deformation of the dorsum of the foot. Regarding the development of the "exostosis" in the *upper* part of the figure, see text.

(Fig. 491) that is comparable to similar findings in the finger joints (compare Fig. 92). Swelling of the soft tissues (effusion, edema, synovial proliferation) is also demonstrable in the metatarsophalangeal joints. A conspicuous phenomenon is the soft-tissue swelling medial to the first metatarsophalangeal joint and lateral to the fifth metatarsophalangeal joint, as well as the separation of the metatarsal heads (Fig. 491). It should be pointed out here that, as a matter of principle, *both* forefeet should be filmed by a *single* exposure on a *single* roentgen film. Only by so doing will it be possible to ascertain precisely any difference in the distance between the metatarsal heads on both sides, the degree of mineralization, and other data. Infection with gas-forming microorganisms (anaerobic cellulitis, gas gangrene; see p. 20) is liable to occur following a trivial injury to the foot or

by way of the bloodstream. More often, however, it is encountered in wounds with extensive laceration of tissues. The roentgenogram is characteristic (Fig. 492).

The *arthritic collateral phenomena*—juxtaarticular decalcification; see p. 12)—in the forefoot (particularly the surroundings of the metatarsophalangeal joints), the metatarsus, and the hindfoot, including the close neighborhood of the ankle joint, show variable radiographic aspects (Figs. 13, 493, and 494). This occurs because in the foot, also, the rule holds good that the more acute or subacute the course of the arthritis, the more spotty the juxtaarticular decalcification and the hazier the bone structure will be. In the chronic stage of arthritis, the prevailing appearance is homogeneous decalcification with thinned but sharply defined cancellous trabeculae. It

Fig. 490 Soft-tissue signs in the ankle joint and its surroundings.

1 and 2 = Anterior and posterior protrusion of the joint cavity produced by intraarticular increase in volume (compare Fig. 516C). The anterior "outpouching" is more frequently demonstrable than the posterior protrusion. The normal course of the capsule is indicated by a *dashed line*. However, it can rarely be identified in the roentgenogram only by a layer of adipose tissue between the synovial membrane and the fibrous joint capsule.

3 = Effusion or other increase in volume in the subtalar joint, corresponding to the *posterior* portion of this joint. The talocalcaneonavicular joint forms the *anterior* portion of the subtalar joint; this portion includes the anterior and middle articular surfaces of the calcaneus and talus as well as the opposite articular surfaces of the talar head and the navicular.

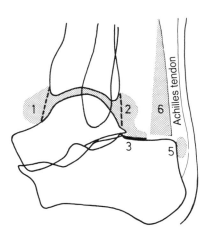

No. 3 can occur alone or in association with nos. 1 and 2, because there exist, as a variant of normal, connections between the talocrural and the subtalar joint (Weston, 1958).

4 = Thickening of soft tissues in the anteroposterior roentgenogram of the ankle joint, due to an intraarticular increase in volume; for example, from a traumatic (sanguineous) effusion (Saunders and Weston, 1971). This finding is demonstrable between the tip of the medial malleolus and the talus.

5 = Swollen retrocalcaneal bursa (see Fig. 563).

6 = Kager's *retromalleolar triangle* (Kager, 1939). This structure is recognizable in lateral roentgenograms as a triangular, retromalleolar, supracalcaneal zone of blackening (narrow base, extending between 10 and 15 cm proximally, its posterior border presenting sharper contours than its anterior border). The triangle owes its origin to adipose tissue in front of the Achilles tendon. Rupture of the Achilles tendon and edematous or sanguineous impregnation of that adipose tissue more or less obliterate the triangle because they render it "equivalent to water" (see Table I, p. 1).

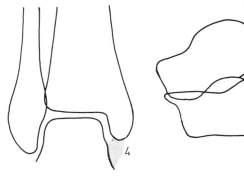

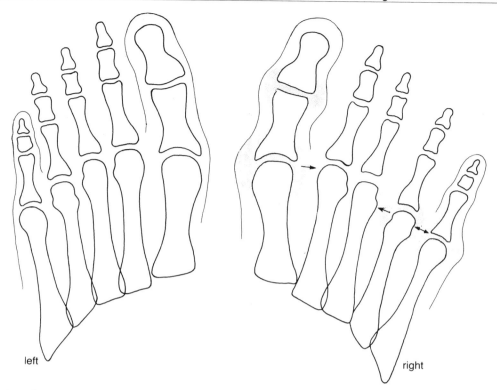

left

right

Fig. 491 **Soft-tissue signs in asymmetrical (oligo-)** arthritis in the region of the right forefoot (in this instance due to clinically diagnosed acute Reiter's syndrome) with separation of the metatarsal heads *(arrows)* and joint-related swelling of soft tissues medial to the first metatarsophalangeal joint on the right as well as lateral to the fifth metatarsophalangeal joint on the right. In addition, fusiform distention of the interphalangeal joint of the right great toe. (The screened densities cannot always be identified; identification is easiest when synovial proliferations are responsible for the intracavitary increase in volume.)

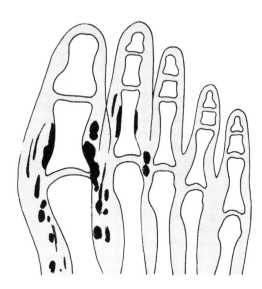

Fig. 492 *Clostridium* **infection in the medial area of the toes and the metatarsus** with marked swelling of soft tissues and partly bubbly diffusion of gas *(black)* between muscles and tendons.

is true that the collateral phenomena are evidence of arthritis only when they are associated with direct and soft-tissue signs of arthritis, but the association of collateral phenomena and soft-tissue signs or their association with direct signs increases the probability that arthritis is present. Not only the typical *Sudeck's syndrome* but also the *transient osteoporosis* (Fig. 18) discussed on page 14 as a variant of the Sudeck's syndrome will require diagnostic differentiation when juxtaarticular decalcification of bone is present (Fig. 493).

The manifold *direct signs of arthritis* to be expected independently of its etiology appear in succession or jointly. Their spectrum can be observed especially during the course of rheumatoid arthritis (Figs. 495 through 500.)

Adult rheumatoid arthritis in the metatarsophalangeal joints consistently shows a tendency to spread from laterally to medially. In contrast, gout (see under this heading) tends to spread in these joints in the reverse direction; i.e., from medially to laterally.

In rheumatoid arthritis, the *initial* erosions in the foot *(early erosions)* often occur in the head of the fifth metatarsal. In this affliction, the erosions not only reflect the capacity of the pannus to destroy the articular cartilage and the bone (Fig. 19) but also may develop as pressure erosions from large subcutaneous rheumatoid nodules (Dalinka and Wunder, 1970). The frequency and extent of the involvement of the second to fifth metatarsophalangeal joints (particularly the second) as well as those of the carpal joints cor-

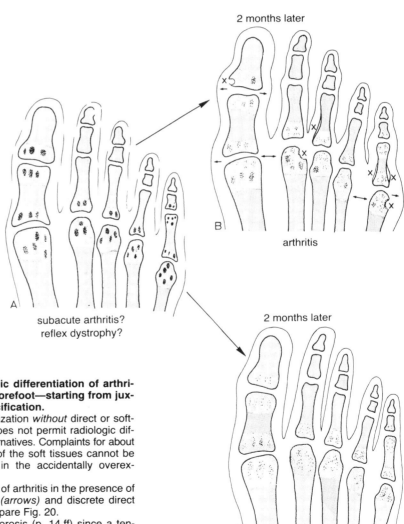

2 months later

arthritis

subacute arthritis?
reflex dystrophy?

2 months later

reflex dystrophy corresponding to
transient osteoporosis

Fig. 493 Roentgenologic differentiation of arthritis in the region of the forefoot—starting from juxtaarticular spotty decalcification.

A = Spotty demineralization *without* direct or soft-tissue signs of arthritis does not permit radiologic differentiation of the two alternatives. Complaints for about 9 weeks. (The contours of the soft tissues cannot be unequivocally assessed in the accidentally overexposed roentgenogram!)

B = Difinite diagnosis of arthritis in the presence of arthritic soft-tissue signs *(arrows)* and discrete direct signs of arthritis (X). Compare Fig. 20.

C = Transient osteoporosis (p. 14 ff) since a tendency for spontaneous remineralization is recognizable in the absence of joint-related soft-tissue swellings or direct signs of arthritis.

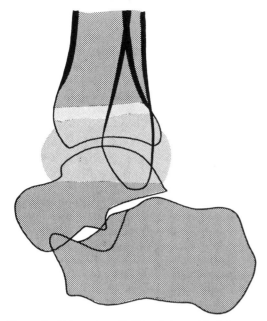

Fig. 494 **Subacute arthritis of the ankle joint** with effusion and collateral decalcification of the juxtaarticular bones.

Note the band-shaped zone of decalcification in the area of the *former* (closed) distal epiphysis of the tibia (compare legend accompanying Fig. 13).

relate with the activity (tendency of progress) of adult rheumatoid arthritis (Larsen, 1976). Radiologic studies of the hands and (fore-) feet must therefore be included among the program of diagnostic information when there is evidence suggestive of rheumatoid arthritis.

On the pages 88 and 89 it was already pointed out that in adult and juvenile rheumatoid arthritis so-called "asymptomatic joints" are encountered, including the metatarsophalangeal joints. Such "asymptomatic joints" reveal roentgen signs of arthritis, although they are not painful. This fact underlines the importance of making roentgenograms of the forefeet, particularly in patients whose rheumatoid arthritis at the onset involves a single large joint so that difficulty will be experienced in making the diagnosis.

In adult rheumatoid arthritis, bony ankyloses are seen with less frequency in the forefoot than in the regions of the metatarsus and the hindfoot (Fig. 499). On the other hand, the forefoot more often shows mutilations of its comparatively smaller bones (Fig. 498).

Faulty positions of the toes and sagging of the transverse and longitudinal arch reflect destructions of the capsuloligamentous apparatus such as usually are to be expected only in the advanced stage of polyarthritis (Fig. 497).

Osteophytes as a secondary osteoarthrotic reaction during the course of arthritis occur especially in

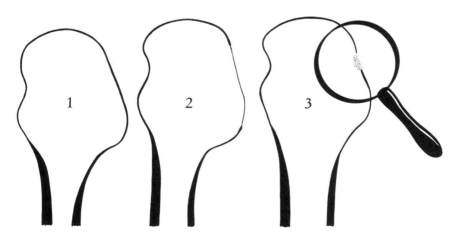

Fig. 495 **Arthritic changes of the marginal subchondral lamella in the metatarsal heads** (here in rheumatoid arthritis).

1 = Normal finding.

2 = Segmental "thinning" (typical site).

3 = Circumscribed change with delicately increased density of cancellous bone underneath the missing marginal lamella.

Note: Bilaterally symmetrical comparison of both sides as well as comparison with the contiguous heads of the metatarsals II to V is imperative. If indicated, use a magnifying loupe.

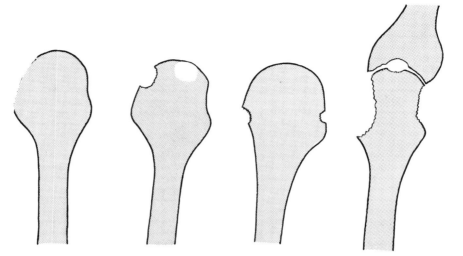

Fig. 496   **Direct signs of arthritis in the metatarsophalangeal joints** (*from left to right:* partial obliteration of the marginal subchondral lamella; erosion and associated arthritic cyst; marginal erosions; destructions; central erosions; narrowing of joint space; faulty position of joint).

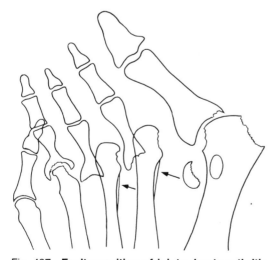

Fig. 497   **Faulty position of joints due to arthritis and sagging of transverse arch in the region of the forefoot** in advanced rheumatoid arthritis (valgus deformity, varus deformity, dislocation). *Arrows* point to delicate lamellar periosteal reactions in two metatarsals. Erosion of the lateral sesamoid bone of the great toe.

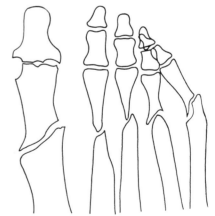

Fig. 498   **Stage of arthritic mutilation** in rheumatoid arthritis of 18 years' standing. Articulating bones of the metatarsophalangeal joints appear "sucked on." Minor signs of inflammation in the interphalangeal joint of the great toe. In rheumatoid arthritis, this joint is more frequently involved than the other interphalangeal joints. Roentgenologic differentiation from neurogenic osteoarthropathy is facilitated by roentgen findings in other joints and the history of polyarthritis extending over years or decades (compare Fig. 543).

the joints near the dorsum of the foot (Fig. 499). As for *rheumatic calcaneopathy,* which can be a decisive extraarticular aid in the diagnosis of inflammatory rheumatic arthropathies, see Fig. 563.

Arthritic signal cysts (see p. 17) in the immediate neighborhood of the ankle joint must also be differentiated from intraosseous ganglia (p. 20, Fig. 21 A) because the surroundings of that joint are a well-known site of predilection for these cystic structures. Fistulas occur not only in the hand but also in the foot in patients with rheumatoid arthritis (*fistulating rheumatism;* Bywaters, 1953). The inflammatory pannus can separate smaller bone fragments from their connection. These fragments become necrotic and remain in situ or are resorbed. From superficial joints—e.g., the metatarsophalangeal joints—such detached necrotic fragments may also be discharged through a fistula. Hence, the presence of fistulas in the vicinity of joints afflicted by rheumatoid arthritis *does not always* indicate a bacterial superinfection of the joint involved but can definitely be part of the clinical picture (though retrograde bacterial invasion by way of the fistula usually may be expected to occur before long).

Juvenile chronic arthritis (p. 88 ff), in comparison with the adult type of the disease, presents specific features, also in the region of the foot. Very often there is a *periosteal reaction* in the nearer and more distant surroundings of the diseased joints (p. 92) and a life-long hypertrophic atrophy of bone with fibrillar cancellous structures (compare Fig. 103). Finally, it shows its character as an *arthritis of the growth period* (p. 92 ff; Figs 501 and 502).

Psoriatic arthritis (p. 93 ff) is characterized by the following roentgenographic findings:

1. The interphalangeal joints of the five toes are frequently involved (Figs. 503 A to F and 504), whereas in rheumatoid arthritis, at most, the interphalangeal joint of the great toe is afflicted regularly. Similarly to the hand (p. 96), in the foot one can also readily distinguish between a *transverse type* and an *axial type* of joint involvement. This means that in the toes, also, there exists a *predominance of*

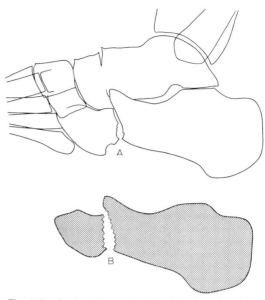

Fig. 499   A = **Involvement of the intertarsal and tarsometatarsal joints** in rheumatoid arthritis. Narrowing and obliteration of the joint space are most conspicuous. With time they lead to the development of the so-called *os tarsale.* Erosions are demonstrable only in the calcaneocuboid joint. The dorsum of the foot shows discrete signs of secondary osteoarthrosis (osteophytes).

B = In joints allowing little mobility, extensive marginal erosion may cause the roentgenologic joint space to appear "widened."

DIP joint involvement and a *concordance of DIP-PIP-MTP involvement* (compare p. 96).
2. At times, exuberant resorption of bone and delayed destruction of cartilage causes the interphalangeal joint space to appear widened (Fig. 503 A).
3. The stage of mutilation *may* be reached in a few years (Figs. 503 B, E, and F and 505 D).
4. In the immediate vicinity of mutilated joints, other

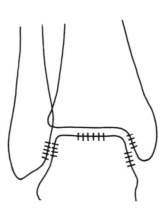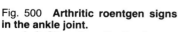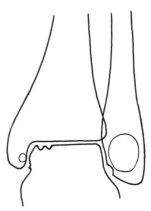

Fig. 500   **Arthritic roentgen signs in the ankle joint.**

Left: Sites of predilection for erosions of the ankle joint in rheumatoid arthritis.

Right: Arthritic narrowing of joint space; erosions; attendant arthritic cysts.

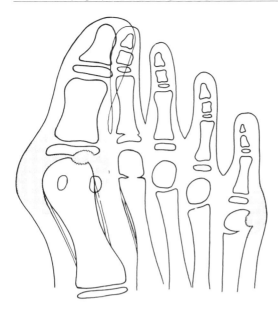

Fig. 501 **Juvenile chronic arthritis** of 2 years' standing. Patient now 10 years old. Swelling and increased density of soft tissues near the 1st and 5th metatarsophalangeal joints. Erosions at 1st metatarsophalangeal joint and head of 5th metatarsal. Lamellar periosteal reactions extending far into the diaphysis and on 1st and 2nd metatarsal.

Valgus deformity of the 1st metatarsophalangeal joint. Roentgen signs of arthritis of the growth period in vicinity of 2nd and 5th metatarsophalangeal joints (premature epiphyseal closure).

joints often undergo bony ankylosis (Fig. 503 E and F).

5.   A striking feature is the tendency to chiefly periosteal proliferations of bone near the joints and at a distance from them, including the ''protuberances'' in the region of the hand that have already been mentioned (Figs. 503 A and D, 504, and 505 A and C). Pronounced ossifying periosteal reactions are observed not only in the forefoot but also in the region of the tarsus and the ankle joint (Fig. 506).

6.   The terminal tufts of the distal phalanges are apt to become resorbed (Figs. 503 A, 504, and 505 B).

7.   The incidence and the radiographic morphology of rheumatic calcaneopathy in psoriatic arthritis are discussed on p. 373 ff. Figure 503 D shows a productive fibroosteitis in one of the sesamoid bones of the great toe.

left   right

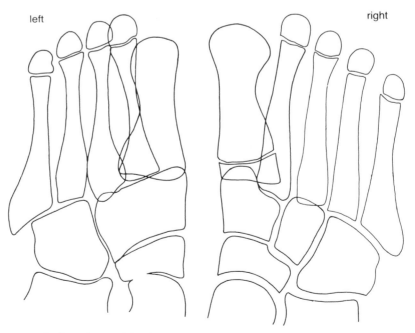

Fig. 502 **Roentgen findings in arthritis of the growth period.** Onset of rheumatoid arthritis in 9th year of life. Patient now 16 years old. *Left foot* shows arthritis of the intertarsal and tarsometatarsal joints (narrowing of joint space, bony ankylosis). In addition, there are signs of arthritic growth disturbance (premature closure of epiphysis of great toe; thinning of the metatarsal shafts).

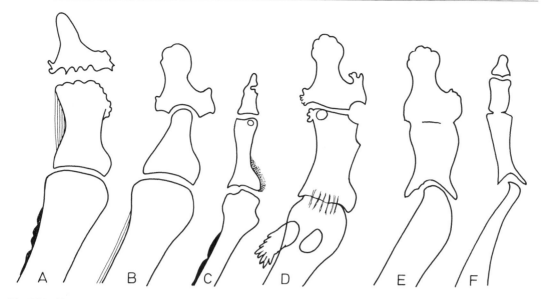

Fig. 503 **Roentgen findings in the forefoot in psoriatic arthritis** (see text). Radiologic diagnosis is based on combination of individual signs and pattern of involvement (compare Figs. 504 and 91).

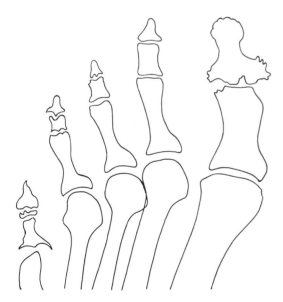

Fig. 504 **According to the roentgenogram (compare Fig. 503) typical psoriatic arthritis** (involvement of the distal interphalangeal joints [in this instance] III, IV, and V; protuberances on the interphalangeal joint of the great toe; mutilation in metatarsophalangeal joint V; osteolysis of terminal tuft V; corresponding, though *asymmetrical,* findings in the joints of the other forefoot *(not shown).* Since the patient does not (yet) suffer from psoriasis, this is a case of **prepsoriatic arthritis.**

8. Arthritis-induced juxtaarticular demineralization (the "arthritic collateral phenomenon") is demonstrable less frequently than in rheumatoid arthritis. Conversely, swelling of soft tissues very frequently is more pronounced in psoriatic than in rheumatoid arthritis (Fig. 507). Almost every other patient gives a history of acute or subacute onset of the arthritis (see p. 95).

Reiter's syndrome affects principally younger males. As a rule it presents a typical triad or tetrad of symptoms (p. 96). The most "dependable" of them is arthritis. Experience teaches that urethritis, conjunctivitis, arthritis and the possible manifestations in the skin, the mucosa, and the nails *may* reveal a very loose temporal connection. In addition, there obviously are rudimentary forms of the disease in which the involvement of the urinary tract and the eyes produces few signs and symptoms and which therefore are easily overlooked by the patient and the physician.

In Reiter's syndrome, involvement of the joints is manifested by a monoarthritis or an asymmetrical oligoarthritis in the lower extremities, and less frequently in the joints of the arms and hands. However, polyarthritic localizations in the lower and upper extremities also are seen, particularly when the disease runs a chronic course, which is to be expected in about every other patient.

The following roentgen findings are either highly suggestive—nearly pathognomonic—of *acute (subacute)* Reiter's syndrome or, less frequently, are the

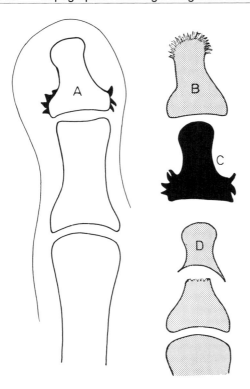

Fig. 505 **Roentgen signs of psoriatic arthritis which are particularly striking in the vicinity of the interphalangeal joint of the great toe.**

A = *Extraarticular protuberances* (see p. 96) and marked swelling of soft tissues in vicinity of interphalangeal joint of great toe.

B = Osteolytic processes in the acra have transformed the terminal tuft into the shape of an *aspergillum (holy-water sprinkler)* (compare Fig. 106).

C = *Eburnation of the phalanx* (Resnick and Broderick, 1977) with protuberances.

D = Fundamental *appearance of mutilation* in interphalangeal joint of great toe (also occurring with other types of chronic arthritis).

Note: Arthritis in Reiter's syndrome also tends to produce periosteal reactions so that protuberances *sometimes* develop in this disease. Periosteal changes similar to protuberances also occur rarely in gout.

first manifestation of psoriatic arthritis. The similarity, if not identity, of certain clinical and radiomorphologic findings in these two diseases was pointed out on p. 96. Four days at the earliest, after the onset of an acute or subacute arthritis of the fingers or toes accompanied by marked swelling of the soft tissues, the roentgenogram reveals a delicate periosteal lamella (Forrester and Kirkpatrick, 1976) to which

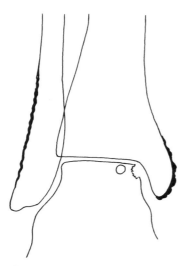

Fig. 506 **Roentgen finding in chronic arthritis of the ankle joint.** Because of the *periosteal reaction* in the malleoli and the distal shaft of the fibula, adult rheumatoid arthritis is less likely than psoriatic arthritis, *chronic* Reiter's syndrome, or peripheral arthritis in ankylosing spondylitis (also compare Fig. 510).

Clinical impression: Psoriatic arthritis.

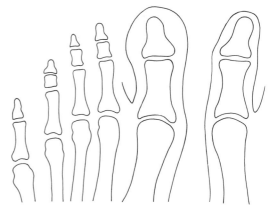

Fig. 507 **Initial acute episode of psoriatic arthritis in the region of the left great toe with erythema and marked swelling of soft tissues.** The differential diagnosis offers little difficulty because (1) the patient is a female (gout rarely afflicts females), (2) there is a 5-year history of psoriasis, and (3) arthritic lesions of the psoriatic type in the hand of this patient (compare Figs. 105 and 106) have been treated for 2 years.

a collateral demineralization supervenes after 1 or 2 weeks (Fig. 508).

Over years and decades, the *chronic* Reiter's syndrome can lead to severe (poly-) arthritic destruction, faulty position of the toes, and even mutilation of the joints of the toes, especially of the metatarsophalangeal joints. These findings, viewed by themselves, cannot be distinguished from the picture of advanced rheumatoid arthritis (Fig. 509). There are, however, two features which, if present, argue *against* the diagnosis of rheumatoid arthritis: "thickened" shafts of small tubular bones that have developed through fusion of periosteal appositions with the compact bone of the diaphysis and metaphysis, and evidence of marked rheumatic calcaneopathy (p. 373 ff).

The **"intestinal arthritides"** were discussed on p. 97 ff. Periosteal reactions in regional enteritis (Crohn's disease), less frequently also in ulcerative colitis, are depicted in Figure 510. The differential diagnosis was discussed on page 98.

Involvement of peripheral joints in ankylosing spondylitis is manifested in a variety of ways. Best known is first the involvement of the large proximal joints (the hip joint being affected more frequently than the shoulder joint; Fig. 304). Secondly, and in addition to this, involvement of the peripheral joints can occur as a mono- and oligoarthritis of the lower extremities (Fig. 511). Thirdly and finally, there occurs a chronic polyarthritis with (asymmetrical) involvement of the joints of the lower and upper extremities (Fig. 109) as well as of the temporomandibular joint. It is of course quite convincing to assign a peripheral arthropathy to ankylosing spondylitis when the diagnosis of this affliction has been settled. On the other hand, it is difficult to place the peripheral pathologic manifestations in the right category when they are demonstrable clinically and in the roentgenogram *before* any characteristic findings appear in the axial skeleton! Particularly in young individuals (in about the second decade and at the beginning of the third decade of life), involvement of the peripheral joints is frequently for years in the forefront of the clinical picture. In these cases, a search should be made serologically not only for the so-called rheumatoid factors but also for the HLA-B27 cell wall antigen (compare pages 89 and 92).

The abbreviation *HLA* means "human leukocyte alloantigen," a special instance of the observa-

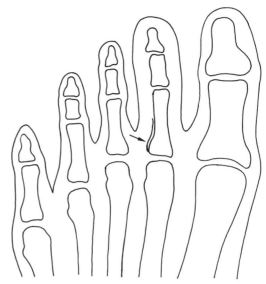

Fig. 508 **Acute monoarticular initial manifestation of arthritis in Reiter's syndrome or—less frequently—in psoriatic arthritis of acute onset.** Roengenologic examination 6 days after onset of the disease. 24-year-old male complaining of pain on urination, slight urethral discharge and a burning sensation in the eyes.

Roentgen finding: marked soft-tissue swelling of the entire second toe; delicate periosteal lamella in the proximal part of the first phalanx of this toe *(arrow).*

Diagnosis: Acute Reiter's syndrome.

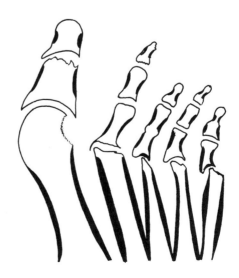

Fig. 509 **Advanced polyarthritis in chronic Reiter's syndrome of 20 years' standing.** Erosion, mutilations, ankylosis, and faulty positions, such as also might have been expected in rheumatoid arthritis of many years standing. Thickened shafts of the 2nd and 5th metatarsals have developed through fusion of lamellar periosteal appositions. These findings are to be expected primarily in chronic Reiter's syndrome and in psoriatic arthritis but are an *extreme rarity* in adult rheumatoid arthritis.

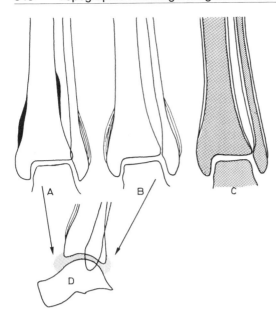

Fig. 510 **Roentgen findings in the ankle joint, tibia, and fibula in regional enteritis (Crohn) or ulcerative colitis.** Arthritic roentgen findings in the ankle joint; e.g., effusion (D). Periosteal reactions which are either lamellar (A, B, D) or massive and fused with the cortex (A, tibia). Roentgenographic appearance of hypertrophic osteoarthropathy Marie-Bamberger (symptomatic pachydermoperiostosis; p. 133 ff) (C). For additional causes of periosteal neoformations of bone surrounding the ankle joint see p. 33 ff.

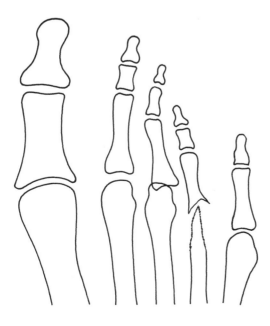

tion that the cell membrane of the nucleated cells (and of the platelets) contains substances that possess antigenic properties with respect to another organism. In the meantime, numerous (1, 2, 3, 4, etc.) histocompatibility antigens have been detected that are genetically determined—hence not acquired but inherited! Their development is governed by a number of loci (A, B, C, D) of the sixth autosome. Meanwhile, diverse diseases have been identified in which certain HLA antigens are more frequently demonstrable than in healthy individuals. Among them are ankylosing spondylitis, Reiter's syndrome, psoriatic arthritis (including sacroiliitis of the "variegated picture" type, see p. 490 ff), regional enteritis (Crohn's disease), and ulcerative colitis, to list only those diseases that are of interest here because of their HLA association.

Between 90 and 95 percent of white and Japanese patients suffering from ankylosing spondylitis possess HLA-B27, which occurs in less than 10 percent of healthy individuals. Up to 80 percent of patients with Reiter's syndrome are HLA-B27 positive. In psoriatic arthritis *associated with* sacroiliitis, HLA-B27 is demonstrable in 70 percent of patients, whereas at most 35 percent of patients with psoriatic arthritis *without* sacroiliitis possess this antigen. HLA-B27 is demonstrable in about 70 percent of patients with Crohn's regional enteritis and ulcerative colitis who present the characteristic roentgen findings of ankylosing spondylitis (see under this heading) in the sacroiliac joints and in the spine (Brewerton and James, 1975; Schattenkirchner et al., 1976; Huaux et al., 1977, and other workers). Hence, the carriers of the inborn HLA-B27 histocompatibility antigen are at considerably greater risk of acquiring ankylosing spondylitis. When an HLA-B27 positive individual is afflicted by Reiter's syndrome, psoriatic arthritis, Crohn's disease, or ulcerative colitis, he or she is also at increased risk of acquiring sacroiliitis of the "variegated picture" type or even fullblown ankylosing spondylitis, as compared with HLA-B27 negative persons. HLA-B27 is therefore a risk factor for the axial skeleton that indicates the genetically determined proneness to develop sacroiliitis of the "variegated picture" type or ankylosing spondylitis.

Fig. 511 **Ankylosing spondylitis with involvement of peripheral joints.** In the foot, the roentgenogram may closely resemble the findings in rheumatoid arthritis (e.g., in Figs. 497, 498, and 500). In the *case sketched here*, the peripheral arthritis is manifested by an appearance that is *atypical* of rheumatoid arthritis; namely (monotopical or oligotopical, see p. 98) mutilation of the 4th metatarsophalangeal joint and faulty position of the 3rd metatarsophalangeal joint of the *right* foot (on the left side, normal roentgen findings). In comparison to involvement of the 2nd to 5th metatarsophalangeal joints, arthritis of the metatarsophalangeal joint of the great toe in ankylosing spondylitis is a rare event.

Ankylosing panarthritis is probably a "malignant" subtype of ankylosing spondylitis starting in adolescence. With time it involves virtually all joints of the extremities and the axial skeleton, leading to bony ankylosis (Fig. 512). Even after ankylosis has occurred, deformations of the articulating bones reveal the onset of the disease in the growth period. Jaccoud's arthritis (and its synonyms) were described on page 98 ff. Figure 513 shows the typical discrepancy between the *severe* malposition of joints and *absent* or *minor* erosive changes in the joint-bearing bones. This discrepancy is due to capsular and pericapsular fibrosis, which characterizes this clinical picture (Murphy and Staple, 1973).

For the **Ehlers-Danlos syndrome,** see the legend accompanying Figure 111.

The **classic collagen diseases** (p. 99 ff) and the **mixed connective tissue disease** (Sharp's syndrome; p. 104 ff) manifest themselves less frequently in the gliding and supporting tissues of the foot than in the hand; the roentgen findings in both instances are identical (Fig. 514).

In **recurrent polychondritis** (p. 105 ff), erosive arthritis is rarely observed but may also occur in the forefoot. Of decisive diagnostic significance, however, is the involvement of the cartilages of the auricle and the nose. In addition to this, special attention should be paid to the question of whether the arthritis is connected with the recurrent polychondritis or constitutes the expression of a *coincidental* inflammatory rheumatic or autoimmune disease. (McAdam et al., 1976).

The roentgenogram of the noncaseating epitheloid cell granulomas of **sarcoidosis** (p. 106 ff) in the joints and bones of the foot (Figs. 515 and 516) is identical to that of the hand. The short tubular bones

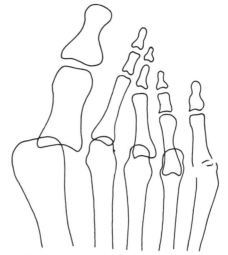

Fig. 513 **Jaccoud's arthritis** (diagnosed clinically, see p. 98 ff). Severe malposition of the metatarsophalangeal joints *without* erosive joint lesions. *The symptomatology and the serology suggest inflammation.* Clinically, the condition must be differentiated from disseminated lupus erythematosus (see legends accompanying Figs. 110 and 111).

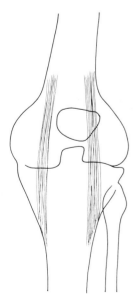

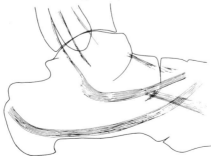

Fig. 512 **Ankylosing panarthritis** (diagnosed clinically, see test). Onset at age 15; patient now 30 years old. The joints illustrated have undergone bony ankylosis. High-grade demineralization of the synostosed bone, remodeling of the cancellous bone into so-called *hypertrophic atrophy* (strengthening of the weight-bearing strands of cancellous bone, extensive resorption of the nonweight-bearing areas of cancellous bone, and thinning of the cortex). Deformation of the intercondylar fossa (compare Fig. 437), of the trochlea tali, and the calcaneal tuberosity, as well as hypertrophic atrophy of bone (see legend accompanying Fig. 13) indicate onset of the disease in the growth period.

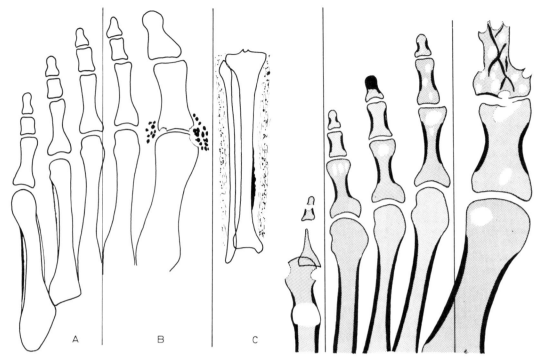

Fig. 514   **Instances of extraarticular (A, C) and articular (B) roentgen findings in the areas of the lower leg and foot in classic collagen diseases and in Sharp's syndrome.**
A, C = Periosteal reactions, most frequently encountered in polyarteritis (nodosa).
B = Arthritis of the metatarsophalangeal joints with grumous localized interstitial calcinosis (diagnosis in the present case: progressive scleroderma).
C = Universal interstitial calcinosis (diagnosis in the present case: dermatomyositis). For the roentgenologic differentiation, see also the legend accompanying Fig. 456.

Fig. 515   **Roentgen findings in sarcoidosis of the region of the forefoot.**
1st digit = Trabecular remodeling; cystic osteolyses, partly with erosion into the joint; incipient acral osteolysis. 2nd to 4th digits = Medullary granulomas have led to circular, heart-shaped, and oval osteolyses which show only a delicate marginal seam, or none. Osteosclerosis in the distal half of 3rd terminal phalanx.
5th digit = Sarcoidosis-induced mutilation, circumscribed expansion in 5th metatarsal by granuloma.

of the hand and foot are the sites of predilection for skeletal sarcoidosis. Less frequently, the disease manifests itself in the carpal and tarsal regions, the long tubular bones, the vertebrae, and the flat bones. At times, the picture is dominated by cystic resorption of bone; in other cases, the "diffuse type" with netlike remodeling of bone and thinning of the cortex prevails (Turek, 1953). Although the cystic resorption of bone *can* lead to severe destruction of the bone, the diffuse form expands the (small) tubular bones more or less evenly (compare Fig. 118). Synovial sarcoidosis most frequently affects the *ankle joint;* this happens independently of whether the disease is accompanied by erythema nodosum (Pavelka, 1979). Especially in middle-aged females, any unilateral or bilateral arthritis of the ankle joint accompanied by erythema nodosum (in which the roentgenogram of the joint may be normal or may reveal an effusion, juxtaarticular demineralization or—infrequently—

erosive changes) should prompt radiologic studies of the thorax (bilateral hilar lymphadenopathy, etc.) and a tuberculin test (negative?).

Prior to diagnosing acute **bacterial arthritis** in the region of the forefoot, one must rule out acute gouty arthritis (podagra), especially in males. In gout, swelling of soft tissues and redness of the skin may extend well beyond the joint proper so that the condition may even be confused with an infectious phlegmon. In addition, *acute* monoarthritis in the foot calls for differentiation between pyogenic infection and monoarticular onset of an inflammatory rheumatic infection; e.g., Reiter's syndrome or psoriatic arthritis.

In *chronic* monoarthritis in the region of the foot, the differential diagnosis should first consider inflammatory rheumatic and tuberculous arthritis. In this connection it is also well to remember that in from 5 to 10 percent of patients with adult rheumatoid arthritis, the disease starts, atypically, in a single joint.

The ankle joint is the most frequent seat of tu-

Fig. 516 **Sarcoidosis of the ankle joint.**

A = Subchondral cyst-like osteolyses, the largest of which shows a sequestrum (the epitheloid cell granuloma having failed to produce resorption of a small portion of bone). The synovial granulomas have led to spotty subchondral demineralization of the three articulating bones and to the development of a band-shaped decalcification in the region of the former distal tibial epiphysis (arthritis of the ankle joint with collateral arthritic phenomena, clinically known for 6 weeks).

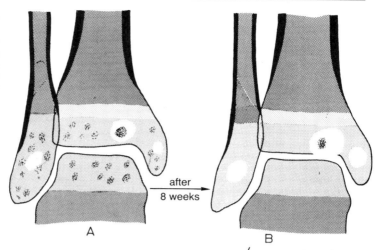

after
8 weeks

A

B

B = After another 8 weeks without adequate therapy the granuloma-induced osteolyses have increased in size. One of them has broken into the ankle joint (circumscribed narrowing of the roentgenologic joint space). The juxtaarticular demineralization has lost its spotty character and now appears to be homogeneous.

C = Lateral roentgenogram at the time of B. Unequivocal evidence of an effusion that bulges forward and backward (compare Fig. 490). Since roentgenologic proof of bilateral hilar lymphadenopathy had been obtained in the meantime, and the tuberculin test had given a negative result, the finding in the ankle joint was classified as sarcoidosis-dependent arthritis. Otherwise a tuberculos infection would have come into question.

C

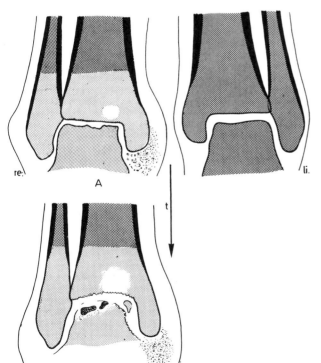

re.

A

t

li.

B

Fig. 517 **Chronic arthritis in the right ankle joint** (progression from A to B; t = time). The additional diagnosis of **ankle tuberculosis** is based on amorphous periarticular calcifications (calcified pus), *very pronounced* demineralization, and breakdown of bone (with dissections in B).

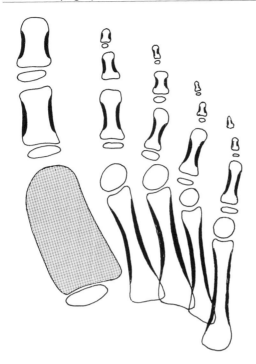

Fig. 518 **Spina ventosa of the 1st metatarsal.** *Differential diagnosis:* See text.

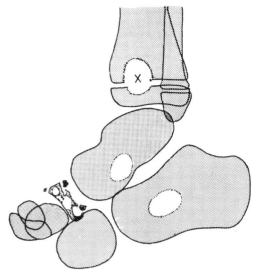

Fig. 519 **Cystic tuberculous skeletal foci** with delicate increased density of the marginal seam. The navicular shows, next to the cystic tuberculous foci, deformation, "crumbling," and increased density (signs of osteonecrosis). The condition should be differentiated roentgenologically from *aseptic* osteonecrosis (Köhler's disease)! Similar considerations apply to entertaining the diagnosis of aseptic osteonecrosis of the head of the 2nd (3rd etc.) metatarsal; i.e. second Köhler's disease, or an osseous tuberculosis localized there.

X = When such a cystlike osteolysis (on both sides of the open epiphysis) occurs as a *single finding,* the condition should be differentiated from benign (epiphyseal) chondroblastoma (see also Figs. 22, and 204).

berculosis in the foot (Fig. 517). It is followed in frequency by the calcaneus (radiologic *differential diagnosis:* principally chronic pyogenic infection, actinomycosis, osteoclastoma, osteolytic osteosarcoma). In children—less frequently in adults—osseous tuberculosis of the metatarsals (metacarpals) and phalanges presents the picture of *spina ventosa* (Fig. 518). Radiologic differential diagnosis is sarcoidosis, syphilitic dactylitis, osteomyelitis of the distal phalanx, enchondroma, and congenital hereditary hemoglobinopathies (sickle cell anemia). *Synovial tuberculosis* of the foot presents a mixed picture of roentgenographic soft-tissue signs, arthritic collateral phenomena, and direct signs. In *osseous tuberculosis,* by contrast, pathogenetic conceptions might lead one to expect that *initially,* destruction of bone, which sometimes presents a cystic appearance, will be in the forefront of the clinical picture (Fig. 519). It is true, however, that in the region of the foot, with its small bones, which are exposed to great static strain, these fundamentally correct conceptions are *not always* in agreement with the actual observations. It should also be emphasized that there is, as a rule, an interval of from three to six months between the onset of discomfort and the first pathologic roentgen findings. With further progression of tuberculosis of the foot, including the ankle joint, detachment of bone and sequestra (Fig. 520) as well as calcified pus (amorphous calcium shadows) are encountered in the

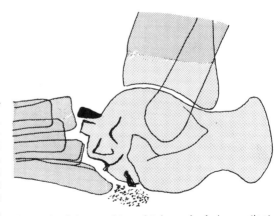

Fig. 520 **Advanced tarsal tuberculosis** in a patient with diabetes mellitus. The condition was misdiagnosed as (neurogenic) diabetic osteoarthropathy. Although static-mechanical "crushing" and "squashing" of the tarsal bones occurs in both diseases, *sequestra* that do not participate in the marked demineralization and the amorphous calcifications immediately dorsal to the tuberosity of the 5th metatarsal *(calcified pus from an abscess)* primarily suggest tuberculosis or chronic bacterial infection.

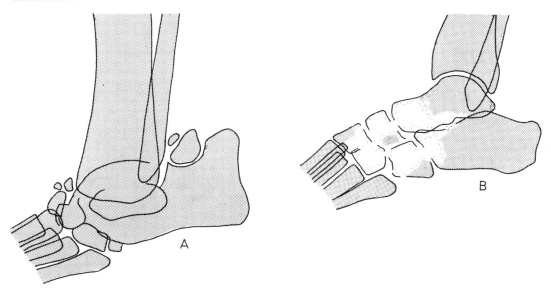

Fig. 521   **Roentgenologic differential diagnosis of advanced tarsal tuberculosis** (compare Fig. 520)

A = **Neurogenic osteoarthropathy** of the entire hindfoot with crushing and squashing of the tarsal bones and the distal portions of tibia and fibula. See the small fragments of bone (also compare Figs. 541 and 542).

B = Roentgenographic appearance of tarsal metastases of a malignant tumor (carcinoma). Extreme "demineralization" of (parts of) tarsal bones.

Fig. 522   A = **Hematogenous osteomylitis (with formation of a Brodie's abscess (in an 8–year–old child** (metaphyseal breakdown with broad sclerotic marginal seam and periosteal lamella). The child complains of intense pain on moving the ankle joint. Serous, hypocellular, bacteriologically sterile aspirate.

Diagnosis: Brodie's abscess of the tibia with sympathetic arthritis (see text) in the ankle joint. (Inspection in front of a good source of light demonstrates the effusion [x] in the ankle joint).

B = Roentgenographic appearance of *osteoid osteoma* in cancellous bone (trochlea tali), which is also apt to trigger a sympathetic arthritis. The calcareous nidus is surrounded by a thin translucent zone; no perifocal sclerosis. Typical increase of pain in the night.

C (talus) = Osteoid osteoma of cancellous bone extending to the surface of the talar neck with swelling of soft tissues. *Arrows* indicate that the three findings illustrated are capable of triggering a *sympathetic ankle arthritis.* A generally produces a serous arthritis. B and C more commonly lead to chronic lymphofollicular synovitis.

Note: Typical of osteoid osteoma are localized pains; they often increase in intensity during the night and are "dramatically" relieved by aspirin.

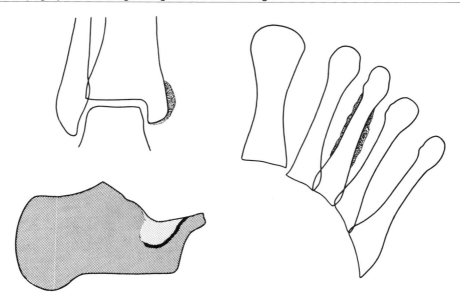

Fig. 523 **Roentgen signs of pyogenic infection of the foot running an insidious course—"peditis"—(in disorder of arterial circulation).** About 4 months previously, slight injury on cutting out an ingrown toenail. Since then moderate pain and swelling in the lateral dorsum of the foot and the ankle. The patient suffers from disorder of the peripheral circulation and diabetes mellitus. *First roentgen examination* about 4 weeks after the injury: *Ossifying periostitis* of the shaft of the 3rd metatarsal and the medial malleolus; *breakdown of bone* in the calcaneus, in part with marginal sclerosis. Incision of the lateral border of the foot and drainage (no discharge of pus). Dissection of the extremity amputated through the lower leg revealed among other lesions empyema in the ankle joint and the joints of the hindfoot. In addition, osteomyelitic foci were encountered in the calcaneus and other bones of the tarsus. The pathologic roentgen findings *(vide supra)* were therefore only the "tip of the iceberg," which is typical of this kind of bacterial infection of the foot, hence the term "peditis."

immediate vicinity of the joints. With inadequate therapy, collapse of the tarsal skeleton follows only later (Figs. 520 and 521). If the *diagnosis of tuberculous arthritis is settled,* the appearance of fistulas, periosteal reactions, and *marked* marginal sclerosis arouses suspicion of *superinfection.*

When a patient complains of pain in the joint *and* one detects, in the neighborhood of the joint, a circumscribed, prevalently metaphyseal breakdown of bone that is delimited by a more or less *broad sclerotic seam* indicating an osteomyelitis (Brodie's abscess [Fig. 522], a plasmacellular osteomyelitis or

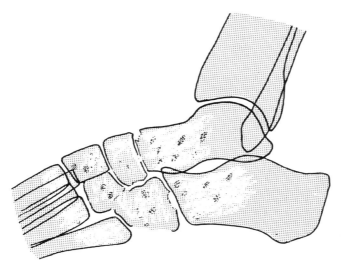

Fig. 524 **Acute pyogenic arthritis of the talus following suppurative tonsillitis.** Roentgenogram obtained 3 weeks after onset of pain, swelling, and reddening of the dorsum of the foot.
Roentgen findings: Major demineralization, in part spotty, and band-shaped subchondrally near the talonavicular joint space. *Narrowing of joint spaces;* partial obliteration of the marginal subchondral lamella; flat *erosions* (compare Fig. 521 B).

possibly the picture of osteoid osteoma—osteoid blastoma complex), it is more likely that one is dealing with a *sterile sympathetic arthritis* (see p. 161) than with a transmitted pyogenic infection of the joint.

Mention should also be made of certain peculiarities of pyogenic infection of the foot: In (elderly) patients with impaired peripheral circulation and/or a diabetic disorder of metabolism, a trivial injury is sometimes followed by an indolent infection that often gradually extends to the entire foot, also involving the supporting and gliding tissues. Owing to the absence of systemic manifestations, a number of weeks or even months usually pass before the patient seeks medical attention and a roentgenogram is obtained. Figure 523 shows such a case in which the roentgenogram revealed only a discrete inflammatory lamellar periosteal reaction in the third metatarsal, a breakdown of bone in the calcaneus, and a periosteal reaction on the medial malleolus. The correct evaluation of these erratic findings prompted an amputation of the lower leg. The operation indeed revealed, besides diverse roentgen-negative tarsal foci, an empyema in the joints of the hindfoot, including the ankle joint, hence a "peditis."

When the circulatory and metabolic conditions are normal, pyogenic infection of the supporting and gliding tissues of the foot (which may be of hematogenous origin (Fig. 524), may follow a perforating injury, or may be due to any other cause) usually remain limited to the original seat of infection or its immediate surroundings. Increasing destruction of joints despite adequate therapy, progressive dense sclerosis of cancellous bone, and local ossifying periostitis suggest transition to a chronic course.

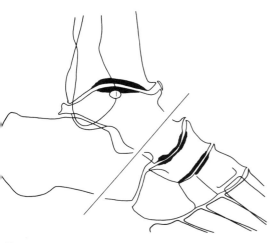

Fig. 525   **Roentgen signs of ankle and intertarsal osteoarthrosis.** *Left:* Eight years previously, fracture of medial malleolus and fibula. Now, advanced (post-traumatic) ankle osteoarthrosis. *Right:* Roentgenographic morphology of intertarsal osteoarthrosis (the osteophytes on the dorsum of the foot are particularly conspicuous).

Extensive phlegmons of the foot not only trigger periosteal reactions in the small tubular bones but at times also lead to demineralization of the foot skeleton, which initially is spotty but subsequently becomes diffuse. Bedside examination must determine whether decalcification is a collateral phenomenon of soft-tissue infection or part of a Sudeck's syndrome developing with such an infection. In these cases, the strong demineralization demonstrable especially in the tarsometatarsal joints (the rounded-oval heads of the metatarsals) is apt to mimic arthritic erosions.

Osteoarthrosis

Regarding osteoarthrosis in the hallux valgus and hallux rigidus, see Figures 487 and 488. Intertarsal osteoarthroses are frequently observed with sagging of the longitudinal arch (flatfoot) but also are observed with other deformities of the foot, including tarsal coalitions (p. 332 ff). For "shaggy foot" see Figure 535. In ankle and subtalar osteoarthrosis, the posterior process of the talus becomes deformed; it is at this process that ligaments for the ankle and the subtalar joint arise or insert. Ankle joint osteoarthrosis is sometimes a direct sequel of injury, or it develops through faulty weight-bearing on this joint after a fracture of the lower leg (Fig. 525). This type of osteoarthrosis can also be due to excessive strain on the cartilage and the capsuloligamentous apparatus of the ankle joint; e.g., in *professional football players.* In this case one often sees, in addition, marked ossifications of the capsule and the ligaments, which develop in avulsions as a repair process and/or are the product of metaplasia taking place in these structures.

Among the best-known **preosteoarthrotic deformities of the foot** are various reconstructed (revascularized) aseptic necroses of bone (Fig. 526): in the navicular—first Köhler's disease; and in the head of the second metatarsal (the other metatarsal heads are seldom involved)—second Köhler's disease (Köhler-Freiberg disease). Less known localizations are the cuneiforms, the sesamoid bones of the great toe, and a possible accessory ossification center in the base of the distal phalanx of the great toe. *Osteochondrosis dissecans* of the trochlea tali (less frequently of the tarsal bones and the metatarsal heads [Fig. 527]) is not only a preosteoarthrotic deformity but occasionally may be confused with a detachment of bone in tuberculosis. The medial side of the trochlea tali is more frequently involved than its lateral side. Osteochondrosis of the trochlea tali, also, is at present predominantly classified among the fatigue fractures (Fig. 527 A; see p. 299 ff; compare the legends accompanying Figs. 527 B and C).

The main sources of blood supply for the talus are vessels that enter the bone from the subtalar region (Haliburton et al., 1958). Dislocations and fracture-dislocations of the talus are therefore attended by the danger of partial or total necrosis of the body

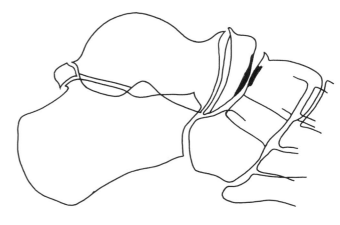

Fig. 526   Specific findings in osteoarthrosis of the foot.

Top: Os naviculare reconstructed after first Köhler's disease with considerable deformation. Moderate osteoarthrosis of the talonavicular and cuneonavicular joints.

Accessory finding: Os trigonum tali with arthrotic deformation (subtalar osteoarthrosis).

Bottom: Status following aseptic necrosis of head of 2nd metatarsal (second Köhler's disease; Köhler-Freiberg disease). Roentgen findings in osteoarthrosis of the 2nd and 3rd distal interphalangeal joints (boxed).

Note: In electrical injuries, there occur aseptic necroses of the metatarsal heads, acral osteolyses in the toes and growth disturbances, depending on the site of exit of the current (site of ground connection). (Kolář and Vrabec, 1960).

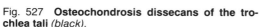

Fig. 527   Osteochondrosis dissecans of the trochlea tali *(black).*

A = In the majority of cases—such as the one illustrated here—the lesion is found at a short distance from the medial edge of the trochlea.

B = Striking deformation of the trochlea tali. Therefore the question arises of whether one is dealing with a persistent ossification center in the trochlea (Ribbing, 1951).

C = Lateral seat of osteochondrosis dissecans, frequently following a known major injury.

Note: It is well known that the osseous bed from which a "joint mouse" has been detached may gradually be smoothed out and become invisible in the roentgenogram. Generally, however, detached fragments of the trochlea do not leave their bed. Therefore, bone shadows in the areas marked by a *circle* are only infrequently displaced "joint mice." More often one is dealing with so-called accessory elements of bone, fragments that have broken off the medial aspects of the malleoli and the anterior edge of the tibia, old avulsions of the capsule and ligaments from the tips of the malleoli, and post-traumatic or degenerative calcifications (ossifications) of the articular soft tissues.

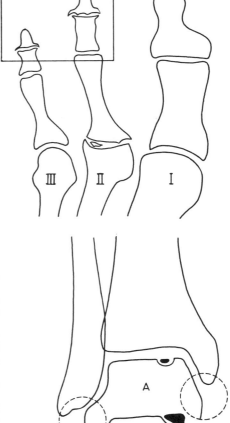

Fig. 528 **Frostbite** of the interphalangeal joint of the great toe terminating in osteoarthrosis (see text). The acral osteolysis that occurs with severe frostbite in the toes (and fingers) takes place in the setting of sloughing soft-tissue necrosis. *Frostbite during the growth period* also leads (in the toes) to shortening and deformation of the distal phalanges as a consequence of frostbite of the growing cartilage.

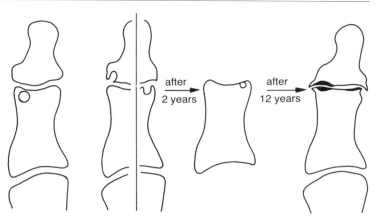

and the trochlea of the talus (p. 377). The multiple other causes of aseptic necrosis of bone (p. 254 ff) likewise are apt to produce necrosis of the talus, the other tarsal bones, and the heads of the metatarsals (Green and Osmer, 1968) and thus can lead to diminished weight-bearing capacity of the necrotic bones with consequent deformation, dissection, and finally ankle joint and *subtalar osteoarthrosis.*

On the other hand, preosteoarthrotic deformations of the articulating bones of the foot skeleton are also known to occur in the (epiphyseal) osteochondrodysplasias (see p. 238 ff). For example, a bilateral symmetrical course of the distal bone contour of the tibial epiphysis from laterocranially to mediocaudally *plus* increased growth of the lateral portion of the talus is considered to be an important roentgen sign in the differential diagnosis of the constitutional systemic osteopathies mentioned above (Leeds, 1960). This deformation, however, also occurs in sickle cell anemia, in hemophilia (see Fig. 536), and in juvenile chronic arthritis. A similar valgus deformity of the trochlea tali develops gradually following segmental resection of the fibula in childhood; for instance, in order to obtain a bone chip (Hsu et al., 1974).

Frostbite of the toe joints, similarly to the fingers (p. 113), manifests itself in the form of cystic defects which are juxtaarticular or may invade the joint (Fig. 528). These defects are to some extent reversible. In addition to this, the small tubular bones show delicate lamellar periosteal reactions that likewise are reversible. These reactions are supposed to be signs of an additional local infection. The defects develop approximately 5 to 12 months after the frostbite has occurred. Their appearance is independent of the degree of frostbite (Blair et al., 1957). Osteoarthrosis that is limited to the joints involved does not develop until years or decades after the frostbite.

Neoplastic synovial chondromatosis (p. 66 ff) occurs but rarely in the region of the foot, as compared with its incidence in the knee and elbow joints. The structures relatively most often affected are the ankle joint and the contiguous tendon sheaths (Figs. 73 and 529). The calcified synovial chondromas immediately attract attention. However, they are only the "visible tip of the iceberg"; the noncalcified chondromas, which usually are much more numerous, are not demonstrable in the plain roentgenogram, although they may be discernible in the form of pressure erosions. Detached capsular chondromas

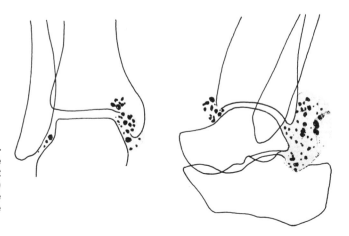

Fig. 529 **Neoplastic synovial chondromatosis of the ankle joint.** Note the massive increase in density of the soft tissues, the numerous (already calcified) synovial chondromas, and the pressure erosion at the medial malleolus and the calcaneus. (Compare Fig. 73.)

occasionally give rise to signs of locking. In addition to this, similarly to other joints, they promote the development of osteoarthrosis.

As for **Kashin-Beck disease,** see p. 114.

Osteoarthropathies

The metatarsophalangeal joint of the great toe (Figs. 530 through 534) is the test joint of **gouty osteoarthropathy** (p. 4 ff). In about 50 percent of gouty patients the *initial* acute attack affects the first metatarsophalangeal joint. During the further course of the disease, as many as three quarters of patients suffer an attack of gout in this joint. Gouty attacks are also observed with appreciable though decreasing frequency in the other joints of the foot (including the ankle joint), in the knee, and also in the carpal region and the fingers. Chronic gout, too, attacks the joints of the lower extremities more frequently than those of the upper extremities. Involvement of the metatarsophalangeal joints in gout extends, as a rule, from the first to the fifth toe. In rheumatoid arthritis,

by contrast, involvement and tendency to extension follow the reverse direction (from the fifth to the first metatarsophalangeal joint).

The tophus (gouty nodule) is the most important hallmark of chronic gout. It is the reflection of a massive deposit of urates. A number of years usually elapse between the initial attack of gout and the demonstrable appearance of tophi. The tophi also develop most frequently about the metatarsophalangeal joint of the great toe (Mertz, 1978). The tophus exerts its destructive effect on the supporting and gliding tissues, though originating in the joint, the subchondral bone marrow, or the paraarticular soft tissues. It not only is a relatively late manifestation of gout but also is indicative of local destruction that commonly is irreversible. The *early diagnosis of gout* as the morbid expression of hyperuricemia must therefore be established by other means. Among these, the differential diagnostic analysis of the initial gouty attack ranks first. The classic attack of gout is conducive to a hyperacute inflammation with heavy collateral edema that extends well beyond the immediate vicinity of the joint. The skin over the strongly swollen great toe is markedly erythematous. Fever and humoral signs

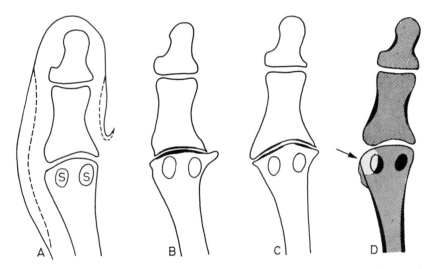

Fig. 530   **Roentgen signs in gout of the region of the right great toe.** Regarding its pathogenesis see p. 41 ff and Fig. 47 (quantity-time quotient of urate precipitation).

A = (Initial) classic hyperacute gouty attack (podagra). Marked reddening and soft-tissue swelling of first digit (normal contours *dashed*); no pathologic roentgen findings in the articulating bones.

B = Hallux rigidus associated with osteoarthrosis (lateral radiographic appearance, see Fig. 488). This finding is also encountered in gouty patients; determination of the level of serum uric acid should therefore never be omitted.

C = Roentgen signs similar to trivial osteoarthrosis of the metatarsophalangeal joint of the great toe. Gout *may* be concealed beneath any appearance of osteoarthrosis of the metatarsophalangeal joint of the great toe, particularly in middle-aged males and in the absence of malposition of this joint! Polyosteoarthrosis of the fingers in males also should prompt, as a matter of principle, determination of serum levels of uric acid.

D = *Arrow* points to a circumscribed increase in translucence with concomitant thinning or obliteration of the cancellous trabeculae (loupe!). This finding may, when associated with corresponding clinical symptomatology, be the early roentgen sign of a tophus in the bone marrow. The delicate oriel-shaped apposition of bone on the mediodistal portion of the metatarsus is a suggestive roentgen sign of gout (S = sesamoid bones of the great toe).

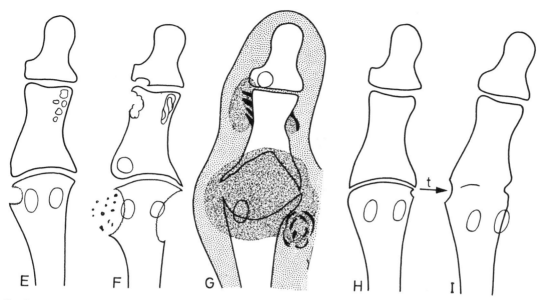

Fig. 531 Continuation of Fig. 530 (gouty osteoarthropathy).

E = Marginal tophaceous defect. In addition, small rounded osteolyses in head of proximal phalanx; these extend to the diaphysis.

F = Halberd shape of metatarsal head due to tophus. In addition, tophaceous defects surrounding interphalangeal joint of the great toe and, in the base of the proximal phalanx, tophaceous calcifications.

G = Tophaceous mutiliation ("cupping") in metatarsophalangeal joint of great toe. The lateral sesamoid bone of the great toe has been destroyed by a tophus (expansion, ballooning, sometimes "eggshell appearance"). Tophus-induced periosteal reaction in the proximal phalanx (tophaceous spine = *medial;* overhanging border of bone = *lateral*). Punched-out defect with a diameter of more than 5 mm in distal phalanx.

H = Chronic gouty arthritis in the metatarsophalangeal joint of the great toe (nonreactive narrowing of joint space, delicate erosion).

I = Findings depicted in H lead to bony ankylosis (t = time course).

Note: Larger tophi are reflected as increases in density within the soft tissues (of toes and fingers); see the legend accompanying Fig. 137. Theoretically, the roentgen findings illustrated are apt to appear, though with less probability, in any finger or toe (Figs. 135 to 139).

Fig. 532. Continuation of Figs. 530 and 531 (gouty osteoarthropathy).

J = Large tophus in the proximal phalanx of the great toe. To be differentiated roentgenologically from enchondroma by definite evidence of gout (periosteal spine with increased density of the surrounding soft tissues = tophus).

K = Oriel-shaped projection of first metatarsal (see legend accompanying Fig. 530 D); increased density of the surrounding soft tissues *without* faulty position of hallux (= tophus).

L = Oriel-shaped projection of first metatarsal in minor degenerative osteoarthrosis of the metatarsophalangeal joint of the great toe; tophaceous spine on the terminal phalanx.

M = Degenerative osteoarthrosis of the first metatarsophalangeal joint with so-called central erosion of the metatarsal head. Degenerative osteoarthrosis of the metatarsophalangeal joint of the great toe should always prompt investigation of the uric acid level in the serum.

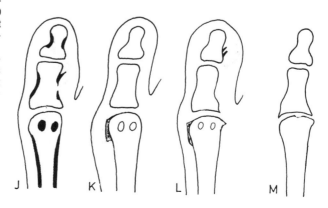

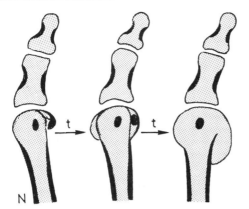

Fig. 533   Continuation of Figs. 530 to 532 (gouty osteoarthropathy).

N = Osteoplastic reaction in head of first metatarsal. Follow-up over a number of years (t) showed that this reaction has led to the so-called mushroom deformity of the metatarsal head (Dihlmann and Fernholz, 1974).

of inflammation indicate the accompanying systemic reaction of the body. Constellations that, in the presence of the local process described, point toward *primary* gout are male sex, middle age, pyknic constitution, adiposity, nephrolithiasis in the history, and the patient's report that the inflammation set in after a copious meal and/or an overindulgence in alcohol. Suspicion of *secondary* gout should be aroused with patients in whom joint complaints appear during the course of polycythemia, chronic myeloid leukemia,

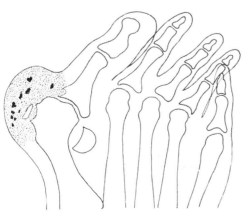

Fig. 534   Severe valgus deformity of the metatarsophalangeal joints I to IV; slight varus of the 5th toe. Erosive changes of contours in head of 1st metatarsal and 1st proximal phalanges, dissection in head of the 1st metatarsal, and heavy, dense swelling of soft tissues with pleomorphic calcium shadows argue against a trivial valgus deformity (compare Fig. 487) and settle the diagnosis of gouty osteoarthropathy.

and other myeloproliferative diseases, or in the setting of chronic renal insufficiency. In these cases, also, the next diagnostic procedure is determination of the uric acid concentration in the serum.

The following is the *differential diagnosis of the first acute gouty attack* in the metatarsophalangeal joint of the great toe:

- *Acute bacterial (pyogenic) arthritis*
- *Phlegmon* (acute cellulitis), because in the gouty attack the swelling very frequently extends to soft tissues at a distance from the joint
- So-called *calcareous peritendinitis* (p. 73 ff)
- *Iatrogenic crystal-induced synovitis* (p. 65 ff) following intraarticular injection of a crystalline corticosteroid
- *Psoriatic arthritis*, acute onset with "sausage toe" (sausage finger; pp. 93 and 95)
- *Articular chondrocalcinosis* presenting the clinical picture of pseudogout (p. 62 ff)
- *Reiter's syndrome*, acute metatarsophalangeal arthritis
- *Rheumatic fever* (acute polyarthritis), if the gouty attack (infrequently) involves several or many joints
- *Ankylosing spondylitis* with acute or subacute involvement of the (metatarsophalangeal) joint
- *Palindromic arthritis* (p. 105) (frequently attacks a single joint)
- *Activated osteoarthrosis* (p. 36 ff)
- Aseptic necrosis of a sesamoid bone of the great toe

Renander disease (Claustre and Simon, 1978) is not only accompanied by intense pain but produces a swelling which, *clinically*, suggests an arthritis in the metatarsophalangeal region. In so-called axial roentgenograms of the sesamoid bones (Fig. 535), the diseased bone presents a crumbled appearance; individual portions of the bone show increased density. Hence, the involved sesamoid bone presents the typical roentgen appearance of osteonecrosis (roentgenologic differential diagnosis: traumatic fracture, osteomyelitis of the sesamoid bone).

Here is the differential diagnosis of chronic gout:

- *Rheumatoid arthritis*
- *Activated polyosteoarthrosis*
- *Erosive polyosteoarthrosis* (p. 38)
- *Psoriatic arthritis*

The *roentgenographic findings* in gout depend on the quantity/time quotient of urate precipitation (Dihlmann and Fernholz, 1969), p. 41 ff). This approach offers a plausible explanation for the formal pathogenesis of the manifold roentgen findings in gouty osteoarthropathy (Figs. 530 through 535).

Insofar as **ochronosis** (p. 44) manifests itself at all clinically and roentgenologically in the joints of the foot (or the hand), it presents the picture of osteoarthrosis.

In addition to the knee and elbow joints, **hemophilia** (p. 44 ff) frequently affects the ankle joints

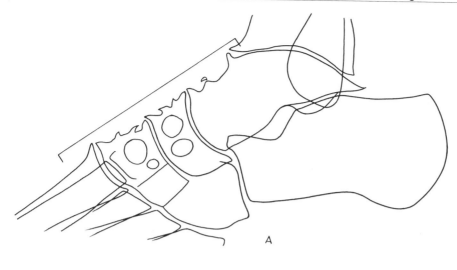

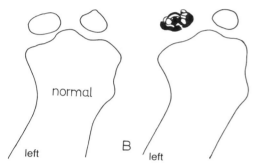

Fig. 535

A = *"Shaggy foot" (marked),* due to osteoarthrotic osteophytes and fibroosteoses in the contour of the dorsum of the foot. The finding is characteristic though not pathognomonic of *gout* (Françon and Leroy, 1962).

B = Roentgenogram of **Renander's disease** (osteonecrosis of one of the metatarsophalangeal sesamoid bones of the great toe). The *clinical* symptomatology may suggest gout. Compare the gouty involvement of a sesamoid bone of the great toe in Fig. 531G.

(Figs. 536, 537, and 538). In the foot, also, the development and the degree of severity of hemophiliac osteoarthropathy are conditioned by the genetically determined diminution in activity of the corresponding coagulation factors. Repeated hemorrhages into the joint give rise to those roentgen findings that, quite generally, determine the roentgenographic appearance of the hemophiliac joint (p. 44 ff). The consequences of intraosseous hemorrhages reveal themselves in the roentgenogram in the form of cystic osteolyses. Intraarticular and subchondral hemorrhages sometimes lead to collapse and fragmentation of the trochlea tali in the sense of aseptic necroses of bone (Fig. 538). Finally, hemophiliac pseudotumor (p. 47) (Fig. 539), disorders of growth, diffuse demineralization, or—in younger hemophiliacs—hypertrophic atrophy of bone have also been observed in the region of the foot. Growth disturbances, deformations, increased density of soft tissues from deposition of hemosiderin and from subchondral cysts occur, in the forefoot, prevalently in the metatarsophalangeal joints (Pavlov et al., 1979).

In the region of the foot, the **congenital hereditary hemoglobinopathies** display the same pathologic lesions that are observed in the supporting and gliding tissues of the hand (p. 119 ff; Fig. 141, nos. 1 to 4). The *tibiotalar slope* sketched in the Figures 536 and 538 as an accompaniment of hemophilia also occurs, as a growth disorder, in sickle cell anemia.

Neurogenic osteoarthropathies (p. 47) in the region of the foot accompany inherited or acquired basic disorders. Diseases in which the majority of neurogenic osteoarthropathies affect the lower extremities were already pointed out on page 49 ff. An important example of these diseases is diabetes mellitus, in which a neurogenic osteoarthropathy is known to occur as a rare late complication. Neurogenic osteoarthropathy in diabetics is *unrelated* to peripheral circulatory disorders in the usual sense of the term, since in these patients the pedal pulses are palpable and the skin is warm and shows no conspicuous pallor or signs of gangrene. Nor do intermittent claudication and calcification of the wall of the metatarsal and phalangeal arteries belong to the picture of neu-

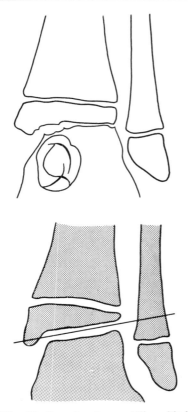

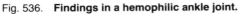

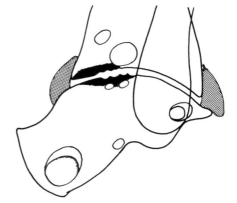

Fig. 537 **Hemophilic ankle joint** of a younger adult. Trochlea tali flattened (growth disturbance); delicate erosions in the tibia and the talus; increased density of the subchondral cancellous bone; larger and smaller cystic osteolyses, not all of them located in the zone of pressure absorption; uncommon *density* of the soft tissues in anterior and posterior to the joint. *In summary:* Mixed picture that cannot be identified as either chronic arthritis with secondary osteoarthrosis or pure osteoarthrosis. The correct diagnosis is suggested by the cystic osteolyses—which are the consequence of hemorrhages into the bone marrow—and the pronounced density of the articular soft tissues, which is produced by the deposition of hemosiderin.

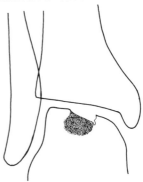

Fig. 536. **Findings in a hemophilic ankle joint.**
Top: Advanced hemophilic osteoarthropathy in an 8-year-old child. Narrowing of joint space and erosion of articular contours in ankle joint. Major cavity in the talus due to resorption following hemorrhages into the bone marrow. These roentgen findings could, among other etiologies, also correspond to a tuberculous affection. However, the history of hemophilia and the **additional** oligoarticular roentgen findings—e.g., in the knee and elbow joints—are guiding factors in making the correct diagnosis.
Bottom: **Tibiotalar slope** due to disordered growth of the distal tibial epiphysis and the trochlea tali in hemophilia with involvement of the ankle joint (regarding differential diagnosis of this growth disturbance see p. 357).

Fig. 538 **Hemophilic ankle joint** of an adult with tibiotalar slope (see Fig. 536) and roentgen signs of partial ischemia of the talus (see p. 44).

rogenic diabetic osteoarthropathy. On the other hand, the symptoms and findings listed are distinctive features of the characteristic disturbances of peripheral circulation in diabetics. Occasionally, however, the two complications occur conjointly. In the foot, the neurogenic osteopathies frequently present a special hallmark in the shape of the so-called perforsting ulcer. These indolent or hardly painful ulcers pave the way for infections which are manifested by ossifying periosteitis, osteomyelitis, or bony ankylosis. In addition to this, fragments of bone are sometimes expelled through the ulcers, and it is only then that some patients feel prompted to seek medical attention.

The earliest roentgenographic findings in neurogenic osteoarthropathies of the foot—e.g., small juxtaarticular defects in the contours of the proximal phalanges and the metatarsal heads measuring between 1 and 5 mm in diameter, are completely indistinctive. They either remain unchanged for a prolonged period of time or increase in size only slowly. In other instances, they are transformed into extensive osteolyses within a few weeks (Pogonowska et al., 1967).

In some studies, the clinical picture was ushered in by spontaneous fractures, fatigue fractures (Fig. 540), and the formation of fragments. These events

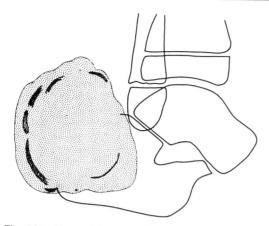

Fig. 539 **Hemophilic pseudotumor.** Disintegration and shell-like expansion of the posterior region of the calcaneus and thickening of soft tissue due to recurrent intraosseous and subperiosteal hemorrhages. Without knowledge of the history of hemophilia the roentgenogram would initially suggest a malignant tumor.

were followed, particularly in the hindfoot, by extensive crumbly disintegration or crushing of the involved bones, with sagging of the arch, subluxations, and dislocations (Figs. 521 A, 541, and 542). These dislocations indicate that in neurogenic osteoarthropathies the ligaments become damaged concomitantly. In the forefoot it is especially the metatarsophalangeal joints that are involved, their articulating bones gradually showing the eroded appearance of "sucked-on sticks of candy" (Figs. 53 and 543). In addition, extensive disintegration of bone may also be seen in the regions of the forefoot and tarsus, sim-

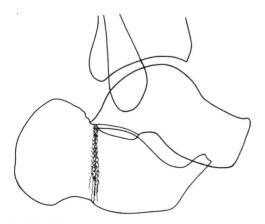

Fig. 540 **Fatigue fracture of the calcaneus** as early sign of neurogenic osteoarthropathy (in the present instance complicating tabes dorsalis). In addition, the dislocation of the talus points to concomitant damage (relaxation) of the capsuloligamentous apparatus.

ilar to the changes described above for the hindfoot (Fig. 564). In individual cases, repair of these destructive lesions has been observed; for example, in neurogenic diabetic osteoarthropathy (Feiereis, 1964; Gondoş, 1968). Calcium shadows in the surroundings of the destroyed bones and joints may be crumbles of bone or paraosseous new bone such as was described on page 47 as an additional feature of neurogenic osteoarthropathies.

In summarizing the roentgen findings to be expected in neurogenic osteopathies of the foot, we must mention three outstanding processes which, to be sure, are variable in extent and duration (Figs. 521 A, and 541 through 544):

1. *Nonreactive osteolysis with a tendency toward being smoothed out,* prevalently in the forefoot and possibly presenting as osteolysis of the acral parts.
2. *Sequestration of bone,* as the result of abnormal brittleness, particularly in the regions of the hindfoot and the metatarsus.
3. *Neoformations of bone* either as neurogenic periosteal, paraosseous, and periarticular ossifications *or* as consequences of a secondary bacterial infection by way of a perforating ulcer of the foot.

(The findings described under items 2 and 3 are summarized under the term "Charcot's joint", see p. 48).

The neurogenic osteoarthropathies of the foot can occur unilaterally or bilaterally (in the latter instance mostly asymmetrically). Bilateral occurrence prevails in the inherited familial osteolyses. Conversely, neurogenic osteoarthropathies as an aftermath of unilateral damage (injury) to peripheral nerves are to be expected only in the extremity involved. The same applies, of course, to posttraumatic osteolyses such as have been seen, for instance, in the neighborhood of the ankle joint following fractures of the distal lower leg (Schüler and Laschner, 1969).

Following extensive burns, not only pyogenic infections are likely to occur in the joints, but also lesions that, on the roentgenogram, are indistinguishable from neurogenic osteoarthropathies or neurogenic paraosteoarthropathies (Figs. 443 and 562). Similar lesions occurring in the knee joint were mentioned on page 311, footnote 23.

The roentgenologic differential diagnosis of osteolytic lesions of the acral parts is described in Figure 146. Most of the findings illustrated there are also observed in the toes.

During the stage of mutilation occurring in a chronic inflammatory (rheumatoid) arthropathy, the roentgen findings in the forefoot may be completely identical to the picture of neurogenic osteolyses. However, the diagnosis presents no difficulty in view of the prolonged history of polyarthritis and the roentgen signs of chronic inflammation in *other* joints of the extremity. When neurogenic osteolyses *start,* for example, in a metatarsophalangeal joint, the roentgenogram gives the impression of arthritic erosions (Fig. 543, 2nd left toe). In most cases, then,

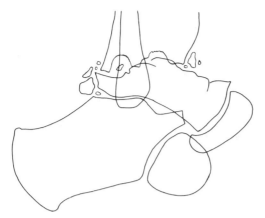

Fig. 541 Neurogenic osteoarthropathy in the region of the hindfoot. Trochlea tali and distal end of tibia appear to be crushed and crumbled. Calcaneus and cuboid slip posteriorly, while talus and navicular slip anteriorly.
Clinically: Painless swelling in the talocrural junction. Deformation of the hindfoot; instability in the ankle joint.

the diagnosis is settled by an inquiry about local pain and also a search for trophic ulcers.

Partially paralyzed children with malformations or nonmalignant tumors of the cord and its meninges sometimes present in the knee and ankle joint the picture of irregularly enlarged epiphyseal plates, narrow epiphyses, and periosteal neoformations of bone. It is supposed that these changes result from continued microtraumas to the metaphysis and epiphysis of these patients, who are still capable of walking but whose sensation of pain is impaired (Gyepes et al., 1965). Figure 545 illustrates such lesions in the ankle joint. Incidentally, it should be remembered that epiphysiolyses and fractures of the metaphysis and diaphysis are characteristic findings in neurogenic osteoarthropathies of the growth period.

The **Ainhum syndrome** (spontaneous dactyloysis, Fig. 60) was mentioned on page 55.

Regarding the differential diagnosis of **massive osteolysis (Graham-Stout)** in the lower leg, compare Figure 444 with Figure 546. Massive osteolysis occurs prevalently in children and young adults. It is true that the pseudarthrosis (of the tibia) illustrated in Figure 546 most frequently occurs in the first year of life but, in principle, can be observed during the entire first decade. Massive osteolysis also may start from the bones of the foot. Congenital pseudoarthrosis involves the long bones of the extremities exclusively.

Amyloidosis (p. 60) manifests itself *predominantly* in the shoulder, the hip, and the hand. In principle, however, the possible roentgen findings (erosions in the vicinity of the capsuloligamentous insertion, articular and periarticular bilaterally symmetrical swellings, and subchondral cystic osteolyses) may be found also in the region of the foot. When this roentgenographic appearance is present in the hand or the foot, the condition must be differentiated from rheumatoid arthritis.

Osteoarthropathy related to hemochromatosis (p. 61 ff) shows nonobjectifiable arthralgia in many joints and a roentgenogram combining (poly-) osteoarthrosis, chondrocalcinosis, and diffuse—hence not joint-related—osteoporosis (Fig. 547). These findings may also be observed in the foot but are more evidential in the hand, the second and third metacarpophalangeal joints being the test joints for osteoarthropathy of hemochromatosis (Fig. 148)! In the foot, also, involvement of the metatarsophalangeal joints, as a manifestation of this iron-storage disease, generally is more frequent than involvement of the other joints of the foot (Laborde et al., 1977).

About 75 percent of the patients suffering from **Wilson's disease** (p. 62) complain of discomfort in the joints (Golding and Walshe, 1977). The following roentgen findings *may* be conspicuous (Fig. 548):

- *Premature* osteoarthrosis (often occurring as early as the third or fourth decade)
- Subchondral fragmentation of bone and bony metaplasia in the articular soft tissues giving the roentgenographic appearance of loose bodies with or without a "mouse bed"

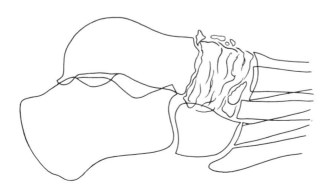

Fig. 542 Neurogenic osteoarthropathy in the tarsus. Cuneiform and navicular have been crushed. Sagging of the longitudinal arch.

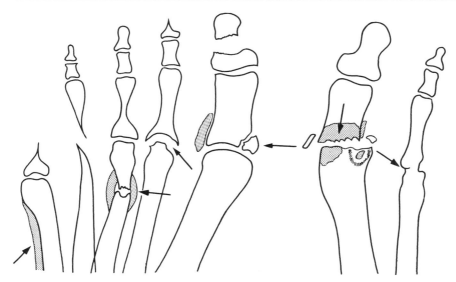

Fig. 543 **Characteristic features and stages of neurogenic osteoarthropathies in the forefoot (synopsis).**
Arrows point to findings which—if isolated—are apt to cause extreme difficulty of differential diagnosis (see Fig. 498). Also, note osteolysis of the acral part of the 2nd distal phalanx on the left.

Note: Periosteal reaction also forms part of the picture of neurogenic osteoarthropathy. However, neurogenic osteoarthropathy *plus* perforating ulcer of the foot (see p. 48) *plus* periosteal reaction renders the diagnosis of superinfection very probable.

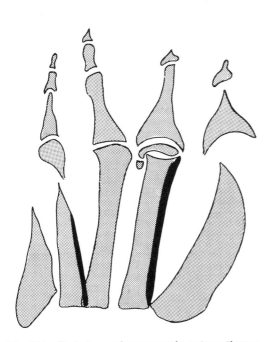

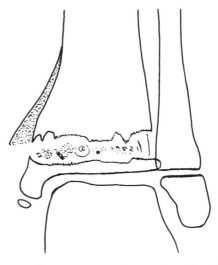

Fig. 544 **End stage of neurogenic osteoarthropathy of the forefoot** after a course of many decades. The causal disease *cannot* be read from the roentgenogram.

Fig. 545 **Consequences of metaphyseal and epiphyseal microtraumas in children with partial paralysis and disturbed sensibility suffering from malformation or nonmalignant tumor of the cord and its meninges** (enlarged zone of epiphyseal growth in the tibia; narrow distal epiphysis of the tibia; periosteal formation of new bone). *Hint for differential diagnosis: Generalized* "enlargement" of the cartilaginous epiphyseal plates and irregular contours of the metaphyses occur in (alimentary, renal, etc.) rickets.

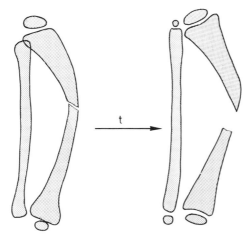

Fig. 546 Follow-up of a congenital pseudoar-throsis of the tibia; for example in von Recklinghausen's neurofibromatosis or fibrous dysplasia.
Development of deformations (t): Bowing of tibia; fatigue fracture which may go on to cure or may pass into a pseudoarthrosis with resorption of bone.
Roentgenographic differentiation from massive osteolysis (Gorham-Stout, see Fig. 444) and idiopathic osteolyses (see legend accompanying Fig. 58).

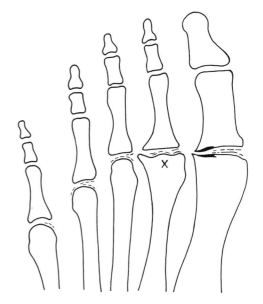

Fig. 547 Metatarsophalangeal chondrocalcinosis in idiopathic hemochromatosis. Osteoarthrosis of 1st metatarsophalangeal joint.
X = Incidental finding of status after aseptic necrosis of 2nd metatarsal head (2nd Köhler's disease, Köhler-Freiberg disease) experienced in the growth period.

- Articular chondrocalcinosis
- Skeletal osteoporosis and rickets (osteomalacia)

In **hyperparathyroidism** (p. 125 ff), radiologic study of the feet is less important for the diagnosis than are roentgenograms of the hands. The roentgen signs of subperiosteal bone resorption (compare Figs. 151 and 549), especially, are less frequently observed in the phalanges of the foot than in the corresponding bones of the hand (Lipson and Williams, 1968). Calcification of the tunica media occurs in the lower extremities with greater frequency than in the upper extremities. Early calcification of the media is observed in the internal iliac artery, the first metatarsal artery (Ritz et al., 1973), and the arteries of the soft tissues in front of and behind the ankle joint (Meema et al., 1976). It should be remembered, however, that calcifications of the arterial walls are completely "nonspecific" findings.

Lipoid-dermatoarthritis (p. 131 ff) shows, also in the foot, the radiographic picture of a chronic bilaterally symmetrical polyarthritis (Gold et al., 1975) which often can lead to severe destruction of the articulating bones within a comparatively short period. For differential diagnosis see page 131.

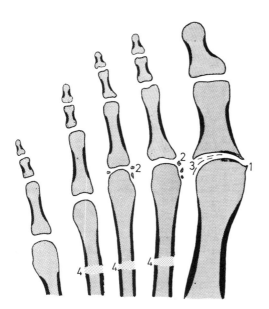

Fig. 548 Full-blown picture of osteoarthropathy in Wilson's disease (young adult).
1 = Discrete osteoarthrosis of 1st metatarsophalangeal joint.
2 = Appearance of loose bodies at the 2nd and 3rd metatarsophalangeal joints without roentgen signs of past aseptic necrosis of bone of the Köhler II type (Köhler-Freiberg disease).
3 = Chondrocalcinosis.
4 = Metatarsal Looser's zones.
Not all items (1 to 4) must be combined to justify the diagnosis! Items 2 and 3 are particularly significant.

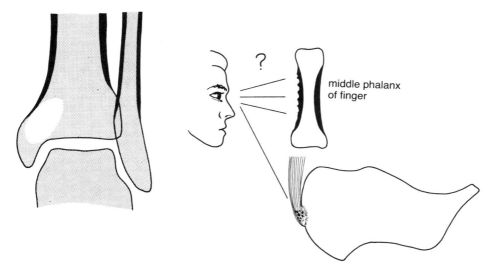

Fig. 549   Oval osteolysis without sclerotic marginal reaction in the medial malleolus.
Roentgenologic differential diagnosis: Brown tumor in so-far-undiagnosed hyperparathyroidism. (Therefore, study the radial side of the middle phalanges of the fingers and the site of insertion of the Achilles tendon. In hyperparathyroidism, insertion defects, often with small calcium shadows, are apt to occur at these sites. Compare Figs. 366 and 563.) Fibrous dysplasia; benign chondroblastoma; osteoclastoma; solitary metastasis.

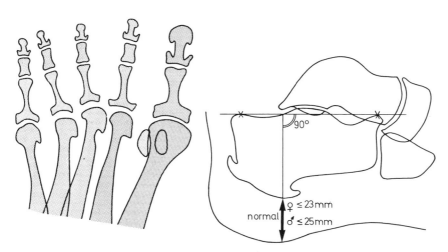

Fig. 550   Roentgen signs of acromegaly in the foot. *Forefoot:* Terminal finger tuft enlarged; distal and middle phalanges thickened; metatarsal heads with "noses"; fibrillar demineralization of the metatarsal heads *(not illustrated).*
Hindfoot: Facultative occurrence of large calcaneal spurs (fibroosteoses). Soft-tissue shadow in the heel of adult white males suffering from acromegaly, >25 mm; of adult females, >23 mm (target–calcaneus distance = 1 m, measuring technique of Kho et al., 1970, which is oriented by the connecting line between the highest anterior and posterior points of the calcaneus and its lowest point). According to Kattan (1975), the soft tissues of the heel may also become thickened by long-term treatment with the antiepileptic agent diphenylhydantoin.

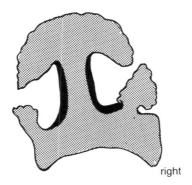

right

Fig. 551 **Excessive remodeling of the distal phalanx of the great toe in acromegaly.**

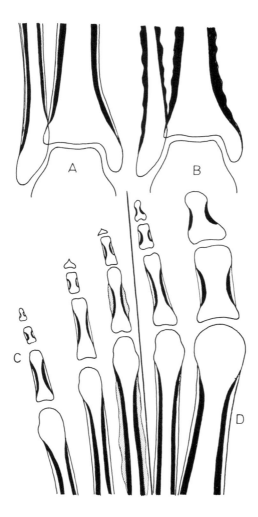

The roentgen findings in **acromegaly** (p. 131 ff) are depicted in Figs. 550 and 551.

The manifold clinical and roentgenologic aspects of **hypertrophic osteoarthropathy** (symptomatic pachydermoperiostosis, Marie-Bamberger syndrome) and **idiopathic pachydermoperiostosis** were discussed on page 133 ff (Figs. 157 through 160 and Fig. 552 with periosteal findings in the lower leg and foot). **Thyroid acropachy** manifests itself in the same way as in the diaphyses of the metacarpals and the phalanges of the fingers (King et al., 1959, p. 136, Fig. 160).

Damage from ionizing rays may be expected in the foot when soft-tissue hemangiomas over an open epiphysis are inappropriately irradiated; i.e., either with an overdose or an inadequate wave length of the effective radiation. The bones show delayed growth and at a later date—following closure of the epiphyses—shortening. In addition, necroses of cartilage and bone have also been observed in the foot as late consequences of radiotherapy (Kolář and Vrabec, 1959). Frequently, though not consistently, an irradiation ulcer was present in the vicinity of the joint involved. The amputations that became necessary have revealed that the roentgen signs of arthritis (erosions, destructions, and narrowing of the joint space) had developed not only by direct extension of a pyogenic arthritis but also by actinic necroses of cartilage and bone.

Neoplasms of the Joints

In the region of the foot, also, the combination of a *palpable, firm,* soft-tissue swelling (increased density in the roentgenogram with pleomorphic calcium shadows and erosion of bone) raises the suspicion of **malignant synovialoma** (Figs. 553, 554, and 555) or soft-tissue chondrosarcoma (a very infrequent affection) and soft-tissue chondroma. Malignant synovialoma develops in the synovial membrane of the joint or in the juxtaarticular soft structures (bursae, tendons, tendon sheaths, fasciae).

In the foot, **pigmented villonodular synovitis** (p. 139 f) frequently has its primary origin in the tendon sheaths and subsequently often erodes the phalanges and the heads of the metatarsals. In this affection, also, there is a circumscribed swelling of the

Fig. 552 **Hypertrophic osteoarthropathy (A, D) and idiopathic pachydermoperiostosis (B, C).** In both processes, the periosteal reactions may be *distinguishable* or may present an *identical* roentgenlogic aspect (compare Fig. 160, "phasic scheme of periosteal reactions"). Acral osteolyses (C), on the other hand, have so far been seen only in idiopathic pachydermoperiostosis (Guyer et al., 1978).

Note: Idiopathic pachydermoperiosteosis has also become known in the literature as the *Touraine-Solente-Golé syndrome.*

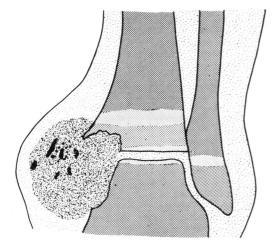

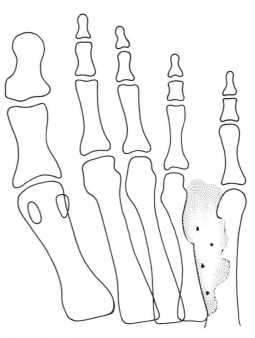

Fig. 553 Firm, nonfluctuating swelling in the medial malleolus increasing for a number of months.
Roentgenologic finding: Destruction of bone; increased density of soft tissue with pleomorphic calcifications **(suspicion of malignant synovialoma).** Atrophy of disuse (demineralization) in vicinity of ankle joint.

Note: In this case, the **firm, nonfluctuating swelling** in the medial malleolus is, also to the radiologist, of crucial importance in the differential diagnosis between malignant synovialoma and tuberculosis.

Fig. 555 Malignant synovialoma (diagnosis confirmed histologically).
Roentgen findings: Increased soft-tissue density standing out against the remaining soft tissues of the foot. Isolated calcium shadows within the zone of increased density. Pressure erosion in the 4th metatarsal; invasion of the 5th metatarsal.
Radiographic diagnosis: Slowly growing malignant tumor originating in the soft tissues. The isolated calcium shadows raise the suspicion of malignant synovialoma.

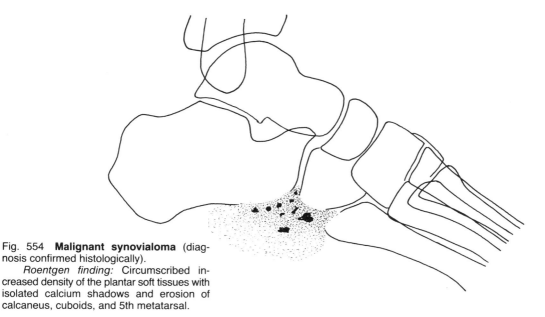

Fig. 554 Malignant synovialoma (diagnosis confirmed histologically).
Roentgen finding: Circumscribed increased density of the plantar soft tissues with isolated calcium shadows and erosion of calcaneus, cuboids, and 5th metatarsal.

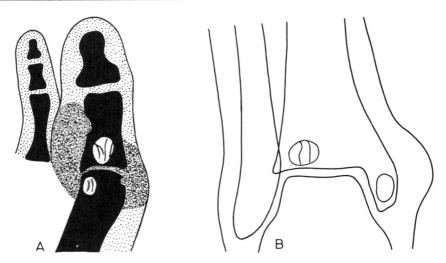

Fig. 556 Roentgen findings in pigmented villonodular synovitis.
A = Homogeneous circumscribed swelling and increased density of soft tissues close to and farther away from the metatarsophalangeal joint of the great toe. Sharply demarcated, trabeculated, cystlike defects of bone; in some parts flat erosions.
No demineralization.
B = Cystic osteolyses in the tibia *and* circumscribed swelling of soft tissues *(without calcium shadows)* in the medial malleolus.

soft tissues in the toes (Fig. 556), but there are no calcium shadows. The swelling is less dense than a gouty tophus. Apart from that, in pigmented villonodular synovitis the discomfort is not as pronounced as it is in gout. Figure 557 shows additional "space-occupying processes" in the regions of the tarsus and the forefoot. For **neoplastic synovial chondromatosis** (p. 66 ff) in the foot see Figures 73 and 529).

Calcification and Ossification of Soft Tissues; Affections of the Fibroosseous Junction and the Bursae

The roentgen findings in **chondrocalcinosis** (p. 62 ff) are recognizable in Figures 547, 548, and 558. The terms **localized (circumscribed) interstitial calcinosis** and **universal interstitial calcinosis** describe calcifications that originate in the *interstitial connective tissue* as circumscribed or continuously extending lesions. Conversely, **pseudotumorous calcinosis** is encountered in *differentiated* tissues; e.g., in bursae, muscles, tendons, and so on. Objections to this sharp demarcation and subclassification were already raised on page 69, where it was pointed out that in the majority of cases the calcinoses are symptomatic findings. Much less frequently, they constitute a separate clinical entity. Figure 559 shows roentgen findings in the forefoot of a patient with chronic uremia

on maintenance hemodialysis. This picture does not allow one to decide with certainty whether exclusively interstitial deposits of calcium are present or whether (very probably) bursae are involved *in addition*. This case demonstrates that classification and localization of calcinoses on the sole basis of the roentgen findings is questionable.

Monotopic bursal calcifications sometimes develop in the wake of chronic, occupational, excessive strain; i.e., continued traumas (Fig. 560). In addition, irregularly shaped calcifications of soft tissues in the foot raise the suspicion of calcified tuberculous pus, including tuberculous bursae. Less frequently, calcifications occur in the vicinity of a pyogenic osteomyelitis or arthritis.

The importance of roentgen findings in the hand and foot in the diagnosis of **pseudohypoparathyroidism** and **pseudopseudohypoparathyroidism** was already mentioned on pages 143 and 145 (Figs. 168 and 561). The feet of these short patients—similarly to their hands—are conspicuous by the shortening of the metatarsals and the deformation of the epiphyses, as well as by calcification of the peri- and extraarticular soft tissues. Larger soft-tissue calcifications are apt to become ossified.

The term **localized traumatic myositis ossificans** denotes calcareous shadows in soft tissues that, in the course of weeks or months, take on an osseous structure. These lesions occur as an aftermath of injuries to the soft structures, with or without involvement of bones and joints. It is rare for these calcareous shadows to develop without any external cause

Fig. 557   **Space-occupying processes in the foot.**

1 = Soft-tissue xanthomas in hyperlipoproteinemia (compare Fig. 166). Of pathognomonic significance is the xanthoma-dependent fusiform bilateral swelling in the Achilles tendon (possibly associated with calcareous lesions and erosion of the calcaneus such as are sketched here).

2 = *Osteitis deformans (Paget's disease)* (compare Fig. 165).

3 = Chronic osteomyelitis **(Brodie's abscess).**

4 = **Chondrosarcoma.** Small *calcium shadows* are visible within destroyed phalanx (Miki et al., 1978).

5 = Pressure erosions due to **nonmalignant soft-tissue tumor** (lipoma, fibroma, neurofibroma; compare Fig. 164).

6 = **Spongy osteoid osteoma** (compare Fig. 164). At times the nidus in the cancellous bone is not visible and can be identified only by angiography.

7 = Painless or painful soft-tissue swelling. Differential diagnosis must consider a *great variety of affections,* among them **paraosseous fasciitis** (p. 68).

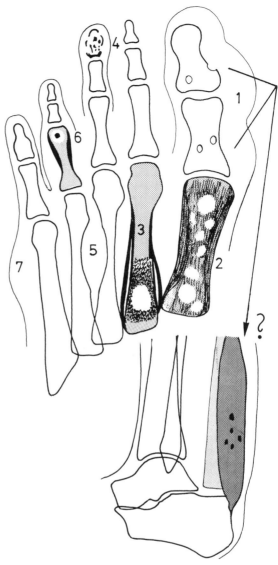

(localized *atraumatic* myositis ossificans). On page 68 the reader will find some diagnostic pointers to avoid confusing an incipient myositis ossificans with an osteoplastic sarcoma of the soft tissue (of the foot). Such possible confusion also includes the juxtaarticular osteosarcomas, which offer a comparatively favorable prognosis (Fig. 74).

Thermal injuries can be followed by calcifications and ossifications—particularly in the elbow, shoulder, knee, and ankle joint—that interfere with the mobility of the joints involved (Fig. 562). To be sure, restriction of articular motion following a thermal trauma may also be the consequence of direct destruction of soft tissues or a complicating infection

of the joint. In rare instances, burns are followed by an aseptic disorganization of the joint which, roentgenologically, resembles the picture of neurogenic osteoarthropathy (p. 311, footnote no. 23).

Progressive myositis ossificans (progressive diaphyseal dysplasia) and its manifestations in the skeleton of the foot were discussed on page 70 (see also Fig. 76). In addition, large anterior and posterior calcaneal spurs should be mentioned. These lesions develop in connection with the progressive pathologic ossification of the tendons and aponeuroses inserting on the calcaneus or arising there.

The fibroosseous affections (p. 72 ff; Figs. 78 and 79) of the foot can best be exemplified by their

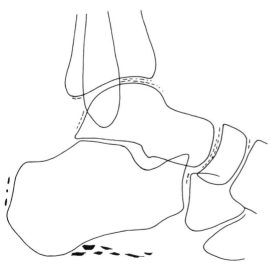

Fig. 558   **Chondrocalcinosis in hyaline cartilage and aponeurotic and tendinous tissue of the foot.**

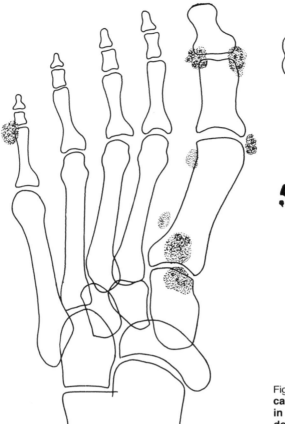

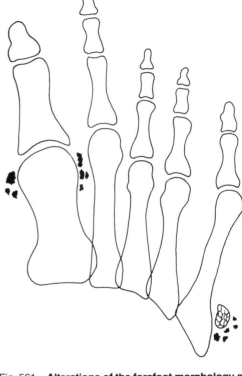

Fig. 561 **Alterations of the forefoot morphology and calcifications as well as ossification of soft tissues in pseudohypoparathyroidism and pseudopseudohypoparathyroidism** (compare Fig. 168).

Fig. 559 **Roentgenographic morphology of calcinosis of the foot** (here in a patient with chronic uremia on maintenance dialysis). Majority of calcium deposits presumably in the interstitial tissue, but calcifications about base of metatarsal and medial cuneiform are typically located in the subtendinous bursa of the tibialis anterior muscle.

Note: The radiologist diagnoses the calcinosis. Its classification—whether an idiopathic entity or a symptomatic finding—requires consideration of the clinical and anamnestic data. The roentgenologic localization of the calcium deposits in a certain anatomic substrate can likewise lead to difficulty (see this figure).

most familiar representative, namely **rheumatic calcaneopathy** (Figs. 563 and 564; also compare Fig. 565), although the pathologic roentgen findings of fibroosteitis can, in principle, be encountered in all tendinous and ligamentous insertions of the foot. Rheumatic calcaneopathy, particularly fibroosteitis, occurs with decreasing frequency in psoriatic arthritis, Reiter's syndrome, ankylosing spondylitis, rheumatoid arthritis, and Jaccoud's arthritis. Figure 566 illustrates varied localizations of reversible circumscribed depositions of calcium—so-called **tendinosis, tendinitis, calcareous peritendinitis** (p. 73)—in the tendons, joint capsules, and bursae of the foot. The characteristic feature of these calcium deposits is their clinical course, which may be either asymptomatic, slightly painful or, at times, assuming the form of a hyperacute inflammation (see p. 74). These calcium deposits differ from sesamoid bones and the so-called accessory ossicles by the typical absence of any structure.

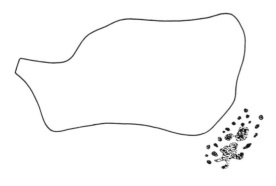

Fig. 560 **Calcifications in the subcutaneous calcaneal bursa** (see text).

Fig. 562 **Extensive periarticular ossifications of soft tissues about the talocrural joint corresponding in roentgenographic appearance to a neurogenic paraosteoarthropathy.** In this case the calcifications or ossifications began 2 months after a thermal injury. Such ossifications leading to extraarticular ankylosis, though, are only encountered in a minority of patients with severe burns.

Fig. 563 **Fibroosseous affections of the calcaneus and other roentgen signs of rheumatic calcaneopathy; ossification of the Achilles tendon.**

1 = Roentgenologic morphology of the *degenerative (reparative)* anterior and posterior calcaneal spur **(fibroostosis).** *Characteristic features:* Pin-shaped, smooth contours; regular structures.

2 = Manifestations of rheumatic calcaneopathy. Characteristic features of **fibroosteitis:** Irregular pin shape or bubble shape; irregular structures and contours, densification in the bordering cancellous bone of the calcaneous. The fibroosteitis illustrated is the productive type (Fig. 79): *On the left* at the origins of the plantar aponeurosis, the flexor digitorum brevis, the abductor hallucis, the abductor digiti quinti, and the ligamentum plantare longum *on the right;* at the origin of the plantar calcaneocuboid ligament. In rare cases, the increased density of the cancellous bone near the fibroosteitis extends far into the calcaneus (Fig. 564). It should also be mentioned that in fibroosteitis, perichondral ossification of the calcaneal apophysis can be expected. In this case a stroke-shaped shadow of calcium stands out against the convexity of the apophysis (Hladik, 1968).

The *precalcaneal bursa* (bursa tendinis calcanei) lies close beneath the posterosuperior edge of the calcaneus between this bone and the Achilles tendon (compare Fig. 490, no. 5). The erosion sketched **("defect due to bursitis of the Achilles tendon")** develops as a result of the pressure exerted by the inflammatory swelling of the bursa and the spreading of the inflammatory process to the calcaneus, which at that site lacks a periosteal sheath. The roentgen signs of bursitis of the Achilles tendon (Rössler, 1896) are also demonstrable in **Haglund's heel** (extremely developed and projecting posterosuperior edge of the calcaneus); in xanthoma of the Achilles tendon (Fig. 557); and—from a pressure erosion—in gout (Gerster et al., 1975). All these affections should enter into the differential diagnosis.

Inflammatory rheumatic **calcaneal periostitis** leads either to neoformation of bone ("cockscomb") or to superficial erosion.

Note: Rheumatic calcaneopathy occurs as an accompaniment, but sometimes also as an *initial manifestation,* of various inflammatory rheumatic arthropathies (see text). The inflammatory rheumatic calcaneopathies differ from inflammatory bacterial affections of the calcaneus by their (as a rule) bilateral occurrence. Bacterial infections commonly originate in the bone marrow and reach the insertions centrifugally (*exception:* osteomyelitis of the calcaneus that develops from a decubitus ulcer of the heel). Inflammatory rheumatic calcaneopathies start from the surface.

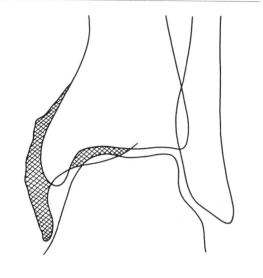

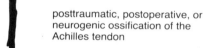

posttraumatic, postoperative, or neurogenic ossification of the Achilles tendon

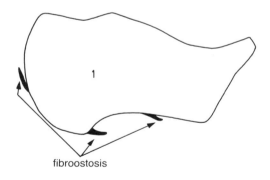

1

fibroostosis

periostitis

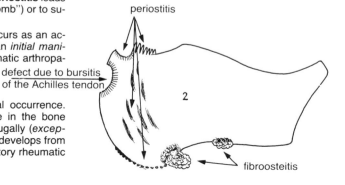

defect due to bursitis of the Achilles tendon

2

fibroosteitis

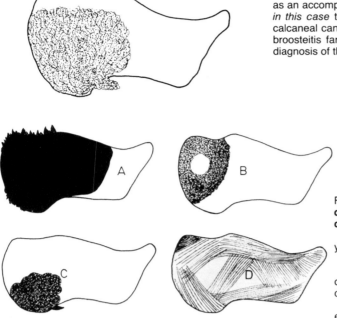

Fig. 564 **Fibroosteitis of the calcaneus** (in this case as an accompaniment of ankylosing spondylitis). Note *in this case* the excessive increase in density of the calcaneal cancellous bone, which extends from the fibroosteitis far into the calcaneus. For the differential diagnosis of this finding, see Fig. 565.

Fig. 565 **Roentgenologic differential diagnosis of fibroosteitis of the calcaneus in Fig. 564.**
A = Osteosarcoma with spicules in a young adult.
B = Brodie's abscess.
C = Osteoplastic metastasis in an incidentally coexisting fibroosteosis at the origin of the plantar aponeurosis.
D = Osteitis deformans (Paget's disease).

Fig. 566 **Structureless reversible calcium deposits** to be classified among the group of so-called calcareous tendinosis, calcareous tendinitis (peritendinitis), etc. (For the nomenclature, see p. 73). *Roentgenologic* differentiation from duplicated, aseptic necrotic (Fig. 535 B), or fractured sesamoid bones *(bone structure sketched in outlines)* and from accessory ossicles (an os peronaeum is shown in the figure). *Clinical* differentiation in the metatarsophalangeal joint of the great toe from gouty attack.

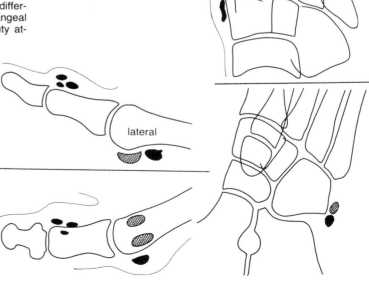

lateral

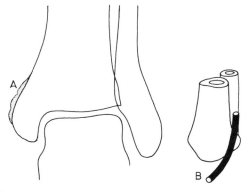

Fig. 567 **Periosteal reaction with typical localization (A) in chronic tenosynovitis of the tibialis posterior muscle** (see text).

B = Distal tibia with the tendon sheath for the tibialis posterior muscle.

Note: The thickened tendon sheath, with or without periosteal reaction, can be visualized in the lateral roentgenogram directly above the ankle joint. The same applies to hygroma of that tendon sheath.

Periosteal reactions on the outer contours of the malleoli are seen in chronic arthritis of the ankle joint (compare Figs. 506 and 510). Among the *extraarticular* processes triggering such periosteal reactions (p. 34 and footnote no. 11), **chronic tenosynovitis of the posterior tibial muscle** should be mentioned in addition. This affection occurs in the setting of rheumatoid arthritis or other inflammatory rheumatic diseases, as a chronic bacterial (tuberculous) or mycotic infection, in pigmented villonodular synovitis, but also as an "idiopathic" disorder (Fig. 567; Norris and Mankin, 1978). It gives rise to pain and swelling in the medial malleolus. In addition, it causes restriction of motion.

Traumas to the Joints

Dislocation of a toe occurs most frequently in the hallux. The dislocation may involve the metatarsophalangeal or the interphalangeal joint. Avulsions of the edge are manifested by small shadows of bone in the soft tissues (Fig. 568). Locking of the sesamoid bones is also a well-known complication. **Dislocations of the metatarsal bones** occur most frequently in Lisfranc's joint or Chopart's joint; the dislocation, hence, involves one or several metatarsals, or the navicular and the cuboid. The first and the fifth metatarsals are dislocated most frequently. Since these joints are heavily strengthened by ligaments, the injury is usually a fracture-dislocation. The first metatarsal may be displaced medially while the other metatarsals, singly or in a group, are dislocated laterally *(divergent dislocation)*. Medial displacement of all metatarsals is termed *homolateral dislocation. Isolated*

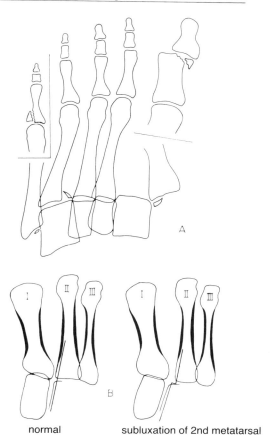

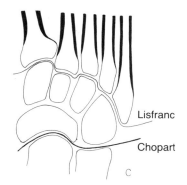

normal   subluxation of 2nd metatarsal

Fig. 568   A = **Injuries to the joints of the forefoot** *(from right to left).* Fracture-dislocation at the interphalangeal joint of the great toe (frequently an open injury because it is usually caused by direct circumscribed violence). Dislocation at the 1st tarsometatarsal joint with small avulsion of bone. Dislocation (subluxation) at the 4th and 5th tarsometatarsal joints (small avulsions of bone). Longitudinal fracture of the base of the 5th proximal phalanx with formation of a step in the articular contour.

B = Roentgenographic diagnosis of subluxation of the 2nd metatarsal (Foster and Foster, 1976) in the dorsoplantar view.

C = Definition of Chopart's joint line and Lisfranc's joint line.

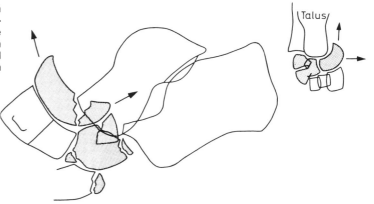

Fig. 569 **Complete dislocation (fracture-dislocation) in Chopart's joint line.** *Arrows* indicate typical direction of dislocation in tarsus and forefoot. Additional small avulsion of tuberosity of 5th metatarsal.

dislocations of one or two metatarsals may also occur. It should be noted that the attributes "lateral" and "medial" denote only the preferential direction of the dislocation, although the metatarsals can, in addition, become displaced dorsally, posteriorly, or even plantarly.

Chopart's joint can suffer a partial or a complete dislocation. In partial dislocation, only the ligaments are torn and the navicular as well as the cuboid (hence, the tarsus and forefoot) are displaced no more than a few millimeters medially or mediodorsally. Possible additional injuries are avulsion of the navicular tuberosity and/or the lateral aspect of the cuboid. Marked displacement occurs only with complete dislocation. The navicular and cuboid, together with the metatarsus and the forefoot, are dislocated mostly mediodorsally and in the direction of the hindfoot (Fig. 569), and less frequently laterally or plantarward. In general, fractures of the navicular and cuboid, but also of the base of the fifth metatarsal and the calcaneus, form part of this injury. Isolated fracture-dislocation of the navicular in the dorsal direction (Fig. 570) follows rupture of the protective dorsal ligaments. The nondislocated lateral and plantar portions of the na-

vicular are compressed and fractured, or are shattered to a large extent.

The dislocations discussed so far are very frequently associated with *additional* avulsions, cracks, major fractures, or even comminuted fractures, hence secondary skeletal injuries. **Pure fractures in the regions of the forefoot and the metatarsus** are only of interest *in this connection* if the fracture lines invade the contiguous joint and thus are apt to favor the development of a *posttraumatic osteoarthrosis* by direct injury to the cartilage, formation of a step, or other deformations. In addition, the mobility of the joint may become impaired if a fracture heals with marked displacement of the fragments. For example, the fragments of a (transverse) fracture of the shaft of the proximal phalanx frequently present an angulation, with the angle open toward the dorsal aspect. This displacement must be corrected to prevent the subsequent formation of a bulge in the sole that will be painful on walking. With shell-like avulsion of the extensor tendons from the dorsal aspects of the distal phalanges, impairment of extension can be prevented only by solid healing of the detached tendon.

Gait disturbances are also the possible consequence of inaccurate reduction of metatarsal fractures. This applies primarily to fractures of several metatarsals, which alter the shape of the plantar arch. In children, injuries to the forefoot, which in adults produce a dislocation (or fracture-dislocation), commonly lead to epiphysiolysis (chondroepiphysiolysis; see p. 384, Fig. 581) or to a fracture of the epiphysis (osteoepiphysiolysis; see p. 384, Fig. 581). Fractures of the small tarsal bones are due to circumscribed violence (blows, kicks, etc.).

Great clinical importance is attached to **fractures of the talus.** *Peripheral* fractures (posterior and lateral process, shearing fractures of the head, fractures of the edge of the trochlea) offer a favorable prognosis if reduction and immobilization are accurately performed. *Increasing displacement of the talus, however,* due to either subtalar (less often talar) dislocations and fracture dislocations or *central* frac-

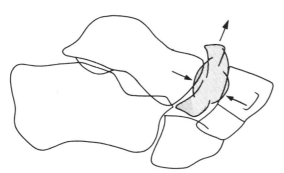

Fig. 570 **Isolated fracture-dislocation of the navicular.** *Arrows* indicate pathway of dislocation and direction of pressure exerted on navicular.

tures of the neck or body of the talus, aggravates the hazard of posttraumatic necrosis of the body and the trochlea (Figs. 571 and 572). This is the consequence of anatomic facts, for the arterial blood supply to the neck and body of the talus is derived from the tarsal sinus (in the calcaneus). The vessels hence enter the

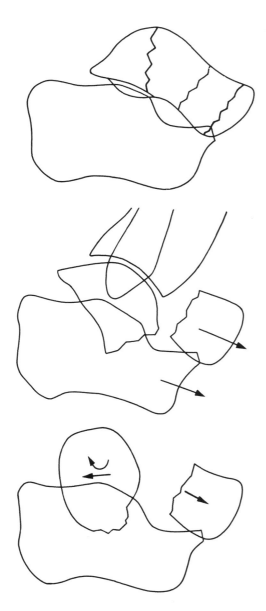

Fig. 571 **Fractures offering a favorable prognosis** *(above)* **and two examples of fracture-dislocation** *(center; below)* **in the junction between body and neck of the talus.** These lesions are apt to trigger an avascular (aseptic) necrosis in the posterior fragment, depending on the extent of the dislocation. The *Arrows* indicate direction of dislocation.

bone from the subtalar region. There is no auxiliary blood supply except by way of the small capsular and ligamental arteries. The head of the talus, on the other hand, is supplied by an artery that reaches it from posterolaterally. In the adult, avascular necrosis is repaired (revascularized) with severe deformation that subsequently leads to osteoarthrosis. Apart from this, any fracture of the talus that has healed with incongruity of the articular surfaces involves the hazard of posttraumatic osteoarthrosis.

Fractures of the talar head often accompany dislocations at the subtalar joint. Other accompaniments of this dislocation are fractures of the navicular, calcaneus, and/or cuboid. Fractures of the posterior process of the talus are frequently observed as a complication of fractures of the calcaneus.

Accurate assessment of an **injury of the calcaneus** requires four roentgenograms:

1. A frontal tibiofibular film of the hindfoot
2. An anteroposterior film of the ankle joint
3. An oblique plantodorsal film (to evaluate the anterior segment of the calcaneus)
4. A so-called axial film of the calcaneus (Fig. 480)

The roentgenograms are made of both the injured and the uninjured leg. If necessary, they are supplemented by tomographs.

The *angle between the tuberosity and the joint (Fig. 573)* is measured in the frontal radiogram. Normally it lies between 30° and 40°. With minor displacements it is in the neighborhood of 25°. Following a major displacement of the calcaneus, the angle approaches zero degrees or even becomes negative.

The *axial angle* is measured in the axial roentgenogram. It encompasses the medial and lateral tangents of the calcaneus and normally amounts to 15° or so. Displacements, axial angulations, and breaks of the wall of the calcaneus increase that angle.

Isolated fracture of the upper distal portion of the calcaneus is most confidently identified in the roentgenogram number 3 *(vide supra)*. It may be difficult or impossible to decide whether an *old,* not consolidated break of the anterior process is present or whether one is dealing with a supernumerary ossicle (second calcaneus), which is apt to occur in this region. The same is true for the differentiation between a break of the posterior process of the talus (Shepherd fracture) and a trigonum.

It would be well to point out here the undesirable sequelae of fractures of the body of the calcaneus, which commonly involve the joint (compare the legend accompanying Fig. 573); namely, painful stiffness of the subtalar joint and posttraumatic osteoarthrosis of the posterior portion of this joint and its anterior portion (the talocalcaneonavicular joint). In addition, traumatic flatfoot may be a troublesome complication of a consolidated fracture of the calcaneus with diminution of the angle between the tuberosity and the joint. Apart from the static complaints caused by the flatfoot, the latter also constitutes a preosteoarthrotic deformity.

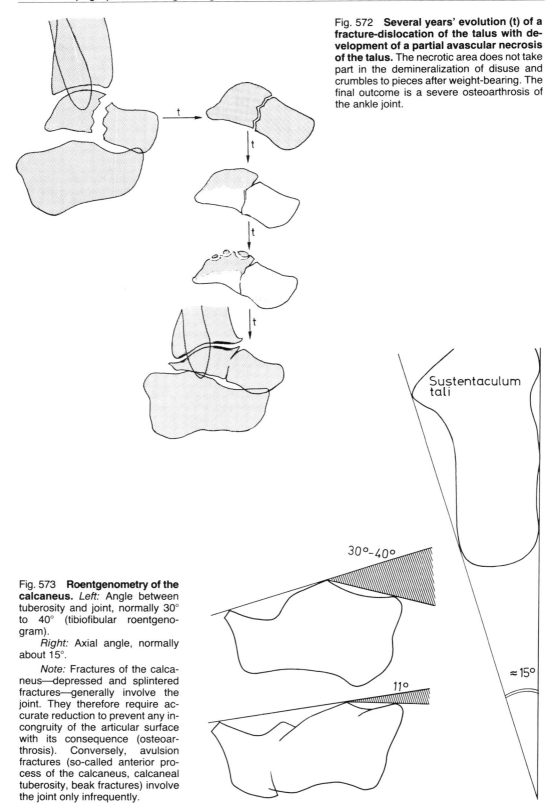

Fig. 572 **Several years' evolution (t) of a fracture-dislocation of the talus with development of a partial avascular necrosis of the talus.** The necrotic area does not take part in the demineralization of disuse and crumbles to pieces after weight-bearing. The final outcome is a severe osteoarthrosis of the ankle joint.

Sustentaculum tali

30°–40°

11°

≈15°

Fig. 573 **Roentgenometry of the calcaneus.** *Left:* Angle between tuberosity and joint, normally 30° to 40° (tibiofibular roentgenogram).

Right: Axial angle, normally about 15°.

Note: Fractures of the calcaneus—depressed and splintered fractures—generally involve the joint. They therefore require accurate reduction to prevent any incongruity of the articular surface with its consequence (osteoarthrosis). Conversely, avulsion fractures (so-called anterior process of the calcaneus, calcaneal tuberosity, beak fractures) involve the joint only infrequently.

Pure ligament injuries can be diagnosed in stress roentgenograms of the ankle joint. (If necessary, a local anesthetic agent is injected into the point of greatest tenderness.) A ligament injury can be inferred from the anteroposterior survey film when the joint is totally dislocated or when avulsions of bone are demonstrable at the sites of the insertion or origin of the ligaments. Shearing injuries in the lateral edge of the talus raise the suspicion of an injury of the collateral ligaments of the fibular malleolus. Widening of the medial portion of the joint space (compare both sides) between the talus and the medial malleolus without fracture of the fibula suggests an injury of the tibial collateral ligament and/or the tibiofibular syndesmosis.

Rupture of the fibular collateral ligaments— commonly caused by a fall with the foot in supination, slight equinus, and internal rotation—leads to lateral instability of the ankle joint. Patients with an undiagnosed injury to the fibular collateral ligaments (anterior talofibular ligament, calcaneofibular ligament, posterior talofibular ligament)—most frequently mistaken for "sprain"—are prone to sudden inversion of the foot ("twisting of the ankle") and recurrent painful irritation in the talocrural joint; osteoarthrosis deformans can develop as a late sequela. In cases of torn ligaments, tilting of the talus

is demonstrable by stress roentgenograms of the foot held in supination, plantar flexion, and inward rotation (Fig. 574). Besides *tipping of the talus, anterior subluxation of the talus* (Fig. 575) also suggests an injury of the fibular collateral ligament of the ankle joint. Quantification (measurement) of the tipping and the anterior subluxation of the talus can replace arthrography on the following premises:

1. Tipping of the talus by $\geq 10°$ is pathologic. To rule out a constitutional ligament weakness, the tipping must also be tested on the contralateral (sound) side. If the angle of tipping is pathologic, a difference between the two sides of $\geq 3°$ in adults and $\geq 6°$ in the years of growth is significant (von Laer et al., 1979); if it correlates with the symptomatology and the clinical findings, it is an indication for surgical intervention.
2. An anterior subluxation of the talus of ≥ 10 mm (Tiedtke et al., 1979) or even 6 mm (Fröhlich et al., 1979) is pathologic and therefore an indication for surgery. Differences of as little as 1 or 2 mm between the injured and the sound side (range of errors in measurement?) may be significant.
3. The measured values of anterior subluxation and tipping of the talus do *not* correlate (Fröhlich et al., 1979). Therefore, both parameters must be tested si-

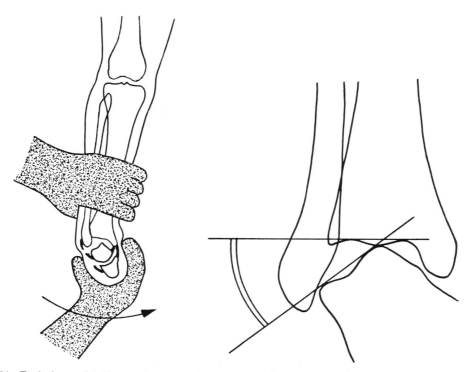

Fig. 574 **Technique of taking a stress roentgenogram with the foot held in varus position to test the fibular collateral ligaments of the malleolus.** (Supination with plantar flexion (−20°) and internal rotation (−20°) after Hördegen, 1970.) Position of the articular tangents for measuring the angle of **talar tipping** (always compare both sides!).

multaneously; i.e., stress roentgenograms with the foot being held in varus or valgus must be made in two planes *if no pathologic finding is demonstrable in one plane.*

4. Localization of the rupture—which of the collateral ligaments is torn?—does not succeed with sufficient certainty using stress roentgenograms with the foot held in varus or valgus (Tiedtke et al., 1979). A pathologic anterior subluxation of the talus may possibly allow the presumption that *at least* the anterior talofibular ligament has been torn.

5. Compared with the stress roentgenographic techniques of holding the foot in a certain position, which are illustrated in Figures 574 and 575, devices commercially available in Germany—e.g., the multipurpose apparatus devised by Professor Scheuba or the Holzrichter-Seiler support (for ascertaining anterior subluxation of the talus)—offer the advantage of giving reproducible results because, with their use, the positioning of the foot and the force applied are clearly defined.

To test the stability of the deltoid (medial) ligament, the examiner fixes the lower leg above the ankle with one hand while the other grasps the talus *without* tilting it and *without* pronating it laterally (Fig. 576). The film is exposed in the attainable end position, and the widths of the medial joint space and the syndesmosis are compared with the uninjured side. If, however, the fibula has been fractured far proximally

or if no fracture has occurred, displacement of the talus *may* be obviated, despite rupture of the ligament and the syndesmosis. In this case, the stress roentgenogram has no evidential value. On the other hand, in distinguishing a simple direct or indirect fracture of the fibula near the ankle joint from a multiple injury (fracture of the fibula plus rupture of the deltoid ligament and the syndesmosis), the significance of this roentgenographic technique remains unimpaired. (Compare *"note"* in Fig. 579).

Most **injuries of the ankle joint** are the result of indirect force. *Fracture-dislocations* occur when the foot is twisted, tilted, or sheared away in any one direction with respect to the lower leg. In *compression fractures,* the traumatizing violence is transmitted from the sole toward the leg.

Fracture-dislocations: The anatomic classification proposed by Weber (1966) focuses the attention of the surgeon and the radiologist on the traumatic lesions in the regions of the fibula and the tibiofibular syndesmosis. Experience teaches that the tibiofibular sydesmosis (the anterior and posterior ligaments), whether it has not been injured or has healed by therapeutic measures, is the decisive criterion for the successful management of fractures of the malleolus. When this fibrotic connection of bones has been damaged by a fracture-dislocation or—as the result of inadequate therapy—can no longer perform its function, valgus osteoarthrosis of the ankle joint is liable to develop.

Type A of Weber's fracture (Fig. 577): the fibula has been injured *distally* to the syndesmosis. The

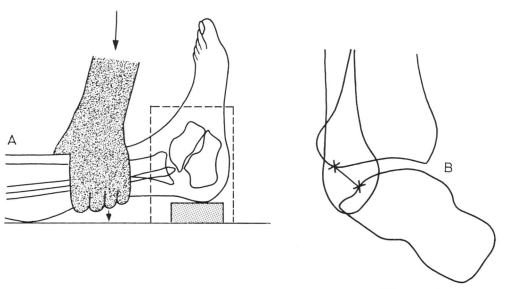

Fig. 575   A = **Stress Roentgenogram** to demonstrate rupture of the fibial collateral ligaments involving *at least* the anterior talofibular ligament (lateral view). With strong pressure upon the distal lower leg *(direction of arrow),* a ligament rupture produces *anterior subluxation of the talus.*

B = $x - x \geq 10$ mm means that rupture of the fibial collateral ligaments, at least of the anterior talofibular ligament, is highly probable. The measuring points (x) are the hindmost and lowest point of the contour of the tibial joint and the nearest point of the talar trochlea.

syndesmosis and the deltoid ligament remain uniformly intact. The roentgenogram demonstrates a transverse fracture of the fibula at the level of the ankle joint, *or* an avulsion from the lateral malleolus or the talus (and possibly the calcaneus), *or* a rupture of the fibular collateral ligaments. (The stress roentgenogram is taken with the foot held in supination, plantar flexion, and internal rotation; see Figs. 574 and 575). As a complication of the part of the tibia, a transverse fracture or a chisel fracture of the medial malleolus, and/or a fracture of the posterior edge (posteromedial Volkmann's triangle) may occur concomitantly.

Type B of Weber's fracture (Fig. 578): The fibula has been injured *at the level of the syndesmosis.* The fibula characteristically presents an oblique fracture, the plane of which generally follows a frontal course; it begins anterodistally at the level of the syndesmosis and runs posterocranially. The syndesmosis is either intact or partly injured. Secondary lesions may be added, such as rupture of the deltoid ligament, or a break of the medial malleolus or the posterior edge of the tibia (posterolateral Volkmann's ligament).

Type C of Weber's fracture (Fig. 579): The course of the fracture of the fibula is oblique, transverse, or transverse with bending of the fragment. The fracture is demonstrable at a variable level *above the ankle joint.* An anterior and posterior lesion of the syndesmosis is *always* present. When additional fractures are demonstrable elsewhere, one *predominantly* encounters avulsions of the syndesmosis from the tibia with a break of the medial malleolus, or else ruptures of the deltoid ligament.

When the fibula fractures *far* proximally (cranially), rupture of the deltoid ligament is more likely to occur than avulsion of the posterior edge of the tibia. *Isolated bursting of the ankle mortise* is a special case of injury that is not accompanied by fracture of the fibula. It either occurs in young individuals with an elastic fibula or there exists a distortion or rupture (dislocation) of the proximal tibiofibular joint. In both instances, the total length of the interosseous membrane is ruptured.

The lesions listed may be accompanied by injuries to the talar trochlea. Such "flake fractures" of the edge of the talus occur when, on suffering the injury, the trochlea tali is braced against the malleoli. When these flakes exclusively concern the cartilage, they cannot be identified in the plain roentgenogram, although at times they are apt to cause considerable discomfort.

The longitudinal compression fractures of the ankle joint also have been classified by Weber (1966) into three types (Fig. 580):

• *Weber's type A compression fracture*—comminuted fracture of the tibia with fracture of the fibula; syndesmosis and trochlea tali intact
• *Weber's type B compression fracture*—commi-

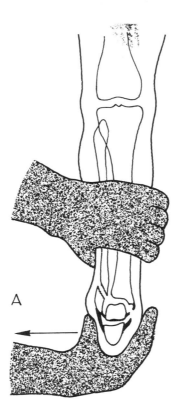
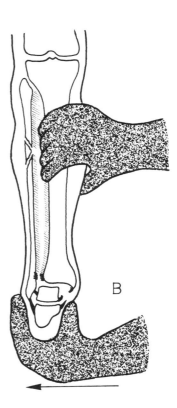

Fig. 576   A = **Stress Roentgenogram with pure lateral displacement of the foot at the ankle joint** to decide whether a known **oblique fracture of the lateral malleolus** about the level of the syndesmosis is accompanied by **rupture of the (medial) deltoid ligament and the syndesmosis** (after Hördegen, 1970).

B = **Stress Roentgenogram with pure lateral displacement of the foot at the ankle joint** to ascertain **rupture of the (medial) deltoid ligament and the tibiofibular syndesmosis** in the **presence of high fracture of the fibula** (after Poigenfürst, 1967). The classification of this fracture of the fibula as a Weber C fracture (p. 383) implies the lesion of the syndesmosis but not the rupture of the deltoid ligament (Fig. 579).

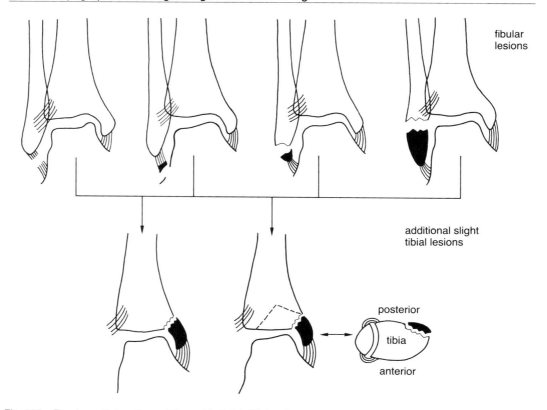

Fig. 577 **Fracture–dislocation of the ankle joint** (Weber fracture, type A).
Principle: The tibiofibular syndesmosis is intact because the lesion of the fibula lies beneath the syndesmosis. Additional bony lesions of the tibia are possible.

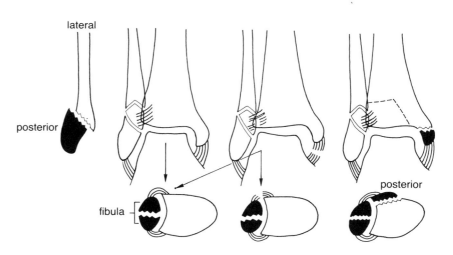

Fig. 578 **Fracture–dislocation of the ankle joint** (Weber fracture, type B).
Principle: The tibiofibular syndesmosis is intact *or* only partially injured because the fibular lesion lies at the level of the syndesmosis. Tibial lesions are possible.

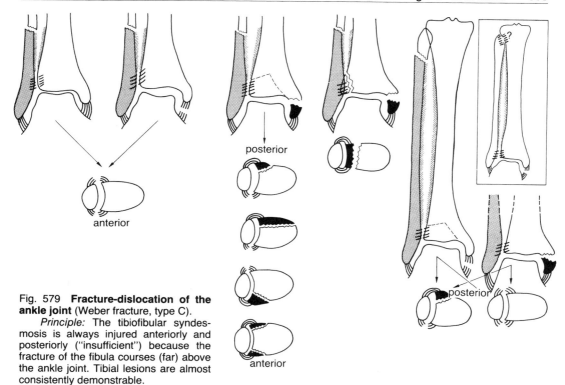

Fig. 579 **Fracture-dislocation of the ankle joint** (Weber fracture, type C).
Principle: The tibiofibular syndesmosis is always injured anteriorly and posteriorly ("insufficient") because the fracture of the fibula courses (far) above the ankle joint. Tibial lesions are almost consistently demonstrable.

insert: So-called **isolated bursting of the ankle mortise** with rupture of the syndesmosis, the deltoid ligament, and the interosseous membrane; distortion or rupture (dislocation) of the ankle joint. Total disruption of the interosseous membrane manifests itself a few days after the trauma by an extensive hematoma in the lower leg.

Note: The integrity or rupture of the anterior and posterior ligaments of the syndesmosis (anterior and posterior tibiofibular ligament) can be directly visualized by computed tomography (Dihlmann, 1982).

nuted fracture of the tibia with fracture of the fibular shaft and the trochlea tali
• *Weber's type C compression fracture*—comminuted fracture of the tibia, fibula not fractured but syndesmosis ruptured

In classifying the **epiphyseal injuries of the long tubular bones** one must, as a general rule, consider

that any trauma to the epiphyseal plate involves the danger of subsequent impairment of longitudinal growth. In addition, the classification should consider the integrity or the involvement of the articular surface (Fig. 581). A traumatic severance of the epiphyseal plate that runs parallel to the course of this plate—hence separating the epiphysis from the shaft of the tubular bone—traverses principally the layer

Fig. 580 **Compression fractures of the ankle joint** (*classification* into types A to C after Weber B. G., 1966).
Principle: Comminuted fractures from longitudinal compression *(heavy arrow)* always lead to disruption of the syndesmosis (rupture of the anterior and posterior tibiofibular ligament) when the fibula does *not* fracture (type C). In types A and B the syndesmosis remains intact because both the tibia and the fibula *or* the tibia, fibula, and trochlea tali (type B) are fractured.

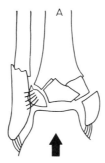 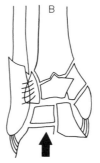 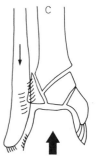

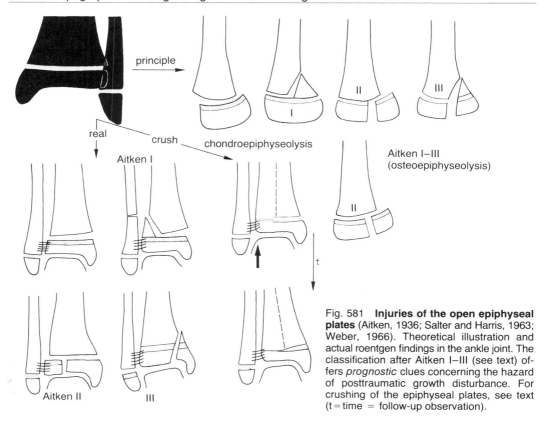

Fig. 581 **Injuries of the open epiphyseal plates** (Aitken, 1936; Salter and Harris, 1963; Weber, 1966). Theoretical illustration and actual roentgen findings in the ankle joint. The classification after Aitken I–III (see text) offers *prognostic* clues concerning the hazard of posttraumatic growth disturbance. For crushing of the epiphyseal plates, see text (t = time = follow-up observation).

of hypertrophic cartilage cells and in any case leaves intact the biologically important zones of the resting and proliferating cartilage cells; i.e., the epiphyseal matrix. Such traumatic severances of the epiphyseal plate offer, therefore, a favorable prognosis with regard to growth disturbance:

1. Chondroepiphyseolysis without involvement of bone
2. Traumatic epiphyseolysis with wedge-shaped break of the metaphysis *(Aitken's type I)*
3. Traumatic epiphyseolysis with the fracture cleft extending through the bony portion of the epiphysis into the neighboring joint *(Aitken's type II)*
4. Fracture traversing the bony epiphysis, the epi-

physeal cartilage, and the shaft of the tubular bone (transepiphyseal-metaphyseal course—Aitken's type III).

Additionally, one distinguishes crushing of the epiphyseal plate, which leads to *localized* premature closure of the epiphysis or, with *complete* premature closure, may lead to shortening of the bone (Salter and Harris, 1963). Such crushing of the epiphyseal plate *cannot* be identified in the roentgenogram, and therefore it is frequently treated as a distortion. On the other hand, it is quite frequent for a crush injury of the epiphyseal plate to be accompanied by a fracture of the osseous epiphysis (Aitken's type II), and then it can be assigned to this category.

Temporomandibular Joint

The articulating bony portions of the temporamandibular joint are, first, the articular surface of the mandibular fossa with the cylindric articular eminence of the temporal bone which lies in front of the fossa, and, second, the condylar process of the mandible, composed of the mandibular head and neck. The rim of the articular disk is attached in its total circumference to the joint capsule. It therefore divides the joint into two compartments and largely compensates for the incongruity of the articulating surfaces.

In the **roentgenologic diagnosis of the temporomandibular joint,** tomography and especially *zonography* is of particular importance because it eliminates the multiple interfering shadows in the vicinity of the joint. The pluridimensional direction of blurring is recommended. For a lateral tomograph, the patient is invited to assume a comfortable prone position and to turn his head until the side to be examined comes to lie close to the film. The "sagittal axes" of both mandibular heads and sockets converge strongly backward and meet approximately in the foramen occipitale magnum. This circumstance, however, is not taken into account and is not compensated for in positioning the patient. Rather it suffices to turn his chin slightly toward the supporting surface so that the condylar process and the ramus of the mandible are brought into one plane. A lateral tomograph then shows the head and neck of the mandible, its coronoid process, and the mandibular notch. A tomograph taken in the frontal plane portrays both joints on a single film (for the focusing technique *vide infra*). The principal indications for this tomographic technique are suspicion of a skeletal injury of the head and neck of the mandible, medial or lateral dislocation of the head and neck of the mandible, and assessment of the width of a bony ankylosis.

Panoramic tomography requires special equipment. In cases of doubt, however, it does not supplant conventional tomography.

The evident advantage of tomography should not lead one to dispence with *survey films prior to* taking tomographs. For the *lateral* view, the conventional roentgenograms of the petrous bone after Schüller are primarily employed. They may be supplemented by contact roentgenograms after Parma. The contact roentgenogram, especially through the open mouth, gives a view of the joint, including the neck of the mandible.

So-called *functional roentgenograms* are indicated principally for stomatological problems. They comprise one lateral roentgenogram after Schüller (if need be, supplemented by tomographs) with the dental arches closely approximated and another one with the mouth maximally opened.

For posteroanterior (suboccipito-nasofrontal) survey films, the following focusing technique is recommended; for example, when there is suspicion of an injury of the articular bones:

The patient lies in a comfortable oblique prone position on the Bucky table or is seated in front of a Bucky device attached to the wall. His mouth is open and his forehead and nose rest against the surface. The roentgen tube is tilted cranially in such a way that the so-called central beam enters at the nuchal hairline and passes through the intercondylar axis to the root of the nose. For tomography in the frontal plane *(vide supra),* the patient is positioned in a similar manner, except that his mouth is closed. The central beam enters perpendicularly, and the patient's forehead and nose are supported in such a way that the posterior border of the ramus of the mandible approximately parallels the surface of the table.

Variants of Normal Shape and Deformities

Figure 582 underscores three typical variants of the normal shape of the temporomandibular joint. The end position of the head of the mandible with the mouth maximally opened is also subject to variation. Even in the complete absence of discomfort and with a normal shape of the temporomandibular joint, the head of the mandible may, on occasion, be encountered in front of the articular eminence (Frommhold and Hielscher, 1962). In the temporomandibular joint, as elsewhere, the diagnosis of an (anterior) dislocation requires the demonstration that the joint is fixed springily in a faulty position (also compare p. 392 under the heading of recurrent dislocation of the temporomandibular joint).

There is no epiphyseal plate in the temporamandibular joint; growth starts from the thick cartilage cover of the condylar process. When this cartilage cover is damaged by inflammatory, obstetric, or other traumatic injuries (which, of course, occur more frequently than in the presence of an epiphyseal plate at distance from the joint), deformation of the condylar process may be the result. There exist, thus, two types of deformities of the condylar process, one congenital and the other acquired.

Hyperplasia of the condylar process (Fig. 583) commonly occurs unilaterally. The thickening and lengthening of the condylar process causes the midline of the mandible to be displaced toward the sound side. Facial asymmetry develops. With such hyperplasia, the condylar process may retain its usual shape despite its increase in size (expansion), or its shape may become irregular. In the latter case, the condition must be differentiated from an osteoma, and the correct diagnosis often can be made only on the basis of the history. Occasionally, such a hyperplasia may be the consequence of a fracture or an arthritis of the temporomandibular joint, possibly experienced during the growth period.

Fig. 582 **Variants of the normal shape of the temporomandibular joint** after Doub and Henny (1953) in the Schüller roentgenogram. Normal shape *(left);* flat type *(center);* convex type *(right).*

In the adult, **osteitis deformans (Paget's disease)** also can lead to expansion of the condylar process. The structural alterations in the diseased condylar process will suggest the correct diagnosis. In **acromegaly** (Fig. 154), the head of the mandible usually does not take part in the deformation of the mandible (increase in size of the mandible with prognathism, abnormal spacing of teeth, possibly increase of the angle between the body and the ramus of the mandible) (Fig. 584). **Hypoplasia** and **aplasia** of the condylar process occur in the setting of certain malformation syndromes; e.g., the Robin syndrome (producing micrognathia) or in mandibulofacial dysostosis and in mucopolysaccharidosis, type I (Hurler-Pfaundler syndrome). Such malformations of the temporomandibular joint may also be the consequence of a local disorder; e.g., an arthritis of the growth period (most frequently **juvenile chronic arthritis**) or a trauma experienced in the growing years (see also Fig. 585). A unilateral underdevelopment causes the middle of the mandible to deviate toward the diseased side. Bilateral hypoplasia and aplasia are followed by the development of a birdlike facies with a receding chin (Fig. 586).

In **von Recklinghausen's neurofibromatosis,** malformations are known to occur in the form of a stumped coronoid process and a slim condylar process of the mandible as well as defects of the floor and the anterior wall of the external auditory canal (Tänzer, 1966).

In children and juveniles, **circumscribed scleroderma** may interfere locally with the growth of the

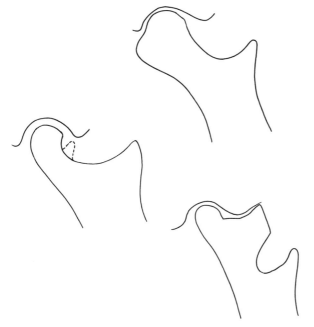

Fig. 583 **Anomalous shapes of the condylar process of the mandible** (lateral tomography). *Left:* Normal shape but *(dashed)* small exostosis of the neck (osteoma). *Upper right:* Hyperplasia of the condylar process (local growth disorder; to be differentiated from *growing* spongy osteoma). Facial asymmetry. *Lower right:* Large exostosis (osteoma) in the region of head and neck. Facial asymmetry.

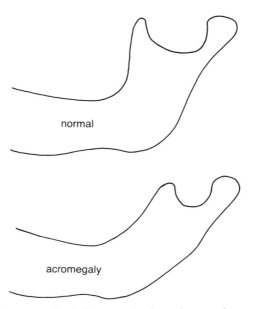

normal

acromegaly

Fig. 584 **Angle between body and ramus in normal individuals and (sometimes) in acromegaly.**

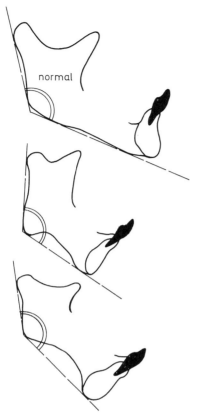

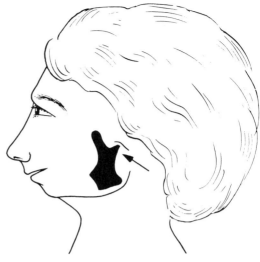

Fig. 586 **Typical birdlike facies (avian facies) with receding chin in mandibular hypoplasia,** in the present case following (cured) juvenile rheumatoid arthritis with involvement of both temporomandibular joints. *Arrow* points to the hypoplastic and deformed condylar process; the socket is flattened. If such patients present additional malformations of the face—e.g., severe deformation of the auricle—one should initially consider a congenital developmental disorder of the first embryonal visceral arch; for example, mandibulofacial dysostosis. In Robin syndrome, the avian facies often regresses spontaneously with advancing age (Smith and Stowe, 1961).

Fig. 585 **So-called antegonial (preangular) depression of the mandible** *(below; center)* in malformation syndromes and following juvenile chronic arthritis, injuries in childhood, hemophilia, and bacterial infections of the surroundings of the temporomandibular joint experienced in childhood (Becker et al., 1976).

neighboring muscles and bones. Unilateral involvement of the face sometimes leads to unilateral maldevelopment of the mandible and unilateral disturbance of dentition (Hoggins and Hamilton, 1969).

The *possible* manifestations of **progressive scleroderma** in the mandibular region are not only an almost uniform widening of the periodontal cleft (Stafne and Austin, 1944) but also osteolyses in the angular area of the mandible (Seifert et al. 1975; Fig. 587).

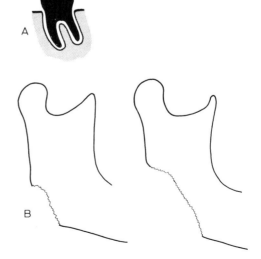

Fig. 587 **Progressive scleroderma.**
   A = Almost even widening of the periodontal cleft.
   B = More or less extensive osteolysis of the mandibular angle.

Arthritis and Its Differential Diagnosis by Radiology

An *acute* inflammation of the temporomandibular joint is suggested by local pain, acute onset of arthrogenic trismus (impaired opening of the mouth), and possibly also swelling in the region of the joint. In addition, the mouth is slightly opened as a reflex protection against the pain. In this position, the interior of the joint has its greatest volume. In unilateral acute arthritis, the mandible deviates toward the unaffected side. In bilateral arthritis, prognathism develops. **Pyogenic arthritis** of the temporomandibular joint owes its origin to hematogenous infection or a local open injury, but it may also develop as a complication of acute otitis media, a furuncle of the auditory canal, a bacterial parotitis, or osteomyelitis of the ramus mandibulae. Such cases require, also in the acute stage of arthritis, a radiographic study which *primarily* will give information about the condition of the tissues in the vicinity of the temporomandibular joint.

In fractures of the base of the skull, the fracture cleft sometimes extends via the anterior wall of the osseous auditory canal into the joint and thus paves the way for infection. Fracture lines through the anterior wall of the auditory canal are identified in roentgenograms of the petrous bone and, better still, in oblique anteroposterior roentgenograms of the temporal bone after E. G. Mayer. With timely diagnosis, modern methods of therapy will as a rule not only prevent the infection from spreading to the temporomandibular joint but will, in the presence of an established purulent infection, obviate its serious sequelae (destruction, ankyloses, and/or disturbed growth) (Fig. 588). It should be added that **syphilis** relatively often gives rise to acute or subacute arthritis of the temporomandibular joint (Sundt, 1948) with ankylosis as a possible late sequel.

Chronic arthritis of the temporomandibular joint is observed primarily in rheumatoid arthritis, in ankylosing spondylitis, and in psoriatic arthritis (Fig. 589). Chronic bacterial arthritis occurs in suppurative cholestatoma of the petrous bone and in chronic osteomyelitis of the mandible. The roentgenogram then will show erosions in the head of the mandible, joint space narrowing, and finally ankylosis (especially in ankylosing spondylitis). It is rare for chronic arthritis—e.g., during the course of rheumatoid arthritis of the *adult*—to destroy the condylar process completely or at least a great part of it (Ludwig and Temming, 1957). This will constitute an arthritic mutilation.

Gout can, in principle, involve any joint, hence also the temporomandibular joint. In this joint, the gouty attack is accompanied by intense local pain, swelling in the region of the parotid gland, and fever. Erosions of the articulating bones, particularly the condylar process, are observed in chronic gout. Tophaceous deposits in the bone marrow sometimes do not lead to resorption of the subchondral cancellous bone but may expand the head of the mandible.

Hyperparathyroidism (secondary hyperparathyroidism in the setting of renal osteopathy) manifests itself in the temporomandibular region by disappearance of the marginal subchondral lamella; by erosion, destruction, or even resorption of the condylar processes; by subchondral cysts; and by narrowing of the joint space, hence by "arthritic" roentgen findings (Dick and Jones, 1973; Cappellini et al., 1978). Local discomfort is slight or absent. Following operations on the parathyroid glands—e.g., subtotal parathyroidectomy for renal osteopathy—recon-

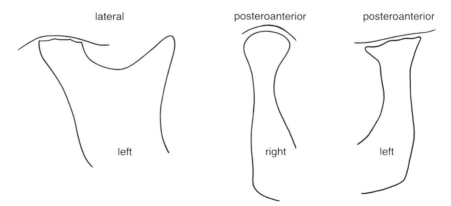

lateral   posteroanterior   posteroanterior

left   right   left

Fig. 588 Status after pyogenic arthritis of the left temporomandibular joint experienced in childhood (lateral and posteroanterior tomography). Destruction and localized disturbance of growth are recognizable. Since clinically, opening of the mouth is considerably impaired, fibrotic ankylosis is likely to be present. Without considering the anamnesis and the clinical finding, it would only be possible to diagnose a roentgenologically demonstrable disturbance of shape and development produced by (inflammatory or traumatic ?) damage to the condylar process incurred during the *growth period.*

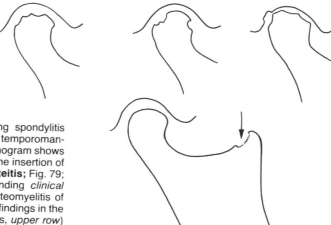

Fig. 589 **Chronic arthritis of the temporomandibular joint** (*upper row:* erosions; narrowing of joint space). The nosological classification of the arthritis (for example, rheumatoid arthritis, ankylosing spondylitis, psoriatic arthritis) is undertaken from clinical points of view and on the basis of the roentgenologic findings in the other joints.

Below: This patient with ankylosing spondylitis complains of unilateral discomfort in the temporomandibular joint on mastication. The roentgenogram shows a normal joint but an erosion *(arrow)* at the insertion of the temporal muscle (**rarefying fibro-osteitis;** Fig. 79; Maes and Dihlmann, 1968). Corresponding *clinical* symptoms are produced by bacterial osteomyelitis of the coronoid process. Identical roentgen findings in the temporamandibular joint (condylar process, *upper row*) may develop in *hyperparathyroidism;* namely: resorption of the marginal lamella, erosions, destruction, subchondral cysts, and even narrowing of the joint space (see text).

struction of the condylar processes may take place (Sellers et al., 1973).

Osteoarthrosis

Generally speaking, disorders of occlusion and articulation promote wear and tear of cartilage and the disk in the temporomandibular joint. In addition, similarly to other joints, constitutional factors (genetically determined "inferiority" of the articular cartilage) play a causative role. Inflammatory secondary osteoarthrosis should also be mentioned in this connection. The disproportion between the strain on the temporomandibular joint and its load capacity that leads to osteoarthrosis, will be illustrated by the following example: The pressure generated by mastication is absorbed by the molars. With unilateral or bilateral loss of the molars, the supporting areas of the joint will collapse. The head of the mandible then sinks deeper into the socket and exerts a chronic traumatic pressure upon the articular cartilage and the disk. Unless the molars are replaced by a prosthesis, osteoarthrosis will develop in the corresponding temporomandibular joint. With time, marginal osteophytes appear, the subchondrally sclerosed head of the mandible loses its roundness, the contours of the mandibular fossa become straightened, and the joint space shows moderate narrowing.

These roentgen signs of osteoarthrosis may also be observed in asymptomatic joints; for example when they are sought in roentgenograms of the petrous bone after Schüller. On the other hand, patients with a roentgenologically normal temporomandibular joint sometimes complain of discomfort which, by anamnestic and clinical findings, suggests the presence

of a degenerative affliction that calls for treatment. In this stage, functional roentgenograms may be helpful in the diagnosis. Schüller roentgenograms or lateral tomographs of each temporomandibular joint are taken in occlusion and with the mouth wide open. If need be, the intermediate phases are also recorded by using a graduated wedge introduced into the mouth. By comparing the two sides, one may establish any diminished excursion of the head of the mandible as an early sign of osteoarthrosis of the temporomandibular joint (Weingraber, 1951). It should be mentioned that impairment of excursions may also be due to a chronic arthritis; it may be demonstrable prior to the appearance of the typical roentgen signs of arthritis *(vide supra)*. However, it is very unlikely that a chronic inflammation of the temporomandibular joint—for example, in rheumatoid arthritis—will manifest itself initially in this joint. The history and the clinical findings must therefore be enlisted to determine the nosological classification of diminished excursion of the head of the mandible that has been demonstrated in the roentgenogram.

It has already been pointed out in the discussion of other joints that **neoplastic synovial chondromatosis** is a preosteoarthritic condition. This disease occurs but infrequently in the temporomandibular joint (Fig. 591). Surgical intervention is, as a rule, necessary before the osteoarthrosis becomes demonstrable in the roentgenogram, because fixed or detached chondromas give rise to pain and lead to dysfunction in the temporomandibular joint. During the course of advanced osteoarthrosis of the temporomandibular joint, *individual* small chondromas also can develop by metaplastic processes in the synovial membrane and, calcified, can be recognized in the roentgenogram.

Fig. 590 **Roentgen signs of advanced temporomandibular osteoarthrosis** (see text) are illustrated *on the left* (Schüller roentgenograms). **Functional roentgenograms** (*center:* mouth closed; *right:* mouth maximally opened) taken in a patient with pronounced left-sided difficulty in chewing reveal limited excursion of the head of the left mandible. With maximal opening of the mouth, the excursion is arrested at the posterior incline of the articular eminence. The shape of the articulating bones, however, is unchanged. On operation, the thickened disk was found to be adherent to the socket; the articular cartilage was moderately roughened.

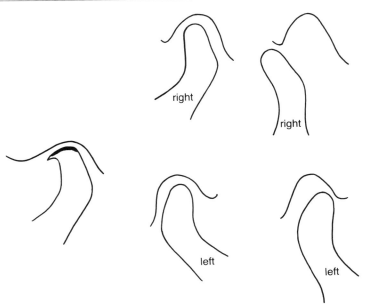

Neoplasms of the Joint

It has already been mentioned that the differential diagnosis between hyperplasia of the condylar process and an osteoma in this location is sometimes difficult (Fig. 583). Osteomas, however, may also originate in the articular eminence. In this case, one recognizes a larger or smaller area of increased density exhibiting a bony structure. This area can—e.g., in tomographs—be demarcated from the condylar process.

The individual components of the temporomandibular gliding tissue (synovial membrane, fibrous capsule, articular disk, articular cartilage) can likewise become the matrix of a benign or malignant mesenchymal neoplasm of the temporomandibular joint. More or less intense pain, *increasing* limitation of motion, and *swelling* indicate the progressiveness of the disorder. Lack of space in the immediate vicinity of the temporomandibular joint—which is squeezed between the condylar process of the mandible, the mandibular fossa, the articular eminence, the zygo-

matic process, and the pars tympanica—explains why early destruction in these bones must be anticipated.

The principal causes of destruction of bone in the immediate vicinity of the temporomandibular joint are **carcinomas** of the external auditory canal and the middle ear, carcinomas of the buccal mucosa which can spread to the temporomandibular joint, and hematogenous **metastases.** The unchecked growth of malignant tumors gives rise to irregular osteolysis. With benign or semimalignant tumors, the destruction of bone appears well demarcated, cystic, or loculated (with **osteoclastoma,** for instance). In addition, with an intraosseous origin of the tumor, the involved area of bone may expand, depending on the nature and rapidity of growth. Only the **osteomas** exhibit primarily a homogeneous intraosseous increase in density (endosteoma) or bulging of the contours (osteochondroma; Fig. 592). Additional information is sometimes obtained from periosteal reactions, circumscribed calcifications in the tumor (**malignant synovialoma?** p. 139) or irregular neoformation of

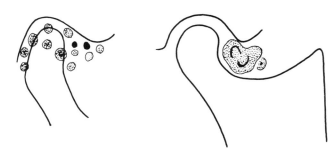

Fig. 591 **Roentgen findings in neoplastic synovial chondromatosis of the temporomandibular joint.**

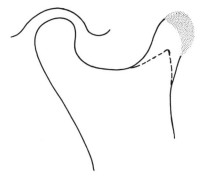

Fig. 592 **Osteochondroma of the coronoid process** (Ramon et al., 1977). The coronoid process is broadened, lengthened, and shows a cap-shaped top of decreased density (in comparison with bone).

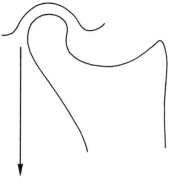

16 months later

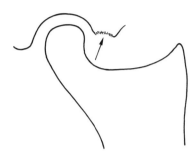

bone in the region or the surroundings of the osteolysis. Moreover, it is the rule for tumors of the glide tissue to erode the bone on both sides of the joint space.

In contrast, neoplasms originating in the contiguous bones destroy the articular abutment on only one side of the interosseous space—for example, the ramus of the mandible with the condylar process—or they exhibit, even in an advanced stage, a larger extent of destruction in a *single* articulating bone. Soft-tissue tumors—for example, a carcinoma of the buccal mucosa spreading to the joint or a juxtaarticular metastasis in the soft tissues—do not follow this rule. Such tumors, however, are generally known and classified prior to involvement of the temporomandibular joint.

Pigmented villonodular synovitis (p. 139 ff) of the temporomandibular joint manifests itself in the early stage by a slowly increasing, painless preauricular swelling while the roentgen findings are still normal. Only in the advanced stage, i.e., after a number of years, are erosive changes in the articulating bones to be expected (Lapayowker et al., 1973; Miyamoto et al., 1977; Fig. 593).

Hemophilic pseudotumor also occurs in the mandible (Brant and Jordan, 1972).

It seems in order at this point to mention **massive osteolysis (Gorham-Stout).** This disorder has been observed in the mandibular region (Heuck, 1979) and sometimes leads to complete resorption of the mandible. In the initial stage, punched-out osteolyses appear in the mandible. Secondary infection from the oral cavity can cause the bone to react with inflammation, which may start in the periosteum. Progressive resorption of bone often leads to spontaneous fracture. If histologic study of a biopsy specimen reveals "connective tissue rich in capillaries" or "highly vascularized granulation tissue" (hemangiomatosis), the diagnosis is settled (Knolle and Meyer, 1965). If the disease starts in the alveolar process, the teeth become loose and fall out. Eventually, the involved

Fig. 593 **Pigmented villonodular synovitis of the temporomandibular joint.** The initial roentgen examination *(above)* gave a normal result although a preauricular swelling and an impairment of mobility attracted clinical attention. Sixteen months later, an erosion of the articular eminence *(arrow)* is demonstrable.

Radiologic differential diagnosis: Chronic (e.g., tuberculous) arthritis of the temporomandibular joint? Pigmented villonodular synovitis? Malignant synovialoma or a malignant tumor in general is less likely because of the slow progression. The *diagnosis* can only be settled by biopsy.

mandibular region is reduced to a bony hook similar to the atrophic senile mandible. On physical examination, the diagnosis of a neurogenic osteolysis then suggests itself. However, the neurologic findings in Gorham-Stout disease are normal.

Another disorder that enters the differential diagnosis is periodontosis, yet the *clinical* picture of this affection includes the presence of an odontal and osseous pocket. In addition, marginal periodontosis becomes arrested after the loss of the involved teeth and the periodontal tissue; i.e., its coordinate morphologic substrate. Conversely, in massive osteolysis the resorption of bone progresses. It is rare for spontaneous arrest to occur prior to extensive disintegration of bone. The mode of spread in massive osteolysis argues against the assumption of a tumor with osteolytic growth: massive osteolysis does not spread radially (cyclically, polycyclically) like a tumor, but along the bony contour; for example, along the al-

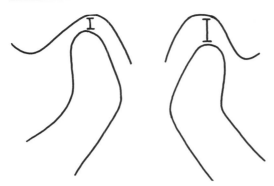

Fig. 594   **Widening of the interosseous space of the temporomandibular joint** (compare both sides!) is the *general* roentgen sign of a major effusion. In this case (Schüller roentgenogram), condition occurred after contusion injury (blow with the fist); hence, traumatic hemorrhage into the joint cavity or serous posttraumatic effusion *(right in the figure)*.

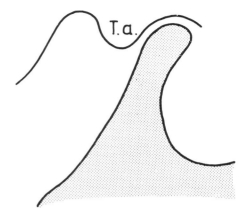

Fig. 595   **Anterior dislocation of the temporomandibular joint** (contact roentgenogram after Parma). The condylar process lies in front of and above the articular eminence (Tuberculum articulare = T.a.)

veolar process. With time it shows a typical "sharpening" (spontaneous fracture) of the involved bone.

Traumas to the Joint

Contusion of the temporomandibular joint is the result of blunt trauma; for example a blow with the fist (e.g., an uppercut). Contusion, and even solely *distortion*, sometimes is followed by a serous or sanguineous effusion which may be visible in the roentgenogram (Fig. 594).

Dislocation of the mandibular head most frequently occurs anteriorly; the head of the mandible glides forward across the articular eminence and then again upward along its anterior aspect (Fig. 595). There it is fixed springily by the muscles of mastication. In unilateral dislocation, the mouth opens and the chin deviates toward the sound side. In bilateral dislocation, the mouth is wide open and the dental arch of the mandible is displaced anteriorly. The mouth cannot be closed. This dislocation can occur *spontaneously* when the mouth is opened extremely wide, such as in yawning, laughing, or vomiting.

Recurrent dislocation develops subsequent to a spontaneous dislocation when the capsular tissue has been grossly overstretched by the initial event and/or when a small articular eminence and a flattened socket pave the way for a renewed dislocation. In childhood and in old age, the articular eminence is flat and low. In these age groups, anterior dislocation is a rare event because the "return" of the dislocated mandibular head is not blocked. *Habitual* dislocation is spoken of when the dislocation occurs each time the mouth is maximally opened, but reduction of the anteriorly dislocated head of the mandible is readily accomplished when the mouth is closed. The patient therefore often fails to notice the dislocated position. This

is why some writers regard habitual dislocation as a "physiologic event" (Reichenbach, 1965); i.e., as a variant (p. 385).

Posterior dislocation of the mandibular head underneath the auditory meatus is an infrequent injury. The mouth then can no longer be opened. Medial or lateral dislocations usually are possible only in connection with fracture of the lower jaw.

In **subluxation of the mandible in front and back of the disk** (Steinhardt, 1963), the head of the mandible changes its position with respect to the articular disk, which is also displaced, though in the reverse direction (discocondylar subluxation or dislocation Fig. 596). This injury is accompanied by disturbed motion in the temporomandibular joint. When the articular head lies *in front* of the disk, dorsal motion in closing the mouth is impaired. At the end of a biting movement, there is no contact between the jaws, and the middle of the lower jaw deviates toward the sound side. When the mandibular head comes to lie *behind* the disk (Figs. 596 and 597), opening of the mouth is impaired and the center of the mandible deviates toward the affected side. In this case, the head of the mandible can no longer slip normally under the articular eminence or in front of it. In both instances, the plain roentgenogram reveals the anomalous position of the mandibular head. The interpretation is based on the history (sudden occurrence while eating, talking, etc.) and the result of the physical examination.

The infrequent **central dislocation of the mandible** comes about by the head of the mandible being thrust into the mandibular fossa. This event is sometimes accompanied by a break of the external auditory meatus and the petrous bone.

Fractures of the mandibular fossa (see also under "central dislocation of the mandible") accompany fractures of the base of the skull that extend to

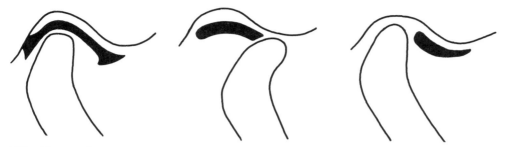

Fig. 596   Changes in position between head of mandible and articular disk. *Left:* Normal topographic relationships between condylar process and disk *(black)* in the temporomandibular joint. *Center:* Situation with "subluxation of the mandible to the front of the disk" *(schematic). Right:* Situation with "subluxation of the mandible to the back of the disk" *(schematic).* See text and Fig. 597.

the temporal bone and reach the mandibular fossa. The intra- and extracapsular fractures of the condyle and the subcondylar fractures of the mandible lie near the temporomandibular joint (Fig. 598). Condylar fractures are subdivided into fractures of the head and those of the neck of the mandible (Fig. 599). The fractures of the mandibular head as well as the subcapital fractures are intracapsular. They have no tendency toward dislocation, but the capital fragment may become necrotic and the devitalized part may be detached. In fractures of the mandibular neck (concerning its *middle portion and its base*), the fracture cleft generally lies outside the capsule. These fractures usually are accompanied by (chiefly medial and anterior) dislocation (Fig. 599).

Fractures of the condylar process are mostly due to indirect trauma. Only bullet injuries and fractures of the zygomatic arch are the consequence of direct violence. Fractures of the condylar process *frequently* occur in connection with fractures of other parts of the mandible, for instance, when it is due to

direct trauma, whereas the (attendant) unilateral or bilateral fracture of the condylar process is produced indirectly by bending or shearing forces. Any fracture of the lower jaw in the region of the chin should prompt an accurate radiographic study of both temporomandibular joints! When the force producing the fracture continues to be exerted, it may bring about a **fracture-dislocation,** depending on the direction of force and the muscle pull. (Less frequently, a primary dislocation is followed by fracture.) The pull of the lateral pterygoid muscle displaces the juxtaarticular fragment medially and anteriorly (Fig. 600), but lateral or posterior displacement is also possible.

Severe dyspnea may be a dramatic *early consequence* of fracture of the mandible. Its causes are as follows: The genioglossus arises from the mental spine in the mandible and spreads out to the tongue in a fanlike fashion. It pulls the tongue anteriorly. When a fracture traverses the protuberance of the chin and when the neck and the ramus of the mandible are concomitantly fractured (Fig. 601 A), the dorsal dis-

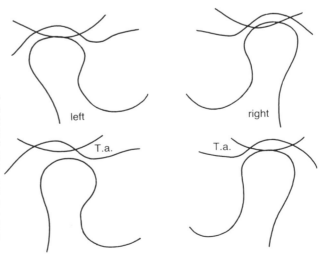

Fig. 597   Acute discocondylar subluxation of the head of the right mandible to the back of the disk (see text). (Contact roentgenogram after Parma). Causal event was biting into a large apple. *Upper row* shows the situation in the mandibular fossa on both sides with the mouth closed. On maximal opening of the mouth *(lower row),* head of the left condylar process slips onto articular eminence (tuberculum articulare; T.a.) whereas head of right condylar process, which has been subluxated to back of disk, remains more or less unchanged in the mandibular fossa.

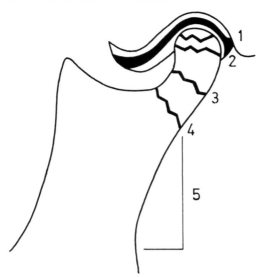

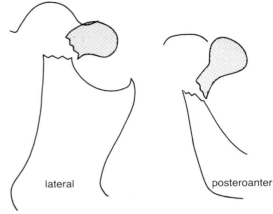

Fig. 600 **Fracture-dislocation of the neck of the mandible.** Proximal fragment is displaced anteriorly and medially (most frequent type of displacement). Mandibular fossa is "empty."

Fig. 598 **Diagram of fractures of the condylar process of the mandible.**
1 = Diacapital fracture. 2 = subcapital fracture. 3 = Fracture of the middle neck. 4 = Fracture of the basal neck. 5 = Region of subcondylar fractures. The intra- or extracapsular position of the fractures is illustrated.

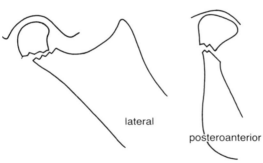

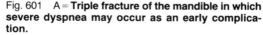

Fig. 599 **Fracture of the neck of the mandible** with medial dislocation and slight anterior tilting of the juxtaarticular fragment (pull of the lateral pterygoid muscle; lateral tomograph and posteroanterior plain roentgenogram).

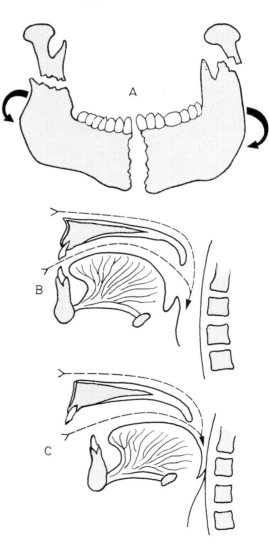

Fig. 601 A = **Triple fracture of the mandible in which severe dyspnea may occur as an early complication.**
      B = Pretraumatic normal nasal and oral airway (arrows).
      C = Mandibular fracture across the mental protuberance, associated with fracture of mandibular neck and ramus, leads to internal rotation and dorsal displacement of fragments of mandibular body with occlusion of pharyngeal airway by tongue: *dyspnea!*

placement of the mandibular fragments and the disconnection of the genioglossus lead to occlusion of the pharynx by the tongue falling backward (Fig. 601 B, C. Gerlock Jr., 1976).

Among the radiologically identifiable *late sequelae* of an injury to the temporomandibular joint are osteoarthrosis and ankylosis. Bony ankylosis is most probably the result of infection of the joint by way of the external auditory meatus. Fibrotic ankylosis could also be conceived to develop as the aftermath of an intraarticular hematoma. The cause and the extent of a possible limitation of motion following a (fracture-) dislocation can be established by functional roentgenograms of the temporomandibular joint. Experience shows, however, that the majority of fractures of the condylar process, even those healed in malposition and/or with deformation, hardly ever lead to impaired mobility of the lower jaw. The temporomandibular joint evidently possesses a high degree of functional adaptability. Posttraumatic disturbances of development and growth following an injury to the junction between bone and cartilage in the condylar process have already been mentioned on page 385.

Answer to question in Figure 3: The part of the metal staple directed toward the fingertips lies dorsally to the middle phalanx.

The Axial Skeleton

The human spine not only carries the head, the shoulder girdle with the arms, and the trunk, but also constitutes the flexible, eccentrically placed axis of the trunk—the *axial skeleton*. The spine thus fulfills a static as well as a dynamic function. Its static carrying and supporting function is reflected by the morphology of its elements—the vertebral bodies and the intervertebral disks—which increase in bulk from cranially to caudally. Its dynamic function of motion depends on coordination of the spine with muscles of the trunk. This coordination not only governs the motions of the spine (inclination, flexion, and rotation) but also determines the posture of the body under the influence of psychosomatic impulses. In so doing, the spine gives expression to the individual's mental and emotional condition. Moreover, the spine protects important structures of the central nervous system, the cord as well as the motor and sensory nerve roots, including the cauda equina, which passes downward from the first or second lumbar vertebra. Finally, the spine houses hematopoietic tissue (red bone marrow) in the meshes of its cancellous bone. These manifold functions make great demands on the morphologic structure of the axial skeleton. To fulfill them, a great number of rigid elements (vertebrae) as well as flexible elements (intervertebral disks, joints, ligaments, and muscles) are combined to build a polymorphous but ingenious structure.

From the functional point of view, the three chief mobile segments of the spine are both a springy axial staff and a link chain whose smallest unit is formed by the **vertebral motor segment** (Junghanns, 1968). The motor segment comprises the motor space between two vertebrae; this space contains in 23 out of 24 cases (exception: C1/C2) the following principal structures (Fig. 602), which can also be assessed roentgenologically: the intervertebral disk (nucleus pulposus, annulus fibrosus); the two end plates composed of hyaline cartilage, which are solidly connected to the intervertebral disk and the vertebral body; the anterior and posterior longitudinal ligament; the elastic right and left ligamentum flavum; the paired intervertebral joints; the thoracic and lumbar interspinous and supraspinous ligaments; the cervical ligamentum nuchae; and the intertransverse ligaments. In addition, the motor segment encompasses parts of the nervous and vascular systems as well as the nerves and muscles.

Pathologic changes of the axial skeleton may lead to dysfunction of the involved motor segment; i.e., decreased mobility (hypomobility, locking of vertebrae, immobility); or increased mobility or loosening of the structures (hypermobility, unstable gliding). They may also impair its bearing capacity. These disorders will be discussed in the following pages. As a general rule, overall mobility in the motor segment depends on the condition of the intervertebral disk, whereas the direction of motion is decisively influenced by the shape and inclination of the articular processes and facets.[29] In addition, the intervertebral joints counteract a pathologic forward slippage of the vertebra.

---

[29] It is true that the articular facets of the intervertebral joints are not in close apposition. This is why certain movements—for example, lateral inclination of the lumbar spine—are, even normally, accompanied by canting of the articular processes.

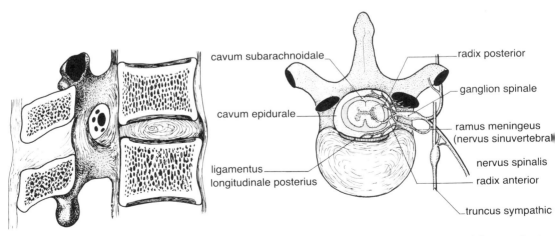

cavum subarachnoidale

cavum epidurale

ligamentus
longitudinale posterius

radix posterior

ganglion spinale

ramus meningeus
(nervus sinuvertebral

nervus spinalis

radix anterior

truncus sympathic

Fig. 602 Macromorphology *(left)* **and special aspects of the sensory innervation** *(right)* **of the vertebral motor segment** (after Peter, 1976). The sinuvertebral nerve receives the sensory fibers for the posterior longitudinal ligament of the spine, the dura mater, the epidural veins, the periosteum, the outer layers of the annulus fibrosus, and the capsules of the intervertebral joints (apophyseal joints) (Théron and Moret, 1978).

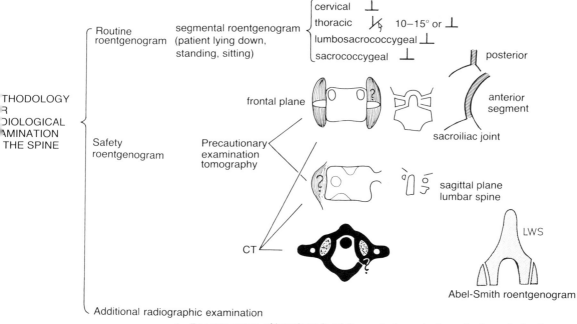

Routine roentgenogram — segmental roentgenogram (patient lying down, standing, sitting)

cervical ⊥
thoracic ⨍ 10–15° or ⊥
lumbosacrococcygeal ⊥
sacrococcygeal ⊥

frontal plane

posterior

anterior segment

sacroiliac joint

Safety roentgenogram — Precautionary examination tomography

sagittal plane lumbar spine

CT

LWS

Abel-Smith roentgenogram

Additional radiographic examination

1. Roentenogram of junctions (occipitocervical, cervicothoracic, thoracicolumbar, lumbosacral) (occipitocervical, cervicothoracic, thoracicolumbar, lumbosacral)
2. Oblique roentgenograms
3. Functional roentgenograms (single film; cineradiography)
4. Total roentgenograms
5. Myeolography — water-soluble contrast medium
   oil-based contrast medium; gas
6. Spinal phlebography
7. Vertebral arteriography
8. Spinal arteriography
9. Discography
10. Stereoscopic views (localization of foreign bodies; compare Fig. 3).

Fig. 603   Radiologic examination of the spine.
Note: For the *lateral* routine film of the thoracic spine and the *lateral* supplementary film of the cervicothoracic junction, the patient is conveniently positioned so that the shoulder girdle next to the focus is rotated between 10° and 15° posteriorly. The upper thoracic segments are thus better demonstrable than with a roentgenogram in the exactly lateral position. For Abel-Smith roentgenograms, see Fig. 605.

Figure 603 illustrates the **methodical radiologic examination of the spine** on the principle of obtaining information *with the least* possible expenditure. In so doing, the radiologist employs a sequence of procedures ranging from:

· **Routine radiologic examination**
· **Precautionary radiologic examination**
· **Supplementary radiologic examination**

The definitions of routine and supplementary radiologic examination are self-evident. Functional roentgenograms and films of the entire spine have already been mentioned on page 3 ff, where the significance of roetgenograms with the patient *standing* and *lying down* has been underscored. Tomography is, in

principle, a precautionary examination. It strengthens or weakens the suspicion of pathologic changes that may have been raised by physical examination or a plain roentgenogram. Tomography permits more distinct recognition of small central osteolyses, delicate defects in the contours of the vertebrae and the sacroiliac joints, the radiographic morphology of the occipitocervical junction, and circumscribed shadows in the perivertebral soft tissues (abscess, tumor tissue, hematoma).

Computed tomography (CT scan) is the technique of choice for *confidently* diagnosing fractures of the vertebral arches. This method of investigation (which requires sophisticated equipment) is indispensable, especially for assessing the arches of the

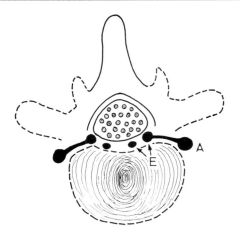

Fig. 604 **Anatomic rationale for spinal phlebography in prolapsed disk** (section through a lumbar disk, *schematically*). Before dorsally or dorsolaterally displaced portions of the disk can exercise any influence on the cauda equina and the nerve roots—demonstrable by myeolography or CT—they compress the medial and lateral eipdural veins (E); recognizable by spinal phlebography (Bücheler et al., 1968; Théron et al., 1978). A = vena lumbalis ascendens.

upper (cervical) vertebrae. In the lumbar spine, CT competes with a focusing technique devised by Abel and Smith (1977) for demonstrating the posterior vertebral elements (Fig. 605). Computed tomography also makes it possible to identify and measure shadows in the perivertbral soft tissues (abscesses, tumors, hematomas, extramedullary hematopoietic tissue) and stenoses of the vertebral canal.

The observer of a segmental roentgenogram receives an abundance of information that must be sorted out before a radiographic diagnosis can be made. Subsequently, the discussion either will start from the

individual pathologic roentgen finding (Fig. 606) or the disease in question, e.g., ankylosing spondylitis, will be described in its context.

Anomalies in the Position of Vertebrae and the Posture of the Spine

It is a matter of principle that, in the lateral roentgenogram, a segmental malposition (extension, dorsal gaping of the intervertebral space [Güntz's sign]) provides more information about *disturbed* mobility than a malposition of entire spinal segments (increased or decreased kyphosis of the thoracic spine, increased or decreased lumbar lordosis, extension of a segment, kyphosis of the lumbar spine, etc.). Monosegmental extension and dorsal gaping of an intervertebral space—hence angular segmental kyphosis with *normal* shape of the vertebral body; compare the definition of gibbus on page 399 (Fig. 607)—develop through reflex muscular pull. They indicate splinting of the segment—in extreme cases, complete obstruction of motion (immobility), which can be evidenced by functional roentgenograms. Similar considerations apply to the abnormal extended position of several vertebrae above a loosened segment (Güntz's sign, Fig. 607).

Segmental malpositions are frequently a clue to retrodisplacement of disk tissue. It is probable that the dorsal gaping of an intervertebral space counteracts compression of the nerve roots by sharply projecting or displacing parts of the disk. However, it also can be that a reflex malposition of the segment is due to other causes; e.g., an inflammatory process, a tumor, or traumatic lesions. Finally, certain affections of the intervertebral joints (p. 464) are liable to produce reflex obstruction of motion.

Gibbus (Figs. 608 and 609) is an angular seg-

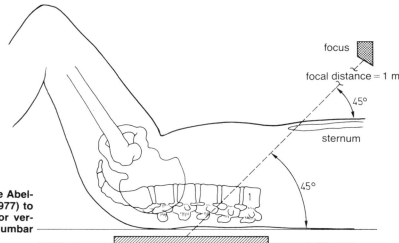

Fig. 605 **Focusing of the Abel-Smith roentgenogram (1977) to demonstrate the posterior vertebral elements in the lumbar spine** (compare Fig. 603).

focus

focal distance = 1 m

45°

sternum

45°

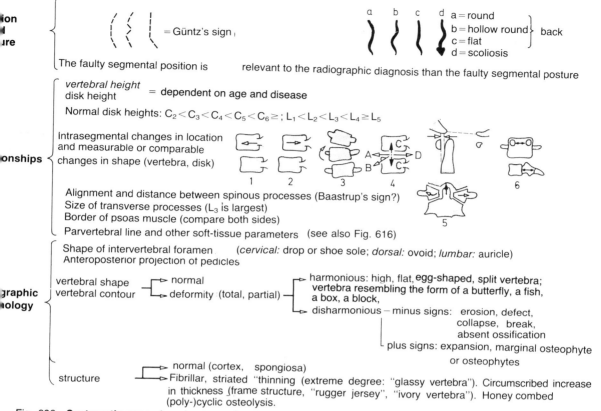

ion
d
ure
$\left\{\begin{array}{l}\end{array}\right.$ = Güntz's sign ¡

a   b   c   d   a = round
b = hollow round } back
c = flat
d = scoliosis

The faulty segmental position is   relevant to the radiographic diagnosis than the faulty segmental posture

$\dfrac{vertebral\ height}{disk\ height}$ = dependent on age and disease

Normal disk heights: $C_2 < C_3 < C_4 < C_5 < C_6 \geq$; $L_1 < L_2 < L_3 < L_4 \geq L_5$

onships

Intrasegmental changes in location and measurable or comparable changes in shape (vertebra, disk)

1   2   3   4   5   6

Alignment and distance between spinous processes (Baastrup's sign?)
Size of transverse processes (L_3 is largest)
Border of psoas muscle (compare both sides)
Parvertebral line and other soft-tissue parameters   (see also Fig. 616)

graphic
ology

Shape of intervertebral foramen   (*cervical:* drop or shoe sole; *dorsal:* ovoid; *lumbar:* auricle)
Anteroposterior projection of pedicles

vertebral shape ⟶ normal
vertebral contour ⟶ deformity (total, partial) ⟶ harmonious: high, flat, egg-shaped, split vertebra; vertebra resembling the form of a butterfly, a fish, a box, a block,
⟶ disharmonious – minus signs: erosion, defect, collapse, break, absent ossification
⌐ plus signs: expansion, marginal osteophyte or osteophytes

structure ⟶ normal (cortex, spongiosa)
⟶ Fibrillar, striated "thinning (extreme degree: "glassy vertebra"). Circumscribed increase in thickness (frame structure, "rugger jersey", "ivory vertebra"). Honey combed (poly-)cyclic osteolysis.

Fig. 606 **Systematic procedure in assessing roentgenograms of the spine.** By testing and judging the physiologic and pathologic parameters listed, the great majority of all pathologic changes in the axial skeleton can be identified.

Note: In the cervical spine, not only lordosis but also overall extension as well as flat-arched overall kyphosis are normal findings.

mental malposition with *changes* in the shape of the vertebral bodies (compare the definition of the dorsally gaping disk space on p. 398). The angulation is primarily anterior. Gibbus is caused by: trauma, bacterial spondylitis, (less frequently) **Scheuermann's disease** (Scheuermann, 1921, Figs. 609 and 610), osteolytic tumors of the vertebral bodies, malformation of the vertebral bodies (posterior hemivertebra), and systemic disorders of endochondral calcification (e.g., osteochondrodysplasias and mucopolysaccharidoses, congenital hypothyroidism, achondroplasia).

Variations in Disk Height

The *normal sequences of the disk heights* in the motor segments of the cervical and lumbar spine can be seen in Figures 606 and 611 A. The increase in disk height is *continuous* and harmonious. An abrupt, *discontinuous* (apparent) *increase* in disk height often

reflects the (actual) *decrease in height* of the next disk *superiorly* (Fig. 611 B)!

Decrease in height of a disk space can be the first roentgen manifestation of an inflammatory, degenerative, or other pathologic process in the disks or the vertebrae.

Ventral Displacement of Vertebrae (Fig 606, no. 1),

In functional roentgenograms of the anteflexed cervical spine, a slight *associated* ventral motion of the superior over the inferior vertebra is a physiologic process (for the conditions in the lumbar spine, compare Fig. 632). A corresponding motion occurs with retroflexion. This leads to the formation of steps in the alignment of the posterior vertebral contours (*physiologic stair-step phenomenon;* Fig. 612 A and B). These steps are equalized as soon as the normal posture—with the hard palate horizontal—is reassumed. This associated movement indicates that the

Fig. 607 **Mono- and oligo-segmental antalgic malpositions assumed by reflex.**

A = Monosegmental extended position of L3/L4.

B = Dorsal gaping of intervertebral space L3/L4 (angular kyphosis without change in shape of the vertebral bodies).

C = Extended position of the vertebral bodies L1–L4 above the degenerated intervertebral disk L4/L5 (Güntz's sign).

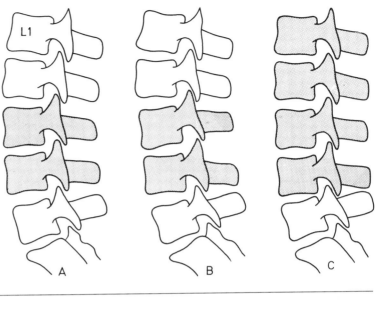

A   B   C

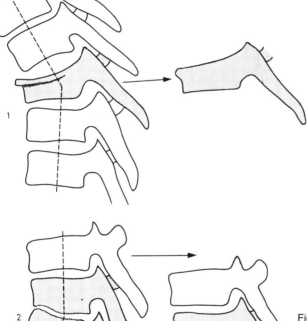

Fig. 608 **Causes of angular segmental malposition with change in shape of the vertebral bodies (gibbus).**

1 = (Hyper-) flexion type of fracture (with unimpaired flexion at the moment of the injury). *Typical roentgen manifestations:* Wedge-shaped vertebra; indentation of the anterior and middle portion of the end plate; formation of a step—"oriel"—in the anterosuperior contour of the vertebral body; contour smoothed out during the healing process *(arrow)*. In a *fresh* fracture, the height of the disk does not usually decrease; rather, the intervertebral space is "widened."

2 = Bacterial spondylitis (evolution with delayed diagnosis and inadequate therapy; *arrow*).

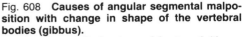

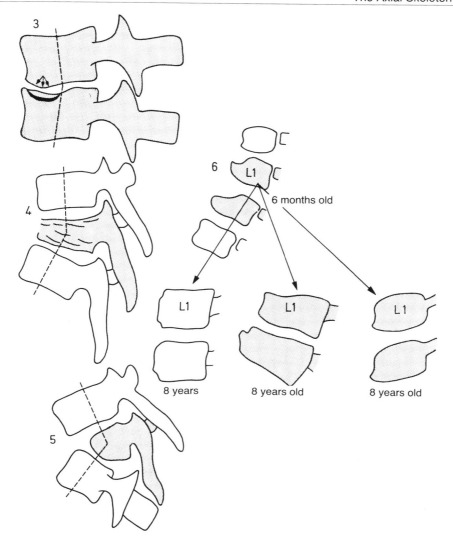

6 months old

8 years   8 years old   8 years old

Fig. 609   **Continuation of Fig. 608.**

3 = Scheuermann's disease (adolescent kyphosis) (see also Fig. 610). With a larger intracancellous prolapse of a disk (Schmorl's nodule), an angular segmental kyphosis and a decrease in disk height may ensue. The *Edgren-Vaino sign,* (Fig. 610 D) which is of importance in the differential diagnosis, has also been illustrated *(arrows).*

4 = Tumor-induced osteolysis. In the present case, the contour of the end plates has been preserved. Generally, there are roentgen signs of a (pathologic) fracture; i.e., changes in the structure of the collapsed vertebral bodies (in the lateral tomograph). Height of the disk space generally not decreased; possibly shadow in the perivertebral soft tissue produced by outward-growing tumorous tissue!

5 = Malformation of vertebral body (posterior hemivertebra).

6 = In the newborn and infant, *uniform vertebral bodies* in the thoracicolumbar junction are *nonspecific indications* of a prenatal growth disorder. This disorder self-corrects during further growth *(left).* In constitutional skeletal diseases, the malformation often persists or even increases. (*Center:* Inadequately treated congenital hypothyroidism. *Right:* Type II mucopolysaccharidosis [Hunter] with persistent infantile ovoid shape of the vertebrae bodies.) Lateral roentgenograms of the thoracic and lumbar spine are therefore an important measure in infancy, early childhood, and school age to diagnose and classify the manifold constitutional skeletal diseases; *for example,* achondroplasia, metatrophic dwarfism, diastrophic dwarfism, congenital spondyloepiphyeseal dysplasia, mucopolysaccharidosis I (Hurler), II (Hunter), III (Sanfilippo), IV (Morquio), VI (Maroteaux-Lamy). (Spranger et al., 1974; Schuster, 1976.)

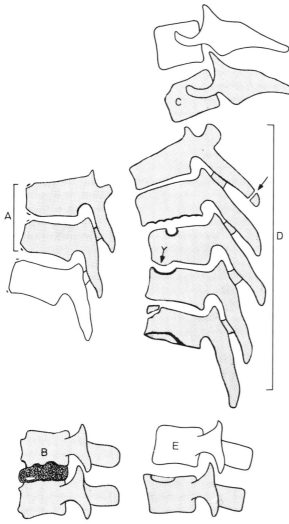

Fig. 610 **Scheuermann's disease (adolescent kyphosis)** begins in prepuberty. Males are prevalently affected. The classic location of Scheuermann's disease is the thoracic spine (T4–T12). It may also occur in the thoracicolumbar junction, the lumbar spine, and less frequently in the cervical spine. The roentgen manifestations of Scheuermann's disease quite generally indicate a lowered weight-bearing capacity of the supporting and pressure-absorbing cartilaginous and osseous end plates of the vertebrae. The disease favors attrition of the disks and the intervertebral joints; it impairs the mobility of the spinal segment involved or leads to loosening of the structure of the diseased segment. An important complication of the decreased weight-bearing capacity are growth disorders of the vertebral bodies (wedge-shaped vertebrae) which lead to early fixation of the kyphosis that affects the lower third of the thoracic spine. Even an angular kyphosis of the gibbus type may occasionally form in serious developmental disorders of the vertebral bodies (see text).

Early roentgen manifestations: Decreased height of the disks, preferentially on their ventral aspects; vertebral bodies slightly wedge-shaped (A).

Roentgen manifestations: Irregular but sharp contours of the end plates. Vacuum phenomenon seen in disk (clue to rupture of the disk, B).

In the cervical spine, flat and wedge-shaped vertebrae develop as well as defects in the edges of the vertebral bodies (C).

D illustrates a combination of roentgen signs in Scheuermann's disease. They favor the development of an arched kyphosis in the lower thoracic spine. The following manifestations are demonstrable from above to below: Wedge-shaped vertebrae; decrease in disk height, more pronounced ventrally; increased anteroposterior diameter of vertebrae; end plate irregular, its density increased; smaller and larger Schmorl's nodules with increased marginal density; retromarginal prolapse of disk (marginal separation); Müller's sign *(arrow)*, i.e., fatigue fracture of the spinous process in pathologic kyphosis (this finding may also be observed in traumatic or inflammatory gibbus); the Edgren-Vaino sign *(tailed arrow)* = a larger Schmorl's nodule is accompanied by "compensatory" circumscribed growth of bone in the opposite end plate. (This is not the case in a spondylitic defect). For roentgen manifestations in Scheuermann's disease see also Fig. 609, no. 3.

E shows deformation of a lumbar vertebral body by a Schmorl's nodule which originally extended as far as the anterior edge of the vertebra; hence it had involved the marginal ridge = the annular apophysis of the vertebral body) and thus interfered with growth of the vertebral body.

Notes: 1. About every second patient with Scheuermann's disease also has slight scoliosis.

2. The roentgen manifestations of Scheuermann's disease can be identified in about 31 percent of the average population (Reinhold, 1966), raising doubts about whether Scheuermann's disease is a pathologic entity at all (Ross, 1963). It is true that evidence of Schmorl's nodules alone does not justify the diagnosis of this disease. Only about one third of individuals with positive roentgen manifestations have complaints that can be related to these findings.

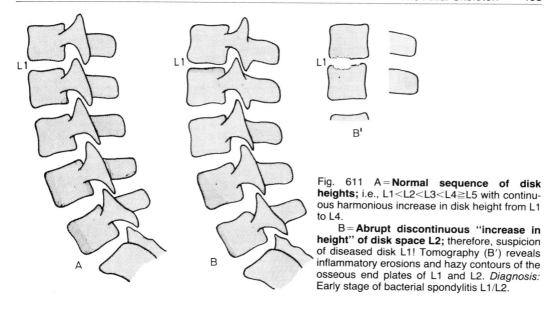

Fig. 611 A = **Normal sequence of disk heights;** i.e., L1<L2<L3<L4≧L5 with continuous harmonious increase in disk height from L1 to L4.

B = **Abrupt discontinuous "increase in height" of disk space L2;** therefore, suspicion of diseased disk L1! Tomography (B') reveals inflammatory erosions and hazy contours of the osseous end plates of L1 and L2. *Diagnosis:* Early stage of bacterial spondylitis L1/L2.

transverse axis of rotation for retroflexion and anteflexion of the cervical spine normally does not lie in the disk space—the center of the motor segment—but more inferiorly. When, in lateral roentgenograms, the intervertebral joint space in the cervical spine is regarded as part of a circular arc, the radius of this virtual arc, and thereby its center—the position of the axis of rotation—can be determined. *In principle, ventral and dorsal motion are most pronounced in that motor segment in which the strongest anteflexion or retroflexion takes place.*

If, in a cervical segment, this premise is fulfilled, an increase in segmental anteflexion (retroflexion) there and an adequate increase in ventral (dorsal) motion in the presence of a normal disk height—*hypermobility* (Erdmann, 1968)—should not be labeled a priori as pathologic, particularly if subsequently the normal posture is reassumed and if young individuals are concerned (see footnote on p. 6)! In the individual case it is, rather, necessary to include the symptomatology in the diagnostic considerations. Conversely, increased ventral or dorsal motions should always be regarded as pathologic *(sign of structural loosening)* when the disk space, which presents a reduced height, is hardly or not at all deformed with extreme anteflexion or retroflexion ("drawer phenomenon"; compare Figs. 632 and 612 D and E). Fixed (obstructed) step formations that are no longer equalized by a change of posture also belong among the pathologic roentgen findings (Fig. 612 F, F'; and G).

Various injuries and their sequelae, which also can lead to ventral displacement of a vertebra, have been classed under the heading of **whiplash injury of the cervical spine** and are still subjects of debate. Erdmann (1973) makes a distinction between *cervi-cal whiplash injury* in the strict sense of the term and *contact traumas (ram injuries) of the anterior skull with cervical angulation.*

1. In whiplash injury, the *abrupt horizontal blow comes from behind;* e.g., by a rear-end collision in driving. Since the cervical spine lies above the backrest, it does *not* take part in the unexpected forward acceleration of the trunk, unless an effective neck support is available. In this instance (neck support present) the forward acceleration is also transmitted to the cervical spine and thus prevents a typical cervical whiplash injury (Erdmann, 1973).

2. The *element of surprise* is essential in the causation of a whiplash injury (humans do not have eyes in the back of their heads). This is why the driver who *causes* a rear-end collision does not suffer a whiplash injury; nor can this type of injury normally occur in a head-on collision. Factors (1) and (2) give rise to a violent, abrupt retroflexion with subsequent anteflexion. These two motions are readily conceivable and evidently have been the reason for coining the metaphoric term "whiplash injury." The real characteristic of this type of injury, however, is neither the retroflexion nor the anteflexion but the sudden shearing movement between the trunk and the neck: two forces become operative in the opposite direction, about perpendicular to the longitudinal axis of the body (Fig. 613). Moreover, these forces occur so close together that a flexion does not take place, or at most it lags behind the shearing motion. The latter occurs jerkily; the backrest conveys a forward acceleration to the trunk while the neck and the head first maintain their original posture. These opposite forces act upon the level of a *single* motor segment. When the shearing force exceeds the tear strength of the soft tissue, they rupture. The cervical whiplash

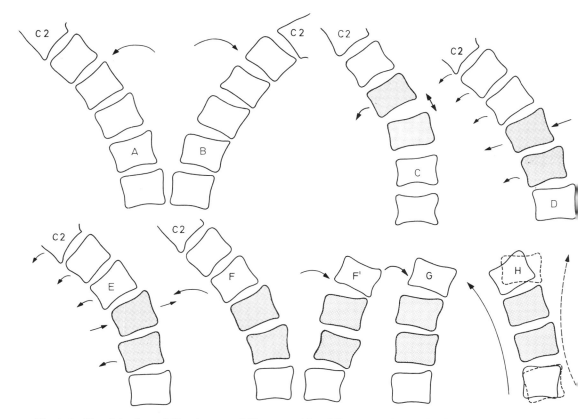

Fig. 612 Physiologic mobility, hypermobility, unstable gliding, and obstruction in functional roentgenograms of the cervical spine.

A, B = *Physiologic* stair-step phenomenon of the posterior contours of the vertebral bodies = *physiologic mobility.*

C = *Hypermobility with normal disk height* in the 4th motor segment (anteflexion and ventral position more pronounced than in the other motor segments). Young adult; no complaints (see text).

D = Reversible *pathologic* ventral displacement of C5 with loss of anteflexion in the 5th segment. With anteflexion of the cervical vertebra in this segment, the disk space becomes only slightly or not at all deformed. The same is true of reversible pathologic dorsal displacement with retroflexion of the cervical spine = *unstable gliding,* drawer phenomenon.

E = Reversible *pathologic* dorsal displacement of C5 with lost anteflexion in the 5th segment in a *roentgenogram with anteflexion* of the cervical spine = *unstable gliding.*

F, G = F and F′ show irreversible stair-step formation with complete segmental obstruction. G shows the irreversible stair-step formation with preserved possibility of retroflexion of the motor segment involved = *obstruction* (F, F′) or *partial obstruction* (F, G).

H = Complete absence of motion *(obstruction; immobility)* in a motor segment without stair-step formation in anteflexion and retroflexion *(sketched one above the other).*

injury therefore causes *primarily* soft-tissue injuries in the region of the cervical spine. The parts involved are the ligaments, the joint capsules, the intervertebral disks (including traumatic prolapse), the cord—traumatic cervical myelopathy in all grades of severity, the nerve roots, and the vessels (occlusion of the vertebral artery by a hematoma of the arterial wall, distortion of the internal carotid by the transverse process of the atlas in abrupt hyperextension with the possible formation of a lacerated intima, of a thrombus and the later development of a traumatic aneu-

rysm). Much less frequent are injuries to the bones; for example, fracture of the vertebral edge, oblique fracture of the spinous process, and fracture of an articular process.

Contact traumas to the anterior skull—*for example,* deceleration injury to the driver in a rear-end collision, the result of a head-on collision, or a trauma to the head from a dive into shallow water—lead to angulation of the cervical spine (hyperflexion, hyperextension, lateral flexion), to rotary injuries, and to axial compression with manifold trauma to the bones

Fig. 613 **Typical unexpected shearing impulse between the head and neck on the one hand and the trunk on the other. In whiplash injury (rear-end collision), this impulse gives rise to characteristic soft-tissue injuries of the cervical spine.**

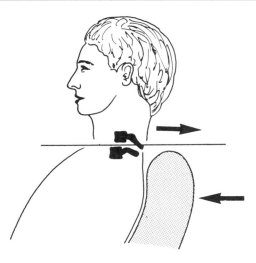

and the soft tissues, depending on the posture of the head at the moment of the accident and the direction of the forces. Besides this, mixed types of whiplash injury and contact trauma occur when the forces operative in the accident are not exhausted by the rear-end collision but, in addition, produce contact injuries to the head with impact on the cervical spine.

The tentative diagnosis of a whiplash injury is based on the history of the trauma, but suspicion may also be raised by the patient's statement that he experienced disorders of swallowing *immediately* after the accident (as the result of a hematoma in the re-

Fig. 614 **With clinical suspicion of a cervical whiplash injury or a contact trauma to the anterior skull with cervical angulation** (anamnesis; bruises on back, neck and skull), particular attention must be paid to the cervical segments marked by a *circle* (dislocation? break of contour? deformation?). A = Sequelae of a shearing or hyperflexion mechanism of any etiology with anteflexed posture of the cervical spine (often better visible than with normal posture; Fig. 4). **In fresh traumas, roentgenograms in retroflexion should be avoided!** (With rupture of the anterior longitudinal ligament there would be danger of cord compression.) At most, roentgenograms to test ligament stability in retroflexion could be made *with caution.*

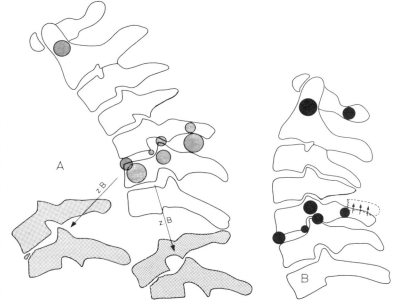

B = Typical locations where results of hyperextension mechanisms of whatever etiology—for instance, a fall head-first into a deep ditch—manifest themselves. The cranial displacement of a broken-off spinous process indicates the extension component of the traumatic event *(arrows).*

Note: In a cervical whiplash and angulation injury, the clinical symptomatology is not definitely related to the roentgen findings. On the one hand, neurologic deficits amounting to complete transverse lesion occur without any injury to bone. On the other, severe dislocations and fractures—e.g., vertebral dislocation with concomitant fracture of the vertebral arch ("saving fracture of the vertebral arch")—which may even lead to widening of the vertebral canal, may take their course without (major) neurologic deficits.

In whiplash injuries and cervical angulations following a contact trauma to the anterior skull, the *lateral view*—best in anteflexion—provides a general survey.

The *anteroposterior view* is most suitable for identifying vertical fractures of the vertebrae and (unilateral) rotary injuries.

Oblique views provide data regarding the condition of (the roots of) the vertebral arches and the articular processes; they allow location of the side of *unilateral* injuries to bone and of malpositions of the articular processes (change in shape of the intervertebral foramen on comparison with the opposite side).

The *transoral view* and possibly conventional tomography, serve principally in judging the odontoid process and the position of the atlantoaxial joint (the indications for computed tomography are discussed on 397).

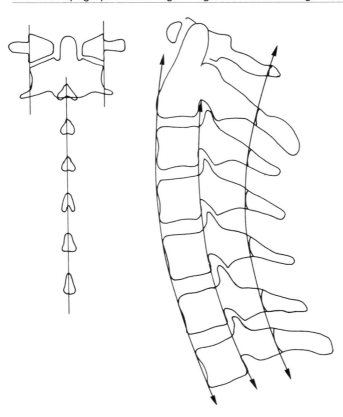

Fig. 615 **Lines of alignment in the cervical spine for identification of faulty positions.** In oblique views, the alignment is tested on the anterior rim of the intervertebral foramen.

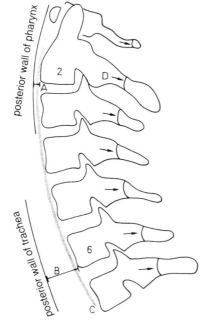

Fig. 616 **Soft-tissue parameters (A to C) and the spinolaminar line (D) in the cervical spine.**

A = *Retropharyngeal width* (measured between the anteroinferior edge of the axis and the posterior wall of the pharynx). Up to 7 mm = normal in children and adults.

B = *Retrotracheal width* (measured between the anteroinferior edge of C6 and the posterior wall of the trachea). Up to 14 mm = normal in children (15 years old and younger); 22 mm in adults (Wholey et al., 1958). A and B are enlarged by hematoma, edema, abscess, or tumor tissue.

C = *Prevertebral fat stripe* (in the roentgenogram a *black stripe* coursing parallel to the anterior longitudinal ligament and reflecting loose, adipose prevertebral connective tissue; Whalen and Woodruff, 1970).

Fracture: Fat stripe displaced anteriorly by hematoma.

Inflammation: Fat stripe with hazy contours, displaced anteriorly or "obliterated."

Tumor: fat stripe displaced anteriorly when, for example, the tumor grows outward from a cervical vertebra.

Opaque foreign body: When located in the pharynx or esophagus, the foreign body is demonstrable in front of the prevertebral fat stripe.

D = *spinolaminar line (arrows),* after von Torklus and Gehle, 1975. Absence of spinolaminar line; e.g., in C1 = dorsal cleft in the arch of the atlas; see Fig. 645. *Broken spinolaminar line* = fracture. *Obliteration or relative thinning of spinolaminar line* = bone tumor growing in junction betwen spinous process and vertebral arch (Tchang, 1974).

Additional information about the existence and extent of a cervical soft-tissue trauma is provided by *deviations of the trachea* and *displacements of the pharynx* (Clark et al., 1979).

gion of the neck and the pharynx). Injuries to the cervical soft tissues can often be demonstrated in the conventional roentgenograms of the cervical spine in four planes. The *full extent* of the soft-tissue damage, and sometimes even its very existence, can as a rule only be recognized in (1) *roentgenograms made with continuous axial distraction* or—in a less complicated manner—(2) a *functional roentgenogram in anteflexion*, or (3) a *roentgenogram to test the stability of the ligaments taken in stressed anteflexion*.

Transoral views as well as frontal and/or lateral tomographs may be required in individual cases to objectify complaints and clinical findings. Figures 614 through 616 indicate those spinal structures that, in whiplash injuries and in cervical angulations following a contact trauma to the skull, must be demonstrated and evaluated with particular care. *Charac-*

teristic injuries to the cervical spine are illustrated in Figures 617 through 619. Repair ossifications in the capsuloligamentous apparatus (corresponding to so-called traumatic localized myositis ossificans, see page 68) and/or the roentgen manifestations of traumatic damage to the intervertebral disk (ossification of the annulus fibrosus, collapse, or full-blown osteochondrosis of the disks involved) sometimes develop as *posttraumatic* events after months or a few years.

Pretraumatic degenerative discopathies (chondrosis, osteochondrosis; see Fig. 674) or osteoarthrotic deformation of the articular processes (apophyseal joint osteoarthrosis, see Fig. 686) may considerably intensify the effects of a whiplash injury or a contact trauma to the anterior skull with cervical angulation on the sensitive structures of the spinal canal, particularly the cord. The same applies to traumatized pa-

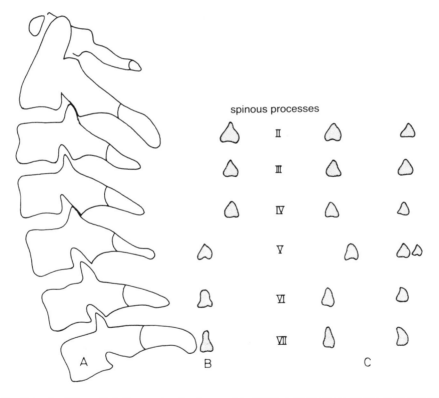

Fig. 617 **Radiologic differential diagnosis of rotary subluxation and fracture of the spinous processes in the cervical spine.** The joint space C2/C3 is normally not recognizable in lateral roentgenograms. The joint spaces of the paired intervetebral joints C3/4–C6/7, however, are visible (compare Figs. 615 and 616). A conspicuous feature of this sketch is that the radiologic joint space C4/C5 is "lacking." Therefore, suspicion is aroused of a rotary malposition of the 4th upon the 5th cervical vertebra. The alignment of the spinous processes should be tested in the anteroposterior roentgenogram (B).

B = Migration of the spinous process C4 *to the left;* hence, rotary subluxation (*synonym:* rotary dislocation) of C4–C5 *to the right.* The malrotated vertebra takes the superior vertebrae with it unless the latter have themselves undergone malrotation (to the opposite side). Causes of cervical rotary subluxation: trauma; atraumatic torticollis; pathologic processes in the vertebral arches and the disks.

C = "Migration" or "double contour" of a spinous process with normal alignment of the superior and inferior spinous processes primarily indicates its fracture. The double contour is better evidence than the migration!

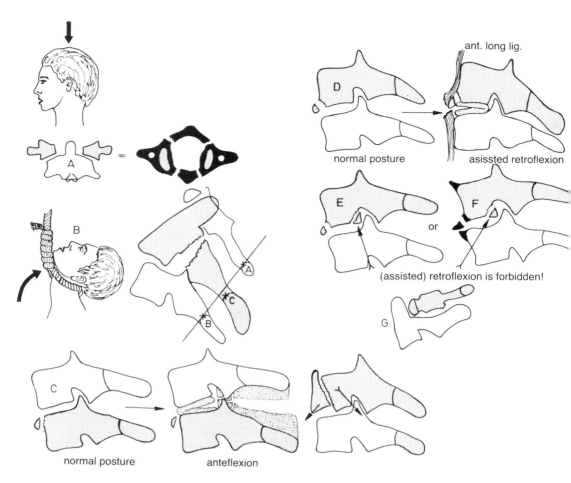

ant. long lig.

normal posture   asissted retroflexion

(assisted) retroflexion is forbidden!

normal posture   anteflexion

Fig. 618 **Typical injuries to the cervical spine:**

A = Quadruple splintered fracture of atlas **(Jefferson fracture)** following axial violence *(arrow)*. The patient had fallen on his head into a deep ditch. *Both* articular surfaces of the atlas are displaced outward and surmount the articular surfaces of the axis by several millimeters. The *lateral roentgenogram* may reveal interposition of the basion (anterior rim of the foramen magnum) between the anterior tubercle of the atlas and the dens (Flournoy et al., 1980).

B = Classic **hangman's fracture** with exactly submental position of the knot *or* caused by some other traumatic hyperextension of the mandible and cranium with respect to the upper cervical spine. This leads to an avulsion fracture of both pedicles of the arch of the axis and anterior dislocation of the body of the axis (Seljeskog and Chou, 1976). With a less severe injury, the avulsion fracture occurs without dislocation. When a tangent to A and B passes ≧ 2mm in front of C, a hangman's fracture must be suspected, whether or not a fracture line is visible in the arch of the axis following a trauma *and* in the presence of a recognizable ventral dislocation of C2 (Swischuk, 1978). *Next diagnostic step:* Computed tomography.

C = **"teardrop" conclusions:**

(1) The vertebra "sheds tears" over the lacerated soft tissues in its motor segment; therefore

(2) a roentgenogram in anteflexion (voluntary or assisted) is indicated. It will provide clues to the presence of traumatic damage to soft-tissue structures.

(3) A broken-off osteophyte of the vertebra—the

cortex is lacking at the fresh fracture site—in a post-traumatic roentgenogram is the same warning sign as the "tear" (see F in this figure).

(4) In a patient with a history of recent trauma, roentgenologic differentiation must be made between "teardrop" and an accessory bone in spondylosis (see p. 457).

(5) The larger the teardrop, the greater is the danger of cord compression by the posterior edge of the vertebral body (see the *tailed arrow*, which indicates the direction of displacement; Schneider and Kahn, 1956).

D = Originally it was supposed that the "tear" indicated a hyperflexion type of cervical trauma. It *may*, however, also be a clue to the hyperextension type. In this case the the film must be taken with (cautiously) assisted retroflexion because the freshly traumatized patient is unable to specify the degree of retroflexion; thus, extensive soft-tissue lacertaions then involve the hazard of cervical cord compression by strong dorsal slipping of the vertebra! When there is suspicion of fracture of the dens, functional roentgenograms are prohibited because they could give rise to fatal displacement of the dens (Schätzker et al., 1971).

E, F = "Tear" with break of the posterior edge *(tailed arrows)* points unequivocally to the hyperextension component of the accident. In *this* case, roentgenograms with retroflexion *must* be avoided!

G = Dorsal dislocation of the atlas without fracture of the dens, or ventral dislocation of C2 following trauma, or congenital anomaly (Patzakis et al., 1974).

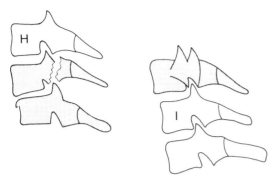

Fig. 619   **Examples of typical injuries to the cervical spine** (continued).

H = *Hyperextension type of injury.* Fracture through the articular processes associated with anterior dislocation of the involved vertebra and axial compression of the anterior end plate of the inferior vertebral body. The slight compression of the anterior end plate suggests that the traumatizing force had not been exhausted by the fracture of the articular processes and the dislocation. These injuries occur preferentially in the middle and inferior segments of the cervical spine.

I = *Unilateral vertebral dislocation* by flexing and rotating force. A single intervertebral joint is visible underneath the dislocated vertebra. In the dislocated vertebra and the motor segments superior to it, two joints each (two pairs of articular processes) are recognizable. Unilateral anterior dislocation of the vertebra can be very inconspicuous. The spinous process of the unilaterally dislocated vertebra migrates toward the side of the dislocation *(not illustrated),* (compare Fig. 617 B; Scher, 1977). For bilateral vertebral dislocation, see Fig. 614 A.

Note: In injuries producing lateral flexion, fractures of the uncinate process—to be differentiated roentgenologically from a persistent ossification center of the uncus (Fig. 678), fractures of the transverse processes (generally C3–C6) and, less frequently, lateral traumatic wedge-shaped vertebrae are apt to occur.

tients with constiutional narrowing of the spinal canal.

A similar group of injuries are the **traumas to the thoracicolumbar spine.** These produce vertebral deformations that indicate the direction of the forces imposed (Fig. 620):

1. *Axial force with free mobility of the spine at the moment of the injury* leads to the *(hyper-) flexion type of fracture without restriction of flexion* (anterior wedge-shaped vertebra, formation of a projecting rim on the anterosuperior edge of the vertebra, Fig. 608, no. 1)

2. When the force mentioned in (1) has a *rotary component,* a lateral wedge-shaped vertebra is the result (Smith et al., 1977).

3. In *axial force with impaired mobility of the spine* from previous tension of the muscles of the trunk, the shearing effect is absent and the force strikes the end plates of the vertebrae predominantly in the axial direction. The explosive force of the nucleus pulpo-

sus then produces more or less extensive breaks of the end plates *(compressed fracture, (hyper-) flexion type of fracture with impaired flexion).*

4. *Extension types of fractures* are due to a fall on the back (on the buttocks). The tensing of the muscles of the back leads to heavy strain on the dorsal segments of the vertebral body (Fig. 620B) and the intervertebral disk.

With extremely abrupt violence and/or diminished resistance of the vertebra, the factors 1 to 4 may also produce a splintered fracture with extensive comminution of vertebrae. Breaking-off of the spinous and transverse processes is often the result of strong muscular pull, hence an indirect effect, or it occurs as a fatigue fracture; e.g., shoveler's fracture of the spinous processes C7–T1(T2). (Fig. 674, see also Fig. 610, no. D). In the film, a broken-off spinous process shows a characteristic "duplication" of its normal contour, or it "migrates" (see Fig. 617 C).

Fractures of the articular processes occur not only in vertebral dislocations but also as the result of direct violence and in association with other vertebral

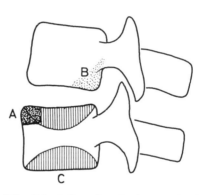

Fig. 620   **Orientation sites in the vertebral bodies of the three mobile segments of the spine relative to the mechanism of trauma:**

A = Area of deformation with flexion (hyperflexion) or a hyperflexion mechanism in the setting of a complex spinal injury. Compare, however, Fig. 618 D to F.

B = Area *(dotted)* in which pathologic extension (hyperextension) most frequently becomes effective.

C = Roentgen manifestations *(dashed areas)* reflecting an axial impact of the traumatizing force or impaired flexibility of the spine (through tensing of muscles) at the moment of the injury. Frequently to be seen in spines with diminished weight-bearing capacity of the vertebrae (osteoporosis, osteomalacia, etc.).

Note: If there is no history or an inadequate history of trauma, the following differential diagnoses must be made.

From A: (Anterior) retromarginal prolapse of the intervertebral disk (Figs. 610 and 640). *From B:* (Infrequent) atraumatic separation of the posterior vertebral edge (dorsal retromarginal prolapse of the disk; see Fig. 678). *From C:* Pathologic fracture in diffuse vertebral metastases or in multiple myeloma (plasmacytoma).

injuries. The same is true of *fractures of the vertebral arches*. These occur more often as secondary injuries in fractures of the vertebral bodies than as isolated events.

The **paravertebral line** (Gupta and Mohan, 1979) is a linear shadow that very frequently can be identified in roentgenograms of the thoracic spine. It runs *on the left, parallel to the vertebrae*, and it usually extends from the fourth to the 11th or 12th thoracic vertebra. The paravertebral line is only rarely present on the right side. It reflects, on the one hand, the border between the posteromedial margin of the (left) lung and its pleural cover, which it meets tangentially, and on the other hand, the denser perivertebral connective tissue. To the left of the paravertebral line and lateral to it, the margin of the descending thoracic aorta is often demonstrable. In persons under age 40, the paravertebral line passes at a distance of about 8 to 10 mm from the lateral borders of the vertebrae; in older individuals, this distance is be-

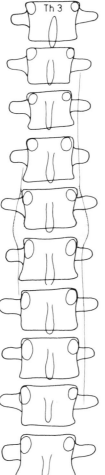

Fig. 621 **Thoracic paravertebral line.** A traumatic perivertebral hematoma has led to circumscribed broadening of the left-sided paravertebral line and to visibility of the right-sided paravertebral line (see text). The fresh (hyper-)flexion type of fracture of the 7th thoracic vertebra was not diagnosed in the lateral film of this patient but only in the lateral tomographs made after discovery of the "pathologic" paravertebral line! A synonym occasionally used for paravertebral line is "paraspinal line."

tween 6 and 15 mm. Broadening of the paravertebral line occurs in various pathologic conditions; for example, with neoplastic enlargement of the mediastinal lymph nodes, with abscesses forming during the course of a bacterial spondylitis (Fig. 697), and also with *perivertebral hematomas from vertebral injuries*. When these lesions are located on the right side or on both sides, displacement of the mediastinal border of the lung may lead to development of a right-sided paravertebral line (Fig. 621). Normally, the right-sided paravertebral line is rarely visible.

The term **spondylolisthesis** (Figs. 622 through 625) refers to a ventral displacement of vertebrae on the basis of a morphologic disorder of the so-called interarticular portion of the vertebral arch (the isthmus of the arch between the superior and inferior articular processes). A prerequisite to the development of spondylolisthesis is either a bone gap—**interarticular spondylolysis** (*synonyms:* spondylolysis, isthmus defect) or an **interarticular dysplasia** (isthmus dysplasia); i.e., lengthening and slimming of the isthmus. Spondylolysis or isthmus dysplasia with or without spondylolisthesis has been described in between 4 and 5 percent of whites, occurring in the fifth and fourth lumbar vertebrae in about 90 percent of cases and much less frequently in the remaining lumbar vertebrae and the cervical spine. Among the Eskimos of Alaska, defects of the vertebral arches, particularly spondylolysis of L5, have been reported in as many as 34 percent of individuals in the fourth decade of life (Stewart, 1953). Spondylolisthesis is not usually present at birth. It develops as a rule in the first decade of life and, in the great majority of cases, it ceases to increase after the completion of growth. At most, degeneration of the intervertebral disk, promoted by the ventral displacement of the vertebrae, can cause an additional slight increase of the displacement after the completion of growth. In some cases, spondylolisthesis does not develop despite a roentgenologically demonstrable spondylolysis or isthmus dysplasia. In other cases, the morphologic disorder of the interarticular portion develops only *unilaterally* or, when the disorder is *bilateral*, only one side becomes loose. In such instances a typical spondylolisthesis does not develop, but a slight rotation of the vertebra, associated with lateral tilting and scoliosis, is observed. There are different opinions concerning the causes of spondylolysis:

1. Spondylolysis is a hereditary congenital malformation (*teratologic spondylolysis and spondylolisthesis*). The condition manifests itself primarily in the fifth lumbar vertebra. In its vicinity, other vertebral malformations occur concomitantly; e.g., a median cleft in the arch and the spinous process (spina bifida occulta, p. 49; Meyerding, 1932). The so-called *dorsal wedge shape (trapezoid shape)* of the fifth lumbar vertebra (Fig. 622 D) is observed more frequently in spondylolisthesis than in patients without this finding (Sim, 1973). Apart from the more or less pronounced dorsal wedge shape, *hypoplasia* of the fifth lumbar

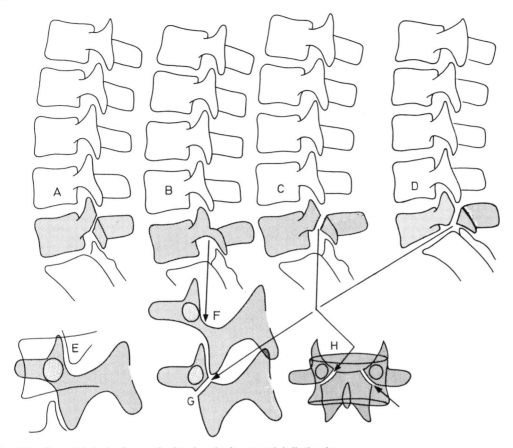

Fig. 622   Spondylolysis, interarticular dysplasia, spondylolisthesis.
A = Interarticular spondylolysis at L5 without slipping of the vertebra. The vertebra is thus divided into an anterosuperior portion (vertebral body, both pedicles of the vertebral arch, superior articular processes) and a posteroinferior portion (inferior articular processes and posterior region of the arch with the spinous process).
B = Dysplasia of the interarticular portions of the vertebral arch of L5 in ventral displacement of the vertebra (spondylolisthesis).
C = Spondylolisthesis of L5 in interarticular spondylolysis.
D = Spondylolisthesis with dorsal wedge-shaped vertebra L5 (see text).
E = Oblique view of the normal lumbar spine *(detail).* Typical Lachapèle's "dog's head." The "eye" of the dog's head is produced by the cortex of the pedicles of the vertebral arch (Brown and Evans, 1973).
F and G = The "dog's head has a lengthened slim neck
neck (F, interarticular dysplasia). The "dog" wears a "collar" (G, spondylolysis).
H = Bilateral spondylolysis in the anteroposterior projection of the lumbar vertebra *(arrows).*

vertebra is sometimes also visible (Frank and Miller, 1979). On studying the *posterior* contours of the vertebral bodies, the shortening of the anteroposterior diameter of the vertebral body (hypoplasia) can, in interarticular spondylolysis, simulate a spondylolisthesis. In fact, there exists only spondylolysis (without ventral displacement). This can be recognized by the normal alignment of the *anterior* vertebral contours (Fig. 626).

2. Spondylolysis develops on the basis of a *hereditary dysplasia of the vertebral arch*. It then occurs as the result of a functionally inferior anomaly of struc-

ture and shape of the interarticular portion (and the articular processes). It reflects a fatigue fracture occurring at the transition from four-legged to two-legged stance and gait in infancy and early childhood (Pfeil, 1975).

3. Cases of *traumatic spondylolysis* have been ascertained in individual patients who, *prior to an accident,* had for other reasons been subjected to a radiologic study of the lumbar spine and in whom an *intact* interarticular portion had been encountered (Sullivan and Bickell, 1960). However, the diagnosis of traumatic spondylolysis requires the greatest reservation

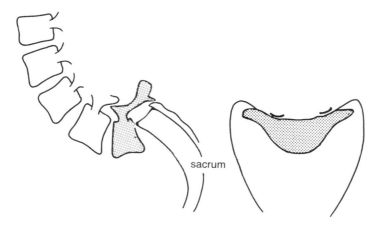

sacrum

Fig. 623 **Extremely severe spondylolisthesis at L5**—so-called **spondyloptosis**—in the lateral view and its projection on the anteroposterior roentgeno-gram (the inverted "Napoleon's hat" configuraton). It is usual for such cases to present only an elongation of the interarticular portion (dysplasia) without spon-dylolysis (formation of a cleft). Note also the common dorsal wedge shape of the slipped vertebra (see text). In women, slipping of the vertebra far ventrally produces narrowing of the parturient canal.

because an asymptomatic spondylolysis or spondyl-olisthesis can, following an accident, manifest itself for the first time by complaints before being detected in the roentgenogram.

4. *Secondary* spondylolysis, and even spondylolis-thesis, have been described with tumorous and osteo-myelitic destruction of the interarticular portion of the vertebral arch (Jaeger, 1935), in Paget's disease of the bone, in neurogenic spondylopathies (Francil-

lon, 1970), in osteomalacia, and in osteogenesis im-perfecta.

5. Spondylolysis occurs as the result of a *stress frac-ture* (in the growth period). It is therefore either as-sociated with a scar or is a pseudoarthrosis. This sup-position is strengthened by four observations. (1) Histologically, interarticular spondylolysis presents a gap in the bone which is filled with fibrotic connec-tive tissue and interspersed with osteocartilaginous

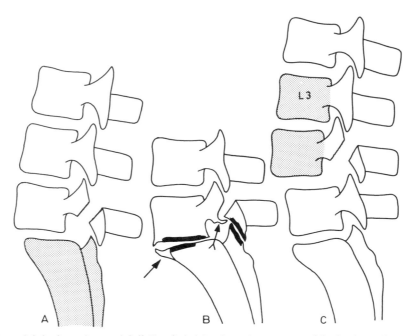

A   B   C

Fig. 624 **Spondylolysis and spondylolisthesis** in lateral roentgenograms of the lumbar spine.
    A = Reflex straightening of the sacrum (pelvis) that counteracts the ventral slipping of the vertebra.
    B = Typical sacral console *(arrow)* and osteophyte in the area of the spondylolysis of L5 *(tailed arrow)*. The lumbosacral intervertebral disk and the intervertebral joints show signs of degeneration (osteochondrosis; apo-physeal joint osteoarthrosis). Spondylolisthesis paves the way for attrition of these elements.
    C = Spondyloretrolisthesis is in L3 (compare Fig. 632). It indicates an additional (degenerative) disk lesion in the lumbar segment L3/4 (see page 415). Usually the slipping vertebra (in this case L4) causes the superior vertebra to take part in the ventral displacement.

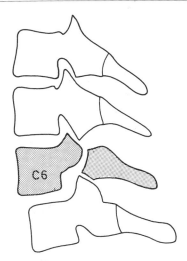

Fig. 625 Interarticular spondylolysis with spondylolisthesis at C6.
Spondylolysis and spondylolisthesis of the cervical spine occur mostly in the 6th vertebra. They are frequently accompanied by a median cleft in the arch and the spinous process (spina bifida occulta); the spinolaminar line of C6 is therefore often absent; see Fig. 616. Deformities of the various portions of the ventrally displaced vertebra (hypoplastic pedicles; lamina; articular processes) and also of the (hyperplastic) articular processes of the two contiguous vertebrae are additional secondary findings in cervical spondylolysis and spondylolisthesis.

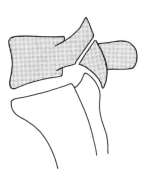

Fig. 626 Solitary interarticular spondylolysis misdiagnosed as spondylolysis with spondylolisthesis.
The 5th lumbar vertebra is not displaced anteriorly (compare the *normal* alignment of the *anterior* contours of vertebrae L5 and S1. Hypoplasia of the body of the 5th lumbar vertebra has led to shortening of its anteroposterior diameter (Frank and Miller, 1979). Comparison of only the *posterior* contours of vertebrae L5 and S1 gives the false impression that the 5th lumbar vertebra is displaced ventrally. Apart from the hypoplasia of the vertebral body, a dorsal wedge shape (trapezoidal shape) of the body of the 5th lumbar vertebra can also be recognized.

islet (Zippel and Runge, 1976). (2) Spondylolysis can occur in the wake of a spinal fusion in the border zone between the ankylosed and the mobile segments of the spine (Harris and Wiley, 1963). (3) Competitive athletes whose sport requires jerky motions of hyperlordosis, and who have been engaged in this sport for a number of years, present spondylolyses with considerably greater frequency than the average population (e.g., 26.5 percent of lumbar spondylolyses, occurring most frequently at L5; Groher 1975). These figures have been ascertained in radiologic studies of such athletes as exhibition gymnasts, divers, javelin throwers, weight-lifters, and trampoline jumpers (Schwerdtner and Schoberth, 1973; Luther and Legal, 1975; Fohler and Schwerdtner, 1975; and other writers). (4) Finally, stress fracture as a pathogenetic factor has been verified by successful treatment of spondylolysis *in childhood:* spondylolysis can disappear—i.e., be cured—by immobilization (Pfeil, 1975; Zippel and Runge, 1976). After discussing the best-known theories on the pathogenesis of spondylolysis, the following fact can be established. In many cases, the interpretation of lumbar interarticular spondylolysis as a stress fracture or its sequela is justified. The occurrence of a stress fracture actually presupposes heavy and prolonged excessive strain on the normally shaped and normally structured segment of bone concerned (compare the increased incidence of spondylolysis in competitive athletes), *or* a malformed—hence dysplastic—interarticular portion of the vertebral arch is unequal to withstanding the normal permanent load present in the two-legged human (compare the familial occurrence of spondylolysis and spondylolisthesis, Léger et al. 1979).

When a ventral displacement of a vertebra is demonstrable in lateral roentgenograms of the lumbar or cervical spine (Fig. 625), the radiologic examiner has to answer the following four questions:

1. Does a typical osseous cleft in the vertebral arch (Fig. 622 G) or an interarticular dysplasia (Fig. 622 F) exist concomitantly? Does one recognize an osteolytic process (tumor, etc.) in the articular portion, or is the slipping result of a change in shape (obliquity, deformation, destruction) of the articular processes acquired in adulthood (pseudospondylolisthesis, Fig. 627)?
2. In which portion of the arch is the recognizable cleft located (in the isthmus, behind the vertebral body, retroisthmic, Fig. 628)?[30]
3. Does the ventrally slipped vertebra (spondylolis-

---

30. For the conventional oblique view of the lumbar spine, the patient is placed in an oblique position of 45° (the intervertebral joint to be filmed close to the film). When ventral slipping of the vertebra is present, it is advisable to tilt the roentgen tube additionally by about 20° audocranially to obtain a distinct view of the interarticular portion of L5. In assessing the intervertebral joints L5/S1, some workers prefer an increase in the patient's oblique position to 45 to 60°.

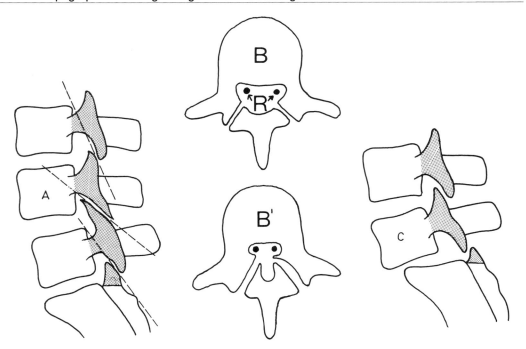

Fig. 627 Lumbar pseudospondylolisthesis, stenosis of the lumbar spinal canal, by apophyseal joint osteoarthrosis dislocation of the intervertebral joint

A = Pseudospondylolisthesis at L4 in apophyseal joint osteoarthrosis of the 4th lumbar segment. It is a matter of debate whether anomalous oblique position of the articular processes in the 4th segment (compare their tangential course) is exclusively the result of the osteoarthrotic deformations in the intervertebral joint or whether a primary deformity (dysplasia) of the articular processes favored the attrition.

B, B' = Osteoarthrotic deformation of the (superior) articular processses may give rise to narrowing of the intervertebral foramina as well as the spinal canal and may cause compression of the nerve roots (r) in the lateral recess of the spinal canal (Epstein et al., 1972). (B = normal finding in L4; B' = apophyseal joint osteoarthrosis of L4, schematically after *computerized tomographs*). The nerve roots are the more readily compressed the greater the *constitutional* narrowness of the spinal canal is! In acromegaly, symptoms on the part of the cauda or the nerve roots may also be produced by thickening of the lamina and/or hypertrophy (thickening) of the ligamentum flavum (Gelman, 1974).

C = Traumatic ventral dislocation of the 5th lumbar vertebra without signs of fracture.

Note: Intermittent claudication does not only occur as a *vascular* disorder in affections of the aortofemoral vessels. There is also a *neurogenic* type of the disease with the same symptomatology in the legs. Patients with neurogenic intermittent claudication often volunteer the information that their complaints are provoked or precipitated by hyperlordosis (for example, in walking downhill or in descending stairs) and that the pain subsides on bending forward. Pathogenetically, neurogenic intermittent claudication of the cauda equina or intermittent compression of the nerve roots has been associated with stenosis of the spinal canal (Verbiest, 1954). Suspicion of neurogenic intermittent claudication should therefore be aroused when the patient reports leg pain on walking (and standing) that subsides on lying down, and when the femoral and pedal pulses are normally palpable and narrowing of the lumbar canal is demonstrable in the roentgenogram (see B' of this figure and Fig. 644).

thesis, pseudospondylolisthesis) show pathologic mobility (to-and-fro displacement—"drawer phenomenon," gliding instability, or hypermobility; see Fig. 632 B) in functional roentgenograms with anteflexion and retroflexion?

4. What is the extent of the spondylolisthesis (measured in degrees or percentages; Figs. 629 and 630)?

The term **pseudospondylolisthesis** (Junghanns, 1930) is applied to a ventral displacement of the vertebra with preserved continuity of the paired pedi-

cles, the paired interarticular portions, and the unpaired lamina of the vertebral arch. The occasionally employed term *"degenerative spondylolisthesis"* is less appropriate. In the great majority of cases, pseudospondylolisthesis occurs as the result of apophyseal joint osteoarthrosis (Fig. 627). However, ventral displacement of the vertebra may also develop following *inflammatory* destruction of the articular processes; for example, in rheumatoid arthritis (Lawrence et al., 1964). Pseudospondylolisthesis does not usually appear before the age of 40. The fourth lumbar

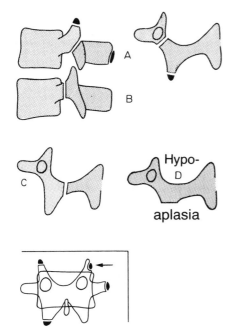

Fig. 628   A = **Spondylolysis** *(synonyms:* isthmus defect, isthmic cleft). B = **Retrosomatic cleft.** C = **Retroisthmic cleft formation.** D = **Deformation of the articular processes.** Compare Figs. 650 G and 687. In addition, the characteristic roentgen findings in persistent apophyses (hence, no traumatic avulsions!) in the articular, transverse, and spinous processes have been sketched in. *Arrow* points to persistent apophysis of the mamillary process at the superior articular process of the lumbar vertebra.

vertebra is most frequently involved (Rosenberg, 1975). The osteoarthrotic deformation of the articular processes—dysplasia of these processes is sometimes a predisposing factor—can cause them to become beveled or flattened (Fig. 627 A). This change in shape favors the ventral slipping of the vertebra. The articular processes, which are deformed (coarsened) by osteoarthrosis, sometimes project into the spinal canal and narrow it. There exist, thus, also acquired stenoses of the spinal canal, apart from the constitutionally determined anomalies in size and shape of the vertebral arch (Verbiest, 1954); for example, shortening of the pedicles and diminution of the interpedicular distance in the lumbar spine, decreasing from cranially to caudally, in achondroplasia. Among the causes of acquired stenosis of the spinal canal in the lumbar region are dorsal prolapse of a disk, apophyseal joint osteoarthrosis with or without pseudospondylolisthesis (Fig. 627 B), and tumorous, inflammatory, and other pathologic processes in the vertebral arch (Cauchoix et al., 1976).

Spondyloretrolisthesis (Dorsal Dislocation of a Vertebra) (Fig. 606, no. 2).

In lateral roentgenograms of the cervical and lumbar spine with normal posture, spondyloretrolisthesis (Figs. 631 and 632 shows a loss in mass of the *caudally* adjacent intervertebral disk because, under the influence of gravitation and by the pull of the elastic ligamentum flavum, the decrease in disk mass leads to approximation of the two adjacent vertebral bodies. *The disk space then decreases in height in the roent-*

Fig. 629   **Roentgenometry of spondylolisthesis (pseudospondylolisthesis) after Meyerding** (1932).
   The end plate of S1 or the vertebra lying inferiorly to the ventrally displaced vertebra is divided into four equal parts. The topographic relationship between the posteroinferior edge of the displaced vertebra and the four quarters of the end plate indicates the degree of ventral displacement. Consequently, there are four degrees of spondylolisthesis (pseudospondylolisthesis).

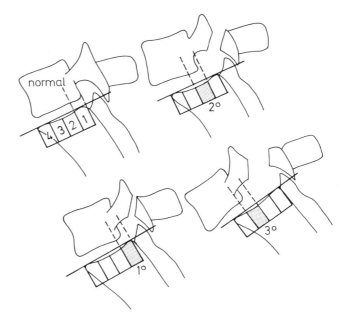

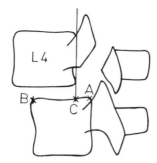

Fig. 630 **Roentgenometry of spondylolisthesis (pseudospondylolisthesis) after Sim** (1973).

The equation $\frac{AC}{AB} \times 100$ provides the percentage of vertebral slipping. In the present case of spondylolisthesis at L4, the vertebra has been dislocated ventrally by 21 percent.

gen picture. Approximation of the two vertebrae, however, is possible only if the corresponding articular processes also are displaced with respect to each other. Since the articular processes possess oblique facets, the inferior articular processes—which lie superiorly in the motor segment—slip posteroinferiorly and necessarily take the vertebral bodies with them dorsally (Fig. 631). This becomes manifest by a stairstep formation in the posterior contours of the

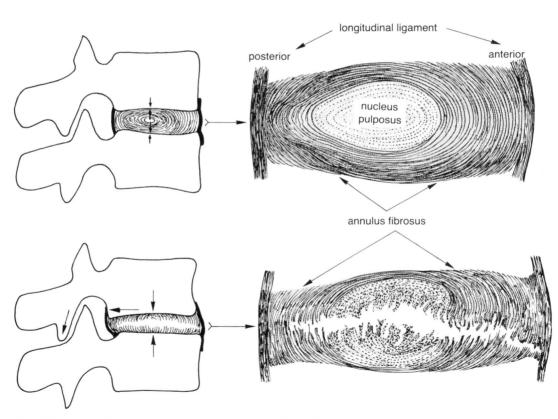

Fig. 631 **Anatomic situation in spondyloretrolisthesis** (for the roentgen findings, see Fig. 632). In the *present case* tears, gaps, and clefts in the nucleus pulposus and the annulus fibrosus have led to brittleness, desiccation, and consequent decrease in volume of the intervertebral disk. Chondrosis has developed. The intervertebral disk thus loses its shock-absorbing function. Under the influence of gravitation and the pull of the elastic ligamentum flavum the two contiguous vertebrae approach each other so that the height of the disk space decreases. The inevitable concomitant approximation of the posterior vertebral elements proceeds along the *oblique* glideway of the left and right intervertebral joints (zygapophyseal junction). The vertebra above the degenerated disk is thus *forced* to slip backward (= spondyloretrolisthesis). By so doing it narrows the corresponding intervertebral foramen (see the *lower part of this figure.*) Nerve root compression with a radicular symptomatology can ensue more readily in the presence of an (incidental) constitutional narrowness of the spinal canal, dorsal vertebral osteophytes, and/or concomitant apophyseal joint osteoarthrosis with deformed articular processes.

vertebral bodies, in which the superior vertebra usually dislocates only a few millimeters posteriorly—*spondyloretrolisthesis* (Figs. 624 C and 632). It should be reemphasized that initially, spondyloretrolisthesis presents only a *loss in mass of the intervertebral disk. This roentgen finding has as yet no pathologic significance for the patient.* Spondyloretrolisthesis, however, assumes the character of a disease either if it

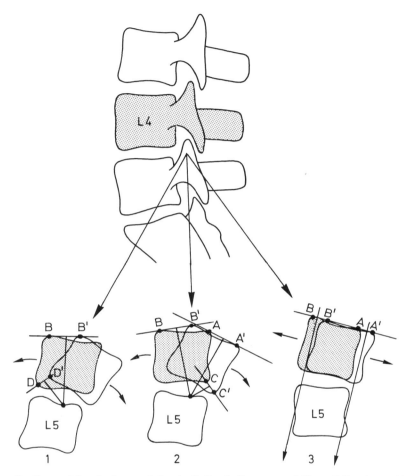

Fig. 632A   **Implications of (lumbar) spondyloretrolisthesis (hypmermobility; gliding instability).**
Above = Spondyloretrolisthesis at L4 in a lateral roentgenogram with normal posture, recognizable by the following signs: The posteroinferior edge of the vertebra L4 surmounts the posterosuperior edge of the vertebra L5 dorsally. The articular processes L4/L5 are mutually displaced with consequent narrowing of the intervertebral foramen L4/L5.
Decrease in height of the intervertebral space L4/L5.
Evaluation: Decrease in mass of disk L4/L5.
Question: Structural loosening in this motor segment?
1 to 3 = Evaluation of the functional roentgenograms with anteflexion and retroflexion by *Euler's principle* to determine the transverse axis of motion (Olssen et al., 1976; Penning et al., 1980). To this end, a tracing of L4 and L5 is made with anteflexion and retroflexion, superimposing the contours of L5. The homologous points A and A', B and B', etc., are connected by a straight line; this line is then divided in two and perpendicular lines are erected upon it. The perpendicular lines intersect in the fulcrum of motion.
Answer to 1 = Spondyloretrolisthesis does not correct itself completely on motion (hypomobility).
Answer to 2 = Spondyloretrolisthesis corrects itself on motion and the vertebra even may slip further ventrally (hypermobility).
Answer to 3 = Gliding instability can be demonstrated in the motor segment L4/L5 with spondyloretrolisthesis at L4; the vertebrae move to and fro with anteflexion and retroflexion ("drawer phenomenon"). There is no fulcrum for this sliding motion; the perpendicular lines erected on the divided straight lines A A', B B', etc. do not intersect.
4 = (see Fig. 632 B). Complete immobility of a motor segment with spondyloretrolisthesis in roentgenograms with anteflexion and retroflexion indicates obstruction of the segment—for example, by dorsal prolapse of a disk—or to immobilizing osteophytes on the vertebrae, etc. (see the caption to Fig. 632 B).

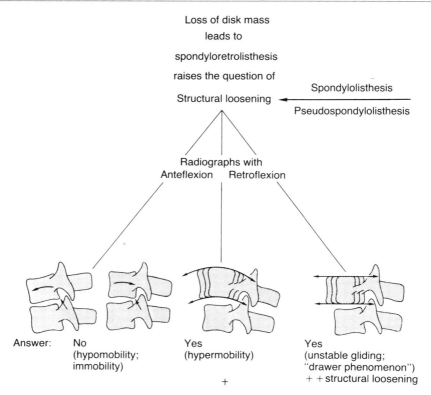

Loss of disk mass
leads to
spondyloretrolisthesis
raises the question of
Structural loosening ⟵ Spondylolisthesis
Pseudospondylolisthesis

Radiographs with
Anteflexion   Retroflexion

Answer: No   Yes   Yes
            (hypomobility;   (hypermobility)   (unstable gliding;
            immobility)   "drawer phenomenon")
                                       +   + + structural loosening

Fig. 632B Implications of (lumbar) spondyloretrolisthesis (continued). This figure illustrates the line of reasoning and the procedure of the radiologic examiner in the presence of decreased disk height (loss in disk mass) on the lateral roentgenogram.

Note: Gliding instability presupposes greater loosening of the segmental structure than hypermobility. Hypomobility of immobility is present when, on anteflexion, the dorsally displaced vertebra moves forward only slightly or not at all (i.e., without complete correction of the spondyloretrolisthesis). This may be related to a variety of causes, among them vertebral osteophytes, dorsal prolapse of the disk (reflex muscular blockage), complete decay of the degenerated disk, severe apophyseal joint osteoarthrosis including capsular ossification of the intervertebral joints. These causes decide whether or not hypomobility and immobility are experienced by the patient as a disease. Spondylolisthesis and pseudospondylolisthesis also raise the question of possible structural loosening.

occurs in association with other pathologic findings or if the process that underlies it is itself a disease that requires treatment.

In the majority of cases, the diffuse degeneration of the disk (loss of turgor, desiccation, brittleness) leads to a decrease in substance of the intervertebral disk. The *incidental* association of spondyloretrolisthesis from chondrosis or osteochondrosis with a constitutional or acquired stenosis of the spinal canal (compare Figs. 627, 643 and 644) may give rise to radicular complaints or manifestations on the part of the cauda equina. When spondyloretrolisthesis occurs as the result of a (major) dorsal prolapse of the disk, a major intracancellous prolapse of disk, perhaps produced by a malignant osteolysis underneath the disk, an inflammatory destruction of the disk, or traumatic damage to the disk (Fig. 669), the complaints in a roentgenologically diagnosed spon-

dyloretrolisthesis can, as a rule, be attributed to the primary disorders listed.

However, pain in spondyloretrolisthesis may also be expected when the dorsally displaced vertebra moves forward on anteflexion and backward again on retroflexion. This structural loosening can be identified by functional roentgenograms taken with anteflexion and retroflexion. It can be ruled out or differentiated between hypermobility or gliding instability when these films are evaluated by Euler's principle (Olsson et. al, 1976; Penning and Blickman, 1980) (Fig. 632 A and B). In the thoracic spine, its connection with the ribs prevents the development of spondyloretrolisthesis.

Figure 633 illustrates a case of so-called **pseudoretrolisthesis** (Dihlmann, 1966a). This finding is always observed in the fifth lumbar vertebra when the assimilation of the first sacral vertebra has produced

Fig. 633 Pseudoretrolisthesis and spondyloretrolisthesis.

A = Pseudoretrolisthesis L5 (end plate S1<L5; the distance between the tip of the articular process S1 and the vertebral arch L5 *(arrow)* is not diminished).

B = "Genuine" spondyloretrolisthesis L5 (end plate S1≈L5; anomalous approximation of tip of the articular process S1 to vertebral arch L5 [*arrow*]).

Note: The decreased height of disk space L5/S1 cannot be relied on for the distinction between spondyloretrolisthesis and pseudoretrolisthesis. Even normally, the 5th intervertebral space is of equal or lower height than the 4th intervertebral space. In addition, in pseudoretrolisthesis the lumbosacral intervertebral disk has a tendency to hypoplasia (i.e., to assimilation).

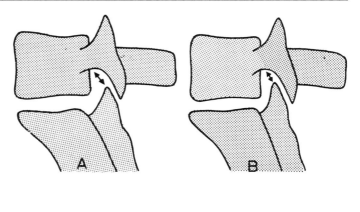

an above average dimunution of its anteroposterior diameter. Pseudoretrolisthesis may be differentiated from "genuine" dorsal dislocation by comparative measurement of the opposite end plates L5 and S1. In addition, in spondyloretrolisthesis the tips of the superior articular processes S1 approach the vertebral arch L5. This is not so in pseudoretrolisthesis. On rare occasions, pseudoretrolisthesis also develops in anomalies of the vertebral bodies (with shortening of their anteroposterior diameter) pertaining to other motor segments.

Rotary Slipping (Fig. 606, no. 3)

Lateral vertebral displacement—rotary slipping in the sense of W. Müller (1931)—has become known principally as an often painful complication of lumbar scoliosis. The uneven load on the spine in scoliosis leads to manifestations of wear and tear in the intervertebral disks and to laxity of the ligaments. This can be recognized in the roentgenogram by the appearance of osteophytes on the vertebrae (apophyseal joint osteoarthrosis, p. 456 ff), especially on the concave side of the scoliosis. In addition, the wear of the intervertebral disk and the laxity of the ligaments manifest themselves by rotary slipping of the vertebra that is observed mostly at the apex of the curvature or underneath it. The rotary component in the laterally slipped vertebra is due to the shape and position of the generally osteoarthrotic articular processes. *The slipped vertebra rotates toward the convex side of the scoliosis.* Roentgenograms in dorsal decubitus therefore show an enlarged projection of the transverse process on the concave side. Conversely, the transverse processes of the slipped vertebra on the convex side appear to be shortened and

reduced in size (Fig. 634) because, among other factors, the rotation has diminished the focal distance.

Scoliosis has multiple causes, but only in a minority of patients does the roentgen picture give information about its etiology. This negative assessment of roentgenologic studies in detecting the cause of a scoliosis is based on the experience that approximately 90 percent of the cases are being classified as "idiopathic." This means that their etiology is so far undetermined. The development and increase of such an **idiopathic scoliosis** are, as a rule, linked to the growth period. After the completion of growth no major increase of the scoliosis is to be expected, since even the possible aggravation from pregnancy or from vertebral osteoporosis in old age is relatively insignificant in comparison with the general tendency to aggravation in the growth period.

Clues to the etiology by physical examination, clinical history, and also radiologic study may be expected in **osteopathic, neuropathic, myopathic, and fibropathic scoliosis.** In this connection it should be pointed out that contrary to idopathic scoliosis, the scoliosis in von Recklinghausen's neurofibromatosis is liable to worsen after the completion of growth. The etiologic significance of vertebral malformations (= osteopathic scoliosis) and massive pleural fibrosis (= fibropathic scoliosis) can be assessed radiographically. In addition, in kyphosis, the roentgenogram can contribute to the important differentiation between *angular* and *arcuate* scoliosis. *Arcuate scoliosis* can, with time, manifest itself clinically and roentgenologically by the spinal *complications* mentioned above—chondrosis, osteochondrosis, apophyseal joint osteoarthrosis, and rotary slipping *(vide supra).*

Severe scolioses of the thoracic spine frequently

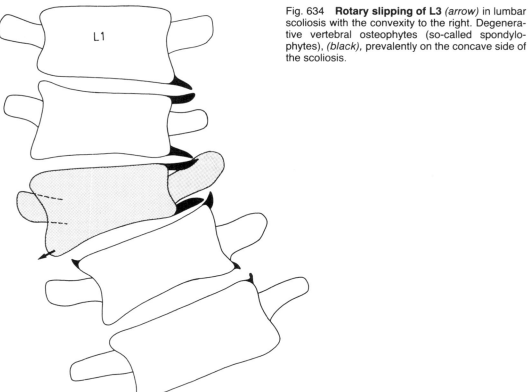

Fig. 634 **Rotary slipping of L3** *(arrow)* in lumbar scoliosis with the convexity to the right. Degenerative vertebral osteophytes (so-called spondylophytes), *(black)*, prevalently on the concave side of the scoliosis.

lead to an increased load on the lesser circulation and the right ventricle. *Angular scoliosis* often points *directly* to a painful process in the vertebrae; for example bacterial spondylitis, tumor, or fracture of a vertebra, but it also occurs in localized vertebral malformations.

Two roentgenologically identifiable causes of scoliosis should be pointed out because of their diagnostic importance: A *painful* scoliosis triggered by reflex can occur in morbid processes which are localized *eccentrically* in the vertebra; *for example,* osteoid osteoma, benign osteoblastoma, aneurysmatic bone cyst, eosinophilic granuloma (histiocytosis X), or focal vertebral osteomyelitis (Mehta and Murray, 1977). This type of scoliosis has its convexity on the side opposite the process (Fig. 635)). It is observed especially in children and young adults.

Fractures of the lumbar transverse processes are sometimes difficult to diagnose because they may be obscured by intestinal gas and thus be less conspicuous. *Unilateral* fractures of the transverse processes often give rise to a scoliosis with its convexity on the side of the fracture. The scoliosis is probably caused by insufficiency of the ipsilateral quadratus lumborum muscle, which originates in the (broken-off)

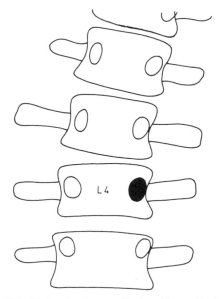

Fig. 635 **Reflex lumbar scoliosis with a pathologic process located eccentrically in the vertebrae** (in the present case osteoid osteoma of the left pedicle of L4; see text; compare Fig. 650).

lumbar transverse processes and also inserts there (Gilsanz et al., 1980; Fig. 636).

The following radiologic studies are necessary in the presence of scoliosis:

1. *Roentgenograms of the spine in two planes,* preferentially including the whole spine and with the patient standing. When the technical facilities for this procedure are lacking, or when the patient is an infant or small child, the roentgenograms are made in dorsal decubitus. In this case, however, at least the pelvic brim and the first thoracic vertebra should be included in the film. For routine follow-ups, the anteroposterior roentgenogram in dorsal decubitus is generally adequate. It is of course essential that already in the initial examination (excepting roentgenograms with the patient standing) a film be taken in dorsal decubitus.

2. A quantitative assessment of the scoliosis is possible by the *roentgenometric techniques of Ferguson and of Cobb* (Fig. 637).

3. To differentiate a *reversible postural scoliosis* from an (initially or very early) *irreversible, fixed structural scoliosis* in infancy and early childhood—hence in the "lying age," an additional stress roentgenogram with the child inclined to the opposite side is made in dorsal decubitus. In this age, the deforming forces of the scoliosis initially affect the intervertebral disks; i.e., those parts of the spine that have not yet ossified; the structural remodeling escapes detection in the conventional anteroposterior roentgenogram. The child should therefore be inclined to the side opposite the scoliosis, and the film should be exposed in this posture. When the scoliosis can be fully corrected, a postural scoliosis is present. In structural scoliosis, correction of the curvature is impeded by muscular contractures, shrinking of the ligaments, and alterations of the intervertebral disks, the vertebral bodies, and the intervertebral joints.

4. An *additional anteroposterior roentgenogram with extension* will show whether traction therapy is still likely to be successful. When the scoliosis does not diminish with extension, traction therapy is not indicated.

Traumatic lateral displacement of the vertebrae is an infrequent finding.

Lateral displacements of vertebrae also occur during the course of **neurogenic spondylopathy** (Fig. 638). The radiographic picture reveals an "anarchic" remodeling (p. 47) of the motor segment involved, that far exceeds the usual consequences of attrition of the intervertebral disks. This finding is typical of neurogenic spondylopathy. Neurogenic osteoarthropathies manifest themselves roentgenologically in two basic manners: osteolysis or Charcot's joint (compare p. 48 ff and Figs. 53 and 54). Figure 638 shows a neurogenic spondylopathy that corresponds to Charcot's joint in the extremities. Bizarre osteophytes, excessive densifications of vertebral cancellous bone as far as so-called ebony vertebra crumbling and disintegration of parts of the vertebra,

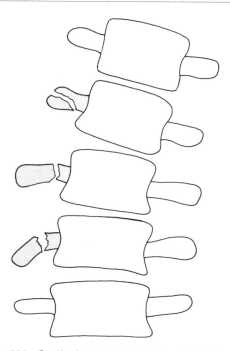

Fig. 636 **Scoliosis accompanying unilateral fracture of transverse processes in the lumbar spine** (see text).

compression of vertebra, *rotary slipping,* and ventral displacement of the vertebra indicate neurogenic damage to the bone and the soft tissues of the vertebral motor segment involved. These alterations develop during the course of months or years, and very infrequently within a few weeks (Feldman et al., 1974). Neurogenic spondylopathy can be the first manifestation of a neurogenic disease of the skeleton!

Nonreactive osteolyses, for example, in the posterior vertebral elements *and* the immediately contiguous ribs (Heyden et al., 1977), are less typical of a neurogenic spondylopathy but should suggest *primarily* Gorham-Stout's massive osteolysis (p. 59)!

Displacement of an Intervertebral Disk (Fig. 606, no. 4)

The normal nucleus pulposus lies like a water cushion between the vertebrae and thus serves the purpose of facilitating segmental mobility. Not being compressible because of its elevated water content, it also carries out bearing and supporting functions. These tasks, however, presuppose that the nucleus pulposus be fixed on all sides by morphologic structures. The annulus fibrosus—which is reinforced anteriorly, anterolaterally, and posteriorly by the two longitudinal ligaments—as well as the cartilaginous and osseous end plates, prevents the nucleus pulposus from moving in any direction. When only one of these restraints gives way, the result is a displacement of the nucleus pulposus in the direction of the damaged

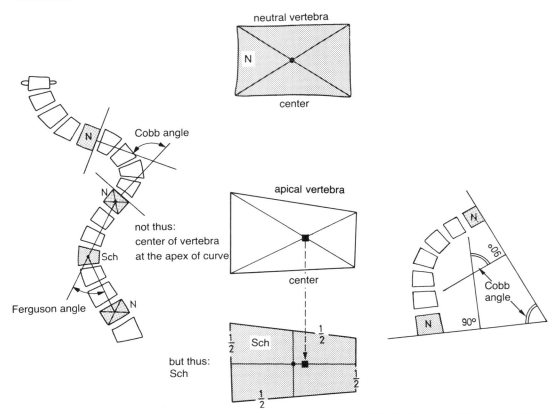

Fig. 637 **Roentgenometry of the scoliotic angle by the methods of J.R. Cobb** *(above left, right)* and A.B. Ferguson *(below left).* Since the two methods produce different scoliotic angles, they cannot be applied alternately!
    Kittleson and Lim (1970) recommended Ferguson's method for scoliotic angles below 50° and Cobb's method for angles above 50°. In follow-up studies, the anteroposterior roentgenograms must *always* be made with the patient standing or *always* with the patient lying down. Both methods start from the **neutral vertebrae** (N). These vertebrae present an approximately parallel projection of the end plates, the greatest inclination with respect to the horizontal line, and the least rotation. After Cobb, perpendiculars are drawn from the inferior end plate of the superior neutral vertebra and from the superior end plate of the inferior neutral vertebra. These perpendiculars intersect, and the complementary angle between them (the scoliotic agle) is measured. For a modification after Luskin (1962) see at the *right.* Ferguson's method starts from the centers of the neutral vertebrae and the center of the vertebrae at the apex of the curve (Sch) (= the vertebra with the most marked wedge shape and/or the strongest rotation). The two lines connecting the three centers form a complementary angle (scoliotic angle).

structure (prolapse or herniation, or its forme fruste: protrusion or bulging disk).

    Anterior prolapse of the disk (Fig. 606, no. 4A) and **lateral prolapse of the disk** following rupture of the annulus fibrosus *and* the anterior longitudinal ligament have no clinical significance, apart from infrequent exceptions (Fig. 639). Even in the roentgenogram, they can be identified only when the displaced part of the disk is calcified. Tears in the anterior and lateral regions of the annulus fibrosus with subsequent displacement of the nucleus have been described as the pathogenetic premise of spondylosis deformans (degenerative vertebral osteophytes), (see under this heading).

    The radiologic picture of separation of the vertebral edge (Niedner, 1932), depicted in Figures 610 D and 640, is of significance in differential diagnosis. This finding is observed primarily in the upper or (less frequently) the lower anterior edge of the vertebra; it occurs with relative frequency in lordotic segments of the spine. In the majority of cases, separation of the ridge reflects a **retromarginal prolapse of the disk** (Fig. 606, no. 4B). In this case, the disk tissue, "exposed to the strain of everyday life" (Schmorl and Junghanns, 1968), makes its way via the more or less solid physiologic connection between the cartilaginous end plate of the vertebra and the bony marginal ridge, following its course. On the other hand, the prolapse may also occur before the bony connection of the marginal ridge and the verte-

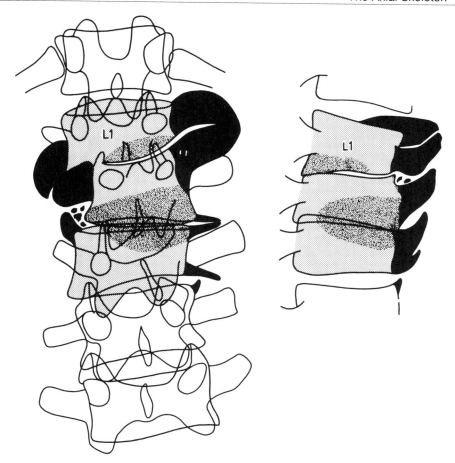

Fig. 638. **Advanced neurogenic spondylopathy** (in tabes dorsalis; the same condition has been observed, for example, with diabetes mellitus, with congenital analgesia and, in the cervical spine, with syringomyelia). A typical feature of neurogenic spondylopathy is the "anarchic" association of fracturelike collapse of the vertebrae (which concomitantly show increased density [sclerosis]) with coarse bony outgrowths. Involvement of the soft tissues is manifested by narrowing or disappearance of the disk space and vertebral displacement (L1 has slipped to the right without a rotary component and L3 presents typical rotary slipping to the right).

(The darker the shade, the denser [more sclerotic] the bone substance.)

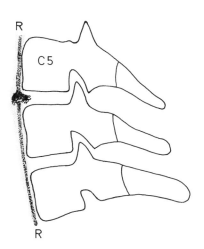

Fig. 639 **Calcified anterior prolapse of the nucleus pulposus C5/C6.** Only the calcification renders the prolapse *directly* visible in the roentgenogram. The circumscribed increase in width of the retropharyngeal space (R) at the level of the involved intervertebral disk is also noticeable. The prevertebral fat stripe lies immediately in front of the anterior vertebral contours (compare Fig. 616).

Clinical features: dysphagia and pain on moving the cervical spine.

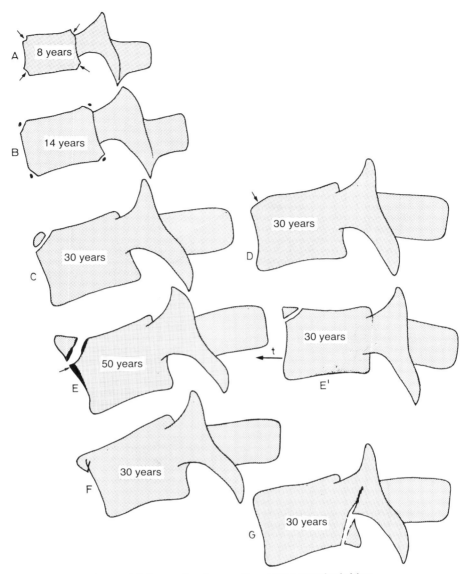

Fig. 640 Radiologic differential diagnosis of separation of the marginal ridge.

A = (Age 8) Appropriately for age, ossification of the marginal vertebral ridge still absent *(arrows)*

B = (Age 14) Physiologic ossification centers in the marginal ridge.

C = (Age 30) Persistent ossification center in the marginal ridge more probable than retromarginal prolapse of disk (no displacement of marginal ridge; smooth contours).

D = (Age 30) Defect of marginal ridge (disturbed ossification of marginal ridge at the upper edge of the vertebral body; *arrow*). This finding occurs most frequently in the cervical spine, either in the setting of Scheuermann's disease or as an idiopathic developmental disorder.

E = (Age 50) Typical radiographic appearance of an "older" separation of the marginal ridge through retromarginal prolapse of the disk (marginal ridge often slightly rotated upward and usually displaced forward; "gaping" cleft between vertebral body and marginal ridge; partially increased density of contours in this area; periosteal lamella *(arrow)*.

E' = (Age 30) This case also presents a slight elevation and rotation of the vertebral edge which has been separated by the prolapse. *Arrow* between E and E' (t = time) indicates that, with time, the separated vertebral edge may not only undergo deformations and sclerosis, but sometimes the separated vertebral ridge may be further displaced.

F = (Age 30) (Hyper-) flexion type of fracture with typical projection; wedge-shaped compression of vertebral body.

G = (Age 30) Posteroinferior separation of the ridge of vertebral body. The radiologic differential diagnosis in this case is fracture (extension type of fracture after fall on the buttocks), because the fracture cleft extends into the vertebral arch. However, *without* an adequate history suggesting the extension mechanism of the injury and without other findings of fracture (e.g., extension of the cleft into the vertebral arch), dorsal retromarginal prolapse of the disk or persistence of the posterior marginal ridge are the more likely initial diagnoses (compare Fig. 678).

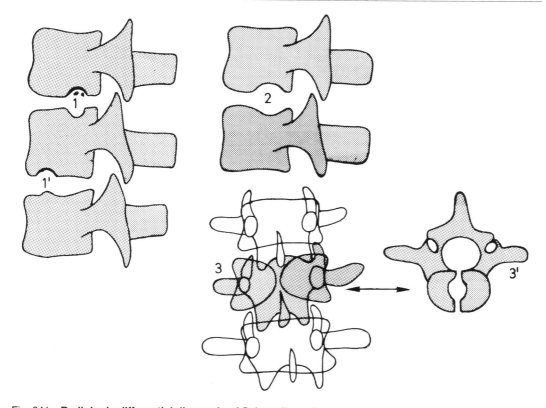

Fig. 641   **Radiologic differential diagnosis of Schmorl's node.**
1, 1′ = Schmorl's node (with or without the Edgren-Vaino sign; see Figs. 609 and 610).
2 = Radiologic aspect of persistent notochord.
3,3′ = Butterfly-shaped vertebra with typical indentation of the *enlarged* vertebral body. *Morphologic gene-sis:* Sagittal cleft of the vertebral body by which the persistent notochord is invaginated (3′).

bral body has become established. The *bony* marginal ridge (the annular apophysis of the vertebral body) can be demonstrated roentgenologically from the second half of the first decade onward. Its fusion with the vertebral body at the different levels of the spine takes place gradually until the completion of growth. Separation of the edge is occasionally visible in several contiguous (lumbar) vertebrae. That is why some speak of persistent vertebral apophyses or this pathogenesis is accepted generally for every separation of vertebral edges. However, the investigations by Niedner (1932) have definitely led to this theory being discarded. Incidentally, the marginal ridge is not responsible for the longitudinal growth of the vertebral body. It is therefore only a secondary ossification center, an apophysis.

Separation of the anterior vertebral ridge is usually not accompanied by complaints. On the other hand, it has acquired clinical significance for two reasons:

1. The loss in mass of the nucleus pulposus *can* lead to a loss in volume of the intervertebral disk owing to the partial retromarginal displacement of the nucleus. The spondyloretrolisthesis described on page 418 ff then develops with all its implications (Fig. 632 A and B).

2. The separation of the vertebral edge is misinterpreted as a sequel to trauma. This erroneous diagnosis is avoided by accurate analysis of the roentgen finding. Retromarginal herniation of the nucleus pulposus at the anterosuperior edge of the vertebra usually leads to *slight elevation* of the separated portion of the marginal ridge. The line of demarcation between the marginal ridge and the vertebral body *is gaping*. The anterosuperior edge of the vertebra, however, is characteristically deformed by the (hyper-) flexion type of fracture with unrestrained mobility at the moment of the trauma:

A. The fracture mechanism forces the broken-off anterior edge into the vertebral body with the subsequent development of a projection (so-called "oriel" [Figs. 608 and 640]). An adequate flexion type of trauma at the time when the marginal ridge has ossified but has not yet fused with the vertebral body gives rise to the development of repair osteophytes on the anterior edge of the vertebra (Keller, 1974).

B. The (hyper-) flexion type of trauma produces a more or less pronounced wedge shape of the vertebra.

The classic **intracancellous prolapsed disk** (Fig. 606, no. 4C) is **Schmorl's node** (Figs. 609, 610, and 641). Like any prolapse of the nucleus pulposus, its development is linked to two premises: *first,* preservation of the explosive force (turgor) of the nucleus pulposus, and *second,* diminished resistance or defects of continuity of the structures that fix the nucleus.[31] Among such "weak spots" are cicatrized gaps for the penetrating vessels, outpouchings at the previous points of exit of the notochord, lumpy foci of necrotic destruction, and finally ontogenic breaks of the fibrous lamellae in the cartilaginous end plates with preservation of their chondrocytes and matrix (Aufdermaur, 1965). Schmorl's nodes occur with particular frequency during the course of Scheuermann's disease (Figs. 609 and 610). These nodes, developing after the completion of growth—i.e., beyond the typical "Scheuermann age"—should always arouse suspicion that malignant metastases, an inflammatory process, or a metabolic disease of the skeleton such as hyperparathyroidism (Resnick and Niwayama, 1978 a) has led to circumscribed resorption of the cancellous bone, beneath a *normal* cartilaginous end plate. The end plate then becomes undermined; it gives way under normal strain and can collapse in these places. Intervertebral disk tissue then penetrates the vertebral body.

Schmorl's nodes usually become visible in the roentgenogram only by their calcification and/or by the reaction of the vertebral cancellous bone, which responds to the collapse by forming a marginal bony shell. This explains why 38 percent of autopsied spines show at least one Schmorl's nodule whereas radiologic studies reveal this deformity in only 13.5 percent (Schmorl, 1928; Schmorl and Junghanns, 1968).

Traumatic damage to the cartilaginous and bony end plates also may force parts of the disk into the vertebral body (so-called traumatic Schmorl's node). For the differential diagnosis between Schmorl's node and (partially) persistent notochord see Figure 641.

The greatest clincial importance is attached to *dorsal displacement of the disk* (Fig. 606, no. 4 D). This may take place either *posteromedially* into the spinal canal or posterolaterally into the intervertebral foramen. Depending on the degree of the displacement, a distinction is made between **dorsal protrusion** and **dorsal prolapse** of the disk. The displaced disk tissue consists of parts of the nucleus pulposus, often also of parts of the annulus fibrosus, and even parts of the cartilaginous end plates. Prolapsed disk is observed most frequently in the lower lumbar spine, where the prolapsed disk acts as a space-occupying process. Posteromedial displacement in the lumbar region gives rise to compression of the cauda equina—though only after reaching a considerable size. In the cervical spine, such displacements produce a chronic cervical myelopathy.[32] A prolapsed disk in the region of the intervertebral foramen may give rise to manifestations of radicular irritation and segmental neurologic defects.

Preliminary conditions for posterior displacement (prolapse) of disk tissue are dorsal tears in the annulus fibrosus—signs of attrition of the disk and, very infrequently, the consequences of a single trauma—*and* a nucleus pulposus that is not completely desiccated and therefore still possesses turgor. The peak incidence of prolapsed lumbar disks associated with complaints therefore lies in the third decade of life (Weber, 1950). The preserved capacity for swelling and the explosive power of the nucleus pulposus (see above) are the chief factors in (dorsal) displacement of parts of the disk. The morphologic prerequisites to protrusion are anomalous extensibility of the annulus fibrosus and smaller tears in this restraining structure (see p. 421).

The symptomatology and the results of clinico-neurologic examination allow, in the majority of cases, diagnosis of a posterior prolapse of the disk. Nevertheless, a plain roentgenogram of the spinal segment and preoperative myelography cannot be dispensed with. The last-named method of investigation will not be taken up in this book. It should, however, be mentioned that myelography is indicated for differentiating between protrusion and prolapse, for accurate preoperative localization of a prolapsed disk, for demonstration of displaced disks in several motor segments, and, finally, for reasons of differential diagnosis.

On page 8 it was pointed out, however, that functional roentgenograms of the lumbar spine (Figs. 9 to 12) also may contribute to the general displacement of the lumbar disks and identification of the level of the lesion. Computed tomography has now entered into competition with myelography and possibly will replace it entirely! CT not only displays the herniated disk but also can depict the congenital or acquired stenosis of the spinal canal by measuring (Dihlmann, 1984).

---

[31] Displacement of the nucleus pulposus undoubtedly precedes the prolapse of the disk. The nucleus squeezes itself through its "burst restraints" (annulus fibrosus, longitudinal ligament, cartilaginous and bony end plate) and can take parts of these structures with it. In addition, the displaced nucleus pulposus—now as Schmorl's nodule—incites a reactive cartilaginous metaplasia in its bed in the vertebra (therefore the term "cartilage node" coined by Schmorl in 1928), as well as the formation of new bone (the shell of Schmorl's node). Histologically, prolapse of the nucleus pulposus does not consist only of nucleus pulposus tissue. Prolapse of the nucleus pulposus and prolapsed disk are therefore synonyms.

---

[32] The manifestations of radicular irritation and deficits as well as "medullary" symptoms (produced by compression of the cauda equina and the spinal cord) have the character of syndromes. They may point to prolapsed disk but they also may be due to a variety of other affections. These problems of differential diagnosis especially concern the neurologist. In any case, the radiologic examination may not only ensure the diagnosis of prolapsed disk but may also reveal different, possibly additional, causes for stenosis of the spinal canal and narrowing of the intervertebral foramen. Figs. 643 and 644).

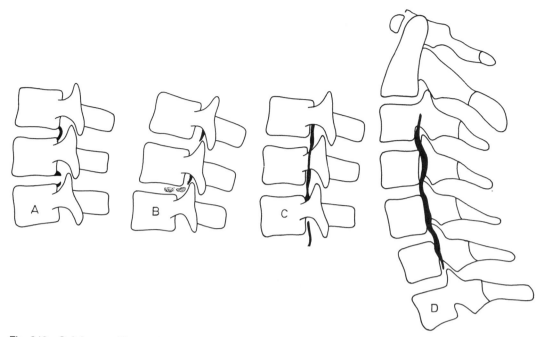

Fig. 642   **Calcium and bone shadows on the anterior aspect of the spinal canal.**
A = Bony spurs, hooks, and ledges on the posterior edges of the vertebrae may be indicative of an "older" dorsal displacement of the disk.

B = Only a calcified dorsal prolapse of the nucleus pulposus is demonstrable in the plain roentgenogram (in the lowest motor segment of this sketch, also accompanied there by spondyloretrolisthesis; see Fig. 632 B). In addition, a partial ossification of the ligamentum flavum with an otherwise normal spine (Voss, 1972) has been illustrated. This finding is usually observed in the thoracicolumbar spine, and much less frequently in the cervical spine (Polgár, 1929; Kamakura et al., 1979). Ossifications of the ligamentum flavum also occur in advanced ankylosing spondylitis.

C, D = Extensive ossification of the posterior longitudinal ligament. Such ligamentous ossification develops, for example, following injuries, in hyperostotic spondylosis, during the course of ankylosing spondylitis, and in endemic or industrial fluorosis (Singh et al., 1962). Still more frequently the cause is undetermined; e.g., in Japan, where ossification of the posterior longitudinal ligament has been encountered among 17% of patients with cervical symptoms (Onji et al., 1967). Such ligamentous ossifications are most often observed in the cervical spine. They occur less frequently in the lumbar and the thoracic spine (Hiramatsu and Nobechi, 1971). Ligamentous ossifications may reach a thickness of 5 mm; they may restrict mobility, depending on their extension. Their course is either asymptomatic or may be accompanied by neurologic defects; for example, as the result of cord compression with the symptoms of a cervical myelopathy.

Suspicion of the presence of an older dorsal displacement of a disk—"older" is used here in contrast to "acute"—is aroused by the development of spurs or hooks on the posterior edges of the vertebral bodies ("sciatic hooks" in the literature of the English-speaking countries; Fig. 642). On lateral roentgenograms, the displacement is projected into the intervertebral foramen. Calcified sequestra of the disk, which have been displaced dorsally, are also demonstrable in a plain roentgenogram.

A *decrease in disk height and spondyloretrolisthesis* also occur in dorsal prolapse of the disk. These manifestations are general signs of a loss in substance of the disk and therefore may also accompany a major prolapse. Dorsal displacement of the disk may be the cause of a correctable postural scoliosis which often has a rotary component. Radicular sciatica, for instance, may give rise to an antaligic scoliosis that relieves the spine of weight; the convexity of the scoliosis lies either on the painful or on the pain-free side, and it even may alternate between the two sides.

In connection with the discussion of the dorsally prolapsed disk, mention should be made once more of the *dorsal gaping of a disk space* and of the *monosegmental extended position* (Fig. 607). These roentgen findings are indicative of a *segmental obstruction of motion*. The latter is produced either by a posteromedial (posterolateral) displacement of the disk (protrusion, prolapse), by other space-occupying processes in the spinal canal and the intervertebral foramen, *or* they develop by reflex as a result of the entrapment of capsular tissue (larger villi, meniscoids) in the intervertebral joint. Finally, loose bodies in the osteoarthrotic intervertebral joint can give

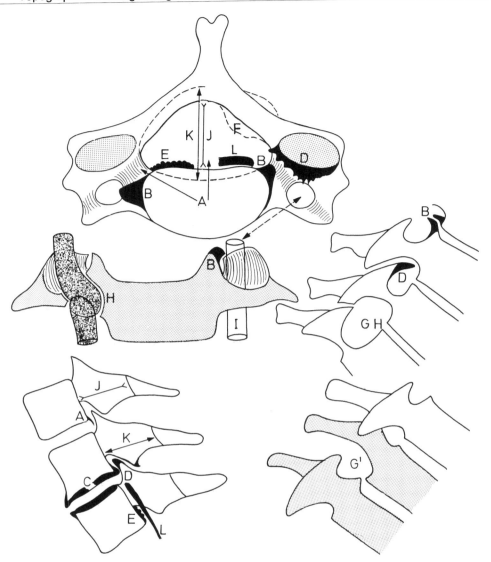

Fig. 643 **Roentgenologically identifiable causes of narrowing or widening of the cervical spinal canal and the intervertebral foramina.** The majority of the pathologic findings discussed here occur also in the thoracic and lumbar spine (compare Fig. 644).

A = Posteromedial and posterolateral disk displacement (protrusion; prolapse). Direct visibility can be achieved by only myelography or discography, unless a delicate, arched bony shell or a spur indicates an "old" displacement—presumptive diagnosis!—or the sequestrated prolapse is calcified (Fig. 642 A and B).

B = Uncovertebral spondylosis (so-called uncovertebral osteoarthrosis). Depending on its size and location, a radicular symptomatology and/or an impact on the vertebral artery and the vertebral sympathetic plexus is *possible*.

C = Intervertebral osteochondrosis with spondyloretrolisthesis and ventral as well as dorsal apposition of a vertebral osteophyte.

D = Apophyseal joint osteoarthrosis (compare Figs. 627, 686, and 687).

E = Development of malignant osteophytes (Fig. 697), illustrated only in the posterior surface of the vertebral body. Theoretically, such osteophytes may develop wherever tumor cells have originated or metastasized in and underneath the periosteum. To be differentiated roentgenologically from chronic fluorosis (see p. 72 ff), which not only produces ossification of ligamentous insertions and entire ligaments but also leads to increased density of the (vertebral) cancellous bone.

F = Bulging or protrusion of the vertebral arch (also applicable to the vertebral body) in Paget's disease of bone, following fractures, in tumors, in acromegaly (Gelman, 1974) and in (chronic) osteomyelitis.

G = Widening of the intervertebral foramen by a slowly growing tumor of the soft tissues (so-called hour-

rise to such faulty positions. Another etiologic factor may be an injury with its impact on the disk and the intervertebral joint. Only *one* of the paired small intervertebral joints is usually involved.

When the cervical spine is concerned *(vide infra)*, the monosegmental extension or the dorsal gaping of the disk space is associated with a rotary malposition (rotary dislocation or rotary subluxation) of the superior vertebra in the segment involved. *The rotary dislocation is demonstrable chiefly by the migration of the cervical spinous process to the side of the triggering intervertebral joint* (Fig. 617). The caudal articular process of the superior vertebra in the involved segment slips anterosuperiorly upon the superior articular process of the next vertebra underneath it. A lateral roentgenogram shows this finding, which additionally is accompanied by an increase in height of the corresponding intervertebral foramen and by double contours of the vertebral body. This cannot always be recognized with certainty in the roentgenogram. It is, however, noticeable that the radiographic joint space in the rotated motor segment is no longer visible, as compared with the superior and inferior intervertebral joints (Fig. 617). The roentgenologic diagnosis of rotary dislocation at the occipitocervical junction, however, is subject to a number of fundamental prerequisites:

1. Any rotation of head and neck must be avoided in positioning the patient for an anteroposterior roentgenogram. In the presence of torticollis, this premise should also be met as far as possible!
2. Even when prerequisite number 1 has been fulfilled, an inadequate position of the atlas and axis[33] with respect to the actual normal attitude of the head is recognizable (Gutmann, 1969; Fig. 645; compare also Fig. 7).
3. One must answer the question of whether "constructional defects" are present; for example, those following congenital asymmetries and/or acquired

---

[33] The occipitocervical junction and the other segments of the cervical spine are those spinal segments in which a radiograph taken in the normal posture already reveals an inadequate position of vertebrae. This is not true for the lumbar spine, for there the vertebrae become interlocked by the shape and position of the articular processes. With *normal* morphology of the vertebrae (i.e., in the absence of malformations or destructions of the articular processes and the interarticular portions of the vertebral arch) reflex deviation of a *single* lumbar vertebra through rotation around its craniocaudal axis is impossible. In addition, functional roentgenograms of the spine have revealed that, in the cervical region, malpositions of vertebrae fixed by reflex (obstruction) usually occur in the end position of possible motion, and therefore alone are particularly conspicuous. In contrast, blocking of lumbar vertebrae often takes place in the intermediate position of the joint so that, in the plain roentgenogram, visible malpositions such as dorsal gaping of the disk space are less frequent there, as compared with the cervical spine.

---

glass tumor; e.g., neurofibroma, meningioma, fibroma, lipoma, herniated meningocele), but also observed in malignant tumors and their metastases. Cervical chordoma *(roentgenologic triad:* vertebral osteolysis; shadow in the perivertebral soft tissues with and without calcifications; destruction of disk) may also lead to widening of the foramen (Hagenlocher and Ciba, 1976). This condition must be differentiated from infectious spondylitis with abscess formation (Firooznia et al., 1976). In the oblique view, congenital absence of a cervical pedicle with the corresponding half of the vertebral arch (G') mimics widening of the pertinent intervertebral foramen (Wilson and Norrell Jr., 1966).

H = Erosion of the vertebra, often with widening of the intervertebral foramen (Barrat, 1974) by circumscribed elongation and torsion or by aneurysm of the vertebral artery.

I = Normal course of the vertebral artery.

J = Constitutionally *shortened* sagittal diameter of the spinal canal (C2–C7≦15mm; C1≦20 mm; focal distance 150 cm). Such shortening, though primarily of the lumbar vertebral arches, also occurs, for example, in achondroplasia. When the sagittal diameter is constitutionally shortened, any additional anrrowing—caused, for instance, by dorsal vertebral osteophytes, ossification of the posterior longitudinal ligament, or sequelae to trauma—has a particularly unfavorable influence! Clinically recognizable compression of the cord, however, is to be expected only when the roentgenologically measurable sagittal diameter of the cervical spinal canal has been narrowed to ≦10 mm; for example, by a dorsal vertebral osteophyte. Between 11 and 13 mm, cord symptoms are likely to occur; with a sagittal diameter>13 mm their appearance is improbable.

K = *Increased* sagittal diameter of the spinal canal *(measured from the middle of the posterior vertebral contour to the nearest point of the spinous process);* for example, due to pressure atrophy of the vertebral body and/or the base of the spinous process. Such as increase indicates an expansive process of the soft tissues in the spinal canal. Pathologic sagittal diameters are:

C1>33 (♂), >30 mm (♀); C2>29 (♂), >26 mm (♀); C3>25 (♂), >23 mm (♀); C4>24 mm (♂), >22 mm (♀); C5>23 (♂), >22 mm (♀); C6>24 mm (♂), >21 mm (♀); C7>23 (♂), >21 mm (♀); all with a focal distance of 150 cm (Boijsen, 1954). In adults, there is no significant age dependence of the width of the spinal canal (Decking and ter Steege, 1975). In children, the sagittal diameters of the spinal canal are approximately identical with those of adults (Wholey et al., 1958).

L = Ossification of the posterior longitudinal ligament (compare Fig. 642 C and D). Hypertrophy of the ligamentum flavum is not demonstrable in the plain roentgenogram; it occurs especially in elderly individuals but also in patients with acromegaly and is likely to narrow the spinal canal with all the clinical consequences to be expected (Beamer et al., 1973; Gelman, 1974; Epstein et al., 1977). In computed tomographs, however, the lumbar ligamentum flavum, its normal configuration, and fibrotic thickening (so-called hypertrophy) are recognizable (Lackner and Schroeder, 1980). The normal thickness of the ligamentum flavum measured in autopsy specimens is between 2 and 4 mm (mean value 2.8 mm). (Dockerty and Love, 1940).

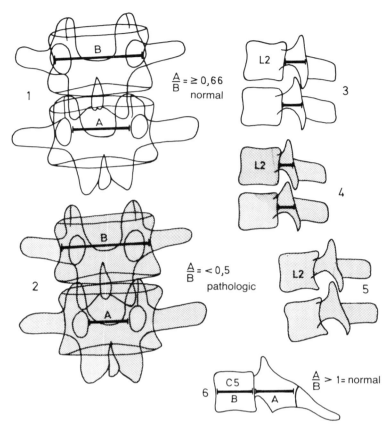

$\frac{A}{B} = \geq 0,66$
normal

$\frac{A}{B} = < 0,5$
pathologic

$\frac{A}{B} > 1 =$ normal

Fig. 644 Roentgenographic diagnosis of stenosis of the spinal canal (1 to 4; 6) and of pathologic dorsal excavation of vertebrae (5). (Compare Fig. 643.)

1 = Measuring technique after Babin et al., 1977. The interpedicular distance in the *lumbar* spine (A) is at least two thirds of the transverse diameter of the vertebra at its narrowest point (B). *(For the sake of clarity, the lines A and B are illustrated in two different vertebrae).*

2 = When A is less than half of B, suspicion that the transverse diameter of the *lumbar* spinal canal is narrowed seems justified.

3 = Radiographic appearance of the normal sagittal diameter in the region of the *lumbar* spinal canal. In *computed tomographs,* stenosis of the lumbar canal can be diagnosed when its sagittal diameter is below 11 to 12 mm, when the interpedicular distance is less than 16 mm, and/or the surface of the lumbar spinal canal amounts to less than 1.45 cm² (Ullrich et al., 1980). *Technical premises of measurement:* Maximal possible correction of lumbar lordosis by positioning the patient with the knee joints flexed; Gantry tilting so that the projection plane is perpendicular to the longitudinal axis of the lumbar spinal canal.

4 = Reduced lumbar sagittal diameter by short pedicles. (Nos. 4 and 5 jointly also in achondroplasia.)

5 = Pathologic dorsal excavation of a vertebra ("scalloping" in the literature of the English-speaking countries).

This finding is encountered (Mitchell et al. 1967):

a) *Localized,* in *slowly* growing, *larger* intraspinal tumors or cysts, in syringomyelia, hydromyelia, extradural gouty tophi (Wald et al., 1979).

b) *Generalized,* in communicating hydrocephalus.

c) In Marfan's syndrome, Ehlers-Danlos' syndrome, and von Recklinghausen's neurofibromatosis.

d) In achondroplasia, Hurler's type I mucopolysaccharidosis, and Morquio's type IV muscopolysaccharidosis.

e) In acromegaly (Bluestone et al., 1971; Baldauf, 1976). An (incidentally detected) "scalloping" therefore prompts additional clinical and roentgenologic studies!

6 = There is suspicion of constitutional narrowing of the *cervical* spinal canal when the quotient of the sagittal diameter of the spinal canal (A) divided by the anteroposterior diameter of the vertebral body (B) is smaller than 1 (normally, it is greater than 1). (Ritter et al., 1975).

Fig. 645　Malpositions of the atlas.

A = Isolated position of atlas, inadequate to the actual normal posture of the head during radiologic examination (rotation to the left; compare Fig. 7, no. 2, 2'; no clue to occipitocervical developmental disturbance; transoral view). *Clinically:* Spontaneous occurrence of painful limitation of motion.

B, C = *Atlas superior* and *atlas inferior*. These malpositions have *no clinical significance* without considering malpositions in the immediate vicinity (anteroposterior view) and without testing mobility by functional roentgenograms with anteflexion and retroflexion. (*Question:* Normal mobility, hypermobility, immobility, partial mobility of the atlas in the superior position?) (Gutmann, 1960.)

Note: In B the spinolaminar line (compare Fig. 616) is absent in the anterior arch of the atlas. This finding is characteristic of a dorsal cleft in the arch of the atlas or an osteolysis in this location.

C = Free projection of the joint space of the intervertebral joints between the axis and C3. Normally this is not the case (compare B and Fig. 617). This finding arouses suspicion of a malposition of the axis.

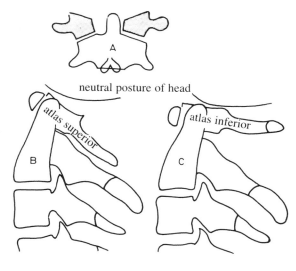

neutral posture of head

disturbances of contours and/or structure (inflammation, osteoarthrosis, tumor, traumatic deformation, etc.) in the morphologic parts accessible to appraisal! Malformations in the occipitocervical junction can mimic malpositions or, as primary asymmetries, can favor the development of malpositions. When the answer to this question is positive or, when reading the roentgenogram, only suspicion is aroused, tomographs should be taken (with consideration of prerequisite number 1).

4. Any identified malposition must also be assessed from the functional point of view with the use of subsequent functional roentgenograms.

The identification, evaluation, and clinical classification of malpositions in the occipitocervical junction and in the remaining cervical spine is therefore closely linked to roentgenometry of this region.

Roentgenometry of the Occipitocervical Junction (Fig. 606, no. 5) and the Spine (Fig. 606, no. 6)

Roentgenometry of the occipitocervical junction and the other spinal segments provides quantitative information that both reveals pathologic alterations as such and indicates the extent of previously diagnosed disorders.

In the occipitocervical junction, congenital as well as acquired malformations and malpositions occur which, in about two thirds of patients, are associated with symptoms on the part of the upper cervical cord and the upper cervical roots, the medulla, the cerebellum, and the 9th to 12th cranial nerves (Dieckmann, 1970). The significance of this statistic for the

individual patient is as follows: Individuals with (1) a short neck, unilateral elevation of the scapula, scoliosis, kyphosis, or similar constitutional anomalies and (2) impairment of head mobility, who additionally (3) complain of pain in the back of the head and the occiput, dizziness, and disturbances of equilibrium, should be subjected to radiologic studies (survey film, tomography) of the occipitocervical junction. This region (occiput, atlas, axis) shows a *developmental lability* that manifests itself by disordered segmentation, dysplasia or apalsia of the individual elements, and a multiple combination of dysrhaphic disorders. Tomography and roentgenometry are indispensable for the accuracte classification of these malformations.

Residues of the phylogenetic segmentation and manifestations of the occipital vertebra are reproduced in Table 5 and in Figure 646. In these cases, additional roentgenograms of the base of the skull should not be omitted, since one might overlook a narrowing of the foramen magnum by an occipital vertebra. Computed tomography of the foramen magnum will also give supplementary information.

Roentgenometric studies have acquired particular importance in the diagnosis of **basilar impression** and **condylar hypoplasia**. In basilar impression, the developmental disorder of the occipital bone leads to an apparent funnel-shaped herniation of the surrounding bones into the foramen magnum. A *genuine* herniation is present in *secondary* basilar impression produced, for instance, by osteomalacia, Paget's disease of bone, hyperparathyroidism, or as a result of bone destruction or inflammation in the vicinity of the foramen magnum. A distinction is made between *anterior basilar impression* by a hypoplastic basioccipital bone (basilar part and clivus) with shortening of the clivus, diminished descent of the thinned basiooccipotal bone, or horizontal orientation of the

Table 5 Residues of phylogenetic segmentation and manifestations of the occipital vertebra (von Torklus and Gehle, 1975). The atlas is not the first but the fifth or sixth primary vertebra. The basioccipital bone develops from fusion of four or five vertebral primordia. The proatlas is the occipital vertebra located above the atlas. A complete occipital vertebra has so far not been observed in the human. Beyond this, however, the occipitocervical junction is a virtually inexhaustible source of malformations!

	In the basiooccipital bone	Basilar transverse cleft (cleft formation in clivus). To be differentiated from sphenooccipital suture, which closes as late as the 12th year of life. Further differentiation from craniopharyngeal (basiopharyngeal) canal. Divided hypoglossal canal. (The hypoglossal canal corresponds to the intervertebral foramen.)
	In the marginal zone of the foramen magnum (ridges, projections, humps)	Arcus praebasiooccipitalis (anterior, paramedian). Condylus tertius (anterior, median, compact, possibly articulating with C1 or C2). Processus basilares (anterior, paramedian). Dystopic os odontoideum (anterior, superior, in the basio—occipital bone). Labia of foramen magnum (posterior, paramedian).
Residues of phylogenetic segmentation and manifestations of the occipital vertebra	As atlantooccipital bony projection, interposition, bridge	Processus paracondylicus (originates laterally in the occipital condyle; stubby, passes toward the free end of the transverse process C1). Beware of confusion with the slender styloid process of the temporal bone! Processus epitransversus (originates in the transverse process C1; passes upward; slim). Ponticulus posterior (hook-shaped in the lateral view; originates in the lateral mass; bridges the groove of the vertebral artery; forms the foramen arcuale).
	In the atlas	Ponticulus lateralis (hook-shaped in the anteroposterior view [tomograph]; passes from the lateral mass to the transverse process C1). It bridges the vertebral artery. Posterior part of the bipartite superior articular facets.
	In the dens	Bergmann's ossiculum terminale in the tip of the dens. (The apical center of ossification develops from the body of the proatlas. It fuses before the age of 12. When the physiologic fusion fails to take place, Bergmann's ossicle develops. When the apical center of the dens does not ossify, the dens becomes bicornuate. Os odontoideum in its proper place (no isolated dens but probably hypoplastic dens with os odontoideum). The latter is presumably a malformed ossiculum terminale which, in the absence of fusion and in the presence of a hypoplastic dens, increases autonomously. Differentiation from "acquired os odontoideum" following inflammatory destruction of the dens in early childhood and "hypertrophic" ossiculum terminale by the clinical history. See also Fig. 646

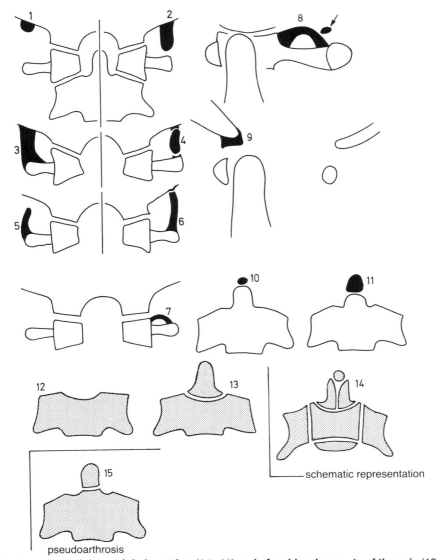

Fig. 646 **Manifestations of the occipital vertebra** (1 to 11) **and of maldevelopments of the axis** (12 to 14).

1 to 4 = Processus paracondylicus.
5, 6 = Processus epitransversus.
7 = Ponticulus lateralis (bridging the vertebral artery).
8 = Foramen arcuale (passage of the vertebral artery) surrounded by the ponticulus posterior.
9 = Condylus tertius (tomograph in the median plane).
10 = Ossiculum terminale and hypoplasia of dens.
11 = Os odontoideum and hypoplasia of dens.

Arrow at 8 points to a small ossicle which also has to be regarded as a manifestation of occipital vertebra (to be differentiated from osseous metaplasia in the ligaments of the occipitocervical junction).

12 = Congenital aplasia or acquired total destruction of the dens from bacterial infection in early childhood.
13 = Persistent intervertebral disk between the body of the atlas (= dens) and the axis.
14 = The axial vertebra has 7 ossification centers (Wackenheim, 1974). Absent fusion and absent ossification account for diverse possible "splits" and deformities.

Note: In **pseudoarthrosis of the dens** (15)—developing at the earliest 3 months after the trauma—the waistline of the dens is preserved. Conversely, the os odontoideum shows no waistline (von Torklus and Gehle, 1975). Both changes are, however, accompanied by ventral and lateral instability (the atlas is movable on the axis). A very uncommon event is the development of a posttraumatic os odontoideum under the following conditions (Fielding and Griffin, 1974): Trauma *in early childhood* (Hawkins et al., 1976); undiagnosed fracture of the dens with subsequent development of a pseudoarthrosis; circulatory disorder of the proximal part of the dens producing a developmental disturbance with formation of an os odontoideum (see Table 5). It is still a matter of debate whether avascular necrosis of the cranial portions of the dens may also be caused by obstruction of the circulation via the ligaments of the tip of the dens (ligamentum apicis dentis; ligamenta alaria). (Tredwell and O'Brien, 1975.)

clivus (platybasia) (Schmidt and Fischer, 1960) on the one hand and *medial (paramedian) basilar impression* on the other. The latter shows a unilateral or bilateral ascent of the lateral portion of the occipital bone toward the foramen magnum; i.e., in the superomedial direction. Moreover, the lateral portion is usually narrowed and thinned; condylar hypolasia may also be present.

Roentgenometric reference lines (Fig. 647) in the survey films lead, as a rule, to the correct diagnosis. However, accurate assessment of the deformations mentioned and their causes (in secondary basilar impression) requires tomographs (with the patient lying on his side for the anterior basilar impression and in dorsal decubitus for the medial basilar

impression). This radiologic examination will also identify the so-called dolichoodontoid ("long dens") and the upward displacement of the dens (in rheumatoid arthritis; see Fig. 709). Both deformities may lead to crossing of the reference lines in Figures 647 C and D.

Condylar hypoplasia—either in the setting of basilar impression or as a solitary unilateral or bilateral finding—may be identified most confidently in tomographs. It can be demonstrated indirectly with use of the angle of the articular axis (Schmidt and Fischer, 1960), also called the *condylar angle* (Fig. 647).

Assimilation of the atlas is the term applied to the bony connection of the entire atlas or parts of it

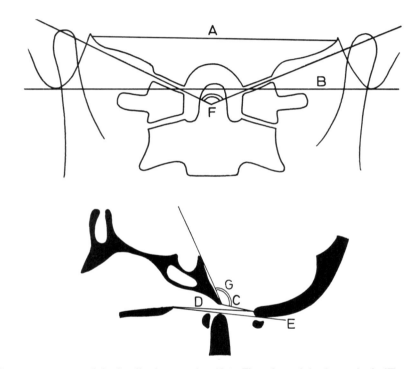

Fig. 647   **Roentgenometry of the basilar impression (A to E) and condylar hypoplasia (F).**
A = *Biventer line* (digastric line) connects the two grooves medial to the mastoids. Normally it is not crossed by the tip of the dens.
B = *Bimastoid line* connects tips of two mastoids. Normally, tip of dens surmounts this line by maximally 10 mm.
C = *Foramen magnum line* (McRae line) from the anterior border (basion) to the posterior border (opisthion) of the foramen magnum. Normally is not crossed by tip of dens.
D = *Palatooccipital line* (Chamberlain line) from the posterosuperior border of the hard palate to the posterior border of the foramen magnum. Tip of dens usually lies close beneath this line (= 1mm ± 3.6 mm).
E = *Palatosuboccipital line* (McGregor line) passes from posterosuperior border of hard palate to lowest point of squama occipitalis. Tip of the dens should not surmount this line by more than 5 mm.
F = *Angle of axis of the atlantoccipital joint (condylar angle;* Schmidt and Fischer, 1960) is normally about 125°. Condylar hypoplasia leads to a change of the angle. With symmetrical structure of the condyles, the intersection of the angle lies approximately in the center of the dens; otherwise it migrates laterally. The angle is determined by tomography.
G = *Boogard's angle* (between the plane of the clivus and the plane of the foramen magnum), normally between 120° and 130°.
For the *intervestibular line* (Wackenheim, 1974) see Fig. 8.

Fig. 648 **Pathologic segmentations of the condyles, the atlas, and the axis and vertebralization of the right occipital condyle** (*schematically* as observed by Schmidt and Fischer, 1960; von Torklus and Gehle, 1970; Wackenheim, 1974).

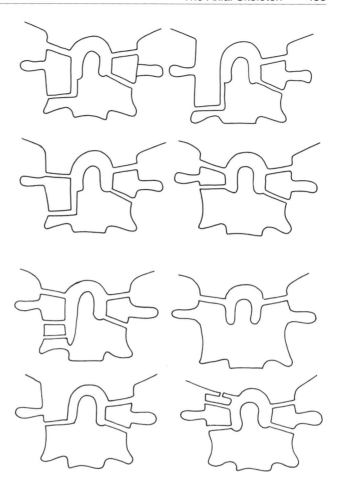

with the occipital bone. This anomaly, much like all the disorders described so far, belongs to the group of the **occipital dysplasias.** However, atlantooccipital fusion may also occur as the result of an inflammatory destruction of the antlantooccipital joints. One of the sequelae of assimilation of the atlas is the ventral dislocation of this vertebra (pp. 5 and 6; Fig. 5).

Among **suboccipital dysplasias** have been observed: Complete or partial aplasia of the arch of the atlas, clefts of the arch of the atlas, dorsal cleft of the spinous process of the axis, dysplasia and aplasia of the dens, fusion of the atlas with the axis (Fig. 648), asymmetrical unilateral segmentations of atlas and axis, and fusion of C2 with C3. The unilateral disorders of segmentation of the atlas and axis—which also may involve the occipital condyles (Fig. 648)—are accompanied by unilateral displacement of the joints superiorly or inferiorly. Since the paired joints between C1 and C2 then no longer lie at the same level but are displaced by the height of a half segment, disorders of motion inevitably result. The location of the displaced joints is approximately horizontal, and their mobility is thereby additionally

impaired. A frequent accompaniment of disordered segmentation of C1/C2 is dysplasia of the dens; for example, bicornuate dens and coarsening of the dens. Aplasia of the dens has been observed in fusion of C1 and C2. The Klippel-Feil syndrome (Fig. 662) (congenital fusion of cervical vertebrae, typical short neck, lowering of the hairline in the back of the head) is the extreme case of disordered segmentation of the upper spine (compare the legend to Fig. 662).

For roentgenometry of the diameter of the spinal canal at its different levels see Figures 643, 644, and 649 and Table 6.

The distinct demonstration of the pedicles of the lumbar and thoracic vertebral arches in the anteroposterior roentgenogram sometimes allows diagnoses of a space-occupying process by recognizing a change in shape of the pedicles without measuring the distance between them. Moreover, it is a well-known fact that the pedicles frequently are the site of hematogenous metastases which produce their partial or complete "obliteration" (Fig. 650).

For the *distance between atlas and dens,* its normal values and the causes and hazards of its increase,

Table 6
A = **normal relationships of the interpedicular distances between two adjacent vertebrae**
(Lindren, 1954).
Examples for application: the interpedicular distance Th 3 can be up to 2 mm greater, equally great, or 1 mm less than the interpedicular distance Th 4; the interpedicular distance at Th 11 is between 2 and 5 mm less than at Th 12; the interpedicular distance at L3 is as great as or up to 3 mm less than the interpedicular distance L4.
B = **Normal relationships of the cervical sagittal diameter of the spinal canal between neighboring cervical vertebrae** (Boijsen, 1954).
Example for application: The sagittal diameter of the spinal canal in lateral roentgenograms at the level of C3 is still normal if it is 1 mm less, equally great, or up to 5 mm greater than that at C4.
Any disturbance of the normal relationships arouses suspicion of a space-occupying process extending in height along one or two vertebrae!

A

C4 $_{2\,mm\,<}^{2\,mm\,>}$ C5
5 $_{2\,mm\,<}^{2\,mm\,>}$ 6
6 $_{3\,mm\,<}^{3\,mm\,>}$ 7
7 $_{3\,mm\,<}^{5\,mm\,>}$ Th1
Th1 $_{1\,mm\,<}^{4\,mm\,>}$ 2
2 $_{1\,mm<}^{3\,mm\,>}$ 3
3 $_{1\,mm\,<}^{2\,mm\,>}$ 4
4 $_{0\,mm\,<}^{2\,mm\,>}$ 5
5 $_{1\,mm\,<}^{1\,mm\,>}$ 6
6 $_{1\,mm\,<}^{1\,mm\,>}$ 7
7 $_{1\,mm\,<}^{1\,mm\,>}$ 8
8 $_{2\,mm\,<}^{0\,mm\,>}$ 9
9 $_{3\,mm\,<}^{0\,mm\,>}$ 10
10 $_{3\,mm\,<}^{0\,mm\,>}$ 11
11 $_{5\,mm\,<}^{2\,mm\,>}$ 12
12 $_{4\,mm\,<}^{1\,mm\,>}$ L1
L1 $_{3\,mm\,<}^{0\,mm\,>}$ 2
2 $_{3\,mm\,<}^{0\,mm\,>}$ 3
3 $_{3\,mm\,<}^{0\,mm\,>}$ 4
4 $_{5\,mm\,<}^{0\,mm\,>}$ 5

B

C1 $_{<2\,mm}^{9\,mm\,>}$ C2
C2 $_{<1\,mm}^{8\,mm\,>}$ C3
C3 $_{<1\,mm}^{5\,mm\,>}$ C4
C4 $_{<2\,mm}^{2\,mm\,>}$ C5
C5 $_{<2\,mm}^{2\,mm\,>}$ C6
C6 $_{<4\,mm}^{3\,mm\,>}$ C7

Fig. 649 **Roentgenometry of the interpedicular distances (transverse diameter of the spinal canal) in children and adults** (values as indicated by Elsberg and Dyke, 1934; Schwarz, 1956). The *upper* limits of the interpedicular distances are reproduced. The *absolute* values obtained by this method are of less importance because their determination is subject to certain factors of uncertainty (focus–film distance used by Elsberg and Dyke = 76 cm; and that used by Schwarz = 91 or 102 cm; individually variable object–film distance, dependent on state of nutrition; correction of kyphosis and lordosis in positioning the patient; errors in determining the minimum interpedicular distance, etc.). As a relative method the course of the values measured is compared with the age related standard scale. Abrupt variations (increased interpedicular distances) of the actual from the theoretical curve or curves directed against the normal direction indicate a (benign) expansive, intra- or extradural space-occupying process with high probability. (*Exceptions:* At the apex of a kyphosis, the pedicles are frequently hypoplastic. With a torsion scoliosis, the measured values become increasingly inaccurate, depending on the degree of the postural defect).

Fig. 650   **Qualitative assessment of the pedicles and the articular processes in anteroposterior roentgenograms of the thoracic and lumbar spine.**

A = Normal projection of the pedicles.

B = Pedicles that are thinned and flattened on the medial aspect or are medially concave raise well-founded suspicion of a space-occupying process in the spinal canal.

C = Complete "obliteration" of a pedicle by an osteolytic process. Differential diagnosis from unilateral aplasia of the pedicle (Bardsley and Hanelin, 1971). With hypoplasia, dysplasia or aplasia of a pedicle, however, one frequently encounters hypertrophy (increase in size, thickening of the cortex, D, E) of the *contralateral* pedicle and increased density of the isthmus of the vertebral arch (Morin and Palacios, 1974; Maldague and Malghem, 1976). Sometimes the roentgen manifestations of rotational instability become visible concomitantly; i.e., the spinous process migrates in the ipsilateral direction.

F = *Unilateral* sclerosis of a pedicle must be differentiated from osteoid osteoma (pain at night!); osteoblastoma; chronic osteomyelitis; osteoma and osteoblastic metastases (particularly) in cancer of the prostate; and neuroblastoma (Wooten et al., 1978). In children one occasionally observes sclerosis of a lumbar pedicle and soliosis on the side opposite a unilateral interarticular spondylolysis with or without spondylolisthesis (Wilkinson and Hall, 1974).

G = **In differentiating an embryologic error of the intervertebral joints from a tumor-induced osteolysis, the following facts should be taken into consideration:** aplasias either concern both articulating processes, or one process is entirely absent while the other is hypoplastic (G). In osteolysis from a metastatic tumor, one articular process is lacking while the fellow process, at least initially, remains preserved. *If the pedicle also is already involved, its contours are (in part) obliterated* (H). **Dysplasias of the articular processes** produce, among other manifestations, a punched-out defect in the articular process or an (angular) deformation (increase in size; coarsening) of the articular processes (Horváth and Massanyi, 1962). Compare also Figs. 628 and 687. Meningiomas may give rise to increased size *and* sclerosis of the articular processes.

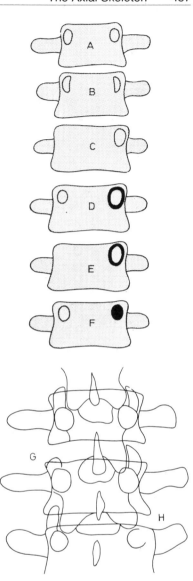

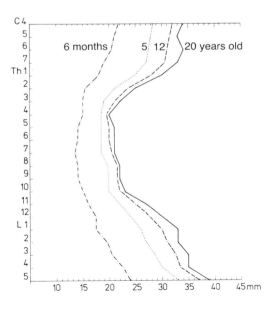

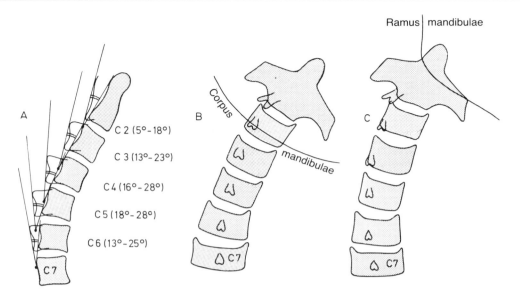

Fig. 651   **Functional roentgen examination of the cervical spine after Buetti-Bäuml** (1954).
A = Motion diagram of the cervical spine (anteflexion; retroflexion). The normal values for adults are indicated. For normal values in children and adolescents, see Fig. 652. *Alternative method:* See Fig. 653.

Methodology: Prior to taking the anteflexion roentgenogram, a tracing of the vertebral bodies is made on transparent paper. Subsequently the tracing of C7 is placed accurately upon the 7th vertebral body in the retroflexion roentgenogram, and the outlines of the 6th cervical vertebra in the retroflexion roentgenogram are sketched onto the tracing. Following this, C6 of the tracing is placed on C6 of the retroflexion roentgenogram, and the position of the 5th cervical vertebra is sketched in. This means that, generally, the inferiorly located vertebral body in the tracing and on the film is superimposed and the contours of the next vertebra superiorly in the retroflexion roentgenogram are sketched onto the tracing. When this procedure has been completed from C7 to C2, tangents are drawn to the posterior contours of the vertebral bodies. The tangents intersect and encompass the angle of excursion in each segment.

B = Principle of functional roentgenograms of the cervical spine to assess maximal *lateral inclination* (without rotating the head).

C = Principle of functional roentgenograms of the cervical spine to assess maximal *rotation* (without voluntary inclination).

Note: The lateral inclination of the cervical spine has a rotatory component; cervical rotation is associated with lateral inclination. Normally, the connecting line of the cervical spinous processes, which deviate by the rotation, describes a harmonious arc on maximal lateral inclination and also on maximal rotation. Segmental lockings manifest themselves by impeding the deviation of the spinous processes. The prominent function of rotation of the axis in lateral inclination becomes evident when the rotation of the axis is blocked (Jirout, 1968). In this case the other cervical vertebrae also lose their ability to rotate, while lateral inclination is not impeded! On lateral inclination, the atlas normally becomes displaced between the axis and the occipital condyles in the direction of inclination. Failure of this displacement to take place or a displacement opposite the direction of inclination is not necessarily pathologic, since atlantooccipital blockage can be recognized (by maximal rotation of the head) only when the atlantoaxial joints are locked. In this position, a transoral roentgenogram taken with the occipital joints flexed *passively* sideward reveals a lateral displacement of the atlas to the side opposite the rotation of the axis. With atlantooccipital blockage this displacement of the atlas is not demonstrable (Lewit, 1970).

see pages 5 and 6. The indications for making *functional roentgenograms of the (cervical) spine* have been listed on page 4 ff. Roentgenograms with anteflexion and retroflexion are taken with the patient standing. Functional roentgenograms of the cervical spine with maximal inclination to the right and the left and with maximal rotation to the right and the left are taken with the patient lying down. In so doing, the patient's shoulders should be fixed (by an assist-

ant, if necessary) so that the motion is performed solely by the cervical spine. Normally, the upper and middle segments show the strongest lateral inclination. This motion, however, may be impeded by a grossly deformed uncinate process (uncovertebral [neurocentral] joint osteoarthrosis; see under this heading). As for the rest, see the captions to Figures 651, 652, and 653.

Fig. 652 Global cervical mobility in children, adolescents, and adults. (Zeitler and Markuske, 1962; Buetti-Bäuml 1954). The data refer to the arithmetic means. Considering the dispersion of the individual values, the differences between individuals of 11 to 14 years of age and those of 15 to 18 have no demonstrable statistical significance. However, in individuals aged 15 to 18 months the range of motion in the motor segment C4/C5 is significantly different from that of adults. For the motion diagrams in the present figure it is also true that the *directional tendency* of the curves is the decisive criterion and that variations of one or more motor segments indicate a change in mobility.

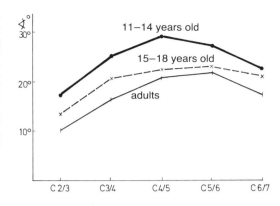

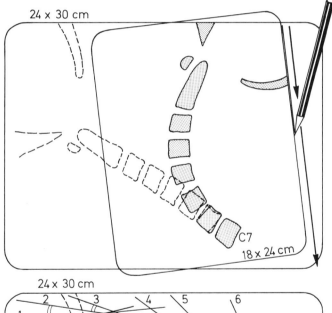

Okz / C1 : 25 – 45°

C1 / C2 : 25 – 45°

C2 / C3 : 5 – 16°

C3 / C4 : 13 – 26°

C4 / C5 : 15 – 29°

C5 / C6 : 16 – 29°

C6 / C7 : 6 – 25°

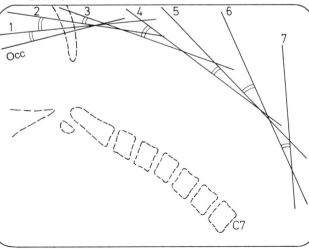

Fig. 653 **Analysis of cervical motion after Penning (1978).** For a roentgenogram of the cervical spine with maximal anteflexion, a film of 24 × 30 cm is employed. For a roentgenogram with maximal retroflexion a film of 18 × 24 cm is used. The smaller film is placed on the larger one, and the vertebral bodies and spinous processes of C7 are superimposed accurately. Subsequently a line is drawn along the *right* border of the 18 × 24 cm film. The same is done for C6 (superimpose both vertebral bodies and spinous processes; draw a line along the right border of the film), and this procedure is repeated for all the remaining vertebrae. The corresponding angles are constructed and measured. The excursions of motion reproduced above in the figure were ascertained in young adults.

Baastrup's syndrome

Normally, the spinous processes of the lumbar spine have no bony contact with each other. In the presence of hyperlordosis, however, such contact between the spinous processes (favored by additional decrease in height of the intervertebral disks) may come about and give rise to reactive formation of new bone and cartilage in the spinous processes. These roentgen findings may also be present with a major decrease in disk height without hyperlordosis. The shape of the spinous processes then becomes changed and appears to be coarsened; abraded surfaces are apt to develop. This so-called **interspinous osteoarthrosis** (Baastrup, 1940) has also been termed *Baastrup's sign* (Basstrup's syndrome) (Fig. 654). With major lordosis of the cervical spine—generally in the setting of severe malformations—the cervical spinous processes may also be in contact. Reactive deformations, however, are usually absent.

Deformities of the Vertebral Bodies, Nonoperative Fusion of Vertebrae

The shape of the vertebral depends on

1. *The genetic construction plan*
2. *The bearing capacity of the vertebra*
3. *The physical activity of the individual*

Errors in the genetic construction plan manifest themselves as deformities and disturbed segmentation of the spine. It is a general rule that *the earlier* in embryonal and fetal life the normal course of development becomes altered, the *more marked* the deformation is and the more it compromises life and the enjoyment thereof.

Figure 655 shows a case of vertebral apalsia (Rathke, 1977). Unilateral *hemivertebrae* (Fig. 656) developing on the left or right side are wedge-shaped and give rise to angular scoliosis (osteopathic sco-

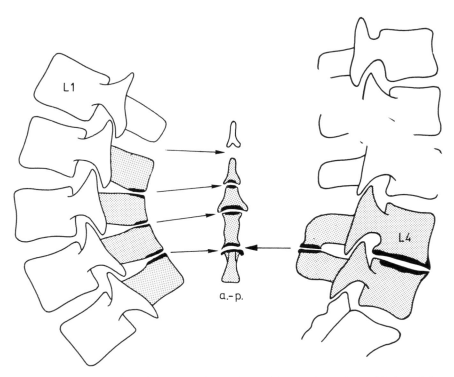

Fig. 654   **Roentgen manifestations in Baastrup's syndrome.** Baastrup's syndrome L2–L5 with hyperlordosis *(left)*. Baastrup's syndrome L4/L5 with severe osteochondrosis in this motor segment *(right)*. In the anteroposterior roentgenogram *(center)*, only the deformed spinous processes are sketched.

Note: Baastrup's syndrome *without* osteochondrosis or hyperlordosis also occurs as a roentgen manifestation of acromegaly.

Fig. 655 **Fundamental radiographic aspect of vertebral aplasia.** The vertebral body is either absent—aplasia in the strict sense—or it (mostly) remains in the cartilaginous state and is deformed (Rathke, 1977). Aplasia is suggested by expansion of the pedicles anteriorly and concretion of the pedicles (computed tomography!). The more caudally the misformed vertebra is located, the greater is the congenital angular kyphosis.

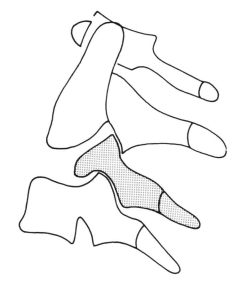

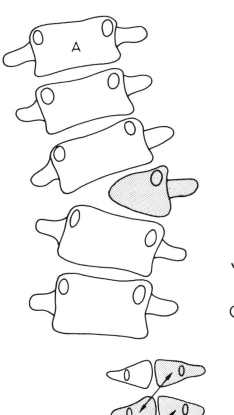

Fig. 656 **Lateral hemivertebra with angular scoliosis (child, A). Morphologic genesis of so-called hemimetameric segmental displacement (B;** Lehmann-Facius, 1925). In the early stage of development of the spine, the primordial halves of the vertebra skip one segment and grow together "wrongly." *Above* and *below* one lateral hemivertebra remains, assuming a lateral wedge shape.

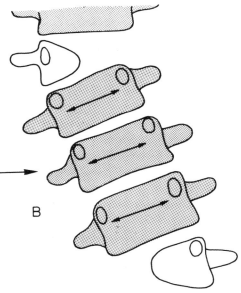

Fig. 657 **Radiographic aspect of the (potential) anterior hemivertebra (A) and the repeatedly observed posterior hemivertebra (B).** The posterior hemivertebra was identified on an elderly individual. Therefore, roentgen signs of disk degeneration are recognizable above and below the hemivertebra.

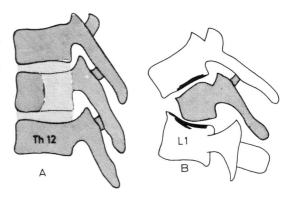

liosis, p. 419). Apart from this type, *posterior* and *anterior hemivertebrae* are known to occur (Fig. 609, no. 5; Fig. 657). A posterior hemivertebra causes the development of congenital angular kyphosis (gibbus). Instances of a persistent notochord, including so-called butterfly vertebra, are shown in Figure 641. The constitutional diseases of the skeleton (osteochondrodysplasias, mucopolysaccharidoses) often are associated with changes in shape of the vertebral bodies; e.g., **vertebra plana, wedge-shaped vertebra, fishhook vertebra** (Figs. 335, 609, no. 6) and/or persistence of the **ovoid infantile shape of the vertebral body** (Fig. 609, no. 6). For monotopical vertebra plana see Figure 658.

So-called (lumbar) **high vertebrae** (Fig. 659) present increased longitudinal height of the vertebrae involved. This can come about when, prior to the completion of growth, some disorder (bacterial spondylitis, congenital fusion of vertebrae, etc.) above these vertebrae leads to a *major* decrease in height of the spinal segment affected. Growth and development of the lumbar vertebral bodies and intervertebral disks are influenced by the physical activity of the individual: immobilized (paralyzed) children have higher vertebrae with convex end plates, lower disks (and more frequently coxa valga) than physically unimpaired children (Houston and Zaleski, 1967). This could offer an additional explanation for the development of high vertebrae underlying a severe bacterial (tuberculous) spondylitis requiring prolonged confinement to bed. (Alternative pathogenetic interpretation: *vide supra.*)

In small children, the anterior contour of the vertebra normally presents depressions (notches) that are produced by the entering vessels. Diseases associated with an increased need for blood or venous stasis in the bone marrow of the vertebrae—e.g., thalassemia major, Gaucher's disease, osteopetrosis (Albers-Schönberg's disease), metastatic neuroblastoma (Mandell and Kricun, 1979)—may, even in later childhood, contribute to the development or the persistence of such anterior vertebral notches (Fig. 660).

Vertebrae with a straightened anterior contour are termed **square vertebrae.** This finding is partic-

ularly conspicuous in the lumbar spine. **Barrel-shaped vertebrae** have a convex anterior contour of the vertebral body. Square and barrel-shaped vertebrae are among the roentgen manifestations of ankylosing spondylitis (p. 485 ff). However, **degenerative square vertebrae** (Fig. 661 B) and straightening of the anterior vertebral contour also occur with systemic diseases of the skeleton that are accompanied by increased plasticity of bone; e.g., osteomalacia (Fig. 661 D). **Codfish vertebrae** also suggest increased vertebral plasticity (Fig. 661 E and 671). The radiologic morphology of the **Paget vertebra** (so-called **ivory vertebra**) and the **hemangiomatous vertebra** is also presented in Figure 661.

Bony fusion of vertebrae destroys the mobility of the spinal segment involved (Figures 662 through 668). Preliminary conditions for the partial or total synostosis of one or more vertebrae are partial or total absence, genetically determined involution, or destruction of one or more intervertebral disks, and possibly also ossifications of the ligaments and the joint capsules. Fused vertebrae may therefore be traced to genetically determined disorders of segmentation or may be acquired conditions. In the individual case, differential diagnosis between dysontogenetic[34] and acquired fusion of vertebrae may be difficult. It should be based on the following rules:

1. Dysontogenetic fusion of vertebrae (Fig. 666) presents a homogeneous structure, occasionally a concave anterior contour, and sometimes a still identifiable hypoplastic intervertebral disk and narrow intervertebral foramina. Its anteroposterior diameter is generally reduced. A bony connection of the vertebral arches is often present. *Synostosis of the spinous processes is proof of its dysontogenetic origin!*
2. **Acquired fusion of vertebrae** most frequently can be traced to inflammatory or traumatic destruction of

---

[34] Dysontogenetic fusion of vertebrae refers to fusion due to disordered development. The synonymous term "congenital fusion" should no longer be employed because genetically induced synostosis of vertebrae can begin or terminate in utero as well as postnatally (Valentin and Putschar, 1936).

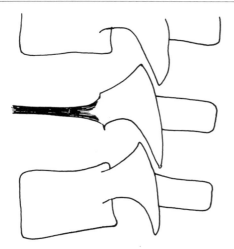

Fig. 658 **Typical vertebra plana** as a monotopical—very infrequently as an oliogotopical—roentgen finding in a 10-year-old child. In the great majority of cases in children, it is a manifestation of histiocytosis X (eosinophilic granuloma). Vertebra plana *osteonecrotica* (Calvé) should therefore be relegated to history. Following effective therapy, the vertebra largely regains its normal shape!

generations in the contiguous motor segments may occur even at a younger age (Fig. 666).

In some cases, roentgenologic differentiation is needed between a *congenital* vertebral synostosis and one acquired in *early* childhood (due, for instance, to a *cured juvenile chronic arthritis*). This disease frequently affects the cervical spine, the sacroiliac, and the temporomandibular joint concomitantly. Apart from the clinical history, radiologic examination of the above joints also reveals the actual cause of a presumptive dysontogenetic fusion of vertebrae or a clinically supposed segmental synostosis of the cervical spine (Klippel-Feil syndrome, Fig. 664) by demonstrating partial or complete ankylosis of the sacroiliac joints, hypoplasia of the mandible, and deformation of its condylar process (birdlike facies, Fig. 586).

In far advanced *ankylosing spondylitis*, not only the external portions of the annulus fibrosus but sometimes also the other regions of the disk are more or less extensively involved in the ossifying process (Fig. 665).

the intervertebral disk (Figs. 666 and 712). Losses of substance in the fused vertebrae, inhomogeneous structures of cancellous bone, and possibly also a perivertebral calcareous shadow in the soft tissues (calcified abscess) suggest an acquired pathogenesis. In senile age, complete attrition of the disk—particularly in the cervical spine—can lead to **age-dependent fusion of vertebrae.** If, in infrequent cases, degenerative bony fusion occurs prior to old age, the condition has been termed **synostosing osteochondrosis** (Fig. 667).

In the thoracic spine, a severe senile kyphopsis (Fig. 668 A) sometimes gives rise to pressure necrosis of the anterior portions of the disk. The result is **partial vertebral synostosis due to senile kyphosis** (Fig. 668 B).

Patients suffering from florid or past Scheuermann's disease infrequently present fusion of the anterior portions of the vertebral bodies in one or more lower segments of the thoracic or thoracolumbar spine. Such fusions may initiate or increase a pathologic curvature (kyphosis; Fig. 668 C). It is a matter of debate whether this **avascular anterior fusion of the thoracolumbar vertebral bodies** forms part of Scheuermann's disease or whether, similarly to the roentgen manifestations of this disease, it must be attributed to a primary constitutional tissue inferiority (Lindemann, 1931; Butler, 1971).

To compensate for the lost mobility, the intervertebral disks above and below a fused vertebra are subjected to increased strain, so that severe disk de-

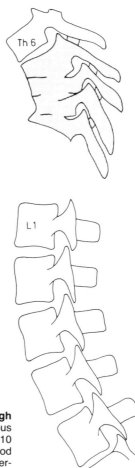

Fig. 659 **Lumbar high vertebra** after tuberculous spondylitis of Th7–Th10 experienced in childhood (cicatricious fusion of vertebrae; gibbus).

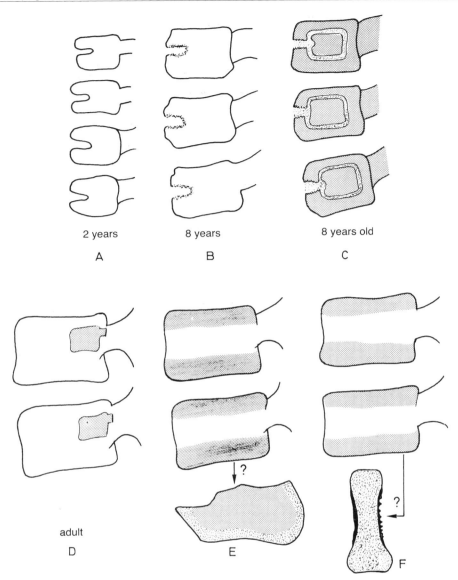

2 years   8 years   8 years old

A   B   C

adult

D   E   F

Fig. 660 **Physiologic (A), pathologic (B) anterior vertebral notch, infantile osteopetrosis Albers-Schön-berg (manifesting early, malignant) (C), phantom vertebra (D), adult osteopetrosis Albers-Schönberg (manifesting late, benign) (E), "rugger jersey" aspect with hyperparathyroidism (in renal osteopathy, F).** The "infantile" phantom vertebra (Teplick et al., 1978) was observed as a sequela of local radiation damage following intravenous injection of Thorotrast in childhood (a similar finding in the pelvic bones is possible). For the radiologic differential diagnosis between E and F, see the "bone in bone" aspect in the cancellous bone (here, the calcaneus) in osteopetrosis (compare Fig. 59) and the subperiosteal resorption of bone (initially) on the radial side of the middle phalanges in hyperparathyroidism (compare Fig. 151). In addition: In E there is a basic tendency toward increase in bone density and in F toward decalcification. In F, the intervertebral disks may be largely "worn," and consequently the intervertebral spaces may be "absent."

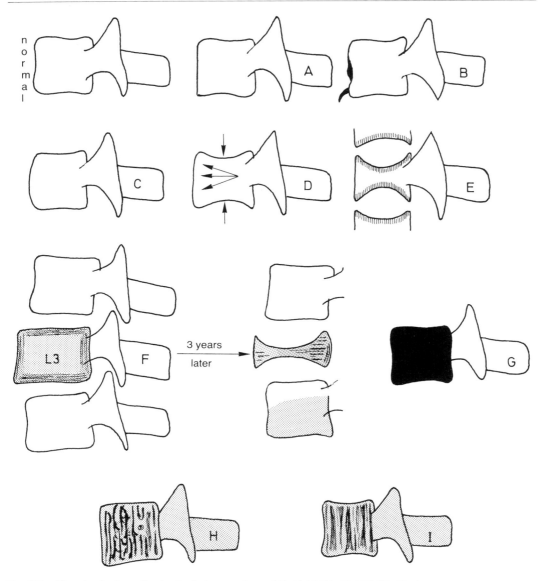

Fig. 661 **Monotopical or oligotopical changes in vertebral contours and structure.**

A = Square vertebra in ankylosing spondylitis.

B = *Degenerative square vertebra.* Usually occurring in connection with degenerative disk disease. (Often) starting with a bulbous formation of new bone in the center of the anterior surface of the vertebra.

C = *Barrel-shaped vertebra* in advanced ankylosing spondylitis.

D = The vertebral deformation sketched indicates the osteomalacic component of an *osteopenic osteopathy.*

E = *Codfish vertebra* in osteopenic osteopathies. In sickle cell anemia, massive vertebral infarcts and ery-throblastic hyperplasia of the bone marrow may reduce the bearing capacity of the involved vertebra to such a degree that it assumed a wedge shape or the appearance of a codfish vertebra (Karayalcin et al., 1976).

F = Paget vertebra (see the "frame structure" and the typical increase in size of the vertebra). Three years later the unresisting vertebra has collapsed. In L4, an equivocal increase in density has developed which, associated with the finding in L3, also suggests Paget's disease.

G = *"Ivory vertebra"* (the increase in bone density is not necessarily homogeneous). Differential diagnosis: Paget's disease; osseous manifestation of clinically known Hodgkin's disease; single osteoblastic metastasis in known or occult carcinoma (most probably of the prostate or the breast), bacterial spondylitis.

H = *Hemangiomatous vertebra* (hemangiohamartoma). Characteristic fibrillar and honeycombed structure; vertebral body possibly slightly enlarged.

I = Characteristics transformation of the cancellous bone in *generalized hyperostosis* (pachydermoperiostosis with and without skin lesions; see p. 133).

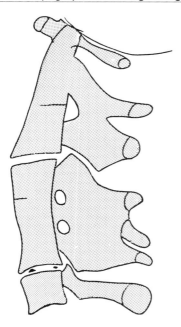

Fig. 662 **Congenital disorder of cervical segmentation (Klippel-Feil syndrome).** In addition, occipital dysplasia. On comparing roentgenograms of the patient in early childhood and juvenile age, the Klippel-Feil syndrome may show a tendency to progression. It is therefore a matter of debate whether it is in fact a disorder of segmentation or whether it reflects a congenital tendency to fusion. The Klippel-Feil syndrome is frequently associated with other malformations; e.g., congenital high scapula (Sprengel's deformity), cervical ribs, and the omovertebral bone (Fig. 663).

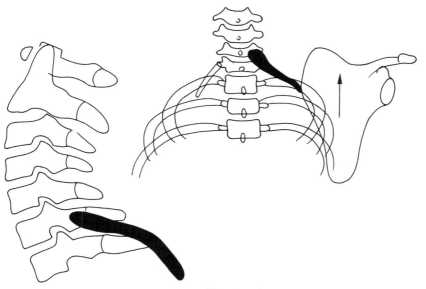

Fig. 663 **Omovertebral bone.** This bony element forms a *unilateral* or *bilateral* bridge between the scapula or its close vicinity and the spinous process, arch, or transverse process of one or more lower cervical vertebrae (Blair and Wells, 1957). The connection of this bone with the scapula and the cervical vertebrae may be osseous, cartilaginous, articular or fibrous. The omovertebral bone resembles the suprascapular bone of lower vertebrates. In the case illustrated the omovertebral bone is associated with high scapula (Sprengel's deformity) and a cervical rib at the right side of C7. Its combination with the Klippel-Feil syndrome is also recognized.

Fig. 664 **Adult female with completely ankylosed neck and birdlike facies** (Fig. 586). Her mother stated that she suffered a "flu with joint swellings" at 4 with stiffening of the neck "as an aftermath." **Typical radiologic picture of cervical synostosis acquired in early childhood following inflammation of the intervertebral joints** (from juvenile rheumatoid arthritis). The intervertebral joints have undergone bony ankylosis. The result is a considerable disturbance of growth and development of the cervical vertebrae (hypoplasia of the vertebral bodies; partial fusion of vertebrae; synostosis of the vertebral arches; hypoplasia of the spinous processes). Compare the close similarity of these findings with the roentgenogram of progressive myositis ossificans in the cervical spine (Fig. 77).

Secondary findings (not illustrated): Partial bony ankylosis of the sacroiliac joints, high vertebra in the lumbar spine, destruction of the condylar processes of both mandibles, and mandibular hypoplasia; hence also radiologic clues to the (meanwhile) cured juvenile chronic arthritis.

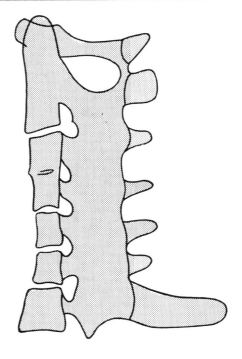

Monosegmental Decrease in Disk Height (Figs. 669 and 670).

By heeding the rule of the successive disk heights (Figs. 606 and 611), one may readily establish a decrease in disk height in any of the intervertebral spaces of the cervical and lumbar spine on lateral roentgenograms. This is also possible in the thoracic spine by taking into account that normally, none of the thoracic disks appears to be considerably thinner in the roentgenogram than its neighboring disks superiorly and inferiorly. The decrease in height reflects—as was mentioned above—a loss in mass of the involved intervertebral disk. This can be related to degenerative disk disease, an inflammatory process, displacement of disk tissue into the neighboring vertebra or dorsal disk displacement or diskectomy. Finally, it should be mentioned that in sacralization of the lowest lumbar vertebra, the corresponding intervertebral disk is often hypoplastic.

Oligo- and Polysegmental Increase in Disk Height

On comparing the craniocaudal diameters of the vertebrae, one often finds that neonates and children have higher intervertebral disks than adults. Diseases that, quite generally, diminish the resistance of the vertebral cancellous and cortical bone can, also in older individuals, give rise to a considerable increase in height of the intervertebral disks (Figs. 661 E and 671). Such ballooning of a disk is sometimes ob-

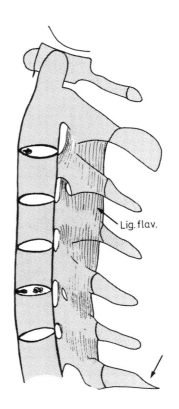

Lig. flav.

Fig. 665 **Bamboo spine appearance of the cervical vertebral column in ankylosing spondylitis of about 25 years' standing.** (The concept "bamboo spine" refers to the anteroposterior roentgen aspect of the lumbar spine in an advanced stage of the disease.) For radiologic differential diagnosis compare Figs. 77, 662, and 664! *Arrow* points to a concentric osteolysis in the spinous process of C7 (occurring also in C6), such as is only observed in ankylosing spondylitis and in adult rheumatoid arthritis (see Figs. 708 and 710).

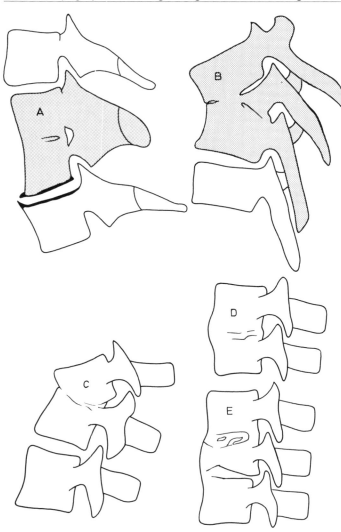

Fig. 666 **Dysontogenetic and acquired vertebral synostosis.** Fused dysontogenetic cervical vertebra (with concomitant synostosis of the spinous processes). Osteochondrosis in the contiguous caudal segment (A). Dysontogenetic vertebral fusion from congenital posterior hemivertebra (B). Inflammatory vertebral fusion following tuberculous spondylitis in the growth period (C and D). Compensatory high vertebra in C (see text). Traumatic vertebral fusion (E).

served in severe vertebral osteoporosis, osteomalacia, Paget's disease (Fig. 661 F), diffuse metastases, and multiple myeloma.

Degenerative Discopathy
(Intervertebral chondrosis, intervertebral osteochondrosis, uncovertebral [neurocentral] joint osteoarthrosis)

Intervertebral chondrosis reflects dehydration of the nucleus pulposus. Tears and clefts make their appearance as the result of desiccation. They can extend as far as the annulus fibrosus and form a pathway for dorsal prolapse of the disk (Fig. 631). These clefts sometimes manifest themselves roentgenologically by the so-called **vacuum phenomenon** (Fig.

672). *A characteristic roentgen finding of chondrosis in the lateral view is the nonreactive decrease in height of the disk space* (compare the physiologic sequences of disk heights, Fig. 606). "Nonreactive" in this connection means the absence of any subdiscal sclerosis of cancellous bone or marginal osteophytes. The decrease in disk height, however, is an equivocal roentgen phenomenon. The younger the patient with a monosegmental decrease in disk height is, the more important and variable are the differential diagnostic problems and inferences (Figs. 669 and 670) that must be considered before the "trivial" roentgenologic diagnosis "intervertebral chondrosis" may be established. The expression "trivial" is intended to point out that chondrosis is a frequent morphologic finding *(attrition of the disk)* that is identifiable with the other aging processes of the organism. On the one hand, its degree and its frequency increase with advancing

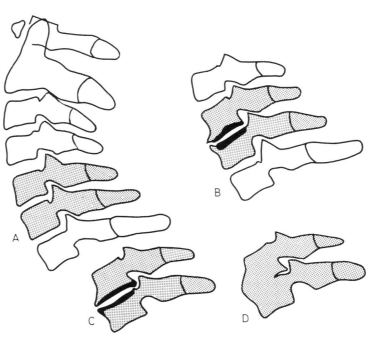

Fig. 667 **Evolution of a case of synostosing disk degeneration.**

A = 40 years old. *Intervertebral chondrosis* (decrease in disk height; spondyloretrolisthesis; slight segmental extension).

B = 49 years old. *Intervertebral osteochondrosis* (The decrease in disk height has become more pronounced. Straightening of the end plates, band-shaped increase in subdiscal density, gross bony marginal elongations, and coarsening of the edges.

C = 52 years old. Increasing osteochondrosis (remodeling of the vertebral bodies as a response to the now absent shock- and pressure-absorbing function of the intervertebral disks).

D = 57 years old. *Synostosing osteochondrosis* (now infrequent finding).

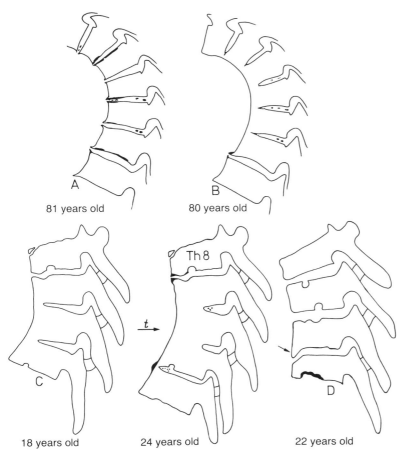

A
81 years old

B
80 years old

C
18 years old

Th 8
24 years old

t

D
22 years old

Fig. 668 **Senile round back and partial vertebral fusions.**

A = Radiologic aspect of typical senile kyphosis.

B = Senile kyphosis with anterior vertebral fusion.

C = Evolution (t) of a progressive **anterior noninflammatory fusion of vertebrae** in a young individual with Scheuermann's disease (see text). In **thalidomide embryopathy,** the peripheral dysmelias recognizable at birth dominate the clinical picture, but in about two thirds of the cases (Ruffing, 1978) spinal lesions are also demonstrable (the teratogenic periods for the extremities and the spine overlap in the first 3 months of fetal development). These represent a phenocopy of Scheuermann's disease, including the postnatal avascular anterior fusion of vertebral bodies.

D = Forme fruste *(arrow)* of noninflammatory anterior fusion of vertebral bodies in Scheuermann's disease (Gougeon et al., 1971)?

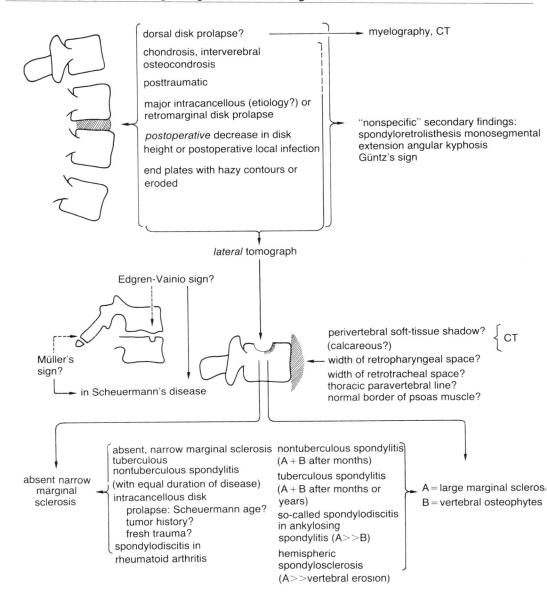

dorsal disk prolapse? ————————→ myelography, CT

chondrosis, interverebral osteocondrosis

posttraumatic

major intracancellous (etiology?) or retromarginal disk prolapse

postoperative decrease in disk height or postoperative local infection

end plates with hazy contours or eroded

"nonspecific" secondary findings: spondyloretrolisthesis monosegmental extension angular kyphosis Güntz's sign

lateral tomograph

Edgren-Vainio sign?

Müller's sign?

└—→ in Scheuermann's disease

perivertebral soft-tissue shadow? (calcareous?) } CT
width of retropharyngeal space?
width of retrotracheal space?
thoracic paravertebral line?
normal border of psoas muscle?

absent narrow märginal sclerosis

absent, narrow marginal sclerosis tuberculous nontuberculous spondylitis (witn equal duration of disease) intracancellous disk
  prolapse: Scheuermann age?
  tumor history?
  fresh trauma?
spondylodiscitis in rheumatoid arthritis

nontuberculous spondylitis (A + B after months)
tuberculous spondylitis (A + B after months or years)
so-called spondylodiscitis in ankylosing spondylitis (A>>B)
hemispheric spondylosclerosis (A>>vertebral erosion)

A = large marginal scleros
B = vertebral osteophytes

Fig. 669 Decrease in height of a disk space and its implications for the roentgenologic technique and diagnosis. For hemispheric spondylosclerosis, a roentgen finding with the character of a syndrome; see Figs. 704 and 705.

Fig. 670 Radiologic differential diagnosis of monosegmental decrease in disk height.
A = Monosegmental decrease in height of a lumbar intervertebral space with spondyloretrolisthesis (plain lateral roentgenogram). *Question:* Can the cause of the loss in mass of the involved intervertebral disk be rendered visible roentgenologically? Therefore lateral tomography (B to F).
B to F = Tomograph shows a defect (with hazy contours) of the end plate of the disk-bearing vertebra.
Radiologic differential diagnosis: (1) *Large fresh Schmorl's node* (20-year-old patient; no history of tumor or trauma). The further evolution (C; t = 13 months) confirms this supposition (marginal sclerosis and the Edgren-Vaino sign [Figs. 609, no. 3; 610 D; 669] are recognizable). (2) *Subdiscal osteolytic metastasis* with fresh break of the end plate and the disk (50-year-old female; radiotherapy for inoperable cancer of the cervix 3 years previously). The ·evolution (t' = 6 months) confirms the diagnosis (D). The progression of the metastasis causes a

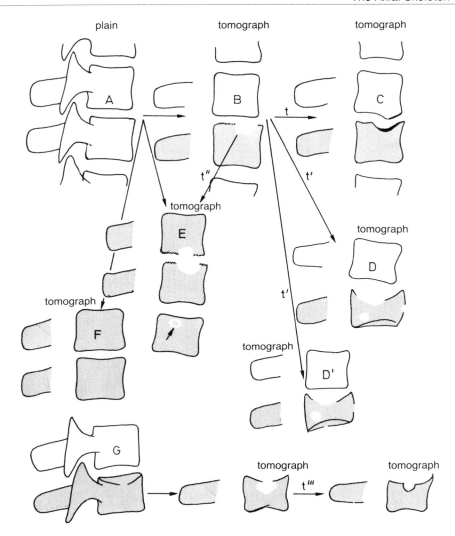

plain   tomograph   tomograph

collapse of the vertebral body in which, additionally, a spherical osteolysis has become visible. The disk space now appears to be "widened." The infrequent causes of vertebral collapse also include primary amyloidosis (Dharmarshi et al., 1978). Massive infiltration with amyloid can also lead to spontaneous fracture of the odontoid process of the axis (Hannon et al., 1975). The evolution of the metastasis in D' is rare and atypical because the disk space shows a decrease in height.

(3) Bacterial spondylitis (E). B was not diagnosed as a bacterial infection, atlhough the poor general condition, subfebrile temperatures, and elevated sedimentation rate would have justified this diagnosis. Repeated tomography after 4 months (t″) revealed erosions of the end plates with hazy contours on *both* sides of the disk space, which had diminished in height; i.e., the characteristic roentgen manifestations of florid bacterial spondylitis. The tuberculous etiology of this case was suggested by a cavity with a small sequestrum in the contiguous vertebra, which had developed in the meantime (*arrow;* see 468). A → the result E would have led directly to the correct diagnosis.

(4) *Intervertebral chondrosis (F).* The tomograph reveals no additional roentgen findings as compared with A. No roentgen manifestations of stenosis of the spinal canal. Radicular or caudal signs and symptoms are an indication for lumbar myelography with a water-soluble contrast medium or for computed tomography!

G = Trauma 3 days previously (fall on the buttocks; 60-year-old patient).Plain roentgenogram reveals an *asymmetrical depression of the end plate.* Tomograph shows in addition a **fresh, traumatic, intracancellous prolapsed disk** (so-called traumatic Schmorl's node). The tomograph t‴, taken 14 months later, shows the prolapse with its characteristic shell-shaped marginal sclerosis. Besides this, a repair osteophyte has developed (see text).

Note: End plates with hazy borders suggest resorptive processes (inflammation, tumor, repair of trauma), but they are not necessarily present in these conditions!

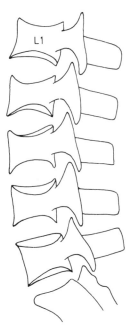

Fig. 671 **Ballooning of the lumbar intervertebral disks ("codfish vertebra") in severe osteoporosis (with additional osteomalacia?).** 78-year-old female.

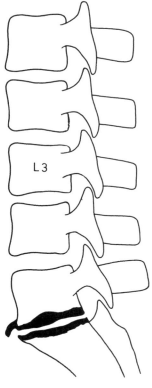

Fig. 673 **Intervertebral chondrosis** L3/L4 with nonreactive decrease in disk height. Above it, several segments are extended by reflex (Güntz's sign). **Intervertebral osteochondrosis** L5/S1 with typical roentgen manifestations (decrease in disk height; subdiscal condensation of bone; marginal vertebral osteophytes).

Fig. 672 **Discal vacuum phenomena**

A = The vacuum phenomenon manifests itself where Sharpey's fibers attach the external portion of the annulus fibrosus to the marginal edge of the vertebral body (→). When these fibers rupture, a vacuum phenomenon may appear at that location, and a vertebral osteophyte may develop in the immediate vicinity (see under Spodylosis deformans).

B = Vacuum phenomenon in advanced intervertebral osteochondrosis (←≺). Discal vacuum phenomena develop with the various manifestations of disk degeneration and—usually in several disks—in spondylopathy of ochronosis (Fig. 50), but also with a vertebral collapse due to a metastatic tumor (Schabel et al., 1979), as well as in bacterial spondylitis. Vacuum phenomena may even become demonstrable in *collapsed vertebrae;* e.g., following corticosteroid therapy (Maldague et al., 1978). Nitrogen gas has been aspirated from vacuum phenomena (Ford et al., 1977).

age. On the other, those intervertebral disks that are exposed to particular (inadequate) strain (*example:* Fig. 666) or that have been damaged previously (*example:* spondylopathy in ochronosis, Fig. 50) have a tendency to degenerate. Secondary nonspecific roentgen manifestations of chondrosis are spondyloretrolisthesis (Fig. 631), segmental extension, and Güntz's sign (Fig. 607), as well as limitation of motion but also hypermobility and gliding instability (compare Fig. 632 B) in functional roentgenograms.

Intervertebral osteochondrosis, as compared with chondrosis, refers to further advanced attrition of the disk. The shock- and pressure-absorbing func-

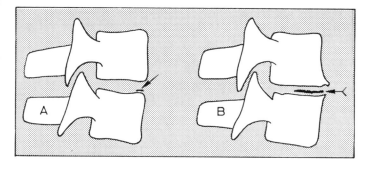

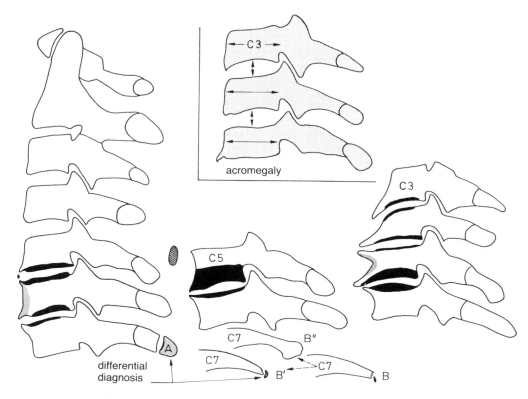

Fig. 674   **Aspects of osteochondrosis and vertebral acromegaly** (compare Fig. 644, no. 5).

Acromegaly: More or less pronounced *increase* in disk height. Increased sagittal diameter of the vertebral body by ventral apposition of bone (most conspicuous in the lower thoracic spine; Finlay and Macdonald, 1954), coarse vertebral osteophytes (Erdheim, 1931). The ventral apposition of bone in osteochondrosis parallels the decrease in height of the disk space; this is not the case in acromegaly (here, the disk—at least initially—is rather higher than normal).

Differential diagnosis from ventral, hence anterior, apposition of bone in hyperostotic spondylosis: In acromegaly the apposition of bone remains limited to the anterior surface of the vertebral body, whereas in hyperostotic spondylosis it is also demonstrable at the level of the disk space (aspect of dripping candle wax, "sugarcoating"; Fig. 681). Apart from this, in the majority of patients acromegaly starts in the third decade of life, whereas hyperostotic spondylosis is encountered in the second half of life. Both pathologic conditions, however, share the tendency to decreased glucose tolerance, amounting to manifest diabetes mellitus. The acromegalic facies and the enlargement of hands and feet are characteristic early signs of acromegaly (Finlay and Macdonald, 1954).

Secondary findings: Osseous metaplasia in the ligamentum nuchae (without clinical significance). Fatigue fracture of C(6)7 or Th 1 (2) in adults; *"shoveler's fracture"* (A). The "corticalization" of the borders of the fracture indicates healing with pseudoarthrosis. Shoveler's fracture in adults takes place in the middle third of the spinous process. In adolescents (between the ages of 14 and 17; B,B'), it is encountered in the tip of the spinous process (most frequently of Th1) and is due to excessive strain of the apophysis that appears at that age in this location (Schmitt and Rücker, 1979). The fracture unites *(dashed arrows)* by bony consolidation with coarsening of the spinous process (B″) or, less frequently, with a pseudarthrosis (B′) as "persistent apophysis." B shows the florid stage (typical history: unaccustomed shoveling, dragging, etc., leads to localized pain). Juvenile and adult shoveler's fracture must be differentiated from "genuine" persistent apophysis of the spinous process (no pain; no history of unaccustomed work; no trauma; no deformation of the spinous process; no caudal dislocation of the persistent apophysis) and from shell-shaped avulsion in acute trauma).

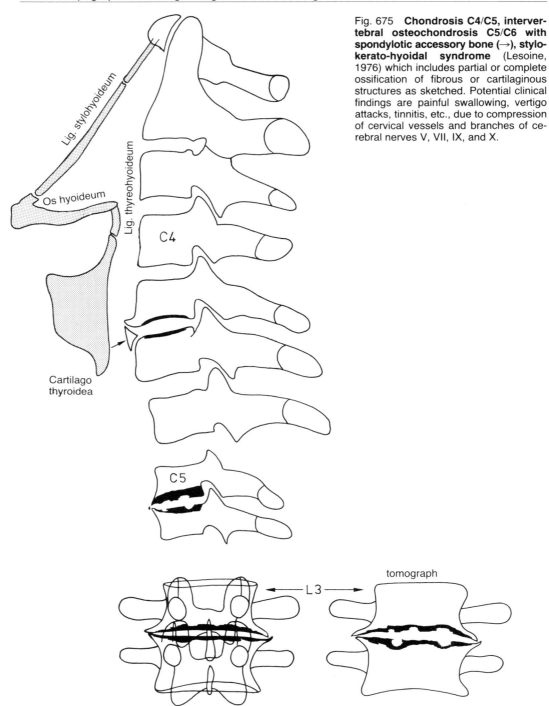

Fig. 675 **Chondrosis C4/C5, intervertebral osteochondrosis C5/C6 with spondylotic accessory bone (→), stylo-kerato-hyoidal syndrome** (Lesoine, 1976) which includes partial or complete ossification of fibrous or cartilaginous structures as sketched. Potential clinical findings are painful swallowing, vertigo attacks, tinnitis, etc., due to compression of cervical vessels and branches of cerebral nerves V, VII, IX, and X.

Fig. 676 **Erosive osteochondrosis.** The condition is generally well demonstrable in lateral roentgenograms of the cervical spine. In the lumbar spine, the contour defects are usually visible only in tomographs. The erosions develop through breaks of the sclerotic, and therefore brittle, subdiscal bone. In general, however, the erosions present no difficulty of differentiation from bacterial spondylitis, provided the aspect of osteochondrosis is otherwise *typical*. Only in *extremely infrequent* cases (compare Lagier and MacGee, 1979) do noninflammatory erosions of erosive osteochondrosis lead to severe destruction of the vertebrae. In this event, roentgenologic diagnosis becomes impossible (compare Fig. 704).

tion of the disk is largely lost. The subchondral ver- tebral cancellous bone shows a reactive, mostly band- shaped increase in density (Figs. 673, 674, and 675). Sharp projections of bone appear on the edges of the vertebrae. Therefore, the radiologic definition of os- teochondrosis is: *decrease in disk height plus subdis- cal condensation of bone plus marginal vertebral os- teophytes* (compare Fig. 679). The neighboring vertebral bodies are remodeled with time; they be- come straightened, rather angular, and coarser. In the cervical spine, their anteroposterior diameter in- creases through apposition of bone to the vertebrae (Fig. 674). The subdiscal sclerosis renders the ver- tebra brittle so that it occasionally breaks (**erosive osteochondrosis,** Fig. 676). In rare cases, the degen- erated crumbling disk is completely resorbed by in- growing vascular and connective tissue. This may lead to more or less pronounced ankylosis of the neigh- boring cervical vertebrae (**synostosing osteochon- drosis,** Fig. 667).

Necrobiotic and necrotic disk tissue is apt to cal- cify. Degeneration of the disk may therefore be ac- companied by calcification. In old people, calcified disks occur with particular frequency in the thoracic spine (Fig. 677 A). Calcification of disks is known to accompany metabolic disorders; e.g., ochronosis (Fig. 50), hyperparathyroidism, idiopathic hemo- chromatosis (Bywaters and Hamilton, 1971; Fig. 677 B), familial and sporadic articular chondrocalcinosis (Fig. 67) and long-term dihydrotachysterol medica- tion (A.T.-10 treatment). It may also follow an in- jury. Deposits of calcium and vacuum phenomena

sometimes reflect a primordial inferiority of the in- tervertebral disk in constitutional diseases of the skeleton; they are already encountered in young in- dividuals (Giedion et al., 1961). In *children and ju- veniles,* discal and paradiscal calcifications, possibly only involving a few segments and occurring most frequently in the cervical spine, are occasionally ac- companied by clinical symptoms of inflammation which often follow a trivial injury (e.g., a fall). The diagnosis of an infectious disease then suggests it- self. Since in such cases, after subsidence of the in- flammatory symptoms, the calcium is generally re- sorbed in the course of months or years, the condition has been compared to so-called calcareous tendinitis (peritendinitis) (Figs. 82 and 83). **Calcareous disci- tis** would then be the correct designation of the dis- ease.

Since the resorption of the precipitated calcium may, as mentioned earlier, last for years while the complaints generally subside after a few weeks, growth disorders of the vertebral bodies (vertebra plana) have been observed as late sequelae of calcareous discitis (Klaus and Nekula, 1975). The calcified disk may prolapse *anteriorly* through the annulus fibrosus and may give rise to dysphagia (Coventry, 1970). *Dorsal* prolapse of the disk also occurs (Mainzer, 1973). In the cervical vertebrae, particular morphologic and developmental conditions lead to **uncovertebral joint osteoarthrosis** (Fig. 678). The uncinate pro- cesses are superolaterally directed, shovel-shaped protuberances on the third to seventh vertebral bodies of the cervical spine. The surface of the vertebral

Fig. 677   Calcification of disks.

A = Calcification of a necro- biotic or necrotic nucleus pulpo- sus in an adult.

B = Calcifications in the exter- nal portions of the annulus fibro- sus; e.g., in *idiopathic hemochro- matosis* (compare with Fig. 682; syndesmophytes in ankylosing spondylitis).

A, B compare with Fig. 67. (Figs. 677 B and 67 are also grouped together under the de- scriptive term "chondrocalci- nosis".)

Note: In chondrocalcinosis, the combination of peripheral joint discomfort and restricted mobility of the spine (from calcified disks) can arouse the clinical suspicion of ankylosing spondylitis. This di- agnosis is proved incorrect by radiologic examination of the spine including the sacroiliac joints.

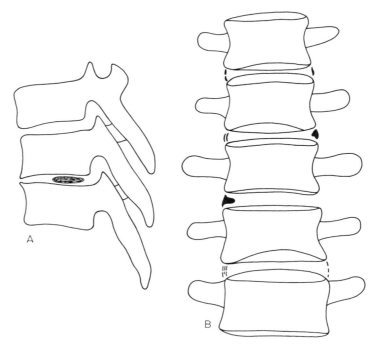

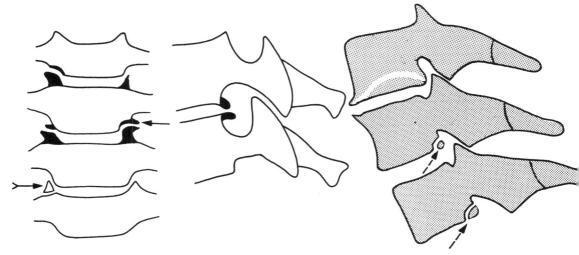

Fig. 678 **Uncovertebral spondylosis** (so-called uncovertebral osteoarthritis) in the three standard views of the cervical spine (anteroposterior, oblique, lateral). In clear-cut uncovertebral spondylosis *(arrow)*, the *pseudocleft in the vertebral body* (Dihlmann and Dörr, 1970) is recognizable in the *lateral* roentgenogram *(right sketch, upper vertebra)*. The pseudocleft allows the inference that the mobility of the segment involved has been completely, or at least largely, abolished. *Tailed arrow* points to a persistent ossification center in the uncinate process (clinical differentiation from fracture and osteochondrosis dissecans). *Dashed arrows* point to detached portions of the posterior marginal ridge of the vertebra. In this case the question arises of whether one is dealing with a dorsal retromarginal prolapsed disk *or* a developmental anomaly of the marginal ridge (persistent ridge) *or* the sequel of a (hyper-)extension type of trauma (compare Figs. 614, 618, and 640). Often it is *not* possible to make the differential diagnosis *exclusively* on the basis of the radiologic morphology *without* consideration of the clinical and historical data *(for example:* does the patient describe a (hyper-) extension type of trauma?).

bodies thus assumes a saddle shape. Developmentally, the uncinate processes are derived from the vertebral arches. In the adult, the intervertebral disks in the vicinity of the uncinate processes present clefts that are invariably directed sideward (Töndury, 1943/43; Harzer and Töndury, 1966). These transverse clefts have been attributed to degenerative processes in the intervertebral disks. In any event, they show a synovial lining and have even been observed in a 1-month-old infant (Stahl and Huth, 1980). Their classification is therefore still open to question (pathologic or physiologic structures?).

The uncovertebral cleavage spaces, however, give rise to an anomalous increase in segmental mobility or occur as the result of increased mobility. Thereby they promote the general attrition of the disk and thus a decrease in disk height. In this way the load is more and more absorbed and transmitted by the uncinate processes, which become deformed under the influence of excessive strain and expand posterolaterally as well as laterally. They may thus come in contact with the contents of the intervertebral foramen; i.e., the vertebral artery and its surrounding synpathetic vertebral plexus (Fig. 643).

Degenerative Discopathy (continued) (Spondylosis deformans, radiologic differential diagnosis of vertebral osteophytes, including diffuse idiopathic skeletal hyperostosis [DISH])

Spondylosis deformans (degenerative vertebral osteophytosis) is the most frequent pathologic roentgen finding in the vertebral column. There can be no doubt about its fundamental pathogenetic relationships to degeneration of the disk. The incidence of spondylosis increases with advancing age. The characteristic radiologic feature of spondylosis is the **submarginal spondylophyte** (Dihlmann, 1979; Fig. 679) at a disk space that shows no decrease in height. The submarginal spondylophyte *starts* its growth immediately beneath the border of the vertebral body—therefore the attribute "submarginal." The base of the spondylophyte gradually becomes broader and expands as far as the edge of the vertebra. The spondylophyte grows on the anterior and lateral surface of the vertebral body in a typical manner; i.e., at first horizon-

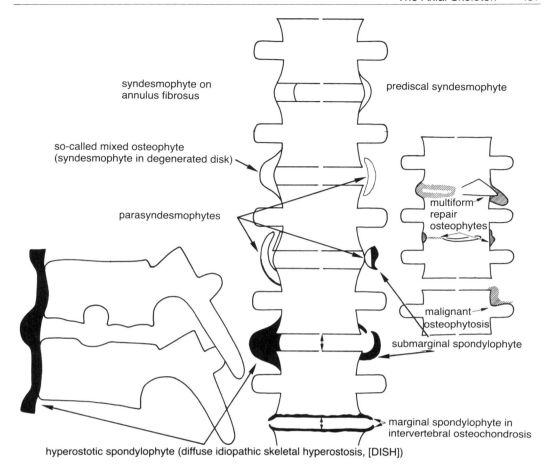

syndesmophyte on annulus fibrosus

prediscal syndesmophyte

so-called mixed osteophyte (syndesmophyte in degenerated disk)

multiform repair osteophytes

parasyndesmophytes

malignant osteophytosis

submarginal spondylophyte

marginal spondylophyte in intervertebral osteochondrosis

hyperostotic spondylophyte (diffuse idiopathic skeletal hyperostosis, [DISH])

Fig. 679   Differential diagnosis of vertebral osteophytes on the basis of their roentgeologic morphology (Dihlmann, 1977).

Note: In the submarginal spondylophytes of spondylosis deformans and the hyperostotic spondylophytes of diffuse idiopathic skeletal hyperostosis (DISH), the neighboring disk space is *generally* of normal height. In DISH, however, this depends on when the finding develops. The earlier (in the second half of life) it appears, the more frequently will the disk height be normal (and vice versa). Marginal spondylophytes in the setting of intervetebral osteochondrosis are associated with a decrease in disk height.

tally and later cranially or caudally. The spondylophyte pushes its way underneath the fibers of the anterior longitudinal ligament of the spine, which serves as its guide rail. In this manner its *handle shape* develops.

According to Schmorl and Junghanns (1968), the spondylophyte indicates stress related fissures and ruptures of Sharpey's fibers, which anchor the annulus fibrosus to the contiguous areas of the vertebral body. Apart from this, a single trauma to the spine without fracture of vertebrae may also lead to tears that trigger the formation of spondylophytes. Aufdermaur (1960, 1978) describes the spondylophytes as resulting from micro- or macrotraumatic tears in the periphery of the intervertebral disks; these tears are

said to favor the bulging of parts of the disks and their being pressed forward. Both theories start from the same assumption; namely, that the break in continuity between the annulus fibrosus and the vertebral body with the resulting pathologic increase in segmental mobility and tensing of the anterior longitudinal ligament by displaced disk tissue gives rise to elevated tensile stress and to overstretching at the insertions of that ligament. The mechanical stimulus at these sites is said to further the activity of the osteoblasts at the insertions of the anterior longitudinal ligament and their immediate surroundings; such increased osteoblastic activity eventually would lead to the development of osteophytes.

In addition, the **spondylotic accessory bone**

(Figs. 679 and 680) forms part of the picture of spondylosis deformans. This is a bony metaplasia within the anterior longitudinal ligament or in its immediate vicinity. The spondylotic accessory bone has no osseous contact with the contiguous vertebral body; its greatest diameter runs in a craniocaudal direction.

Spondylophytes also develop in intervertebral osteochondrosis (p. 452). Originally, they form on the edge of the vertebra and therefore have been termed **marginal spondylophytes** (Fig. 679; Dihlmann, 1977). Morphologically, they are analogous to the marginal osteophytes of the (peripheral) joints in osteoarthrosis.

Dorsal spondylophytes develop less frequently than spondylophytes on the anterior or lateral surface of the vertebral body. This difference is probably related to anatomic conditions, since the posterior longitudinal ligament inserts primarily in the disk and only with delicate strands of fibrous tissue in the vertebral body. The pathogenetic preconditions for the development of dorsal submarginal spondylophytes are therefore absent *(vide supra)*. Dorsal prolapse of the disk, however, may lead to the formation of dorsal spondylophytes (Fig. 642 A), and osteochondrosis may give rise to dorsal marginal spondylo-

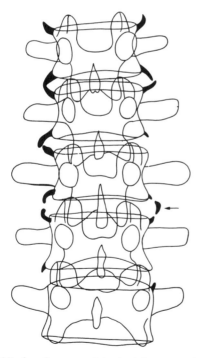

Fig. 680   Lumbar spondylosis deformans showing, among other anomalies, a spondylotic accessory bone *(arrow)*. Spondylosis deformans commonly appears first, and is most noticeable, in the thoracicolumbar junction—hence the junction between a spinal segment with greater one and one with lesser mobility. The same applies to the syndesmophytes of ankylosing spondylitis (see p. 485 ff).

phytes (Fig. 643 C). In gross pathologic specimens, dorsal marginal osteophytes commonly manifest themselves by a bony ridge along the entire posterior edge of the vertebral body.

The coarse **hyperostotic spondylophyte** that expands far laterally and/or anteriorly as well as the "sugar-iced" apposition of bone on the anterior surface of the vertebra (Fig. 681) is a characteristic roentgen manifestation of **diffuse idiopathic skeletal hyperostosis (DISH)** (Ott, 1953). Other writers speak of *ankylosing hyperostosis of the spine* (Forestier and Rotés-Quérol, 1950; Forestier et al., 1969). DISH reflects a constitutionally occasioned mode of reaction that is evidenced by "exuberant" bony metaplasia of tight fibrous tissue, hence an **osteoplastic diathesis** (Dihlmann, 1967/1978; Forestier and Lagier, 1971; Resnick et al., 1975). This tendency to ossification—which has a preference for the male sex—commonly manifests itself as late as the second half of life (for exceptions see De Sèze and Claisse, 1960) and is not limited to the peripheral portions of the intervertebral disk and the perivertebral connective tissue, including the anterior and posterior longitudinal ligament. The tendency to ossification is also demonstrable in the joint capsules; for example, in the intervertebral joints, the costovertebral joints (Vernon-Roberts et al., 1974), and the sacroiliac joints (Dihlmann and Freund, 1968), in the ligaments, and in the tendinous insertions of the trunk and the extremities. The changes in the tendinous insertions are typical, sometimes voluminous, fibroosteoses (p. 72 ff). Persons with DISH present with comparable frequency, a number of other chronic degenerative disorders such as diabetes mellitus or a tendency to hyperglycemia (Boulet and Mirouze, 1954; Ott et al., 1963; Schoen et al., 1969; Lequesne et al., 1970), gout, or at least hyperuricemia (Schilling et al., 1965), and the roentgen manifestations of Scheuermann's disease or at least a conspicuous number of Schmorl's nodes (Aufdermaur, 1965; Vernon-Roberts et al., 1974). A case of DISH associated with plantar hyperkeratosis has been observed by Beardwell (1969).

The **syndesmophytes** (Figs. 679 and 682) are among the most impressive roentgen manifestations of ankylosing spondylitis. With this disease, in the majority of cases (61 percent) they appear first in the thoracicolumbar junction (Dihlmann, 1968a). In ankylosing spondylitis, the syndesmophytes reflect a systemic reaction which, in its fully developed state, produces the so-called *bamboo spine* (Fig. 682). Development of the syndesmophytes, however, is related to the patient's age. When the disease begins in juvenile age (Schilling et al., 1969), syndesmophytes are sparsely formed or entirely lacking (Fig. 682 C). Forestier and associates (see Sicard and Forestier, 1931; Forestier and Robert, 1934) have introduced the term "syndesmophyte" to delimit the vertebral osteophytes in ankylosing spondylitis terminologically as well as clinically from other kinds of vertebral osteophytes.

In ankylosing spondylitis, the stiffening verte-

Fig. 681 **Vertebral roentgen findings in diffuse idiopathic skeletal hyperostosis (DISH)** *(apposition of bone = black).*

Note: DISH spondylosis is the prominent and most constant feature of a constitutional tendency to "exuberant" ossification of the vertebral and extravertebral tight fibrous connective tissue that affects the entire body. In the great majority of cases, this *osteoblastic diathesis* manifests itself only in the second half of life. It involves the thoracic spine primarily, and less frequently the cervical and lumbar spine. Concerning the difficulty of differentiating roentgenologically between DISH and anklylosing spondylitis starting after the 50th year of life—i.e., in presenile or senile age—see p. 486 ff. It should be noted that in DISH, also, the sacroiliac joint spaces sometimes appear to be "obliterated" because the joint capsule undergoes massive ossification under the influence of the osteoblastic diathesis (Dihlmann and Freund, 1968). Exuberant ossification of the ligamental apparatus in the region of the costovertebral joints gives rise to *hyperostosis of the heads of the ribs* (see x in the figure). This hyperostosis also reflects a constitutional tendency to "exuberant" ossification of the fibrous connective tissue; it appears isolated or in connection with DISH (Fischer and Stecher, 1972). It is a *rule* that, in the middle and lower thoracic spine, hyperostotic spondylophytes develop primarily on the right side and have a coarser shape than on the left side (*reason:* right-handedness? Left-sided course of the thoracic aorta whose pulsations restrict the growth of the spondylophytes?). (Shapiro and Batt, 1960.)

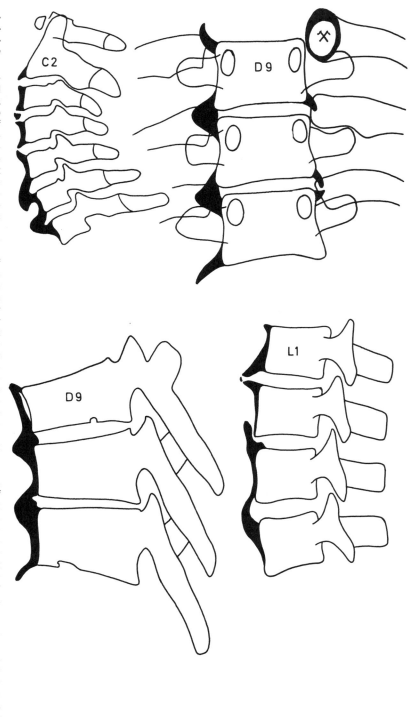

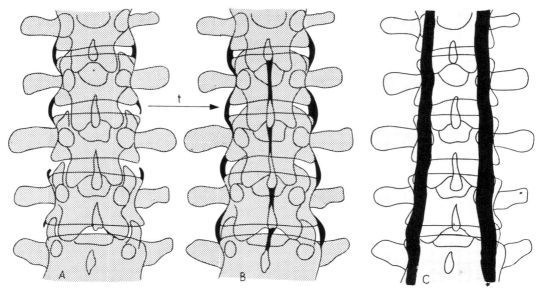

Fig. 682   **Syndesmophytes; bamboo spine; ankylosis of the intervertebral joints in ankylosing spondylitis.**

A, B = Follow-up study (t) of a case of ankylosing spondylitis in the lumbar spine. Initially (A), there are only isolated syndesmophytes—more pronounced in the upper lumbar spine than in its lower part. *Years later* (B): So-called bamboo spine; intervertebral joints ossified; ossification of the supraspinal and interspinal ligaments. C = Juvenile ankylosing spondylitis; 20-year-old patient in whom the disease began at the age of 15. No syndesmophytes (p. 486 ff) but extensive ossification of the intervertebral joints and the ligamentum flavum ("double-track tramway rails"); *marked* vertebral osteoporosis.

bral osteophytes grow in the external lamellae of the annulus fibrosus and in the space between the intervertebral disk and the anterior longitudinal ligament. Contrary to popular opinion, syndesmophytes do *not* develop through ossification of the anterior longitudinal ligament. At most, especially in aged individuals, this ligament may be involved in pathologic ossification in the advanced stage of ankylosing spondylitis (Fig. 683), together with the entire intervertebral disk. The syndesmophyte may be identified roentgenologically by a characteristic feature that results from its direction of growth: the syndesmophyte generally expands along the longitudinal axis of the spine, hence axially. Exceptions occur, however, when the syndesmophyte develops in a previously degenerated disk. Such syndesmophytes lose their harmonious, axially directed shape and bulge slightly in a lateral and/or anterior direction. Krebs (1931) has termed these structures **mixed osteophytes.** The attribute "mixed" indicates that they are an association of syndesmophytes *and* spondylophytes.

Syndesmophytes also occur as individual findings following an injury to the spine, in subligamental vertebral osteomyelitis (p. 474), and in ochronotic spondylopathy. These new bone formations, therefore, are not specific for ankylosing spondylitis but are only one among the possible reactions of the damaged axial skeleton (Dihlmann and Maes, 1970).

In adults, **familial hypophosphatemia** (familial hyperphosphaturia, so-called vitamin D–resistant rickets or osteomalacia, or familial vitamin D resistance, [Stanbury et al., 1959; Blackard et al., 1962;

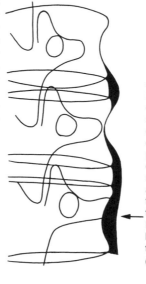

Fig. 683   **In ankylosing spondylitis the anterior longitudinal ligament does not ordinarily ossify.** Only in cases where a constitutional osteoblastic diathesis happens to be present or in aged patients does ossification of the annulus at the marginal ridge and of the space anterior to the disk spread to the anterior longitudinal ligament. In the oblique view of the lumbar spine, the vertebra then loses its "waistline" *(arrow).*

Fig. 684 **Psoriatic spondylitis with lumbar parasyndesmophytes and (in the present patient) unilateral sacroiliac involvement** (sacroiliitis of the "variegated picture" type; see under this heading). Affection of the spine in Reiter's syndrome leads to identical findings ("spondylitis of Reiter's syndrome").

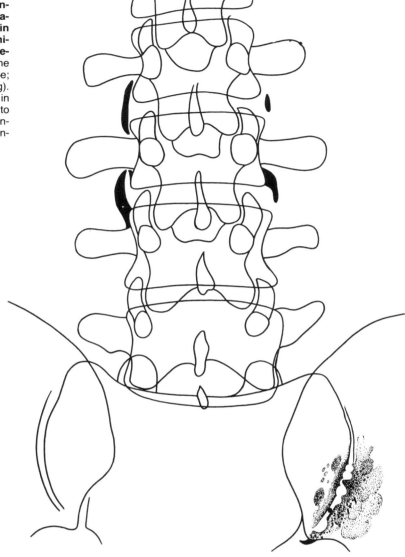

Moser and Fessel, 1974; Patton, 1976]) is *sometimes* associated with bony hooks resembling syndesmophytes, with ossification of the capsules of the intervertebral joints, and even with pathologic destruction of the sacroiliac joints leading to ankylosis. Marked fibroosteoses, and *primarily* the concomitantly identifiable Looser's zones in the skeleton, are signsposts for the diagnosis of this disorder of tubular reabsorption, which generally is of hereditary nature but may also occur sporadically. (Humoral signs of the full-blown disease picture are hypophosphatemia, normal calcium levels in blood, elevated alkaline phosphatase, and normal levels of parathyroid hormone). In **idiopathic** or **postoperative hypoparathyroidism,**

the mobility of the spine may also be considerably restricted by bony hooks resembling hyperostotic spondylophytes, syndesmophytes, or parasyndesmophytes (see under this heading). The diagnostically decisive roentgen findings in these cases (Adams and Davies, 1977) are absence of sacroiliitis, presence of marked fibroosteoses, ossifications of ligaments in the pelvic region and the extremities, and symmetrical calcifications in the basal ganglia. Perivertebral ossifications with the roentgenologic appearance of syndesmophytes also occur in **hereditary (chronic) hyperphosphatemia** (osteoectasis with hyperphosphatasia; McNulty and Pim, 1972). However, increase in alkaline serum phosphatase, osteoporosis, tendency to fractures, cortical thickening and bending of the long tubular bones, and increased thickness of the calvarium facilitate the correct diagnosis. (Radiologic differential diagnosis: fibrous dysplasia, Paget's disease—the term "juvenile Paget's disease" is a synonym for hyperphosphatasia—van Buchem's disease—endosteal hyperostosis, Camurati-Engelmann's diaphyseal dysplasia, osteogenesis imperfecta). In addition, the etiologic interpretation of vertebral osteophytes requires consideration of all the diseases and intoxications—e.g., chronic fluorine intoxication—that have been described on p. 72 as possible causes of ligament ossifications (in the spine).

The term **parasyndesmophyte** (Figs. 679 and 684) has been introduced by the present author (Dihlmann, 1968a) to characterize those vertebral osteophytes that indicate the involvement of the spine in Reiter's syndrome and in psoriatic arthritis. The distinction of parasyndesmophytes from syndesmophytes in ankylosing spondylitis was undertaken not only on the grounds of (radiologic) morphology but also for prognostic reasons! In the presence of a genetic predisposition, patients with chronic recurrent Reiter's syndrome or psoriatic arthritis may develop lesions in the skeleton of the trunk that cannot be differentiated clinically and roentgenologically from ankylosing spondylitis, and which lead to ankylosis of the spine. These patients present syndesmophytes that expand from one vertebra to the next. When, however, the involvement of the spine during the course of Reiter's syndrome or psoriatic arthritis (Bywaters and Dixon, 1965) *with or without concomitant sacroiliitis* (see under this heading) manifests itself by parasyndesmophytes, the prognosis with reference to discomfort and the risk of ankylosis is more favorable, because the parasyndesmophytes do not grow from one vertebral body to the other. They either have bony contact with a *single* vertebra or they develop in the perivertebral connective tissue *without* bony connection with the adjacent vertebral bodies. The mobility of the spine, therefore, is not at all, or only slightly, impaired by the parasyndesmophytes. Spondylitis in Reiter's syndrome and "psoriatic spondylitis" consequently offer a better prognosis than ankylosing spondylitis. When syndesmophytes develop concomitantly with the parasyndesmophytes (Schilling and Schacherl, 1967) or when follow-up films show that parasyndesmophytes are being transformed into syndesmophytes (Killebrew et al., 1973), more intense pain and marked limitation of spinal mobility are to be expected.

Parasyndesmophytes are observed in the lumbar spine—preferentially in the anteroposterior roentgenogram—in the thoracicolumbar junction, and in lateral films of the cervical spine. Three different morphologic types of parasyndesmophytes may be differentiated roentgenologically (Dihlmann, 1977; Figs. 679 and 684):

1. The steerhorn type
2. The elongated bony hook with sharp or hazy

contours, expanding paradiscally and paravertebrally
3. The paradiscal ossicle (which cannot be differentiated by its radiologic morphology from the spondylotic accessory bone; see p. 458).

However, to *settle* the diagnosis of parasyndemophytes with all the resultant diagnostic and prognostic inferences, *at least two* of the types described should be identifiable! Appearance of parasyndesmophytes may antedate the appearance of psoriatic skin lesions (Sundaram and Patton, 1975).

The **repair osteophyte** (Fig. 679) replaces—repairs—tissues of the disk and the vertebral body that have been destroyed by inflammation, trauma, or other processes. Therefore its configuration is not as characteristic and constant as that of the spondylophytes, syndesmophytes, or parasyndesmophytes. Its shape and its radiologic morphology adapt themselves to the existing situation. The repair osteophyte, therefore, is a multiform bony structure.

In **malignant osteophytosis** (Fig. 679), vertebral osteophytes are formed by the vertebral periosteum when a (sub-) periosteal metastasis or a developing malignant tumor stimulates the formation of new bone. The radiographic appearance resembles a spicule or a cockscomb.

Roentgenologic and Clinical Implications of Disk Degeneration

Spondylosis deformans, uncovertebral (neurocentral) joint osteoarthrosis intervertebral chondrosis, and intervertebral osteochondrosis undoubtedly are pathologic roentgen findings. However, this does not mean that every carrier of such lesions experiences them as a morbid event and complains of discomfort. Apart from this, the climate influences the clinical manifestations of disk degeneration. In warm and sunny climates, disk degeneration gives rise to less complaints than in cold and moist regions (Lawrence, 1975). It is true, however, that patients with pains in the neck, shoulder, and arm, as well as those suffering from low back pain or sciatic discomfort without radicular manifestations present signs of disk degeneration with greater frequency than people without such lesions of the intervertebral disks (Lawrence, 1969). The literature, therefore, describes degenerative disease of the disk as a *potential disorder* that *may* give rise to local discomfort, subjectively experienced restriction of vertebral motion, and pain, as well as other symptoms in remote areas, either cranially or caudally to the degenerated disk. For that reason, clinical syndromes have been described in connection with disk degeneration, the designation of which depends on their localization, their chief symptoms, and the duration of the complaints. These syndromes have an acute or an insidious onset and subsequently run a chronic course.

Among these morbid conditions are the **local cervical syndrome**, the **cervicobrachial syndrome**, the **cervicocephalic syndrome**, the **cervicomedul-**

lary **syndrome** (cervical myelopathy), the (infrequent) **thoracic syndrome,** and the **lumbar syndrome.** When these syndromes have been *diagnosed clinically,* a subsequent roentgen examination is indispensable, not only to establish a radiologically identifiable disk degeneration but also to demonstrate or to rule out such conditions as, *for example,* bacterial inflammation of the vertebrae and disks, inflammatory rheumatic affections of the spine, primary or metastatic tumors, (post-) traumatic lesions, vertebral malformations, and disorders of the intervertebral joints.

Occasionally it is necessary to perform a radiologic examination of *extravertebral* morphologic structures that can be assessed roentgenologically. On the one hand, such an examination serves to diagnose or to rule out the coincidence of disk degeneration and independent extravertebral lesions. On the other, discogenic extravertebral lesions can become independent to such a degree that eventually they decide the course of the disease and require treatment of their own (Krämer, 1978). "Syndrome" means, also in the skeleton, that identical complexes of signs and symptoms may have multiple causes!

The submarginal spondylophyte growing anteriorly and laterally to the vertebral body only very infrequently gives rise to complaints. However, isolated cases have been observed in the cervical spine in which large anterior (hyperostotic) spondylophytes, have obviously mechanically produced dysphagia (particularly difficulty in swallowing) and hoarseness (Heck, 1956; Gribovsky, 1966). It has been demonstrated on the operating table that large lumbar spondylophytes occasionally lead to circumscribed painful irritation of the peritoneum and of ileal loops with local hyperemia and increased thickness of tissues, as well as to painful elongation of the ureter (Rawat et al., 1975). Following removal of the spondylophyte the complaints subsided. Aneurysms of the abdominal aorta may manifest themselves indirectly by resorption of anterior spondylophytes and hyperostotic spondylophytes, and by erosion of the anterior surface of the vertebral body (Chaiton et al., 1979). Mechanical damage to the cord—grouped together clinically under the concept of cervical myelopathy—due to *dorsal spondylophytes* is only to be expected when, coincidentally, a concomitant constitutional narrowness of the spinal canal is present (compare the legend to Fig. 643 J). The same applies to ossifications of the posterior longitudinal ligament (Figs. 642 C and D).

Uncovertebral joint osteoarthrosis can, similarly to a posterolateral prolapsed disk and cervical spondylarthrosis deformans, encroach upon the intervertebral foramen (Figs. 643 A, B, and D) and can give rise to *radicular symptoms.* Moreover, these disorders may have a mechanical impact on the vertebral artery and its accompanying sympathetic vertebral plexus. Apophyseal joint osteoarthrosis may exert a similar effect (Fig. 643 D; Harzer and Töndury, 1966).

Circulatory disorders of the vertebral artery manifest themselves by *manifold* and *equivocal* symptoms, among them headaches (if episodic, called cervical migraine), attacks of giddiness, visual disturbances (e.g., scintillating scotomas), auditory disturbances (e.g., tinnitus), and difficulty in swallowing. A typical feature of this cervicocephalic syndrome is that *certain* movements or postures of the head precipitate, aggravate, or eliminate the complaints! Apart from these symptoms, the patients frequently give a history of (additional) complaints referable to the local cervical syndrome, such as pains in the back of the neck and the shoulders that appear or worsen in certain positions, limitation of cervical motion, and tightness of the musculature of neck and shoulders. In all the cases listed, the possible cervical etiology must be elucidated radiologically in four planes (sagittal, lateral, oblique from the right, oblique from the left). When the question of surgical intervention (extirpation of the uncus, uncoforaminectomy) arises, angiography of the vertebral arteries is also mandatory.

The motion of the three mobile segments of the spine takes place by the "collective principle," since each motor segment contributes its part in the range of motion of the spinal segment concerned. This practical division of function, however, has biologic disadvantages as soon as the motor function in one or a few segments is impaired; for example, by *intervertebral chondrosis* or *osteochondrosis.* When, for instance, the mobility in one or more motor segments is abolished or considerably diminished, the neighboring motor segments either compensate for this by increased mobility *or* their mobility is likewise impaired by reflex. An originally mono- or oligosegmental disorder has an impact on the entire spinal section:

1. *Limited mobility of a motor segment developing chronically (i.e., insidiously) has a variety of causes.* Vertebral osteophytes that bridge a disk, *complete* degenerative or traumatic destruction of a disk (crumbling, attrition, rupture, wear and tear), acquired (and congenital) synostosis of vertebral bodies, ossification of capsules and ligaments, and destruction of the intervertebral joints are examples of the manifold causes of segmental hypomobility and immobility. Diminution and complete loss of mobility in a motor segment due to pathologic changes of morphology—whether a congenital condition or developing gradually over a prolonged period—do not usually cause discomfort. The complaints of the patient, who in most cases does not subjectively experience the slowly progressing loss of function of a *single* motor segment, refer as a rule to the mobile segments and adjoining superiorly and inferiorly (Jenkner and Dossi, 1977). There, the segmentally distributed autochthonous musculature of the back—including all the muscles innervated by the dorsal branches of the spinal nerves—is forced to perform *extra work* of a static *(isometric)* nature to maintain the erect posture; for example, in the presence of a

monosegmental extended position or with an angular kyphosis. The extra load, however, also has a substantial dynamic *(isotonic)* component that serves to maintain the physiologic global mobility of the spinal segment involved. The additional muscular work can lead to myalgic decompensation of the muscles mentioned *(vide infra)*. This decompensation becomes manifest by pain and muscular tightness. It indicates, in principle, a disproportion between functional demands and functional efficiency of the muscles concerned. The compensatory extra strain upon the contiguous intervertebral disks from muscular overwork furthers their attrition. This supposition has been confirmed in principle, since the roentgen manifestations of disk degeneration are encountered more frequently in heavy workers (miners, etc.) than in control groups of comparable age without heavy physical work (Lawrence, 1969; Billenkamp, 1972). Finally, in the avascular intervertebral disk of the adult there exists no exertional hyperemia. The *compensatory hypermobility* of the adjacent motor segments therefore passes gradually into a *pathologic hypermobility (structural loosening) with spondyloretrolisthesis*. It eventually terminates in hypomobility or even immobility of this motor segment as the expression of an enforced position of comfort assumed by reflex (see below under 3) and/or as the result of advanced attrition of the disk that has developed in the meantime. In this manner the hypomobility or immobility that once has developed in a motor segment (or which is of congenital nature, Fig. 666A) extends over the years and decades more and more cranially and/or caudally in the part of the spine concerned.

2.   With **acute (-short-term) onset of immobilization (obstruction) of one or more motor segments,** the afferent nerve impulses pass via the sinuvertebral nerve (Fig. 602). Therefore it is primarily the dorsal prolapse of the disk and canted malpositions of the intervertebral joints with "strangulation" of synovial folds and so-called *meniscoids* (Zukschwerdt et al., 1960) that give rise to such *antalgic segmental positions of comfort*. They are the result of reflex tightening of the autochthonous muscles of the back, which leads to a segmental impairment of motion. Scoliosis in sciatica and torticollis are the best known *clinical* examples of the corresponding *postures* of comfort. Among the roentgenologically identifiable mono- or oligosegmental *positions* of comfort—"posture" refers to spinal segments and "position" to individual motor segments—are (pages 398 and 399):

·   The monosegmental extended position (Fig. 607 A)
·   The dorsal gaping of the disk space (Fig. 607 B)
·   The extended position of several motor segments *above* a disk space in which the roentgen signs of a loss in disk mass are recognizable (Fig. 607 C, Güntz's sign).

Güntz's sign and the other positions of comfort triggered by reflex can also have causes that are different from displaced disk tissue or malpositions of the intervertebral joints. They develop *acutely*—for example, by a trauma—or *chronically* (insidiously)—for example, with structural loosening in chondrosis and osteochondrosis by a growing tumor and inflammatory processes as soon as these exert their influence on the nerve roots or the sinuvertebral nerve.

The teleological characterization of the mono- or oligosegmental malpositions described as antalgic positions of comfort illustrates that any active or passive change of the pathologic positions of the vertebrae produces considerable pain. Only the elimination of the pain by physiotherapeutic procedures, manual therapy, operation, etc., or the interruption of the afferences and their reflex consequences by medication, local anesthesia, or neural therapy can bring about the regression of these malpositions and hence can eliminate the cause as well as the consequence of the pain.

3.   *Structural loosening* means, in principle, "individualization" of the motor function in the segment involved; it is in contradiction to the collective principle of construction and motion of the spine. Structural loosening is counteracted by a reflex increase in tone of the corresponding musculature ("reflex hypertonia"). The latter places a pertinent unphysiologic strain on the muscles involved so that with time the blood flow and thereby the exchange of matter between the capillaries and muscle tissue becomes impaired. The blood supply to the muscle is inadequate; hypoxia and lactacidosis (Peter, 1976) ensue. Ischemia, hypoxia, and acidosis are known to be potential sources of pain in the musculature; they may become manifest in the form of myalgia when the muscles involved are subjected to a *trifling additional strain* such as bending down, lifting a load, uncoordinated sudden movements, local chilling (drafts), etc. In a form of vicious circle, the muscle pain in turn increases the muscle tone by reflex, and the initially protective increase in muscle tone eventually terminates in an enforced sustained contraction. This is a condition which, physiologically, is analogous to the boardlike rigidity of the abdominal muscles in acute appendicitis or following the perforation of a gastroduodenal ulcer. The discogenic structural loosening, however, not only is experienced by the patient as myalgia but also manifests itself by the consequences of another morphologic fact: sensory branches from the dorsal ramus of the spinal nerves penetrate the back muscles on their way to the corresponding dermatomes. The enforced tensing of the muscles leads to mechanical entrapment of these nerves (Peter, 1976), putting them, so to speak, in a straitjacket. The result is segmentally radiating pain. The "cry" of the diseased intervertebral disk thus reaches the surface (of the skin)!

Apart from the painful muscular manifestations triggered by reflex, complaints also develop by direct irritation of the sensory endings of the sinuvertebral nerve. Adequate stimuli in the morphologic structures (compare Fig. 602) supplied by this nerve can give rise there, for example, to stretching and distortion that occur with structural loosening. This supposition is confirmed by (intentional) provocation of pain by injection into the disk—discography. (distention sign; Krämer, 1978). By this procedure one tests whether local and irradiating pains are in fact precipitated by the roentgenologically diagnosed lesions of the disk. This provocation of pain has acquired importance in *preoperative* diagnosis because an intervertebral disk that remains *asymptomatic* following intradiscal injection, is not eligible for surgical treatment, however severe the degenerative changes visible in the roentgenogram may be (Krämer, 1978).

The *potential* sequelae of pathologically restricted segmental mobility and pathologically increased segmental mobility—structural loosening—have been described in the foregoing on the basis of current knowledge. However, there can be no doubt that this description is fundamentally correct. As a matter of fact, treatment of these disorders of vertebral function must avail itself of the physiologic concepts described if it is to eliminate the complaints. Existing chondrosis or osteochondrosis of course remains unchanged. Chondrosis, intervertebral osteochondrosis, and uncovertebral spondylosis thus rank as disease factors the radiologic examiner must consider.

Methodologic premises for this heuristic discernment are: an anteroposterior view and oblique (cervical) views with anteflexion and retroflexion; i.e., only one additional roentgenogram as compared with the conventional radiologic program!

Osteoarthrosis of the Apophyseal (Intervertebral) Joints, the Costovertebral Joints, and the Lumbosacral Assimilation Joints

Degenerative lesions in these joints present no fundamental difference from osteoarthrosis of the joints of the extremities. Narrowing of the radiologic joint space, subchondral band-shaped condensation of the cancellous bone, and marginal osteophytes indicate the deforming nature of these signs of attrition. In addition, a few qualitative and quantitative details are to be mentioned:

Osteoarthrosis of the intervertebral joints has been termed **spondylarthrosis deformans.** One must consider development of this condition by taking into account the cooperation between the intervertebral disk and the two associated intervertebral joints (see p. 396). In so doing, some contradictory aspects emerge:

On the one hand, study of roentgenograms of the cervical spine regularly reveals that motor segments with marked osteochondrosis show no, or only minor, spondylarthrotic changes, and vice versa. In

advanced osteochondrosis, the discogenic segmental limitation of motion evidently "spares" the intervertebral joints, and vice versa. On the other hand, the diminished height of the intervertebral disk in degeneration of this element gives rise to an anomalous position of the articular processes of the two associated intervertebral joints (Fig. 685). In addition, loss—or even the limitation—of the shock-absorbing function of the disk in degeneration leads to increased strain on the intervertebral joints. The result of the discogenic segmental structural loosening is increased mobility of the intervertebral joints that presents a risk of excessive and inappropriate demands on their mechanical function and thereby furthers the development of spondylarthrosis. Finally, it should be mentioned that pseudospondylolisthesis develops on the basis of spondylarthrosis (Fig. 627 A). In this case, attrition of the intervertebral joints may lead to structural loosening in the region of the disk. This unbiased enumeration of apparent or "genuine" contradictions in the pathogenesis of spondylarthrosis should also interest the radiologic examiner. The chief interest, however, of course attaches to the roentgen manifestations of spondylarthrosis in the different segments of the spine (see Figs. 627 A, 686, and 687).

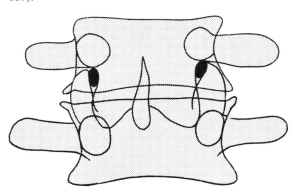

Fig. 685 **"Telescoping subluxation" of the lumbar vertebral joints** (Reinhardt, 1957) as a clue to the influence of degeneration of the intervertebral disk on the position of the articular processes in the same segment. Characteristic features are the "holes" *(shaded black)*. For these holes to develop in the anteroposterior roentgenogram, the caudally directed articular process must have a lateral concavity. The articulating surface of the articular process—which passes upward—must lie in the sagittal plane; it must expand laterally, and its tip must reach the transverse process; i.e., it must be displaced cranially. Apart from this, the decrease in height of the degenerated disk is an important preliminary condition for the upward slipping of the articular process. In tomographs taken in the recumbent position, the cranial circumference of the lightened oval is not usually entirely complete. In the contrary case—when the "hole" has a complete osseous border—one may assume that the joint capsule has been entirely worn away and that the tip of the canal articular process has "bored" itself into the transverse process.

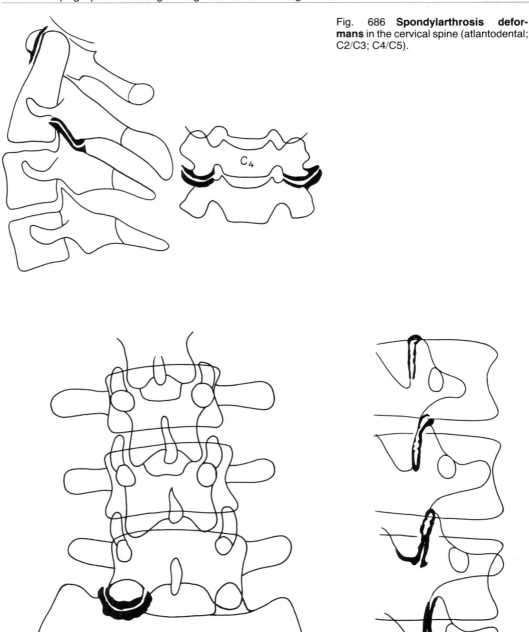

Fig. 686 **Spondylarthrosis deformans** in the cervical spine (atlantodental; C2/C3; C4/C5).

Fig. 687 **Osteoarthrosis of the apophyseal joints (so-called spondylarthrosis deformans) of the lumbar spine.** *Left:* Right-sided lumbosacral spondylarthrosis. Dysplasias of the lumbosacral articular processes—as sketched in the figure—favor the development of spondylarthrosis in the lumbosacral junction. These dysplasias are characterized by a club-shaped structure of the caudal articular processes, which gradually become embedded in the sacrum. The joint space frequently courses in the frontal plane. In the present case, the development of osteoarthrosis on the *right* side was obviously favored by the slight lumbar scoliosis (compare Figs. 628 D and 650 G).

Right: Osteoarthrosis of the apophyseal joints in an oblique view of the lumbar spine. Note the capsular ossifications and compare them with the roentgen findings in the intervertebral joints encountered in ankylosing spondylitis (Fig. 749).

Fig. 688   **Radiographic characteristics of osteoar-throsis in the costovertebral joints.**
Th 11: Costotransverse osteoarthrosis.
Th 12: Osteoarthrosis of the head of the rib a few years (t) after dislocation at the right costovertebral joint Th 12.

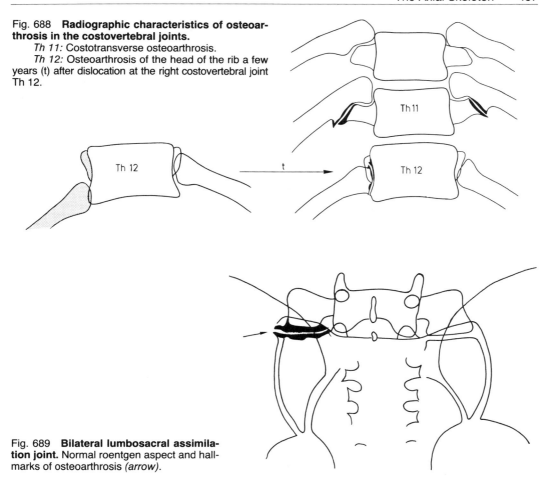

Fig. 689   **Bilateral lumbosacral assimilation joint.** Normal roentgen aspect and hallmarks of osteoarthrosis *(arrow).*

The costovertebral joints are differentiated into the *joint of the costal head* and the *costotransverse joint.* The former connects the head of the rib to the vertebral body and the adjacent intervertebral disk, whereas the latter connects the articular facet of the costal tubercle with the transverse process of the vertebra. Costovertebral osteoarthrosis manifests itself much more frequently in the roentgenogram than **costotransverse osteoarthrosis** and less frequently than **osteoarthrosis of the costal head** (Fig. 688). Costotransverseosteoarthrosis shows beak-shaped elongations of the straightened articular surfaces and subchondral densifications (Fig. 688). In addition, the capsuloligamentous apparatus partakes in the attrition of the costovertebral joints, and fibroosteoses or ligament calcifications are formed. The latter are particularly conspicuous in the lateral costotransverse ligament of the first ribs. Ossifications of capsule and ligaments, however, in the region of the costovertebral joints are also observed without roentgen signs of degeneration in these joints (Hohmann, 1968). Such ossifications also develop during the course of ankylosing spondylitis (Fig. 751).

In the lumbosacral junction, nearthroses **(lumbosacral assimilation joints)** may develop in transitional vertebrae. In these joints, the unilateral or bilateral shovel-shaped transverse process of the last lumbar vertebra articulates with the sacrum. Figure 689 shows the radiologic characteristics of such a neoarthrosis and its osteoarthrosis.

Infections of the Spine

Spinal infections manifest themselves *roentgenologically* by three different findings:

1. Infectious spondylitis
2. Vertebral osteomyelitis
3. Migrating spondylitis

The microorganisms are disseminated to the bone marrow primarily through the arterial bloodstream. Infections may also start from the intervertebral disk, which in the early growth period may still be supplied by blood vessels, and from the prediscal space (between the anterior longitudinal ligament and the annulus fibrosus), which is permanently vascularized. It is a matter of debate whether microorganisms may also be disseminated by the *venous circulation*. Clinical observations (Lame, 1956) to the effect that bacterial infections following operations in the lower pelvis and metastases of urologic carcinomas frequently lodge in the vertebrae have attracted attention to the so-called vertebral venous system. This venous system interconnects the superior and inferior vena cava but, unlike the circulation in the azygos veins, it is not influenced by increases in intrathoracic or intraabdominal pressure. It forms a valveless network that extends along the spine (external and internal vertebral venous plexus) and terminates cranially in the dural sinus (Batson, 1957). A *direct implantation* of microorganisms may occur during operations on the disk (Bösch, 1965; Greiner, 1974), by puncture of the disk for discography (Vogelsang, 1973), and also as a complication of paravertebral lumbar anesthesia of the sympathetic chain by spinal puncture or peridural anesthesia. With the three last-named interventions, infection starts from the (incorrectly) punctured intervertebral disks or from the perivertebral connective tissue (Sewcz and Preuss, 1970). Finally, infection of the spine also may follow an open injury such as a gunshot wound.

Infectious spondylitis is conventionally divided into tuberculous and nonspecific bacterial spondylitis. Tuberculous spondylitis generally becomes manifest between 6 and 12 months after hematogenous dissemination. In some cases, the latency period between dissemination (possibly indicated by exudative pleurisy) and clinical manifestation may be prolonged up to two years. The early hematogenous focus in the bone marrow is most frequently located in the vicinity of the vertebral end plates. This location governs the radiologic appearance of both tuberculous spondylitis [35] and nonspecific bacterial infection. Either the inflammatory destruction of bone in the vicinity of the end plates soon spreads to the disk, or disk tissue prolapses into the inflammatory focus in the bone (Fig. 690). The lateral roentgenogram then reveals a conspicuous decrease in height of the intervertebral disk involved (see p. 401; Figs. 669 and 670). When concomitant haziness of the contour or a contour defect in the vertebral body is already demonstrable, *lateral* tomography of the involved vertebral region should be performed without delay.

Concerning the radiologic differentiation between tuberculous and nonspecific bacterial spondylitis, it must be mentioned here that tuberculous infections of the vertebrae develop more frequently in

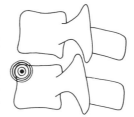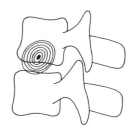

Fig. 690 **Localizations of bacterial infections of the bone marrow which can be identified relatively early by radiology.** The stratified circles and ellipses indicate the continuous spread of the process (*on the right: through the disk*).

a few areas than nonspecific bacterial disseminations. When, therefore, study by tomography is not limited to the suspect motor segment but, for example, includes the two or three motor segments superiorly and inferiorly, the probability of demonstrating a clinically asymptomatic bone lesion (breakdown) increases (Fig. 670). The radiologic diagnosis of *tuberculous* spondylitis is thereby considerably facilitated and becomes more probable.

Monosegmental decrease in disk height in a lateral film of the spine *with or without* haziness of the end plates, *without* contour defects, *without* vertebral osteophytes, and *without* subdiscal, band-shaped condensation of the vertebral cancellous bone—hence a **monosegmental nonreactive decrease in disk height**—should definitely arouse suspicion of spondylitis! In children and juveniles—at an age when degenerative changes are not to be expected—it nearly always evidences bacterial infection. In adulthood, monosegmental nonreactive decrease in disk height without contour defects should arouse suspicion of an infectious etiology. This suspicion is corroborated by certain historical data and clinical findings (Table 7); it becomes verified or invalidated by tomography (Figs. 670, 691, and 692). As a bacterial infection of the vertebra progresses (Fig. 693), increasingly larger portions of the intervertebral disk and the vertebral substance undergo destruction and become resorbed (dissolved). This process leads to progressive decrease in disk height, destructive deformation of the adjacent vertebrae with formation of sequestra, and malposition—mostly angular kyphosis (gibbus) or angular scoliosis—and the development of an abscess.

Sequestra (Fig. 694) and abscesses can be identified roentgenologically; sequestra are most confidently demonstrable on tomographs (Fig. 695). An abscess must have a larger volume to become visible as a shadow in the conventional roentgenogram; computed tomography is therefore advisable. Pus may manifest itself by calcium shadows. Small fragments of bone, for instance, become apparent at some distance from the spondylitis, and precipitated calcium is recognizable in *inspissated* pus. Indirect demonstration of an abscess is possible with the aid of cer-

---

[35] Tuberculous infection of the bone marrow leads to necrosis and death of the contiguous cancellous trabeculae. Although dead bone does not decalcify in response to a local inflammatory disorder of circulation (see under arthritic collateral phenomena), its cells are resorbed. Resorption, however, takes a great deal of time. This biologic phenomenon explains why tuberculous lesions of bone, their progression, and their healing quality are radiographically demonstrable relatively late as well as why tuberculous skeletal lesions usually are more extensive than would be presumed from the roentgen findings.

Table 7 **Diagnostic procedure for the early identification of a spinal infection (spondylitis).** The term "infection" refers here primarily to the colonization of tuberculous and nontuberculous microorganisms. In much rarer instances, the recommended diagnostic procedure will detect a fungal or parasitic infection; e.g. actinomycosis or echinococcosis. The latter findings are "rarities."

Localized pain in the spine (spontaneous pain, tenderness on palpation, pain on compression in the longitudinal axis)

Roentgenogram:	Monosegmental nonreactive narrowing of disk space with or without indistinct contours of the end plates.
Anamnesis, clinical findings:	Exudative pleurisy; tuberculosis of organs or the skeleton; fever; elevated sedimentation rate; local or systemic bacterial infection in the recent past ("dissemination disease"); interventions (operations) on the spine or the organs of the lower pelvis.
Lateral tomography:	Poorly defined borders of the end plate(s) and/or contour defect(s) with and without sequestra, possibly additional bone lesions (osteolyses, cavities with or without sequestra) in the adjacent vertebrae.
Roentgen diagnosis:	Infectious spondylitis. Etiologic classification by anamnesis (*vide supra*), serologic methods, culture, and animal experiment following puncture or vertebral biopsy.

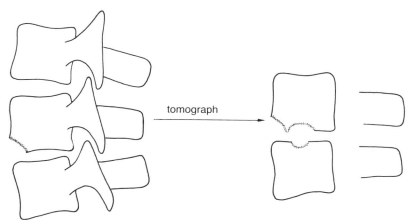

Fig. 691 **Nonreactive decrease in disk height plus spondyloretrolisthesis plus erosion of the anterior vertebral edge = bacterial spondylitis.** Tomography only assists in the accurate "quantitative" assessment of the infection; i.e., it *may* demonstrate additional inflammatory erosions, such as here in both end plates.

tomograph

Fig. 692 **The combined roentgen findings of "non-reactive decrease in disk height plus spondyloretrolisthesis in the lumbar spine in a young male has been the reason for taking a lateral tomograph.** When the tomograph reveals hazy contours *(above)* or erosions *(below)* of the end plates, the diagnosis of **bacterial spondylitis** is settled. *Exceptions:* If the patient suffers from rheumatoid arthritis or ankylosing spondylitis, one must first consider destruction of the disk ("discitis" see p. 474) or of the disk *and* the vertebra (spondylodiscitis; see the footnote on p. 474 by inflammatory rheumatic granulation tissue, compare p. 508 (see also Andersson's lesion during the course of ankylosing spondylitis).

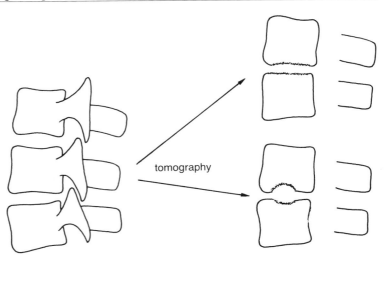

tomography

tain roentgen signs which depend on its location (Figs. 696, 697, 698, and 699). Sequestra and abscesses occur *primarily* with tuberculous spondylitis, and in individual cases, this statistical statement permits a presumptive diagnosis. However, neither roentgen finding proves the tuberculous etiology of a spondylitis, since sequestra as well as abscesses are also occasionally found in nonspecific bacterial infections of the vertebrae.

The *tendency to healing* in infectious spondylitis is demonstrable by four roentgen findings:

1. Smoothing and sharp outlines of the defects
2. Perifocal sclerosis of the cancellous bone.
3. Development of repair osteophytes (Fig. 679)
4. Bony fusion of vertebrae (Figs. 659 and 666 C and D).

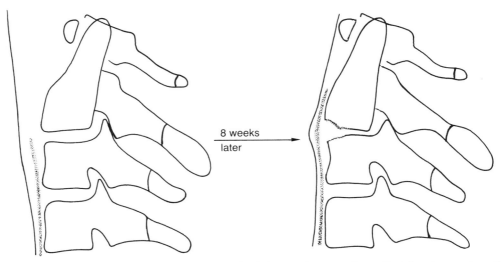

8 weeks later

Fig. 693 **Nonspecific bacterial spondylitis following injury to the posterior wall of the pharynx by a fishbone.** About 1 week after the injury intense pains persist, both spontaneously and on swallowing. The lateral roentgenogram reveals that the posterior wall of the pharynx has been forced away from C2 and C3; the prevertebral fat stripe is displaced anteriorly and in part obliterated (compare Fig. 616 C). No changes in the vertebral contours and the disk space C2/C3. Eight weeks later, the swelling of the soft tissues has largely resolved under antibiotic therapy. However, a decrease in disk height and erosions in C2 and C3 are now demonstrable.

Inference: The nonspecific bacterial infection of the retropharyngeal space due to injury by a fishbone has spread to the vertebral bodies C2 and C3 and to the intervertebral disk C2/C3.

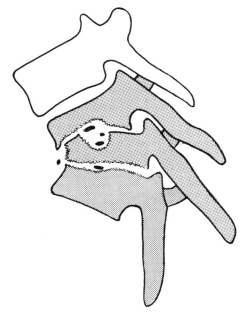

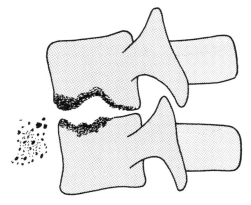

Fig. 696 **Suspicion of an "older" abscess in a case of known tuberculous spondylitis:** Numerous calcium shadows and small fragments of bone (calcium precipitates in an inspissating abscess?) have appeared in the prevertebral region.

Fig. 694   Advanced florid tuberculous spondylitis with sequestra and formation of a gibbus (angular kyphosis of three vertebrae with deformation of the vertebral bodies; see p. 398).

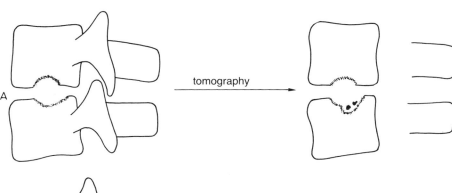

tomography

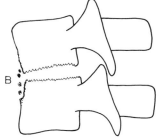

Fig. 695 **Infectious spondylitis (A).** The lateral survey film identifies the inflammatory process (nonreactive decrease in disk height; spondyloretrolisthesis; erosions of the end plates). The tomograph shows, as additional findings, a few sequestra; therefore a tuberculous spondylitis appears to be more likely than a nonspecific bacterial infection (see also Table 7 on p. 469).

Infectious spondylitis (B), recognizable by decrease in disk height, ill-defined end plates, angular kyphosis with deformed vertebral bodies (=gibbus). Melting away of the vertebral edges with small sequestra. The sequestra suggest a tuberculous etiology.

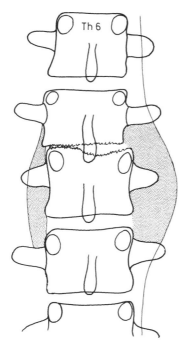

Fig. 697 **Tuberculous spondylitis in the thoracic spine.** Radiologic aspect in the anteroposterior roentgenogram. Abscess formation is indicated by the fusiform broadening of the left paravertebral line and by circumscribed visibility of the right paravertebral line (compare Fig. 621, p. 410).

Perifocal sclerosis of the cancellous bone surrounding the destroyed vertebral region indicates a fundamental reaction of bone; i.e., the formation of a "defensive wall" against any pathogenic agents, whether they be microorganisms, cancer cells, or a sustained injury (in this case: callus formation occurs). Perifocal sclerosis of the cancellous bone may increase to form the so-called *ivory vertebra* (Fig. 661 G). From the footnote on page 468 one may infer that in nonspecific bacterial spondylitis, perifocal sclerosis of the cancellous bone develops earlier and is more pronounced than in tuberculous infection. The more manifest the third and fourth roentgen signs, the farther advanced are the stabilization and cicatrization of the bacterial inflammation.

In nonspecific bacterial spondylitis, the four processes mentioned run their course over a few months (Fig. 700). In tuberculous spondylitis, their course may require many months or even years, depending on the extent of vertebral destruction at the onset of treatment, but this information is of little importance in the differential diagnosis between tuberculous and nonspecific bacterial infection, since it can be established only in retrospect. In a case of diagnosed and treated tuberculous or nonspecific spondylitis, however, it may help in estimating the effectiveness of therapy and thus the prognosis for its duration. Furthermore, it is known that some vertebral infections—e.g., *Brucella* spondylitis—have a particularly marked tendency to form repair osteophytes.

The term **malum suboccipitale** denotes a tuberculous infection of the cervicooccipital junction that formerly offered an unfavorable or at least doubtful prognosis. The condition involves not only the occipital condyles but also the atlas, the axis, and the joints as well as the ligaments of this region. The destruction of bone is followed by faulty positions; e.g., ventral dislocation of the atlas (Fig. 5). The more extensive the destruction in the region of the occipital bone, the earlier may the roentgen manifestations of destruction in the first and second cervical vertebra *and* their joints be interpreted as being of tuberculous nature. Involvement of this region by adult rheumatoid arthritis is not, as a rule, to be expected until late in the disease. Therefore, rheumatoid arthritis cannot escape the notice of the radiologic examiner, provided he does not confine himself to reading the roentgenogram but also examines the patient!

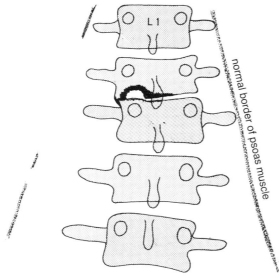

Fig. 698 **Tuberculous spondylitis known and treated for many years.** The extensive "obliteration" of the border of the psoas muscle is indicative of the psoas abscess that has developed in the meantime.

Differential diagnosis of the "obliterated" psoas border: Hematoma (traumatic; accompanying a coagulopathy); abscess (spondylitis; paranephritic; appendicitis that has perforated into the retroperitoneal space); malignant retroperitoneal tumor (primary or metastatic); lodgment of an echinococcus.

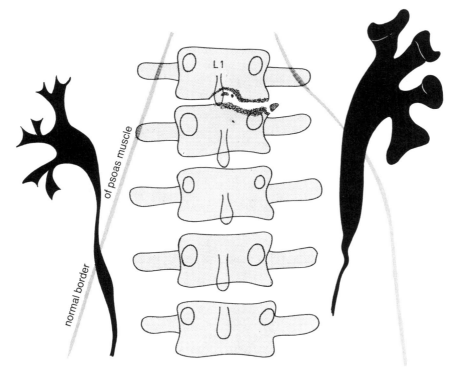

Fig. 699 **Tuberculous spondylitis L1/L2 with large left-sided psoas abscess.** Note the broadening and projection of the border of the psoas muscle and the *left-sided* hydronephrosis on excretory urography.

Note: The border of the psoas major muscle does not normally cross the imaginary upward prolongation of the sacroiliac joint space at the level of L3.

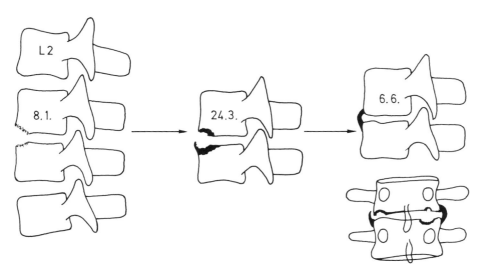

Fig. 700 **Stabilization of a nonspecific bacterial spondylitis treated with antibiotics in the course of 5 months.** The first roentgenogram was taken about 1 month after a paravertebral sympathetic block with a local anesthetic. This therapeutic procedure evidently led to the inoculation of pathogenic microorganisms.

Following surgery for a prolapsed disk, the surgically treated motor segment may present lesions that have the radiologic appearance of bacterial spondylitis. The initial symptoms of this infection often occur as early as a few weeks after the operation (Busse et al., 1976). Diminished disk height, haziness and erosions of the end plates, perifocal sclerosis of the cancellous bone as well as repair osteophytes, and eventually partial or complete fusion of vertebrae are demonstrable in the radiograph and justify diagnosis and treatment of this **postoperative nonspecific bacterial inoculation spondylitis.** In such cases, the surgical wound may heal by primary intention or (when infected) by secondary intention (Stern and Crandall, 1959).

Postoperative roentgen findings that manifest themselves only a number of months after the operation by recurrent discomfort and which are *not* produced by renewed prolapse of the disk have occurred. The surgical wound has healed primarily and there is no fistulation or abscess formation. The sedimentation rate may be normal or slightly elevated. Roentgenologically, however, the finding is consistent with bacterial spondylitis *(vide supra)*. Nevertheless, needle biopsies, reoperations, or autopsies with cultures and histologic study have failed to provide a clue to local infection (Lowman and Robinson, 1966). It has therefore been suggested that operations on the disk are apt to be followed by nonbacterial (sterile) inflammations due to **aseptic necrosis in the discovertebral field of operation,** which has been produced by the surgical trauma (Kaganas, 1964; Lowman and Robinson, 1966; Greiner et al., 1974; Busse et al., 1976).

The term **"discitis,"** which refers to an inflammatory process in the intervertebral disk, presupposes a vascularized disk. Vascularization frequently persists in the growth period, especially in children, and inflammation again becomes possible in old age, when blood vessels have grown into a degenerated disk. Calcareous discitis in (small) children has already been mentioned (Fig. 83). In principle, however, a bacterial spondylitis may also develop by way of the bloodstream and may lead to decrease in height of the disk space and to antalgic extension of the involved spinal segment. Usually, the inflammatory process quickly spreads to the contiguous vertebral body. This manifests itself particularly in tomographs by haziness and/or erosion of the contours of the end plates. In most cases, therefore, the bacterial discitis is already a "spondylodiscitis" (spondylitis[36]).

Inflammatory rheumatic diseases such as adult rheumatoid arthritis sometimes give rise to a "genuine" discitis (see p. 481). Inflammatory rheumatic granulation tissue may grow into the disk space (Bywaters, 1974) and may destroy the intervertebral disk

without producing destruction of the vertebra. This condition may be demonstrated by tomography. When, however, the granulation tissue attacks the disk *and* the contiguous vertebral body, **inflammatory rheumatic spondylodiscitis** develops (Dihlmann and Nebel, 1980). This condition is characterized by a decrease in disk height, haziness of the end plates (see *"note"* in Fig. 670), erosions of the end plates, *and* absent or minimal vertebral osteophytes (Figs. 708 and 711). For spondylodiscitis in ankylosing spondylitis see p. 508 ff.

Sarcoidosis (p. 106 ff) may also attack the spine, though this is an extremely infrequent event. The following roentgen findings, which usually occur in several motor segments, have been observed: Osteolyses with marginal sclerosis, defects of the end plates, decrease in disk height, vertebral collapse, pathologic fracture of the dens, perivertebral soft-tissue shadows, and osteoblastic vertebral foci (Goobar et al., 1961; Zener et al., 1963; Berk and Brower, 1964; Brun et al., 1966; Uehlinger and Wurm, 1976; Brodey et al., 1976; Stump et al., 1976; Zimmermann and Leeds, 1976). Involvement of the axial skeleton in sarcoidosis does not occur without concomitant (hilar) lymphadenopathy, but it may be the only skeletal manifestation of the disease! The great variety of the roentgen findings listed *sometimes* calls for differential diagnosis from infectious (especially tuberculous) spondylitis. Similar considerations can be obtained in differentiating tuberculous sacroiliitis from sacroiliac sarcoidosis. In the final analysis, the diagnosis must be settled by cultural examination and histologic study.

The destructive osteoarthropathy in **chondrocalcinosis** has been described on p. 64 ff. This metabolic disorder seldom manifests itself by destructive lesions in the spine (Villiaumey et al., 1974; Cottin et al., 1980). The roentgenologic aspect is that of infectious spondylitis.

Gout also may lead to discovertebral destructions that present the roentgenologic appearance of infectious spondylitis (Vinstein and Cockerill, 1972). It may also erode the pedicles and the vertebral bodies by an epidural tophus (Wald et al., 1979).

In **hyperparathyroidism,** lesions resembling inflammatory or tumorous destruction have been observed in the spine (Freyschmidt and Hehrmann, 1978). **Recurrent polychondritis** sometimes causes erosions of the end plates with perifocal vertebral sclerosis (Johnson et al., 1973).

Vertebral osteomyelitis results from bacterial infection of the vertebra *without* involvement of the contiguous intervertebral disk(s). The inflammation thus is located in the vertebral arch or in the vertebral processes. The bacterial focus has the appearance of an osteolytic area possibly surrounded by a (delicate) seam of increased density. (Lateral) tomographs sometimes reveal sequestra in bone that has broken down; such sequestra escape detection in survey films. Suspicion of tuberculosis (tuberculous vertebral osteomyelitis) is aroused by sequestra as well as by oli-

---

[36] In the German literature, bacterial diseases with involvement of the vertebrae and disks are termed *spondylitis*. The designation *spondylodiscitis* is reserved for involvement of the vertebrae and disks in inflammatory rheumatic diseases.

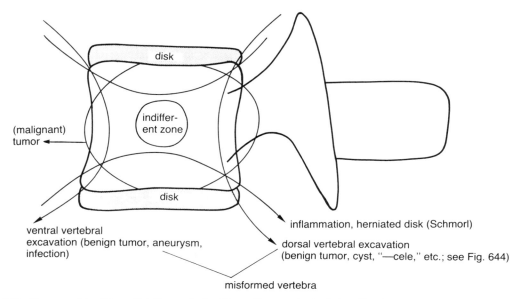

ventral vertebral
excavation (benign tumor, aneurysm,
infection)

inflammation, herniated disk (Schmorl)

dorsal vertebral excavation
(benign tumor, cyst, "—cele," etc.; see Fig. 644)

misformed vertebra

Fig. 701   **Topographic differential diagnosis facilitates the nosological classification of pathologic changes of vertebral contours and vertebral structure.** Lesions that are centrally located in the vertebral body—osteolyses and osteoblastic foci—may be of tumorous or of inflammatory origin. They therefore lie in the indifferent radiologic zone. When they expand and reach the surface of the vertebral body, an inflammatory process will traverse the barrier of the cartilaginous end plate, whereas, with the exception of chordoma, tumor cells as a rule fail to do so and will involve the intervertebral disk.

The following *working hypothesis* is therefore applicable: Destruction of the vertebral body plus decrease in disk height indicates inflammation. Destruction (or even collapse) of the vertebral body *without* adequate trauma and *without* conspicuous osteoporosis argues for neoplasm! The cartilaginous barrier is absent on the anterior, lateral, and posterior surfaces of the vertebral body. This is why tumor tissue or an inflammatory process can break through there; both can give rise to a perivertebral soft-tissue shadow in the roentgenogram. Pathologic vertebral excavations develop under the influence of chronic pressure, but also by inflammatory erosion. They can also indicate a vertebral malformation (compare Fig. 644, no. 5).

gotopic foci, and also by the association of vertebral infection and spondylitic processes in other motor segments (concomitant affection of the vertebra and the intervertebral disk). The clinical history (Table 7, p. 469) may also be of assistance in differentiating between tuberculous and nonspecific bacterial osteomyelitis of vertebrae. The more central (i.e., remote from the disk) the site of osteolysis in the vertebral body, the more difficult, or even impossible, becomes the radiologic differential diagnosis between inflammation and tumorous or tumorlike lesions (Fig. 701).

Migrating spondylitis is a rare bacterial inflammatory process in the spine that has been observed in (mixed) tuberculous infection (Glogowski, 1959) as well as with nonspecific bacterial inflammation (Dihlmann, 1967; 1978). The ascent or descent of a tuberculous (or nonspecific bacterial) abscess is easy to discern when it collects and expands between the vertebrae and the anterior longitudinal ligament (Fig. 702). More difficult to interpret from the pathogenetic point of view is the subligamental spread of an infection that runs its course without abscess forma-

tion (Forstmann, 1956). Such spread can trigger the development of vertebral osteophytes in the external portion of the disk, which resemble the syndesmophytes of ankylosing spondylitis and which also may involve the sacroiliac joints. Moreover, bacterial infection sometimes spreads in the perivertebral region and even leads to inflammation and eventually to bony ankylosis of intervertebral joints. The result are roentgen findings that have to be differentiated from ankylosing spondylitis and that offer diagnostic difficulty in any event (Fig. 703).

Hemispheric Spondylosclerosis— A Polyetiologic Syndrome

The roentgen findings in degenerative disk disease show quantitative and qualitative varieties. The disk may, for instance, be completely crushed and resorbed so that a more or less extensive synostosis of the contiguous vertebrae results. This finding—**synostosing osteochondrosis**—occurs prevalently in the cervical spine (Figs. 667 and 704). The marginal osteophytes of intervertebral osteochondrosis at times

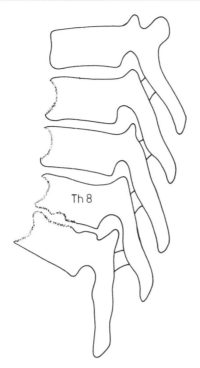

Th 8

Fig. 702 **Migrating spondylitis** developing on the basis of a (known) tuberculous spondylitis of Th8/Th9 through subligamental spread of the infection (or the pus). This finding was previously termed "anterior superficial tuberculous spondylitis" (Schulthess, 1904).

develop into coarse hyperostotic spondylophytes under the influence of a constitutional osteoblastic diathesis (see p. 458) that is present coincidentally in the patient (see the legend to Fig. 679). The increased density of the subdiscal bone renders it more brittle than the normal tridimensional trabecular system. The bone may break under the influence of axial (physiologic) forces so that (small) erosions become visible in the upper and lower vertebral contours— **erosive osteochondrosis,** (Figs. 676 and 704) (Lagier et al., 1979). In the cervical spine, these erosions are—together with the characteristic roentgen findings of osteochondrosis—already visible in lateral survey films, whereas in the lumbar spine they can in most cases be detected only in tomographs (Fig. 676). In *extremely infrequent* cases, extensive destructive phenomena occur in the vertebral bodies adjacent to a degenerated disk, which have the aspect of an infectious spondylitis (Fig. 704). These findings may be differentiated only on the operating table or by autopsy (Williams et al., 1968; Martel et al., 1976; Lagier and MacGee, 1979). They are beyond the limits of radiographic diagnosis! The same is true of the *extremely rare* invasion of the disk by a metastatic malignancy, in which expanding tumor tissue may produce a diagnostically misleading soft-tissue shadow (Hubbard and Gunn, 1972; Resnick and Niwayama, 1978 a,b). Chordoma likewise breaks

through the disk into the surrounding tissues (perivertebral soft-tissue shadow with or without encrusted calcium), (Firootnia et al., 1976).

The most variable morphologic feature of disk degeneration is subdiscal sclerosis of the cancellous bone (Fig. 704). It constitutes an adaptive thickening of the cancellous trabeculae, which develops as the result of the decreased elasticity of the degenerated disk.

Figures 704 through 707 illustrate an additional finding in the vertebrae that the present author has termed **hemispheric spondylosclerosis.** This condition presents the following radiologic features (Figs. 705 and 706):

In the area of hemispheric spondylosclerosis *no* scoliosis, *no* kyphoscoliosis, and *no* pathologically increased kyphosis (convex curvature of the back) are found. Faulty positions and faulty postures that could involve an excessive static-mechanical strain on circumscribed portions of the disk and the soft tissues are therefore not demonstrable.

The presence of a convex increase in vertebral density resembling a dome or a helmet *above* an intervertebral disk is indispensable for the diagnosis. The convex area of increased density is located in the anterior or middle third of the vertebral body. At times, the posterior third of the vertebral body is also involved with preservation of the convex shape of the sclerosis.

Vertebrae of predilection are (in decreasing order of frequency) L4, L5, and L3, as well as the thoracicolumbar junction and the middle cervical spine. In about 80 percent of the cases there develops a periosteal reaction or a circumscribed ossification of the anterior longitudinal ligament develops where the sclerotic area meets the anterior contour of the vertebra. Eighty-five percent of patients show a small erosion at the base of the hemispheric spondylosclerosis. Apparently this finding is the result of disk tissue invading the brittle and sclerosed vertebra. Multiple erosions are less frequently observed. Follow-up studies reveal that the hemispheric sclerosis usually precedes the erosion mentioned above. In nearly 90 percent of patients with hemispheric spondylosclerosis, a decrease in height of the adjacent disk space is encountered. In about 80 percent of the patients, vertebral osteophytes develop on the anterior edge(s) of the vertebrae. Almost three quarters of the patients present formation of new bone at the base of the sclerosis (see no. 6 in Fig. 705). In nearly two thirds of the cases, increased density of the cancellous bone develops below the hemispheric spondylosclerosis in the vertebral body next to the disk. Unlike the constant hemispheric shape above the disk, this area of increased thickness has a *multiform* appearance. It may be convex, triangular, spherical, band-shaped, narrow, or broad, and it rarely involves the entire vertebra. Sometimes—in about one-third of the cases—small erosions are visible in this *infradiscal* sclerotic area.

Nearly 30 percent of patients with hemispheric spondylosclerosis present a spondyloretrolisthesis. In

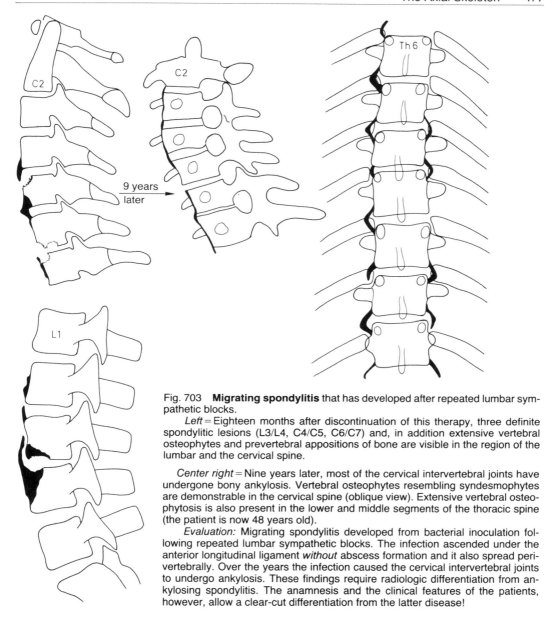

Fig. 703 **Migrating spondylitis** that has developed after repeated lumbar sympathetic blocks.

Left = Eighteen months after discontinuation of this therapy, three definite spondylitic lesions (L3/L4, C4/C5, C6/C7) and, in addition extensive vertebral osteophytes and prevertebral appositions of bone are visible in the region of the lumbar and the cervical spine.

Center right = Nine years later, most of the cervical intervertebral joints have undergone bony ankylosis. Vertebral osteophytes resembling syndesmophytes are demonstrable in the cervical spine (oblique view). Extensive vertebral osteophytosis is also present in the lower and middle segments of the thoracic spine (the patient is now 48 years old).

Evaluation: Migrating spondylitis developed from bacterial inoculation following repeated lumbar sympathetic blocks. The infection ascended under the anterior longitudinal ligament *without* abscess formation and it also spread perivertebrally. Over the years the infection caused the cervical intervertebral joints to undergo ankylosis. These findings require radiologic differentiation from ankylosing spondylitis. The anamnesis and the clinical features of the patients, however, allow a clear-cut differentiation from the latter disease!

only about 20 percent of the cases does the roentgenogram demonstrate an unequivocal etiology of hemispheric spondylosclerosis; e.g., (tuberculous) spondylitis, osteoid osteoma, ankylosing spondylitis, metastatic carcinoma, or a dorsal prolapse of the disk. In the majority of cases, degenerative disk disease is believed to be the cause, although so far no satisfactory explanation for the pathogenesis and localization of the condition has been provided. About 50 percent of the cases, for instance, concern the fourth lumbar vertebra). In addition, females are affected about 2.5 times more frequently than males. The average age for both sexes is between the 40th and 45th years of life. At times, a regressive tendency of the area of increased density has been observed (Renier et al., 1968; Martel et al., 1976; Dihlmann, 1981).

The varied observations in hemispheric spondylosclerosis and their results (Knetsch, 1967; Renier et al., 1968; Pohl and Kränzlein, 1973; Glimet et al., 1975; Martel, 1977a; Sauser et al., 1978) may be summarized as follows: Hemispheric spondylosclerosis in one or more vertebrae is a potentially reversible, painful vertebral process that may have a variety of causes—inflammation, degeneration, or tumor. From the etiologic point of view, the condition is a syndrome, and its diagnosis is a problem. The con-

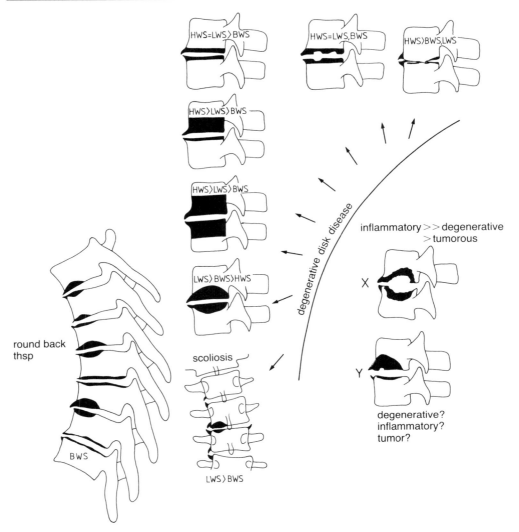

Fig. 704   **Varieties of degenerative disk disease** *(intervertebral ostochondrosis, left;* compare Figs. 667, 674, and 676).

X = Very infrequent *extreme type of erosive osteochondrosis* which cannot be differentiated roentgenologically from infectious spondylitis and from the sequelae of the likewise very infrequent invasion of the disk by a tumor (e.g., metastatic carcinoma; chordoma).

Y = *Hemispheric spondylosclerosis* with the character of a syndrome.

stant morphology of the affection, its preference for certain vertebrae (primarily L4 and L5), and its prevalent occurrence in females are remarkable features that so far have not been irrefutably explained. The frequently difficult differential diagnosis between a noninflammatory (degeneration, tumor) and an inflammatory (infectious) pathogenesis prompts the examiner to utilize clinical (see Table 7) as well as serological and chemical laboratory studies (elevated sedimentation rate without any other cause, leukocytosis, etc.). Arguments in favor of an infectious etiology are the extent and the coalescence of the ero-

sions *along* the end plate of the involved vertebra and/or the subjacent vertebra (Fig. 707), the "melting away" of the anterior edge(s) of the vertebra (mostly demonstrable in a lateral roentgenogram), and sequestra within the hemispheric spondylosclerosis or in the vertebra underneath it. The identification of these diagnostically decisive roentgen manifestations requires a lateral tomograph of the vertebra! When a dorsal prolapse of the disk at the same level as the hemispheric spondylosclerosis can be demonstrated by myelography, an inflammatory pathogenesis is very unlikely. Computed tomography is instrumental in

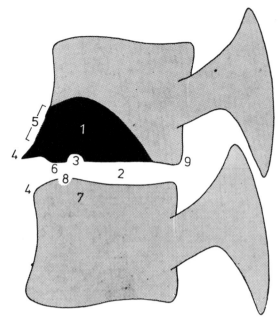

Fig. 705 **Distribution of features in hemispheric spondylosclerosis of the spine** (Dihlmann, 1981).

1 = Typical hemispheric or helmet shape of hemispheric spondylosclerosis with its center in the anterior portions of the vertebra or, less frequently, expanding into the posterior third of the vertebral body—100 percent.

2 = Decrease in disk height—87 percent.

3 = At least one very small erosion in the base of the sclerosis—85 percent.

4 = Vertebral osteophyte(s) (spondylophytes or repair osteophytes; see Fig. 679)—81 percent.

5 = Smooth or denticulate periosteal reaction at the anterior contour of the vertebra or ossification of the anterior longitudinal ligament along the sclerosis—79 percent.

6 = Caudally directed new bone formation at the anterior base of the sclerosis—74 percent.

7 = *Multiform* spondylosclerosis of the subjacent vertebra—64 percent. (Hence, in 36 percent of the observations this infradiscal spondylosclerosis was absent!).

8 = Erosion(s) in the region of the *infradiscal* end plate = 36 percent.

9 = Spondyloretrolisthesis = 29 percent.

diagnosing or ruling out a paravertebral abscess. A glance at the sacroiliac joints determines whether hemispheric spondylosclerosis of a vertebra has developed in connection with ankylosing spondylitis. The syndromic character of the condition should in every case prompt the examiner to exhaust all diagnostic possibilities, including biopsy!

Rheumatoid Arthritis of the Spine

Adult rheumatoid arthritis of the spine generally becomes manifest only in an advanced stage of the disease. In the great majority of cases the disease then has been known for years or decades and has already led to severe destruction in the joints of the extremities (*exception:* initial lateral atlantoaxial arthritis in adult rheumatoid arthritis; see Van Kerckhove, 1970). The age of the patients with spinal involvement would suggest degenerative lesions in the disks and the intervertebral joints; their age, the prolonged duration of the disease, and possibly also the treatment have led to vertebral osteoporosis or have contributed to its development. These changes are additional factors in producing the radiographic picture of rheumatoid arthritis of the spine. In principle, any segment of the spine can be affected by rheumatic arthritis, but the

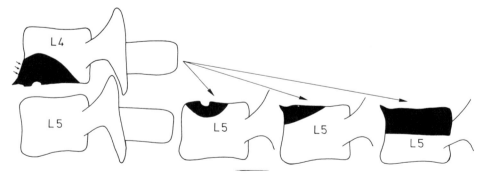

Fig. 706 **Hemispheric spondylosclerosis** (sketched in the vertebra of predilection = L4). Characteristic features are the hemispheric, helmet-shaped or cupola-shaped vertebral scleroses above a disk space of normal or diminished height and the erosion of the end plate, which is *small* in comparison with the sclerotic area! Apposition of bone on the anterior contour of the vertebra at the level of the sclerosis *(arrows)*, the caudally directed formation of new bone on the corresponding end plate in front of the erosion, and the multiform (or absent) sclerosis of the cancellous bone in the contiguous *caudal* vertebra are possible roentgen manifestations.

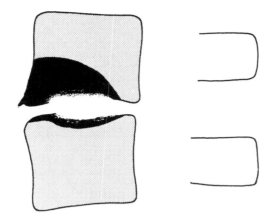

Fig. 707 **Tuberculous spondylitis mimicking the radiologic appearance of hemispheric spondylosclerosis.**
A remarkable feature is the erosion of both vertebrae along the end plates. This tomographic finding arouses suspicion of an infectious pathogenesis of the hemispheric spondylosclerosis. The suspicion may be corroborated by clinical manifestations, by demonstration of an abscess, and/or by biopsy.
Note: Some cases that are completely identical to the finding in Fig. 706 show a constantly elevated sedimentation rate. This arouses suspicion of an infection by microorganisms of low pathogenicity.

risk of its developing in the cervical spine is particularly great. Experience has shown that adult rheumatoid arthritis behaves as if this spinal segment were the fifth extremity. When, therefore, a cervical syndrome makes its appearance in a patient with rheumatoid arthritis, an anteroposterior roentgenogram and a lateral one with anteflexion must immediately be taken. By so doing, the morphology of the inflammatory rheumatic destructions and their sequelae in the occipitoatlantoaxial region and in the subaxial area is evidenced (Fig. 708). However, to estimate their clinical and prognostic significance, a neurologic examination is necessary. Occasionally, the deleterious pathogenesis is detected only at autopsy (Webb et al., 1968—bilateral thrombosis of the vertebral artery; Nakano et al., 1978).

Occipitoatlantoaxial region: *Ventral dislocation* of the atlas (*synonyms:* ventral subluxation of the atlas, anterior atlantoaxial subluxation) is diagnosed when, in adults, the atlas-dens distance exceeds 3 mm and when, in children and juveniles, the cleft between atlas and dens is greater than 4 mm (Figs. 5 and 708 A). Ventral dislocation of the atlas has a variety of causes, among them rheumatoid arthritis, other inflammatory rheumatic affections—for example, ankylosing spondylitis (Martel and Page, 1960)— bacterial infections, metabolic disorders, malformation syndromes, isolated disturbance of occipitocervical development, traumas, and so on (see pp. 6 and 8). An important preliminary condition for the devel-

opment of ventral dislocation of the atlas is insufficiency of the transverse ligament of the atlas, a ligament that passes behind the odontoid process. Such ligamental insufficiency develops in rheumatoid arthritis when granulation tissue appears at the ligamentous insertions, when the ligament atrophies, or is destroyed by granulation tissue and/or when the posterior surface of the dens becomes eroded. Insufficiency of the transverse ligament allows the atlas to slip forward by a distance of about 5 mm (Ball and Sharp, 1971). Ventral displacement of the atlas exceeding this distance is possible when, *in addition,* the alar ligaments have become insufficient and inflammatory destruction of the capsules and articular surfaces of the median and lateral atlantoaxial joints has supervened. The atlas then often slips so far anteriorly that it both tips and glides: the anterior arch of the atlas tips caudally and inferiorly while the posterior arch of the atlas moves cranially, and the dens of the axis "ascends" and sometimes even crosses the foramen magnum line (Fig. 647 C).

This *upward displacement of the dens* (Fig. 709), however, may also occur *without* ventral dislocation of the atlas (Martel and Page, 1960; Rana et al., 1973). The same is true of *deformations of the odontoid process* (Fig. 709) by granulation tissue in rheumatoid arthritis. On the one hand, the deformations favor the displacement in the atlantoaxial region and, on the other, they may protect the medulla from the adverse effects of upward displacement of the dens; for example, when partial or complete destruction of the dens has occurred or even when it only becomes "pointed" (Rosenberg et al., 1978).

Anterior and/or posterior, lateral, or all-round erosions of the dens (Fig. 709) involve the danger of (pathologic) fracture (Chevrot et al., 1978; Park et al., 1979). Reactive polymorphic bony excrescenses in the dens may also develop in rheumatoid arthritis, in psoriatic arthritis, in ankylosing spondylitis, and in DISH (Dirheimer, 1977; Fig. 709 C).

Dorsal dislocation (subluxation) and transverse (lateral) dislocation (subluxation) of the atlas (Figs. 8, 709A) are additional possibilities of displacement of this vertebra. They result from severe inflammatory destruction of the joints, the joint-bearing bones, and the ligaments of the occipitoatlantoaxial region (Burry et al., 1978). Thus, dorsal dislocation of the atlas becomes possible only following extensive or even complete osteolysis of the dens, its (pathologic) fracture, or destruction of the anterior arch of the atlas (Frigaard, 1978).

Quantitative and qualitative analysis of the inflammatory destructions in the joints of the occipitoatlantoaxial region and the manifold resulting, frequently combined, malpositions requires additional studies by tomography, particularly with a view to the necessary surgical intervention. Depending on the clinical problem and the suspicion aroused by survey films, the tomographs are taken with the patient in the recumbent (Figs. 7 and 8) or the side-lying position, or in both planes.

Fig. 708 **Radiologic spectrum of possible findings in the cerivcal spine affected by adult rheumatoid arthritis.**

A = Ventral dislocation of the atlas (frequently recognizable only in roentgenograms taken with anteflexion, as in the present case).

B = Erosion of the dens.

C = Rheumatoid spondylodiscitis.

D = Bony ankylosis of the intervertebral joints (often recognizable only in tomographs).

F = Rheumatoid discitis (or chondrosis).

G, G' = Discitis *or* osteochondrosis *and* roentgenologically invisible arthritis of the intervertebral joints, which produces ventral slipping of C6 (G'); spondylodiscitis (G).

H = Typical picture of osteochondrosis (coincidence!).

I = Osteolysis of the spinous process.

See also the stepladder phenomenon at the anterior edges of the vertebrae!

Note: The majority of the radiologic findings sketched (A, B, C, D, E, F, G, I) can also be due to ankylosing spondylitis and other inflammatory rheumatic arthropathies. H = coincidental disk degeneration.

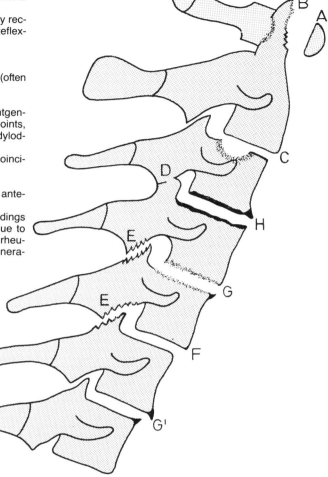

Subaxial region (C3 to C7; Fig. 708): In the cervical spine, inflammatory rheumatic granulations develop not only in the intervertebral but also in the so-called uncovertebral joints (Ball and Sharp, 1971; p. 455 ff). From the latter joints the destruction by granulation tissue may spread to the entire intervertebral disk and the vertebral body. The result is **rheumatic discitis or spondylodiscitis** (see the footnote on p. 474). Arthritis of the intervertebral joints often can be diagnosed only in tomographs by erosions of the contours of the joints and inflammatory destruction of the articular processes. In adult rheumatoid arthritis, these processes seldom lead to bony ankylosis (Cabot and Becker, 1978) but much more frequently to segmental instability that is manifested by ventral slipping of vertebrae (pseudospondylolisthesis, p. 414 ff) or, with concomitant disk disease, by spondyloretrolisthesis (p. 415 ff). In the cervical spine, involvement of the intervertebral joints by adult rheumatoid arthritis occurs in a more or less generalized manner. The vertebrae at the different levels slip variably forward. Their anterior edges present the *stepladder phenomenon* (Fig. 708; Schilling et al., 1963).

In the spinous process C7, less frequently also in the spinous processes superiorly and inferiorly (Peter et al., 1964), adult rheumatoid arthritis (occasionally also ankylosing spondylitis) leads to deformations (osteolysis of the spinous processes). The spinous process then has a beak-shaped or shovel-shaped appearance, or it gives a "sucked-on" impression (Figs. 708 I and 710). These deformations are produced by the inflammatory granulation tissue that starts from the ligamentous insertions of the spinous processes

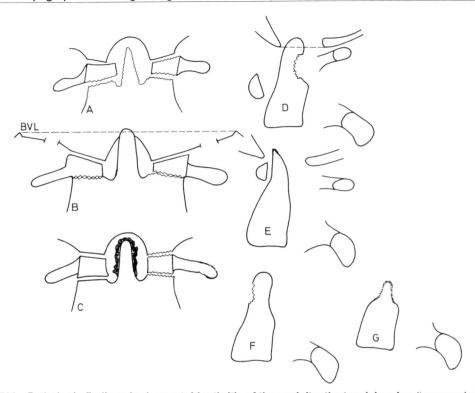

Fig. 709   Pathologic findings in rheumatoid arthritis of the occipitoatlantoaxial region (tomographs).
A = Subluxating arthritis of the atlantooccipital and the lateral atlantoaxial joints; severe erosion of the dens.
B = Upward dislocation of the dens in severe lateral atlantoaxial arthritis. The biventer line (BVL; see Fig. 647 A) is crossed by the tip of the dens.
C = "Crowned" dens (Dirheimer, 1977). These and other new bone formations originate in the dens or in the anterior arch of the atlas. They are encountered in rheumatoid arthritis, ankylosing spondylitis, psoriatic arthritis, and DISH. *Radiographic differential diagnosis:* Manifestations of the occipital vertebra and bony metaplasias in the ligaments of the cervico-occipital junction (Fig. 646).
D, E = Upward displacement of the dens in severe ventral dislocation of the atlas (D) or without ventral dislocation of the atlas (E), accompanied by advanced lateral atlantoaxial arthritis. Erosion of the dens.
D, E, F, G = Instances of inflammatory erosion of the dens.

and from inflamed "interspinous" cervical bursae, which are physiologic structures (Bywaters, 1978).

Thoracic and lumbar spine: As in the cervical spine, involvement of the lumbar intervertebral joints by rheumatoid arthritis leads to segmental instability. In the thoracic spine, however, the connection with the ribs prevents the vertebrae from slipping. There, arthritic granulation tissue derived from diseased costovertebral joints (Cohen et al., 1978) may invade the intervertebral disk and the adjacent end plates, giving rise to *rheumatoid discitis* and *spondylodiscitis* (Bywaters, 1974 and 1978). Rheumatoid nodules and inflammatory rheumatoid granulation tissue also develop in the bone marrow, the vertebral ligamentous insertions, and the connective tissue of the disk (Baggenstoss et al., 1952; Lorber et al., 1961; Shichikawa et al., 1978). Contributory causes in the development of discovertebral destruction during the course of rheumatoid arthritis are: the above-mentioned instability in the motor segments whose intervertebal joints are affected by rheumatoid arthritis, the vertebral osteoporosis to be expected in patients with longstanding rheumatoid arthritis, and age-dependent degeneration of the disks (Lawrence et al., 1964; Martel, 1977b; Resnick, 1978). This is why the pathogenesis of these lesions (inflammatory rheumatic, degenerative with pathologic inhibition of the osteophytic reactions, mechanical from osteoporosis) is still a subject of debate. However, the typical radiologic appearance of (spondylo-) discitis in rheumatoid arthritis (Fig. 711)—i.e., *marked* decrease in disk height with *or without* minimal spondylophytes, absent or moderate subdiscal vertebral sclerosis, slight or absent erosions of the end plate—is universally recognized (Pučar et al., 1969; and others).

Late in the disease, the pathologic discovertebral findings either terminate in partial or complete bony fusion of the vertebrae (Fig. 712) *or* present the

Fig. 710 **Osteolysis of the spinous process C7** (less frequently also above and below this vertebra) in rheumatoid arthritis and ankylosing spondylitis.

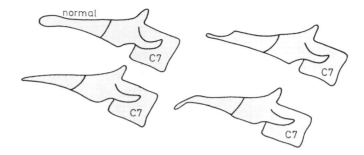

radiologic aspect of "osteoporotic" compression of the vertebrae *or* are consistent with the radiographic picture of bacterial spondylitis. In an individual case, the etiologic interpretation therefore can offer diagnostic difficulties. As a matter of fact, in patients with rheumatoid arthritis—even in those not treated with corticosteroids—hematogenous infections of the peripheral joints (Karten, 1969) are known to occur with above average frequency, and pyogenic infections of the intervertebral and uncovertebral joints of the cervical spine have been observed (Ball and Sharp, 1971). Moreover, the inflammatory rheumatoid granulation tissue can grow out of the disk space. In this case— for example, in the thoracic spine—the paravertebral line is broadened (Fig. 621) or, in the cervical spine, the prevertebral fat stripe changes (Fig. 616 and 639). In connection with the discovertebral destructions,

these roentgen findings may be misinterpreted as the expression of an abscess or, conversely, actual bacterial infections in patients with rheumatoid arthritis may be made minimized as rheumatic discitis or spondylodiscitis!

Juvenile chronic arthritis generally attacks the axial skeleton in an early or intermediate stage of the disease, at times even initially (Kölle, 1975). In the cervical spine the same fundamental lesions occur as those seen in the adult type of the disease (Fig. 713). Among them are ventral dislocation of the atlas, arthritic changes in the joints of the occipitoatlantoaxial region and the subaxial intervertebral joints, as well as erosions of the dens (Mäkelä et al., 1979). It is true, however, that in juvenile chronic arthritis there is a stronger tendency for the intervertebral joints to become ankylosed than in the adult disease (Fig. 714).

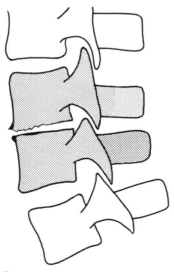

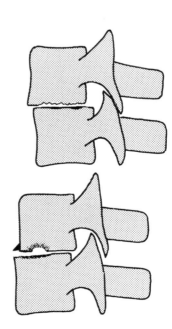

Fig. 711 **Lumbar spondylodiscitis in rheumatoid arthritis.** Note the characteristic association of *marked* decrease in disk height and *minor* or even *absent* spondylophytes.

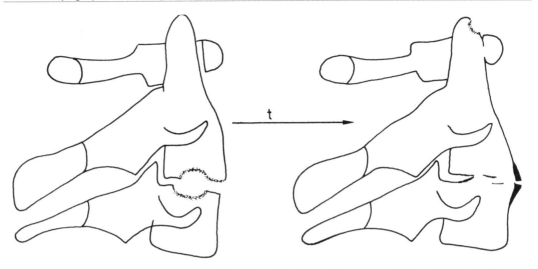

Fig. 712 **Development of an inflammatory fused vertebra during the course of rheumatoid arthritis spondylodiscitis C2/C3** (t = 6 years). In addition, (infrequent) bony ankylosis in the medial atlantoaxial joint and erosion of the dens have supervened. (Compare Fig. 666 C and D = acquired vertebral fusion).

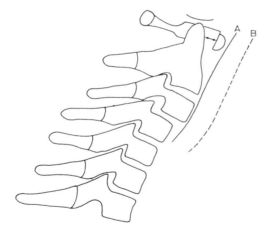

Fig. 713 **Ventral dislocation of the atlas (↔) and arthritis of the intervertebral joints C3/C4 with ventral slipping of C3 in florid juvenile chronic arthritis** (patient aged 14 years).

A = Normal course of the posterior pharyngeal wall; see Fig. 616. A similar *radiologic finding* may occur in Grisel's syndrome (infectious torticollis; nasopharyngeal torticollis; Fig. 6, p. 6). In this case, however, the width of the retropharyngeal space (see Fig. 616 A) is generally increased (B; by edema or abscess formation). In addition, see the footnote on p. 6 (cervical hypermobility in children between the ages of 1 and 7 as a variant normal).

Ankylosis of the intervertebral joints acquired in the (early) growth period has sequelae that throughout life offer a retrospective clue to rheumatoid arthritis experienced in childhood. The bony fusion of the intervertebral joints, for example, not only impairs their mobility but also interferes to a considerable degree with the growth and development of the intervertebral disks, the vertebral bodies, the laminal arches, and the spinous processes (Schacherl, 1974; Dihlmann and Friedmann, 1977). Figures 664 and 715 show the characteristic radiologic aspect of rheumatoid lesions in the cervical spine detected in the adult but acquired in childhood. The radiologic differential diagnosis may be inferred from Figure 662 (Klippel-Feil syndrome) and Figure 77 (progressive myositis ossificans). Inflammatory rheumatic spondylodiscitis occurs less frequently in juvenile chronic arthritis than in the adult form of the disease.

The infrequent **lipoid-dermatoarthritis** (p. 131 ff) also involves the intervertebral joints; the articular processes of which may become eroded. Ventral dislocation of the atlas and erosions of the dens are known to occur in this disease (Schwarz and Fish, 1960; Gold et al., 1975). The same is true of ankylosing sacroiliitis (Martel et al., 1961), destruction of the symphysis pubis, and erosive lesions in the costovertebral joints.

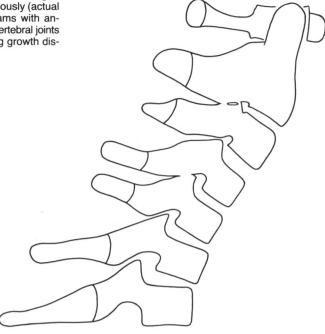

Fig. 714 **Juvenile chronic arthritis.** In the setting of this disease, cervical arthritis 7 years previously (actual age = 14 years). Functional roentgenograms with anteflexion reveal bony ankylosis of the intervertebral joints C2/C3 and C4/C5, as well as the resulting growth disturbance of disks and vertebrae.

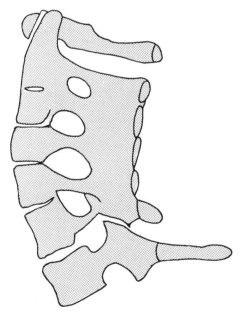

Fig. 715 **Juvenile inflammatory rheumatic cervical synostosis** (onset of juvenile chronic arthritis at the age of 4; present age 38 years). In comparison with Fig. 664, there is a conspicuous dysplasia of the vertebral arch behind the vertebral body, which has led to increased size of the intervertebral foramina and to elongation of the sagittal diameter of the spinal canal.

Ankylosing Spondylitis

Ankylosing spondylitis is the classic inflammatory rheumatic disease that leads to stiffening of the spine (see footnote on p. 80). Although involvement of the axial skeleton, including the joints of pelvis and thorax, is the predominant and most consistent manifestation of the disease, 50 percent of patients with ankylosing spondylitis also report problems involving the peripheral and even the temporomandibular joints. The insertions of tendons and ligaments may be affected in the form of fibroosteitis (see p. 73 ff), and bursae may be involved (see Achilles bursitis, Fig. 563). Finally, visceral localizations of the disease have been described (iridocyclitis, aortitis, carditis, cystic fibrosis of the upper lobe of the lungs, and pleural fibrosis [Davies, 1972]). On the other hand, (renal) amyloidosis, the cauda equina syndrome (Russell et al., 1973), and central nervous manifestations (in ventral dislocation of the atlas) have been known as complications. Ankylosing spondylitis is a disease with preference for males; about 70 to 90 percent of patients with clinically diagnosed (hence known) ankylosing spondylitis are males.

The morbidity of ankylosing spondylitis has been reported as approximately 1.0 per thousand, but this statistic has been questioned, given our current knowledge about the association of the HLA-B27 antigen (see p. 348 ff) with ankylosing spondylitis. Since this antigen occurs with about the same frequency in males and in females, the risk of becoming afflicted with ankylosing spondylitis is therefore approximately identical for both sexes. In addition, clinical and radiologic studies on HLA-B27 positive blood donors have shown that the incidence of ankylosing spondylitis among this group varies between 0.8 and 1.7 percent (Thorel et al., 1978). It is therefore probable that the actual morbidity corresponds to the lowest percentages (Calin and Fries, 1975; Krüger and Schattenkirchner, 1980). Evidently there are—particularly in females (Dequeker et al., 1978)—abortive forms of ankylosing spondylitis and "benign" evolutions. In these forms, the disease does not invade the sacroiliac joints, nor does one see bony sacroiliac ankylosis—to say nothing of bamboo spine.

The age of onset in ankylosing spondylitis is of great clinical and roentgenologic significance because the patient's age also affects the clinical and radiologic findings. The manifestations of ankylosing spondylitis vary according to the age of onset and by the developmental stage of the patient; i.e., the biologic background (Schilling, 1978).

Juvenile ankylosing spondylitis, as the term indicates, starts before completion of the 16th year

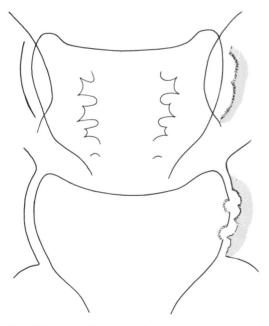

Fig. 716   **Juvenile ankylosing spondylitis with unilateral sacroiliitis.** In survey films taken in dorsal decubitus *(above)*, garland-shaped pseudodilatation and subchondral iliac sclerosis are the prominent features. In the tomograph *(below)* one also recognizes sacral erosions and delicate osseous burgeons which grow from the ilium into the joint space (articular cartilage), hence corresponding to the "variegated picture" type of sacroiliitis (see text).

of life. This is the case in about 10 percent of patients. In the great majority of persons diseased at this age, radiologic signs and symptoms occur primarily in the peripheral joints. Characteristically the patient reports "low back pain" in the lumbosacroiliac region when arising after remaining for some time in the resting position although this symptom usually makes its appearance only at puberty. It should prompt an examination of the sacroiliac joints. Typically, this low back pain arouses the patient late in the night or early in the morning. The patient is compelled to get out of bed and walk about until the pain subsides and sleep can be resumed.

The following constellations raise suspicion of *(juvenile)* ankylosing spondylitis (Schilling, 1974, 1978):

1. Male sex
2. Monoarthritis or oligoarthritis of the lower extremities
3. Inflammatory rheumatic calcaneopathy (p. 373 ff)
4. History of iridocyclitis
5. Familial predisposition; e.g., father suffering from ankylosing spondylitis and/or presence of the HLA-B27 antigen.

Roentgen examination of the sacroiliac joints should be the next diagnostic step in these cases, in order to search for unilateral or bilateral sacroiliitis. The sacroiliitis is basically, of the "variegated picture" type (see p. 490 ff). Survey films of the sacroiliac joints often show the so-called pseudodilatation (see p. 489) as a prominent feature (Fig. 716). Between the 10th and the 16th years of life, the sacroiliac joints are difficult to judge in survey films, because discrete pathologic changes must be detected. At this age the contours of the ilium are mostly hazy or cannot be confidently evaluated (Dihlmann, 1967, 1978). The incipient ossification of the sacral wings is the cause of additional possibilities of error, so that tomography of the sacroiliac joints in dorsal decubitus is as a rule indispensable!

Radiologic study of the sacroiliac joints is supplemented by *clinical* function tests of the spine. In *juvenile* ankylosing spondylitis, roentgen examination of the (lumbar) spine, initially and in the intermediate stage, provides little reliable information because experience has shown that the body is capable of forming syndesmophytes only from the third decade of life upward (see p. 458 ff, Figs. 679 and 682)! *Prior to the 20th year of life,* ankylosis of the spine develops exclusively as the result of disease of the intervertebral joints.

At least 80 percent of all cases of ankylosing spondylitis start between the 16th and the 40th years of life—**adolescent** and **adult ankylosing spondylitis.** The peak incidence of the disease lies in the third decade. The rules for early diagnosis and assessment of the evolution set forth later in this section are applicable in these cases.

Presenile (beginning in the fifth and sixth decades) and **senile ankylosing spondylitis** comprise about 5 percent of the cases. The aging processes, especially in the intervertebral disks, influence the shape of the syndesmophytes. The typical syndesmophytes develop only in a healthy disk! Instead, the so-called *mixed osteophytes* (p. 460; Fig. 679) make their appearance in the fifth decade and later. These are types intermediate between sydesmophytes and spondylophytes (Krebs, 1931), which are observed primarily when ankylosing spondylitis begins after the 40th year of life or when the disease starts earlier and continues actively into this period of life with the formation of syndesmophytes. In the second half of life, the human body has a basic tendency toward ossification of tight fibrous connective tissue. This is why at this age the syndesmophytes may be associated with ossification of the anterior longitudinal ligament (Fig. 683), although they grow, in principle, by pathologic ossification in the external portion of the annulus fibrosus and *between* the annulus fibrosus and the anterior longitudinal ligament. Difficulties of radiographic differentiation between ankylosing spondylitis and DISH (see p. 458 ff) may be encountered when a patient with ankylosing spondylitis that starts at senile or presenile age is the coincidental carrier of a constitutional attribute which the present author has termed *osteoplastic diathesis* (p. 458; see the caption to Fig. 681). This constitution-dependent "exuberant" ossification of tight fibrous connective tissue usually becomes manifest only in the second half of life. When, by chance, ankylosing spondylitis also manifests itself at the same period, three factors can make the differentiation between DISH and ankylosing spondylitis impracticable:

1.   Experience has shown that in old age the mode of reaction that leads to sacroiliitis of the "variegated picture" type disappears. At this age, bony fusion of the sacroiliac joints in ankylosing spondylitis takes place primarily through ossification of the anterior capsule of the sacroiliac joints and the ventral sacroiliac ligaments. These ligamentous ossifications are located like a "board" anterior to the preserved sacroiliac joint space (Fig. 717 A) and "obliterate" it in survey films.
2.   In DISH, the (anterior) sacroiliac joint capsule and its reinforcing ligaments very frequently participate in the ossification of the tight fibrous connective tissue (Dihlmann and Freund, 1968). This is also why the sacroiliac joints *sometimes* appear in the roentgenogram to be "obliterated," hence to have undergone bony ankylosis.
3.   In the spine, particularly its thoracic and lumbar segments, the osteoblastic diathesis modifies the development of syndesmophytes by spreading of the pathologic ossification to the anterior longitudinal ligament (Fig. 717 B).

In these (infrequent) cases, the diagnosis cannot be established on the basis of the roentgenograms alone. The definitive diagnosis depends on *clinical* findings (inflammatory serology, HLA-B27 antigen, extravertebral skeletal and visceral manifestations of an-

kylosing spondylitis, or a diabetic and hyperuremic metabolic situation which is often present in DISH), as well as the constitutional type (prevalently leptosomal in ankylosing spondylitis and prevalently pyknic in DISH).

(Early) roentgenologic diagnosis and assessment of evolution in ankylosing spondylitis (*exceptions: juvenile* and *senile* cases; see under these headings) are accomplished by adherence to the following nine rules (Dihlmann, 1979). These rules allow, in addition, the radiologic differential diagnosis of diseased sacroiliac joints and ankylosing affections of the spine.

Rule 1: In about 99 percent of patients with ankylosing spondylitis, the earliest roentgen manifestations appear in the sacroiliac joints. In only 1 percent of cases do other roentgen manifestations— e.g., syndesmophytes (Dihlmann, 1965a), square vertebrae (Louyot, 1954), or even spondylodiscitis (Andersson's lesion)—antedate the changes in the sacroiliac joints (Dihlmann, 1968a).

Comment: Rule 1 quantifies a fact established by experience. It does not, however, admit the inference that ankylosing spondylitis originates in the sacroiliac joints and that it ascends from there to involve the spine. Such suppositions have at most a medicohistorical background. Romanus (1953), for instance, proposed the "mechanistic" theory to the effect that ankylosing spondylitis or its unknown pathogen would be triggered by a nonspecific inflammation of the prostate and the seminal vesicles and from there would spread continuously along the spine by way of the venous circulation and the lymphatics. The therapeutic suggestion by Scott (1936) to extirpate the sacroiliac joints as the supposed primary seat of ankylosing spondylitis reflects similar views. The following observations argue against the continuous ascent of the disease along the spine: The pathologic demonstration of *focal* lesions in the entire spine (Fraenkel 1903, 1904, 1907; Aufdermaur, 1953), the occasional occurrence of the earliest syndesmophytes in the cervical spine, and the regular initial manifestation of the syndesmophytes in the thoracicolumbar junction (Dihlmann, 1968). Ankylosing spondylitis therefore should be considered as a systemic reaction of the spine that concomitantly involves the entire axial skeleton but which has a predilection for certain parts (sacroiliac joints, thoracicolumbar junction, atlantoaxial region [Schilling et al., 1963; Reid and Hill, 1978; Sorin et al. 1979]).

Rule 2: In about 10 percent of patients, ankylosing spondylitis manifests itself at the outset unilaterally in the sacroiliac joints before, months or years later, pathologic roentgen findings also become visible in the contralateral sacroiliac joint.

Comment: This statement (Dihlmann, 1976a) refers to a mean value which also considers the patient's age at the onset of the disease. As a matter of fact, unilateral involvement of the sacroiliac joints in juvenile ankylosing spondylitis (Fig. 716) considerably exceeds 10 percent. In addition, evidence of

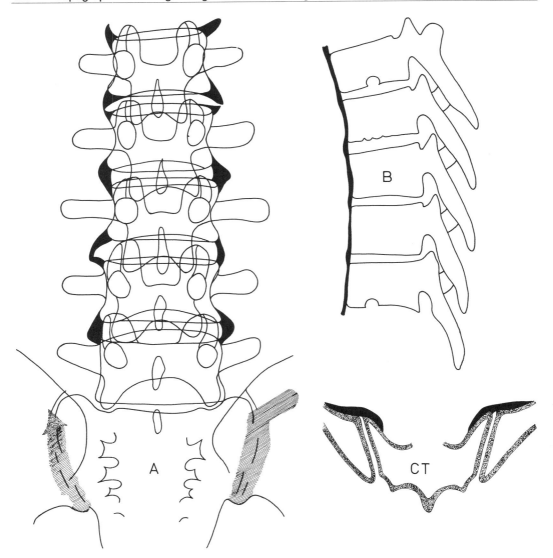

Fig. 717   **67-year-old patient in whom hyperostotic spondylosis cannot be differentiated from senile ankylosing spondylitis by radiology alone.** Old age in association with a coincidentally present constitutional osteoplastic diathesis (see text) has led to boardlike, thick ossification of the anterior sacroiliac joint capsule and its reinforcing ligaments. This has led to "obliteration" of the sacroiliac joint space in the survey film taken in dorsal decubitus (A). The computed tomograph (CT) shows, however, that the joint space proper has been preserved, hence is not ossified. Some of the vertebral osteophytes have the aspect of syndesmophytes; others resemble mixed osteophytes; and still others appear to be hyperostotic spondylophytes (A). Hence, they cannot be definitely classified (see text). In B, the thoracic spine presents ossifying processes which also have involved the anterior longitudinal ligament.

unilateral or bilateral sacroiliitis (Fig. 718) depends on the interval between the onset of complaints and the initial roentgen examination. The greater the interval, the more likely bilateral involvement of the sacroiliac joints becomes.

Rule 3: There is no single roentgen manifestation in the sacroiliac joints that would be proof

of ankylosing spondylitis. There are, however, pathologic roentgen signs that are encountered only in these joints and are observed in ankylosing spondylitis as well as in other affections. Among these is the so-called pseudodilatation of the sacroiliac joint space.

Comment: Forestier (1939) described sacroiliac

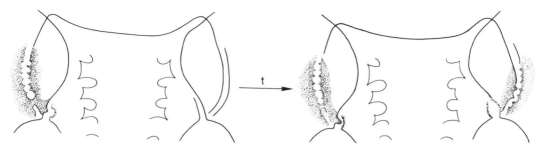

Fig. 718   **Unilateral sacroiliitis in ankylosing spondylitis, followed in the course of 16 months (t) by bilateral involvement of the sacroiliac joints.**

pseudodilatation (Fig. 719 B) as a roentgen manifestation of ankylosing spondylitis. Since then it has become known that this roentgen sign is also encountered in diseases of the sacroiliac joints that are not related etiologically to ankylosing spondylitis; for example, gout (Dihlmann, 1976, 1978), osteomalacia, hyperparathyroidism (Dihlmann and Müller, 1973), bacterial infections, and metastatic tumors. ''Genuine'' widening of the radiologic sacroiliac joint space is due to traumatic rupture of the capsule and the ligaments. The joint space appears widened, and its contours are smooth. Pseudodilatation appears along the articular contours of the ilium and the sacrum following marginal resorption of bone. It has the aspect of a wreath, pursues a flat-arched course, and involves smaller or larger segments of the joint.

Rule 4: Ankylosing spondylitis encompasses all the potential reactions of the sacroiliac joints.

Therefore it can present roentgen findings that otherwise are associated with quite different affections of the sacroiliac joints. Among them are dissection (described as a radiographic indicator of bacterial infections), triangular ilial sclerosis—known as a decisive feature of hyperostosis triangularis ilii (formerly termed osteitis condensans ilii), and ossifications of the sacroiliac capsules and ligaments (heretofore interpreted as repair ossifications of these structures that followed excessive strains and traumas) (Fig. 720).

Comment: The various roentgen manifestations of ankylosing spondylitis in the sacroiliac joints may be classified as (1) signs of destruction, (2) signs of sclerosis, or (3) signs of ankylosis (Fig. 721). Among the *signs of sacroiliac destruction* (Fig. 721 A to F) are ill-defined articular contours, hazy structure of the subchondral cancellous trabeculae (particularly

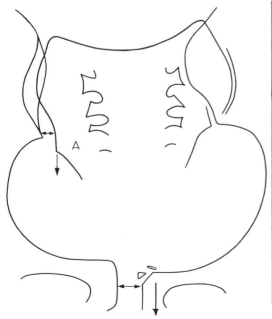

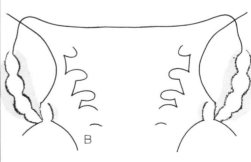

Fig. 719   **Radiologic morphology of "genuine" traumatic widening and pseudodilatation of the sacroiliac joint space.**
A = Traumatic rupture of the right sacroiliac joint and the symphysis pubis. *Arrows* indicate the direction of dislocation of the articulating bones.
B = Pseudodiliatation of the sacroiliac joints in ankylosing spondylitis. The marginal resorption of bone has produced a garland-shaped appearance.

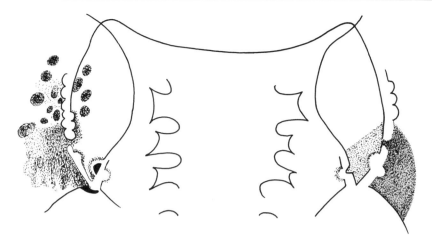

Fig. 720 **Bilateral sacroiliitis in ankylosing spondylitis presenting the following conspicuous roentgen manifestations of importance in differential diagnosis: Dissection; triangular ilial sclerosis; ossification of capsule and ligaments at the inferior border of the right sacroiliac joint (see rule no. 4 in text).**

recognizable on the side of the ilium), garland-shaped pseudodilatation, pseudodilatation with preservation of the subchondral marginal lamella (visible only in the "earlobe region" of the joint space), as well as erosions and dissections. The erosions usually develop earlier in the contour of the ilium than on the side of the sacrum. As long as they have not expanded to the borders of the articular surfaces, they present themselves as oval or rounded translucences *within* the smooth contours of the radiologic joint space. The terms "string of beads" or "rosary" are used to characterize small erosions lined up one behind another at corresponding sites of the ilium and the sacrum. Unilateral erosions lying one behind the other, for example in the ilium, resemble a saw blade or the perforated edge of a postage stamp.

The shape of the *signs of sacroiliac sclerosis* (Fig. 721, G to I) is particularly variable. These signs occur as diffuse (amorphous), band-shaped subchondral (similar to osteoarthrosis), spherical, spotty, and triangular increases of thickness in the surroundings of the joint. Following bony ankylosis of the sacroiliac joints, sclerosis of the cancellous bone regresses with time.

The *signs of sacroiliac ankylosis* (Fig. 721 J and K) reflect ossifying processes in the articular cartilage, the joint capsule, and its reinforcing ligaments. Initially, small burgeons of cartilage develop, measuring only a few millimeters in width and in length, as well as slim bony bridges that connect the ilium with the sacrum. With time they enlarge and become fused with one another. In addition, destruction of the cartilage leads to narrowing of the joint space. The final result is complete bony ankylosis of the sacroiliac joints. Below the linea terminalis, ossifications of capsule and ligaments present themselves as bony hooks. Above this line, they show a striated structure (provided they are sufficiently thick). At the superior border of the joint (at the reflection between the anterior and the posterior portion of the capsule) they form the so-called "star sign" (Hart and Robinson, 1959).

"Phantom joint" is the term applied to parts of the articular contour that remain visible following the advent of bony ankylosis. Star sign and phantom joints are nonspecific roentgen manifestations of *acquired* sacroiliac ankylosis. Therefore they are also useful in differentiating acquired ankylosis from agenesis of the sacroiliac joint (Fig. 722).

The manifold roentgen signs of ankylosing spondylitis described show an individual simultaneity and succession as well as an individual predominance of one or the other features prior to the monotonous picture of bony ankylosis. No diagnostic advances were therefore to be expected from attempts at staging the sacroiliac affection in ankylosing spondylitis. At most, complete bony ankylosis can be contrasted with the preceding alterations.

Rule 5: The characteristic radiologic feature of ankylosing spondylitis is the "variegated" sacroiliac picture (sacroiliitis of the "variegated picture" type).

Comment: The term "variegated sacroiliac picture" (Dihlmann 1970a, 1974, 1976a) has been applied to the *simultaneous triad* of destructive changes in the sacroiliac joints (erosions, pseudodilatation, etc., see Fig. 721), multiform sclerosis of the subchondral cancellous bone, *and* initially discrete signs of ankylosis (intraarticular burgeoning of bone, transarticular bony bridges) (Fig. 723). This simultaneity of signs of sacroiliac destruction, sclerosis, and discrete ankylosis reflects a mode of reaction that is characteristic of ankylosing spondylitis and therefore can be expected from the outset. However, the "variegated" sacroiliac picture becomes visible in the roentgenogram *at least* 4 months after complaints commence. For the rest, the following principle holds good: The earlier the stage of the disease, the greater the diagnostic significance of the "variegated" picture and the urgency of taking tomographs of the sacroiliac joints to identify the variegated picture at all! For conventional tomography the patient assumes the recumbent position, the sections filmed measure between 4 and 9 cm, and the distance between the in-

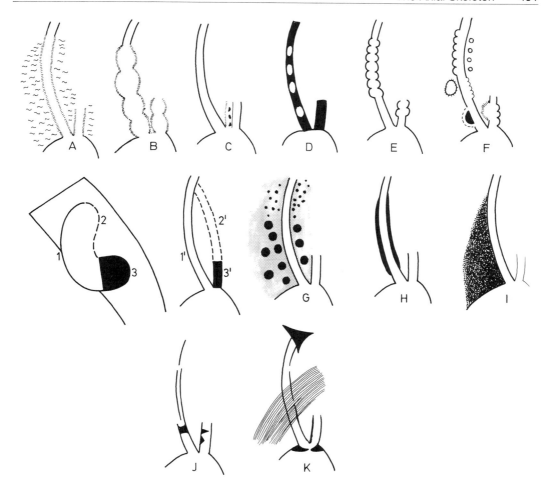

Fig. 721 **Schematic illustration of the individual signs of destruction (A to F), of sclerosis (G to I), and of ankylosis (J, K) in ankylosing spondylitis. Correlation of anatomic and roentgenologic features of the sacroiliac joint (view of the sacroiliac articular surface—1, 2, 3. Projection of the right sacroiliac joint in a survey film taken in dorsal decubitus—1', 2', 3' 1 = 1', 2 = 2', 3 = 3').**

A = Ill-defined (hazy) articular contours and subchondral cancellous structures.

B = Garland-shaped pseudodilatation.

C = pseudodilatation with preserved marginal subchondral lamella (usually only demonstrable in the "earlobe region"; see 3, 3').

D = Erosions on the ilial and sacral sides of the sacroiliac joint. They have, however not yet expanded to the anterior (1) border of the joint but appear as rounded or oval translucences in the radiologic joint space, which presents smooth contours.

E, F = erosions with the shape of a "string of beads," a "rosary," a "saw blade," or the "perforated edge of a stamp"; smaller or larger spherical osteolyses; dissection.

G = Diffuse (amorphous), dotted, spherical sclerosis of the subchondral cancellous bone.

H = Band-shaped sclerosis of the subchondral cancellous bone.

I = Triangular sclerotic area in the ilium.

J = Phantom joint; uniform narrowing of the joint space; bony bridge between the two articulating bones; burgeons of bone *(listed from top to bottom)*.

K = Star sign (see text); very voluminous ossification of capsule and ligaments (passing *in front* of the sacroiliac joint). Capsular ossification at the inferior border of the joint *(listed from top to bottom)*.

Note: Sacroiliitis in ankylosing spondylitis presents, in this individual case, a variable simultaneousness and succession of all the possible modes of reaction on the part of the sacroiliac joints!

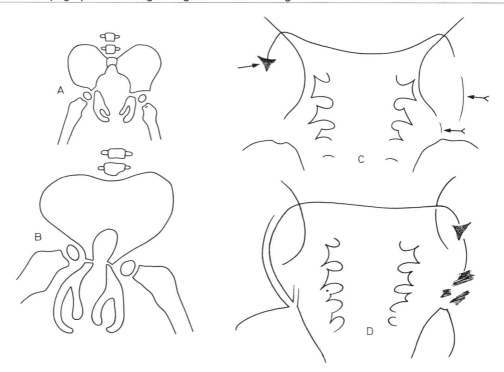

Fig. 722   **Radiologic differential diagnosis between agenesis and acquired fusion of the sacroiliac joints.**
A, B = Excessive reduction of the tail segment has, among other anomalies, led to agenesis of the sacroiliac joints. Such caudal regression *(synonyms:* caudal dysplasia; caudal hypoplasia) gives rise not only to agenesis of the caudal spine but also to maldevelopment or underdevelopment of the pelvis and legs. In addition, the condition may be accompanied by variable disturbances of innervation of the smooth and the striated musculature, and by malformation of the urogenital system and the intestinal tract. It is likely that children of diabetic mothers are more frequently afflicted with caudal regressions than the normal population (Schönenberg, 1971).

C = Bilateral bony ankylosis of the sacroiliac joints occurring after the completion of growth. The **star sign** *(arrow)* and preserved parts of the marginal subchondral lamella **(phantom joint;** *tailed arrows)* indicate that the condition is an *acquired* ankylosis and not an agenesis. The star sign develops by ossification of the anterior joint capsule at its upper posterior reflection. Hence, the sacroiliac joint extends no farther cranially then the site of the star sign.

D = pelvis obliquely contracted by unilateral bony ankylosis of the sacroiliac joints acquired in the *growth period.* Radiologic manifestations of acquired sacroiliac ankylosis are: Star sign, Phantom joint and increased thickness of scars in the cancellous bone *(listed from top to bottom).* These findings make it possible to differentiate this condition from congenital oblique contracture of the pelvis (Naegele's pelvis) in unilateral aplasia of the sacral wing.

dividual sections in an adult is 1 cm (Fig. 724 and 725). So-called oblique views of the sacroiliac joints are of *no significance* in the early diagnosis of ankylosing spondylitis! The sacroiliac joints can be confidently assessed in survey films taken with the patient in the supine or prone position, provided the examiner is familiar with their morphologically determined projected appearance: the posteroinferior part of the sacroiliac joint (the so-called ear lobe of its articular surface) presents medially and inferiorly, mostly in the orthograde view, in the form of a slit. The anterior border of the joint expands with its convexity lateralward.

In contrast to the anterior border of the joint, its posterosuperior and posteromedial borders are not always demonstrable. When these borders are visible, however, they pass from the upper pole of the joint to the ear lobe and lie medially (in the direction of the sacrum) to the lateral-convex anterior border of the joint (Fig. 721).

An alternative to survey films of the sacroiliac joints with the patient supine which lends support to the diagnosis is tomography of these joints in the manner described above.

The diagnostic significance of the "variegated" picture of the sacroiliac joints becomes manifest on

Fig. 723 **Bilateral sacroiliitis of the "variegated picture" type in ankylosing spondylitis.** Compare the additional information by tomographs.

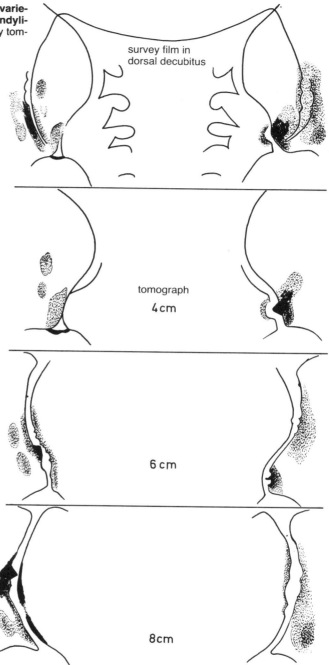

survey film in
dorsal decubitus

tomograph
4 cm

6 cm

8cm

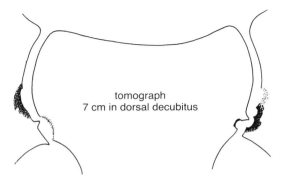

Fig. 724 **"Variegated" picture of the sacroiliac joints** coincidentally demonstrable by a conventional tomograph. See also the delicate intraarticular bone burgeons. Zonography—tomography with a smaller blurring angle and greater laminar thickness—is *not* appropriate for the exploration of the sacroiliac joints; the same applies to the use of the simultaneous-section cassette!

comparing sacroiliitis of the "variegated picture" type with bacterial sacroiliitis. Bacterial infection follows three stages. Initially, destructive lesions are conspicuous in the contours of the joint and in the subchondral area. The second stage is the phase of stabilization and repair. It is recognized by multiform sclerosis of the subchondral cancellous bone. The (third) cicatricial stage finally leads to partial or complete ankylosis, depending on the degree of destruction. This successive triad in bacterial infection of the sacroiliac joints (Fig. 726) is therefore opposed to the simultaneous triad of signs in sacroiliitis of the "variegated picture" type. This statement applies to bacterial infections of *acute* onset in which the radiologic examination is performed without an intervening

period of many months. In addition, there is a second type of sacroiliac infection which has an insidious onset and runs a *chronic* course (temperature elevations slight or absent, moderate complaints). This form includes most cases of tuberculous sacroiliitis but also some of the nonspecific bacterial type (Feldmann et al., 1981). In these instances, radiologic examination of the sacroiliac joints is often delayed for months. Roentgen signs of *spontaneous* stabilization (i.e., subchondral sclerosis) and spontaneous cicatrization—hence ankylosing processes—are then often already visible. Therefore, every case of *unilateral* sacroiliitis of the "variegated picture" type must also be differentiated from chronic bacterial sacroiliitis; e.g., by serologic tests for Brucellosis, by skeletal

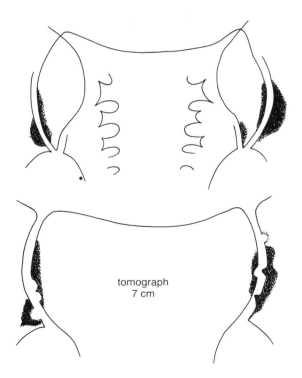

tomograph
7 cm

Fig. 725 **Equivocal sclerosis of** the subchondral cancellous bone in the **survey film; clear-cut demonstration of the "variegated" picture of the sacroiliac joints in the tomograph.** Note the simultaneous triad of erosions, sclerosis of the cancellous bone, and intraarticular bone burgeons in the tomograph. *Conclusion:* Only tomography provides the decisive information!

Fig. 726 **Evolution of an acute febrile nonspecific bacterial sacroiliitis developing by bloodstream dissemination as the aftermath of a peritonsillar abscess and treated with antibiotic agents.** On January 7 and on March 4 there is a preponderance of signs of destruction (compare Fig. 721). On May 3, perifocal sclerosis of the cancellous bone has come to the fore as a radiologic sign of stabilization. Repair processes have led to resorption of necrotic bony elements. On November 12 (almost complete) bony ankylosis of the sacroiliac joint has taken place.

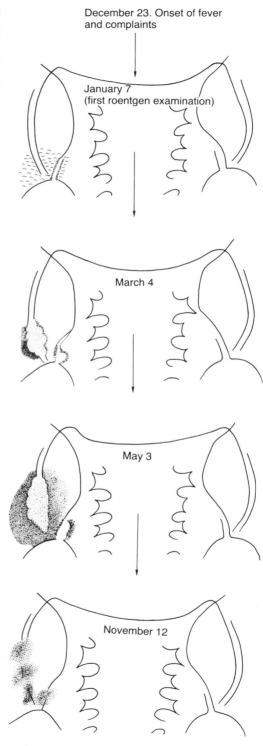

December 23. Onset of fever and complaints

January 7
(first roentgen examination)

March 4

May 3

November 12

scintigraphy and by radiologic examination of the thorax. (Every second case of tuberculous sacroiliitis is associated with at least two tuberculous foci of different loclization; Feldmann et al. 1981; see also p. 498 ff)!

Rule 6: The "variegated" picture of the sacroiliac joints is not diagnostic of ankylosing spondylitis, but it narrows the radiologic differential diagnosis to a few entities that can be distinguished by clinical means. Among them are chronic Reiter's syndrome, psoriatic arthritis, enteropathic sacroiliitis in ulcerative colitis, Crohn's regional enteritis, Whipple's intestinal lipodystrophy, Behçet's disease, hyperparathyroidism or renal osteopathy, and the possible sacroiliac lesions in patients with tetraplegia and paraplegia.

Comment: The identical "variegated picture" of the sacroiliac joints in ankylosing spondylitis, chronic Reiter's syndrome, psoriatic arthritis, ulcerative colitis (Fig. 728), and regional enteritis, in Behçet's disease (p. 96; Dilsen, 1975), and in Whipple's intestinal lipodystrophy[37] (Eyler and Doub, 1956; Kelly and Weisiger, 1963) underscores common features of these diseases, which also may manifest themselves by the HLA-B27 antigen. The majority of these diseases are, in fact, associated with this antigen, though with variable frequency (p. 348). It was not least the joint association with HLA-B27 and the sacroiliitis of the "variegated picture" type which caused the introduction of the concept of **"seronegative spondarthritis"** (Moll et al., 1974; Wright, 1978, 1979). The diseases listed—the seronegative spondarthritides (*synonym:* seronegative spondarthropathies)—have been defined as diseases in which the rheumatoid factors (p. 87) and the subcutaneous rheumatoid nodules are absent and which tend to develop into a polyarthritis with asymmetrical involvement of joints and with a preference for the lower extremities and the sacroiliac joints (sacroiliitis of the "variegated picture" type); the full-blown picture of ankylosing spondylitis may ensue. Besides this, the individual spondarthritides present "overlapping" symptoms in the eyes, the skin, the mucous membranes, the intestines, the urogenital system, and the blood vessels (thrombophlebitis). The frequent association of the seronegative spondarthritides with the HLA-B27 antigen has already been mentioned. This association as well as observations concerning the simultaneous occurrence of *different* types of spondarthritis in the *same family* suggest that, on the one hand, these diseases originate in a genetically prepared soil and, on the other, that little known or unidentified environmental factors initiate their clinical manifestation.

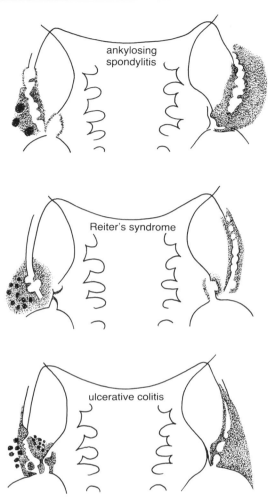

Fig. 727 **"Variegated" sacroiliac picture in three different diseases associated with HLA-B27.** Despite the individual variability of the simultaneous occurrence of the various signs of destruction, sclerosis, and ankylosis, the criteria of the "variegated" sacroiliac picture are noticeable (compare Fig. 721).

Hyperparathyroidism or *renal osteopathy* may give rise to marginal resorption of bone (erosions, pseudodilatation) in the articular surfaces of the sacroiliac joints, to a reactive increase in thickness of the cancellous trabeculae, and to necrosis of the articular cartilage (Dihlmann and Müller, 1973). Calcium salts sometimes precipitate in the necrotic articular cartilage. In addition, the latter is replaced by fibrous connective tissue, and bony trabeculae sprout into the devitalized articular cartilage. Eventually, bony fusion of the sacrum and ilium develops, provided the patients live to this date or parathyroidectomy has been performed (Fig. 728; Steinbach et al., 1961). The processes described produce the "variegated"

---

[37] The rarity of Behçet's and Whipple's diseases and the resulting scarcity of cases reported in the literature heretofore have prevented a conclusive statement of whether the association of these diseases with HLA-B27 and sacroiliitis is statistically significant (compare Bussière et al., 1980).

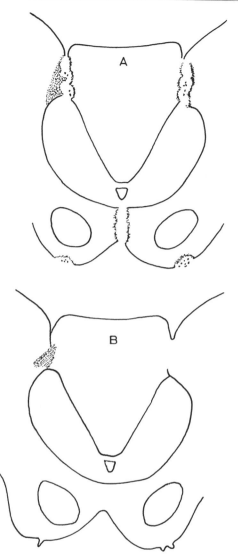

Fig. 728   Primary hyperparathyroidism prior to (A) and following parathyroidectomy (B).

A = Radiologic criteria of the "variegated" sacroiliac picture and ossifications of cartilage in both sacroiliac joints. Pseudodilatation of the symphysis pubis. Hyperparathyroid defects of the tendinous insertions; calcifications of the ischiocrural tendons in both ischia (compare Fig. 366).

B = One year after parathyroidectomy the three connections of the pelvic bones have undergone synostosis. The insertion defects in the ischia are filled with bone. The ossifying processes have partly spread to the tendons.

picture" in the roentgenogram of the sacroiliac joints. The nosological classification of a diagnosed "variegated sacroiliac picture" therefore requires, as a matter of principle, determination of the serum levels

of calcium and phosphate! Similar or even identical roentgen manifestations in the sacroiliac joints, including bony fusion and ossifying processes in the external portions of the annulus fibrosus (syndesmophytes), have been observed in chronic hyperphosphatemia and hypophosphatemia (see p. 461). In such infrequent cases, concomitantly present Looser's zones provide a *radiologic* hint of the diagnostic and therapeutic procedures required.

Neurogenic paraosteoarthropathies (p. 52 ff)—i.e., ectopic calcifications and ossifications in muscles, tendons, fasciae, ligaments, and joint capsules—are known to occur in individuals with a paraplegia or tetraplegia, and occasionally also in hemiplegic patients (Rosin, 1975). Defects in the bones or even extensive osteolyses sometimes develop near pressure sores or in the vicinity of decubitus ulcers (Fig. 57). In addition to these manifestations, bony ankylosis is observed in the sacroiliac joints and the symphysis pubis. In the sacroiliac joints, ankylosis has the aspect of the "variegated picture." Erosions, pseudodilatation, increased thickness of the subchondral cancellous bone and bony bridges, as well as narrowing of the joint space and even bony transformation of the joint and capsular ossification are visible in 50 percent of patients on the average, but occasionally with greater or lesser frequency (Lodge, 1956; Liberson and Mihaldzic, 1965; Bhate et al., 1979; Khan et al., 1979). Changes in the sacroiliac joints may appear as early as three months after the advent of paralysis (Wright et al., 1965); their incidence increases with the duration of the paralysis. Discrete syndesmophytes and ossification of the interspinous and supraspinous ligaments have rarely been observed in the spines of paralyzed patients (Bhate et al., 1979). No relationship has been established between the occurrence of decubitus ulcers or urinary tract infections and alterations of the sacroiliac joints and the spine (lumbar spine, thoracicolumbar junction) (Abel, 1950; Liberson and Mihaldzic, 1965; Catterall et al., 1967). Typing of the paralyzed individuals revealed no association between the incidence of the pathologic findings in the axial skeleton and that genetic risk factor HLA-B27 (Bhate et al., 1979), (p. 348 ff). The etiology of the ossifying processes in the sacroiliac joints, the symphysis pubis and the joints and soft tissues of the paralyzed extremities therefore remains obscure. Long-term immobilization and the absence of weight-bearing cannot be—as has been suggested—the essential cause for the sacroiliac remodeling, because these changes and all the other pathologic findings develop in only some of the patients. So far it has not been clarified whether the concomitant occurrence of ankylosing spondylitis and *familial Mediterranean fever* (p. 296) is due to coincidence or to association of the two diseases (Camus, 1965; Heller et al., 1966; Lejeune et al., 1975; Caroit et al., 1980). There appears to be no relationship between the HLA-B27 antigen and familial Mediterranean fever (Chaouat et al., 1977). The "variegated sacroiliac picture" has been observed in cases of coincident or associated familial Mediterranean fever (*synonym:* periodic disease) and sacroiliitis or ankylosing spondylitis (compare Heller et al., 1966; Brodey and Wolff, 1975).

Radiologic Differential Diagnosis of the "Variegated Sacroiliac Picture"

Destructive phenomena—from hazy joint contours, erosions, and pseudodilatation to dissection and formation of sequestra—can be traced primarily to inflammatory processes, among them bacterial sacroiliitis. This affection usually follows hematogenous spread of microorganisms to the synovial membrane or the juxtaarticular bone marrow. However, infections may also invade the sacroiliac joints by direct spread from a contiguous lesion; for example, a gluteal abscess produced by an intramuscular injection, infected soft tissues of the pelvis (following an obstetric tear of the vagina or extirpation of the rectum), an open pelvic injury, or a psoas abscess. Similarly to infectious spondylitis, nonspecific bacterial sacroiliitis in the sacroiliac joints is distinguished, for practical purposes, from sacroiliac tuberculosis.

Acute **nonspecific bacterial sacroiliitis** (Figs. 726 and 729) is most frequently due to infection with pyogenic cocci. These cases are often preceded by a disseminating focus of infection; e.g., suppurative tonsillitis. Following a short interval, the patients are taken ill with fever, inflammatory hematologic changes, and serologic signs of inflammation. They report pain in the sacroiliac region, which sometimes causes difficulty in walking (limping). Acute suppurative sacroiliitis is occasionally accompanied by symptoms that refer to an affection of the lower urinary tract or mimic an "acute abdomen." The first pathologic roentgen manifestations in these cases are to be expected after about 2 to 3 weeks: haziness of the juxtaarticular cancellous structures, narrowing of the joint space, and erosions. Scintigraphy with bone-

scanning radioisotopes, however, reveals a pathologic tracer accumulation after only a few days. The process then runs its course in the form of the "succeeding triad" described on p. 494—the destructive phase is succeeded by stabilization with sclerosis of the subchondral cancellous bone, and finally by the cicatricial stage with partial or complete bony ankylosis of the sacroiliac joint. The "star sign" and the "phantom joint" have already been mentioned as roentgen manifestations of *acquired* sacroiliac ankylosis (Fig. 722 C and D). Bacteria sacroiliitis in the growth period may give rise to *oblique contracture of the pelvis* (Fig. 722 D)—assuming that the bacterial affection involved a single sacroiliac joint. In hematogenous sacroiliitis a single joint is involved in the great majority of cases. A bacterial infection of both sacroiliac joints should therefore always arouse suspicion that the inflammatory process has spread to these joints as a result of contiguity; for example, from an abscess or an extensive infection of the surrounding soft tissues (anamnesis).

Conversely, nonspecific bacterial infections of the sacroiliac joints may start insidiously with pain and may pursue a *chronic* course (Fig. 729). The differential diagnosis then must take into account sacroiliac tuberculosis but also ankylosing spondylitis (in which about 10 percent of cases begin with unilateral involvement of the sacroiliac joints) (see rule 5, p. 490 ff).

Tuberculous sacroiliitis (Figs. 730 and 731) manifests itself clinically six months after hematogenous dissemination—at the earliest. The onset of dissemination can be determined, for example, by the advent of an exudative pleurisy. In addition, the tuberculous etiology of a sacroiliitis can be presumed in all probability when active pulmonary tuberculosis needing therapy or another tuberculous affection of the skeleton is present *concomitantly*. Sequestra (tomography), abscess formation in the pelvic area (atypical soft-tissue shadows in the lower pelvis, extensive crumbly or pasty calcium shadows within the

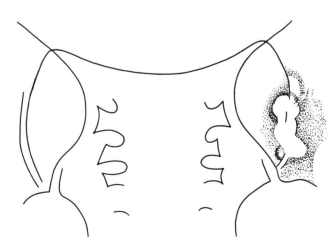

Fig. 729 Six months previous, incision of an abscess in the left gluteal region caused by an intramuscular injection. Since that time continuing subfebrile temperature and "boring" pain in the left sacroiliac area. The survey films show extensive inflammatory destructions in the left sacroiliac joint and a slight increase in density of the cancellous bone in the surroundings of the joint.

Evaluation: Still **florid, chronic nonspecific bacterial sacroiliitis** on the left side, probably due to direct spread of the gluteal abscess.

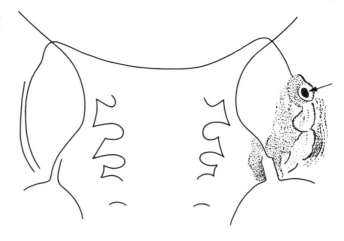

Fig. 730 **Advanced left-sided destructive sequestrating** *(arrow)* **inflammatory process in the sacroiliac joint.**

Two years previously, exudative pleurisy; since then, under supervision because of a pulmonary "shadow." For the last 5 months, left-sided low back pain radiating to the left thigh and the left inguinal region. Altogether there is no doubt about the presence of **sacroiliac tuberculosis.**

involved sacroiliac joint or in the soft tissues of the pelvis) and cutaneous fistulas with concomitant destruction of the sacroiliac joint are also dependable indicators of tuberculosis. Bacterial sacroiliac infections are characterized by far-reaching destructions, as compared with inflammatory rheumatic affections of these joints including rheumatoid arthritis, possible sacroiliac involvement in gout, lipoid-dermatoarthritis, or recurrent polychondritis (p. 105 ff; Braunstein et al., 1979). Bacterial infection of the sacroiliac joints tends to "bury itself" in the joint-bearing bones or spreads "in depth" from the articulating bones to the sacroiliac joint (Fig. 731). In practice it is therefore safe to follow *Brocher's rule,* which states that six and more *flat* erosions, which frequently are in a line like a string of beads (tomography), rule out sacroiliac tuberculosis and suggest the presence of ankylosing spondylitis or some other type of sacroiliitis associated with HLA-B27.

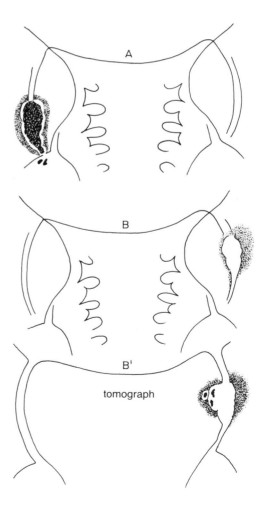

Fig. 731 **Radiologic aspects of tuberculous sacroiliitis.**

A = in addition to contour defects, the roentgenogram is characterized by inspissated and calcified *intra articular* pus. Also individual *extraarticular* calcium shadows in the lower pelvis.

B, B' = The survey film (B) shows circumscribed destructions with perifocal increase in density of the cancellous bone. Only the tomograph (B') reveals a sequestrating process in the wing of the sacrum which has invaded the sacroiliac joint.

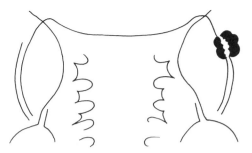

Fig. 732 Circumscribed sacroiliitis; i.e., an area of increased density with cyclic or polycyclic borders on both sides of the sacroiliac joint space, eroded contours, possibly a small dissection which sometimes is revealed only by tomography (compare Fig. 733).

In advanced adult rheumatoid arthritis, the sacroiliac joint spaces may be indiscernible or barely discernible in survey films because of the marked osteoporosis. Alternatively, they may have undergone bony ankylosis as a consequence of the disease. At times, erosions and joint space narrowing are recognizable prior to this stage, particularly in tomographs. In **adult rheumatoid sacroiliitis,** however, any indication of sclerosis is consistently absent, unless different causes (osteoarthrosis, repair ossification of capsuloligamental damage from excessive strain) have led to the development of sclerosis.

Circumscribed sacroiliitis (Dihlmann and Schuler, 1963; Dihlmann 1964a, 1965c; Figs. 732 and 733) is an inflammatory disease of unknown etiology. It manifests itself on both sides of the sacroiliac joint space as an area of increased density with cyclic or polycyclic borders. The joint contour shows superficial erosions, at times also a small dissection. Complete ossification of the joint space in the area of circumscribed sacroiliitis is not to be expected. The condition (Fig. 733) must be differentiated from repair ossification of the anterior sacroiliac joint capsule damaged by excessive strain and from hyperostosis triangularis ilii. Hyperostosis triangularis in the ilium has a characteristic triangular shape (p. 505 ff). Repair ossifications of capsular damage from excessive strain lie prevalently in front of the sacroiliac cleft, which is bridged by them; less frequently the repair ossifications also involve the posterior portions of the capsule. Erosions and dissection do not occur in the capsular ossifications.

Focal nonspecific bacterial osteomyelitis of the pelvis is frequently located in the immediate vicinity of the sacroiliac joint. The condition reflects the sequelae of hematogenous lodgment of microorganisms with little pathogenicity in the bone marrow and runs its course without a clear-cut clinical symptomatology so long as it does not invade the contiguous sacroiliac joint. In the latter case it leads to partial or complete bony ankylosis of the joint. The various, though characteristic, radiologic aspects of

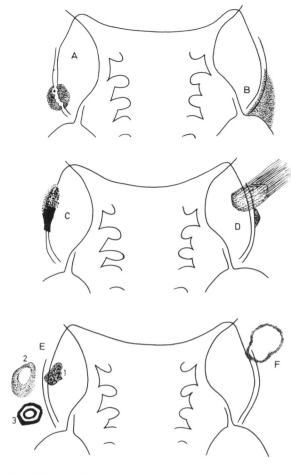

Fig. 733 Radiologic differential diagnosis of circumscribed sacroiliitis.

A = **Circumscribed sacroiliitis** (compare Fig. 732).

B = **Hyperostosis triangularis ilii** (see Figs 740 to 742).

C, D = **repair ossification of damage to the anterior sacroiliac joint capsule and its reinforcing ligaments from excessive strain** (see also Figs. 71, 339, and 739). Big bulge (C) "obliterating" the joint space or flat ossification of capsule and ligaments; the contours of the joint space then "shimmer" through the area of increased density (D).

E = Radiologic morphology of **focal nonspecific bacterial osteomyelitis of the pelvis.** Irregular, rounded, or oval area of increased density which here is located in the posterior iliac spine (E1). (Scar? Differential diagnosis from solitary osteoblastic pelvic metastasis; e.g., by anamnesis or skeletal scintigraphy); or rounded focus of increased density with concentric or eccentric breakdown (E2); or rounded, or polygonal focus of increased density with double contour (E3). When the florid inflammation invades the contiguous sacroiliac joint, partial or complete bony ankylosis develops.

F = **Juxtaarticular rounded osteolysis with thin, continuous marginal sclerosis** (type of bone cyst; nonossifying osseous fibroma or enchondroma).

focal pelvic osteomyelitis—which, as a rule, originates in the ilium—are illustrated in Fig. 733 E 1–3.

The radiologic lesions of the sacroiliac joint in unilateral or bilateral avascular necrosis of the apophysis of the sacral wing—so-called **sacral osteochondrosis** (Rogers and Cleaves, 1935; Dihlmann 1964b; Fig. 734)—impress one as being destructive. This disorder of apophyseal ossification in the wing of the sacrum manifests itself between the 16th and 20th years of life; i.e., at the time of physiologic ossification and fusion of the apophysis. *The apophysis has the appearance of being fragmented, thickened, and delimited by hazy borders.* The contour of the ilium, in contrast, remains smooth. This is an important radiologic feature in differentiating between sacral osteochondrosis—some writers also speak of sacral osteochondritis, which is incorrect from the pathogenetic point of view—and sacroiliitis in ankylosing spondylitis. In fact, sacroiliitis of the "variegated picture" type, and also other types of different etiology, are characterized by the *early* appearance of erosions in the contour of the ilium or by *concomitant* erosions in the ilial as well as the sacral aspect of the joint. Prior to diagnosing sacral osteochondrosis, which is a self-limited condition and therefore offers a favorable prognosis, one should make it a matter of principle to rule out the other inflammatory rheumatic diseases that are apt to attack the sacroiliac joints.

Damage to the sacroiliac joints from excessive strain involves the articular cartilage, the capsuloligamental apparatus, and the subchondral bone. **Osteoarthrosis of the sacroiliac joints** (Fig. 736) is the classic affection of the articular cartilage caused by excessive strain. Preliminary conditions for the development of the radiologic characteristics of osteoarthrosis are damage to the articular cartilage *as well as* preserved mobility of the joint. Since the sacroiliac joints physiologically possess little mobility, osteoarthrosis of the sacroiliac joints is diagnosed less frequently than degeneration of the articular cartilage can be evidenced by histologic study. The roentgen manifestations of sacroiliac osteoarthrosis are consistent with those encountered in osteoarthrosis of other joints; i.e., joint space narrowing, band-shaped increase in density of the cancellous bone, debris cysts, and marginal osteophytes. The osteoarthrotic osteophytes grow in prolongation of the articular surfaces. When they project into the soft tissues of the pelvis, they are recognizable in plain roentgenograms as pointed marginal spurs in the caudal region of the joint. In contrast to capsuloligamentous ossifications of the sacroiliac joints *(vide infra)*, they do not bridge the joint space.

Damage to the capsuloligamentous apparatus of the sacroiliac joints due to excessive strain manifests itself clinically and roentgenologically as **pelvic loosening** and **pelvic rigidity** (Dihlmann, 1963, 1965b). During the course of the menstrual cycle and during pregnancy, hormonal influences lead to loosening of the capsuloligamentous apparatus of the sacroiliac joints. The result is increased mobility and thereby increased vulnerability of the pelvic connections. Parturition also promotes damage to the fibrous sacroiliac structures. In addition, unilateral excessive strain on the sacroiliac capsule and ligaments is to be expected with thoracicolumbar scoliosis, deformation of the pelvis, chronic diseases of the hip joint, and shortening of a leg. Bilateral damage from excessive strain may occur as the result of a change in pelvic posture, in adiposity of the abdominal wall, and in pareses and contractures of the muscles that stabilize the pelvis. Finally, the capsuloligamentous apparatus may also be damaged by trivial traumas of everyday life; for example, a slip on the staircase or a fall. Histologic study in these cases has shown tears, avulsions, and hemorrhages in the sacroiliac capsule

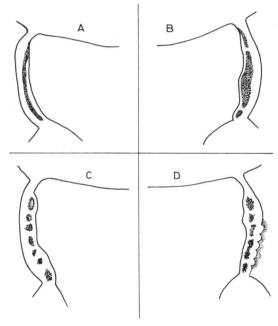

Fig. 734 Normal (A, B) and pathologic (C, D) ossification of the apophysis of the sacral wing—the lateral part of the sacrum—between the 16th and 20th years of life.

A, B = *Normal ossification of the apophysis;* beginning fusion with the other parts of the sacrum. The ossified apophysis has a denser appearance than the contiguous bones. This phenomenon is frequently observed in apophyseal ossifications—in whatever place.

C = Fragmented apophyseal ossification centers with hazy contours on both sides (illustrated only on the right side). The contours of the ilium, however, are always *smooth. Clinically:* Low back pain for the last year (present age 17); no serologic signs of inflammation. Spinal mobility normal.

Diagnosis: **Sacral osteochondrosis** (see text).

D = Roentgen manifestations of sacral osteochondrosis *plus* erosions in the ilium = ankylosing spondylitis or sacroiliitis of different etiology.

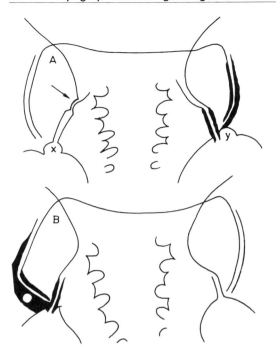

Fig. 735 Osteoarthrosis of the sacroiliac joint.
A = Typical roentgen manifestation of osteoarthrosis of the left sacroiliac joint (see text).
X = paraglenoidal sulcus in the ilium and the sacrum; at Y only in the ilium. This groove, which is a variant of normal, forms the point of attachment for the fibrous anterior joint capsule. **Accessory sacroiliac joint** between the posterior iliac spine and the posterior surface of the sacral wing *(arrow)*.
B = Osteoarthrosis of the right sacroiliac joint in dysplasia of the sacrum (sacral scoliosis; malformation of the right wing of the sacrum).

and ligaments. The result of these injuries is either increased (nonphysiologic) mobility of the joint involved—pelvic loosening—or the development of repair ossifications in the capsule and ligaments, which produce irreversible fusion of the sacrum and ilium—pelvic rigidity. Pelvic loosening, particularly, is frequently accompanied by discomfort (low back pain). The survey film of the pelvis in dorsal decubitus already provides hints about pelvic loosening or rigidity. Capsular damage to the sacroiliac joints from excessive strain—and even more, traumatic rupture or inflammatory bacterial destruction of the sacroiliac soft tissues—may give rise to a typical malposition

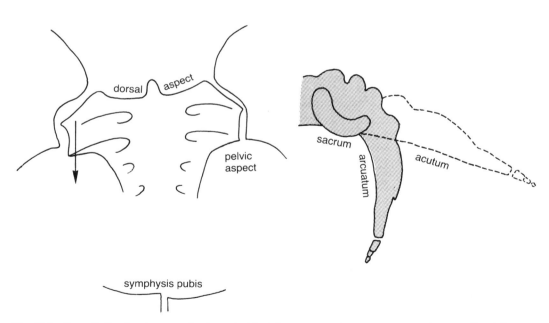

Fig. 736 Sacrolisthesis. As a result of a coincidental sacrum acutum or arcuatum, the sacroiliac joints are projected *axially*. This is why the sacrolisthesis in the right sacroiliac joint (dorsoventral displacement *(arrow)* and spreading of the joint space) is already recognizable in this survey film of the pelvis with the patient in dorsal decubitus. The descended right side of the sacrum has taken with it the *left* ilium across the not loosened *left* sacroiliac joint; this causes the *left* horizontal pubic ramus to descend.
With a normally shaped sacrum, one can try to obtain the axial projection of the sacroiliac joints by producing an "artificial" hyperlordosis of the lumbar spine. This is achieved by placing the patient on a thick, firm cushion. Alternatively, the sacrolisthesis can be identified by computed tomography (Fig. 742). Data beyond sacrolisthesis are provided by radiologic function tests of the pelvic connections (Fig. 737).

1. Survey film of the pelvis in dorsal decubitus:

Suspicion of pelvic loosening?

Suspicion of pelvic rigidity?

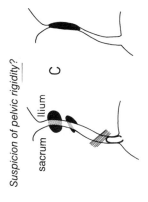

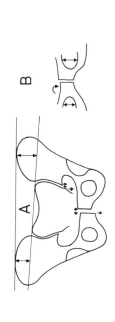

2. Survey film of the pelvis with the patient standing, following unilateral loading with 5 kg for 10 minutes: *signs of pelvic loosening or of incomplete pelvic rigidity?* = as compared with the findings in the roentgenogram no. 1 (A, B)

3. Two spots films of the symphysis with alternation of weighted leg:

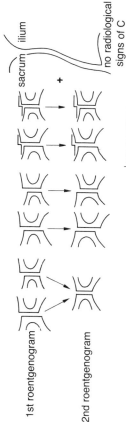

Pelvic loosening

1st roentgenogram

2nd roentgenogram

unilateral mobility   *bilateral mobility*

impaction?
The asymmetrically positioned horizontal rami of the os pubis are not displaceable on alternation of the weight-bearing leg. The sacro-iliac joint, however, presents signs suspicious of loosening (see 1A) without ossification of capsule and ligaments (see 1C).

no radiological signs of C

Pelvic rigidity

incomplete
Despite roentgen signs of pelvic rigidity, the asymmetrically positioned horizontal rami of the os pubis are still displaceable on alternation of the weight-bearing leg

complete
The asymmetrically positioned horizontal rami of the os pubis are *not* displaceable on alternation of the weight-bearing leg. In addition, there are roentgen signs of pelvic rigidity.

Fig. 737   **Radiologic function tests of the pelvic connections** (sacroiliac joints, symphysis pubis) Trostzer (1938), Schapals (1971) and Dihlmann (1973).

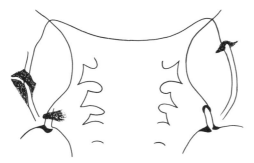

Fig. 738   Roentgen findings in repair ossifications of the sacroiliac capsule and ligaments (see also Figs. 71, 733 C and D, and 739). These ossifications are observed following damage due to excessive strain or major trauma, and also in ankylosing spondylitis, in which they form part of the "variegated" sacroiliac picture and hence are accompanied by erosions, multiform subchondral sclerosis, and intraarticular osseous burgeons and bridges.

of the joint, because the weight of the trunk forces the sacrum into the pelvis. This **sacrolisthesis** (Figs. 736 and 742 C) is manifested by a staircase formation between the sacrum and the ilium at the level of the linea arcuata. Additional pathologic findings illustrated in Figures 737 A and B also points to morbid loosening of the pelvic connections.

Repair ossification of the damaged *anterior* sacroiliac joint capsule leads to varied but characteristic roentgen manifestations (Dihlmann, 1963; Figs. 71, 733 C and D, 737, 738, and 739). Ossifying processes in the *posterior* part of the sacroiliac capsule are much less frequently identified in survey films than in tomographs and with use of computed tomography (Fig. 742 C). The same is true of calcifications and ossifications of the interosseous sacroiliac ligaments which pass through the retroarticular space (Fig. 739).

Before therapeutic measures are begun, an exact

quantitative and qualitative radiologic analysis of the soft-tissue damage in the regions of the sacroiliac joints and the symphysis pubis should be performed with use of so-called functional roentgenograms. This postulate refers not only to the evaluation of damage to the capsuloligamentous apparatus related to excessive strain but, still more explicitly, to pelvic loosening or rigidity caused by a major trauma; e.g., dislocation of the sacroiliac joints, vertical fractures in the immediate vicinity of the ilium and sacrum, fracture of the anterior pelvic ring, and ruptures of the symphysis pubis. On the one hand, these injuries probably will cause severe disruptions of the sacroiliac capsule and ligaments with permanent loosening. On the other hand, severe traumatic damage to the gliding tissues, including the articular cartilage, can be followed by **posttraumatic noninflammatory (abacterial) bony ankylosis of the sacroiliac joints.**

Radiologic Function Tests of the Pelvic Articulations (Sacroiliac Joints, Symphysis Pubis)

Principle of the method: The symphysis pubis lies on the long lever arm of the sacroiliac joints. Since the sacrum is fixed, and depending on the length of the lever arm, excursions in these joints are therefore transmitted to the symphysis pubis to a larger extent and cause the latter to move in the longitudinal direction of the body. An approximately equally strong pathologic loosening of *both* sacroiliac joints manifests itself in survey films of the pelvis by an axial projection of the pelvic ring; one then looks into the pelvic ring from above, as one does in an axial roentgenogram of the symphysis. This assumption is, however, only justified when, on positioning the patient for the survey film of the pelvis, the lumbar lordosis has been corrected. With pathologic loosening of *one* sacroiliac joint or asymmetrical loosening of *both* these joints, the structure of the symphysis pubis also becomes loosened, since its ligamentous reinforcement is inadequate. Such loosening manifests itself by the horizontal rami of the pubis being displaceable relative to each other. A slight displacement of about 1 mm is still physiologic; in the later stages of pregnancy and post partum, however, the potential displacement may be even greater.

Explanation of the investigative procedure and the roentgen sketches in Figure 737:

1.   The following *suspicious signs of loosening* of the pelvic connections (A, B) and of *bony hooks bridging the joint space* (C) are searched for in a survey film of the pelvis with the patient supine:

A.   Divergent tangents to the pelvic brim and the cranial contour of the sacrum? Step forma-

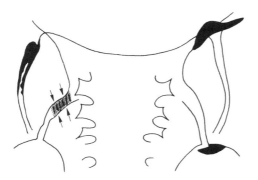

Fig. 739   Repair ossifications of the sacroiliac capsuloligamental apparatus (continued). Note also the ossified interosseous sacroiliac ligaments *(arrows).*

tion between sacrum and ilium at the linea arcuata? Gaping of the inferior part of the sacroiliac joint space? Step formation at the superior and inferior border of the symphysis pubis, widening of the symphyseal cleft?

B.   Rotation of one half of the anterior pelvic ring (asymmetrical obturator foramina) and different level of those parts of the os pubis that bear the symphysis?

C.   Typical forms of projection of damages to the sacroiliac capsule and ligaments that have led to repair ossification; when the joint space is *completely* bridged, immobilization of the joint ensues (pelvic rigidity).

2.   When roentgen manifestations suggestive of pelvic loosening or pelvic rigidity are encountered in the survey film, *and/or* the clinical findings and the patient's complaints arouse a suspicion of pelvic loosening, a second survey film of the pelvis is made *with the patient standing* and following (unilateral) weight-bearing for 10 minutes. To this end, the patient holds a 5 kg weight in his hand and walks about for 10 minutes. Pelvic loosening or incomplete pelvic rigidity manifests itself by a modification of the roentgen signs A and B (see roentgenogram no. 1).

3.   Two fluoroscopic spot examinations with alternation of the weight-bearing leg (first examination with the patient standing on his left leg with his right leg raised; second examination with the patient standing on his right leg with his left leg raised, or in the reverse order). These radiologic studies can ascertain whether a pelvic loosening diagnosed on survey films 1 and 2 exhibits *unilateral*[38] or *bilateral mobility,* whether one is dealing with an *impaction* of the loosened sacroiliac joint (*without* ossification of capsule and ligaments) or whether a pelvic rigidity is incomplete or complete.

Hyperostosis triangularis ilii (Dihlmann, 1976b, c)—formerly known as osteitis condensans ilii—is characterized by triangular projection of an area of increased iliac density in the immediate vicinity of the sacroiliac joint (Fig. 740). In about 50 percent of cases, the sacrum also presents an area of increased density of extremely variable shape (Fig. 741). Hyperostosis triangularis has a marked predilection for females in the 4th and 5th decades of life, hence in the childbearing age; it occurs unilaterally or bilaterally. Females with hyperostosis triangularis have more commonly borne children than those without

---

[38] Commonly it is the sacroiliac joint *contralateral* to the descended or rotated horizontal ramus of the pubis that becomes loosened. The reason is that the sacrum, which is displaced caudally in the loosened sacroiliac joint, takes with it caudally the contralateral ilium, including the symphysis together with the non-loosened sacroiliac joint (Fig. 737, A and B). *Bilateral* loosening (see Fig. 737, "*bilateral mobility*") may be diagnosed only when the horizontal rami of the pubis can be displaced to a greater extent relative to each other (Kamieth, 1958a, b), when the distance between the tangents to the ilium and the sacrum increases *bilaterally* on weight-bearing, and when additional radiologic signs of *bilateral* loosening are demonstrable (Fig. 737 A and B).

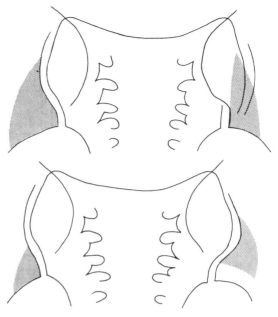

Fig. 740   **Hyperostosis triangularis ilii.** Triangular hyperostoses of variable size. Their demonstration depends on the projection of the sacroiliac joints in roentgenograms taken in dorsal decubitus.

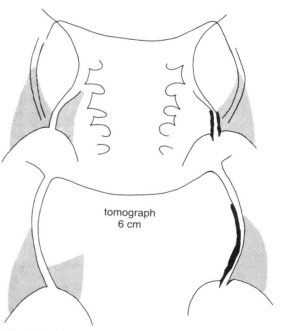

tomograph
6 cm

Fig. 741   **Hyperostosis triangularis ilii (continued).** Polymorphous increase of density in the sacrum *(left).* It is primarily the tomograph that detects the *concomitant* roentgen manifestations of sacroiliac osteoarthrosis *(right).*

this anomaly (Peña Arrebola et al., 1975). Histologic studies have shown that the condition is *not* an osteitis or osteomyelitis but a noninflammatory transformation of cancellous into compact bone and that, in addition, so-called mosaic structures are indicative of increased remodeling of bone. The majority of patients with triangular hyperostosis complain of low back pain. It is, however, hardly probable that noninflammatory remodeling of bone gives rise to the discomfort. The latter is due rather to conditions that can be demonstrated histologically, clinically, and by radiologic examination in most patients suffering from hyperostosis; namely, sacroiliac osteoarthrosis and pelvic loosening (Kamieth, 1958b). This non-coincidental association of hyperostosis triangularis ilii and damage from excessive strain (osteoarthrosis affects the articular cartilage and pelvic loosening affects the capsuloligamental apparatus) arouses the suspicion that triangular hyperostosis, also, is the result of excessive strain on the sacroiliac joints. The frequently observed reversibility of triangular hyperostosis (Dihlmann, 1976c), which is either spontaneous or follows arthrodesis, makes it unlikely that the condition is a general feature of sacroiliac osteoarthrosis. Degeneration of the articular cartilage is an irreversible process. In individual cases, a very solid repair ossification of the ventral sacroiliac ligaments can lead to a triangular zone of increased density. The latter lies, however, *in front* of the sacroiliac joint (Dihlmann, 1967, 1978). In contrast, conventional and computed tomography (Dihlmann et al., 1979) have shown that triangular hyperostosis develops within the bone. On studying macerated transverse sections of the ilium and computed tomographs of normal sacroiliac joints, one recognizes a small triangular zone of increased density in the anterior corner of the ilial joint (sclerosis of the anterior corner of the ilial joint; Fig. 742) which is not demonstrable on survey films and in conventional tomographs. When one imagines this triangular zone to be three-dimensional, it has the shape of a pyramid; i.e., it tapers cranially. In the roentgenogram, a pyramid is projected in principle as a triangle. When a person is standing on both legs, the center of pressure on the sacroiliac joints lies in that physiologic zone of increased density at the anterior corner of the ilial joint (Pauwels, 1965). This is why, even under normal conditions, cancellous bone is remodeled into compact bone that has a greater weight-bearing capacity. The compressive load in the sacroiliac joints *may* increase—for example, as the result of pathologic hypermobility in pelvic loosening or through loss of the pressure-absorbing articular cartilage in sacroiliac osteoarthrosis. On the other hand, the anterior corner of the ilial joint *may* coincidentally be the seat of a disease which leads to "softening" of bone; for example Paget's osteitis deformans (Fig. 743) or systemic affections that reduce the weight-bearing capacity of the skeleton; e.g., marble bone disease (Albers-Schönberg) or hyperparathyroidism. The result is an adaptive reaction of the bone. Phys-

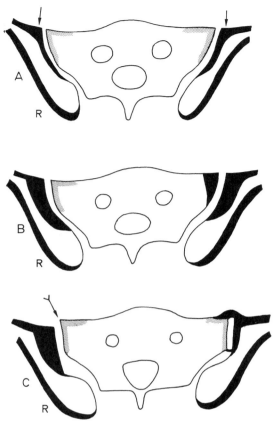

Fig. 742 Computed tomography of the sacroiliac joints (Dihlmann et al., 1979).

A = *Physiologic* triangular area of increased density at the anterior corner of the ilial part of joint *(arrows)*.

B = Hyperostosis triangularis ilii, at the *left* associated with hyperostosis of the sacrum.

C = besides the right-sided hyperostosis triangularis illii (R = right side), sacrolisthesis *(tailed arrow)* and ossification of the anterior and posterior capsules of the left sacroiliac joint are demonstrable.

iologic sclerosis of the anterior corner of the ilial joint increases with preservation of its shape and becomes visible on survey films and in tomographs; hyperostosis triangularis ilii—damage to the anterior corner of the ilial joint from excessive strain—has developed, or the triangular projection of an area of increased density in the sacroiliac joint accompanies one of the osteopathies mentioned above.

The foregoing clarification of the pathogenesis of hyperostosis triangularis ilii may be of heuristic interest. More important for practical purposes are clear instructions concerning the radiologic differentiation of that condition from sacroiliitis of the "variegated picture" type. It is well to remember here rule 4 (p. 489 ff), which states that the shape of sacroiliac sclerosis in ankylosing spondylitis is subject to great variations and that therefore triangular increases in density of the ilium are apt to occur in the setting of the "variegated" sacroiliac picture. Occasionally, triangular sclerosis of the ilium becomes so prominent in the radiologic morphology that delicate marginal erosions and bony bridges—the other diagnostic components of the "variegated" sacroiliac picture—cannot be identified on survey films (Fig. 743). The following constellation should therefore prompt tomographic study of the sacroiliac joints:

1. *Young* male (remember the preference of triangular hyperostosis for females) *with triangular sclerosis of the ilium*
2. *Pain in the lumbosacral region* (so-called low back pain) *increasing in the late hours of the night*
3. *Elevated sedimentation rate* without any other definite cause.

In this way the detection or the absence of the "variegated" sacroiliac picture can become the decisive diagnostic factor. However, in cases of triangular sclerosis of the ilium even tomography of the sacroiliac joints cannot always prevent *false positive* radiologic diagnoses of the "variegated" sacroiliac picture. The reasons are: It is true that hyperostotic bone transmits the load better than cancellous bone, but it is more brittle than the latter and tends to break. Histologic studies have shown that in the region of such microtraumas the fragments of bone become replaced by highly cellular inflammatory connective tissue (Dihlmann, 1981). This is manifested in the roentgenogram, particularly in tomographs, by erosion of the articular contour. In addition, the radiologic joint space may appear to be narrowed by the *accompanying* osteoarthrosis of the sacroiliac joint *(vide supra)*, and at times even small bony bridges traverse the circumscribed areas of devitalized articular cartilage. In these cases, tomographs present the "variegated" sacroiliac picture. This signifies that the limits of radiologic differential diagnosis have been reached! The hazard of misdiagnosing the "variegated" sacroiliac picture arises when, in these instances, the radiologic examiner relies exclusively on tomographic studies and fails to include the results of clinical, serological, and anamnestic investigations and data in the diagnostic considerations (see p. 485 ff).

Rule 7: The syndesmophyte is the characteristic intervertebral osteophyte of ankylosing spondylitis.

Comment: In 61 percent of the patients with ankylosing spondylitis, the *first* sydesmophytes develop in the thoracicolumbar junction (Dihlmann, 1966a, b). Therefore, the roentgenogram of the lumbar spine should on principle include not only the two sacroiliac joints but also the 12th, and if possible even the 11th thoracic motor segment. In the radiologic diagnosis, the syndesmophytes must be differentiated from the other intervertebral and vertebral osteophytes. The characteristic radiologic morphology of the syndesmophytes, parasyndesmophytes, spondylophytes, and repair osteophytes has therefore been illustrated side

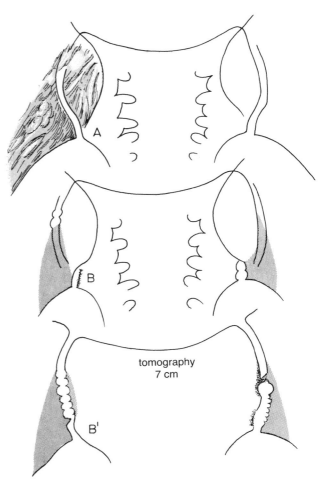

Fig. 743   **Triangular iliac area of increased density in Paget's osteitis deformans (A) and in ankylosing spondylitis (B, B').** The radiologic differentiation of hyperostosis triangularis ilii from Paget's disease offers no difficulty (see the fibrillar transformation of the cancellous bone in the ilium, also outside the triangular area of increased density). Besides the triangular sclerosis of the cancellous bone, the survey film of case B shows discrete destructive phenomena. Only tomography (B') reveals the characteristic "variegated" sacroiliac picture of ankylosing spondylitis or the other types of sacroilliitis associated with the HLA-B27 antigen (see rule no. 6 in text).

by side in Figure 679 (compare Figs. 680 through 684; see also p. 456 ff). Among the diseases associated with HLA-B27, ulcerative colitis and regional enteritis (Crohn's disease) may be accompanied not only by sacroiliitis but also by syndesmophytes. They may therefore present the full-blown picture of ankylosing spondylitis. When, on the other hand, Reiter's syndrome and psoriatic arthritis involve the axial skeleton with or without sacroiliitis,

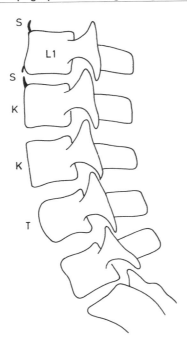

Fig. 744 **Square vertebra (K), barrel-shaped vertebra (T), and syndesmophytes (S) in ankylosing spondylitis** *(synopsis).* Square vertebrae *may* precede the appearance of syndesmophytes. Barrel-shaped vertebrae, however, are indicative of an advanced stage of the disease.

syndesmophytes are encountered in some cases but parasyndemophytes in others (McEwen et al., 1971). This carries prognostic significance for the patient (p. 462 ff).

Rule 8: During the course of ankylosing spondylitis the spine may also present destructive changes; namely, box-shaped vertebrae, barrel-shaped vertebrae, the Romanus lesion, and Andersson's lesion.

Comment: **Square vertebra**—"squaring phenomenon"—is identified in the lateral roentgenogram of the lumbar spine by its *straightened* anterior contour (Figs. 661 A, and 744). In the cervical and thoracic spine, straightened anterior vertebral contours also occur as a normal variant. Therefore, they have not the same diagnostic significance in these places as in the lumbar spine. The **barrel-shaped vertebra** (Dihlmann 1966b; Figs. 661 C and 744) is characterized in the thoracic as well as the lumbar spine by its *convex* anterior contour. Figure 745 presents observations concerning the development of the square and the barrel-shaped vertebrae. For the radiologic differentiation between the two anomalies see Fig. 661 and page 442.

Romanus and Ydén (1952) have described a small contour defect in the anterior (superior and inferior)

marginal border of the vertebral body—**Romanus lesion; anterior spondylitis** (Fig. 745). This defect also occurs less frequently in the superior or inferior *posterior* edge of the vertebral body so that, in general terms, one also speaks of marginal spondylitis (Schilling, 1974). The defect of the vertebral edge is usually surrounded by a perifocal increase in density of the cancellous bone. Such sclerosis of the vertebral edge occasionally develops without a defect—**shiny corner** (Zvaifler and Martel, 1960). The Romanus lesion is observed in about 10 percent of patients with ankylosing spondylitis; it is therefore a comparatively infrequent manifestation of this disease. This fact alone argues against the assumption that anterior spondylitis *generally* precedes the formation of syndesmophytes or that the bony repair of the defect in anterior spondylitis takes place by the development of syndesmophytes (Ball, 1971).

Andersson (1937) was the first to point out that during the course of ankylosing spondylitis, destructions involving the disks and the spine sometimes occur. Believing that these destructive lesions and those of bacterial spondylitis were radiologically similar, if not identical, clinicians have referred to a **spondylodiscitis** that develops during the course of ankylosing spondylitis. Alternatively—and unfortunately for the enuring treatment, they have assumed that an additional (coincidental) bacterial (i.e., tuberculous) spondylitis had been superimposed upon a known ankylosing spondylitis. Contrary to these beliefs, morphologic analysis of spondylodiscitis by radiologic examination, as well as reported histologic findings (compare Bywaters and Ohlsen, 1968; Sutherland and Matheson, 1974; Dihlmann and Delling, 1978) have shown that *two types* of spondylodiscitis evidently occur in ankylosing spondylitis: the "inflammatory type" and the "noninflammatory type" (Figs. 746 and 747).

"Inflammatory" spondylodiscitis presents a circumscribed defect of one or two contiguous vertebral bodies. The vertebral defect is surrounded by a *broad* perifocal area of increased density, and the corresponding disk may show a decrease in height. Spines with (several) "inflammatory" foci of spondylodiscitis are conspicuous by the paucity or absence of syndesmophytes. The "inflammatory type" develops primarily during the first 9 years of the disease (Dihlmann and Delling, 1978).

The "noninflammatory type" usually develops at a still later date. It reflects a fatigue fracture through the disk or a pseudoarthrosis in the osteoporotic, stiffened spine. This information, derived from histologic studies, is strengthened by the radiologic appearance: the fatigue fracture may extend posteriorly to the ankylosed articular processes of the intervertebral joints (Fig. 747 B). Extensive vertebral destructions without a major increase in density of the surrounding cancellous bone contrast with a slight decrease in disk height—or even none. At times the disk space even appears to be "widened" (Fig. 748).

Since the term **Andersson's lesion** is neutral from

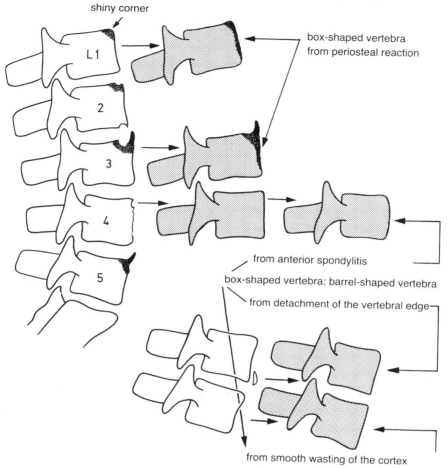

shiny corner

box-shaped vertebra
from periosteal reaction

from anterior spondylitis

box-shaped vertebra; barrel-shaped vertebra

from detachment of the vertebral edge

from smooth wasting of the cortex

Fig. 745 **Pathogenesis of the square and barrel-shaped vertebra, manifestations of anterior spondylitis (see L2–L4)," shiny corner" (see L1).**

the pathogenetic point of view, it is more appropriate for characterizing the discovertebral destruction in ankylosing spondylitis than is the term "spondylodiscitis," which basically presupposes inflammatory processes. The incidence of Andersson's lesion varies between a few percent and 28 percent, depending on the radiologic technique (survey film, tomography) and the nature of the subjects (Jacqueline, 1965). The lower thoracic spine and the lumbar spine are the sites of predilection for Andersson's lesion. The condition may run an asymptomatic course and may become stabilized through the formation of intervertebral osteophytes; occasionally it gives rise to local discomfort or even leads to signs of compression in the cord or the cauda equina.

Courtois and colleagues (1980) have employed the neutral term *"erosive spondylopathy"* to describe oligotopical destructions resembling Andersson's lesion with and *without*

ankylosing spondylitis as a process of unknown etiology, though excluding its infectious or tumorous genesis.

Rule 9: Pathologic changes in the intervertebral and costovertebral joints as well as in the spinal ligaments have no practical significance in the early radiologic diagnosis of ankylosing spondylitis.

Comment: In the majority of patients with ankylosing spondylitis, the stiffening process in the *intervertebral joints* manifests itself radiologically by ossification of the capsule; erosions can much less frequently be identified (Fig. 749). It is true that a delicate capsular ossification immobilizes the joint, but the radiologic joint space—the indicator of the thickness of the articular cartilage—remains temporarily unchanged. By taking into account the unclear depicton of the (lumbar) intervertebral joints in anteroposterior, lateral, and even oblique views, it is

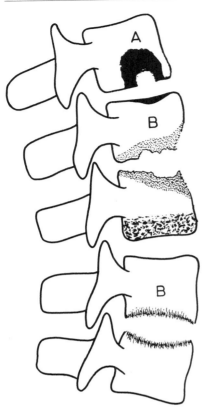

Fig. 746 **Radiologic morphology of Andersson's lesion in ankylosing spondylitis** *(synopsis)*.
A = "Inflammatory type"; B = "noninflammatory type" (see text). The other roentgen findings in ankylosing spondylitis have not been illustrated.

easy to understand that delicate capsular ossifications escape notice quite readily. On the other hand, capsular ossifications (Fig. 687), and even flat erosions in the (lumbar) intervertebral joints, also occur in osteoarthrosis of the spine (Dihlmann, 1968a). In oblique views of the lumbar spine, also, such roentgen findings as hazy contours and narrowing of the joint space require the greatest caution when being interpreted as pathologic. Joints are optimally demonstrable when the articular surfaces are met tangentially by the roentgen beam. Even in oblique views of the lumbar spine this will not always be the case, let alone when all intervertebral joints of the same side are filmed concomitantly. The reason is that the variable shape and alignment of the articular processes from one motor segment to the other and the physiologic incongruity of their articular surfaces interfere with their optimal radiologic demonstration (Dihlmann, 1968a). Only bony ankylosis of the intervertebral joints is readily demonstrable in the roentgenogram (Fig. 747 A and B), but at this stage ankylosing spondylitis is no longer susceptible to early diagnosis!

The *costovertebral joints* are divided into the joint of the head of the rib and the costotransverse joint.

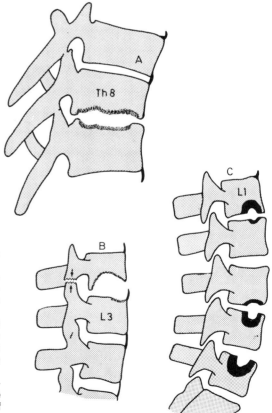

Fig. 747 **Andersson's lesions in ankylosing spondylitis** (continued).
A = Ankylosing spondylitis of many years' standing. The discovertebral destruction in Th8/Th9 is identified roentgenologically as being noninflammatory (compare Fig. 746 A).
B = Noninflammatory Andersson's lesion in L2/L3 with a history of many years and almost complete stiffening of the spine. See also the fracture cleft through the ankylosed articular processes (*arrows;* compare text).
C = Inflammatory type of Andersson's lesion involving several segments of the lumbar spine. Five years' anamnesis; typical "variegated" appearance of the sacroiliac joints; so far only one syndesmophyte (Th12/L1).

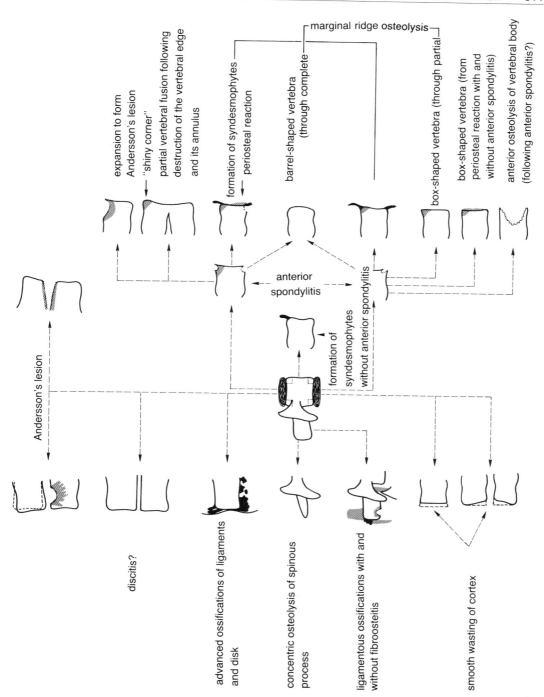

Fig. 748 **Schematic synopsis of the destructive and osteoblastic lesions of the spine in ankylosing spondylitis** (illustrated in lateral roentgenograms of the spine). For concentric osteolysis of the spinous process see also Figs 665 and 710.

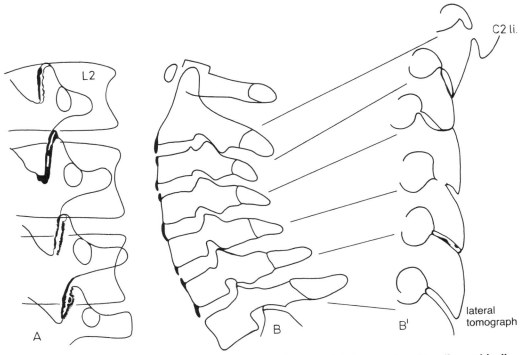

Fig. 749 Lesions of the intervertebral joints in ankylosing spondylitis recognizable radiographically.
A = Oblique view of the lumbar spine. The periarticular and intraarticular roentgen manifestations resemble those encountered in apophyseal joint osteoarthrosis (Fig. 687). Note particularly the capsular ossifications in both diseases.
B = Longstanding ankylosing spondylitis with cervical syndesmophytes. Involvement of the intervertebral joints cannot be definitely identified in this lateral roentgenogram. The cervical spine is completely ankylosed.
B′ = Lateral tomography of the left intervertebral joints. Ossifications of the joint capsule are the prominent feature.

In the roentgenogram, ankylosing spondylitis manifests itself primarily in the joints of the heads of the ribs (costovertebral joints in the strict sense). In these joints, the disease leads in the first place to ossification of the capsule and the ligaments, and much less frequently to erosions of the articular surfaces (Fig. 750). Initially, however, these changes can be identified with some assurance only in the paired joints Th1 to Th3 and Th10 to Th12. Apart from this, ossification of the capsule and ligaments also occurs in degenerative lesions, and even without osteoarthrosis of the costovertebral joints. The capsuloligamentous ossifications illustrated in Figure 750 can therefore be assessed as radiologic evidence of ankylosing spondylitis only in conjunction with the appearance of syndesmophytes.

The anteroposterior roentgenogram of the thoracic spine suffices only conditionally for the demonstration of the costotransverse joints because it allows assessment of the costotransverse joints of only the *lower* half of the thoracic spine. *Williams' focusing technique,* on the other hand, affords a distinct projection of (most of) the costotransverse joints. To this end, the patient is placed on his back and the roentgen tube is tilted cephalad between 20° and 40° (Hohmann and Gasteiger, 1970). The central beam is then directed toward the sixth thoracic vertebra, its site of entrance being the xiphoid process. The more pronounced the thoracic kyphosis, the more the tube should be tilted. Roentgenograms by the Williams technique not only permit more accurate assessment of the involvement of the costotransverse joints by osteoarthrosis (Fig. 688) but also permit demonstration of erosive lesions in inflammatory diseases; e.g., lipoid-dermatoarthritis (Gold et al., 1975). However, the number of joints of the costal heads freely projected in Williams roentgenograms is about the same as in conventional anteroposterior roentgenograms. It should be added here that in traumatic disruption of the costovertebral joint Th1, the apex of the lung is often clouded by the attendant hematoma (compare with the opposite side).

In principle, any ligament of the spine may ossify during the course of ankylosing spondylitis. This

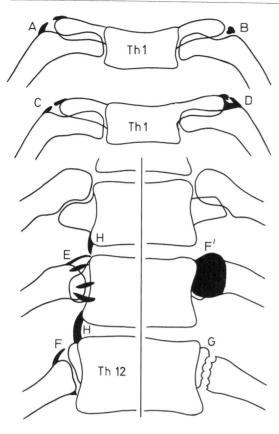

Fig. 750 **Roentgen findings in the costovertebral joints in ankylosing spondylitis.**

A, B, C = Ossifying processes in the lateral costo-transverse ligament occur in ankylosing spondylitis, in degenerative arthropathies, and without known etiology (damage due to excessive strain?).

D = Ligamentous *and* intraarticular ossifying processes.

E, F = Hook-shaped capsular ossifications can be interpreted as roentgen manifestations of ankylosing spondylitis only when syndesmophytes (H) are present concomitantly, because they also occur in osteoarthrosis and from unknown causes (excessive strain on the capsule?).

F′ = Complete ossification of capsule and joint in ankylosing spondylitis (total ankylosis). For the radiologic aspect of hyperostosis of the costal head (in hyperostotic spondylosis), see Fig. 681.

G = Inflammatory erosion of the articular surfaces (infrequently demonstrable finding).

is a late finding that has no significance in the diagnosis of the disease (Figs. 665 and 682 B and C).

Symphysis pubis

Differential diagnosis of pathologic roentgen manifestations in the symphysis pubis is based on the width of the symphyseal cleft, the contours, and the cancellous structures of each os pubis. Assessment of the symphysis on survey films of the pelvis is sometimes supplemented by the axial view to demonstrate the anterior and posterior aspect of the os pubis. For functional roentgenograms see Figure 737.

Congenital diastasis of the pubic bones—**symphyseal diastasis** (Fig. 751)—occurs with exstrophy of the bladder, epispadias, hypospadias, anal atresia, developmental disorders of the abdominal and pelvic musculature, and in cleidocranial dysplasia. The more distinct the diastasis, the less is the morphologic adaptation of the bilateral public contours—the cartilaginous symphyseal abutment.

Unilateral **aplasia** or **hypoplasia** of the **os pubis** (Ehalt, 1943) is an infrequent finding. When detected in an adult, this condition must be differentiated from advanced **osteolysis of the pubis** by a metastatic tu-

mor, especially when the anamnesis arouses such a suspicion. Osteolysis of the pubis is also known to occur in massive osteolysis (Gorham-Stout) and in paraplegia (neurogenic osteolysis of the pelvis) (Fig. 57). Sometimes paraplegia is followed only by erosions of the symphysis, narrowing of the symphyseal cleft, and development of bony bridges (Bhate et al., 1979).

Traumatic **ruptures of the symphysis** frequently present attendant avulsions of bone which are projected into the gaping symphyseal cleft (Fig. 719). In obstetric traumas this is usually not the case because disruption of the loosened symphysis is more likely to occur than avulsion of bone from its site of attachment. The processes of gestatory loosening occasionally manifest themselves by a vacuum phenomenon in the symphyseal cavity. This cavity in the fibrocartilaginous disk can be demonstrated at autopsy in the majority of adult individuals. Avulsions of bone from the symphysis (following an injury to the pelvis) must be differentiated from persistent apophyseal centers of ossification; *most* of the latter occur symmetrically in both pubic bones (Fig. 752).

In pelvic injuries, including those incurred during labor, a marked asymmetrical position of the pubic bones and/or a gaping symphyseal cleft on the

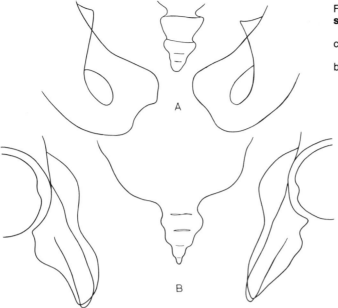

Fig. 751 **Congenital diastasis of the symphysis.**
A = Operation for hypospadias in childhood (present age 51).
B = Diastasis in exstrophy of the bladder (adult).

survey film of the pelvis suggest an additional injury to the sacroiliac region (rupture of capsule and ligaments, vertical fracture of the sacral wing and the ilium) (Fig. 753). A radiologic function study of all pelvic articulations should then be performed (Fig. 737), unless this is too taxing to the patient. In fractures of the anterior pelvic ring, a concomitant injury to the symphysis may often manifest itself *at a later date* by irregular narrowing of the symphyseal space and/or ligament ossification (Fig. 754). The anomalies remaining after obstetric damages to the symphysis are often not only the asymmetrical position of the horizontal rami of the os pubis but also irregular contours and increased density of the cancellous bone in the vicinity of the symphysis.

Multiparas mostly have a wider and more irregular symphyseal cleft—measuring more than 6 mm—than women of childbearing age who are childless or who have delivered only one child. In multiparas, a symphyseal joint with a synovial membrane frequently develops (Dihlmann, 1967/1978).

Asymmetries on weight-bearing from *unilateral* pelvic affections, may be congenital or acquired in the (early) growth period; for example, congenital dislocation of the hip, destructive bacterial coxitis, sacroiliitis, and osteomyelitis of the anterior pelvic ring. These disorders, which may also be related to paralysis of muscles, give rise to hypoplasia of the ipsilateral os pubis that forms the symphysis, and even

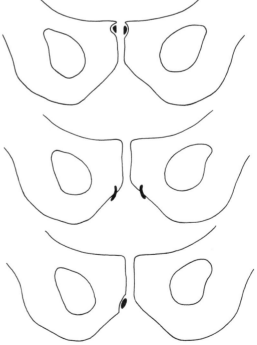

Fig. 752 **Persistent ossification centers in the symphyseal region (demonstrated among persons in the 4th decade of life).**

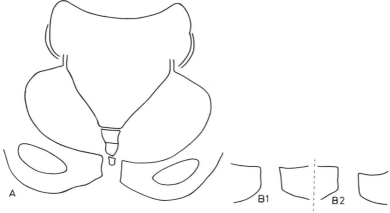

Fig. 753 **Rupture of the symphysis at labor,** recognizable by the gaping symphyseal cleft (A), and the asymmetrical position of the horizontal rami of the pubis, which are extensively displaceable in functional roentgenograms of the symphysis (B1, B2; see Fig. 737, no. 3). Since her delivery, the patient complains of right-sided sciatic pain radiating to the posterior aspect of the thigh. This aroused suspicion of an obstetric damage to the sacroiliac soft tissues on the right side. Subsequent complete radiologic function studies of the pelvic articulations (Fig. 737, nos. 1–3) provided evidence of additional obstetric damage (tears, avulsions) to the right-sided capsuloligamental apparatus of the sacroiliac joint (see p. 501 ff). In the present case, this information could *not* be obtained from the plain roentgenogram of the pelvic articulations.

to underdevelopment of the entire half of the pelvis involved. In these cases, in which the bony abutment of the symphysis has developed asymmetrically, there ensues **loosening of the symphysis** that manifests itself radiologically by an asymmetrical level of the horizontal rami of the os pubis. Consequently, the rami may be displaced with respect to each other in

the longitudinal direction of the body, or half of the pelvis may rotate around its transverse axis (Fig. 737 A and B) so that a stairstep formation measuring more than 1 or 2 mm develops.

Three sets of data are important to the principal clinical evaluation of the symphyseal step formation:

1. Persons with asymmetrical pubic bones have no pain in the region of the symphysis but very often suffer from low back pain, provided the anomaly is not the sequel of an injury or of inflammatory destruction of the symphysis.
2. Approximately every fifth adult individual presents an asymmetrical position of the pubic bone on survey films of the pelvis (Kamieth and Reinhardt, 1955) in the absence of unilateral pubic hypolasia *(vide supra)* of whatever origin. Females are involved about seven times more frequently than males.
3. Patients with destructive diseases of the sacroiliac joints (tuberculosis, nonspecific bacterial inflammations, tumors, etc.) almost invariably show an asymmetrical position of the horizontal rami of the pubes.

These observations reveal that in the majority of cases a symphyseal stairstep is proof of pathologic loosening of the sacroiliac joints! The symphysis is in fact located on the long lever arm of these joints, and any anomalous mobility of the sacroiliac joints is necessarily transmitted to the symphysis pubis. The absence of a fibrous capsule in the symphysis and the paucity of reinforcing ligaments then inevitably lead to gradual loosening of the symphysis. The mechanical relationships between the sacroiliac joints and the symphysis as well as the radiologic function study of

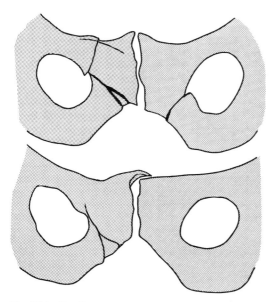

Fig. 744 **Posttraumatic lesions of the symphysis following fracture of the anterior pelvic ring.**

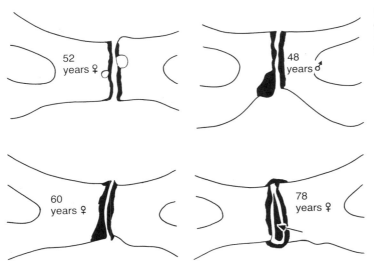

Fig. 755 **Degenerative lesions of the symphysis pubis,** including calcification of the fibrocartilaginous disk *(arrow)*.

these articulations have been described on page 504 ff.

The increased mobility of the symphysis pubis and the strain to which it is exposed in labor promote attrition of the cartilage so that the same lesions as in osteoarthrosis are apt to appear. The symphyseal cleft narrows and may disappear entirely. The density of the subchondral cancellous bone increases, and osteophytic spurs develop on the pubic bones. In addition, one occasionally encounters rounded translucences in the subchondral area, which are interpreted as debris cysts or as equivalents of Schmorl's vertebral nodes. A vacuum phenomenon as well as calcifications and ossifications of the fibrocartilage and the ligaments may be present (Fig. 755). With the physiologic and pathologic loosening processes in mind, **degenerative lesions of the symphysis** are to be expected particularly in females, though they also occur in males, if much less frequently.

Ochronosis manifests itself in the symphysis pubis as a metabolic disorder that promotes attrition. Contour defects, narrowing of the symphyseal cleft, sclerosis of the cancellous bone, marginal spurs, and hazy cancellous structures are observed (Fig. 756).

Articular chondrocalcinosis is identified in the symphysis pubis with much greater frequency than in the sacroiliac joints (Fig. 757). In addition, calcifications of the symphysis are known to occur in **idiopathic hemochromatosis** and in **hyperparathyroidism.** The latter disease, as well as advanced **renal osteopathy,** also gives rise to pseudodilatation of the symphyseal cleft with hazy borders, due to marginal resorption of bone—similarly to the processes in the sacroiliac joints (Fig. 728 A). Following surgical cure of primary hyperparathyroidism, the pseudodilatation may largely regress, or it may eventuate in a synostosis (Fig. 728 B).

Inflammatory processes of the symphysis pubis are the result of local bacterial infection or occur in

the setting of an inflammatory systemic rheumatic disease. Infections by microorganisms usually spread from one os pubis to the symphysis and subsequently to the opposite os pubis. Less frequently, they start initially from the symphysis.

Owing to its clinical manifestations, *acute* hematogenous osteomyelitis presents hardly any difficulties in differential diagnosis. The pathologic scintigram precedes the pathologic roentgen findings in the bone! The initial stage of *chronic* infections of the symphysis must be differentiated from an osteolytic osteosarcoma. In the flat bones, reactive bone changes

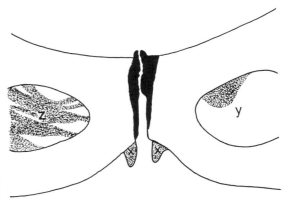

Fig. 756 **Ochronotic affection of the symphysis** (radiologic aspect of symphyseal degeneration). In addition, extensive bilateral fibroosteosis of the gracilis muscles (x); fibroosteosis at the origin of the obturator externus (y); and ossification of the obturator membrane (z). Compare also Figs. 357 and 378. The frequency and magnitude of fibroosteosis in ochronosis have already been mentioned on p. 44.

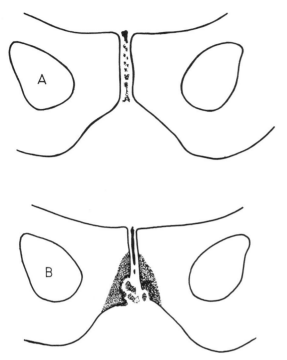

Fig. 757 **Chondrocalcinosis of the symphysis pubis.**
A = Calcium pyrophosphate precipitates in the fibrocartilage of the symphysis.
B = Destructive lesions of the symphysis accompanied by fragmentation of bone in chondrocalcinosis.

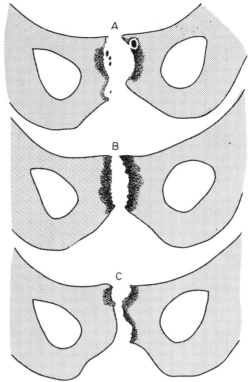

Fig. 758 **Roentgen findings in florid, chronic inflammatory destruction of the symphysis.** The nosological classification (A = tuberculosis, B = nonspecific bacterial osteomyelitis, C = gummatous destruction) can in most cases be effected only with consideration of the anamnesis, the clinical findings, the results of serologic investigation, etc., or even by biopsy. Sequestration and calcium shadows in the soft tissues are more in favor of tuberculous than of nonspecific bacterial infection.

originate less frequently in the periosteum than in the cancellous bone and manifest themselves as sclerosis of the cancellous bone that surrounds and infiltrates the demineralized and destroyed areas. Since *tuberculosis of the os pubis and the symphysis* initially causes hardly any discomfort, in most cases the first radiologic examination already reveals, apart from the destructions, a reactive increase in density of the cancellous bone. The roentgen finding, therefore, renders the differential diagnosis between chronic hematogenous osteomyelitis and tuberculosis of the symphysis extremely difficult or even impossible. Fistulas, sequestrations (dissections) and calcifications of soft tissues suggest tuberculosis rather than chronic osteomyelitis. Experience has shown that other tuberculous skeletal lesions are frequently concomitantly demonstrable—a fact that facilitates the differential diagnosis in these cases (skeletal scintigraphy!) Figure 758 presents the roentgen findings in tuberculosis of the symphysis, in chronic destruction of the symphysis versus osteomyelitis, and in tertiary (gummatous) syphilis. For the radiologic differential diagnosis of sclerosis of the cancellous bone in the vicinity of the symphysis, see Figure 759.

The writers who first described so-called **osteitis**

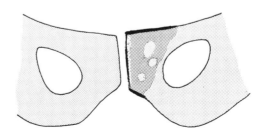

Fig. 759 **Paget's disease (osteitis deformans) of the os pubis.** The radiologic differentiation from chronic osteomyelitis and an osteoblastic metastasis is based *primarily* on the uniform increase in size of the bone involved, which is the result of the uniform periosteal formation of new bone in Paget's disease.

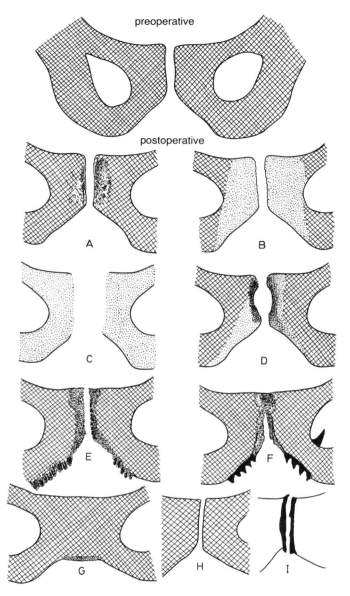

preoperative

postoperative

A

B

C

D

E

F

G

H

I

Fig. 760 **Osteitis pubis: clinical courses, end stages.**

A = Symphyseal contours ill-defined. In the subchondral space diffuse, in part spotty, demineralization and hazy structures of cancellous bone.

B = The changes depicted in A—especially decalcification—have extended as far as the ischium.

C = Considerable decalcification giving rise to "widening of the symphyseal cleft."

D = Erosion as direct cause of A and B.

E = Repair stage recognizable by increase in density of the subchondral cancellous bone. In addition, bony trabeculae grow into the symphseal cleft (which has been narrowed by the increase in density). Roentgen manifestations of productive fibroosteitis in the ischium.

F = Progression of E.

G = Healing by synostosis (may also develop directly after D).

H = Except for narrowing of the symphyseal cleft, the picture has returned to normal (for example, directly after C).

I = Degenerative lesions of the symphysis as a late condition (e.g., after A–D).

Note: Chronic bacterial infections of the symphysis and the surrounding bones, as well as the aseptic circulatory disorder in this region (an equivalent of Sudeck's syndrome; see text), present an identical radiologic picture! Besides this, compare their radiologic resemblance with Fig. 761 (os pubis syndrome).

pubis (Legueu and Rochet, 1923; Fig. 760) emphasized the relationship between this disease and prostatectomy, but it is a rare complication that occurs in only a small percentage of prostatectomized patients. Discomfort in the symphysis usually starts between 4 and 12 weeks after (suprapubic, transvesical, or perineal) prostatectomy. Less frequently, the disorder follows resection of the prostate by transurethral electrocautery, inguinal herniorrhaphy, plastic operations on the vagina, abdominosacral extirpation of rectum, delivery, abortion, or even extraction of a ureteral calculus with a snare. A blunt injury of the pelvis may also be responsible. The pain *may* be accompanied by a rise in temperature and an elevated sedimentation rate; it also may radiate to the inguinal region and the medial aspect of the thigh.

The *roentgen manifestations* to be expected a number of weeks after the onset of pain are hazy contours and a spotty or diffuse demineralization of an ill-defined structure in the surroundings of the symphysis, which at times extends so far as the ischium. During the further evolution of the disorder, the demineralization may assume such proportions that it gives the impression of widening of the symphysis.

Contour erosions, and possibly even sequestrations and dissections, complete the picture.

After a number of months, repair processes occur (recalcification, increased density of the cancellous bone), sometimes eventuating in narrowing of the symphyseal cleft or even in partial or complete synostosis. Sharply defined contour defects and increased densities of the cancellous bone may result. Ossifications of tendinous insertions of the productive fibroosteitis type (compare Fig. 79 with Fig. 760 E and F) appear in the florid stage and increase in density during the course of healing. The clinical picture and the initial roentgen findings leave no doubt about the inflammatory pathogenesis and the bacterial etiology of osteitis pubis. Conspicuous though infrequent attendant findings such as osteomyelitis of the ischium with demonstration of microorganisms (Arlet et al., 1978), suppurative coxarthritis (Katzenstein, 1934; Friedenberg, 1950) and infectious lumbar spondylitis suggest that osteitis pubis is a (subacute) osteomyelitis. In some cases, this assumption has been confirmed by histologic studies. In other cases, however, no inflammatory histologic substrate was demonstrable, so that osteitis pubis has also been interpreted as aseptic, ischemic necrosis of bone or as the result of a local circulatory disturbance similar to Sudeck's syndrome (Lame and Chang, 1954; Eickelmann, 1976). In an individual case, when the patient gives a history of a malignant tumor, a metastatic osteolysis in the vicinity of the symphysis must be ruled out. However, as a rule, metastases occur only unilaterally; if bilateral, they are asymmetrical. In addition, the (infrequent) osteolytic metastases of a prostatic carcinoma are accompanied by an increase in the concentration of acid phosphatase in the serum.

The terms **"gracilis syndrome," "os pubis syndrome,"** or **"posttraumatic osteonecrosis of the pubis"** have been applied to chronic damage related to excessive strain that affects the origin of the gracilis, adductor longus, and adductor brevis muscles and also involves the symphysis pubis (Schneider, 1964; Rispoli, 1965; Luschnitz et al., 1967). The muscles mentioned are anchored in a relatively small

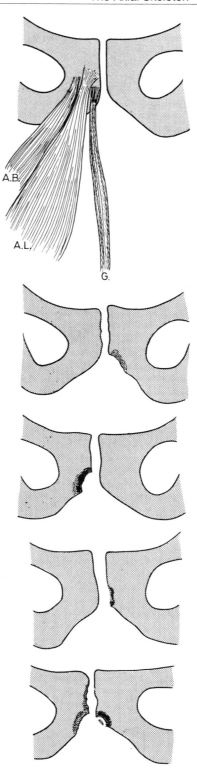

Fig. 761 **So-called os pubis syndrome (gracilis syndrome; posttraumatic osteonecrosis of the pubis in competitive athletes, particularly soccer players).**

Above: Origins of the gracilis muscle (G), the abductor longus (A.L.), and the abductor brevis (A.B.) as pathogenetic factors.

Below: Minor roentgen manifestations of symphyseal loosening (asymmetrical level of the pubic bones), sometimes also developmental anomaly of the parts of the os pubis which form the symphysis (age of patient!). In addition, erosions at the origin of the gracilis muscle and its surroundings; delicate or marked perifocal increase in density of the cancellous; bone fragments. For radiologic differential diagnosis, see Figs. 378, 758, 760, and 762.

region of the os pubis by tendons whose attachments occupy a small sectional area. Athletes (for example, football players, hurdlers, and fencers) sometimes complain of pain that originates in the symphyseal area and radiates to the inguinal region and the lower abdomen. This pain heralds a damage from excessive strain to the tendinous insertions and the symphysis. The condition *may* manifest itself unilaterally or bilaterally in the roentgenogram by the findings illustrated in Figure 761; i.e., asymmetrical position of the pubic bones (loosening of the symphysis), erosions, or only an irregular contour (Schneider et al., 1976) and furthermore by necrotic bone fragments (Spring, 1977) and sclerosis of the cancellous bone. Fibroosteoses occur in the repair stage.

Among the inflammatory rheumatic diseases apt to involve the symphysis pubis, ankylosing spondylitis and adult rheumatoid arthritis are the most significant. The initially painless involvement of the symphysis—**symphysitis of ankylosing spondylitis**—is a late finding (Fig. 762) that often manifests itself by a rarefying fibroosteitis of the arcuate ligament of the pubis. Marginal bone resorption may give rise to pseudodilatation of the symphyseal cleft. The contour defects are surrounded by increased density

of the cancellous bone. With time, trabeculae grow into the symphyseal cleft, and the cleft narrows and eventually undergoes synostosis. Symphyseal changes accompanying ankylosing spondylitis are no more frequently observed in females than in males. For parasymphyseal lesions in ankylosing spondylitis see Figure 378C. Rheumatoid arthritis manifests itself in the symphysis pubis by erosions and by increased density of the subchondral cancellous bone—**rheumatoid symphysitis**. Complete ossification occurs only infrequently.

Manubriosternal Synchondrosis (Upper Thoracic Synchondrosis)

Radiologic examination of the manubriosternal synchondrosis comprises a lateral survey film and *tomography in the prone position*. In the oblique posteroanterior roentgenogram of the sternum, on the other hand, minor pathologic changes very easily escape detection. The upper thoracic synchondrosis is sub-

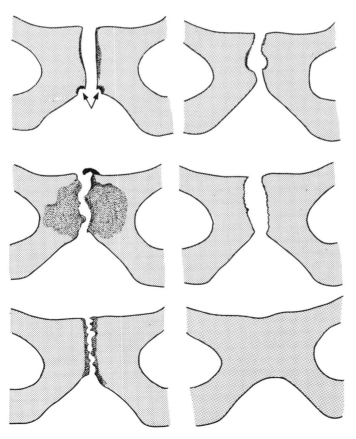

Fig. 762 **Involvement of the symphysis pubis in ankylosing spondylitis.** Rarefying fibroosteitis of the arcuate ligament of the pubis is often an early radiologic manifestation *(arrows)*. Note: affections of synchondroses (connections of bones without synovial membrane) are characterized by their reactions (compare Figs. 758, 760, 761, 762). The etiologic diagnosis by radiography, therefore, must be supported by clinical and anamnestic data!

Fig. 763 **Radiologic diagnosis of manubriosternal synchondrosis.**

A = Normal roentgen findings (variants of normal) in tomographs of the upper sternal synchondrosis (taken in the prone position).

B = Trivial anomalous roentgen finding ("cartilage node"; see text).

C to F = Chronic inflammatory lesions (erosions with ill-defined contours and more or less broad marginal increase in density; tendency to synostosis). Differential diagnosis by clinical criteria and/or nosologically unequivocal roentgen findings of, e.g., rheumatoid arthritis or ankylosing spondylitis in other sites. The radiologic morphology of finding E (major destruction; slight perifocal sclerosis of the cancellous bone) would also suggest tuberculosis. However, a destructive process in the synchondrosis with swelling of the soft tissues might also be a so-called chondrosis-perichondrosis (F, H; see text).

G = Lateral roentgenogram of the synchondrosis; normal finding.

I = Degenerative lesions of the synchondrosis. A similar lateral radiograph is sometimes also encountered in ankylosing spondylitis.

J = Inflammatory destruction of the synchondrosis with subluxation (here in rheumatoid arthritis).

K = Large osteolysis near the synchondrosis with nonfluctuating swelling of the soft tissues. No erythema. Well-founded suspicion of primary or metastitic malignant tumor.

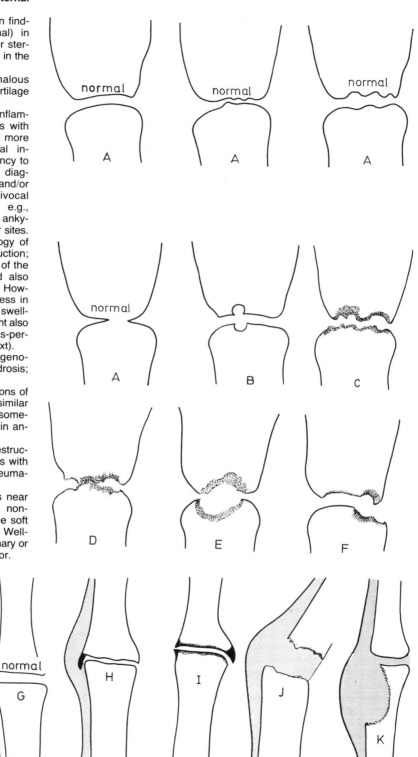

ject to numerous variations that concern the course of the cleft—plane-parallel, oblique, concave, convex, biconvex, S-shaped, etc.—as well as its width and its contours. Normal upper thoracic synchondroses may present smooth, irregular, or eroded contours (Fig. 763 A). Partially or completely synostosed synchondrosis is also a known variant (Candardjis et al., 1978a). Such cases usually concern a spontaneous fusion, because the incidence of synostosis increases with advancing age (Cameron and Fornasier, 1974).

The biologic variability of the upper sternal synchondrosis also manifests itself by accessory synchondroses of the body of the sternum—multipartite sternum—and by displacement of the segments. In the latter instances, a synchondrosis has developed between the segments of the body rather than between the manubrium and the body of the sternum. Circumscribed depressions of the fibrocartilage into the cancellous bone of the manubrium and the body of the sternum resemble Schmorl's nodes in the roentgenogram and should not be mistaken for inflammatory erosions (Fig. 763 B).

Erosions are of pathologic significance when they have ill-defined borders and/or are surrounded by a perifocal, more or less broad but definitely not shell-shaped area of sclerosis. In addition, attendant joint space narrowing or a tendency to synostosis, as well as larger destructions with subluxation (lateral roentgenogram!) suggest florid **inflammatory processes in the upper sternal synchondrosis.** When ankylosing spondylitis, Reiter's syndrome (Candardjis et al.,

1978b), psoriatic arthritis (Kormano et al., 1975), rheumatoid arthritis, or recurrent polychondritis (MacAdam et al., 1976) are known to be present, local pain, tenderness, and sometimes edema usually justify radiologic examination. When the roentgenogram reveals the pathologic findings sketched in Fig. 763, the nosological classification offers no difficulty. However, in the absence of a known systemic disease, the etiologic classification of destructive lesions in the upper thoracic synchondrosis presents considerable difficulty; for example, the differential diagnosis between a tuberculous or a nonspecific bacterial infection of the synchondrosis and so-called **manubriosternal chondritis-perichondritis (chondrosis-perichondrosis).** This very rare condition is probably due to trauma from excessive strain (Fig. 763 F and H). In any event, inflammatory granulation tissue is not demonstrable (Reiter, 1956; Köhler and Zimmer, 1967). When the skin over a destroyed upper sternal synchondrosis is warm and erythematous, a bacterial infection is the most probable explanation. Larger osteolyses with marked swelling of soft tissues without erythema and fluctuation are suggestive of a **neoplasm** (Fig. 763 K).

Degenerative lesions of the synchondrosis may be recognized by osteophytes on its posterior and anterior aspect, a band-shaped increase in density of the subchondral sternal cancellous bone, and bone bridges inside the synchondrosis (Fig. 745 I). Injuries to the sternum may lead to dislocation of the upper thoracic synchondrosis—**synchondrolysis** (Gelehrter, 1958). These dislocations occur from direct massive trauma (thrust, blow, fall, impact), as an attendant injury in severe fractures of the thoracic spine (Busch, 1966), and indirectly through sudden maximal muscular contraction; for example, in tetanus infection. Indirect violence in gymnastics, particularly in exercises on the parallel bars, also may lead to synchondrolysis (Kläber, 1979). Dislocation of the fractured synchondrosis or fracture-dislocation of a synostosed synchondrosis is detected in the exactly lateral roentgenogram of the sternum.

Tomographs of the sternum taken in the prone position permit assessment of the sternocostal joints. Figure 764 presents degenerative lesions of these joints.

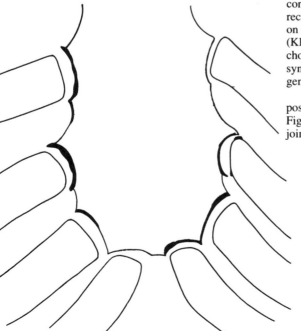

Fig. 764 Tomograph of the body of the sternum. Some of the sternocostal articulations show degenerative changes (subchondral increase in density; elongation of the articulating surfaces). The xiphoid process lies at a different level and therefore does not appear in the tomograph.

Note: **Tietze's syndrome** is diagnosed clinically by a tender, or even spontaneously painful, bulge of the parasternal costal cartilage. The 2nd to 4th ribs are primarily involved. The roentgen finding is normal (negative) because the noncalcified costal cartilage behaves like soft tissue with regard to the roentgen beam, so that its structure cannot be assessed.

Bibliography

Anatomy, radiologic anatomy (see also under Trauma); methodology of taking radiograms; roentgenometry (see also under Variants of normal).

Bernau, A.: Orthopädische Röntgendiagnostik—Einstelltechnik. München: Urban and Schwarzenberg, 1982.

Bernau, A.: Tübinger Lagerungsgerät für Défilé-Aufnahmen der Patella. Z Orthop 119:78–79, 1981.

Dihlmann, W.: Röntgenaufnahmen in der Rheumatologie. Aktucl Rheumatol 7:228–230, 1982.

Dihlmann, W., G. Nebel: Computed tomography of the hip joint capsule. J Comput Assist Tomogr 7:278–285, 1983.

Dunlap, K., A.R. Shands Jr., L.C. Hollister JR., J.S. Gaul Jr., H.A. Streit: A new method for determination of torsion of the femur. J Bone Joint Surg 35A:289–311, 1953.

Elgeti, H., R. Grote, G. Giebel: Bestimmung der Tibiatorsion mit der axialen Computertomographie. Unfallheilkunde 83:14–19, 1980.

Elssasser, U., N. Walker: Zur Bestimmung der Torsion des Schenkelhalses. Z Orthop 111:926–933, 1973.

Engelhardt, P.: Juvenile Hüftkopflösung und Koxarthrose. Morphologie und Prognose im Langzeitverlauf 1922–1982. Stuttgart: Ferdinand Enke Verlag, 1984.

Gekeler, J.: Die Hüftkopfepiphysenlösung. Radiometrie und Korrekturplanung. Stuttgart: Ferdinand Enke Verlag, 1977.

Grote, R., H. Elgeti, D. Saure: Bestimmung des Antetorsionswinkels am Femur mit der axialen Computertomographie. Röntgenblätter 3:31–42, 1980.

Gutjahr, G.: Die Röntgendiagnostik der Schulterluxation und ihrer knöchernen Begleitverletzungen. Röntgenblätter 36:225–233, 1983.

Häfner, H., C.J. Wirth: Experimentelle Untersuchungen zur Erklärung des Lachman–Testes. In: Kapselbandläsionen des Kniegelenkes. Experimentelle Grundlagen der Diagnostik und Therapie. M. Jäger, M.H. Hackenbroch and H.J. Refior. (Eds). Stuttgart: Georg Thieme Verlag, 1981, p. 123–128.

Harris Jr., J.H., C.K. Loh, H.C. Periman, C.T. Rotz Jr.: The roentgen diagnosis of pelvic extraperitoneal effusion Radiology 125:343–350, 1977.

Hellige, R., K. Gretenkord, B. Tillmann: Funktionelle Anatomie des oberen und unteren Sprunggelenkes. Orthop Praxis 17:299–304, 1981.

Hepp, W.R.: Radiologie des Femoro-Patellargelenkes. Stuttgart: F. Enke, 1983.

Hinck, V.C., W.M. Clark, Jr., C.E. Hopkins: Normal interpediculate distances (minimum and maximum) in children and adults. Am J Roentgenol 97:141–153, 1966.

Kattan, K.R., M.J. Pais: Some borderlands of the cervical spine. Part 1: normal (and nearly normal) that may appear pathologic. Skeletal Radiol 8:1–6, 1982.

Keats, T.E., J.M. Joyce: Metaphyseal cortical irregularities in children: a new perspective on a multi–focal growth variant. Skeletal Radiol 12:112–118, 1984.

Krepler, P., R. Mazoch, W. Schwägerl, E. Schuster: Diagnosis and relevance of suspected dysplasia of the hip joint, radiologic investigation starting with the age of 3 months. Arch Orthop Trauma Surg 101:29–37, 1982.

Lequesne, M., J. Becker, M. Bard, J. Witvoet, M. Postel: Capsular constriction of the hip: arthrographic and clinical considerations. Skeletal Radiol 6:1–10, 1981.

Levene, G., S.A. Kaufman: The diagnostic significance of roentgenologic soft tissue shadows in the pelvis. Amer J Roentgenol 79:697–704, 1958.

Levinsohn, E.M., W.P. Bunnell, H.A. Yuan: Computed tomography in the diagnosis of dislocations of the sternoclavicular joint. Clin Orthop 140:12–16, 1979.

Lingg, G., D. von Torklus: Röntgenzeichen der azetabulären Hüftdysplasie beim Erwachsenen. Radiologe 21:291–295, 1981.

Lorenz, R., V. Fiedler: Der Navikularefettstreifen (NFS). Bedeutung für die Erkennung von Frakturen des Os naviculare. Fortschr Röntgenstr 137:286–290, 1982.

Neugebauer, H.: Cobb oder Ferguson. Eine Analyse der beiden gebräuchlichsten Röntgenmeβmethoden von Skoliosen. Z Orthop 110:342–356, 1972.

Niethard, F.U.: Das Hüftgelenk im frontalen Strahlengang. Ein Beitrag zur röntgenologischen Erfassung der Hüft–kopf–Pfannen–Relation. Z Orthop 120:821–827, 1982.

Mino–Murcia, M., R.J. Wechsler, R.E. Brennan: Computed tomography of the iliopsoas muscle. Skeletal Radiol 10:107–112, 1983.

Norell, H.G.: Roentgenologic visualization of the extracapsular fat. Its importance in the diagnosis of traumatic injuries of the elbow: Acta Radiol (Stockh) 42:205–210, 1954.

Peterson, H.A., R.A. Klassen, R.A. McLeod, A.D. Hoffmann: The use of computerized tomography in dislocation of the hip and femoral neck anteversion in children. J Bone Joint Surg 63B:198–208, 1981.

Poigenfürst, J.: Röntgendiagnostik der Verletzungen des oberen Sprunggelenkes. Hefte Unfallhlkd 92:9–11, 1967.

Reiser, M., N. Rupp, P.M. Karpf, St. Feuerbach, O. Paar: Erfahrungen mit der CT-Arthrographie der Kreuzbänder des Kniegelenkes. Ein Bericht über 512 Untersuchungen. Fortschr Röntgenstr 137:372–379, 1982.

Reiser, M., N. Rupp, P.M. Karpf, St. Feuerbach, H. Anacker: Evaluation of the cruciate ligaments by CT. Europ J Radiol 1:9, 1981.

Resnick, D., J.D. Newell, J. Guerra Jr., L.A. Danzig, G. Niwayama, T.G. Goergen: Proximal tibiofibular joint: anatomic-pathologic–radiographic correlation. Am J Roentgenol 131:133–138, 1978.

Rodriguez, M., J. Suezawa, H.A.C. Jacob: Experimentelle Untersuchungen zur Diagnose des Kniebandapparates. In: Kapselbandläsionen des Kniegelenkes. Experimentelle Grundlagen der Diagnostik und Therapie. M. Jäger, M.H. Hackenbroch and H.J. Refior (Eds). Stuttgart: Georg Thieme Verlag, 1981, p. 93–97.

Rogers, S.L., D.W. MacEwan: Changes due to trauma in the fat plane overlying the supinator muscle: a radiological sign. Radiology 92:954–958, 1969.

Rubin, S.A., R.L. Gray, W.R. Green: The scapular "Y": an aid in shoulder trauma. Radiology 110:725–726, 1974.

Ryder, C.T., L. Crane: Measuring femoral anteversion: the problem and a method. J Bone Joint Surg 35A:321–328, 1953.

Schild, H., H.A. Müller, H. Wagner, W. Bätz: Betrachtungen zur sog. "Radius–Capitulum–Achse." Fortschr Röntgenstr 136:177–181, 1982.

Schindlmaisser, H., R. Kotz: Röntgenologische Beurteilung der Pfannenbodendicke des Hüftgelenkes. Wien Med Wochenschr 122:430–432, 1972.

Schneider, R.: Die intertrochantere Osteotomie bei Coxarthrose. Berlin: Springer, 1979.

Tillmann, B.: Die Beanspruchung des menschlichen Hüftgelenkes III. Die Form der Facies lunata. Z Anat Entwickl Gesch 128:329–349, 1969.

Töndury, G.: Zur Anatomie und Entwicklungsgeschichte der Wirbelsäule mit besonderer Berücksichtigung der Altersveränderungen der Bandscheiben. Schweiz Med Wochenschr 85:825–827, 1955.

Töndury, G.: Entwicklung, Bau und Altersveränderungen der Zwischenwirbelscheiben unter spezieller Berücksichtigung der Halsregion. Therapiewoche 10:432–438, 1960.

Torg, J.S., W. Conrad, V. Kalen: Clinical diagnosis of anterior cruciate ligament instability in the athlete. Amer J Sports Med 4:84–93, 1976.

Trueta, J.: The three types of acute haematogenous osteomyelitis. A clinical and vascular study. J Bone Jt Surg 41:671–680, 1959.

Vouge, M.: Interapophysolaminar spaces (IALS) of the lumbar spine and their utility in the diagnosis of narrow lumbar canal. In: Wackenheim, A., E. Babin (Eds). The narrow lumbar canal. Radiologic signs and surgery. Berlin: Springer, 1980 p. 23–25.

Wiberg, G.: Studies on dysplastic acetabula and congenital subluxation of the hip joint with special reference to the complication of osteoarthritis. Acta Orthop Scand 12:319–410, 1941.

Variants of normal; variants, deformities, and their causes and sequelae visible in the roentgenogram (see also under Osteoarthrosis); local and systemic (constitutional) malformations; congenital disorders of bone structure (see also under Roentgenometry; Inflammation).

Athreya, B.H., H.R. Schumacher: Pathologic features of a familial arthropathy associated with congenital flexion contractures of fingers. Arthritis Rheum 21:429–437, 1978.

Blauth, W., M. Blauth: Zur Theorie und Praxis der angeborenen Unterschenkelpseudarthrosen. Z Orthop 119:36–53, 1981.

Blinder, G., Y. Barki, M. Pezt, J. Bar–Ziv: Widespread osteolytic lesions of the long bones in basal cell nevus syndrome. Skeletal Radiol 12:196–198, 1984.

Boven, F., M. de Boeck, R. Potvliege: Synovial plicae of the knee on computed tomography. Radiology 147:805–809, 1983.

Caffey, J.: The early roentgenographic changes in essential coxa plana: their significance in pathogenesis. Am J Roentgenol 103:620–634, 1968.

Calver, R., V. Venugopal, J. Dorgan, G. Bentley, T. Gimlette: Radionuclide scanning in the early diagnosis of Perthes' disease. J Bone Joint Surg 63B:379–382, 1981.

Canigiani, G., J. Wickenhauser, W. Czech: Beitrag zur Osteochondrosis dissecans im Foramen supratrochleare. Fortschr Röntgenstr 117:66–68, 1972.

Christ, F., G. Anders: Die Röntgenmorphologie der Arthrogryposis multiplex congenita. Fortschr Röntgenstr 135:592–596, 1981.

Cremin, B., J.M. Connor, P. Beighton: The radiological spectrum of fibrodysplasia ossificans progressiva. Clin Radiol 33:499–508, 1982.

Dähnert, W., J. Ahlers, J. Rudiger: Ungewöhnliche Muskelvariante zur Differentialdiagnose in einem Weichteiltumor. Röntgenblätter 36 (1983) 425–427.

Deák, P.: Die Akroosteosklerose. Fortschr Röntgenstr 89:59–66, 1958.

Deutsch, A.L., D. Resnick, G. Campbell: Computed tomography and bone scintigraphy in the evaluation of tarsal coalition. Radiology 144:137–140, 1982.

Dunaway, C.L., J.P. Williams, B.G. Brogdon: Case report 222 (sacral and coccygeal supernumerary ribs [pelvic ribs]). Skeletal Radiol 9:212–214, 1983.

Engelhardt, P.: Juvenile Hüftkopflösung und Koxarthrose. Stuttgart: Ferdinand Enke Verlag, 1984.

Fischer, E.: Akroosteosklerose der Finger, eine normale geschlechts–und altersabhängige endostale Reaktion. Fortschr Röntgenstr 137:384–388, 1982.

Fotter, R., J. Lammer, G. Ritter: Szintigraphische 5–Jahres–Studie bei Kindern mit M. Perthes. Diagnostische Aussagen und therapeutische Konsequenzen. Fortschr Röntgenstr 137:141–146, 1982.

Garces, M.A., J.K. Muraskas, E.K. Muraskas, M. Abdel–Hammed: Hereditary onycho–osteo–dysplasia (HOOD Syndrome): report of two cases. Skeletal Radiol 8:55–58, 1982.

Gardiner, T.B.: Osteochondritis dissecans in three members of one family. J Bone Joint Surg 37B:139–141, 1955.

Gekeler, J.: Die Hüftkopfepiphysenlösung. Radiometrie und Korrekturplanung. Stuttgart: Ferdinand Enke Verlag, 1977.

Glöckler, W.T., M. Langer, K.A. Schumacher, W. Mutschler, R. Langer: Nichtinvasive radiologische Diagnostik der Chondropathia patellae. Unfallheilkunde 84:194–199, 1981.

Goldenberg, R.R., E.L. Wild: Chondromalacia fabellae. J Bone Joint Surg 34A:688–690, 1952.

Goldman, A.B., D. Davidson, H. Pavlov, P.G. Bullough: "Popcorn" calcifications: a prognostic sign in osteogenesis imperfecta. Radiology 138:351–358, 1980.

Gore, D.R.: Iatrogenic avascular necrosis of the hip in young children. J Bone Jt Surg 56A:493–502, 1974.

Graf, R.: Grundprinzipien der sonographischen Hüftgelenks–dysplasie bei Säuglingen. Orthop Praxis 19:933–941, 1983.

Greenspan, A., A. Norman: The "pelvic digit"—an unusual developmental anomaly. Skeletal Radiol 9:118–122, 1982.

Griffiths, H., J. Wandtke: Tibiotalar tilt—a new slant. Skeletal Radiol 6:193–197, 1981.

Haglund, P.: Die hintere Patellakontusion. Zbl Chir 53:1757–1760, 1926.

Hanstein, F., H. Meffert, E. Schumann: Über die Skelettelemente des zweiten Kiemenbogens. Radiol Diagn 23:285–294, 1982.

Hardaker, W.T., Jr., T.L. Whipple, F.H. Bassett, III: Diagnosis and treatment of the plica syndrome of the knee. J Bone Joint Surg 62A:221–225, 1980.

Harrison, R.B., T.E. Keats: Epiphyseal clefts. Skeletal Radiol 5:23–27, 1980.

Hehne, H.-J.: Das Patellofemoralgelenk. Funktionelle Anatomie—Biomechanik—Chondromalazie und operative Therapie. Stuttgart: F. Enke, 1983.

Heitzeberg, H., I. Reiner–Theisen: Die Ossifikation der Korako–Klavikularbänder. Röntgenblätter 31:512–515, 1978.

Henßge, J.: Die talo-kalkaneale Knochenbrücke. Z Orthop 94:88–93, 1961.

Hepp, W.R.: Radiologie des Femoro-Patellargelenkes. Stuttgart: F. Enke, 1983.

Hepp, W.R.: Zur Bestimmung der Dysplasie des Femoro–Patellargelenkes. Z Orthop 120:259–267, 1982.

von Hessling, P.: Einseitig doppeltes Sitzbein. Fortschr Röntgenstr 138:494, 1983.

Hsu, L.C.S., J.P. O'Brien, A.C.M.C. Yau, A.R. Hodgson: Valgus deformity of the ankle in children with fibular pseudarthrosis. Results of treatment by bone-grafting of the fibula. J Bone Surg 56A:503–510, 1974.

Imhäuser, G.: Die physiologische intrapelvine Vorragung des Hüftpfannenbodens. (Ein Beitrag zur Entwicklung des Hüftgelenkes). Z Orthop 81:161–179, 1952.

Ishikawa. H., K. Hirohota, D. Kashiwagi: A case report of patella cubiti. Z Rheumatol 35:407–411, 1976.

Jacobsen, S.T., A.H. Crawford: Congenital vertical talus. J Pedr Orthop 3:306–310, 1983.

Kämmerer, K., W. Dihlmann, D. Dörstelmann: Rudimentärzeichen der tuberösen Skerose am Skelett. Fortschr Röntgenstr 115:306–312, 1971.

Kaibara, N., K. Takagishi, I. Katsuki, M. Eguchi, S. Masumi, A. Nishio: Spondyloepiphyseal dysplasia tarda with progressive arthropathy. Skeletal Radiol 10:13–16, 1983.

Keats, T.E.: The distal anterior femoral metaphyseal defect: an anatomic variant that may simulate disease. Am J Roentgenol 121:101–102, 1974.

Kosowicz, J.: The carpal sign in gonadal dysgenesis. J Clin Endocrinol Metab 22:949–952, 1962.

Laasonen, E.M.: Das Syndrom der polyzystischen Osteodysplasie mit progressiver Demenz. Fortschr Röntgenstr 122:313–316, 1975.

Laasonen, E.M., U. Lahdenranta: Lipomembranous polycystic osteodysplasia with progressive dementia. J Comput Assist Tomogr 5:580–582, 1981.

Lawson, J.P., J.A. Ogden, E. Sella, K.W. Barwick: The painful accessory navicular. Skeletal Radiol 12:250–262, 1984.

Le Minor, J.M.: Sésamoides bipartita du gros orteil. Étude de 750 clichés radiographiques. Radiologie J Cepur 4:169–172, 1984.

Lingg, G.L. Hering: Computertomographie der Chondropathia patellae. Experimentelle und klinische Ergebnisse. Fortschr Röntgenstr 139:663–668, 1983.

Lingg, G., L. Hering: Computertomographie und pathogenes Potential der Plica parapatellaris medialis. Fortschr Röntgenstr 140:561–566, 1984.

Löser, H.: Erkennungsmerkmale der Alkoholembryopathie. Dtsch Ärztebl 79:34–39, 1982.

Lombardo, S.J., A.C. Retting, R.K. Kerlan: Radiographic abnormalities of the iliac apophysis in adolescent athletes. J Bone Joint Surg 65A:444–446, 1983.

Mäkelä, P., O. Järvi, P. Hakola, P. Virtama: Radiologic bone changes of polycystic lipomembranous osteodysplasia with sclerosing leukoencephalopathy. Skeletal Radiol 8:51–54, 1982.

Mangieri, J.V.: Peroneal–nerve injury from an enlarged fabella. J Bone Joint Surg 55A:395–397, 1973.

Mau, H., J. Dietz: Chondrolyse—Protrusion—Pubertätshüftsteife. Z Orthop 121:160–167, 1983.

Nehrkorn, O.: Ungewöhnliche Apophysenentwicklungsstörung des linken Sitzbeins. Fortschr Röntgenstr 101:100, 1964.

Nixon, J.E.: Bilateral Madelung's disease of the wrist: a familial condition? J Royal Soc Med 76:313–315, 1983.

Nüvemann, M., H. Contzen: Die Hypoplasie der Tuberositas tibiae. Ein ausreichend häufiges Röntgenzeichen für das Vorliegen einer Chondropathia patellae? Unfallhlkd 84:334–337, 1981.

Outerbridge, R.E.: Further studies on the etiology of chondromalacia patellae. J Bone Joint Surg 46B:179–190, 1964.

Pavlov, H., A.B. Goldman, R.H. Freiberger: Infantile coxa vara. Radiology 135:631–640, 1980.

Penttinen, R., E. Sipola, K. Kouvalainen, S. Similä, M. Remes: An arthropathic form of osteogenesis imperfecta. Acta Paediatr Scand 69:263–267, 1980.

Pipkin, G.: Lesions of the suprapatellar plica. J Bone Joint Surg 32A:363–369, 1950.

Resnick, D.: Talar ridges, osteophytes, and beaks: a radiologic commentary. Radiology 151:329–332, 1984.

Ritter, G.: Der Morbus Perthes in der Szintigraphie–Frühdiagnose, Verlauf und therapeutische Konsequenzen. Z Orthop 120:850–859, 1982.

Sarno, R.C., B.L. Carter, M.S. Bankoff, M.C. Semine: Computed tomography in tarsal coalition. J Comp Ass Tomogr 8:1155–1160, 1984.

Schacherl, M., F. Schilling: Zur Differentialdiagnose erworbener und angeborener Carpalsynostosen. Fortschr Röntgenstr 102:68–77, 1965.

Schnyder, P.A.: Osseous changes of osteopathia striata associated with cranial sclerosis. Skeletal Radiol 5:19–22, 1980.

Schumacher, K.A., W. Th. Glöckler, W. Mutschler, K. Rittmeyer: Zur Manifestation der Chondropathia patellae im Röntgennativbild. Fortschr Röntgenstr 131:636–639, 1979.

Sheth, K.J., G.C. Bernhard: The arthropathy of Fabry disease. Arthritis Rheum 22:781–783, 1979.

Slanina, J.: Fabella distalis: a new sesamoid bone. Radiol Clin 25:274–277, 1956.

Strauss, J.: Formabweichung des Schienbeinkopfes bei der Femoropatellararthrose. Z Orthop 112:716–718, 1974.

Théron, J.: Angiography in Legg–Calvé–Perthes disease. Radiology 135:81–92, 1980.

Tillmann, B., H. Brade: Morphologische und biomechanische Untersuchungen an der Facies articularis patellae. Orthop Prax 16:462–467, 1980.

Tredwell, S.J., D.F. Smith, P.J. Macleod, B.J. Wood: Cervical spine anomalies in fetal alcohol syndrome. Spine 7:331–334, 1982.

Twigg, H.L., R.C. Rosenbaum: Duplication of the clavicle. Skeletal Radiol 6:281, 1981.

Waldenström, H.: On necrosis of the joint cartilage by epiphyseolysis capitis femoris. Acta Chir Scand 67:936–946, 1930.

Wiberg, G.: Roentgenographic and anatomic studies on the femoropatellar joint. With special reference to chondromalacia patellae. Acta Orthop Scand 12:319–410, 1941.

Inflammation; arthritis; autoimmune diseases and their radiologic differential diagnosis (see also under Osteoarthropathy; Calcifications of soft tissues; Radiologic anatomy; Trauma); sternocostoclavicular hyperostosis.

Amor, B., S. Laoussadi: Physiopathologie du syndrome de Fiessinger–Leroy–Reiter et affections apparentées. I. Facteurs d'environnement: les facteurs infectieux. Rev Rhum 49:553–558, 1982.

Amor, B.: Reiter's syndrome and reactive arthritis. Clin Rheumatol 2:315–319, 1983.

Amor, B., H. Bouchet, F. Delrieu: Enquête nationale sur les arthrites réactionelles de la Société Française de Rhumatologie. Rev Rhum 50:733–743, 1983.

Anderson, R.B., B.B. Dorwart: Pneumarthrosis in a shoulder infected with serratia liquefasciens: case report and literature review. Arthritis Rheum 26:1166–1168, 1983.

Aptekar, R.G., O.J. Lawless, J.L. Decker: Deforming non–erosive arthritis of the hand in systemic lupus erythematosus. Clin Orthop 100:120–124, 1974.

Arnett, F.C., W.B. Bias, M.B. Stevens: Juvenile–onset chronic arthritis. Clinical and roentgenographic features of a unique HLA–B27 subset. Am J Med 69:369–376, 1980.

Arlart, I., G. Bargon: Periostale Knochenneubildung bei Colitis ulcerosa im jugendlichen Alter. Fortschr Röntgenstr 135:577–582, 1981.

Bäckdahl, M.: The caput ulnae syndrome in rheumatoid arthritis. A study of the morphology, abnormal anatomy and clinical picture. Acta Rhumatol Scand Suppl 5:1, 1963.

Barnes, L., G.P. Rodnan, T.A. Medsger Jr., D. Short: Eosinophilic fasciitis. A pathologic study of twenty cases. Am J Pathol 96:493–507, 1979.

Barry, M., L. Katz, L. Cooney: An unusual articular presentation of progressive systemic sclerosis. Arthritis Rheum 26:1041–1043, 1983.

Beaulieu, A., R. Roy, G. Mathon, et al.: Psoriatic arthritis: risk factors for patients with psoriasis—a study based on histocompatibility antigen frequencies. J Rheumatol 10:633–636, 1983.

Begemann, M.: Das HLA–System des Menschen. Med Klin 77:15–23, 1982.

Beraneck, L., J. Crouzet: Hyperostose sterno–costo–claviculaire. A propos d'un cas avec hyperostose vertébrale. Rev Rhum 50:247, 1983.

Bird, H.A., W. Esselinckx, A. St. J. Dixon, A.G. Nowat: An evaluation of criteria for polymyalgia rheumatica. Ann Rheum Dis 38:434–439, 1979.

Bleck, E.E.: Idiopathic chondrolysis of the hip. J Bone Joint Surg 65A:1266–1275, 1983.

Blocka, K.L.N., L.W. Bassett, D.E. Furst, P.J. Clements, H.E. Paulus: The arthropathy of advanced progressive systemic sclerosis. A radiographic survey. Arthritis Rheum 24:874–884, 1981.

Bocanegra, T.S., L.R. Espinoza, P.H. Bridgeford, F.B. Vasey, B.F. Germain: Reactive arthritis induced by parasitic infestation. Ann Intern Med 94:207–209, 1981.

Bolton, R.P., G.M. Wood, M.S. Losowsky: Acute arthritis associated with Clostridium difficile colitis. Br Med J 283:1023–1024, 1981.

Bookbinder, S.A., N.A. Fenske, G.B. Clement, L.R. Espinoza, B.F. Germain, F.B. Vasey: Clavicular hyperostosis and acne arthritis. Ann Intern Med 97:615–616, 1982.

Bourgeois, P., L. Bocquet, M. Grossin, H. Olivier, M.F. Kahn: Ostéoarthropathie destructrice rapide de la hanche au cours d'une cirrhose biliaire primitive. Données cliniques, radiologiques et anatomopathologiques. Rev Rhum 48:437–439, 1981.

Brock, J.G., H.C. Meredith: Case report 102 (osteomyelitis of hallux sesamoid). Skeletal Radiol 4:236–239, 1979.

Bruk, M.I.: Articular and vascular manifestations of polymyalgia rheumatica. Ann Rheum Dis 26:103–116, 1967.

Bywaters, E.G.L.: Still's disease in the adult. Ann Rheum Dis 30:121–133, 1971.

Cabanel, G., X. Phelip, J.P. Gras, D. Mouries, P. Couderc: Lésions osseuses macro–géodiques au cours de la polyarthrite rhumatoide. Rev Rhum 40:259–263, 1973.

Camus, J.P., A. Prier, B. Cassouy: L'hyperostose sterno–costo–claviculaire. Rev Rhum 47:361–363, 1980.

Canoso, J.J., M. Saini, J.A. Hermos: Whipple's disease and ankylosing spondylitis simultaneous occurrence in HLA–B27 positive male. J Rheumatol 5:79–84, 1978.

Carr, R.D., E.B. Heisel, T.D. Stevenson: CRST syndrome. Arch Dermatol 92:519–525, 1965.

Carty, H., M. Maxted. J.A. Fielding, P. Gulliford, R. Owen: Isotope scanning in the "irritable hip syndrome". Skeletal Radiol 11:32–37, 1984.

Catoggio, L.J., R.M. Bernstein, C.M. Black, G.R.V. Hughes, P.J. Maddison: Serological markers in progressive systemic sclerosis: clinical correlations. Ann Rheum Dis 42:23–27, 1983.

Cros, D., T. Gamby, G. Serratrice: Acne rheumatism. Report of a case. J Rheumatol 8:336–339, 1981.

David–Chaussé, J., J. Dehais, M. Boyer, M.L. Darde, Y. Imbert: Les infections articulaires chez l'adulte atteintes périphériques et vertébrales a germes banals et a bacilles tuberculeux. Rev Rhum 48:69–76, 1981.

David–Chaussé, J.: Le devenir des arthrites réactionelles. Rev Rhum 50:799–806, 1983.

Davis, D.E., F.J. Viozzi, O.F. Miller, R.C. Blodgett: The musculoskeletal manifestations of acne fulminans. J Rheumatol 8:317–320, 1981.

Delamere, J.P., R.M. Baddeley, K.W. Walton: Jejuno–ileal bypass arthropathy: its clinical features and associations. Ann Rheum Dis 42:553–557, 1983.

De Valderrama, J.A.F.: The "observation hip" syndrome and its late sequelae. J Bone Joint Surg 45B:462–470, 1963.

Dihlmann, W.: Beurteilung von Therapieeffekten bei Arthritiden mit röntgenologischen Methoden? In: Spontanverlauf und Therapiebeurteilung rheumatischer Erkrankungen. M. Franke, W. Müller (Eds). Darmstadt: Steinkopff, 1983 p.115–118.

Doury, P.: Epidemiologische Studie des Fiessinger–Leroy–Reiter–Syndroms. In: Das Fiessinger–Leroy–Reiter–Syndrom, H. Kayser and F. Delbarre (Eds). Bielefeldt: Lab. Français Thérap., 1977.

Dubois, E.L., L. Cozen: Avascular (aseptic) bone necrosis associated with systemic lupus erythematosus. JAMA 174:966–971, 1960.

Dubois, E.L., D.L. Tuffanelli: Clinical manifestations of systemic lupus erythematosus. Computer analysis of 520 cases. JAMA 190:104–111, 1964.

Duncan, J.W., R. Nasca, J. Schrantz: Idiopathic chondrolysis of the hip. J Bone Joint Surg 61A:1024–1028, 1979.

Dunn, E.C., D.W. Jones, S. Mattingly, W.M. Robinson, R. William: The prognosis in palindromic rheumatism. Ann Rheum Dis 40:206–207, 1981.

Eckardt, J.J., J.C. Ivins, H.O. Perry, K.K. Unni: Osteosarcoma arising in heterotopic ossification of dermatomyositis: case report and review of the literature. Cancer 48:1256–1261, 1981.

Enna, C.D., R.R. Jacobson, R.O. Rausch: Bone changes in leprosy: a correlation of clinical and radiographic features. Radiology 100:295–306, 1971.

Esdaile, J.M., H. Tannenbaum, D. Hawkins: Adult Still's disease. Am J Med 68:825–830, 1980.

d'Eshougues, J.R., B. Delcambre, D. Defrance: Les manifestations articulaires de la maladie de Whipple. Rev Rhum 43:565–573, 1976.

Espinoza, L.R., F.B. Vasey, S.W. Gaylord, C. Dietz, L. Bergen, P. Bridgeford, B.F. Germain: Histocompatibility typing in the seronegative spondylarthropathies: a survey. Semin Arthritis Rheum 11:375–381, 1982.

Fassbender, H.G.: Pathomechanismen der Osteoarthrose. Aktuel Rheumatol 9:91–98 1984 (Sonderheft).

Foster, D.R., W.M. Park, I.W. McCall, D.J. Ward: The supinator notch sign in rheumatoid arthritis. Clin Radiol 31:195–199, 1980.

Fritzler, M.J., T.D. Kinsella, E. Garbutt: The CREST syndrome: a distinct serologic entity with anticentromere antibodies. Am J Med 69:520–526, 1980.

Gerster, J.C., P. Anani, P. de Goumoens, M. Pellation: Lytic lesions of the femoral neck in rheumatoid arthritis simulating pigmented villonodular synovitis or malignancy. Clin Rheumatol 1:30–34, 1982.

Greenstein, A.J., H.D. Janowitz, D.B. Sachar: The extra–intestinal complications of Crohn's disease and ulcerative colitis: a study of 700 patients. Medicine 55:401–412, 1976.

Hamza, M., A. Hubault, A. Ryckewaert: Les manifestations articulaires de la maladie de Behçet. Rev Rhum 42:527–531, 1975.

Hanson, V.: From Still's disease and JRA to JCPA, JCA, and JA: medical progress or biased ascertainment? J Rheumatol 9:819–820, 1982.

Hayden, C.K., Jr., L.E. Swischuk: Paraarticular soft–tissue changes in infections and trauma of the lower extremity in children. Am. J. Roentgenol 134:307–311, 1980.

Heinicke, M.H., M.H. Zarrabi, P.D. Gorevic: Arthritis due to synovial involvement by extramedullary haematopoiesis in myelofibrosis with myeloid metaplasia. Ann Rheum Dis 42:196–200, 1983.

Heuck, F.: Ungewöhnliche Form der Osteoarthropathie bei einer Psoriasis–Erythrodermie. Radiologe 22:572–580, 1982.

Hohmeister, R.: Eosinophile Fasziitis. Fortschr Med 100:1670–1672, 1982.

Holzmann, H., N. Hoede, K. Hahn, D. Eißner: Knochenbefunde bei Psoriasis. Arch Dermatol Res 262:191–196, 1978.

Huang, T.L., C. Fossier, R.D. Ray, L. Ghosh: Intra–articular rheumatoid nodule of the knee joint associated with recurrent subluxation of the patella. A case report. J Bone Joint Surg 61A:438–440, 1979.

Hutter, R.V.P., F.W. Foote, Jr., K.C. Francis, N.L. Higinbotham: Parosteal fasciitis. A self–limited benign process that simulates a malignant neoplasm. Am J Surg 104:800–807, 1962.

Hyer, F.H., N.L. Gottlieb: Rheumatic disorders associated with viral infection. Semin Arthritis Rheum 8:17–31, 1978.

Immelman, E.J., S. Bank, H. Krige, I.N. Marks: Roentgenologic and clinical features of intramedullary fat necrosis in bones in acute and chronic pancreatitis. Am J Med 36:96–105, 1964.

Ingram, J.T.: The significance and management of psoriasis. Br Med J II:823–828, 1954.

Ingram, A.J., M.S. Clarke, C.S. Clark, Jr., W.R. Marshall: Chondrolysis complicating slipped capital femoral epiphysis. Clin Orthop 165:99–109, 1982.

Isemein, L., A.M. Fournier: Sur les altérations radiologiques du poignet observées dans les formes de début de la polyarthrite chronique évolutive. Sem Hôp Paris 10:560–564, 1954.

Jäger, M., J.M. Schmidt: Subluxation im proximalen Tibiofibulargelenk auf dem Boden einer Synovialitis bei chronischer Polyarthritis. Aktuel Rheumatol 6:103–105, 1981.

James, D.G., E. Neville, L.S. Carstairs: Bone and joint sarcoidosis. Semin Arthritis Rheum 6:53–81, 1976.

Jayson, M.I.V., D. Rubenstein, A. St., J. Dixon: Intra–articular pressure and rheumatoid geodes (bone "cysts"). Ann Rheum Dis 29:496–502, 1970.

Jirik, F.R., H.B. Stein, A. Chalmers: Clavicular hyperostosis with enthesopathy, hypergammaglobulinemia, and thoracic outlet syndrome. Ann Intern Med 97:48–50, 1982.

Jüngling, O.: Über Ostitis tuberculosa multiplex cystoides, zugleich ein Beitrag zur Lehre von den Tuberkuliden des Knochens. Bruns' Beitr Klin Chir 143:401–475, 1928.

Karasick, S., D. Karasick: Case report 188 (sternocostoclavicular hyperostosis). Skeletal Radiol 8:74–76, 1982.

Kaushansky, K., G.A.M. Finerman, A.D. Schwabe: Chronic destructive arthritis in familial Mediterranean fever: the predominance of hip involvement and its management. Clin Orthop 155:156–161, 1981.

Keiser, H., F.L. Ruben, E. Wolinsky, I. Kushner: Clinical forms of gonococcal arthritis. N Engl J Med 279:234–240, 1968.

Kelly, A.P., R.E. Burns: Acute febrile ulcerative conglobate acne with polyarthralgia. Arch Dermatol 104:182–187, 1971.

Keysser, M., J. Weber: Wirbelsäulenbeteiligung beim Behçet–Syndrom (BS). Aktuel Rheumatol 9:169–171, 1984.

Kozlowski, K., R. Anderson, A. Tink: Multifocal recurrent periostitis. Report of two cases. Fortschr Röntgenstr 135:597–602, 1981.

Küster, R.M.: Chronische (Poly–) Arthritis bei Kindern und Jugendlichen. Therapiewoche 31:363–376, 1981.

Kuttnig, M., R. Kurz, G. Ritter, R. Fotter, G. Breisach: Die Coxitis Fugax. Monatsschr. Kinderhlkd 129:688–691, 1981.

Kvien, T., K.H.M. Høyeraal, E. Kåss: Diagnostic criteria of rheumatoid arthritis in children. Proposed criteria for controlled clinical studies. Scand J Rheumatol 11:187–192, 1982.

Lämmle, B., U. Steiger, H. Schärer, E. Schröder, H. Thölen: Morbus Still des Adulten. Bericht über zwei Fälle. Schweiz Med Wochenschr 113:138–144, 1983.

Lambert, J.R., V. Wright: Psoriatic spondylitis: a clinical and radiological description of the spine in psoriatic arthritis. Q J Med N S 46:411–425, 1977.

Laravoire, P., H. Ott: Polyarthrite sévère chez un patient atteint d'une hypogammaglobulinémie. Rev Rhum 47:571–575, 1980.

Lazarus, G.S., L.A. Goldsmith, R.E. Rocklin, R.S. Pinals, J.P. de Buisseret, J.R. David, W. Draper: Pyoderma gangrenosum, altered delayed hypersensitivity, and polyarthritis. Arch Dermatol 105:46–51, 1972.

Le Goff, P., R. Jaffres, C. Schwarzberg, A. Brousse, J.P. Leroy: Arthrite chronique destructrice du genou d'origine sarcoidosique associée a des géodes des os longs. Rev Rhum 49:647–652, 1982.

Lehman, T.J.A., V. Hanson, H. Kornreich, R.S. Peters, A.D. Schwabe: HLA–B27–negative sacroiliitis: a manifestation of familial Mediterranean fever in childhood. Pediatr 61:423–426, 1978.

Leirisalo, M., G. Skylv, M. Kousa, L.M. Voipio–Pulkki, H. Suoranta, M. Nissilä, L. Hvidman, E.D. Nielsen, A. Svejgaard, A. Tiilikainen, O. Laitinen: Follow-up study on patients with Reiter's disease and reactive arthritis, with special reference to HLA–B27. Arthritis Rheum 25:249–259, 1982.

Lequesne, M., S. de Sèze: Les coxites rhumatismales isolées (monarthrites de la hanche). Diagnostic par la méthode des critères et des exclusions. Rev Rhum 37:53–62, 1970.

LeVine, M.E., W.O. Dobbins III: Joint changes in Whipple's disease. Semin Arthritis Rheum 3:79–93, 1979.

Leskinen, R.H., B.V. Skrifvars, L.S. Laasonen, K.J. Edgren: Bone lesions in systemic lupus erythematosus. Radiology 153:349–352, 1984.

Lièvre, J.A., J.P. Camus, C. Bénichou, V. May, Mme. J.A. Lièvre: La polyarthrite stéatonécrotique et l'ostéolyse stéatonécrotique. Rev Rhumat 32:167–174, 1965.

Loreck, D., P. Schulze, M. Miehe: Röntgenmorphologische Befund am Skelettsystem bei der Psoriasis arthropathica. 1. Mitteilung: Hand—und Fußskelett, andere Gelenke. Radiol diagn 22:651–662, 1981. 2. Mitteilung: Ileosakralgelenke, Wirbelsäule, extraartikuläre Manifestationen. Radiol Diagn 22:742–754, 1981.

Luzar, M.J., J.H. Caldwell, H. Mekhjian, F.B. Thomas: Yersinia enterocolitica infection presenting as chronic enteropathic arthritis. Arthritis Rheum 26:1163–1165, 1983.

Magyar, É., A. Talerman, M. Fehér, H.W. Wouters: Giant bone cysts in rheumatoid arthritis. J Bone Joint Surg 56:121–129, 1974.

Mannerfelt, L., M. von Raven: Die Ätiologie und Bedeutung der Radiuskrypte im rheumatischen Handgelenk. Verh Dtsch Ges Rheumatol 5:94–96, 1978.

Mannerfelt, L.: Das unbehandelte rheumatische Handgelenk—natürliche Entwicklung und Verlauf. Aktuel Rheumatol 8:137–140, 1983.

Martel, W., K.J. Stuck, A.M. Dworin, R.G. Hylland: Erosive osteoarthritis and psoriatic arthritis: a radiologic comparison in the hand, wrist, and foot. Am J Roentgenol 134:125–135, 1980.

Marx, W.J., D.J. O'Connell: Arthritis of primary biliary cirrhosis. Arch Intern Med 139:213–216, 1979.

Mathies, H.: Die Terminologie der primär chronischen Polyarthritis. Klin Wochenschr 48:513–518, 1970.

Meijers, K.A.E., D.M. Paré, H. Loose, F. Eulderink, D.R. Siewertsz van Reesema: Periarteritis nodosa and subperiosteal new bone formation. J Bone Joint Surg 64B:592–596, 1982.

Melish, M.E.: Kawasaki Syndrome: a new infectious disease? J Infect Dis 143:317–324, 1981.

Meneghello, A., M. Bertoli: Neuropathic arthropathy (Charcot's joint) in dialysis patients. Fortschr Röntgenstr 141:180–184, 1984.

Meyer, O., T. Haim: Les anticorps anticentromère. Valeur diagnostique et pronostique. Nouv Presse Méd 11:2891–2894, 1982.

Miller, J.L., K. Soltani, C.D. Tourtellotte: Psoriatic acroosteolysis without arthritis. A case study. J Bone Joint Surg 53A:371–374, 1971.

Mohr, W.: Gelenkkrankheiten. Diagnostik und Pathogenese makroskopischer und histologischer Strukturveränderungen. Stuttgart: Georg Thieme Verlag, 1984.

Moll, J.M.H., I. Haslock, I.F. Macrae, V. Wright: Associations between ankylosing spondylitis, psoriatic arthritis, Reiter's disease, the intestinal arthropathies, and Behçet's syndrome. Medicine (Baltimore) 53:343–364, 1974.

Mueller, C.E., J.F. Seeger, W. Martel: Ankylosing spondylitis and regional enteritis, Radiology 112:579–581, 1974.

Müller–Brodmann, W., Y. Pfisterer, K.M. Goebel: Differentialdiagnose der seronegativen Oligoarthritis. Inn Med 11:65–74, 1984.

Neuwelt, C.M., D.G. Borenstein, R.P. Jacobs: Reiter's syndrome: a male and female disease. J Rheumatol 9:268–272, 1982.

Niederle, N., C.G. Schmidt, S. Seeber: Neurologische Krankheitsbilder bei malignen Erkrankungen. Tumor Diagn Therapie 3:61–67, 1982.

O'Dell, J.R., P.A. Andersen, J.R. Hollister, S.G. West: Anterior tibial mass: an unusual complication of popliteal cysts. Arthr Rheum 27:113–115, 1984.

O'Malley, B.P., I. Anderson, F.D. Rosenthal: Bone lesions in systemic acne (acne fulminans). Br J Dermatol 100:703, 1979.

Osial, T.A., Jr., A. Avakian, V. Sassouni, A. Agarwal, T.A. Medsger, Jr., G.P. Rodnan: Resorption of the mandibular condyles and coronoid processes in progressive systemic sclerosis (scleroderma). Arthr Rheum 24:729–733, 1981.

Otte, P., H. Schiller, F. Schilling: Arthritis und Spondyl-arthritis bei Akne fulminans. Aktuel Rheum 7:33–35, 1982.

Paice, E.W., F.W. Wright, A.G.S. Hill: Sternoclavicular erosions in polymyalgia rheumatica. Ann Rheum Dis 42:379–383, 1983.

Park, W.M., D. Ward, J. Ball, A. Bane: Rheumatoid disease and rib defects. Ann Rheum Dis 30:466–475.

Pastershank, S.P., D. Resnick: "Hook" erosions in Jaccoud's arthropathy. J Can Assoc Radiol 31:174–175, 1980.

Paus, B.: Tumour, tuberculosis, and osteomyelitis of the spine. Differential diagnostic aspects. Acta Orthop Scand 44:372–382, 1973.

Persigehl, M., H. Hövels–Gürich, G. von Bernuth: Neben-wirkung am Skelettsystem bei Behandlung mit Prostaglandin E. Fortschr Röntgenstr 141:427–430, 1984.

Pitt, P., E.B.D. Hamilton, E.H. Innes, K.D. Morley, B.E. Monk, G.R.V. Hughes: Sarcoid dactylitis. Ann Rheum Dis 42:634–639, 1983.

Pönkä, A., J. Martio, T.U. Kosunen: Reiter's syndrome in association with enteritis due to campylobacter fetus ssp. jejuni. Ann Rheum Dis 40:414–415, 1981.

Queneau, P., A. Gabbai, B. Perpoint, et al.: Acro–ostéolyses au cours de la lèpre. A propos de 19 observations personnelles. Rev Rhum 49:111–119, 1982.

Resnick, D., G. Niwayama, R.D. Coutts: Subchondral cyst (geodes) in arthritic disorders: pathologic and radiographic appearance of the hip joint. Am J Roentgenol 128:799–806, 1977.

Resnick, D.: Sternocostoclavicular hyperostosis. Am J Roentgenol 135:1278–1280, 1980.

Resnick, D., V. Vint, N.L. Poteshman: Sternocostoclavicular hyperostosis. A report of three new cases. J Bone Joint Surg 63A:1329–1332, 1981.

Richter, R., F.J. Krause: Primäre Diaphysentuberkulose der langen Röhrenknochen. Fortschr Röntgenstr 139:549–552, 1983.

Ringel, R.E., J.I. Brenner, P.J. Haney, J.E. Burns, A.L. Moulton, M.A. Berman: Prostaglandin–induced periostitis: a complication of long–term PGE$_1$–infusion in an infant with congenital heart disease. Radiology 142:657–658, 1982.

Rodnan, G.P., A.G. DiBartolomeo, T.A. Medsger Jr., E.L. Barnes: Eosinophilic fasciitis—report of six cases of a newly recognized scleroderma–like syndrome. Clin Res 23:443a, 1975.

Rohlfing, B.M., C.M. Basch, H.K. Genant: Acroosteolysis as the sole skeletal manifestation of rheumatoid vasculitis. Br J Radiol 50:830–833, 1977.

Rosenthal, J., M.D. Benson: Diffuse fasciitis and eosinophilia with symmetric polyarthritis. Arch Intern Med 92:507–509, 1980.

Rosner, I.A., D.E. Richter, T.L. Huettner, G.H. Kuffner, J.J. Wisnieski, C.G. Burg: Spondylarthropathy associated with hidradenitis suppurativa and acne conglobata. Ann Intern Med 97:520–525, 1982.

Schaaf, R.E., N. Jacobs, F.M. Kelvin, H.A. Gallis, O. Akwari, W.M. Thompson: Clostridium septicum infection associated with colonic carcinoma and hematologic abnormality. Radiology 137:625–627, 1980.

Schattenkirchner, M., K. Krüger, P. Herzer: B27–positive Krankheiten. Ein neues Konzept in der Rheumatologie. Münch Med Wochenschr 122:1725–1728, 1980.

Schattenkirchner, M.: Serologische und immunologische Befunde bei ankylosierender Spondylitis. Aktuel Rheumatol 79–81, 1982.

Schidlow, D.V., D.P. Goldsmith, J. Palmer, N.N. Huang: Arthritis in cystic fibrosis. Arch Dis Child 59:377–379, 1984.

Schilling, F., M. Schacherl: Röntgenmorphologie des chronischen Reiter-Syndroms. In: Das Fiessinger–Leroy–Reiter–Syndrom. H. Kaiser and F. Delbarre (Eds). Bordeaux and Bielefeld, 1977.

Schilling, F., M.L. Stadelmann: Klinik und Röntgenmorphologie der Arthritis psoriatica. In: Psoriasis–Psoriasis-arthritis. Colloquia rheumatologica 18. H.J. Albrecht. München-Gräfelfing: Dr. E. Banaschewski–Verlag, 1984, p. 29–47.

Schneider, P.: Palindromer Rheumatismus (Palindrome Arthritis). Aktuel Rheumatol 6:183–187, 1981a.

Schneider, P.: Viral bedingte Arthritiden beim Menschen. Münch Med Wochenschr 123:1891–1894, 1981b.

Seebacher, C., E. Köstler, B. Gebhardt: Zur Ätiologie und Pathogenese des Morbus Reiter. Dermatol Monatsschr 167:287–292, 1981.

Serre, H., G. Kalfa, A. Brousson u. 3 Mitarb.: Manifestations ostéo–articulaires de la brucellose. Aspects actuels. Rev Rhum 48:143–148, 1981.

Severini, A., M. Bellomi, G. Cozzi, L. Bellegotti, A. Lattuada: Rib erosion: late complication of long-standing biliary drainage catheters. Radiology 150:666, 1984.

Shimizu, T., G.E. Ehrlich, G. Inaba, K. Hayashi: Behçet's disease (Behçet's syndrome). Semin Arthritis Rheum 8:223–260, 1979.

Shulman, L.E.: Diffuse fasciitis with hypergammaglobulinemia and eosinophilia: a new syndrome? J Rheumatol Suppl 1:46, 1974.

Shulman, L.E.: Diffuse fasciitis with eosinophilia: a new syndrome? Trans Assoc Am Physicians 88:70–86, 1975.

Simkin, P.A., J.D. Brunzell, D. Wisner, et al.: Free fatty acids in the pancreatitic arthritis syndrome. Arthritis Rheum 26:127–132, 1983.

Sonozaki, H., S. Furusawa, H. Seki, T. Kurokawa, A. Tateishi, K. Kabata: Four cases with symmetrical ossifications between the clavicles and the first ribs of both sides. Kanto J Orthop Traum 5:244–247, 1974.

Sonozaki, H. and 15 co-workers: Clinical features of 22 cases with ''inter–sterno–costo–clavicular ossification''. A new rheumatic syndrome. Arch Orthop Traum Surg 95:13–22, 1979.

Sonozaki, H., H. Mitsui, Y. Miyanaga, K. Okitsu, M. Igarashi, Y. Hayashi, M. Matsuura, A. Azuma, K. Okai, M. Kawashima: Clinical features of 53 cases with pustulotic arthro–osteitis. Ann Rheum Dis 40:547–553, 1981.

Stadelmann, M.L., F. Schilling: Typeneinteilung der Arthritis psoriatica. Verh Dtsch Ges Rheumatol 7:423–426, 1981.

Steere, A.C., S.E. Malawista, D.R. Snydman, et al.: Lyme arthritis. An epidemic of oligoarticular arthritis in children and adults in three Connecticut communities. Arthritis Rheum 20:7–17, 1977.

Steere, A.C., A. Gibofsky, M.E. Patarroyo and 3 co-workers: Chronic Lyme arthritis. Clinical and immunogenetic differentiation from rheumatoid arthritis. Ann intern Med 90:896–901, 1979.

Steere, A.C., N.H. Bartenhagen, J.E. Craft and 7 co-workers: The early clinical manifestations of Lyme disease. Ann Intern Med 99:76–82, 1983b.

Steere, A.C., R.L. Grodzicke, A.N. Kornblatt and 6 co-workers: The spirochetal etiology of Lyme disease. N Engl J Med 308:733–740, 1983b.

Stein, H.B., O.L.A. Schlappner, W. Boyko, R.H. Gourlay, C.E. Reeve: The intestinal bypass arthritis–dermatitis syndrome. Arthritis Rheum 24:684–690, 1981.

Stephan, U., H.G. Wiesemann: Zystische Fibrose beim Jugendlichen und Erwachsenen. Dtsch Ärztebl 81:3504–3510, 1984.

Steven, M.M., A. Cats: Diffuse fasciitis. Clin Rheumatol 3:282–284, 1984.

Stovell, P.B., S.C. Ahuja, A.E. Inglis: Pseudarthrosis of the proximal femoral epiphysis in juvenile arthritis. A. case report. J Bone Joint Surg 57A:860–861, 1975.

Stursberg, H.: Über verstümmelnde Gelenkentzündung. Dtsch Med Wochenschr 61:5–7, 1935.

Theiss, B., U.W. Schnyder, A. Böni, F. Wagenhäuser: Intra-familiäre Untersuchungen bei Psoriasis–Arthritis. Z Rheumaforschg 28:403–424, 1969.

Theiss, B.: Zur Differentialdiagnose der Gelenkerkrankungen bei Psoriatikern. Dtsch Med Wochenschr 96:300–303, 1971.

Thompson, M., E.G.L. Bywaters: Unilateral rheumatoid arthritis following hemiplegia. Ann Rheum Dis 21:370–377, 1962.

Thorel, J.B., J.J. Baron, Ph. Dessauw, P. Deshayes: La cirrhose biliaire primitive vue par le rhumatologue. A propos de deux observations. Rev Rhum 48:341–346, 1981.

Tillmann, K., G. Binzus: Der Energiestoffwechsel der Gelenke bei Arthrose und Arthritis und seine medikamentöse Beeinflußbarkeit. Verhandlungen der Deutschen Orthopädischen Gesellschaft, 55. Kongreß. Ferdinand. Stuttgart: Enke Verlag, 1969, p. 221–227.

Tilly, G., M. Audran, M.F. Le Bodic, et al.: Ostéite condensante de l'extrémité interne de la clavicule. A propos d'un nouveau cas. J Radiol Électrol 59:223–226, 1978.

Tomlinson, I.W., M.I.V. Jayson: Erosive Crohn's arthritis. J Royal Soc Med 74:540–542, 1981.

Trentham, D.E., A.T. Masi, G.F. Bale: Arthritis with an inflammatory dermatosis resembling Sweet's syndrome. Report of a unique case and review of the literature on arthritis associated with inflammatory dermatoses. Am J Med 61:424–432, 1976.

Trnavsky, K., M. Zbojanova, F. Vlcek: Rheumatoid type of psoriatic arthritis. Clin Rheumatol 2:133–137, 1983.

Trueta, J.: The three types of acute haematogenous osteomyelitis. A clinical and vascular study. J Bone Joint Surg 41B:671–679, 1959.

Ueda, K., A. Saito, H. Nakano, M. Aoshima, M. Yokota, R. Muraoka, T. Iwaya: Cortical hyperostosis following long–term administration of prostaglandin E_1 in infants with cyanotic congenital heart disease. J Pediatr 97:834–836, 1980.

Velasco Dominguez, E., F. Garcia Velasco, J.L. Arranz Velasco: Quiste gigante de Baker de origen tuberculoso. Rev Esp Reum 6:171–177, 1979.

Wagenhäuser, F.J.: Diagnose und Differentialdiagnose rheumatischer Krankheiten. Stuttgart: H. Huber, Bern, 1967.

Weinberger, A., S. Berliner, J. Pinkhas: Articular manifestations of essential cryoglobulinemia. Semin Arthritis Rheum 10:224–229, 1981.

Weinberger, A., S. Berliner, J. Pinkhas: Spine manifestations in essential cryoglobulinaemia. Rheumatol Rehabil 21:27–30, 1982.

Weston, W.J.: The soft-tissue signs of the enlarged ulnar bursa in rheumatoid arthritis. J Can Assoc Radiol 24:282–287, 1973.

Weston, W.J.: Traumatic effusions of the ankle joint and posterior subtaloid joint. Brit J Radiol 31:445–447, 1958.

Willkens, R.F., F.C. Arnett, T. Bitter, A. Calin and 4 co-workers: Reiter's syndrome. Evaluation of preliminary criteria for definite disease. Arthritis Rheum 24:844–849, 1981.

Windom, R.E., J.P. Sanford, M. Ziff: Acne conglobata and arthritis. Arthritis Rheum 4:632–635, 1961.

Winfield, J., A. Young, P. Williams, M. Corbett: Prospective study of the radiological changes in hands, feet, and cervical spine in adult rheumatoid disease. Ann Rheum Dis 42:613–618, 1983.

Wright, V., J.M.H. Moll: Seronegative polyarthritis. Amsterdam: North–Holland Publ. Comp. 1976.

Yancey, C.L., C. Zmijewski, B.H. Athreya, R.A. Doughty: Arthropathy of Down's syndrome. Arthritis Rheum 27:929–934, 1984.

Yurdakul, S., H. Yazici, Y. Tüzün, H. Pazarli, B. Yalçin, M. Altaç, Y. Özyazgan, N. Tüzüner, A. Müftüoğlu: The arthritis of Behçet's disease: a prospective study. Ann Rheum Dis 42:505–515, 1983.

Zeidler, H.: Pathologisch–klinisch–chemische Befunde und pathologische Immunphänomene. Therapiewoche 32:803–827, 1982.

Osteoarthrosis (see also under Deformities; Anatomy).

Bene, É., P. Temesváry, M. Szilágyi, F. Pera: Ergebnisse einer klinischen und radiologischen Reihenuntersuchung der Bewegungsorgane bei Bergleuten in Ungarn. Z Rheumatol 43:117–123, 1984.

Bugnion, J.P.: Lésions nouvelles du poignet. Pseudokystes nécrobiotiques, kystes par herniations capsulaires, arthrite chronique dégénérative par ostéochondrose marginale. Acta Radiol Suppl 90 Stockholm 1951.

Carstens, C.: Untersuchungen zur mechanischen Beanspruchung der Osteophyten des arthrotischen Femurkopfes. Z Orthop 120:698–701, 1982.

Danielsson, L., J. Hernborg: Morbidity and mortality of osteoarthritis of the knee (gonarthrosis) in Malmö, Sweden. Clin Orthop 69:224–226, 1970.

Ehrlich, G.E.: Osteoarthritis beginning with inflammation. Definitions and correlations. JAMA 232:157–159, 1975.

Fassbender, H.G.: Die Bedeutung entzündlicher Prozesse bei der Osteoarthrose. Z Rheumatol 42:145–151, 1983.

Goldberg, R.P., J.I. Zulman, H.K. Genant: Unilateral primary osteoarthritis of the hand in monoplegia. Radiology 135:65–66, 1980.

Jacqueline, F.: Résorptins osseuses massives et brusques au cours des coxarthroses destructrices rapides. Étude radiologique et anatomique. Rev Rhum 46:619–627, 1979.

Lange, S., K. Mechsner, Ph. Langenscheidt: Die sekundäre Arthrose nach operativ versorgten Sprunggelenksfrakturen. Fortschr Röntgenstr 140:69–74, 1981.

Lequesne, M., M. Fallut, R. Coulomb, J.L. Magnet, J. Strauss: L'arthropathie destructrice rapide de l'épaule. Rev Rhum 49:427–437, 1982.

Lingg, G., G. Nebel: Röntgenologische Frühdiagnostik der Koxarthrose. Beziehungen zwischen Knorpelläsion und Femurkopfosteophytose (einschließlich des sogenannten Plaquezeichens). Z Rheumatol 41:57–62, 1982.

Mohr, W.: Gelenkkrankheiten. Diagnostik und Pathogenese makroskopischer und histologischer Strukturveränderungen Stuttgart: G. Thieme, New York, 1984.

Nilsson, B.E., L.G. Danielsson, S.A.J. Hernborg: Clinical feature and natural course of coxarthrosis and gonarthrosis. In: Management of degenerative joint diseases. A. Bjelle (Ed). Scand J Rheumatol Suppl 43:13–21, 1982.

Otte, P.: Ätiologische und pathogenetische Vorstellungen bei der Arthrose. Z Rheumatol 42:242–248, 1983a.

Otte, P.: Arthrose: Pathogenetisches Konzept und Interpretation der Symptome. Aktuel Rheumatol 8:54–58, 1983b.

Pauwels, F.: Über die Verteilung der Spongiosadichte im coxalen Femurende und ihre Bedeutung für die Lehre vom funktionellen Bau des Knochens. Gegenbaurs Morphol Jahrb 95:35–54, 1955.

Pauwels, F.: Atlas zur Biomechanik der gesunden und kranken Hüfte. Prinzipien, Technik und Resultate einer kausalen Therapie. Berlin: Springer, 1973.

Rose, C.P., W.P. Cockshott: Anterior femoral erosion and patello–femoral osteoarthritis. J Can Assoc Radio 33:32–34, 1982.

Sheth, K.J., C.G. Bernhard: The arthropathy of Fabry disease. Arthritis Rheum 22:781–783, 1979.

Thomas, W.: Über die Ätiologie der Daumensattelgelenksarthrose und deren Behandlung durch eine spezielle Endoprothese. Z Orthop 115:699–707, 1977.

Wright, V.: The management of degenerative joint disease—an introduction In: Management of degenerative joint diseases. A. Bjelle (Ed). Scand J Rheumatol [Suppl] 43:7–11, 1982.

Osteoarthropathies (avascular, due to vitamin deficiency, electrical injury, hemoglobinopathy, due to hormones, coagulopathies, drugs, metabolic disorders, myelogenic, neurogenic, radiogenic, renal, thermal); osteolysis syndrome; massive osteolysis; neurogenic paraosteoarthropathy; lipoid-dermatoarthritis; pachydermoperiostosis (hypertrophic osteoarthropathy, Marie-Bamberger syndrome); paraneoplastic diseases (see also under Tumors); bone marrow necrosis; congenital pseudarthrosis.

Abel, M.S., G.R. Smith: The case of the disappearing pelvis. Radiology 111:105–106, 1974.

Arlart, I., G. Bargon: Periostale Knochenneubildung bei Colitis ulcerosa im jugendlichen Alter. Fortschr Röntgenstr 135:577–582, 1981.

Arlet, J., B. Mazieres, Cl. Netry: Osteonecrosis of the femoral head and pregnancy. Clin Rheumatol 1:95–103, 1982.

Armstrong, R.D., A.J. Crisp, R. Grahame, D.L. Woolf: Hypertrophic osteoarthropathy and purgative abuse. Br Med J 282:1836, 1981.

Ballou, S.P., M.A. Khan, I. Kushner: Diffuse intervertebral disk calcification in primary amyloidosis. Ann Intern Med 85:616–617, 1976.

Barrow, M.V., K. Holubar: Multicentric reticulohistiocytosis. A review of 33 patients. Medicine 48:287–305, 1969.

Baumann, F., H. Ilse: Ein Beitrag zur Osteochondrosis dissecans des Os naviculare manus. Therapiewoche 28:4466–4471, 1978.

Bensen, W.G., C.A. Laskin, H.A. Little, A.G. Fam: Hemochromatotic arthropathy mimicking rheumatoid arthritis. A case with subcutaneous nodules, tenosynovitis, and bursitis. Arthritis Rheum 21:844–848, 1978.

Benz, H.J.: Die Entwicklung der Epiphysen und Knochenkerne bei der hämophilen Arthropathie des Ellenbogens. Fortschr Röntgenstr 133:305–311, 1980.

Bertoli, C.L., J. Stassi, M.D. Rifkin: Ainhum—an unusual presentation involving the second toe in a white man. Skeletal Radiol 11:133–135, 1984.

Bessler, W.: Roentgenographic and scintigraphic findings in idiopathic aseptic necrosis of the femoral head. In: Idiopathic ischemic necrosis of the femoral head in adults. W.M. Zinn. (Ed). Stuttgart: G. Thieme, 1971, pp. 145–151.

Bjelle, A., O. Hassler, E. Hägg, G. Lindström: Arthropathy in haemochromatosis. Clinical survey and a morphological study of synovial and synovial sheath membranes. Aktuel Rheumatol 7:148–153 (spec. issue).

Blender, W.: Röntgenologische Veränderungen der Hand nach Erfrierung III. Grades. Fortschr Röntgenstr 133:674–675, 1980.

Bloch-Michel, H., M. Benoist, J. Peyron: Ostéonécroses aseptiques au cours de la corticothérapie du pemphigus. Rev Rhum 26:648–659, 1959.

Bobechko, W.P., W.R. Harris: The radiographic density of avascular bone. J Bone Jt Surg 42B: 626–632, 1960.

Böhm, G., U. Pittrich; Malum perforans pedis—aufgrund einer Strahlenspätschädigung des Plexus lumbosacralis. Med Welt 30:480–481, 1979.

Böhmer, R., H.P. Missmahl: Amyloidosen. Dtsch Ärztebl 78:2173–2178, 1981.

Bonavita, J.A., M.K. Dalinka: Shoulder erosions in renal osteodystrophy. Skeletal Radiol 5:105–108, 1980.

Bouillet, R., Vermeulen: Présentation de deux cas de nécrose aseptique partielle de la tête du fémur, attribuée à un traitement cortisonique prelongé. Acta Orthop Belg 29:531–538, 1963.

Brower, A.C., R.M. Allman: Pathogenesis of the neurotrophic joint: neurotraumatic vs. neurovascular. Radiology 139:349–354, 1981.

Bruckner, F.E., B.E. Kendall: Neuroarthropathy in Charcot–Marie–Tooth disease. Ann Rheum Dis 28:577, 1969.

Brunt, P.W.: Unusual cause of Charcot joints in early adolescence (Riley–Day-syndrome). Br Med J 4:277–278, 1967.

Butt, W.P.: The radiology of infection. Clin Orthop 96:20–30, 1973.

Camus, J.P., J. Crouzet, A. Prier, A.C. Koeger: L'ostéomalacie hypophosphorémique de tumeurs du tissu conjonctif. Rev Rhum 49:301–306, 1982.

Canigiani, G., G. Pusch: Radiologischer Beitrag zur aseptischen Kopfnekrose im Humerus—und Femurbereich. Radiologe 9:222–226, 1969.

Carbonell-Abelló, J., J. Font, J. Coll, J. Vivancos, J.M. Planas: Amiloidosis y afección articular. Rev Esp Reum 7:187–193, 1980.

Catterall, R.D., V. Wright, J.B. Cook: Arthritis and genital infection in paraplegic patients. Br J Vener Dis 43:81–88, 1967.

de Ceulaer, K., M. Forbes, D. Roper, G.R. Serjeant: Non–gouty arthritis in sickle cell disease: report of 37 consecutive cases. Ann Rheum Dis 43:599–603, 1984.

Chalmers, A., W.J. Reynolds, D.G. Oreopoulos and 3 co-workers: The arthropathy of maintenance intermittent peritoneal dialysis. Can Med Assoc J 123:635–638, 1980.

Chaouat, D., J. Lambrozo, A. Baffet, D. Vignaud: Ostéonécrose aseptique bilatérale de la tête fémorale au course d'une acromégalie. Rev Rhum 51:215–217, 1984.

Cirincione, R.J., B.E. Baker: Tendon ruptures with secondary hyperparathyroidism. A case report. J Bone Joint Surg 57A:852–853, 1975.

Claustre, J., L. Simon: Aspects de la pathologie sésamoidienne du premier métatarsienne. Rev Rhum 45: 479–486, 1978.

Cornelius III, C.E., W.B. Shelley: Pincer nail syndrome. Arch Surg 96:321–322, 1968.

Crasselt, C.: Die Akroosteolyse. 1. Teil: Zur Differential–diagnose der generalisierten Akroosteolyse. Z Orthop 93:540–564, 1960.

Crasselt, C.: Die Akroosteolyse. 2. Teil: Zur Differential–diagnose der lokalisierten Akroosteolyse und die Ätiologie des Akroosteolysesyndroms. Z Orthop 94:33–50, 1961.

Dalinka, M.K., V. Stewart, J.S. Bomalaski, M. Halpern, M.E. Kricun: Periarticular calcifications in association with intra–articular corticosteroid injections. Radiology 153:615–618, 1984.

Dambacher, M.A.: Die Diagnostik des primären Hyperparathyreoidismus. Aktuel Rheumatol 8:34–37, 1983.

Damson III, T.C., C.S. Resnik, J. Guerra Jr., C. Vint, M.H. Weisman, D. Resnick: Hand and wrist arthropathies of hemochromatosis and calcium pyrophosphate deposition disease: distinct radiographic features. Radiology 147:377–381, 1983.

Delrieu, F., C. Marty, C.L. Benhamou, M. Forest, C.J. Menkes, B. Amor: Monoarthrites révélatrices de tumeurs osseuses de voisinage. Étude de 5 cas. Rev Rhum 51:137–144, 1984.

Denman, A.M., L. Szur, B.M. Ansell: Joint complaints in polycythaemia vera. Ann Rheum Dis 23:139–144, 1964.

Destouet, J.M., W.A. Murphy: Guitar player acroosteolysis. Skeletal Radiol 6:275–277, 1981.

Diggs, L.W.: Bone and joint lesions in sickle–cell disease. Clin Orthop 52:119–143, 1967.

Dihlmann, W.: Glukocorticoidnebenwirkungen am Stütz–und Gleitgewebe. Fortschr Röntgenstr 103:308–314, 1965.

Dihlmann, W.: CT analysis of the upper end of the femur: the asterisk sign and ischaemic bone necrosis of the femoral head. Skeletal Radiol 8:251–258, 1982.

Dihlmann, W., M. Heller: Asterisk-Zeichen und adulte ischämische Femurkopfnekrose. Fortschr Röntgenstr (in press).

Doury, P., F. Eulry, S. Pattin, M. Fromantin, D. Gautier, J. Bernard, F. Tabaraud, Ch. Masson, P. Dano: L'hyperparathyroidisme familial et récidivant. A propos de 7 adénomes chez 3 membres d'une même famille. Revue de la litterature. Rev Rhumat 50:99–103, 1983.

Drevet, J.G., D. Blanc, Y. Laborde, J. Vincent, X. Phelip, G. Cabanel: Les paralysies crurales par hématome de la fosse iliaque interne, au cours des traitements anticoagulants. Intérêt du traitement chirurgical précoce. Rev Rhum 48:403–411, 1981.

Ellenberg, M.: Diabetic foot. NY State J Med 73:2778–2781, 1983.

Estouet, J.M., W.A. Murphy: Acquired acroosteolysis and acronecrosis. Arthritis Rheum 26:1150–1154, 1983.

Eyanson, S., M.D. Benson: Erosive arthritis in hereditary amyloidosis. Arthritis Rheum 26:1145–1149, 1983.

Fam, A.G., A.J. Lewis, D.H. Cowan: Multiple myeloma and amyloid bone lesions complicating rheumatoid arthritis. J Rheumatol 8:845–850, 1981.

Feller, E.R., H.R. Schumacher: Osteoarticular changes in Wilson's disease. Arthritis Rheum 15:259–266, 1972.

Finby, N., A.G. Bearn: Roentgenographic abnormalities of the skeletal system in Wilson's disease (hepatolenticular degeneration). Amer J Roentgenol 79:603–611, 1958.

Fisher, D.E., W.H. Bickel, K.E. Holley: Histologic demonstration of fat emboli in aseptic necrosis associated with hypercortisonism. Mayo Clin Proc 44:252–259, 1969.

Fisher, D.E.: The role of fat embolism in the etiology of corticosteroid–induced avascular necrosis. Clinical and experimental results. Clin Orthop 130:68–80, 1978.

Forgács, S.: Bones and joints in diabetes mellitus. The Hague: M. Nijhoff Publ., 1982.

Frager, D.H., K. Subbarao: The "bone within a bone". JAMA 249:77–79, 1983.

Freyschmidt, J., R. Hehrmann: Primärer Hyperparathyreoidismus als Differentialdiagnose von schweren Skelettdestruktionen Röntgenblätter 31:495–502, 1978.

Gama, C., J.B.B. Meira: Occupational acro–osteolysis. J Bone Joint Surg 60A:86–90, 1978.

Genant, H.K., L.L. Heck, L.H. Lanzl, K. Rossmann, J.V. Horst, E. Paloyan: Primary hyperparathyroidism. A comprehensive study of clinical, biochemical and radiographic manifestations. Radiology 109:513–524, 1973.

Ghozlan, R., M. Dupuis, L. Antebi: Ostéonécrose de la tête fémorale au cours d'une maladie de Waedenström. Rev Rhum 48:721–723, 1981.

Glimcher, M.J., J.E. Kenzora: The biology of osteonecrosis of the human femoral head and its clinical implications. I. Tissue biology. II. The pathological changes in the femoral head as an organ and in the hip joint. III. Discussion of the etiology and genesis of the pathological sequelae; comments on treatment. Clin Orthop 138:284–309, 1979; 139:283–312, 1979; 140:273–312, 1979.

Golding, D.N., J.M. Walshe: Arthropathy in Wilson's disease. Study of clinical and radiological features in 32 patients. Ann Rheum Dis 36:99–111, 1977.

Goldman, A.B., H. Pavlov, P. Bullough: Case report 137 (primary amyloidosis involving the skeletal system). Skelet Radiol 6:69–74, 1981.

Gondos, B.: The pointed tubular bone. Its significance and pathogenesis. Radiology 105:541–545, 1972.

Grandjean, P., G. Thomsen: Reversibility of skeletal fluorosis. Br J Ind Med 40:456–461, 1983.

Gregg, P.J.: The use of radioisotopes in aseptic bone necrosis. In: Aseptic bone necrosis. (Eds.) A. Evans, D.N. Walder. London: Ciria Underwater Engineering Group, 1977, p. 77–83.

Griffin, C.N. Jr.: Severe erosive arthritis of large joints in chronic renal failure. Skeletal Radiol 12:29–33, 1984.

Güell-González, J.R., O.M. de Acosta, et al.: Bone lesions in congenital generalised lipodystrophy. Lancet II:104–105, 1971.

Guigan, L., A. Fleming: Osteonecrosis of the humerus related to pregnancy. Ann Rheum Dis 42:597–599, 1983.

Hall, F.M., M. Segall–Blank, H.K. Genant, F.O. Kolb, L.E. Hawes: Pseudohypoparathyroidism presenting as renal osteodystrophy. Skeletal Radiol 6:43–46, 1981.

Hall, F.M., R.P. Goldberg, E.J. Kasdon, H. Glick: Posttraumatic osteolysis of the pubic bone simulating a malignant lesion. J Bone Joint Surg 66A:121–126, 1984.

Hamilton, E.B.D., E.G.L. Bywaters: Joint symptoms in myelomatosis and similar conditions. Ann Rheum Dis 20:353–363, 1961.

Hansoti, R.C., N.J. Shah: Cirrhosis of liver simulating congenital cyanotic heart disease. Circulation 33:71–77, 1966.

Hehrmann, R., E. Keck: Erkrankungen der Nebenschilddrüsen. Dtsch Ärztebl 79:42–48, 1982.

Heilbrun, N., W.G. Kuhn Jr.: Erosive bone lesions and soft–tissue ossifications associated with spinal cord injuries (paraplegia). Radiology 48:579–593, 1947.

Heimann, W.G., R.H. Freiberger: Avascular necrosis of the femoral and humeral heads after high–dosage corticosteroid therapy. N Engl J Med 263:672–675, 1960.

Heller, M., W. Dihlamnn: Computertomographie der Paget–Koxopathie. Forstschr Röntgenstr 138:427–434, 1983.

Hernandez, R.J., A.K. Poznanski: Distinctive appearance of the distal phalanges in children with primary hypothyroidism. Radiology 132:83–84, 1979.

Heuck, F., M. Euchenhofer: Röntgenbefunde einer Paraosteoarthropathie nach Intensivbehandlung infolge Intoxikation. Radiologe 14:470–477, 1974.

Heuck, F.H.W., H. Treugut: Die "Hüftkopfnekrose" bei metabolischen und hormonellen Osteopathien–eine radiologisch–morphologische Analyse. Radiologe 24:319–337, 1984.

Horn, V., D. Spohrová, Z. Bozděch, M. Macek, T. Foukal: Primäres Tumoramyloid im Knochen. Z Orthop 121:137–141, 1983.

Houpt, J.B., B. Alpert, M. Lotem u. 4 Mitarb.: Spontaneous osteonecrosis of the medial tibial plateau. J Rheumatol 9:81–90, 1982.

Hungerford, D.S.: Early diagnosis of ischemic necrosis of the femoral head. Johns Hopkins Med J 137:270–275, 1975.

Irnell, L., I. Werner, L. Grimelius: Soft tissue calcification in hyperparathyroidism. Acta Med Scand 187:145–151.

Jayson, M.I.V., K. Lloyd–Jones, D.C. Berry, M. Bromige: Resorption of the mandible in vinyl chloride acro-osteolysis. Arthritis Rheum 19:971, 1976.

Johnson, C., C.B. Graham, F.K. Curtis: Roentgenographic manifestations of chronic renal disease treated by periodic hemodialysis. Am J Roentgenol 101:915–926, 1967.

Joseph, B., V. Chacko: Acro-osteolysis associated with hypertrophic pulmonary osteoarthropathy and pachydermoperiostosis. Radiology 154:343–344, 1985.

Kavanaugh, J.H.: Multiple myeloma, amyloidarthropathy, and pathological fracture of the femur. A case report. J Bone Joint Surg 60A:135–137, 1978.

Kidd, G.S., M. Schaaf, R.A. Adler, M.N. Lassman, H.L. Wray: Skeletal responsiveness in pseudohypoparathyroidism. A spectrum of clinical disease. J Med 68:772–781, 1980.

Kiraly, III. J.F., M.S. Wheby: Bone marrow necrosis. Am J Med 60:361–368, 1976.

Kirkwood, J.R., M.B. Ozonoff, H.L. Steinbach: Epiphyseal displacement after metaphyseal fracture in renal osteodystrophy. Am J Roentgenol 115:547–554, 1972.

Klotz, O.: Studies upon calcareous degeneration. I. Reprocess of pathological calcification. J Exp Med 7:633–675, 1905.

Klümper, A., E. Uehlinger, V. Lohmann, S. Weller, M. Strey: Femurkopfinfarkte nach Glucocorticoidbehandlung. Dtsch Med Wochenschr 92:1108–1111, 1967.

Knickerbocker, W.J., N.F. Quenville: Widespread marrow necrosis during pregnancy. Skeletal Radiol 9:37–40, 1982.

Kohler, E., D. Babbitt, B. Huizenga, T.A. Good: Hereditary osteolysis: A clinical, radiological and chemical study. Radiology 108:99–105, 1973.

Koischwitz, D., H.J. Marsteller, K. Lackner, G. Brecht, Th. Brecht: Veränderungen der Hand–und Fingerarterien bei der Vinylchloridkrankheit. Fortschr Röntgenstr 132:62–68, 1980.

Kolář, J., H. Zidková, M. Vohralik, F. Stryhal, F. Horáček: Langfristige Teilremission des Gorhamschen Syndroms. Fortschr Röntgenstr 134:214–215, 1981.

Kricun, M.E., D. Resnick: Patellofemoral abnormalities in renal osteodystrophy. Radiology 143:667–669, 1982.

Kricun, M.E., D. Resnick: Elbow abnormalities in renal osteodystrophy. Am J Roentgenol 140:577–579, 1983.

Kröpelin, T., D.P. Mertz: Rückbildung von Gichttophi unter Langzeitbehandlung mit Allopurinol. Med. Klin 67:614–618, 1972.

Krokowski, E.: Röntgenologische Zeichen der osteoporotisch bedingten Veränderung von Knochenstruktur und Körperstatik. Aktuel Rheumatol 8:1–5, 1983.

Kuhlencordt, J., H.P. Kruse, J. Franke: Diagnostischer Wert der Lamina dura alveolaris bei generalisierten Knochenerkrankungen. Fortschr Röntgenstr 134:401–407, 1981.

Lafferty, F.W.: Pseudohyerparathyroidism. Medicine 45:247–260, 1966.

Lagier, R., C.A. Bouvier, N. van Strijthem: Skeletal changes in congenital fibrinogen abnormalities. Skeletal Radiol 5:233–239, 1980.

Lagier, R., U. Steiger: Hip arthropathy in ochronosis: Anatomical and radiological study. Skeletal Radiol 5:91–98, 1980.

Lagier, R., W. Mac Gee: Spondylodiscal erosions due to gout: anatomico–radiological study of a case. Ann Rheum Dis 42:350–353, 1983.

Laragh, J.H., H.O. Heinemann, F.E. Demartini: Effect of chlorothiazide on electrolyte transport in man. Its use in the treatment of edema of congestive heart failure, nephrosis and cirrhosis. JAMA 166:145–152, 1958.

Lee, C.K., H.T. Hansen, A.B. Weiss: The "silent hip" of idiopathic ishemic necrosis of the femoral head in adults. J Bone Joint Surg 62A:795–800, 1980.

Le Mignon, L., M. Simon, R. Fauchet, G. Edan, M. Le Reun, P. Brissot, B. Genetet, M. Bourel: An HLA–A11 association with the hemochromatosis allele? Clin Genet 24:171–176, 1983.

Leu, W.J., U. Brunner: Osteolysierende Hämangiomatose nach Trauma. Gorham–Syndrom, "Syndrome of disappearing bone". Dtsch Med Wochenschr 106:1424–1428, 1981.

Lewis, V.L., T.E. Keats: Bone end sclerosis in renal osteodystrophy simulating osteonecrosis. Skeletal Radiol 8:275–278, 1982.

Lotz, W., M. Ebert, E. Fasske: Die massive Osteolyse (Gorham–Stout–Syndrom) mit lokaler Neurofibromatose. Überlegungen zu einem seltenen Krankheitsbild mit kasuistischem Beitrag. Fortschr Röntgenstr 137:55–62, 1982.

Lynch, C., A. Pont, S.I. Weingarden: Heterotopic ossification in the hand of a patient with spinal cord injury. Arch Phys Med Rehabil 62:291–293, 1981.

Mabille, J.P., M. Gaudet, J.F. Charpin: Ostéonécrose de la tête humérale au cours de l'encéphalopathie bismuthique. Sem Hôp Paris 57:389–391, 1981.

McFarland, P.H., H.M. Frost: A possible new cause for aseptic necrosis of the femoral head. Henry Ford Hospital Med Bull 9:115–122, 1961.

McGuigan, L.E., J.P. Edmonds, D.M. Painter: Pubic osteolysis. J Bone Joint Surg 66A:127–129, 1984.

Marcus, N.D., W.F. Enneking, R.A. Massam: The silent hip in idiopathic aseptic necrosis. Treatment by bone–grafting. J Bone Joint Surg 55A:1351–1366, 1973.

Mathias, K., U. Ludwig: Idiopathische multizentrische Osteolyse mit Kraniodysplasie und Schwachsinn: Ein neues Syndrom? Fortschr Röntgenstr 127:255–261, 1977.

Meema, H.E., D.L. Schatz: Simple radiologic demonstration of cortical bone loss in thyrotoxicosis. Radiology 97:9–15, 1970.

Meema, H.E., D.G. Oreopoulos, G.A. deVeber: Arterial calcifications in severe chronic renal disease and their relationship to dialysis treatment, renal transplant, and parathyroidectomy. Radiology 121:315–321, 1976.

Meneghello, A., M. Bertoli: Neuropathic arthropathy (Charcot's joint) in dialysis patients. Fortschr Röntgenstr 141:180–184, 1984.

Merle d'Aubigné, R., M. Postel, A. Mazabraud, P. Massias, J. Gueguen: Idiopathic necrosis of the femoral head in adults. J Bone Joint Surg 47B:612–633, 1965.

Mertz, D.P.: Rheumatische Syndrome bei Hypothyreose. Krankenhausarzt 53:526–530, 1980.

Mitnick, J.S., F.B. Axelrod, N.B. Genieser, M. Becker: Aseptic necrosis in familial dysautonomia. Radiology 142:89–91, 1982.

Mohr, W., D. Wessinghage, P. Heimstädt: Morphologie des Knorpels bei der alkaptonurischen Arthropathie. Aktuel Rheumatol 4:205–212, 1979.

Morein, G., Z. Goldschmidt, M. Pauker, M. Seelenfreund, J.B. Rosenfeld, A. Fried: Spontaneous tendon ruptures in patients treated by chronic hemodialysis. Clin Orthop 124:209–213, 1977.

Morgan, A.G., W.C. Walker, M.K. Mason, H. Herlinger, M.S. Losowsky: A new syndrome with hepatocellular carcinoma. Gastroenterology 63:340–345, 1972.

Murray, R.O.: Iatrogenic lesions of the skeleton. Am J Roentgenol 126:5–22, 1976.

Neuberger, A., C. Rimington, J.M.G. Wilson: Studies on alcaptonuria. 2. Investigations on a case of human alcaptonuria. Biochem J 41:438–448, 1947.

Nguyen, V.C., W.M. Sennott, G.S. Knox: Neonatal hyperparathyroidism. Radiology 112:175–176, 1974.

Norman, A., G.C. Steiner: Radiographic and morphological features of cyst formation in idiopathic bone infarction. Radiology 146:335–338, 1983.

Orkin, M., R.W. Goltz, R.A. Good, A. Michael, I. Fisher: A study of multicentric reticulohistiocytosis. Arch Dermatol 89:619–654, 1964.

Oster, H.: Die familiäre Dysautonomie. Dtsch Med Wochenschr 82:2038–2040, 1957.

Ott, A.: Hochgradige Osteoarthropathie nach Poliomyelitis. (Zugleich ein Beitrag zur Ätiologie der Arthropathia mutilans). Fortschr Röntgenstr 87:135–137, 1957.

Palmer, A.K., R.N. Hensinger, J.M. Costenbader, D.R. Bassett: Osteonecrosis of the femoral head in a family with hyperlipoproteinemia. Clin Orthop 155:166–171, 1981.

Palmers, P.E.S., J.E.P. Thomas: Osteopetrosis with unusual changes in the skull and digits. Br J Radiol 31:705–708, 1958.

Paolaggi, J.B., J.M. Le Parc, M. Durigon and 4 co-workers: Ostéonécroses cortisoniques: acquisitions tirées de l'observation chez l'homme et confrontation avec les résultats de l'expérimentation animale. Rev Rhum 47:719–729, 1980.

Parker, L.N., S.Y. Wu, M.K. Lai, M.B. Ramadan, R.K. Rajan, A.M. Yusi: The early diagnosis of atypical thyroid acropachy. Arch Intern Med 142:1749–1751, 1982.

Petrie, J.G.: A case of progressive joint disorders caused by intensivity to pain. J Bone Joint Surg 35B 399–401, 1953.

Phemister, D.B.: Changes in bones and joints resulting from interruption of circulation. 1. General considerations and changes resulting from injuries. Arch Surg 41:436–472, 1940.

Reinhardt, K.: Der diabetische Fuß. Diabetische Arthropathien und Osteopathien. Stuttgart: Ferdinand Enke Verlag, 1983.

Resnick, D., M. Oliphant: Hemophilia-like arthropathy of the knee associated with cutaneous and synovial hemangiomas. Report and review of the literature. Radiology 114:323–326, 1975.

Ritz, E., J. Bommer, B. Krempien, O. Mehls: Osteopathie und Wachstumsstillstand des kindlichen Skeletts bei Urämie. Med Welt 26:2321–2324, 1975.

Robinson, S.C., J.P. Sweeney: Cauda equina lipoma presenting as acute neuropathic arthropathy of the knee. A case report. Clin Orthop 178:210–213, 1983.

Rosenthal, D.I., J.A. Scott: Biomechanics important to interpret radiographs of the hip. Skeletal Radiol. 9:185–188, 1983.

Rossak, K.: Ein Beitrag zur Myositis ossificans circumscripta neurotica. Z Orthop 94:576–581, 1961.

Rougdot–Thoraval, F., M. Halphen, D. Larde, M. Galliot, J. Crymer, F. Galacteros, D. Dhumeaux: Evaluation of liver iron content by computed tomography: its value in the follow–up of treatment in patients with idiopathic hemochromatosis. Hepatology 3:974, 1983.

Rutishauser, E., A. Rohner, D. Held: Experimentelle Untersuchungen über die Wirkung der Ischämie auf den Knochen und das Mark. Virchows Arch Patholo Anat 333:101–118, 1960.

Schild, H., G. Neuhaus, F. Gerlach: Dactylolysis spontanea (Ainhum). Z Orthop 119:320–322, 1981.

Schilling, F., B. Knick, H. Kuck: Hyperostosis generalisata mit Cutis verticis gyrata und ihre Differentialdiagnose (Akromegalie, hypertrophische Osteoarthropathie und Pachydermoperiostose) Dtsch Arch Klin Med 207:456–491, 1961.

Schilling, F.: Gicht—Diagnose, Differentialdiagnose und Therapie. Ärztl Fortbildg 16:36–47, 1967.

Schlansky, R., K.A. Kucer, R.J. DeHoratius, J.L. Abruzzo, N.M. Smukler: Arthritis and distal tuft resorption associated with keratosis palmaris et plantaris. Arthr Rheum 24:726–728, 1981.

Schmidt, K.L., H.W. Leber, G. Schütterle: Arthropathie bei primärer Oxalose—Kristallsynovitis oder Osteopathie? Dtsch Med Wochenschr 106:19–22, 1981.

Sella, E.J., A.H. Goodman: Arthropathy secondary to transfusion hemochromatosis. J Bone Joint Surg 55A:1077–1081, 1973.

Seymour, E.Q.: Osteolysis of the clavicular tip associated with repeated minor trauma to the shoulder. Radiology 123:56, 1977.

Sherry, D.D., R.R.L. Rothstein, R.E. Petty: Joint contractures preceding insulin–dependent diabetes mellitus. Arthritis Rheum 25:1362–1364, 1982.

Simon, L., L. Bertrand, H. Michel, F. Blotman, J. Claustre: Ostéonécrose, éthylisme et stéatose hépatique. Rev Rhum 42:103–108, 1975.

Singer, F.: Zur Mononatriumuratkristallablagerung im Femur-kopf bei Osteonekrose. Aktuel Rheumatol 7:177–181, 1982.

Singh, M., A.R. Nagrath, P.S. Maini: Changes in trabecular pattern of the upper end of the femur as an index of osteoporosis. J Bone Jt Surg 52A:457–467, 1970.

Stremmel, W., G. Strohmeyer: Wilsonsche Krankheit. Störungen im Stoffwechsel der Schwermetalle, Teil II. Dtsch Arztebl 78:2125–2131, 1981.

Strohmeyer, G., W. Stremmel: Hämochromatose und Hämosiderosen. Störungen im Stoffwechsel der Schwermetalle, Teil I. Dtsch Ärztebl 78:1775–1780, 1981.

Šváb, V.: Knochen–und Gelenkveränderungen durch Hitze und Kälte. In: Handbuch der Medizinischen Radiologie Bd.V/1, L. Diethelm, F. Heuck, O. Olsson, K. Ranniger, F. Strnad, H. Vieten, A. Zuppinger. (Eds). Berlin: Springer, 1976, pp. 307–344.

Tishler, J.M.: The soft-tissue and bone changes in frostbite injuries. Radiology 102:511–513, 1972.

Todd, R.C., M.A.R. Freeman, C.J. Pirie: Isolated trabecular fatigue fractures in the femoral head. J Bone Jt Surg 54B:723–728, 1972.

Tyler, T., H.D. Rosenbaum: Idiopathic multicentric osteolysis. Am J Roentgenol 126:23–31, 1976.

Uehlinger, E.: Pathologische Anatomie der Therapieschäden. Verhdlg Dtsch Ges Innere Med Kongr 67:457–472, 1961.

Vidal, J.J., J. Ruiz, T. Santiago, P. Sanjuro, C. Moure: Case report 106 (ichthyosiform erythroderma associated with osteolysis of the terminal tufts of the hands [and feet]). Skeletal Radiol 4:251–252, 1979.

Vilar, J., J.L. Parra, E. Monzo: Case report 124 (pseudotumor of fibula secondary to thrombocytopenic purpura) Skeletal Radiol 5:197–199, 1980.

Virchow, R.: Ein Fall von allgemeiner Ochronose der Knorpel und knorpelähnlichen Theile. Arch Pathol Anat 37:212–219, 1866.

Vogl, A., S. Goldfischer: Pachydermoperiostosis. Primary or idiopathic hypertrophic osteoarthropathy. Am J Med 33:166–187, 1962.

Warin, R.P., C.D. Evans, M. Hewitt, A.L. Taylor, C.H.G. Price, J.H. Middlemiss: Reticulohistiocytosis (lipoid dermato-arthritis). Br Med J 1:1387–1391, 1957.

Watson Jones, R., R.E. Roberts: Calcification, decalcification, and ossification. Br J Surg 21:461–499, 1933/34.

Watt, I., H. Middlemiss: The radiology of gout. Clin Radiol 26:27–36, 1975.

Weizman, Z., A. Tennenbaum, S. Yatziv: Interphalangeal joint involvement in Gaucher's disease, type I, resembling juvenile rheumatoid arthritis. Arthritis Rheum 25:706–707, 1982.

Wills, M.R., C.Y.C. Pak, W.G. Hammond, F.C. Bartter: Normocalcemic primary hyperparathyroidism. Am J Med 47:384–391, 1969.

Wilson, S.A.K.: Progressive lenticular degeneration: a familial nervous disease associated with cirrhosis of the liver. Brain 34:295–509, 1912.

Winfield, J., T.C.B. Stamp: Bone and joint symptoms in Paget's disease. Ann Rheum Dis 43:769–773, 1984.

Woodward, H.R., D.P.K. Chan, J. Lee: Massive osteolysis of the cervical spine. A case report of bone graft failure. Spine 6:545–549, 1981.

Wriedt–Elfgang, K.: Klinik der Thalassämien. Monatsschr Kinderheilkd 127:707–708, 1979.

Zea–Mendoza, A.C., A. Alonso–Ruiz, A. Garcia–Vadillo, A. Moreno–Caparrós, J. Beltrán–Gutierrez: Poems syndrome with neuroarthropathy and nodular regenerative hyperplasia of the liver. Arthritis Rheum 27:1053–1057, 1984.

Zolla–Pazner, S., S.S. Pazner, V. Lanyi, M. Meltzer: Osteonecrosis of the femoral head during pregnancy. JAMA 244:689–690, 1980.

Enthesopathies (fibroosteosis, fibroosteitis); diseases of bursae and tendons; calcifications of soft tissues (see also under Autoimmune diseases) including chondrocalcinosis and crystalinduced synovitis; ossifications of soft tissues (see also under Neurogenic paraosteoarthropathy); carpal tunnel syndrome (unless discussed elsewhere under the headings of its causes); synovial cysts.

Adamson III, T.C., C.S. Resnik, J. Guerra Jr., V.C. Vint, M.H. Weisman, D. Resnick: Hand and wrist arthropathies of hemochromatosis and calcium pyrophosphate desposition disease: distinct radiographic features. Radiology 147:377–381, 1983.

Albert, J., R. Lagier: Enthesopathic erosive lesion of patella and tibial tuberosity in juvenile ankylosing spondylitis. Anatomico–radiological study of a case with tibia bursitis. Fortschr Röntgenstr 139:544–548, 1983.

Amendola, M.A., G.M. Glazer, F.P. Agha, et al.: Myositis ossificans circumscripta: computed tomographic diagnosis. Radiology 149:775–779, 1983.

Anderson, D.E., J.K. Davidson, M.E. Catto: Case report 227 (primary hyperoxaluria [oxalosis]). Skeletal Radiol 9:266–271, 1983.

Baldursson, H., E.B. Evans, W.F. Dodge, W.T. Jackson: Tumoral calcinosis with hyperphosphatemia. A report of a family with incidence in four siblings. J Bone Joint Surg 51A:913–925, 1969.

Bard, H., D. Kuntz, D. Molle, J. Witvoet, A. Ryckewaert: Étude du métabolisme du phosphore dans un cas de calcinose tumorale. Rev Rhum 51:63–68, 1984.

Bassiouni, M., M. Kamel: Bilharzial arthropathy. Ann Rheum Dis 43:806–809, 1984.

Bayerl, W., K. Fischer: Das Pronator teres Syndrom. Klinik, Pathogenese und Therapie des nicht traumatischen Kompressionssyndroms des Nervus medianus in Höhe des Ellenbogengelenkes. Handchirurgie 11:91–97, 1979.

Binder, A.I., D.Y. Bulgen, B.I. Hazleman, J. Tudor, P. Wraight: Frozen shoulder: an arthrographic and radionuclear scan assessment. Ann Rheum Dis 43:365–369, 1984.

Bishop, A.F., J.M. Destouet, W.A. Murphy, L.A. Gilula: Tumoral calcinosis: case report and review. Skeletal Radiol 8:269–274, 1982.

Bjelle, A., U. Edvinsson, Å. Hagstram: Pyrophosphate arthropathy in two Swedish families. Arthritis Rheum 25:66–74, 1982.

Boillat, M.A., J. Garcia, L. Velebit: Radiological criteria of industrial fluorosis. Skeletal Radiol 5:161–165, 1980.

Bonavita, J.A., M.K. Dalinka, H.R. Schumacher, Jr.: Hydroxyapatite deposition disease. Radiology 134:621–625, 1980.

Bourqui, M., T.L. Vischer, P. Stasse, C. Docquier, G.H. Fallet: Pyrophosphate arthropathy in the carpal and metacarpophalangeal joints. Ann Rheum Dis 42:626–630, 1983.

Bray, J.F.: The "inverted V" sign of pneumoperitoneum. Radiology 151:45–46, 1984.

Chafetz, N., H.K. Genant, F.T. Hoaglund: Ischiogluteal tuberculous bursitis with progressive bony destruction. J Can Assoc Radiol 33:119–120, 1982.

Cone III, R.O., D. Resnick, L. Danzig: Shoulder impingement syndrome: radiographic ekaluation. Radiology 150:29–33, 1984.

Cosendai, A., J.C. Gerster, T.L. Vischer, et al.: Arthropathies destructrices liées à la chondrocalcinose articulaire. Etude clinique et métabolique de 16 cas. Schweiz Med Wochenschr 106:8–14, 1976.

Dekel, S., T. Papaioannou, G. Rushworth: Idiopathic carpal tunnel syndrome caused by carpal stenosis. Br Med J 1:1297–1299, 1980.

Diepp, P.A., D.V. Doyle, E.C. Huskisson, D.A. Willoughby, P.R. Crocker: Mixed crystal deposition disease and osteoarthritis. Br Med J 1:150, 1979.

Dihlmann, W.: Periarthropathia calcificans (röntgenologisch–histologische Synopsis, Terminologie). Z Rheumatol 40:261–263, 1981.

Doury, P., S. Pattin: Un diagnostic différentiel difficile des spondylodiscites: les discarthroses érosives et pseudopottiques. Rev Rhum 48:64–68, 1981.

Eade, A.W.T., A.J. Swannel, N. Williamson: Pyrophosphate arthropathy in hypophosphatasia. Ann Rheum Dis 40:164–170, 1981.

Engelstad, B.L., L.A. Gilula, M. Kyriakos: Ossified skeletal muscle hemangioma: radiologic and pathologic features. Skeletal Radiol 5:35–40, 1980.

Eulert, J., A. Apoil, P. Dautry: Zur Pathogenese und operativen Behandlung der sogenannten Periarthritis humeroscapularis. Z Orthop 119:25–30, 1981.

Françon, F.: Une nouvelle entité clinique: la bursite ischiatique. Rev Rhum 33:253–258, 1966.

Frössler, H., F. Osmers: Bilaterale manschettenförmige venöse Stauungsossifikation am Oberschenkel. Fortschr Röntgenstr 124:496–498, 1976.

Garancis, J.C., H.S. Cheung, P.B. Halverson, D.J. McCarty: "Milwaukee shoulder"—association of microspheroids containing hydroxyapatite crystals, active collagenase, and neutral protease with rotator cuff defects. III. Morphologic and biochemical studies of an excised synovium showing chondromatosis. Arthritis Rheum 24:484–491, 1981.

Gerster, J.C., R. Lagier, G. Boivin: Olecranon bursitis related to calcium pyrophosphate dihydrate crystal deposition disease. Clinical and pathologic study. Arthritis Rheum 25:989, 1982.

Gilsanz, V., B.H. Bernstein: Joint calcification following intraarticular corticosteroid therapy. Radiology 151:647–649, 1984.

Gloor, H.J., O. Wetterwald, B. Truniger: Medikamentöse Fluorose bei Myelom. Schweiz Med Wochenschr 110:807–812, 1980.

Hadjipavlou, A., P. Lander, R. Boudreau, H. Srolovitz, M. Paleyew: Pagetoid changes in a heterotopic center of ossification. J Bone Joint Surg 63A:1339–1341, 1981.

Hajiroussou, V.J., M. Webley: Familial calcific periarthritis. Ann Rheum Dis 42:469–470, 1983.

Halverson, P.B., H.S. Cheung, D.J. McCarty, J. Garancis, N. Mandel: "Milwaukee shoulder"—association of microspheroids containing hydroxyapatite crystals, active collagenase, and neutral protease with rotator cuff defects. II. Synovial fluid studies. Arthritis Rheum 24:474–483, 1981.

Halverson, P.B., H.S. Cheung, D.J. McCarty: Enzymatic release of microspheroids containing hydroxyapatite crystals from synovium and of calcium pyrophosphate dihydrate crystals from cartilage. Ann Rheum Dis 41:527–531, 1982.

Halverson, P.B., J.C. Garancis, D.J. McCarty: Histopathological and ultrastructural studies of synovium in Milwaukee shoulder syndrome—a basic calcium phosphate crystal arthropathy. Ann Rheum Dis 43:734–741, 1984.

Hamilton, E.B.D., E.G.L. Bywaters: Joint symptoms in myelomatosis and similar conditions. Ann Rheum Dis 20:353–363, 1961.

Homma, W., A. Rütt: Die familiäre Calcinosis interstitialis. (Eine Langzeitstudie über 20 Jahre). Z Orthop 120:774–779, 1982.

Hug, I., J.M. Mihatsch: Die primäre Oxalosis. Fallmitteilung mit radiologisch–pathologisch–anatomischer Korrelation und Literaturübersicht. Fortschr Röntgenstr 123:153–162, 1975.

Jansen, H.H.: Kortikoidschäden aus pathologisch–anatomischer Sicht. Therapiewoche 17:1907–1913, 1967.

Kattapuram, S.V.: Case report 181 (calcified popliteal cyst [Baker cyst]). Skeletal Radiol 7:279–281, 1982.

Koebke, J., W. Thomas, H.J. Winter: Zur Bedeutung des Knochenspornes an der Basis des zweiten Mittelhandknochens für die Pathogenese der Daumensattelgelenksarthrose. Z Orthop 121:108–112, 1983.

Luska, G., H. Zeidler, H.St. Stender: Chondrocalcinose (Pseudogicht). Fortschr Röntgenstr 121:574–583, 1974.

Martijn, A., C.J.P. Thijn: Radiologic finding in primary hyperoxaluria. Skeletal Radiol 8:21–24, 1982.

McCarty, D.J., P.F. Pepe, S.D. Solomon, J. Cobb: Inhibition of human erythrocyte pyrophosphatase activity by calcium, cupric and ferrous ions. Arthritis Rheum 13:336, 1970.

McCarty, D.J., P.B. Halverson, G.F. Carrera, B.J. Brewer, F. Kozin: "Milwaukee shoulder"—association of microspheroids containing hydroxapatite crystals, active collagenase, and neutral protease with rotator cuff defects. I. Clinical aspects. Arthritis Rheum 24:464–473, 1981.

McKee, P.H., N.G. Liomba, M.S.R. Hutt: Tumoral calcinosis: a pathological study of fifty–six cases. Br J Dermatol 107:669–674, 1982.

Men, J., J.K. van der Korst: Calcifying supracoracoid bursitis as a cause of chronic shoulder pain. Ann Rheum Dis 43:758–759, 1984.

Meneghello, A., M. Bertoli: Tendon disease and adjacent bone erosion in dialysis patients. Br J Radiol 56:915–920, 1983.

Milazzo, S.C.: Chondrocalcinosis and other crystal induced arthropathies. Aust NZJ Med 8, Suppl I:152–154, 1978.

Nebel, G., W. Dihlmann: Ossification des Ligamentum pectineale Cooperi. Fortschr Röngenstr 131:110–111, 1979.

Neviaser, J.S.: Arthrography of the shoulder joint. Study of the findings in adhesive capsulitis of the shoulder. J Bone Joint Surg 44A:1321–1330, 1962.

Neviaser, J.S.: Adhesive capsulitis and the stiff and painful shoulder. Orthop Clin North Am 11:327–331, 1980.

Nidecker, A., H. Hartweg: Seltene Lokalisationen verkalkender Tendopathien. Fortschr Röntgenstr 139:658–662, 1983.

O'Dell, J.R., P.A. Andersen, J.R. Hollister, S.G. West: Anterior tibial mass: an unusual complication of popliteal cysts. Arthritis A Rheum 27:113–115, 1984.

Pavlov, H., M.A. Heneghan, A. Hersh, A.B. Goldman, V. Vigorita: The Haglund syndrome: initial and differential diagnosis. Radiology 144:83–88, 1982.

Petersson, C.J., C.F. Gentz: Ruptures of the supraspinatus tendon. The significance of distally pointing acromioclavicular osteophytes. Clin Orthop 174:143–148, 1983.

Phelps, P., A.D. Steele, D.J. McCarthy Jr.: Compensated polarized light microscopy. JAMA 203:166–170, 1968.

Rathbun, J.B., I. Macnab: The microvascular pattern of the rotator cuff. J Bone Joint Surg 52B:540–553, 1970.

Reichenberger, M., J. Löhnert: Osteosis cutis multiplex. Hautarzt 22:73–77, 1971.

Resnick, D., G. Niwayama: Entheses and enthesopathy. Anatomical, pathological, and radiological correlation. Radiology 146:1–9, 1983.

Richards, A.J., E.B.D. Hamilton: Destructive arthropathy in chondrocalcinosis articularis. Ann Rheum Dis 33:196–203, 1974.

Rosenbaum, L.H., J.J. Nicholas, B.S. Slasky, D.L. Obley, L.D. Ellis: Malignant myositis ossificans: occult gastric carcinoma presenting as an acute rheumatic disorder. Ann Rheum Dis 43:95–97, 1984.

Schmidt, K.L., H.W. Leber, G. Schütterle: Arthropathien bei primärer Oxalose—Kristallsynovitis oder Osteopathie? Dtsch Med Wochenschr 106:19–22, 1981.

Schreiber, S., P. Dupont: Apetite–induced acute bursitides triggered by parathyroidectomy. Clin Rheumatol 2:315–319, 1983.

Schwartz, G., T. Vischer, I. Papageorgiou, W. MacGee: A propos d'un cas de chondrocalcinose vertébrale avec tetraparésie. Rhumatol 32:247–249, 1980.

Smathers, R.L., C.B. Stelling, T.E. Keats: The destructive wrist arthropathy of pseudogout. Skeletal Radiol 7:255–258, 1982.

Stark, P., H.E. Hildebrandt–Stark: Calcific tendinitis of the piriform muscle. Fortschr Röntgenstr 138:111–112, 1983.

Thickman, D., A. Bonakdar–Pour, M. Clancy, J.V. Orden, H. Steel: Fibrodysplasia ossificans progressiva. Am J Roentgenol 139:935–941, 1982.

Tillmann, B., W. Thomas: Anatomie typischer Sehnenansätze,—ursprünge und Engpässe. Orthop Praxis 18:910–917, 1982.

Uhthoff, H.K.: Calcifying tendinitis, an active cell–mediated calcification. Virchons Arch [Pathol Anat] 366:51–58, 1975.

Uhthoff, H.K., K. Sarkar, J.A. Maynard: Calcifying tendinitis. A new concept of its pathogenesis. Clin Orthop 118:164–168, 1976.

Uhthoff, H.K., K. Sarkar, I. Hammond: Die Bedeutung der Dichte und der Schärfe der Abgrenzung des Kalkschattens bei der Tendopathia calcificans. Radiologe 22:170–174, 1982.

Vero, F., G.F. Machacek, F.H. Bartlett: Disseminated congenital osteomas of the skin with subsequent development of myositis ossificans. Report of a case in an infant. JAMA 129:728–734, 1975.

Wepfer, J.F., J.G. Reed, G.M. Cullen, W.P. McDevitt: Calcific tendinitis of the gluteus maximus tendon (gluteus maximus tendinitis). Skeletal Radiol 9:198–200, 1983.

Wolfe, M.S., E.R. North: Extravasation of injected calcium solution leading to calcifications in the upper extremity of the neonate. J Bone Joint Surg 65A:558–559, 1983.

Space-occupying processes; tumors, tumorlike lesions (including xanthoma and pigmented villonodular synovitis), their diagnosis, radiologic differential diagnosis and their complications (see also under Pachydermoperiostosis; Paraneoplastic diseases).

Adler, C.P., A. Klümper: Röntgenologische und pathologischanatomische Aspekte von Knochentumoren. Radiologe 17:355–392, 1977.

Arzimanoglu, A.: Bilateral arborescent lipoma of the knee. A case report. J Bone Jt Surg 39A:976–979, 1957.

Bloom, R., J.N. Pattinson: Osteochondromatosis of the hip joint. J Bone Jt Surg 33B:80–84, 1951.

Blümlein, H., P. Puls, H.M. Schneider, Th. Wunderlich: Benigne und maligne Gelenkchondromatose. Beitrag zur Klinik und Histologie der Erkrankung. Z Orthop 118:8–14, 1980.

Brower, A.C., J.E. Culver Jr., T.E. Keats: Diffuse cystic angiomatosis of bone. Report of two cases. Am J Roentgenol 118:456–463, 1973.

Bufkin, W.J.: The avulsive cortical irregularity. Am J Roentgenol 112:487–492, 1971.

Campbel, A.J., I.P. Wells: Pigmented villonodular synovitis of a lumbar vertebral facet joint. J Bone Joint Surg 64A:145–146, 1982.

Cayla, J., Y. Chaouat, Cl. Labrousse, F. Coste: La forme décalcificante de la chondromatose de la hanche. A propos de 3 observations. Rev Rhum 32:646–653, 1965.

Christ, F., H.D. Siemes, R. Stiens: Pelvine Knochenangiome. Fortschr Röntgenstr 140:79–83, 1984.

Denis, F., G.W.D. Armstrong: Scoliogenic osteoblastoma of the posterior end of the rib. A case report. Spine 9:74–76, 1984.

Döhler, R., H.L. Poser, D. Harms, H.R. Wiedemann: Systemic lipomatosis of bone. A case report. J Bone Joint Surg 64B:84–87, 1982.

Freyschmidt, J., D. Saure, S. Dammenhain: Der fibröse metaphysäre Defekt (fibröser Kortikalisdefekt, nicht ossifizierendes Knochenfibrom). I. Mitteilung: Untersuchung zur Häufigkeit. Fortschr Röntgenstr 134:169–177, 1981.

Freyschmidt, J., H. Ostertag, D. Saure: Der fibröse metaphysäre Defekt (fibröser Kortikalisdefekt, nicht–ossifizierendes Knochenfibrom). 2. Mitteilung: Zur Differentialdiagnose. Fortschr Röntgenstr 134:392–400, 1981.

Glass, T., A.S.E. Mills, R.E. Fechner, R. Dyer, W. Martin III, P. Armstrong: Giant-cell reparative granuloma of the hands and feet. Radiology 149:65–68, 1983.

Gmeinwieser, J., U. Gullotta, M. Reiser, Y. Saida, D. Mack: Extramedulläre Hämatopoese als Ursache paravertebraler Tumorbildungen im Thorax. Fortschr Röntgenstr 137:68–72, 1982.

Griffiths, H.J., K. Robinson, T.A. Bonfiglio: Aggressive fibromatosis. Skeletal Radiol 9:179–184, 1983.

Haacke, H., M.R. Parwaresch: Spontaneous rupture of the Achilles tendon—a sign of hyperlipoproteinaemia (HLP) type II. Klin Wochenschr 57:397–400, 1979.

Hoessly, M., R. Lagier: Anatomico–radiological study of intraosseus epidermoid cysts. Fortschr Röntgenstr 137:48–54, 1982.

Holtz, U., E. Gerstenberg: Zur Isomorphie primärer und sekundärer Knochengeschwülste im Röntgenbild. Rontgenblatter 28:553–559, 1975.

Jacobs, J.E., P. Kimmelstiel: Cystic angiomatosis of skeletal system. J Bone Joint Surg 35A:409–464, 1952.

Jonasch, E.: Das Kniegelenk. Diagnose und Therapie seiner Verletzungen und Erkrankungen. Berlin: De Gruyter, 1964.

Kissling, R., K.-G. Tan: Echinococcus cysticus im Knochen. Fortschr Röntgenstr 141:470–471, 1980.

Köster, R., H. Jansen: Generalisierte Hämangiomatose des Skeletts mit Organbefall. Fortschr Röntgenstr 134:69–74, 1981.

Lafferty, F.W.: Pseudohyperparathyreoidism. Medicine 45:247–260, 1966.

Lequesne, M., J.L. Nicolas, M. Kerboull, M. Postel: La synovite villo–nodulaire de la hanche. Étude de six cas. Int. Orthop 4:133–144, 1980.

van Linthoudt, D., R. Lagier: Calcaneal cysts. A radiological and anatomico–pathological study. Acta Orthop scand 49:310–316, 1978.

Lodwick, G.S.: Solitary malignant tumors of bone. The application of predictor variables in diagnosis. Semin Roentgenol 1:293–313, 1966.

Lyall, A.: Massive extramedullary bone–marrow formation in a case of pernicious anemia. J Pathol 41:469–472, 1935.

Madewell, J.E., B.D. Ragsdale, D.E. Sweet: Radiologic and pathologic analysis of solitary bone lesions. Part I: internal margins. Radiol Clin North Am 19:715–748, 1981.

McCarthy, E.F., T. Matsuno, H.D. Dorfman: Malignant fibrous histiocytoma of bone: a study of 35 cases. Hum Pathol 10:57–70, 1979.

McCarthy, E.F., S. Matz, G.C. Steiner, H.D. Dorfman: Periosteal ganglion: a cause of cortical bone erosion. Skeletal Radiol 10:243–246, 1983.

Melhem, R.E., T.J. Saber: Erosion of the medial cortex of the proximal humerus. A sign of leukemia on the chest radiograph. Radiology 137:77–79, 1980.

Monsees, B., W.A. Murphy: Distal phalangeal erosive lesions. Arthritis Rheum 27:449–455, 1984.

Murphy, W.A., M.J. Siegel, L.A. Gilula: Arthrography in the diagnosis of unexplained chronic hip pain with regional osteopenia. Am J Roentgenol 129:283–287, 1977.

Myers, B.W., A.T. Masi, S.L. Feigenbaum: Pigmented villonodular synovitis and tenosynovitis: a clinical epidemiologic study of 166 cases and literature review. Medicine 59:223–238, 1980.

Niederle, N., C.G. Schmidt, S. Seeber: Neurologische Krankheitsbilder bei malignen Erkrankungen. Tumor Diagn Therapie 3:61–67, 1982.

Norman, A., H.D. Dorfman: Osteoid–osteoma inducing pronounced overgrowth and deformity of bone. Clin Orthop 110:233–238, 1975.

Pelker, R.R., J.C. Drennan, M.B. Ozonoff: Juvenile synovial chondromatosis of the hip. A case report. J Bone Joint Surg 65A:552–554, 1983.

Pirschel, J.: Zur Differentialdiagnose primärer und sekundärer Sternumtumoren. Fortschr Röntgenstr 135:197–203, 1981.

Poussa, M., T. Holmström: Intraosseous lipoma of the calcaneus. Report of a case and a short review of the literature. Acta Orthop Scand 47:570–574, 1976.

Ragsdale, B.D., J.E. Madewell, D.E. Sweet: Radiologic and pathologic analysis of solitary bone lesions. Part II: periosteal reactions. Radiol Clin North Am 19:749–783, 1981.

Reiser, M., U. Gullotta, St. Feuerbach, Th. Biehl, K. Glas: Die computertomographische Diagnostik des Meniskusganglion. Fortschr Röntgenstr 133:671–672, 1980.

Salzer, M., M. Salzer–Kuntschik: Ganglien mit Knochenbeteiligung. Arch Orthop Unf Chirurgie 64:87–99, 1968.

Schabel, S.I., L. Tyminski, R.D. Holland, G.M. Rittenberg: The skeletal manifestations of chronic myelogenous leukemia. Skeletal Radiol 5:145–149, 1980.

Schäfer, H.: Das Meniskusganglion. Früherkennung durch Ausmessung standardisierter Arthrogramme. Fortschr Röntgenstr 136:505–514, 1982.

Schajowicz, F., M. Clavel Sainz, J.A. Slullitel: Juxta–articular bone cysts (intra–osseous ganglia). Clinicopathological study of eighty-eight cases. J Bone Joint Surg 61B:107–116, 1979.

Séruzier, E., J.L. Simonin, C. Ducastelle, J. Hémet., N. Biga, J.M. Thomine, P. Deshayes: Ostéome ostéoïde avec synovite a propos de deux observations. Rev Rhum 43:521–526, 1976.

Shapiro, L., C.S. Baraf: Subungual epidermoid carcinoma and keratoacanthoma. Cancer 25:141–152, 1970.

Sim, F.H., D.C. Dahlin, J.C. Ivins: Extra–articular synovial chondromatosis. J Bone Joint Surg 59A:492–495, 1977.

Stelling, C.B., W. Martin, R.E. Fechner, B.A. Alford, D.V. Strider: Case report 150 (Solitary bone cyst with cementum–like bone production) Skeletal Radiol 6:213–215, 1981.

Stoker, D.J., J. Pringle: Case report 205 (Chordoma of the mid–cervical spine) Skeletal Radiol 8:306–310, 1982.

Weitzman, G.: Lipoma arborescens of the knee. Report of a case J Bone Jt Surg 47A:1030–1033, 1965.

Trauma (major trauma, persistent trauma, fatigue trauma, traumas of the growth period; see also under Radiologic anatomy); posttraumatic and

postoperative changes (see also under Osteoar-
throsis); sympathetic reflex dystrophies.

Acquaviva, P., A. Schiano, P. Harnden, D. Cros, G. Serratrice: Les algodystrophies: terrain et facteurs pathogéniques. Résultats d'une enquête multicentrique portant sur 765 observations. Rev Rhum 49:761–766, 1982.

Albert, J., H. Ott: Three brothers with algodystrophy of the hip. Ann Rheum Dis 42:421–424, 1983.

Amor, B., F. Tallet, D. Raichvarg, B. Guenee, et al.: Algodystrophie et anomalies métaboliques. Rev Rhum 49:827–833, 1982.

Arlet, J., P. Ficat, R. Durroux, R. Girou de Gercourt: Histopathologie des lésions osseuses et cartilagineuses dans l'algodystrophie sympathique réflexe de genou. A propos de 16 observations. Rev Rhum 48:315–321, 1981.

Arlet, J., P. Ficat: Phlébographie transosseuse, pression intramédullaire et oxymetrine du sang osseux au cours des algodystrophies sympathiques réflexes. Rev Rhum 49:883–885, 1982.

Artz, T.D., J.L. Posch: The carpometacarpal boss. J Bone Joint Surg 55A:747–752, 1973.

à Wengen, H.C.: Zum Kahnbeinbruch der Hand und seine unfallmedizinische Bedeutung. Stuttgart: H. Huber, Bern, 1971, S. 1.

Borden, IV, S.: Roentgen recognition of acute plastic bowing of the forearm in children. Am J Roentgenol 125:524–530, 1975.

Cahill, B.R.: Osteolysis of the distal part of the clavicle in male athlets. J Bone Joint Surg 64A:1053–1058, 1982.

Crowe, J.E., L.E. Swischuk: Acute bowing fractures of the forearm in children: a frequently missed injury. Am J Roentgenol 128:981–984, 1977.

Curtis, D.J., E.F. Downey, Jr.: A simple first metacarpophalangeal stress test. Radiology 148:855–856, 1983.

Curtiss, P.H., Jr., W.E. Kincaid: Transitory demineralisation of the hip in pregnancy. A report of three cases. J Bone Joint Surg 41A:1327–1333, 1959.

de Carvalho, A., F. Illum, J. Jørgensen: Calcification simulating peroneus longus tendinitis. Skeletal Radiol 12:37–39, 1984.

Dengel, H.: Radiologische Untersuchungsmethoden des oberen Sprunggelenkes, insbesondere der tibio–fibularen Bandläsion. Röntgen–Ber 13:53–62, 1984.

Dihlmann, W., W. Thomas: Diagnostischer Algorithmus für die transitorische Hüftosteoporose–unter Einbeziehung der Computertomographie. Fortschr Röntgenstr 138:214–219, 1983.

Echtermeyer, V., H.J. Oestern: Kompartment–Syndrom. Ätiologie–Pathophysiologie–Lokalisation–Diagnostik–Therapie Hefte Unfallheillkd 162:75–96, 1983.

Edelstein, G., R.G. Levitt, D.P. Slaker, W.A. Murphy: Computed tomography of Tietze syndrome. J Comput Assist Tomogr 8:20–23, 1984.

Eklof, O., C. Hugosson, S. Lindham: Normal variations and posttraumatic appearances of the tuberosity of ischium in adolescence. Ann Radiol 22:77–84, 1979.

Fenton, R.L.: The naviculo–capitate fracture syndrome. J Bone Joint Surg 38A:681–684, 1956.

Frank, E.: Die traumatische Subluxation des Speichenköpfchens bei Kindern. Aktue Chir 2:21–34, 1967.

Foster, S.C., R.R. Foster: Lisfranc's tarsometatarsal fracture-dislocation. Radiology 120:79–83, 1976.

Friedman, A.P., F.T. Velcek, J.O. Haller, H. Nagar: Clavicular periostitis: an unusual complication of percutaneous subclavian venous catheterization. Radiology 148:692, 1983.

Gerlock Jr., A.J.: The flared mandible sign of the flail mandible. Radiology: 117:299–300, 1976.

Gutjahr, G.: Die Röntgendiagnostik der Schulterluxation und ihrer knöchernen Begleitverletzungen. Rontgenblatter 36:225–233, 1983.

Hackenbruch, W., B. Noesberger: Die Kapselbandläsion am Sprunggelenk. Ther Umsch 33:433–439, 1976.

Haines, J.F.: Bilateral rupture of the Achilles tendon in patients on steroid therapy. Ann Rheum Dis 42:652–654, 1983.

Harley, J.D., L.A. Mack, R.A. Winquist: CT of acetabular fractures: Comparison with conventional radiography. Am J Roentgenol 138:413–417, 1982.

Harrison, R.B., T.E. Keats, C.J. Frankel, R.L. Anderson, P. Youngblood: Radiographic clues to fractures of the unossified medial humeral condyle in young children. Skeletal Radiol 11:209–212, 1984.

Hausel, M.: Ergebnisse bei der operativen Therapie von Talusfrakturen. Krankenhausarzt 53:415–422, 1980.

Hill, H.A., M.D. Sachs: The grooved defect of the humeral head. A frequently unrecognized complication of dislocations of the shoulder joint. Radiology 35:690–700, 1940.

Hunder, G.G., P.J. Kelly: Roentgenologic transient osteoporosis of the hip. A clinical syndrome? Ann Intern Med 68:539–552, 1968.

Jend, H.H., M. Daase, M. Heller, D. Holzrichter: Zur Diagnostik von Bandverletzungen des oberen Sprunggelenks mit gedrückten Aufnahmen. Fortschr Röntgenstr 139:540–543, 1983.

Judet, R., J. Judet, E. Letournel: Fractures of the acetabulum: Classification and surgical approaches for open reduction. Preliminary report. J Bone Joint Surg 46A:1615–1646, 1675, 1964.

Lagier, R.: Posttraumatic Sudeck's dystrophy localized in the metatarso-phalangeal region. An anatomico–radiological study of a case. Fortschr Röntgenstr 138:496–499, 1983.

Lee, B.S., R. Kaplan: Turret exostosis of the phalanges. Clin Orthop 100:186–189, 1974.

Lequesne, M., B. Mauger: Cent algodystrophies décalcificantes de la hanche chez 74 malades. Rev Rhum 49:787–792, 1982.

Letournel, E.: Acetabulum fractures: classification and management. Clin Orthop 151:81–106, 1980.

Lev–Toaff, A.S., D. Karasick, V.M. Rao: "Drooping shoulder"—nontraumatic causes of glenohumeral subluxation. Skeletal Radiol 12:34–36, 1984.

Longstreth, P.L., L.R. Malinak, C.S. Hill, Jr.: Transient osteoporosis of the hip in pregnancy. Obstet Gynecol 41:563–569, 1973.

Louis, D.S., R.H. Hartwig, A.K. Poznanski: Case report 116 (carpal fusion following ischemic contracture of the forearm). Skeletal Radiol 5:127–128, 1980.

Luschnitz, E., W. Beyer: Die seltene traumatische Epiphysenlösung am Os ischii. Fortschr Röntgenstr 105:589–590, 1966.

Machan, F.G.: Die perilunäre Luxation der Hand und ihre Begleitverletzungen. Zbl Chir 104:161–170, 1979.

Marx, F., J. Kolář, J. Kácl, L. Paleček, V. Potocký: Skelettveränderungen als Folge posttraumatischer Gefäßzustände. Fortschr Röntgenstr 96:82–86, 1962.

Moss, G.D., A. Goldman, M. Sheinkop: Case report 219 (bilateral stress fractures of the distal ends of the radii). Skeletal Radiol 9:148–150, 1982.

Murphy, W.A., M.J. Siegel: Elbow fat pads with new signs and extended differential diagnosis. Radiology 124:659–665, 1977.

Murray, W.T., P.R. Meuller, D.I. Rosenthal, R.R. Jauerneck: Fracture of the hook of the hamate. Am J Roentgenol 133:899–903, 1979.

Nance, E.P., Jr., J.J. Kaye: Injuries of the quadriceps mechanism. Radiology 142:301–307, 1982.

Newberg, A., L. Wales: Radiographic diagnosis of quadriceps tendon rupture. Radiology 125:367–371, 1977.

Niethard, F.U., R. Plaue: Experimentelle Untersuchungen über die Grenzen der röntgenologischen Darstellung von Schienbeinkopfbrüchen. Fortschr Röntgenstr 125:136–140, 1976.

Ogden, J.A.: Injury to the growth mechanisms of the immature skeleton. Skeletal Radiol 6:237–253, 1981.

Plaue, R.: Die Diagnostik der lateralen Kapselbandschäden des oberen Sprunggelenkes. Arch Orthop Unf–Chir. 63:135–152, 1968.

Prager, P.J.: Differential diagnosis and radiological work–up in bilateral lateral atlantoaxial luxation. Eur J Radiol 3:309–313, 1983.

Reichen, A., R. Marti: Die frische fibulare Bandruptur—Diagnose, Therapie, Resultate. Arch Orthop Unfall–Chir 80:211–222, 1974.

Rosen, R.A.: Transitory demineralization of the femoral head. Radiology 94:509–512, 1970.

Rosenthal, D.I., A.E. Rosenberg, A.L. Schiller, R.J. Smith: Destructive arthritis due to silicone: a foreign–body reaction. Radiology 149:69–72, 1983.

Sagel, J.: Fracture of sesamoid bones. A report of two cases. Am J Surg 18:507–509, 1932.

Schild, H., H.A. Mueller, G. Schreiber: Das Halbmondzeichen bei distaler Humerusfraktur. Röntgenblätter. 34:417–420, 1981.

Schild, H., H.A. Mueller, H.J. Klotter: Transskaphoidale, transkapitale Luxationsfraktur ("Naviculo–Capitate–Fracture Syndrome")—eine seltene Handwurzel–Kombinationsverletzung. Röntgenblätter. 36:299–302, 1983.

Schild, H., H.A. Mueller, H.J. Klotter, F.P. Kuhn: Die traumatische Knochenverbiegung (sog. Bowing-Fracture)—eine besondere Skelettverletzung. Röntgenblätter. 36:241–243, 1983.

Schild, H., H. Weigand: Anatomie und Röntgenologie der normalen und verletzten Hüftpfanne. Rötgenblätter 37:228–235, 1984.

Schmitt, H.G.: Pagetoider Umbau des Knochens (Remaniement pagétoide). Fortschr Röntgenstr 87:269–270, 1957.

Seiler, H., D. Holzrichter: Zur standardisierten Diagnose der "Ligamentären Außenknöchelfrakturen". Chir Praxis 22:667–674, 1977.

Sherman, S.B., A. Greenspan, A. Norman: Osteonecrosis of the distal pole of the carpal scaphoid following fracture—a rare complication. Skeletal Radiol 9:189–191, 1983.

Smith, G.R., J.W. Loop: Radiologic classification of posterior dislocations of the hip: refinements and pitfalls. Radiology 119:569–574, 1976.

Steinbrocker, O., T.G. Argyros: The shoulder-hand syndrome: present status as a diagnostic and therapeutic entity. Med Clin North Am 42:1533–1553, 1958.

Szántó, D.: Verbreiterung des retrosternalen Weichteilschattens beim Tietze–Syndrom. Fortschr Röntgenst 139:456–457, 1983.

Telaranta, T., K.A. Solonen, K. Tallroth, J. Nickels: Bone cysts containing silicone particles in bones adjacent to a carpal silastic implant. Skeletal Radiol 10:247–249, 1983.

Tevar, J.P.: Osteoporosis transitoria (algodistrofia) de la cadera. Rev Esp Reumatol 7:24–31, 1980.

Tietze, A.: Ueber eine eigenartige Häufung von Fällen mit Dystrophie der Rippenknorpel. Berl Klin Wochenschr 58:829–831, 1921.

Vogel, H., J. Thomä, K.H. Jungbluth: Nativdiagnostik der Schultereckgelenkssprengung. Röntgenblätter 33:564–570, 1980.

Volkmann, R.: Die ischaemischen Muskellähmungen und Kontrakturen. Cbl. Chir. 8:801–803, 1981.

Weigand, H., D. Sarfert, C.H. Schweickert, H.J. Walde: Die reine traumatische Hüftluxation des Erwachsenen. Analyse von 24 nachunterschten Fällen. Unfallheillkd 81:20–27, 1978.

Müller, We.: Allgemeine Diagnostik und Soforttherapie bei Bandverletzungen am Kniegelenk. Unfallheillkd 83:389–397, 1980.

Wenger, D.R., B.T. Jeffcoat, J.A. Herring: The guarded prognosis of physeal injury in paraplegic children. J Bone Joint Surg 61A:241–246, 1980.

Weh, L., G. Dahmen, T. Gärtner, K. Pressler, O. Algermissen: Die pathogene Relevanz der Plika parapatellaris medialis. Teil 1: Korrelation klinischer und arthrographischer Befunde zur Plika parapatellaris medialis. Aktuel Rheumatol 7:238–242, 1982.

Weh, L., W. Eickhoff: Innervationsstörungen der Musculus quadriceps bei Chondropathia patellae. Eine kritische Revision des gültigen Chondropathia–Konzeptes. Z Orthop 121:171–176, 1983.

Weiner, D.S., I. Macnab: The "fabella syndrome": an update. J Pediatr Orthop 2:405–408, 1982.

Whyte, M.P., W.A. Murphy, M.D. Fallon, T.J. Hahn: Mixed–sclerosing–bone–dystrophy: report of a case and review of the literature. Skeletal Radiol 6:95–102, 1981.

Spine, including sacroiliac joints; symphysis pubis; manubriosternal synchondrosis (see also the reference relating to individual diseases, etc.).

Aufdermaur, M.: Juvenile kyphosis (Scheuermann's disease): radiography, histology, and pathogenesis. Clin Orthop 154:166–174, 1981.

Beamer, Y.B., J.T. Garner, C.H. Shelden: Hypertrophied ligamentum flavum. Clinical and surgical significance. Arch Surg 106:289–292, 1973.

Begemann, M.: Das HLA–System des Menschen. Med Klinik 77:15–23, 1982.

Brower, A.C., E.F. Downey Jr.: Kümmell disease: report of a case with serial radiographs. Radiology 141:363–364, 1981.

Bruna, J., V. Janečka: Ausgeprägte retropharyngoösophageale Abszeese. Fortschr Röntgenstr 117:33–38, 1972.

Canoso, J.J., M. Saini, J.A. Hermos: Whipple's disease and ankylosing spondylitis simultaneous occurrence in HLA–B27 positive male. J Rheumatol 5:79–84, 1978.

Chance, G.Q.: Note on a type of flexion fracture of the spine. Br J Radiol 21:452–453, 1948.

Cintron, E., L.A. Gilula, W.A. Murphy, J.A. Gehweiler: The widened disk space: A sign of cervical hyperextension injury. Radiology 141:639–644, 1981.

David–Chaussé, J., J. Dehais, M. Boyer, M.L. Darde, Y. Imbert: Les infections articulaires chez l'adulte atteintes périphériques et vertébrales a germes banals et a bacilles tuberculeux. Rev Rhum 48:69–76, 1981.

De Sèze, S., Cl. Guérin, Mme. Rameau–Vareille: Les formes pseudo–pottiques de la discarthrose lombaire. Discarthrose lombaire avec érosions pseudo–pottiques des plateaux vertébraux. Sem Hôp Paris 34:498–508, 1958.

De Sèze, S., Cl. Guérin, Mme Rameau: Les formes érosives et géodiques "pseudo–pottiques" de l'arthrose lombaire. Rev Rhum 26:161–167, 1959.

Dihlmann, W.: Hyperparathyreoidismus und Discus intervertebralis. Fortschr Röntgenstr 135:353, 1981.

Duquesnoy, B., A. Thévenon, J.L. Siame, C.L'Hermine, B. Delcambre: Phénomène du vide intravertébral: ostéonécrose vertébrale ou simple tassement ostéoporotique? A propos de quatre cas. Rev Rhum 49:35–37, 1982.

El–Khoury, G.Y., D.K. Yousefzadeh, M.H. Kathol, G.M. Mulligan: Pseudospondylolysis. Radiology 139:72, 1981.

Espinoza, L.R., F.B. Vasey, S.W. Gaylord, C. Dietz, L. Bergen, P. Bridgeford, B.F. Germain: Histocompatibility typing in the seronegative spondyloarthropathies: a survey. Semin Arthritis Rheum 11:375–381, 1982.

Feldberg, M.A.M., P.R. Koehler, P.F.G.M. van Waes: Psoas compartment disease studied by computed tomography. Analysis of 50 cases and subject review. Radiology 148:505–512, 1983.

Feldmann, J.L., C.J. Menkès, B. Amor, A. Chevrot, F. Delbarre: L'ostéonécrose vertébrale de l'adulte. A propos de 4 cas. Rev Rhum 48:773–780, 1981.

Fielding, J.W., R.N. Hensinger, R.J. Hawkins: Os odontoideum. J Bone Joint Surg 62A:376–383, 1980.

Frenay, J., N. Lambooy: Syndrome de la queue de cheval secondaire à un spondylolisthésis par atteinte lombaire basse d'une polyarthrite chronique évolutive. Neurochirurgie (Paris) 20:431–440, 1974.

Fried, K.: Die Dysspondylien: ein Beitrag zum M. Scheuermann. Radiologe 22:412–418, 1982.

Gekeler, J.: Morbus Scheuermann. Zum Krankheitsbild und Krankheitswert der Osteochondrosis spinalis adoloscentium. Dtsch Med Wochenschr 106:1585–1591, 1981.

Gerster, J.C.: Plantar fasciitis and Achilles tendinitis among 150 cases of seronegative spondarthritis. Rheumatol Rehabil 19:218–222, 1980.

Hinck, V.C., C.E. Hopkins, W.M. Clark: Sagittal diameter of the lumbar spinal in children and adults. Radiology 85:929–937, 1965.

Hukuda, S., T. Mochizuki, M. Ogata, K. Schichikawa: The pattern of spinal and extraspinal hyperostosis in patients with ossification of the posterior longitudinal ligament and the ligamentum flavum causing myelopathy. Skeletal Radiol 10:79–85, 1983.

Inoue, N., S. Motomaru, Y. Murai, Y. Tsukamoto, H. Nakata, K. Ito, M. Ijichi: Computed tomography in calcification of ligamenta flava of the cervical spine. J Comput Assist Tomogr 7:704–706, 1983.

Isu, T., H. Abe, T. Ito, et al.: Atlantoaxial dislocation in neurofibromatosis—report of three cases. Neurol Surg 10:785–791, 1982.

Jelsma, R.K., P.T. Kirsch, J.F. Rice, L.F. Jelsma: The radiographic description of thoraco–lumbar fractures. Surg Neurol 18:230–236, 1982.

Keysser, M., J. Weber: Wirbelsäulenbeteiligung bei Behçet–Syndrom (BS). Aktuel Rheumatol 9:169–171, 1984.

Khan, M.A.: Axial arthropathy in Whipple's disease. J Rheumatol 9:928–929, 1982.

Klaus, E., J. Chudáček: Zur Röntgendiagnose der Bandscheibenverkalkungen im Kindesalter. Fortschr Röntgenstr 140:200–203, 1984.

Koeger, A.C., Cl. Merlet, A. Prier, F. Mignon, J.P. Camus, Y. Le Quintrec: Manifestations articulaires de la maladie de Whipple. Un cas avec sacro–iliite et coxopathie destructrice. Sem Hôp Paris 59:1237–1241, 1983.

Koss, J.C., M.K. Dalinka: Atlantoaxial subluxation in Behçet's syndrome. Am J Roentgenol 134:392–393, 1980.

Kudo, H., K. Iwano, H. Yoshizawa: Cervical cord compression due to extradural granulation tissue in rheumatoid arthritis. J Bone Joint Surg 66B:426–430, 1984.

Kuntz, D., B. Naveau, T. Bardin, T. Drueke, R. Treves, A. Dryll: Destructive spondylarthropathy in hemodialyzed patients. A new syndrome. Arthritis Rheum. 27:369–375, 1984.

Ladd, J.R., J.T. Cassidy, W. Martel: Juvenile ankylosing spondylitis. Arthritis Rheum 14:578–590, 1971.

Lardé, D., D. Mathieu, J. Frija, A. Gaston, N. Vasile: Spinal vacuum phenomenon: CT diagnosis and significance. J Comput Assist Tomogr 6:671–676, 1982.

Lardé, D., D. Mathieu, J. Frija, A. Gaston, N. Vasile: Vertebral osteomyelitis: disk hypodensity on CT. Am J Roentgenol 139:963–967, 1982.

Larsen, J.L., D. Smith: The lumbar spinal canal in children. Part I: the sagittal diameter. Eur J Radiol 1:163–170, 1981.

Lochead, J.A., I.M. Chalmers, W.H. Marshall, B. Larsen, V.M. Skanes, R.H. Payne, J.M. Barnard: HLA–B27 haplo–types in family studies of ankylosing spondylitis. Arthritis Rheum 26:1011–1016, 1983.

Macnab, I.: The traction spur. An indicator of segmental instability. J Bone Joint Surg 53A:663–670, 1971.

Mallas, E.G., P. Mackintosh, P. Asquith, T. Cooke: Histocompatibility antigens in inflammatory bowel disease. Their clinical significance and their association with arthropathy with special reference to HLA–B27 (W27). Gut 17:906–910, 1976.

Manaster, B.J., A. Norman: CT diagnosis of thoracic pedicle aplasia. J Comput Assist Tomogr 7:1090–1091, 1983.

Markowitz, R.I., J.B. Mendel: Retropharyngeal bleeding in hemophilia. Br J Radiol 54:521–523, 1981.

Mathias, K., R. Fürmaier: Sakrokokzygeale Agenesie mit lumbaler Dysgenesie. Fortschr Röntgenstr 125:187–188, 1976.

Michel, J.L., J. Bouzat, A. Rivoal u. 4 Mitarb.: La dissection gazeuse du corps vertébral ou phénomène du vide intrasomatique vertébral. Arguments physiopathologiques. J Radiol 63:479–484, 1982.

Mironov, A., F. Ziegler: Unterschiedliche Stadien von Hyperostose der Rippenköpfchen bei Spondylosis hyperostotica. Fortschr Röntgenstr 139:416–420, 1983.

Mixter, W.J., J.S. Barr: Rupture of the intervertebral disc with involvement of the spinal sternal. N Engl J Med 211:210–215, 1934.

Moilanen, A., U. Yli–Kerrtula, A. Vilppula: Cervical spine involvements in Reiter's syndrome. Fortschr Röntgenstr 141:84–87, 1984.

Nebel, G., L. Hering, G. Lingg: Die adulte generative und senile degenerative Hyperostosis triangularis ilii. Fortschr Röntgenstr 135:478–481, 1981.

Neugebauer, H.: Spondylolisthese und Dornfortsatz. Z Orthop 12:381–388, 1960.

Pietilä, K., I. Hakasalo: Ein auf dem thorako-lumbalen Gebiet befindlicher, einen paravertebralen Abszeß simulierender Weichteilschatten. Fortschr Röntgenstr 113:248, 1970.

Prohaska, E.: Isolated sacroiliitis as monosymptomatic form of ankylosing spondylitis—a possible cause of chronic back pain. Clin Rheum Dis 3:33–37, 1984.

Quinnell, R.C., H.R. Stockdale: Flexion and extension radiography of the lumbar spine: a comparison with lumbar discography. Clin Radiol 34:405–411, 1983.

Ravichandran, G.: A radiologic sign in spondylolisthesis. Am J Roentgenol 134:113–117, 1980.

Redlund–Johnell, I.: Atlanto–occipital dislocation in rheumatoid arthritis. Acta Radiol (Stockh) 25:165–168, 1984.

Redlund–Johnell, I., H. Pettersson: Vertical dislocation of the C1 and C2 vertebrae in rheumatoid arthritis. Acta Radiol (Stockh) 25:133–141, 1984.

Resnik, C.S., L.V. Smithson, J.A. Bradshaw, I. Yaghmai: The two–eyed Scotty dog: a normal anatomic variant. Radiology 149:680, 1983.

Richter, R., P. Michels, Fr.J. Krause: Die Schambeintuberkulose und ihre Differentialdiagnose. Aktuel Rheumatol 7:126–134, 1982.

Rosenthal, R.E., W.A. Spickard, R. Markham, R.K. Rhamy: Osteomyelitis of the symphysis pubis: a separate disease from osteitis pubis. Report of three cases and review of the literature. J Bone Joint Surg 64A:123–128, 1982.

Rosner, I.A., D.E. Richter, T.L. Huettner, G.H. Kuffner, J.J. Wisnieski, C.G. Burg: Spondyloarthropathy associated with hidradenitis suppurativa and acne conglobata. Ann Intern Med 97:520–525, 1982.

Saternus, K.S.: Die Begutachtung des Schleudertraumas der Halswirbelsäule. Aktuel Traumatol 12:4–11, 1982.

Schattenkirchner, M.: Serologische und immunologische Befunde bei ankylosierender Spondylitis. Aktuel Rheumatol 7:79–81 (Sonderheft), 1982.

Schild, H., W. Menke, F.P. Kuhn: Arachnoiditis ossificans der LWS. Rontgenblatter 36:158–159, 1983.

Shahriaree, H., K. Sajadi, S.A. Rooholamini: A family with spondylolisthesis. J Bone Joint Surg 61A:1256–1258, 1979.

Skaane, P., K.J. Klott: Die peridentale Aureole (crowned odontoid process) bei der vorderen Atlantodentalarthrose. Fortschr Röntgenstr 134:62–68, 1981.

Sonnabend, D.H., T.K.F. Taylor, G.K. Chapman: Intervertebral disc calcification syndromes in children. J Bone Joint Surg 64B:25–31, 1982.

Stelling, C.B.: Anomalous attachment of the transverse process to the vertebral body: an accessory finding in congenital absence of a lumbar pedicle. Skeletal Radiol 6:47–50, 1981.

Storms, G.E.M.G., M.W.M. Kruijsen, H.J. van Beusekom, et al.: Pathological fracture of the odontoid process in rheumatoid arthritis. Neth J Med 23:120–122, 1980.

Strohmeyer, G., M. Buñata: Medikamentös bedingte Fluorose. Z Rheumatol 40:138–141, 1981.

Tena, X., R. Rodriguez, T. Perez, J. Ballina, A. Rodriguez: L'hyperostose sternale. Rev Rhum 50:554–555, 1983.

Vilppula, A.H., T.U.A. Jussila, A.M.L. Kokko: Atlanto–axial dislocation in an 18–year–old female with yersinia arthritis. Clin Rheumatol 3:239–241, 1984.

Vogelsang, H., H. Deutschmann: Ausgedehnte meningeale Verkalkung im Thorakalbereich bei tuberkulöser Meningitis adhaesiva. Fortschr Röntgenstr 136:611–612, 1982.

Weir, D.C.: Roentgenographic signs of cervical injury. Clin Orthop 109:9–17, 1975.

Westermark, N., G. Forssman: The röntgen diagnosis of tuberculous spondylitis. Acta Radiol 19:207–214, 1938.

Wiltse, L.L., R.B. Winter: Terminology and measurement of spondylolisthesis. J Bone Joint Surg 65A:768–772, 1983.

Winfield, J., D. Cooke, A.S. Brook, M. Corbett: A prospective study of the radiological changes in the cervical spine in early rheumatoid disease. Ann Rheum Dis 40:109–114, 1981.

Wiseman, M.J.: Dislocation of the manubriosternal joint in rheumatoid arthritis. Ann Rheum Dis 40:307–308, 1981.

Wright, V., J.M.H. Moll: Seronegative polyarthritis. Amsterdam: North–Holland Publ. Comp., Oxford 1976.

Yazici, H., M. Tuzlaci, S. Yurdakul: A controlled survey of sacroiliitis in Behçet's disease. Ann Rheum Dis 40:558–559, 1981.

Ziza, J.M., J.P. Bouvet, L. Auquier: Cervicalgie aigue sous–occipitale d'origine calcique. Rev Rhum 49:549–551, 1982.

Bibliography

Anatomy, radiologic anatomy (see also under Trauma); methodology of taking radiograms; roentgenometry (see also under Variants of normal).

Ahlbäck, S.: Osteoarthrosis of the knee. A radiographic investigation. Acta radiol. (Stockh.), Suppl. 277 (1968)

Andrén, L., S. von Rosen: The diagnosis of dislocation of the hip in newborns and the primary results of immediate treatment. Acta radiol. (Stockh.) 49 (1958) 89-95

Bessler, W., M. E. Müller: Zur Röntgendiagnose der Coxa valga und Coxa vara. Radiol. clin. (Basel) 32 (1963) 538–548

Bledsoe, R. C., J. L. Izenstark: Displacement of fat pads in disease and injury of the elbow. A new radiographic sign. Radiology 73 (1959) 717–724

Bloom R. A.: The metacarpal sign. Brit. J. Radiol. 43 (1970) 133–135

Clementschitsch, F.: Mitteilung einer symmetrischen Aufnahme beider Kiefergelenke in posterior-anteriorer Richtung. Z. Stomat. 39 (1941) 817–822

Edinger, A., H. Gajewski, H. Gepp: Röntgen-Ganzaufnahmen der Wirbelsäule. Fortschr. Röntgenstr. 84 (1956) 365–371

Fassbender, C. W., E. Hipp, E. A. Hühn: Klinische Gesichtspunkte zur Bedeutung und zur Technik nuklearmedizinischer Methoden bei Hüftkopfnekrosen. Z. Orthop. 107 (1969) 75–93

Ficat, P.: Pathologie fémoro-patellaire. Masson, Paris 1970.

Fick, R.: Hdb. der Anatomie und Mechanik der Gelenke unter Berücksichtigung der bewegenden Muskeln. I. Teil. Fischer, Jena 1904

Fredensborg, N., B. E. Nilsson: The joint space in normal hip radiographs. Radiology 126 (1978) 325–326

Frommhold, W., W. Hielscher: Röntgenkinematographische Studien zur Form der Kondylenbahn des Kiefergelenkes. Fortschr. Röntgenstr. 96 (1962) 103-108

Göb, A.: Die Diagnostik von Verletzungsfolgen und Entwicklungsstörungen am hinteren Pfannendach. Z. Orthop. 89 (1958) 528-540

Grashey, R., R. Birkner: Atlas typischer Röntgenbilder vom normalen Menschen. Mit Berücksichtigung der Varietäten und Fehlerquellen sowie der Aufnahmetechnik, 10. Aufl. Urban & Schwarzenberg, München 1964

Grote, R., H. Elgeti, D. Saure: Bestimmung des Antetorsionswinkels am Femur mit der axialen Computertomographie. Röntgen-Blätter 33 (1980) 31–42.

Haage, H.: Die Arthrographie des Handgelenkes. I. Radiologe 6 (1966) 50–57

Hall, F. M.: Radiographic diagnosis and accuracy in knee joint effusions. Radiology 115 (1975) 49–54

Hart, V. L., V. Gaynor: Roentgenographic study of the carpal canal. J. Bone Jt Surg. 23 (1941) 382-383

Heuser, H.: Über die Erkrankungen des Kiefergelenkes im Röntgenbild. Dtsch. zahnärztl. Z. 18 (1963) 1407-1415

Hilgenreiner, H.: Zur Frühdiagnose und Frühbehandlung der angeborenen Hüftgelenkverrenkung. Med. Klin. 21 (1925) 1385–1389, 1425–1429

Hipp, E.: Die Gefäße des Hüftkopfes. Anatomie, Angiographie und Klinik. Enke, Stuttgart 1962

Holmgren, B. S.: Flüssiges Fett im Kniegelenk nach Trauma. Acta radiol. (Stockh.) 23 (1942) 131–137

Hördegen, K. M.: Technik und Indikationen gehaltener Röntgenaufnahmen von Gelenken in der Unfallpraxis. Röntgenpraxis 23 (1970) 221–236

Imhäuser, G.: Die physiologische intrapelvine Vorragung des Hüftpfannenbodens. (Ein Beitrag zur Entwicklung des Hüftgelenkes). Z. Orthop. 81 (1952) 161–179

Insall, J., E. Salvati: Patella position in the normal knee joint. Radiology 101 (1971) 101–104

Kalman, M. A.: Radiologic soft tissue shadows in the pelvis: Another look. Amer. J. Roentgenol. 130 (1978) 493–498

Kessler, I., Z. Silberman: An experimental study of the radiocarpal joint by arthrography. Surg. Gynec. Obstet. 112 (1961) 33–40

Köhnle, H.: Röntgenstereoverfahren. In: Handbuch der medizinischen Radiologie, Bd. III, hrsg. von L. Diethelm, O. Olsson, F. Strnad, H. Vieten, A. Zuppinger. Springer, Berlin 1967 (S. 220–361)

Kölbel, R., G. Bergmann, A. Rohlmann: Eine Röntgenaufnahmetechnik zur reproduzierbaren Darstellung des femoropatellaren Gleitlagers (FPG). Z. Orthop. 117 (1979) 60–66

Kopits, E.: Ein sicheres Verfahren zur Frühdiagnose der angeborenen Hüftverrenkung. Z. Orthop. 69 (1939) 167-173

Lange, F.: Die Diagnose der Coxa vara und Coxa valga. Z. orthop. Chir. 41 (1921) 135–146

Leach, R. E., T. Gregg, F. J. Siber: Weight-bearing radiography in osteoarthritis of the knee. Radiology 97 (1970) 265–268

Lequesne, M.: Die Erkrankungen des Hüftgelenkes beim Erwachsenen. I. Bau, Funktion und Untersuchung des Hüftgelenkes. Fol. Rheum. 17 a (J. R. Geigy, Basel) (1967)

Lusskin, R.: Curves and angles. A comparison of scoliosis measurement. Clin. Orthop. 23 (1962) 232–235

McMaster, M.: The natural history of the rheumatoid metacarpophalangeal joint. J. Bone Jt Surg. 54 B (1972) 687–697

Melzer, E.: Röntgenologische Untersuchungstechnik und Diagnostik der kindlichen Hüfte. Röntgen-Bl. 30 (1977) 91–96

Müller, M. E.: Die hüftnahen Femurosteotomien unter Berücksichtigung der Form, Funktion und Beanspruchung des Hüftgelenkes, 2. Aufl. Thieme, Stuttgart 1971

Papadopulos, J. S., G. L. Malahias: Hüftgelenkspaltbreite: Ist der Seitenvergleich für Diagnostik auswertbar? Arch. orthop. Unfall-Chir. 77 (1973) 44–51

Peic, St.: Die Köhlersche Tränenfigur und ihre Bedeutung in der Röntgendiagnostik. Fortschr. Röntgenstr. 114 (1971) 305–316

Pipkin, G.: Lesions of the suprapatellar plica. J. Bone Jt Surg. 32 A (1950) 363–369

Raspe, R.: Ein neues Verfahren zur Herstellung von Röntgen-Ganzaufnahmen der Wirbelsäule (,,3-Phasen-Technik"). Fortschr. Röntgenstr. 85 (1956) 106–110

Rau, W. S., G. Kauffmann: Röntgendiagnostik des Knorpelschadens am Kniegelenk. Radiologe 18 (1978) 451–458

Rau, W. S., II.-J. Hehne, M. Schlageter: Die Chondromalacia patellae - Arthrographische Beobachtungen zur Genese und Diagnose. Fortschr. Röntgenstr. 130 (1979) 644–652

Ravelli, A.: Anatomisch-röntgenologische Handgelenkstudien. Z. Orthop. 86 (1955) 70–89

Rippstein, J.: Zur Bestimmung der Antetorsion des Schenkelhalses mittels 2 Röntgenaufnahmen. Z. Orthop. 86 (1955) 345–360

Saxer, U.: Femurschaftfrakturen. In: Die Frakturbehandlung bei Kindern und Jugendlichen, hrsg. von B. G. Weber, Ch. Brunner, F. Freuler. Springer, Berlin 1978 (S. 272-297)

Schinz, H. R., W. E. Baensch, W. Frommhold, R. Glauner, E. Uehlinger, J. Wellauer: Lehrbuch der Röntgendiagnostik, 6. Aufl. Bd. I. Thieme, Stuttgart 1965

Schwetlick, W.: Die kindliche Luxationshüfte. Diagnose und Therapie. Arthrographisch-röntgenkinematographische Untersuchungen, 2. Aufl. Enke, Stuttgart 1976

Slater, S.: An evaluation of the metacarpal sign (short fourth metacarpal). Pediatrics 46 (1970) 468–471

Swischuk, L. E.: Anterior displacement of C2 in children: Physiologic or pathologic? A helpful differentiating line. Radiology 122 (1977) 759–763

Terry jr., D. W., J. E. Ramin: The navicular fat stripe. A useful roentgen feature for evaluating wrist trauma. Amer. J. Roentgenol. 124 (1975) 25–28

Titze, A.: Zur Diagnostik der Seitenbandverletzungen des Kniegelenkes. Fortschr. Röntgenstr. 85 (1956) 257–258

Tönnis, D., D. Brunken: Eine Abgrenzung normaler und pathologischer Hüftpfannendachwinkel zur Diagnose der Hüftdysplasie. Auswertungen von 2294 Pfannendachwinkeln kindlicher Hüftgelenke. Arch. Orthop. Unfal-Chir. 64 (1968) 197–228

Trueta, J., M. H. M. Harrison: The normal vascular anatomy of the femoral head in adult man. J. Bone Jt Surg. 35 B (1953) 442–461

Urist, M. R.: Fracture-dislocation of the hip joint. The nature of the traumatic lesion, treatment, late complications, and end results. J. Bone Jt Surg. 30 A (1948) 699–727

Weston, W. J.: The extrasynovial and capsular fat pads on the posterior aspect of the knee joint. Brit. J. Radiol. 44 (1971) 277–283

Wilhelm, M.: Röntgendiagnostik zur Begutachtung von Verletzungsfolgen, Entwicklungsstörungen und Arthrosen des Hüftgelenks. Röntgen-Bl. 26 (1973) 537–543

Willich, E., M. Englert: Das Metakarpalzeichen. Fortschr. Röntgenstr. 119 (1973) 443–450

Wolf, H.G.: Röntgendiagnostik beim Neugeborenen und Säugling. Maudrich, Wien 1959

Zeitler, E.: Praxis der röntgenologischen Wirbelsäulen-Funktionsdiagnostik. Röntgen- u. Lab.-Prax. 14 (1961) 81–92

Zeitler, E., H. Dietz: Röntgenologische Funktionsdiagnostik der Lendenwirbelsäule und ihre Leistungsfähigkeit bei der Diagnose und Lokalisation lumbaler Bandscheibenhernien. Fortschr. Röntgenstr. 102 (1965) 489–501

Zsernaviczky, J.: Zur Röntgendiagnostik der sogenannten angeborenen Hüftluxation. Z. Orthop. 111 (1973) 914–919

Zsernaviczky, J., G. Türk: Über ein neues Röntgenzeichen in der Frühdiagnostik der kongenitalen Hüftdysplasie. Z. Orthop. 112 (1974) 460–465

Zsernaviczky, J., G. Türk: Der β-Winkel. Ein diagnostisches Zeichen für Frühdiagnose der angeborenen Hüftdysplasie. Fortschr. Röntgenstr. 123 (1975) 131–133

Variants of normal; variants, deformities, and their causes and sequelae visible in the roentgenogram (see also under Osteoarthrosis); local and systemic (constitutional) malformations; congenital disorders of bone structure (see also under Roentgenometry; Inflammation).

Ablow, R. C., Y. E. Hsia, I. K. Brandt: Acrodysostosis coinciding with pseudohypoparathyroidism and pseudo-pseudohypoparathyroidism. Amer. J. Roentgenol. 128 (1977) 95–99

Afshani, E., B. R. Girdany: Atlanto-axial dislocation in chondrodysplasia punctata. Report of the findings in two brothers. Radiology 102 (1972) 399-401

Albright, F., C. H. Burnett, P. H. Smith, W. Parson: Pseudohypoparathyroidism - an example of „Seabright-Bantam syndrome". Report of three cases. Endocrinology 30 (1942) 922-932

Andrén, L., G. Theander: Tarsoid and gonoid malformations of upper limbs. Radiologe 15 (1975) 53–58

Ankerhold, J.: Der Scheibenmeniskus. Chir. Praxis 15 (1971) 413–419

Arndt, J.: Grundlagen zur Röntgenmorphologie des Erwachsenenkniegelenks. VEB Fischer, Jena 1965 (S. 1–107)

Bathfield, C. A., P. H. Beighton: Blount disease. A review of etiological factors in 110 patients. Clin. Orthop. 135 (1978) 29–33

Bauer, R.: Die möglichen Ursachen der dorsalen Cuneiforme-„Exostose". Arch. orthop. Unfall-Chir. 63 (1968) 29–37

Baumgartl, F.: Das Kniegelenk. Erkrankungen, Verletzungen und ihre Behandlung mit Hinweisen für die Begutachtung. Springer, Berlin 1964

Becker, M. H., P. J. Coccaro, J. M. Converse: Antegonial notching of the mandible: An often overlooked mandibular deformity in congenital and acquired disorders. Radiology 121 (1976) 149–151

Beighton, P., J. Craig: Atlanto-axial subluxation in the Morquio syndrome. Report of a case. J. Bone Jt Surg. 55 B (1973) 478–481

Bergstrand, I., O. Norman: Die Krankheiten des Hüftgelenks im Kindesalter. Radiologe I (1961) 76–89

Bjerkreim, I.: Secondary dysplasia and osteoarthrosis of the hip joint in functional and in fixed obliquity of the pelvis. Acta orthop. scand. 45 (1974) 873–882

Blount, W. P.: Tibia vara. Osteochondrosis deformans tibiae. J. Bone Jt Surg. 29 (1937) 1–29

Brill, C. B., J. S. Rose, L. Godmilow, S. Sklower, K. Hirschhorn: Spastic quadriparesis due to C1-C2 subluxation in Hurler syndrome. J. Pediat. 92 (1978) 441–443

Cattell, H. S., D. L. Filtzer: Pseudosubluxation and other normal variations in the cervical spine in children. A study of one hundred and sixty children. J. Bone Jt Surg. 47 A (1965) 1295–1309

Cigtay, O. S., V. J. Mascatello: Scapular defects: A normal variation. Amer. J. Roentgenol. 132 (1979) 239–241

Cleveland, R. H., V. Gilsanz, R. H. Wilkinson: Congenital pseudarthrosis of the radius. Amer. J. Roentgenol. 130 (1978) 955–957

Cockshott, W. P.: The coracoclavicular joint. Radiology 131 (1979) 313–316

Conway, J. J., H. R. Cowell: Tarsal coalition: Clinical significance and roentgenographic demonstration. Radiology 92 (1969) 799–811

De Cuveland, E.: Zur Differentialdiagnose inkonstanter Skelettelemente der Hand. Fortschr. Röntgenstr. 83 (1955) 847–849

Diller, W., G. Lamoth: Carpaltunnelsyndrom durch atypisches Knochenelement. Fortschr. Röntgenstr. 105 (1966) 123–124

Dörr, W. M.: Hüftdysplasie. Therapiewoche 19 (1969) 797–801

Dörr, W. M.: Funktionelle und konservative Behandlungsverfahren der sog. angeborenen Hüftluxation. Orthop. Prax. 6 (1970) 111-116

Dörr, W. M.: Zur Gelenkkontrastdarstellung der sogenannten „angeborenen Hüftluxation". Die Abgrenzung der echten Luxation von den übrigen Luxationsstufen, insbesondere von der „Forme intermédiaire". In: Verhandlungen der Deutschen Orthopädischen Gesselschaft, 57. Kongreß. Enke, Stuttgart 1971 (S. 167-169)

Doub, H. P., F. A. Henny: Radiological study of the temporomandibular joints. Radiology 60 (1953) 666–674

Dume, Th., W. Schulte-Brinkmann, A. Sturm jr.: Osteopoikilie mit Hyperostose. Dtsch. med. Wschr. 96 (1971) 422–428

Dunnick, N. R., G. L. Head, G. L. Peck, F. W. Yoder: Nevoid basal cell carcinoma syndrome: Radiographic manifestations including cystlike lesions of the phalanges. Radiology 127 (1978) 331–334

Dykes, R. G.: Kirner's deformity of the little finger. J. Bone Jt Surg. 60 B (1978) 58–60

٭b, K.: Über das Vorkommen freier und gestielter Knochenkörper in der Fossa olecrani und ihre Beziehungen zum Foramen supratrochleare. Arch. klin. Chir. 185 (1936) 482–492

Fendel, H.: Rolle der Hand bei Skeletdysplasien. Radiologe 16 (1976) 273–277

Freyer, B.: Beobachtung einer Fabella im medialen Gastroknemiuskopf. Fortschr. Röntgenstr. 92 (1960) 469–470

Gelberman, R. H., P. B. Salamon, J. M. Jurist, J. L. Posch: Ulnar variance in Kienböck's disease. J. Bone Jt Surg. 57 A (1975) 674–676

Glass, R. S., W. M. Barnes, D. U. Kells, S. Thomas, C. Campbell: Ossicles of knee menisci. Report of seven cases. Clin. Orthop. 111 (1975) 163–171

Goldman, A.B., T. Hallel, E. M. Salvati, R. H. Freiberger: Osteochondritis dissecans complicating Legg-Perthes disease. A report of four cases. Radiology 121 (1976) 561–566

Goldman, A. B., R. Schneider, W. Martel: Acute chondrolysis complicating slipped capital femoral epiphysis. Amer. J. Roentgenol. 130 (1978) 945–950

Gross, F., H. Hainke, Kh. Idelberger: Die Antetorsion des coxalen Femurendes bei ausschließlich funktioneller Behandlung der Hüftdysplasie. Arch. Orthop. Unfall-Chir. 65 (1969) 293-312

Harrison, R. B., M. B. Wood, T. E. Keats: The grooves of the distal articular surface of the femur—a normal variant. Amer. J. Roentgenol. 126 (1976) 751–754

Heidenblut, A.: Doppelseitig persistierender Schaltknochen am hinteren Rand des Acetabulum (Os acetabuli posterius bilaterale). Fortschr. Röntgenstr. 99 (1963) 109–111

Heim, M., H. Roux, J. L. San Marco, Ph. Vague, R. Simonin: Un nouveau cas de chéiroarthropathie au cours du diabète juvénile. Rev. franç. Endocr. 17 (1976) 403–405

Henssge, J.: Fuß und Fußgelenke. In: Handbuch der medizinischen Radiologie, Bd. IV/2, hrsg. von L. Diethelm, O. Olsson, F. Strnad, H. Vieten, A. Zuppinger. Springer, Berlin 1968 (S. 546–638)

Henssge, J.: Diskussionsbemerkung zur Arbeit von J. Steinhäuser: ,,Weitere Beobachtungen kugelförmiger Knöchelgelenke bei angeborenen Fußwurzelsynostosen", Z. Orthop. 112 (1974) 433. Z. Orthop. 113 (1975) 426–427

Hofer, H.: Morbus Perthes. I. Ätiologie und Klinik. Chir. Praxis 17 (1973) 265–278

Hoffa, A.: Die angeborene Coxa vara. Dtsch. med. Wschr. 31 (1905) 1257–1260

Höffken, W.: Eine Varietät Ulna und ihre Täuschungsmöglichkeit. Fortschr. Röntgenstr. 76 (1952) 259–260

Hopf.: Die angeborenen Veränderungen des Unterarmes und der Hand. In: Handbuch der Orthopädie, Bd. III, hrsg. von G. Hohmann, M. Hackenbroch, K. Lindemann. Thieme, Stuttgart 1959 (S. 419–506)

Houston, C. S.: The radiologist's opportunity to teach bone dynamics. J. Canad. Ass. Radiol. 29 (1978) 232–238

Hultén, O.: Über anatomische Variationen der Handgelenkknochen. Ein Beitrag zur Kenntnis der Genese zwei verschiedener Mondbeinveränderungen. Acta radiol. (Stockh.) 9 (1928) 155–168

Imhäuser, G.: Zur Pathogenese und Therapie der Jugendlichen Hüftkopflösung. Z. Orthop. 88 (1957) 4–41

Imhäuser, G.: Die Jugendliche Hüftkopflösung bei steilem Schenkelhals. Z. Orthop. 91 (1959) 403–413

Imhäuser, G.: Frühdiagnose und Frühbehandlung der jugendlichen Hüftkopflösung. Therapiewoche 19 (1969) 810–813

Imhäuser, G.: Kugelförmige Knöchelgelenke bei angeborenen Fu wurzelsynostosen. Beitrag zur Form-Funktions-Beziehung. Z. Orthop. 108 (1970) 247–258

Jack, E. A.: Bone anomalies of the tarsus in relation to ,,peroneal spastic flat foot". J. Bone Jt Surg. 36 B (1954) 530–542

Jackson, D.: Acquired vertical talus due to burn contractures. A report of two cases. J. Bone Jt Surg. 60 B (1978) 215–218

Johanning, K.: Coxa vara infantum. I. Clinical appearance and aetiological problems. Acta orthop. scand. 21 (1951/52) 273–299

Jonasch, E.: 12 Fälle von Osteopoikilie. Fortschr. Röntgenstr. 82 (1955) 344–353

Jost, R., E. Straub: Pseudohypoparathyreoidismus. Eine Übersicht zur Differentialdiagnose aus Anlaß einer eigenen Beobachtung. Mschr. Kinderheilk. 120 (1972) 319–324

Kamhi, E., G. D. MacEwen: Osteochondritis dissecans in Legg-Calvé-Perthes disease. J. Bone Jt. Surg. 57 A (1975) 506–509

Katz, J. F., R. S. Siffert: Skeletal maturity in Legg-Calvé-Perthes disease. Determination based on bone age of carpal centres. Int. Orthop. (SICOT) 1 (1977) 227–230

Keats, T. E., R. B. Harrison: Hypertrophy of the talar beak. Skelet. Radiol. 4 (1979) 37–39

Kemp, H. S., J. L. Boldero: Radiological changes in Perthes' disease. Brit. J. Radiol. 39 (1966) 744–760

Kemp, H. B. S., J. A. Cholmeley, J. K. Baijens: Recurrent Perthes' disease. Brit. J. Radiol. 44 (1971) 675–681

Kessel, L., M. Rang: Supracondylar spur of the humerus. J. Bone Jt Surg. 48 B (1966) 765–769

Kirner, J.: Doppelseitige Verkrümmungen des Kleinfingerendgliedes als selbständiges Krankheitsbild. Fortschr. Röntgenstr. 36 (1927) 804–806

Kleinsorge, H., E. Böttger: Das Gorlin-Cohen-Syndrom (frontometaphysäre Dysplasie). Fortschr. Röntgenstr. 127 (1977) 451–458

Klippel, M., T. Trenaunay: Du noevus variqueux ostéo-hypertrophique. Arch. gén. Méd. 3 (1900) 641-672

Klümper, A., H. Wendt, S. Weller, E. Plötner: Entwicklung einer Melorheostose. Fortschr. Röntgenstr. 103 (1965) 572–583

Kolb, F. O., H. L. Steinbach: Pseudohypoparathyroidism with secondary hyperparathyroidism and osteitis fibrosa. J. clin. Endocr. 22 (1962) 59–70

Kopits, S. E., M. N. Perovic, V. McKusick, R. A. Robinson, J. A. Bailey III: Congenital atlantoaxial dislocations in various forms of dwarfism. J. Bone Jt Surg. 54 A (1972) 1349–1350

Kossoff, J., A. Naimark, M. Corbett: Case report 85 (meniscus ossicles). Skelet. Radiol. 4 (1979) 45–46

Kozlowski, K., E. Rupprecht: Klinik und Röntgenbild der Osteochondrodysplasien und Mukopolysaccharidosen. Akademie-Verlag, Berlin 1972

Langenskiöld, A., E. B. Riska: Tibia vara (osteochondrosis deformans tibiae). A survey of seventy-one cases. J. Bont Jt Surg. 46 (1964) 1405–1420

Larson, E. H., J. Reimann: Calvé Perthes disease. Acta orthop. scand. 44 (1973) 426–438

Leeds, N. E.: Epiphyseal dysplasia multiplex. Amer. J. Roentgenol. 84 (1960) 506–510

Legg, A. T.: An obscure affection of the hip-joint. Boston med. surg. J. 162 (1910) 202–204

Leszczyński, St.: Radiologische Untersuchungen in Fällen von Turner-Syndrom. Ergebnisse von 32 Beobachtungen. Fortschr. Röntgenstr. 97 (1962) 200–212

Levinson, E. D., M. B. Ozonoff, P. M. Royen: Proximal femoral focal deficiency (PFFD). Radiology 125 (1977) 197–203

Lindemann, K.: Das erbliche Vorkommen der angeborenen Coxa vara. Z. Orthop. 72 (1941) 326–352

Lindemann, K.: Zur Morphologie der Coxa vara congenita. Z. Orthop. 78 (1949) 47–62

Lockitch, G., S. A. Fellingham, C. D. Elphinstone: Mseleni joint disease: A radiological study of two affected families. S. Afr. med. J. 47 (1973) 2366–2376

Maroteaux, P., M. Lamy, J. Bernard: La dysplasie spondylo-epiphysaire tardive. Description clinique et radiologique. Presse méd. 65 (1957) 1205–1208

Mau, H.: Wesen und Bedeutung der enchondralen Dysostosen. Thieme, Stuttgart 1958

von Mauch, O.: Schaltknochen im Akromio-Klavikulargelenk. Fortschr. Röntgenstr. 83 (1955) 733

Meythaler, K., G. L. Bach: Das Os styloides ulnae. Unter besonderer Berücksichtigung der chronischen Polyarthritis. Eular, Basel 1979

Mickelson, M. R., G. Y. El-Khoury, J. R. Cass, K. J. Case: Aseptic necrosis following slipped capital femoral epiphysis. Skelet. Radiol. 4 (1979) 129–133

von Muralt, R. H.: Supinationsbehinderung des Vorderarms. Fortschr. Röntgenstr. 81 (1954) 497–503

Murray, R. O., J. McCredie: Melorheostosis and the sclerotomes: A radiological correlation. Skelet. Radiol. 4 (1979) 57–71

Nebel, G., G. Lingg: Sind die Formvarianten der Patella nach Wiberg Präarthrosen? Radiologe 21 (1981) 101–103

Ortolani, M.: Frühdiagnose und Frühbehandlung der angeborenen Hüftgelenksverrenkung. Kinderärztl. Prax. 19 (1951) 404–407

Otte, P.: Das Wesen der Perthesschen Erkrankung unter besonderer Berücksichtigung der Pathogenese und des röntgenologischen Bildes. Verhandlungen der Deutschen Orthopädischen Gesellschaft, 54. Kongreß. Enke, Stuttgart 1968 (S. 140–158)

Otte, P., H. A. Seybold: Die Rolle der Coxa Valga als präarthrotischer Faktor. Z. Orthop. 112 (1974) 597–599

Papadopulos, J. S.: Osteolytische Druckdefekte am Schenkelhals und Hüftkopfkern bei extremer Spreizbehandlung. Z. Orthop. 110 (1972) 182–186

Passarge, E., U. Wendel, W. Wöhler, H. W. Rüdiger: Krankheiten infolge genetischer Defekte im lysosomalen Mucopolysaccharid-Abbau. Die Mucopolysaccharid-Speicherkrankheiten. Dtsch. med. Wschr. 99 (1974) 144-158

Ponseti, I.V.: Legg-Perthes' disease. Observation on pathological changes in two cases. J. Bone Jt Surg. 38 A (1956) 739–750

Poznanski, A. K., E. A. Werder, A. Giedion: The pattern of shortening of the bones of the hand in PHP and PPHP - a comparison with brachydactyly E, Turner syndrome, and acrodysostosis. Radiology 123 (1977) 707–718

Psenner, L., E. Schönbauer: Das Krankheitsbild der tuberösen Sklerose mit besonderer Berücksichtigung der röntgenologischen Symptomatik. Fortschr. Röntgenstr. 89 (1958) 301–318

Ravelli, A.: Über eine eigenartige Form des sternalen Schlüsselbeinendes (,,Fischmaulform"). Fortschr. Röntgenstr. 82 (1955) 827–828

Ravelli, A.: Persistierende Apophyse am Proc. coracoides. Fortschr. Röntgenstr. 84 (1956) 500–502

Ribbing, S.: Hereditäre multiple Epiphysenstörungen und Osteochondrosis dissecans. Acta radiol. (Stockh.) 36 (1951) 397–404

Richin, P. F., A. Kranik, L. van Herpe, S. L. Suffecool: Congenital pseudarthrosis of both bones of the forearm. J. Bone Jt Surg. 58 A (1976) 1032-1033

Robichon, J., J. P. Desjardins, M. Koch, C. E. Hooper: The femoral neck in Legg-Perthes' disease. Its relationship to epiphysial change and its importance in early prognosis. J. Bone Jt Surg. 56 B (1974) 62–68

Rompe, G.: Die Arthrogryposis multiplex congenita und ihre Differentialdiagnose. Thieme, Stuttgart 1968

Rosenbloom, A. L., J. L. Frias: Diabetes mellitus, short stature and joint stiffness - a new syndrome. Clin. Res. 22 (1974) 92

Rossak, K., K. Parsch, K.-P. Schulitz: Die Behandlung der Hüftgelenksluxation bei Myelomeningocelen. Arch. orthop. Unfall-Chir. 67 (1970) 199–210

Rubin, P.: On organizing a dynamic classification of bone dysplasias. Arthr. and Rheum. 7 (1964) 693–708

Rubinstein, H. M.: Thiemann's disease. A brief reminder. Arthr. and Rheum. 18 (1975) 357–360

Ruiz-Torres, A., M. Ali, H.-J. Merker, J. Schneider, R.-D. Staud: Zur Frage der Arthrogryposis multiplex. Med. Klinik 71 (1976) 2243–2247

Schaaf, J., A. Wagner, G. Schwarz: Röntgenuntersuchungen bei Patienten mit Pseudohypoparathyreoidismus und Pseudo-Pseudohypoparathyreoidismus. I. Röntgensymptome. Forschr. Röntgenstr. 105 (1966) 877–886

Schlegel, K. F.: Hackenfuß beim Neugeborenen. Dtsch. med. Wschr. 97 (1972) 1572

Schmidt, H., S. Braun: Zur Ätiologie des Pfannenrandknochens am Hüftgelenk (Os ad acetabulum). Med. Welt 1961, 1843–1847

Schuster, W.: Verdacht auf angeborene Skeletdysplasie. Welche Skeletteile sollen geröntgt werden? Radiologe 16 (1976) 270–272

Schwarz, G.: Pseudohypoparathyreoidismus. In: Nebenschilddrüse und endokrine Regulationen des Calciumstoffwechsels. Spontan-Hypoglykämie. Glucagon, hrsg. von J. Kracht. Springer, Berlin 1968 (S. 45–50)

Smith, J. L., F. R. Stowe: The Pierre Robin syndrome (glossoptosis, micrognathia, cleft palate). A review of 39 cases with emphasis on associated ocular lesions. Pediatrics 27 (1961) 128–133

Spech, H. J., A. J. Olah: Symptome und neuere Befunde beim Pseudohypoparathyreoidismus. Med. Klin. 69 (1974) 387–394

Spranger, J.: Internationale Nomenklatur konstitutioneller Knochenerkrankungen. (Die Pariser Nomenklatur). Fortschr. Röntgenstr. 115 (1971) 283–287

Spranger, J.: Generalisierte Skeletdysplasien, Nosologie, Häufigkeit und praktische Bedeutung. Radiologe 16 (1976a) 257–261

Spranger, J. W., H.-R. Wiedemann: The genetic mucolipidoses. Diagnosis and differential diagnosis. Humangenetik 9 (1970) 113–139

Spranger, J. W., L. O. Langer jr., H.-R. Wiedemann: Bone dysplasias. An atlas of constitutional disorders of skeletal development. Fischer, Stuttgart 1974

Srivastava, K. K., V. L. Kochhar: Congenital absence of the carpal scaphoid. A case report. J. Bone Jt Surg. 54 A (1972) 1782

Stögmann, W., W. Oser: Das röntgenologische Erscheinungsbild des Pseudohypoparathyreoidismus und Pseudo-Pseudohypoparathyreoidismus und seine Pathogenese. Fortschr. Röntgenstr. 120 (1974) 192-200

Taillard, J., A. Mégevand, P. Scholder-Hegi, E. Morscher: Die Epiphyseolysis capitis femoris. Acta rheum. Geigy 21 (1964)

Tänzer, A.: Die Veränderungen am Schädel bei der Neurofibromatosis Recklinghausen. Versuch einer Einteilung. Fortschr. Röntgenstr. 105 (1966) 50–62

Thiemann, H.: Juveline Epiphysenstörungen. Forschr. Röntgenstr. 14 (1909) 79–87

Thomas, G.: Die dysplastische Hüftpfanne. Ihre Biomechanik und ihre operativen Behandlungsmethoden. In: Bücherei des Orthopäden, Bd. I, hrsg. von M. Lange. Enke, Stuttgart 1969

Valdueza, A. F.: The nail-patella syndrome. A report of three families. J. Bone Jt Surg. 55 B (1973) 145–162

Velasco Dominguez, E., F. Garcia Velasco, R. Velasco Dominguez, J. Crespo Pinilla, A. Marañón Cabello: Neuropatia por inclusión del nervio mediano en el anillo osteofibroso formado por la apófisis supraepitroclear y la cinta fibrosa de Struthers. Rev. esp. Reum. 5 (1978) 241–252

Viehweger, G.: Oberarm. In: Handbuch der medizinischen Radiologie, Bd. IV/2, hrsg. von L. Diethelm, O. Olsson, F. Strnad, H. Vieten, A. Zuppinger. Springer, Berlin 1968 (309–342)

Waldenström, H.: The first stages of coxa plana. J. Bone Jt Surg. 20 (1938) 559–566

Walker, N.: Klinik und radiologische Kriterien der sekundären Coxa vara congenita. Z. Orthop. 111 (1973) 847–857

Walker, N.: Primäre und sekundäre Coxa vara congenita (C.v.c.) - Differentialdiagnostische Untersuchungen. Z. Orthop. 112 (1974) 589–594

Walter, E.: Die Familiäre, kongenitale radio-ulnare Synostose. Fortschr. Röntgenstr. 129 (1978) 241-245

Weyers, H.: Erbliche Gelenkleiden. In: Handbuch der medizinischen Radiologie, Bd. V/3, hrsg. von L. Diethelm, O. Olsson, F. Strnad, H. Vieten, A. Zuppinger. Springer, Berlin 1968 (S. 407–511)

Wise, D., H. J. Wallace, E. H. Jellinek: Angiokeratoma corporis diffusum. A clinical study of eight affected families. Quart. J. Med. 31 (1962) 177–205

Witt, H.: Die differentialdiagnostische Bedeutung der unvollständigen Hyperphalangie des Daumens für die Begutachtung. Fortschr. Röntgenstr. 103 (1965) 487–490

Wolf, E. L., W. E. Berdon, J. R. Cassady, D. H. Baker, R. Freiberger, H. Pavlov: Slipped femoral capital epiphysis as a sequela to childhood irradiation for malignant tumors. Radiology 125 (1977) 781–784

Wood, B. P., G. P. Reading: Case report 30 (Longitudinally bracketed diaphysis [„delta phalanx" anomaly] Skelet. Radiol. 1 (1977) 259–260

Wynne-Davies, R.: A family study of neonatal and late-diagnosis congenital dislocation of the hip. J. med. Genet. 7 (1970) 315–333

Inflammation; arthritis; autoimmune diseases and their radiologic differential diagnosis (see also under Osteoarthropathy; Calcifications of soft tissues; Radiologic anatomy; Trauma); sternocostoclavicular hyperostosis.

Anderson, J., A. M. Stewart: The significance of the magnitude of the medial hip joint space. Brit. J. Radiol. 43 (1970) 238–239

Ansell, B.: Chronic arthritis in childhood. Ann. rheum. Dis. 37 (1978) 107–120

Ansell, B. M., E. G. L. Bywaters: Growth in Still's disease. Ann. rheum. Dis. 15 (1956) 295–319

Ansell, B. M., P. A. Kent: Radiological changes in juvenile chronic polyarthritis. Skelet. Radiol. 1 (1977) 129–144

Ansell, B. M., R. A. D. Wigley: Arthritic manifestations in regional enteritis. Ann. rheum. Dis. 23 (1964) 64–72

Arlet, J., P. Ficat, R. Durroux, J. F. Gourdou: Observations anatomo-cliniques de coxites rhumatismales isolées. Rev. Rhum. 38 (1971) 107-115

Aufdermaur, M.: Pathologische Anatomie der peripheren Gelenke bei der progredient chronischen Polyarthritis (PCP) und bei der Spondylitis ankylopoetica Bechterew (Sp.a.). Radiol. clin. biol. (Basel) 43 (1974) 292–303

Avila, R., D. G. Pugh, C. H. Slocumb, R. K. Winkelmann: Psoriatic arthritis: A roentgenologic study. Radiology 75 (1960) 691–702

Bachmann, F., R. Foroutan, P. W. Hartl: Der informative Fall: Rezidivierende Polychondritis. Therapiewoche 26 (1976) 6306–6312

Bachmann, H. J., O. Schriever, W. Havers: BCG-Osteomyelitis und BCG-Arthritis als Komplikationen nach BCG-Impfung. Med. Klin. 72 (1977) 1814–1817

Baker, S. B., D. R. Robinson: Sympathetic joint effusion in septic arthritis. J. Amer. med. Ass. 240 (1978) 1989

Ball, J. A. I. Grayzel: Arteritis and localised periosteal new bone formation. J. Bone Jt Surg. 46 B (1964) 244–250

Baum, J.: Infection in rheumatoid arthritis. Arthr. and Rheum. 14 (1971) 135–137

Beneke, G.: Pathologische Anatomie der rheumatoiden Arthritis. Therapiewoche 21 (1971) 709–721

Berens, D. L., R.-K. Lin: Roentgen diagnosis of rheumatoid arthritis. Thomas, Springfield/Ill. 1969

Berens, D. L., L. M. Lockie, Ru-Kan Lin, B. M. Norcross: Roentgen changes in asymptomatic joints in rheumatoid arthritis. Arthr. and. Rheum. 9 (1966) 491

Bernstein, C., W. D. Loeser, L. E. Manning: Erosive rib lesions in paralytic poliomyelitis. Radiology 70 (1958) 368-372

Beyer, A., A. Stecken: Ossale Veränderungen beim Klippel-Tren-
aunay-P.-Weber-Syndrom. Fortschr. Röntgenstr. 97 (1962) 45–
51

Bjarnason, D. F., D. M. Forrestier, R. L. Swezey: Destructive arthritis of the large joints. A rare manifestation of sarcoidosis. J.
Bone Jt Surg. 55 A (1973) 618–622

Bjersand, A. J.: New bone formation and carpal synostosis in scleroderma. A case report. Amer. J. Roentgenol. 103 (1968) 616–
619

Bland, J. H., W. M. Eddy: Hemiplegia and rheumatoid hemiarthri-
tis. Arthr. and Rheum. 11 (1968) 72–78

Bleifeld, C. J., A. E. Inglis: The hand in lupus erythematosus. J.
Bone Jt Surg. 56 A (1974) 1207–1215

Böni, A.: Die progredient chronische Polyarthritis. In: Klinik der
rheumatischen Erkrankungen, hrsg. von R. Schoen, A. Böni, K.
Miehlke. Springer, Berlin 1970 (S. 139–180)

Bohrer. S. P.: Tuberculous synovitis with widening of the intercondylar notch of the distal femur. Brit. J. Radiol. 42 (1969) 703–
704

Bouvier, M., P. Queneau, J. Brun. Les formes ostéoarticulaires de
la sarcoidose. Schweiz. Rdsch. Med. 61 (1972) 631–646

Braun-Falco, O.: Neuere Aspekte zur Pathogenese der Hauterschei-
nungen bei Psoriasis vulgaris. Hautarzt 27 (1976) 363-374

Braun-Falco, O., G. Rassner: Psoriasis arthropathica aus dermato-
logischer Sicht. Therapiewoche 19 (1969) 261–265

Brewerton, D. A.: HLA-B27 and the inheritance of susceptibility to
rheumatic disease. Arthr. and Rheum. 19 (1976) 656–668

Brewerton, D. A., D. C. O. James: The histocompatibility antigen
(HL-A27) and disease. Semin. Arthr. and Rheum. 4 (1975) 191–
207

Brodey, P. A., S. M. Wolff: Radiographic changes in the sacroiliac
joints in familial Mediterranean fever. Radiology 114 (1975) 331–
333

Brower, A.C., D. E. Sweet, T. E. Keats: Condensing osteitis of the
clavicle. A new entity. Amer. J. Roentgenol. 121 (1974) 17–21

Brown, I.: A study of the „capsular" shadow in disorders of the hip
in children. J. Bone Jt Surg. 57 B (1975) 175–179

Burkhart, J. M., J. Jowsey: Parathyroid and thyroid hormones in the
development of immobilization osteoporosis. Endocrinology 81
(1967) 1053–1062

Bywaters, E. G. L.: The relation between heart and joint disease
including „rheumatoid heart disease" and chronic postrheumatic
arthritis (type Jaccoud). Brit. Heart J. 12 (1950) 101–131

Bywaters, E. G. L.: Fistulous rheumatism. A manifestation of rheumatoid arthritis. Ann. rheum. Dis. 12 (1953) 114–121

Bywaters, E. G. L.: Discussion. Arthr. and Rheum. 9 (1966) 645–
646

Bywaters, E. G. L.: Lesions of bursae, tendons and tendon sheaths.
Clin. rheum. Dis. 5 (1979) 883–925

Bywaters, E. G. L., B. M. Ansell: Arthritis associated with ulcerative colitis. A clinical and pathological study. Ann. rheum. Dis.
17 (1958) 169–183

Bywaters, E. G. L., B. M. Ansell: Monoarticular arthritis in children. Ann. rheum. Dis. 24 (1965) 116–122

Caffey, J., F. N. Silverman: Pediatric X-ray diagnosis, 5. Aufl.
Yearbook Medical Publishers. Chikago 1967

Camus, J.-P.: Spondylarthrite ankylosante et maladie périodique.
Rev. Rhum. 32 (1965) 614–616

Canigiani, G., K. Zweymüller: Skelettveränderungen im Spätstad-
ium der Dermatomyositis. Radiol. clin. biol. 41 (1972) 99–114

Carter, M. E.: Sacro-iliitis in Still's disease. Ann. rheum. Dis. 21
(1962) 105–120

Castillo, B. A., R. A. El Sallab, J. T. Scott: Physical activity, cystic
erosions, and osteoporosis in rheumatoid arthritis. Ann. rheum.
Dis. 24 (1965) 522–527

Catterall, R. D., V. Wright, J. B. Cook: Arthritis and genital infection in paraplegic patients. Brit. J. vener. Dis. 43 (1967) 81–88

Christoph, R., E. Genth, C. Klemm, E. Uehlinger, W. Hartl: Po-
lyostische, plasmazelluläre Osteomyelitis unter dem Bilde der
chronischen Polyarthritis. Therapiewoche 27 (1977) 2731–2743

Clark, R. L., C. A. Muhletaler, S. I. Margulies: Colitic arthritis.
Clinical and radiographic manifestations. Radiology 101 (1971)
585–594

Collins, L. C., M. D. Lidsky, J. T. Sharp, J. Moreland: Malposition
of carpal bones in rheumatoid arthritis. Radiology 103 (1972) 95–
98

Compston, J. E., M. F. Laker, J. S. Woodhead, J.-C. Gazet, L. W.
L. Horton, A. B. Ayers, H. J. Bull, T. R. E. Pilkington: Bone
disease after jejuno-ileal bypass for obesity. Lancet 1978//II, 1–4

Cooke, C. L., D. S. Owen jr.: Gonococcal arthritis. Med. Aspects
Hum. Sex. 7 (1973) 151–157

Cowan Collins, L., M. D. Lidsky, J. T. Sharp, J. Moreland: Malposition of carpal bones in rheumatoid arthritis. Radiology 103
(1972) 95–98

Dalinka, M. K., J. F. Wunder: Unusual manifestations of rheumatoid arthritis. Radiology 97 (1970) 393–395

Dihlmann, W.: Pleuropulmonale Äquivalente per primär chronischen Polyarthritis. Deutscher Röntgenkongreß 1966, Teil A.
Thieme, Stuttgart 1967 (S. 75–78)

Dihlmann, W.: Der Processus styloideus - ein röntgenologischer In-
dikator für chronische rheumatische Polyarthritiden. Fortschr.
Röntgenstr. 109 (1968 a) 199–202

Dihlmann, W.: Ein röntgenologisches Frühzeichen der Arthritis. Der
Schwund der subchondralen Grenzlamelle. Z. Rheumaforsch. 27
(1968 b) 129–132

Dihlmann, W.: Über die Arthritis reformans. Fortschr. Röntgenstr.
111 (1969) 245–251

Dihlmann, W.: Die praktische Bedeutung und Problematik der
Röntgenfrühsymptome - dargestellt am Nørgaard-Zeichen der
chronischen rheumatischen Polyarthritis. Fortschr. Röntgenstr. 112
(1970) 247–253

Dihlmann, W.: Zur Differentialdiagnose der Gelenkerkrankungen
bei Psoriatikern. Dtsch. med. Wschr. 96 (1971) 557

Dihlmann, W.: A systematic approach to the radiological diagnosis
of arthritic diseases. In: Chronic forms of polyarthritis, hrsg. von
F. J. Wagenhäuser. Huber, Bern 1976 a (S. 87–98)

Dihlmann, W.: Röntgenmorphologische Befunde bei kindlicher
rheumatoider Arthritis. Verh. dtsch. Ges. Rheum. 4 (1976 b) 60–
69

Dihlmann, W.: Fortschritte in der Röntgendiagnostik des chronisch-
entzündlichen Gelenkrheumatismus. In: Fortschritte auf dem Gebiete des chronisch-entzündlichen Gelenkrheumatismus (PCP) hrsg.
von H.-J. Holtmeier, H. Franke. Thieme, Stuttgart 1977 (S. 36–
49)

Dihlmann, W., M. Cen: Die ankylosierende dysostotische Arthritis.
Fortschr. Röntgenstr. 110 (1969) 246–248

Dihlmann, W., H.-J. Fernholz: Die sympathische Arthritis - Beitrag
zur Plasmazellenosteomyelitis. Fortschr. Röntgenstr. 129 (1978)
26–33

Dihlmann, W., E. Peter: Die diagnostische Bedeutung des glokken-
förmigen Femurkopfes. Fortschr. Röntgenstr. 102 (1965) 306–
309

Dihlmann, W., G. Liebaldt, W. Undeutsch: Die Kapillarausspros-
sung als Reparationsprinzip bei örtlichen Strahlenschäden. Strahlentherapie 114 (1961) 552–564

Dirheimer, Y.: The craniovertebral region in chronic inflammatory
rheumatic diseases. Springer, Berlin 1977

Eastmond, C. J., J. C. Woodrow: The HLA system and the arthropathies associated with psoriasis. Ann. rheum. Dis. 36 (1977)
112–120

Edeiken, J., A. F. DePalma, H. Moskowitz, V. Smythe: „Cystic"
tuberculosis of bone. Clin. Orthop. 28 (1963) 163–168

Ehrlich, G. E.: Antecubital cysts in rheumatoid arthritis - A corol-
lary to popliteal (Baker's) cysts. J. Bone Jt Surg. 54 A (1972)
165–169

Elke, M.: Dystrophische Rippenveränderungen bei Sklerodermie.
Fortschr. Röntgenstr. 99 (1963) 717–719

El-Khoury, G. Y., M. R. Mickelson: Chondrolysis following slipped
capital femoral epiphysis. Radiology 123 (1977) 327–330

Exner, G. U.: Die plasmacelluläre Osteomyelitis. Langenbecks Arch.
klin. Chir. 326 (1970) 165–185

Eyler, W. R., H. P. Doub: Extraintestinal roentgen manifestations
of intestinal lipodystrophy. J. Amer. med. Ass. 160 (1956) 534–
536

Farman, J., E. L. Effman, V. Grnja: Crohn's disease and periosteal
new bone formation. Gastroenterology 61 (1971) 513–522

Fassbender, H. G.: Estra-articular processes in osteoarthropathia
psoriatica. Arch. Orthop. Traumat. Surg. 95 (1979) 37–46

Favez, G.: Die Sarkoidose. Dtsch. med. Wschr. 100 (1975) 2574–
2579

Fischer, M.: Röntgenmorphologie der Arthritis psoriatica. Akt.
rheumatol. 2 (1977) 109–114

Fischer, M., D. Konietzko: Röntgenologische und dermatologische Untersuchungen zur Diagnostik der Arthritis psoriatica. Z. Haut-u. Geschl.-Kr. 52 (1977) 679–684

Fitzgerald, P., F. O. C. Meenan: Sarcoidosis of hands. J. Bone Jt Surg. 40 B (1958) 256–261

Flenker, I., D. Ricken: Pseudo-LE and Sharp-Syndrom - zwei neue immunpathologische Krankheitsbilder. Diagnostik 10 (1977) 861–864

Forrester, D. M., J. Kirkpatrick: Periostitis and pseudoperiostitis. Radiology 118 (1976) 597–601

Fotopoulos, J. P. E. Scull, R. R. Roy: Arthritis mutilans. Report of an unusually extensive case. Conn. med. J. 22 (1958) 552–557

Fritze, E., W. Schroeder, H. Dickmans: Rheumatische Reaktionslage und Pneumokoniose. Rundherdpneumokoniose bei Rheumatismus nodosus. Z. Rheumaforsch. 21 (1962) 61–70

Ganguli, P. K.: Radiology of bone and joint tuberculosis with special reference to tropical countries. Asia Publishing House, London 1963

Gelman, M. I., J. R. Ward: Septic arthritis: A complication of rheumatoid arthritis. Radiology 122 (1977) 17–23

Giedion, A.: Weichteilveränderungen und radiologische Frühdiagnose der akuten Osteomyelitis im Kindesalter. Fortschr. Röntgenstr. 93 (1960) 455–466

Girgis, F. L., A. W. Popple, F. E. Bruckner: Jaccoud's arthropathy. A case report and necropsy study. Ann. rheum. Dis. 37 (1978) 561–565

Glick, E. N.: Asymmetrical rheumatoid arthritis after poliomyelitis. Brit. med. J. 1967/III, 26–28

Goldbloom, R. B., P. B. Stein, A. Eisen, J. B. McSheffrey, B. St. J. Brown, F. W. Wiglesworth: Idiopathic periosteal hyperostosis with dysproteinemia. A new clinical entity. New Engl. J. Med. 274 (1966) 873–878

Gondos, B.: The pointed tubular bone. Its significance and pathogenesis. Radiology 105 (1972) 541–545

González Lanza, M., E. Brito Brito, F. Garcia-Cossio, C. Sáez de la Calzada, C. Moro Serrano, C. Castro Alcaide: Artritis de Jaccoud, presentación de tres casos y revisión de la literatura. Rev. esp. Reum. 3 (1976) 20–32

Gordon, E. J., A. W. Perlman, N. Shechter: Diffuse inflammation of cartilage. A case report of a hitherto unreported entity. J. Bone Jt Surg. 30 A (1948) 944–956

Grashey, R., R. Birkner: Atlas typischer Röntgenbilder vom normalen Menschen. Mit Berücksichtigung der Varietäten und Fehlerquellen sowie der Aufnahmetechnik, 10. Aufl. Urban & Schwarzenberg, München 1964

Gray, M. S., T. Philp: Syphilitic arthritis. Diagnostic problems with special reference to congenital syphilis. Ann. rheum. Dis. 22 (1963) 19–25

Green, N., J. C. Osmer: Small bone changes secondary to systemic lupus erythematosus. Radiology 90 (1968) 118–120

Grelier, J. M., J. G. Hardin: Synovial cyst of sternoclavicular joint as mediastinal mass. Ann. intern. Med. 83 (1975) 525–526

Griffiths, H. J., A. A. Rossini: A case of lipoatrophic diabetes. Radiology 114 (1975) 329–330

Grisel, P.: Enucléation de l'atlas et torticolis naso-pharyngien. Presse méd. 38 (1930) 50–53

Gristina, A. G., G. D. Rovere, H. Shoji: Spontaneous septic arthritis complicating rheumatoid arthritis. J. Bone Jt Surg. 56 A (1974) 1180–1184

Grokoest, A. W., A. I. Snyder, C. Ragan: Some aspects of juvenile rheumatoid arthritis. Bull. rheum. Dis. 8 (1957) 147–148

Gschnait, F., E. Ita: Harnsäurewerte im Serum von Patienten mit Psoriasis vulgaris. Wien. klin. Wschr. 90 (1978) 309–311

Gumpel, J. M., C. J. Johns, L. E. Shulman: The joint disease of sarcoidosis. Ann. rheum. Dis. 26 (1967) 194–205

Hamza, M., A. Hubault, A. Ryckewaert: Les manifestations articulaires de la maladie de Behçet. Rev. Rhum. 42 (1975) 527–531

Hansen, H. H.: Über eine besondere Verlaufsform der Psoriasis arthropathica. Verh. dtsch. Ges. Path. 47 (1963) 203–205

Harders, H.: Beitrag zur Kenntnis eines rheumatischen Syndroms mit allgemeinem Befall des Knorpels. Schweiz. med. Wschr. 84 (1954) 712–715

Hardinge, K.: The etiology of transient synovitis of the hip in childhood. J. Bone Jt Surg. 52 B (1970) 100–107

Harris, R. D., H. L. Hecht: Suprapatellar effusions. A new diagnostic sign. Radiology 97 (1970) 1–4

Harris, N. H., W. H. Kirkaldy-Willis: Primary subacute pyogenic osteomyelitis. J. Bone Jt Surg. 47 B (1965) 526–532

Haux, J.-P., R. Flasse, M. de Bruyere, C. Nagant de Deuxchaisnes: HLA B 27 in regional enteritis with and without ankylosing spondylitis or sacroiliitis. J. Rheum. Suppl. 3 (1977) 60–63

Heimstädt, P.: Rezidivierende Polychondritis. Akt. rheumatol. 1 (1976) 35–40

Heimstädt, P.: Ein Fall von sterno-kosto-klavikulärer Hyperostose. Verh. dtsch. Ges. Rheum. 5 (1978) 334–335

Heine, J., G. Leitz: Schmerzhafte einseitige Hüftgelenkserkrankung bei Säuglingen und Kleinkindern. Med. Welt 23 (1972) 1194–1196

Heller, H., J. Gafni, D. Michaeli, N. Shahin, E. Sohar, G. Ehrlich, I. Karten, L. Sokoloff: The arthritis of familial Mediterranean fever (FMF). Arthr. and Rheum. 9 (1966) 1–17.

Hench, P. S., E. F. Rosenberg: Palindromic rheumatism. A „new", oft recurring disease of joints (arthritis, periarthritis, para-arthritis) apparently producing no articular residues - Report of thirty-four cases; its relation to „angioneural arthrosis", „allergic rheumatism" and rheumatoid arthritis. Arch. intern. Med. 73 (1944) 293–321

Hennemann, H. H.: Die Diagnose der Autoaggressionskrankheiten. diagnostik 2 (1969) 297–301

Hermodsson, I.: Roentgen appearances of arthritis of the hip. Acta radiol. (Stockh.) 12 (1972) 865–881

Herness, D., M. Makin: Articular damage in familial mediterranean fever. Report of four cases. J. Bone Jt Surg. 57 A (1975) 265–267

Herzer, R.: Ausgeprägte ossäre Protuberanzen der Malleoli tibiales bei „Arthritis psoriatica". Fortschr. Röntgenstr. 114 (1971) 281–282

Hirschberg, M., R. Biehler: Lepra der Knochen. Derm. Z. 16 (1909) 415–438, 490–508

Hladik, M: Vorzeitige entzündliche perichondrale Verkalkung und Verknöcherung im Kindesalter. Fortschr. Röntgenstr. 108 (1968) 758–760

Hoggins, G. S., M. C. Hamilton: Dentofacial defects associated with scleroderma. Oral Surg. 27 (1969) 734–736

Hornstein, O. P.: Klinische Pathologie der Haut bei rheumatischen Erkrankungen. Z. Rheumaforsch. 26 (1967) 273–290

Houli, J., J. Rezek: Articular diseases in ulcerative colitis, regional ileitis and Whipple's disease. Acta rheum. scand. 11 (1965) 291–298

Huskisson, E. C.: Psoriatic arthropathy. Proc. roy. Soc. Med. 60 (1967) 6–8

Ignaczak, T., L. R. Espinoza, O. S. Kantor, K. Osterland: Jaccoud arthritis. Arch. intern. Med. 135 (1975) 577–579

Isemein, L., A.-M. Fournier: Contribution a l'étude radiologique des polyarthrites évolutives a début. Rev. Rhum. 19 (1952) 1016–1026

Jayson, M. I. V., A. St. J. Dixon, P. Yeoman: Unusual geodes („bone cysts") in rheumatoid arthritis. Ann. rheum. Dis. 31 (1972) 174–178

Jensen, O. A., F. Jensen: Relapsing polychondritis. A histopathological and histochemical study of the first Danish case. Acta path. microbiol. scand. 69 (1967) 357–371

Johnson, T. H., N. Mital, G. P. Rodnan, R. J. Wilson: Relapsing polychondritis. Radiology 106 (1973) 313–315

Jones, G.: Radiological appearances of disuse osteoporosis. Clin. Radiol. 20 (1969) 345–353

Jüngling, O.: Ostitis tuberculosa multiplex cystica (eine eigenartige Form der Knochentuberkulose). Fortschr. Röntgenstr. 27 (1919–1921) 375–383

Kaplan, H.: Sarcoid arthritis. A review. Arch. intern. Med. 112 (1963) 924–933

Karagevrekis, C., G. Gauthier, J. Fabre: Main parkinsonienne et arthrite rhumatoide. Schweiz. Rdsch. Med. 61 (1972) 787–796

Kastert, J., E. Uehlinger: Skelettuberkulose. Mit einem Beitrag über allgemeine Pathologie und pathologische Anatomie der Skelettuberkulose. In: Handbuch der Tuberkulose, Bd. IV, hrsg. von J. Hein, H. Kleinschmidt, E. Uehlinger. Thieme, Stuttgart 1964 (S. 443–538)

Keipert, J. A., P. E. Campbell: Recurrent hyperostosis of the clavicles: An undiagnosed syndrome. Aust. paediatr. J. 6 (1970) 97–104

Kelly III, J. J., B. B. Weisiger: The arthritis of Whipple's disease. Arthr. and Rheum. 6 (1963) 615–632

Kelly, P. J., W. J. Martin, M. B. Coventry: Bacterial (suppurative) arthritis in the adult. J. Bone Jt Surg. 52 A (1970) 1595–1602

Kienböck, R.: Über schwere infantile Polyarthritis chronica und ihre Folgezustände. Allgemeiner Wachstumsstillstand und Mikromelie, „Pseudo-Achondroplasie". Fortschr. Röntgenstr. 30 (1922/23) 1–31, 258–283

King jr., B. G., S. Novy, E. B. Evans: Palindromic rheumatism: An unusual cause of the inflammatory joint. J. Bone Jt Surg. 56 A (1974) 142–144

Klemperer, P., A. D. Pollack, G. Baehr: Diffuse collagen disease. Acute disseminated lupus erythematosus and diffuse scleroderma. J. Amer. med. Ass. 119 (1942) 331–332

Klopfer, F.: Die Distensionsluxation im Röntgenbild. Fortschr. Röntgenstr. 73 (1950) 357–361

Klotz, H. G., J. Thurner, N. Stefenelli: Gonokokkenpolyarthritis Med. Klin. 69 (1974) 1271–1273

Köhler, A., E. A. Zimmer: Grenzen des Normalen und Anfänge des Pathologischen im Röntgenbild des Skelets, 11. Aufl. Thieme, Stuttgart 1967

Köhler, H., E. Uehlinger, J. Kutzner, T. R. Weihrauch, L. Wilbert, R. Schuster: Sterno-kosto-klavikuläre Hyperostose - ein bisher nicht beschriebenes Krankheitsbild. Dtsch. med. Wschr. 100 (1975) 1519–1523

Köhler, H., E. Uehlinger, J. Kutzner, T. B. West: Sternocostoslavicular hyperostosis: Painfull swelling of the sternum, clavicles, and upper ribs. Report of two new cases. Ann. intern. Med. 87 (1977) 192–194

Kölle, G.: Klinisches Bild und Verlauf der juvenilen rheumatoiden Arthritis und des Still-Syndroms. Mschr. Kinderheilk. 118 (1970) 488–493

Kölle, G.: Die juvenile rheumatoide Arthritis (juvenile chronische Polyarthritis) und das Still-Syndrom. Eine klinische und Katamnestische Dokumentation. Rheumaforum 4. Braun, Karlsruhe 1975

Kölle, G.: Klinischer Verlauf und Prognose der kindlichen rheumatoiden Arthritis (juvenile chronische Polyarthritis) und ihrer Sonderformen. Verh. dtsch. Ges. Rheum. 4 (1976) 4–12

Korting, H. C., W. Tröscher: Arthritis und Erythema nodosum als typische Manifestationen einer Yersinia-enterocolitica-Infektion. Med. Welt (Stuttg.) 29 (1978) 1754–1758

Krokowski, E.: Die Osteoporose aus radiologischer Sicht: Entwicklung einer neuen Theorie. Radiologe 16 (1974) 54–62

Kruse, H.-P., F. Kuhlencordt, J.-D. Ringe: Ergebnisse einer Langzeittherapie der primären Osteoporose mit Natriumfluorid. Dtsch. med. Wschr. 103 (1978) 248–252

Kühne, H.: Wachstumsstörung bei Sklerodermie. Bruns Beitr. klin. Chir. 189 (1954) 447–454

Kutzner, J., H. Köhler, E. Uehlinger: Sterno-kosto-klavikuläre Hyperostosis. Fortschr. Röntgenstr. 123 (1975) 446–449

Lambert, J. R., V. Wright: Serum uric acid levels in psoriatic arthritis. Ann. rheum. Dis. 36 (1977) 264–267

Larsen, A.: The value of individual joints for radiologic assessment of rheumatoid arthritis. Scand. J. Rheum. 5 (1976) 119–123

Latchaw, R. E., G. W. Meyer: Reiter disease with atlanto-axial subluxation. Radiology 126 (1978) 303–304

Lejeune, E., A. Daumont, J. P. Deplante: Association maladie périodique - spondylarthrite ankylosante. Nouv. Presse méd. 4 (1975) 2949–2950

Lenoch, F., A. Vonková, V. Králík, O. Vojtíšek: Befall des Hüftgelenkes bei der primär chronischen Polyarthritis. Z. Rheumaforsch. 25 (1966) 343–350

Lentz, M. W., F. R. Noyes: Osseous deformity from osteomyelitis variolosa. A case report. Clin. Orthop. 143 (1979) 155–157

Leriche, R.: The problem of osteo-articular diseases of vasomotor origin. Hydrarthrosis and traumatic arthritis: Genesis and treatment. J. Bone Jt Surg. 10 (1928) 492–500

Levine, A. H., M. J. Pais, H. Berinson, P. S. Amenta: The soleal line: A cause of tibial pseudoperiostitis. Radiology 119 (1976) 79–81

Levine, M. E., W. O. Dobbins III: Joint changes in Whipple's disease. Semin. Arthr. Rheum. 3 (1973) 79–93

Ludwigs, N., R. Temming: Arthritis mutilans mit besonderer Beteiligung von Kiefer- und Zwischenwirbelgelenken. Fortschr. Röntgenstr. 87 (1957) 784–785

Lundberg, M., S. Ericson: Changes in the temporomandibular joint in psoriasis arthropathica. Acta derm.-venereol. (Stockh.) 47 (1967) 354–358

McAdam, L. P., M. A. O'Hanlan, R. Bluestone, C. M. Pearson: Relapsing polychondritis: Prospective study of 23 patients and a review of the literature. Medicine 55 (1976) 193–215

McBrine, C. S., M. S. Fisher: Acrosclerosis in sarcoidosis. Radiology 115 (1975) 279–281

Mac Ewan, D. W., J. S. Dunbar: Early radiologic recognition of pus in the joint of children. J. Canad. Ass. Radiol. 12 (1961) 72–77

Maes, H. J., W. Dihlmann: Befall der Temporomandibulargelenke bei der Spondylitis ankylopoetica. Fortschr. Röntgenstr. 109 (1968) 513–516

Magyar, É., A. Talerman, M. Fehér, H. W. Wouters: Giant bone cysts in rheumatoid arthritis. J. Bone Jt Surg. 56 B (1974) 121–129

Martel, W., J. T. Hayes, I. F. Duff: The pattern of bone erosion in the hand and wrist in rheumatoid arthritis. Radiology 84 (1965) 204–214

Martel, W., J. F. Holt, J. T. Cassidy: Roentgenologic manifestations of juvenile rheumatoid arthritis. Amer. J. Roentgenol. 88 (1962) 400–423

Mason, R. M., C. G. Barnes: Behçet's syndrome with arthritis. Ann. rheum. Dis. 28 (1969) 95–103

Masshoff, W., K. H. Täger: Fokale Lipodystrophie im Knochenmark. Dtsch. med. Wschr. 100 (1975) 88–87

Mattingly, S.: Palindromic rheumatism. Ann. rheum. Dis. 25 (1966) 307–317

Maurer, R. C., I. J. Larsen: Acute necrosis of cartilage in slipped capital femoral epiphysis. J. Bone Jt Surg. 52 A (1970) 39–50

Meema, H. E.: Recognition of cortical bone resorption in metabolic bone disease in vivo. Skelet. Radiol. 2 (1977) 11–19

Meredith, H. C., G. M. Rittenberg: Pneumarthropathy: An unusual radiographic sign of gram-negative arthritis. Radiology 129 (1978) 642

von Meyenburg, H.: Ueber Chrondromalacie. Schweiz. med. Wschr. 17 (1936) 1239–1240

Miller, L. D., M. B. Stevens: Skeletal manifestations of polymyalgia rheumatica. J. Amer. med. Ass. 240 (1978) 27–29

Mills, K. L. G.: Transitory synovitis of the hip in children. Postgrad. med. J. 40 (1964) 190–192

Mitjá Piferrer, J., J. A. del Olmo Bru, J. Granados Durán, J. Rotés Querol, J. Muñoz Gómez, M. Centellas Portella, A. Brancós Cunill: Sindrome de Behçet. Revisión a propósito de 11 casos. Rev. esp. Reum. J. (1976) 177–188

Moll, J. M. H., V. Wright: Psoriatic arthritis. Semin. Arthr. Rheum. 3 (1973) 55–78

Mortensson, W., O. Eklöf, H. Jorulf: Radiologic aspects of BCG-osteomyelitis in infants and children. Acta radiol. Diagn. 17 (1976) 845–855

Moule, N. J., J. S. R. Golding: Idiopathic chondrolysis of the hip. Clin. Radiol 25 (1974) 247–251

Müller, W.: Immundiagnostik der chronischen Polyarthritis. Immun. u. Infekt. 4 (1976) 70–78

Murphy, W. A., T. W. Staple: Jaccoud's arthropathy reviewed. Amer. J. Roentgenol. 118 (1973) 300–307

Nakata, H., W. J. Russel: Chest roentgenograms in rheumatoid arthritis: Hiroshima-Nagasaki. Amer. J. Roentgenol. 108 (1970) 819–824

Niederecker, K.: Die sympathische Coxitis. In: Handbuch der Orthopädie, Bd. IV/1, hrsg. von G. Hohmann, M. Hackenbroch, K. Lindemann. Thieme, Stuttgart 1961

Noetzli, M.: Über weniger auffällige Röntgenveränderungen bei primächronischer Polyarthritis. Radiol. clin. (Basel) 32 (1963) 525–532

Noonan, C., D. T. Odone, E. P. Engleman, S. D. Splitter: Roentgenographic manifestations of joint disease in systemic lupus erythematosus. Radiology 80 (1963) 837–843

Nøgarrd, F.: Earliest roentgenological changes of polyarthritis of the rheumatoid type: rheumatoid arthritis. Radiology 84 (1965) 325–329

Norris, S. H., H. J. Mankin: Chronic tenosynovitis of the posterior tibial tendon with new bone formation. J. Bone Jt Surg. 60 B (1978) 523–526

O'Connell, D. J., R. M. Bennett: Mixed connective tissue disease -

clinical and radiological aspects of 20 cases. Brit. J. Radiol. 50 (1977) 620–625

O'Connell, D. J., W. J. Marx: Hand changes in primary biliary Cirrhosis. Radiology 129 (1978) 31–35

O'Hanlan, M., L. P. McAdam, R. Bluestone, C. M. Pearson: The arthropathy of relapsing polychondritis. Arthr. and Rheum. 19 (1976) 191–194

Otte, P.: Das Krankheitsbild der „flüchtigen Coxitis". Z. Rheumaforsch. 26 (1967) 474–481

Ozonoff, M. B., F. J. Flynn jr.: Roentgenologic features of dermatomyositis of childhood. Amer. J. Roentgenol 118 (1973) 206–212

Palmer, D. G.: Synovial cysts in rheumatoid disease. Ann. intern. Med. 70 (1969) 61–68

Pankovich, A. M., M. M. Jevtic: Coccidioidal infection of the hip. J. Bone Jt Surg. 55 A (1973) 1525–1528

Pavelka, K.: Zur Frage der Gelenk-Sarkoidose. Z. Rheumatol. 38 (1979) 90–98

Peterson Jr., C. C., M. L. Silbiger: Reiter's syndrome and psoriatic arthritis. Their roentgen spectra and some interesting similarities. Amer. J. Roentgenol. 101 (1967) 860–871

Pilger, E., H. Schmidberger, G. Klein, P. Schmid: Salmonellenspondylitis der oberen Halswirbelsäule. Akt. Rheumatol. 2 (1977) 177–182

Pool, Jr., W. H.: Cartilage atrophy. Radiology 112 (1974) 47–50

Poppe, H.: Die Röntgendiagnostik entzündlicher Knochen- und Gelenkerkrankungen. Chirurg 41 (1970) 198–203

Rabinowitz, J. G., J. Twersky, M. Guttadauria: Similar bone manifestations of scleroderma and rheumatoid arthritis. Amer. J. Roentgenol 121 (1974) 35–44

Rassner, G.: Lupus erythematodes und Hydralazin-Syndrom. Dtsch. med. Wschr. 91 (1966) 1391-1392

Ravelli, A.: Zum Röntgenbild des proximalen Schienbeindrittels. Fortschr. Röntgenstr. 82 (1955) 48–52

Reichmann, S.: Roentgenologic soft tissue appearances in hip joint disease. Acta Radiol. Diagn. 6 (1967) 167–176

Resnick, D.: Rheumatoid arthritis of the wrist: Why the ulnar styloid? Radiology 112 (1974) 29–35

Resnick, D.: Pyarthrosis complicating rheumatoid arthritis. Radiology 114 (1975) 581–586

Resnick, D., T. W. Broderick: Bony proliferation of terminal toe phalanges in psoriasis. The „ivory" phalanx. J. Canad. Ass. Radiol. 28 (1977) 187–189

Resnick, D., J. T. Gmelich: Bone fragmentation in the rheumatoid wrist: Radiographic and pathologic considerations. Radiology 114 (1975) 315–321

Resnick, D., J. F. Scavulli, T. G. Goergen, H. K. Genant, G. Niwayama: Intra-articular calcification in scleroderma. Radiology 124 (1977) 685–688

Roberts, M. E. T., V. Wright, A. G. S. Hill, A. C. Mehra: Psoriatic arthritis. Follow-up study. Ann. rheum. Dis. 35 (1976) 206–212

Rodnan, G. P.: The nature of joint involvement in progressive systemic sclerosis (diffuse scleroderma). Clinical study and pathologic examinations of synovium in twenty-nine patients. Ann. intern. Med. 56 (1962) 422–439

Rodnan, G. P., T. A. Medsger jr.: The rheumatic manifestations of progressive systemic sclerosis (scleroderma). Clin. Orthop. 57 (1968) 81–93

Rohe, K., M. Bierther, D. Wessinghage: Zur Pathogenese der Arthritis psoriatica. Z. Orthop. 118 (1980) 300–310

Rothenberger, W., W. Stoll: Zur Klinik und Pathogenese der Panchondritis. Med. Welt (Stuttg.) 25 (1974) 744–749

Ruderman, R. J., F. E. Ward: HLA-B27 in black patients with ankylosing spondylitis. Lancet 1977/I. 610

Rutishauser, E., J. P. Bugnion: Neue Befunde am Handgelenk. Schweiz. Z. Path. 14 (1951) 477–478

Rutishauser, E., F. Jacqueline: Die rheumatischen Koxitiden. Eine pathologisch-anatomische und röntgenologische Studie. Docum. rheum. 16 (J. R. Geigy, Basel 1959)

Sargent, E. N., A. F. Turner, G. Jacobson: Superior marginal rib defects. An etiologic classification. Amer. J. Roentgenol. 106 (1969) 491–505

Saunders, C. G., W. J. Weston: Synovial mass lesions in anteroposterior projection of the ankle joint. J. Canad. Ass. Radiol. 22 (1971) 275–277

Schacherl, M. H. Holzmann: Zur Polyarthritis bei progressiver Sklerodermie. Fortschr. Röntgenstr. 107 (1967) 485–493

Schacherl, M. A. Reihl: Röntgenmorphologie der kindlichen rheumatoiden Arthritis im Erwachsenenalter (am Beispiel der Hände). Verh. dtsch. Ges. Rheum. 4 (1976) 70–87

Schacherl, M. F. Schilling: Zur Differentialdiagnose erworbener und angeborener Carpalsynostosen. Fortschr. Röntgenstr. 102 (1965) 68–77

Schacherl, M., F. Schilling: Röntgenbefunde an den Gliedma-ßengelenken bei Polyarthritis psoriatica. Z. Rheumaforsch. 26 (1967) 442–450

Schaller, J., R. J. Wedgwood: Juvenile rheumatoid arthritis: A review. Pediatrics 50 (1972) 940–953

Schattenkirchner, M., W. Schürer, K. Diem, S. Scholz, E. D. Albert: Die Bedeutung der Histokompatibilitäts-Antigene (HLA-Antigene) für die Rheumatologie. Akt. Rheumatol. 1 (1976) 23–24

Schilling, F.: Die symptomatischen Arthritiden. Heilkunst 83 (1970) 1–6

Schilling, F.: Spondylitis Ankylopoetica. Die sogenannte Bechterewsche Krankheit und ihre Differentialdiagnose (einschließlich Spondylosis hyperostotica, Spondylitis psoriatica und chronisches Reiter-Syndrom). In: Handbuch der medizinischen Radiologie, Bd. VI/2, hrsg. von L. Diethelm, F. Heuck, O. Olsson, K. Ranniger, F. Strnad, H. Vieten, A. Zuppinger. Springer, Berlin 1974 (S. 452–689)

Schilling, F.: Yersinia-Arthritis. Dtsch. med. Wschr. 101 (1976) 1515–1519

Schriber, R. A., H. Firooznia: Extensive phalangeal cystic lesions. Sarcoidosis limited to the hands and feet Arthr. and Rheum. 18 (1975) 123–128

Schumacher jr., H. R.: Joint involvement in progressive systemic sclerosis (scleroderma): A light and electron microscopic study of synovial membrane and fluid. Amer. J. clin. Path. 60 (1973) 593–600

Seifert, M. H., J. C. Steigerwald, M. M. Cliff: Bone resorption of the mandible in progressive systemic sclerosis. Arthr. and Rheum. 18 (1975) 507–512

Selmes, J., P. Dreyfus: La main inflammatoire. Gaz. méd. Fr. 76 (1969) 3335–3344

Sewell, J. R., B. Liyanage, B. M. Ansell: Calcinosis in juvenile dermatomyositis. Skelet. Radiol. 3 (1978) 137–143

Shagrin, J. W., B. Frame, H. Duncan: Polyarthritis in obese patients with intestinal bypass. Ann. intern. Med. 75 (1971) 377–380

Shapiro, R. F., D. Resnick, J. J. Castles, R. D'Ambrosia, P. R. Liscomb, G. Niwayama: Fistulization of rheumatoid joints. Spectrum of identifiable syndromes. Ann. rheum. Dis. 34 (1975) 489–498

Sharp, G. C., W. S. Irvin, E. M. Tan, R. G. Gould, H. R. Holman: Mixed connective tissue disease - an apparently distinct rheumatic disease syndrome associated with a specific antibody to an extractable nuclear antigen (ENA). Amer. J. Med. 52 (1972) 148–159

Sholkoff, S. D., M. G. Glickman, H. L. Steinbach: Roentgenology of Reiter's syndrome. Radiology 97 (1970) 497–503

Siegmeth, W., R. Eberl: Organmanifestationen und Komplikationen bei der chronischen Polyarthritis. Documenta Geigy. Ciba-Geigy, Basel 1976

Sills, E. M.: Errors in diagnosis in juvenile rheumatoid arthritis. Johns Hopk. med. J. 133 (1973) 88–95

Sohar, E., J. Gafni: Familial mediterranean fever and its articular manifestations. Clin. rheum. Dis. 1 (1975) 195–209

Sohar, E., J. Gafni, M. Pras, H. Heller: Familial mediterranean fever. A survey of 470 cases and review of literature. Amer. J. Med. 43 (1967) 227–253

Soila, P.: Roentgen manifestations of adult rheumatoid arthritis with special regard to the early changes. Acta rheum. scand., Suppl. 1 (1958)

Spritzer, H. W., A. L. Weaver, H. S. Diamond, E. L. Overholt: Relapsing polychondritis. Report of a case with vertebral column involvement. J. Amer. med. Ass. 208 (1969) 355–357

Staeffen, J., R. Terme, G. Laborie, C. Séries, B. Pachebat: Arthropathies destructrices au cours d'une maladie de Whipple diagnostiquée par duodénoscopie. Sem. Hôp. Paris 54 (1978) 117–120

Stafne, E. C., L. T. Austin: A characteristic dental finding in acrosclerosis and diffuse scleroderma. Amer. J. Orthodont. 30 (1944) 25–29

Stecher, R. M.: Ankylosis of the finger joints in rheumatoid arthritis. Ann. rheum. Dis. 17 (1958) 365–375

Stŕeda, A., R. Bardfeld: Über den Einfluß der juvenilen primärchronischen (rheumatoiden) Arthritis auf die Gestaltung des Hüftgelenkes. Z. Rheumaforsch. 23 (1964) 265–275

Streuli, R., G. Pouliadis: Periostale Knochenneubildung beim Morbus Crohn. Schweiz. med. Wschr. 108 (1978) 518–522

Sundt, H.: Arthro-syphilis congenita tardiva et acquisita et arthrometasyphilis. Acta derm.-venerol. (Stockh.) Suppl. 20 (1948)

Teske, H.-J., H. Chüden: Die Atlasverschiebung als Folgezustand entzündlicher Veränderungen oder operativer Eingriffe im Nasen-Rachen-Raum (Krankheitsbilder nach Grisel und Hadley). Fortschr. Röntgenstr. 113 (1970) 519–522

Thiers, G., H. Holzmann, G. Böhm, K. Hahn, D. Eissner: Die psoriatische Knochenmanifestation. Akt. rheumatol. 5 (1980) 189–195

Thorel, J. B., B. Cavelier, J. C. Bonneau, J. L. Simonin, C. Ropartz, P. Deshayes: Étude d'une population porteuse de l'antigène HLA B27 comparée a celle d'une population témoin non B27 a la recherche de la spondylarthrite ankylosante. Rev. Rhum. 45 (1978) 275–282

Thould, A. K., A. G. Stansfield, H. Wykeham Balme: Chronic atrophic perichondritis. Ann. rheum. Dis. 24 (1965) 563–568

Tittor, W., G. Schwalbach: Die primäre biliäre Zirrhose. Klinikarzt 8 (1979) 313–320

Turek, S.: Sarcoid disease of bone at the ankle joint. J. Bone Jt Surg. 35 A (1953) 465–468

Udoff, E. J., H. K. Genant, F. Kozin, M. Ginsberg: Mixed connective tissue disease: The spectrum of radiographic manifestations. Radiology 124 (1977) 613–618

Uehlinger, E.: Die pathologische Anatomie der hämatogenen Osteomyelitis. Chirurg 41 (1970) 193–198

Uehlinger, E.: Bone changes in rheumatoid arthritis and their pathogenesis. In: Rheumatoid Arthritis. Pathogenic Mechanisms and Consequences in Therapeutics, hrsg. von W. Müller, H.-G. Harwerth, K. Fehr, Academic Press, London 1971 (S. 25–26)

Uehlinger, E., K. Wurm: Skelettsarkoidose. Literaturübersicht und Fallbericht. Fortschr. Röntgenstr. 125 (1976) 111–122

Vainio, K.: The rheumatoid foot. A clinical study with pathological and roentgenological comments. Ann. Chir. Gynaec. Fenn. 45 (1956), Suppl. 1, p. 1–107

Vernon-Roberts, B., C. G. Barnes, P. A. Revell: Synovial pathology in Behçet's syndrome. Ann. rheum. Dis. 37 (1978) 139–145

Wackenheim, A.: Roentgen Diagnosis of the Craniovertebral Region. Springer, Berlin 1974

Wagenhäuser, F. J.: Klinik der progredient chronischen Polyarthritis der Erwachsenen. Med. Welt (Stuttg.) 19 (1968) 2323–2334

Watson, R. C., I. Cahen: Pathological fracture in long bone sarcoidose. Report of a case. J. Bone Jt Surg. 55A (1973) 613–617

Weissmann, B. N., A. S. Rappoport, J. L. Sosman, P. H. Schur: Radiographic findings in the hands in patients with systemic lupus erythematosus. Radiology 126 (1978) 313–317

Wenger, D. R., M. R. Mickelson, I. V. Ponsetti: Idiopathic chondrolysis of the hip. Report of two cases. J. Bone Jt Surg. 57 A (1975) 268–271

Wessinghage, D.: ,,Rheumatische" Beschwerden bei peripheren Nervenkompressionssyndromen. Therapiewoche 22 (1972) 2533–2538

Weston, W. J., D. G. Palmer: Soft tissues of the extremities. A radiologic study of rheumatic disease. Springer, Berlin 1978

Weyers, H.: Über Ostitis multiplex cystoides im frühen Kindesalter. Fortschr. Röntgenstr. 85 (1956) 316–320

Whipple, G. H.: A hitherto undescribed disease characterized anatomically by deposits of fat and fatty acids in the intestinal and mesenteric lymphatic tissues. Bull. Johns Hopk. Hosp. 18 (1907) 382–391

Williams, M. H., P. J. H. S. Sheldon, G. Torrigiani, V. Eisen, S. Mattingly: Palindromic rheumatism. Clinical and immunological studies. Ann. rheum. Dis. 30 (1971) 375–380

Williams jr., R. C.: Dermatomyositis and malignancy: A review of the literature. Ann. intern. Med. 50 (1959) 1174–1181

Winter, W., F. Kammerhuber: Seltene Lokalisation von Knochenveränderungen bei progressiver (diffuser) Sklerodermie. Fortschr. Röntgenstr. 122 (1975) 364–366

Winter, T. Q., K. D. Pearson: Systemic sporotrixosis. Radiology 104 (1972) 579–583

Winterbauer, R. H.: Multiple telangiectasia, Raynaud's phenomenon, sclerodactyly, and subcutaneous calcinosis: a syndrome mimicking hereditary hemorrhagic telangiectasia. Bull. Johns Hopk. Hosp. 114 (1964) 361–383

Wissler, H.: Über eine besondere From sepsisähnlicher Krankheiten (Supsepsis hyperergica). Mschr. Kinderheilk. 94 (1944) 1–15

Wissler, H.: Subsepsis allergica. Ergebn. inn. Med. Kinderheilk. 23 (1965) 202–220

Wolf, G., G. Canigiani, E. Deimer: Knochenveränderungen im Rahmen der Sklerodermie. Fortschr. Röntgenstr. 112 (1970) 523–530

Woodlief, R. M.: Superior marginal rib defects in traumatic quadriplegia. Radiology 126 (1978) 673–674

Wright, D.: Psoriatic arthropathy. Proc. roy. Soc. Med. 60 (1967) 8–9

Wright, V., W. Reed: The link between Reiter's syndrome and psoriatic arthritis. Ann. rheum. Dis. 23 (1964) 12–21

Yune, H. Y., V. A. Vix, E. C. Klatte: Early fingertip changes in scleroderma. J. Amer. med. Ass. 215 (1971) 1113–1116

Zawadzki, Z. A., T. G. Benedek: Rheumatoid arthritis, dysproteinemic arthropathy, and paraproteinemia. Arthr. and Rheum. 12 (1969) 555–568

Osteoarthrosis (see also under Deformities; Anatomy).

Abelanet, R., M. Forest, M. Postel, M. Kerboull, J.-P. Roux, M. Daudet-Monsac: Les aspects anatomo-cliniques des coxopathies destructrices rapides. A propos de 172 observations. Arch. Anat. path. 22 (1974) 165–182

Acheson, R. M., A. B. Collart: New Haven survey of joint diseases. XVII. Relationship between some systemic characteristics and osteoarthrosis in general population. Ann. rheum. Dis. 34 (1975) 379–387

Ahlbäck, S.: Osteoarthrosis of the knee. A radiographic investigation. Acta radiol. (Stockholm), Suppl. 277, 1968

Ahlbäck, S. S. Mattsson: Patella alta and gonarthrosis. Acta radiol. Diagn. 19 (1978) 578–584

Arnoldi, C. C., H. Linderholm, H.. Müssbichler: Venous engorgement and intraosseous hypertension in osteoarthritis of the hip. J. Bone Jt Surg. 54 B (1972) 409–421

Arnoldi, C. C., H. Linderholm, Ä. Vinnerberg: Skeletal and soft tissue changes in the lower leg in patients with intracalcanean hypertension. Acta. chir. scand. 138 (1972) 25–37

Bandi, W.: Die Arthrose des femoro-patellaren Gelenkes und ihre Therapie. Hefte Unfallheilk. 110 (1972) 181–186

Bandi, W.: Vorverlagerung der Tuberositas tibiae bei Chondromalacia patellae und femoro-patellarer Arthrose. In: Knorpelschaden am Knie, hrsg. von C. Burri, A. Rüter. Springer, Berlin 1976 S. 175–186

Bouchard, C. J.: Du rôle pathogenic de la dilatation de l'estomac et des relations clinique de cette maladie avec divers accidents morbides. Bull. Mém. Soc. méd. Hôp. Paris 1884, 3e série, 226–240

Burri, C., A. Rüter: Knorpelschaden am Knie. Springer, Berlin 1976

Chapchal, G.: Die Bedeutung der Fehlbelastung in der Genese der Arthrosen. In: Ursachen rheumatischer Krankheiten. In: Rheumatismus in Forschung und Praxis, Bd. III, hrsg. von W. Belart. Huber, Bern 1966 (S. 110–119)

Chu Chang-jen, Tsui Te-yu: Pathogogic study of metacarpointerphalangeal joints in Kaschin-Beck disease. Chin. med. J. 4 (1978) 309–318

Coste, F., J. Forestier: Hémiplégie et nodosités d'Heberden contralatérales. Bull. Mém. Soc. méd. Hôp. Paris 51 (1935) 772–775

Cotta, H.: Präarthrose und präarthrotische Deformität. Eine Studie zur Erweiterung des Begriffs von Hackenbroch. Z. Orthop. 112 (1974) 8–23

Cotta, H., W. Puhl: Pathophysiologie des Knorpelschadens. In: Knorpelschaden am Knie, hrsg. von C. Burri, A. Rüter. Springer, Berlin 1976 (S. 1–22)

Crain, D. C.: Interphalangeal osteoarthritis. Characterized by painful, inflammatory episodes resulting in deformity of the proximal and distal articulations. J. Amer. med. Ass. 175 (1961) 1049–1053

Danielsson, L. G.: Incidence and prognosis of coxathrosis. Acta orthop. scand., Suppl. 66 (1964)

Dick, W., H. R. Henche, E. Morcher: Der Knorpelschaden nach Patellafraktur. Arch. orthop. Unf.-Chir. 81 (1975) 65–76

Dihlmann, W.: Über ein besonderes Coxarthrosezeichen (Pseudofrakturlinie) im Röntgenbild (Kritik des sogenannten Mach-Effektes). Fortschr. Röntgenstr. 100 (1964) 383–388

Dihlmann, W.: Fortschritte in der Röntgendiagnostik des chronisch-entzündlichen Gelenkrheumatismus. In: Fortschritte auf dem Gebiete des chronisch-entzündlichen Gelenkrheumatismus (PCP), hrsg. von H.-J. Holtmeier, H. Franke. Thieme, Stuttgart 1977 (S. 36–49)

Dihlmann, W., W. Frik: Das Plaquezeichen am Hüftgelenk. (Spezielle, weniger beachtete Röntgenbefunde am Stütz- und Gleitgewebe 2). Fortschr. Röntgenstr. 114 (1971) 297–304

Dihlmann, W., A. Hopf: Das Wiberg-Zeichen als Hinweis auf gestörte Hüftgelenksmechanik. (Spezielle, weniger beachtete Röntgenbefunde am Stütz- und Gleitgewebe 3). Fortschr. Röntgenstr. 115 (1971) 572–581

Dihlmann, W., G. Nebel, G. Lingg: Marginale Osteophyten als röntgenologisch-klinische Indikatoren der Femoropatellararthrose. Fortschr. Röntgenstr. 131 (1979) 632–635

Doppman, J. L.: The association of patellofemoral erosion and synovial hypertrophy: A diagnostic entity. Radiology 82 (1964) 240–245

Ehrlich, G. E.: Inflammatory osteoarthritis - I. The clinical syndrome. J. chron. Dis. 25 (1972a) 317–328

Ehrlich, G. E.: Inflammatory osteoarthritis - II. The superimposition of rheumatoid arthritis. J. chron. Dis. 25 (1972b) 635–643

Finsterbusch, A., B. Friedman: Early changes in immobilized rabbits knee joints: A light and electron microscopic study. Clin. Orthop. 92 (1973) 305–319

Friedebold, G.: Die posttraumatische Arthrose. Hefte Unfallheilk. 110 (1972) 127–140

Gresham, G. E., U. K. Rathey: Osteoarthritis in knees of aged persons. Relationship between roentgenographic and clinical manifestations. J. Amer. med. Ass. 233 (1975) 168–170

Hackenbroch, M.: Die Arthrosis deformans der Hüfte. Grundlagen und Behandlung. Thieme, Leipzig 1943

Heberden, W. (the Elder): Commentaries on history and cure of diseases, 2. Aufl. Payne, London 1802 (S. 148–149)

Heine, J.: Über die Arthritis deformans. Virchows Arch. path. Anat. 260 (1926) 521–663

Herzog, A.: Scheinfrakturen bei der Arthritis deformans coxae. Röntgenpraxis 5 (1933) 174–177

Horváth, F., T. Kákosy: Arthrose des distalen radioulnaren Gelenkes bei Motorsägenbetreibern. Fortschr. Röntgenstr. 131 (1979) 54–59

Horváth, F., L. Kéry, P. Sillár: Röntgenmorphologie einiger Struktur- und Formveränderungen im lateralen Schenkelhalsdrittel. Z. Orthop. 112 (1974) 294–299

Kidd, K. L., J. B. Peter: Erosive Osteoarthritis. Radiology 86 (1966) 640–647

Lancourt, J. E., J. A. Cristini: Patella alta and patella infera. Their etiological role in patellar dislocation, chondromalacia, and apophysitis of the tibial tubercle. J. Bone Jt Surg. 57 A (1975) 1112–1115

Lequesne, M., S. de Sèze, J. Amouroux: La coxarthrose destructrice rapide. Rev. Rhum. 37 (1970) 721–733

Liebeskind, D.: Berufskrankheiten im Röntgenbild. Barth, Leipzig 1970

Lindemann, K.: Die juvenile Arthritis deformans des Großzehengrundgelenkes (Hallux rigidus). Z. Orthop. 64 (1936) 391–403

McEwen, C.: Osteoarthritis of the fingers with ankylosis. Arthr. and Rheum. 11 (1968) 734–744

Mintz, G., A. Fraga: Severe osteoarthritis of the elbow in foundry workers. Arch. environm. Hlth. 27 (1973) 78–80

Munoz Gomes, J., J. Rotés Querol, J. Granados Duran: Arthropathie interphalangienne destructive. Rev. Rhum. 39 (1972) 373–378

Mutter, K., K. F. Schlegel: Zur Ätiologie der Koxarthrose. Eine radiologische Studie. Z. Orthop 113 (1975) 402–405

Otte, P.: Über das Wachstum der Gelenkknorpel. Hüthig. Heidelberg 1965

Otte, P.: Degeneration des Gelenkknorpels. Klinische und radiologische Aspekte. Münch. med. Wschr. 110 (1968) 2677 bis 2683

Otte, P.: Das Wesen der Coxarthrose und die Prinzipien ihrer Behandlung. Dtsch. med. J. 20 (1969) 341–346

Otte, P.: Die Pathophysiologie der Arthrosen. Therapiewoche 21 (1971) 2723–2725

Otte, P.: Pathophysiologische Grundlagen präarthrotischer Faktoren. Z. Orthop. 112 (1974) 541–547

Otte, P.: Die aktivierte Arthrose. In: Das rheumatische Gelenk Pathologie, Diagnose, Therapie, Red. W. Dihlmann, H. Mathies. Sharp & Dohme, München 1976

Pauwels, F.: Die kausale Therapie der Coxarthrose. Dtsch. Ärztebl. 73 (1976) 2795–2802

Perry, G. H., M. J. G. Smith, C. G. Whiteside: Spontaneous recovery of the joint space in degenerative hip disease. Ann. rheum. Dis. 31 (1972) 440–448

Peter, J. B.: Discussion. Arthr. and. Rheum. 9 (1966) 450 u. 463

Peter, J. B., C. M. Pearson, L. Marmor: Erosive osteoarthritis of the hands. Arthr. and Rheum. 9 (1966) 365–388

Puls, P.: Aktivierung und Progredienz der Koxarthrose durch partielle Hüftkopfnekrosen. Z. Orthop. 112 (1974) 690–694

Radi, I.: L'arthrose érosive des doigts. Rev. Rhum. 37 (1970) 119–123

Ruckes, J., F. Schuckmann: Über die Topik der Capillaren im Stratum synoviale des Kniegelenkes in Abhängigkeit vom Lebensalter unter besonderer Berücksichtigung der Arthrosis deformans. Frankfurt. Z. Path. 72 (1962) 243–255

Rüter, A. Retropatellare Arthrose (Diagnose und Therapieübersicht). In: Knorpelschaden am Knie, hrsg. von C. Burri, A. Rüter. Springer, Berlin 1976 (S. 137–155)

Rütt, A.: Die röntgenologische Differenzierung der sogenannten „epiphysären Hüfte" und der epiphysären Coxarthrose. Arch. orthop. Unfall-Chir. 79 (1974) 54–65

Sauer, G.: Die „beetartigen Erhabenheiten" am Schenkelhals Z. Anat. 104 (1935) 285–294

Schacherl, M., F. Schilling: Die destruierende Polyarthrose. Fortschr. Röntgenstr. 113 (1970) 551–560

Schneider, P. G., H. Lichte: Arthrosis deformans nach ultraphysiologischen Gelenkbelastungen. Z. Orthop. 107 (1970) 287–303

Siguda, D.: Die Chondropathia patellae. Therapiewoche 25 (1975) 5631–5673

Smukler, N. M., J. Edeiken, V. J. Guiliano: Ankylosis in osteoarthritis of the finger joints. Radiology 100 (1971) 525–530

Spranger, M.: Die therapeutische Ruhigstellung als Präarthrose. Z. Orthop. 112 (1974) 574–576

Sutro, C.: Scallop-like defects in the anterior cortices of the femora. Co-existence with osteoarthritis of the knee. Bull. Hosp. Jt Dis. (N.Y.) 25 (1964) 57–63

Tillmann, K., G. Binzus: Der Energiestoffwechsel der Gelenke bei Arthrose und Arthritis und seine medikamentöse Beeinflußbarkeit. Verhandlungen der Deutschen Orthopädischen Gesellschaft, 55. Kongreß. Enke, Stuttgart 1969 (S. 221–227)

Uehlinger, E.: Die posttraumatische Arthrose. Hefte Unfallheilk. 110 (1972) 111–123

Utsinger, P. D., D. Resnick, R. F. Shapiro, K. B. Wiesner: Roentgenologic, immunologic, and therapeutic study of erosive (inflammatory) osteoarthritis. Arch. intern. Med. 138 (1978) 693–697

Vincelette, P., C. A. Laurin, H. P. Lévesque: The footballer's ankle and foot. Canad. med. Ass. J. 107 (1972) 872–877

Weingraber, H.: Die Funktionsprüfung in der Röntgenfrühdiagnostik der Kiefergelenkserkrankungen. Fortschr. Röntgenstr. 74 (1951) 84–86

Weiss, K.: Degenerative Gelenkerkrankungen. In: Handbuch der medizinischen Radiologie, Bd. V/3, hrsg. von L. Diethelm, O. Olsson, F. Strnad, H. Vieten, A. Zuppinger. Springer, Berlin 1968 (S. 543–602)

Wiberg, G.: Studies on dysplastic acetabula and congenital subluxation of the hip joint with special reference to the complication of osteoarthritis. Acta chir. scand., Suppl. 58 (1939)

Wiberg, G.: Roentgenographic and anatomic studies on the femoropatellar joint with special reference to chondromalacia patellae. Acta orthop. scand. 12 (1941) 319–410

Wise, D., H. J. Wallace, E. H. Jellinek: Angiokeratoma corporis diffusum. A clinical study of eight affected families. Quart. J. Med. 31 (1962) 177–205

Osteoarthropathies (avascular, due to vitamin deficiency, electrical injury, hemoglobinopathy, due to hormones, coagulopathies, drugs, metabolic disorders, myelogenic, neurogenic, radiogenic, renal, thermal); osteolysis syndrome; massive osteolysis; neurogenic paraosteoarthropathy; lipoid-dermatoarthritis; pachydermoperiostosis (hypertrophic osteoarthropathy, Marie-Bamberger syndrome); paraneoplastic diseases (see also under Tumors); bone marrow necrosis; congenital pseudarthrosis.

Ahlbäck, S., G. C. H. Bauer, W. H. Bohne: Spontaneous osteonecrosis of the knee. Arthr. and Rheum. 11 (1968) 705–733
Ahlberg, Å. K. M.: On the natural history of hemophilic pseudotumor. J. Bone Jt Surg. 57 A (1975) 1133–1136
Ahuja, S. C., P. G. Bullough: Osteonecrosis of the knee. A clinicopathological study in twenty-eight patients. J. Bone Jt Surg. 60 A (1978) 191–197
Aichroth, P., A. C. Branfoot, E. C. Huskisson, L. W. Loughridge: Destructive joint changes following kidney transplantation. Report of a case. J. Bone Jt Surg. 53 B (1971) 488–494
Alarcón-Segovia, D., L. E. Ward: Marked destructive changes occuring in osteoarthritic finger joints after intra-articular injection of corticosteroids. Arthr. and Rheum. 9 (1966) 443–449
Albert, J., W. Bruce, A. C. Allen, H. Blank: Lipoid dermatoarthritis. Reticulohistiocytoma of the skin and joints. Amer. J. Med. 28 (1960) 661–667
Amstutz, H. C., E. J. Carey: Skeletal manifestations and treatment of Gaucher's disease. Review of twenty cases. J. Bone Jt Surg. 48 A (1966) 670–701
Ansell, B. M., E. G. L. Bywaters: Histiocytic bone and joint disease. Ann. rheum. Dis. 16 (1957) 503–510
Baldauf, G.: Das Skelett des Akromegalen im Röntgenbild. Röntgenpraxis 29 (1976) 255–267
Balzereit, F., A. Tänzer: Paraartikukäre Ossifikation als Problem in der Intensivpflege. Verh. dtsch. Ges. inn. Med. 74 (1968) 890–893
Bauer, J., R. Kienböck: Zur Kenntnis der Knochen- und Gelenksveränderungen bei Alkaptonurie. Osteoarthrosis alcaptonurica (ochronotica). Fortschr. Röntgenstr. 40 (1929) 32–42
Bauer, R.: Osteomyelitis urica. Fortschr. Röntgenstr. 108 (1968) 266
Beck, R. E.: Roentgenographic findings in the complications of diabetes mellitus. Amer. J. Roentgenol. 82 (1959) 887–896
Bernhard, G. C., G. T. Hensley: Amyloid arthropathy. Arthr. and Rheum. 12 (1969) 444–453
Blair, J. R., R. Schatzki, K. D. Ott: Sequelae to cold injury in one hundred patients. Follow-up study four year after occurence of cold injury. J. Amer. med. Ass. 163 (1957) 1203–1208
Bland, J. H., J. W. Frymoyer: Rheumatic syndromes of myxedema. New Engl. J. Med. 282 (1970) 1171–1174
Blanford, A. T., S. P. Keane, D. J. McCarty, J. W. Albers: Idiopathic Charcot joint of the elbow. Arthr. and Rheum. 21 (1978) 723–726
Bluestone, R., E. G. L. Bywaters, M. Hartog, P. J. L. Holt, S. Hyde: Acromegalic arthropathy. Ann. rheum. Dis. 30 (1971) 243–258
Bohne, W., G. Muheim: Spontane Osteonekrose des Kniegelenkes. Z. Orthop. 107 (1969) 384–402
Bohrer, S. P.: Growth disturbances of the distal femur following sickle cell bone infarcts and/or osteomyelitis. Clin. Radiol. 25 (1974) 221–235
Boldero, J. L., H. S. Kemp: The early bone joint changes in haemophilia and similar blood dyscrasias. Brit. J. Radiol. 39 (1966) 172–180
Brant, D. D., H. H. Jordan: Radiologic aspects of hemophilic pseudotumors in bone. Amer. J. Roentgenol. 115 (1972) 525–539

Brass, H.: Metabolische Osteopathien mit besonderer Berücksichtigung der renalen Osteopathie. Therapiewoche 26 (1976) 6251–6258
Brinn, L. B., M. T. Khilnani: Epidermolysis bullosa with characteristic hand deformities. Radiology 89 (1967) 272–274
Brodey, P. A.: Multicentric reticulohistiocytosis: A rare cause of destructive polyarthritis. Radiology 114 (1975) 327–328
Bronsky, D.: Hyperparathyroidism with Albright's osteodystrophy: Case report and a proposed new classification of parathyroid disease. J. clin. Endocr. 31 (1970) 271–276
Brown, G. A., W. R. Osebold, I. V. Ponseti: Congenital pseudarthrosis of long bones. A clinical, radiographic, histologic and untrastructural study. Clin. Orthop. 128 (1977) 228–242
Brunner, W.: „Subakute Polyarthritis" bei Bronchuskarzinom - ein paraneoplastisches Syndrom. Schweiz. med. Wschr. 97 (1967) 611–612
Bücheler, E., H. L. Klammer: Ossäre hämophile Pseudotumoren. Fortschr. Röntgenstr. 120 (1974) 468–473
Buge, A., A. Hubault, G. Rancurel: Les arthropathies de l'intoxication par le bismuth. Rev. Rhum. 42 (1975) 721–729
Buhtz, P., K. Mölleken: Generalisierte Amyloidose mit Arthropathie. Z. ges. inn. Med. 29 (1974) 594–597
Bywaters, E. G. L., A. Sr. J. Dixon, J. T. Scott: Joint lesions of hyperparathyroidism. Ann. rheum. Dis. 22 (1963) 171–187
Calabro, J. J.: Cancer and arthritis. Arthr. and Rheum. 10 (1967) 553–567
Campbell, W. L., F. Feldman: Bone and soft tissue abnormalities of the upper extremity in diabetes mellitus. Amer. J. Roentgenol. 124 (1975) 7–16
Cappellini, G., P. Pavlica, G. Stasi, R. Tonti, G. Viglietta: Temporo-mandibular joint changes in renal osteodystrophy. Radiol. clin. (Basel) 47 (1978) 330–333
Cegla, U. H.: Zur Bedeutung und Pathogenese von Trommelschlegelfingern. Dtsch. med. Wschr. 98 (1973) 2143–2144
Červeňanský, J., Š. Sitaj, T. Urbánek: Alkaptonuria and ochronosis. J. Bone Jt Surg. 41 A (1959) 1169–1182
Chandler, G. N., V. Wright: Deleterious effect of intra-articular hydrocortisone. Lancet 1958/II; 661–663
Chandler, G. N., D. T. Jones, V. Wright, S. J. Hartfall: Charcot's arthropathy following intra-articular hydrocortisone. Brit. med. J. 1959/I, 952–953
Chawla, S.: Cranio-skeletal dysplasia with acro-osteolysis. Brit. J. Radiol. 37 (1964) 702–705
Cheney, W. D.: Acro-osteolysis. Amer. J. Roentgenol. 94 (1965) 595–607
Chevrot, A., G. Pallardy, G. Ledoux-Lebard: Manifestations squelettiques de l'hyperthyroidie. J. Radiol. Électrol. 59 (1978) 167–173
Clouse, M. E., H. F. Gramm, M. Legg, T. Flood: Diabetic osteoarthropathy. Clinical and roentgenographic observations in 90 cases. Amer. J. Roentgenol. 121 (1974) 22–34
Cole, G. J.: Ainhum. An account of fifty-four patients with special reference to etiology and treatment. J. Bone Jt Surg. 47 B (1965) 43–51
Courey, W. R., R. C. Pfister: The radiographic findings in renal tubular acidosis. Analysis of 21 cases. Radiology 105 (1972) 497–503
Crecelius, W.: Ein Beitrag zum Krankheitsbild der Osteopathia dysplastica familiaris. Fortschr. Röntgenstr. 76 (1952) 196–202
Crosby, W. H., A. D. Dawson, P. K. Hench, E. R. Korn, P. V. Sacks, P. Saltman, L. T. Yam: Hemochromatosis (iron-storage disease). J. Amer. med. Ass. 228 (1974) 743–752
Daumont, A., J.-P. Deplante, M. Bouvier, E. Lejeune: L'ostéonécrose des condyles fémoraux chez l'adulte. A propos de 30 cas personnels. Rev. Rhum 43 (1976) 27–35
David-Chaussé, J., N. Ducassou: Les Hémarthroses des coagulapathies autres que l'hémophilie. Bordeax méd. 4 (1971) 43–69
Delling, G.: Endokrine Osteopathien. Verh. dtsch. Ges. Path. 58 (1974) 176–192
De Séze, S., M. Phankim-Koupernik: Syndrome du canal carpien d'origine goutteuse (3 cas.). Rev. Rhum 31 (1964) 9–12
De Séze, S., J. Solnica, D. Mitrovic, L. Miravet, H. Dorfmann: Joint and bone disorders and hypoparathyroidism in hemochromatosis. Semin. Arthr. and Rheum. 2 (1972) 71–94
Dick, R., D. N. Jones: Temporo-mandibular joint changes in patients undergoing chronic haemodialysis. Clin. Radiol. 24 (1973) 72–76

Diem, E., G. Wolf, R. Oppolzer: Zur Kenntnis der nicht-familiären sogenannten sporadischen Acropathia Ulceromutilans der unteren Extremitäten (Bureau-Barrière-Syndrom). Z. Haut- u. Geschl.-Kr. 50 (1975) 13–24

Dieterich, H.: Die subchondrale Herderkrankung am Metacarpale III. Arch. klin. Chir. 171 (1932) 555–567

Dihlmann, W.: Richtungweisende Röntgenzeichen bei der disseminierten Lipogranulomatose (Morbus Farber). Fortschr. Röntgenstr. 117 (1972) 47–51

Dihlmann, W.: Das Blutergelenk - die Osteoarthropathie bei angeborenen Blutgerinnungsstörungen. Fortbild. Rheum. 3 (1974a) 62–74

Dihlmann, W.: Über den Einfluß von Knochenerkrankungen auf die Gelenkmorphologie (Lunatummalazie und sakroiliakale Pseudoerweiterung bei der renalen Osteopathie). Verh. dtsch. Ges. Rheum. 3 (1974b) 164–167

Dihlmann, W.: Röntgendiagnostik der Sakroiliakalgelenke und ihrer nahen Umgebung, 2. Aufl. Thieme, (Stuttgart) 1978

Dihlmann, W., H. J. Fernholz: Gibt es charakteristische Röntgenbefunde bei der Gicht? Dtsch. med. Wschr. 94 (1969) 1909–1911

Dihlmann, W., H. J. Fernholz: Radiological signs of gout. Germ. med. Mth. 15 (1970) 211–213

Dihlmann, W., H. J. Fernholz: Osteoplastische Reaktionen bei chronischer Gicht. Fortschr. Röntgenstr. 120 (1974) 216–218

Dihlmann, W., H. Greiling, R. Kisters, H. W. Stuhlsatz: Biochemische und radiologische Untersuchungen zur Pathogenese der Alkaptonurie. Dtsch. med. Wschr. 95 (1970) 839–844

Dinkel, L.: Veränderungen des Fußskelets bei Diabetes mellitus. Fortschr. Röntgenstr. 110 (1969) 223–234

Dinkel, L.: Ein Beitrag zur neurogenen Osteopathie. Radiologe 12 (1972) 101–102

Doerr, W.: Idiopathische Hüftkopfnekrose und Hyperurikämie. Verh. dtsch. Ges. Path. 58 (1974) 408–411

Dorfmann, H., M. F. Kahn, S. de Sèze: Les lupus iatrogènes: état actuel de la question. I. Étude clinique et principaux produits incriminés. Nouv. Presse méd. 1972/I, 2907–2912

Dorfmann, N., M. F. Kahn, S. de Sèze: Les lupus iatrogènes: état actuel de la question.: II. Physiopathologie des lupus induits. Nouv. Presse méd. 1972/1, 2967–2970

Dorfmann, H., J. Solnica, D. Mitrovic, P. Dreyfus: Veränderungen an Knochen und Gelenken bei der Hämochromatose. Münch. med. Wschr. 111 (1969) 1396 bis 1401

Dorwart, B. B., H. R. Schumacher: Joint effusions, chondrocalcinosis and other rheumatic manifestations in hypothyroidism. A clinicopathologic study. Amer. J. Med. 59 (1975) 780–790

Doyle, F. H.: Radiological patterns of bone disease associated with renal glomerular failure in adults. Brit. med. Bull. 28 (1972) 220–224

Dreyfuss, J. R., M. J. Glimcher: Epephyseal injury following frostbite. New Engl. J. Med. 253 (1955) 1065–1068

Duncan, T. R.: Validity of the sesamoid index in the diagnosis acromegaly. Radiology 115 (1975) 617–619

Dymock, I. W., E. B. D. Hamilton, J. W. Laws, R. Williams: Arthropathy of haemochromatosis. Clinical and radiological analysis of 63 patients with iron overload. Ann. rheum. Dis. 29 (1970) 469–476

Edeiken, J., P. J. Hodes: Roentgen Diagnosis of Diseases of Bone, 2. Aufl. Bd. I u. II. Williams & Wilkins, Baltimore 1973

Edeiken, J., P. J. Hodes, H. I. Libshitz, M. H. Weller: Bone ischemia. Radiol. Clin. N. Amer. 5 (1967) 515–529

Ehricht, H. G.: Die Osteolyse im lateralen Claviculaende nach Preßluftschaden. Arch. orthop. Unfall-Chir. 50 (1959) 576–582

Eichler, J.: Tumorähnliche Knochenveränderungen bei Hämophilie. Fortschr. Röntgenstr. 104 (1966) 103–107

Eichler, J.: Knochennekrosen bei Fettstoffwechselstörungen. Orthop. Prax. 11 (1975) 758–764

Engh, C. A., J. L. Hughes, R. C. Abrams, J. W. Bowerman: Osteomyelitis in the patient with sickle-cell disease. Diagnosis and management. J. Bone Jt Surg. 53 A (1971) 1–15

Erbe, W., G. Stephen, H. Böttcher: Das Muster der Skelettveränderungen bei der Akromegalie. Fortschr. Röntgenstr. 122 (1975) 317–322

Espinoza, L. R., I. Spilberg, C. K. Osterland: Joint manifestations of sickle cell disease. Medicine 53 (1974) 295–305

Farman, J., J. Twersky, S. Fierst: Ulcerative colitis associated with hypertrophic osteoarthropathy. Amer. J. dig. Dis. 21 (1976) 130–135

Feiereis, H.: Arthropathie bei Diabetes Mellitus und Adie-Syndrom. Internist. Prax. 4 (1964) 183–195

Feindt, W.: Beitrag zur Röntgendiagnose von Dekompressionsfolgen am Skelett. Arbeitsmed. Sozialmed. Präventivmed. 9 (1974) 14–16

Feldman, F., A. M. Johnson, J. F. Walter: Acute axial neuroarthropathy. Radiology 111 (1974) 1–16

Fetterman, L. E., R. Hardy, H. Lehrer: The clinico-roentgenologic features of ainhum. Amer. J. Roentgenol. 100 (1967) 512–522

Fischer, V., C. Dietschi: Die idiopathische Hüftkopfnekrose des Erwachsenen bei Hyperurikämie und Dyslipidämie. Münch. med. Wschr. 114 (1972) 1937–1941

Fisher, M. S.: An unusual change in acromegaly. Skelet. Radiol. 3 (1978) 177–178

Fochem, K.: Zum Röntgenbild der Osteoarthropathia diabetica. Radiol. clin. biol. (Basel) 40 (1971) 281–290

Forgács, S.: Stages and roentgenological picture of diabetic osteoarthropathy. Fortschr. Röntgenstr. 126 (1977) 36–42

François, J.: Dystrophie dermo-chondro-cornéenne familiale. Bull. Acad. roy. Méd. Belg. 14 (1949) 135–171

Françon, F., J. Leroy: Le „pied hérissé" hors de la goutte. Rev. Rhum. 29 (1962) 12–17

Fried, K.: Neurotrophische Osteoarthropathien als Folge einer Unterbrechung der peripheren Nerven. Radiol. diagn. (Berl.) 10 (1969) 77–85

Fried, K.: Beitrag zum Verlauf und zur Pathogenese der neurotrophischen Osteoarthropathien. Fortschr. Röntgenstr. 113 (1970) 560–575

Fried, K., N. Kalná: Multiple neurotrophische Arthropathie als Folge einer Polyradikulomyelitis. Fortschr. Röntgenstr. 132 (1980) 447–449

Friedrich, H.: Über ein noch nicht beschriebenes, der Perthesschen Erkrankung analoges Krankheitsbild des sternalen Clavikelendes. Dtsch. Z. Chir. 187 (1924) 385–398

Fries, G.: Zur Röntgen-Diagnostik osteoradionekrotischer Hüftveränderungen nach Röntgen-Radiumbestrahlung weiblicher Genitalkarzinome. Strahlentherapie 132 (1967) 113–127

Frostberg, N.: On bone defects in terminal phalanges. Acta radiol. (Stockh.) 21 (1940) 126–142

Frymover, J. W., J. Bland: Carpal-tunnel syndrome in patients with myxedematous arthropathy. J. Bone Jt Surg. 55 A (1973) 78–82

Ganz, R.: Avaskuläre Nekrose des proximalen Tibiaendes bei Gicht. Z. Orthop. 109 (1971) 881–888

Gerstenbrand, F., M. Liebe-Kreutzder, W. Bruha: Periartikuläre Ossifikationen beim traumatischen apalischen Syndrom. Zur Klinik, Pathogenese und Therapie. Arch. orthop. Unfall-Chir. 67 (1970) 173–186

Gilula, L. A., J. Bliznak, T. W. Staple: Idiopathic nonfamilial acroosteolysis with cortical defects and mandibular ramus osteolysis. Radiology 121 (1976) 63–68

Gimlette, T. M. D.: Thyroid acropathy. Lancet 1960/I, 22–24

Glynn, J. J., M. L. Clayton: Sapring effect of hemiplegia on tophaceous gout. Ann. rheum. Dis. 35 (1976) 534–535

Gohel, V. K., M. K. Dalinka, J. Edeiken: Ischemic necrosis of the femoral head simulating chondroblastoma. Radiology 107 (1973) 545–546

Gold, R. H., A. L. Metzger, J. M. Mirra, H. J. Weinberger, K. Killebrew: Multicentric reticulohistiocytosis (lipoid dermatoarthritis). An erosive polyarthritis with distinctive clinical, roentgenographic and pathologic features. Amer. J. Roentgenol. 124 (1975) 610–624

Goldberg, A., I. Brodsky, D. McCarty: Multiple myeloma with paramyloidosis presenting as rheumatoid disease. Amer. J. Med. 37 (1964) 653–658

Goldberg, L. S., R. Fisher, E. A. Castronova, J. J. Calabro: Amyloid arthritis associated with Waldenstrom's macroglobulinemia. New Engl. J. Med. 281 (1969) 256–257

Golding, D. N.: The musculo-skeletal features of hypothyroidism. Postgrad. med. J. 47 (1971) 611–614

Golding, J. S. R., J. E. MacIver, L. N. Went: The bone changes in sickle cell anaemia and its genetic variants. J. Bone Jt Surg. 41 B (1959) 711–718

Gondos, B.: Roentgen observations in diabetic osteopathy. Radiology 91 (1968) 6–13

Gordon, D. A., W. Pruzanski, M. A. Ogryzlo, H. A. Little: Amyloid arthritis simulating rheumatoid disease in five patients with multiple myeloma. Amer. J. Med. 55 (1973) 142–154

Gore, D. R.: Iatrogenic avascular necrosis of the hip in young children. J. Bone Jt Surg. 56 A (1974) 493–502

Gorham, L. W.: Circulatory changes associated with osteolytic and osteoblastic reactions in bone. The possible mechanism involved in massive osteolysis: An experimental study. Arch. intern. Med. 105 (1960) 47–64

Gorham, L. W., A. P. Stout: Massive osteolysis (acute spontaneous absorption of bone, phantom bone, disappearing bone). Its relation to hemangiomatosis. J. Bone Jt Surg. 37 A (1955) 985–1004

Götting, H.: Röntgenologische Frühform der atrophischen Osteoarthrosis syringomyelica der Schulter mit Verlaufskontrolle. Fortschr. Röntgenstr. 78 (1953) 623

Grauthoff, H., P. Hofmann, K. Laackner, H. H. Brackmann: Hämophiler Pseudotumor und Iliacushämatom; radiologische und klinische Befunde. Fortschr. Röntgenstr. 129 (1978) 614–620

Greenfield, G. B.: Radiology of Bone Diseases. Lippincott, Philadelphia 1969

Greenfield, G. B.: Bone changes in chronic adult Gaucher's disease. Amer. J. Roentgenol. 110 (1970) 800–807

Greiling, H., E. Peter, B. Schuler: Zur Pathogenese der hypercholesterinämischen Xanthomatose. Dtsch. med. Wschr. 89 (1964) 1887–1891

Grosse, K.-P., B. Neidhardt, G. Seiler, K. Th. Schricker, G. Dorn: Kongenitaler Faktor-VII-Mangel. Klin. Pädiat. 186 (1974) 29–33

Grossman, R. E., G. T. Hensley: Bone lesions in primary amyloidosis. Amer. J. Roentgenol. 101 (1967) 872–875

Gunn, D. R., W. B. Young: Myositis ossificans as a complication of tetanus. J. Bone Jt Surg. 41 B (1959) 535–540

Guyer, P. B., F. J. Brunton, M. W. G. Wren: Pachydermoperiostosis with acro-osteolysis. A report of five cases. J. Bone Jt Surg. 60 B (1978) 219–223

Gyepes, M. T., D. H. Newbern, E. B. D. Neuhauser: Metaphyseal and physeal injuries in children with spina bifida and meningomyeloceles. Amer. J. Roentgenol. 95 (1965) 168–177

Haas, H. G.: Knochenstoffwechsel-und Parathyreoidea-Erkrankungen. Ihre Erforschung mittels Calciuminfusionen. Thieme, Stuttgart 1966

Hackenbroch jr., M. H., V. Fischer, K. Matzen: Ätiologische Beurteilung aseptischer Hüftkopfnekrosen aufgrund blutserologischer Stoffwechselparameter. Münch. med. Wschr. 120 (1978) 795–798

Hadler, N. M., W. A. Franck, N. M. Bress, D. R. Robinson: Acute polyarticular gout. Amer. J. Med. 56 (1974) 715–719

Hannon, R. C., C. Limas, O. S. Cigtay, H. L. Twigg: Bone and joint involvement in primary amyloidosis. J. Canad. Ass. Radiol. 26 (1975) 112–115

Harris, B. K., H. A. Ross: Hemarthrosis as the presenting manifestation of myeloproliferative disease. Arthr. and Rheum. 17 (1974) 969–970

Hasselbacher, P., H. R. Schumacher: Bilateral protrusio acetabuli following pelvic irradiation. J. Rheumatol. 4 (1977) 189–196

Haverbusch, T. J., A. H. Wilde, W. A. Hawk jr., A. L. Scherbel: Osteolysis of the ribs and cervical spine in progressive systemic sclerosis (scleroderma). J. Bone Jt Surg. 56 A (1974) 637–640

Heath, D. A., D. J. Martin: Periosteal new bone formation in hyperparathyroidism associated with renal failure. Brit. J. Radiol. 43 (1970) 517–521

Heintz, R.: Nieren-Fibel für Klinik und Praxis. 2. Aufl. Thieme, Stuttgart 1968

Heiple, K. G., M. R. Cammarn: Diabetic neuroarthropathy with spontaneous peritalar fracture-dislocation. A report of two cases. J. Bone Jt Surg. 48 A (1966) 1177–1181

Heller, M., J.-D. Ringe: Ungewöhnliche Lokalisation einer Paraosteoarthropathie (POA) an den Sternoklavikulargelenken. Fortschr. Röntgenstr. 130 (1979) 114–115

Herrmann, J., F. T. Zugibe, F. E. Gilbert, J. M. Opitz: Arthrodento-osteo-dysplasia (Hajdu-Cheney syndrome). Review of a genetic „acro-osteolysis" syndrome. Z. Kinderheilk. 114 (1973) 93–110

Heuck, F.: Case report (massive osteolysis [vanishing bone disease, Gorham disease] of mandible). Skelet. Radiol. 3 (1979) 241–243

Heyden, G., L. G. Kindblom, J. Möller Nielsen: Disappearing bone disease. A clinical and histological study. J. Bone Jt Surg. 59 A (1977) 57–61

Hirsch, J. H., F. C. Killien, R. H. Troupin: The arthropathy of hemochromatosis. Radiology 118 (1976) 591–596

Holland, C., H. Werner: Über Osteolysen. Arch. orthop. Unfall-Chir. 60 (1966) 317–339

Hollister, D. W., D. L. Rimoin, R. S. Lachman, A. H. Cohen, W. B. Reed, G. W. Westin: The Winchester syndrome: A nonlysosomal connective tissue disease. J. Pediat. 84 (1974) 701–709

Holstein, J., H.-G. Heinrich: Gelenkveränderungen im Röntgenbild bei Thrombopathie. Beitrag zur röntgenologischen Differentialdiagnose der Hämophilie. Fortschr. Röntgenstr. 93 (1960) 783–786

Horejschi, W., G. Brandt, B. Kaduk: Das Hämochromatose-Syndrom. Inn. Med. 4 (1977) 81–87

Horváth, F.: Röntgenmorphologie des Caisson-bedingten Knochenmarkinfarktes. (Über die Verbindung zwischen akuter Arthralgie und Knochenmarkinfarkt). Fortschr. Röntgenstr. 129 (1978) 33–40

Hutcheson, J.: Peripelvic new bone formation in hemophilia. Report of three cases. Radiology 109 (1973) 529–530

Ingwersen, O. S.: Congenital indifference to pain. Report of a case. J. Bone Jt Surg. 49 B (1967) 704–709

Jakob, A.: Ein Beitrag zur Differentialdiagnose der enossalen Verkalkung, insbesondere des Knocheninfarkts. Fortschr. Röntgenstr. 74 (1951) 77–83

Jansen, H. H.: Kortikoidschäden aus pathologisch-anatomischer Sicht. Therapiewoche 17 (1967) 1907–1913

Jensen, P. S.: Hemochromatosis: A disease often silent but not invisible. Amer. J. Roentgenol. 126 (1976) 343–351

Johnson, H. M., I. L. Tilden: Reticulohistiocytic granulomas of the skin associated with arthritis mutilans. Arch. Derm. 75 (1957) 405–417

Kaiser, W., N. Zöllner: Lesch-Nyhan-Syndrom. Ein kongenitaler Defekt im Purinstoffwechsel mit den klinischen Zeichen einer Gicht und zentralnervösen Störungen. Dtsch. med. Wschr. 95 (1970) 1077–1080

Karayalcin, G., J. Dorfman, F. Rosner, A. J. Aballi: Radiological changes in 127 patients with sickle cell anemia. Amer. J. med. Sci. 271 (1976) 133–144

Kattan, K. R.: Thickening of the heel-pad associated with long-term Dilantin therapy. Amer. J. Roentgenol. 124 (1975) 52–56

Katz, G. A., J. B. Peter, C. M. Pearson, W. S. Adams: The shoulder-pad sign—a diagnostic feature of amyloid arthropathy. New Engl. J. Med. 288 (1973) 354–355

Katz, J.: Recurrent avascular necrosis of the proximal femoral epiphysis in the same hip in Gaucher's disease. Case report. J. Bone Jt Surg. 49 A (1967) 514–518

Keitel, W., R. Fuchs, G. Weber, G. Lutze: Ungewöhnliche Gelenkbeteiligung bei Sichelzellanämie. Z. ges. inn. Med. 31 (1976) 998–1000

Kho, K. M., A. D. Wright, F. H. Doyle: Heel pad thickness in acromegaly. Brit. J. Radiol. 43 (1970) 119–125

Kindermann, G., F. Weber, H. Wenderoth: Ungewöhnliche Knochenschäden nach Cortison. Med. Klin. 64 (1969) 1919 bis 1923

King, L. R., H. Braunstein, D. Chambers, R. Goldsmith: A case study of peculiar soft-tissue and bony changes in association with thyroid disease. J. clin. Endocr. 19 (1959) 1323–1330

Klein, W., F. Huth: Die Gelenkkapsel bei idiopathischer hypertropher Osteoarthropathie. Z. Orthop. 114 (1976) 177–182

Kleinberg, D. L., I. S. Young, H. S. Kupperman: The sesamoid index. An aid in the diagnosis of acromegaly. Ann. intern. Med. 64 (1966) 1075–1078

Klümer, A., V. Lohmann, E. Uehlinger, S. Weller, M. Strey: Aseptische Knochennekrosen des Oberschenkelkopfes nach Glucocorticoidbehandlung. Fortscher. Röntgenstr. 107 (1967) 96–112

Klümper, A., M. Strey, S. Weller, U. Roth, P. Bildstein: Neurogene Osteolysen. Defekte an Fußknochen nach traumatischer Schädigung peripherer Nerven. Röntgenstr. 108 (1968a) 62–71

Klümper, A., M. Strey, S. Weller, U. Roth, H. Müller-Bergh: Neurogene Osteolysen bei Diabetes mellitus. Fortschr. Röntgenstr. 108 (1968b) 221–233

Knolle, G., D. Meyer: Massive Osteolyse im Bereich des Unterkiefers infolge Hämangiomatosis des Knochens. Dtsch. Zahn-, Mund- u. Kieferheilk. 45 (1965) 433–463

Kohler, E., D. Babbitt, B. Huizenga, T. A. Good: Hereditary osteolysis. A clinical, radiological and chemical study. Radiology 108 (1973) 99–105

Kolář, J., R. Vrabec: Gelenkknorpelschäden nach Röntgenbestrahlung. Fortschr. Röntgenstr. 90 (1959) 717–721

Kolář, J., R. Vrabec: Röntgenologische Knochenbefunde nach der Hochstromverletzung. Fortschr. Röntgenstr. 92 (1960) 385–394

Kolář, J., R. Vrabec: Strahlenbedingte Knochenschäden. In: Handbuch der Medizinischen Radiologie Bd. V/1, hrsg. von L. Diethelm, F. Heuck, O. Olsson, K. Ranniger, F. Strnad, H. Vieten, A. Zuppinger. Springer, Berlin, 1976 (S. 389–512)

Kolář, J., L. Jirásek, R. Vrabec: Berufsbedingte Knochenveränderungen durch äußere Strahlenbelastung. Fortschr. Röntgenstr. 103 (1965) 584–589

Kolář, J., R. Vrabec, J. Chyba: Arthropathies after irradiation. J. Bone Jt Surg. 49 A (1967) 1157–1166

Kolb, F. O., H. L. Steinbach: Pseudohypoparathyreoidism with secondary hyperparathyreoidism and osteitis fibrosa. J. clin. Endocr. 22 (1962) 59–70

Koletsky, S., R. M. Stecher: Primary systemic amyloidosis. Involvement of cardiac valves, joints and bones, with pathologic fracture of the femur. Arch. Path. 27 (1939) 267–288

Kraft, E., E. Spyropoulos, N. Finby: Neurogenic disorders of the foot in diabetes mellitus. Amer. J. Roentgenol. 124 (1975) 17–24

Krause, W., H. G. Lasch: Die Hämophilie. Med. Klin. 64 (1969) 367–373

Krempien, B.: Stoffwechsel und Struktur des Knochengewebes bei chronischer Niereninsuffizienz. Verh. dtsch. Ges. Path. 58 (1974) 156–175

Krempien, B., O. Mehls, E. Ritz: Morphologische Untersuchungen zur Pathogenese der urämischen Epiphysenlösung. Verh. dtsch. Ges. Path. 57 (1973) 468

Krosch, H.: Ein Fall von periostaler Hyperostose. Fortschr. Röntgenstr. 83 (1955) 546–553

Kuhlencordt, F., J. Kracht: Chronischer Hyperparathyreoidismus mit C-Zellenhyperplasie der Schilddrüse. Überlegungen zur Einteilung der Hyperparathyreoidismus. Dtsch. med. Wschr. 93 (1968) 2411 bis 2415

Kuntz, J. L., L. Asch: Ostéocondensation diffuse au cours d'une drépanocytose. Rev. Rhum. 45 (1978) 145–149

Laborde, J. M., D. L. Green, A. D. Askari, A. Muir: Arthritis in hemochromatosis. A case report. J. Bone Jt Surg. 59 A (1977) 1103–1107

Lamy, M., P. Maroteaux: Acro-osteolyse dominante. Arch. franç. Pediat. 18 (1961) 693–702

Landbeck, G., A. Kurme: Die hämophile Kniegelenksarthropathie. Ein Beitrag zur Behandlung von Kniegelenkblutungen und ihren Folgezuständen. Mschr. Kinderheilk. 118 (1970) 29–41

Landgraf, F.-K.: Die Apophysitis acromialis, eine Osteochondropathie seltener Lokalisation. Fortschr. Röntgenstr. 81 (1954) 797–800

Laurent, J., P. Meunier, P. Courpron, C. Edouard, J. Bernard, G. Vignon: Recherches sur la pathogénie des nécroses aseptiques de la tête femorale. Evaluation du terrain osseux sur 35 biopsies iliaques étudièes quantitativement. Nouv. Presse méd. 14 (1973) 1755–1760

Lehman, C. A., M. H. Schreiber: Autonomous hyperparathyroidism in patients on maintenance home dialysis. Amer. J. Roentgenol. 127 (1976) 377–380

Lequesne, M.: La nécrose de la tête femorale avec chondrolyse rapide. J. belge Rhum. 27 (1972) 152–161

Lesch, M., W. L. Nyhan: A familial disorder or uric acid metabolism and central nervous system function. Amer. J. Med. 36 (1964) 561–570

Lévy, Ph., A. Bonnin, R. Ghozlan, F. Delrieu, A. Chevrot: Ostéonécrose primitive du condyle interne du génou du sujet âgé. J. Radiol. 53 (1972) 440–444

Lièvre, J.-A., A. Chaput, J.-P. Camus: Pycnodysostose de Maroteaux et Lamy (une observation). Rev. Rhum. 31 (1964) 282–286

Lindenfelser, R., W. Dihlmann, H. Mann, P. Plache, R. Wilmen: Resorptives Riesenzellgranulom und sekundärer Hyperparathyreoidismus. Fortschr. Röntgenstr. 121 (1974) 584–590

Lingg, G., G. Heinemeier: Morbus Friedrich—Aseptische Knochennekrose des sternalen Klavikulaendes. Beobachtung von 6 Fällen. Fortschr. Röntgenstr. 134 (1981) 74–77

Lipson, R. L., L. E. Williams: The „connective tissue disorder" of hyperparathyroidism. Arthr. and. Rheum. 11 (1968) 198–205

Lithner, F.: Skin lesions of the legs and feet and skeletal lesions of the feet in familial amyloidosis with polyneuropathy. Acta med. scand. 199 (1976) 197–202

Löhr, W.: Die Verschiedenheit der Auswirkung gleichartiger bekannter Schäden auf den Knochen Jugendlicher und Erwachsener, gezeigt an Epiphysenstörungen nach Erfrierungen und bei der Hämophilie. Zbl. Chir. 57 (1930) 898–909

Love, R. R., W. Kaboth: Sichelzellanämie. Eine Übersicht über klinische Symptome und Therapie beim Erwachsenen. Med. Klin. 71 (1976) 2103–2111

Lovell, R. R. H., G. B. D. Scott: Hypertrophic osteo-arthropathy in polyarteritis. Ann. rheum. Dis. 15 (1956) 46–50

Maas, D., H. Schubothe, J. Sennekamp, E. Genth, G. Maerker-Alzer, M. Droese, P. W. Hartl, K. Schumacher: Zur Frage einer Induzierbarkeit des Pseudo-LE-Syndroms durch Arzneimittel. Vorläufige Ergebnisse von Erhebungen bei 58 Fällen. Dtsch. med. Wschr. 100 (1975) 1555–1557

McCormick, C. C.: Case report 20. (Sezary's syndrome—mycoses fungoides group). Skelet. Radiol. 1 (1977) 183–184

McLaughlin, G. E., D. J. McCarty jr., B. L. Segal: Hemarthrosis complicating anticoagulant therapy. Report of three cases. J. Amer. med. Ass. 196 (1966) 1020–1021

Mähr, G., K. Rommel, W. Knoth: Paramyloidose mit Karpaltunnelsyndrom bei Bence-Jones-Plasmozytom. Dtsch. med. Wschr. 91 (1966) 2166–2170

Marcus, N. D., W. F. Enneking, R. A. Massam: The silent hip in idiopathic aseptic necrosis. Treatment by bone-grafting. J. Bone Jt Surg. 55 A (1973) 1351–1366

Marder, V. J., N. R. Shulman: Clinical aspects of congenital factor VII deficiency. Amer. J. Med. 37 (1964) 182–194

Martel, W.: The overhanging margin of bone: A roentgenologic manifestation of gout. Radiology 91 (1968) 755–756

Martel, W., B. H. Sitterley: Roentgenologic manifestations of osteonecrosis. Amer. J. Roentgenol. 104 (1969) 509–522

Martel, W., M. R. Abell, I. F. Duff: Cervical spine involvement in lipoid dermato-arthritis. Radiology 77 (1961) 613–617

Massry, S. G., R. Bluestone, J. R. Klinenberg, J. W. Cobum: Abnormalities of the musculoskeletal system in hemodialysis patients. Semin. Arthr. and. Rheum. 4 (1975) 321–349

Mau, H.: Idiopathische Hüftkopfnekrose Erwachsener. Z. Orthop. 101 (1966) 18–34

Maurer, R. M., O. L. Langford: Rothmund's syndrome. A cause of resorption of phalangeal tufts and dystrophic calcification. Radiology 89 (1967) 706–708

Mazières, B., R. Durroux, E. Jambon, G. Bouteiller, J. Arlet: Densification osseuse et Nécrose de la tête fémorale par thésaurismose a la polyvinyl-pyrrolidone. (Discussion diagnostique avec l'histiocytose X). Rev. Rhum. 47 (1980) 257–265

Meema, H. E., D. G. Oreopoulos, S. Rabinovich, H. Husdan, A. Rapoport: Periosteal new bone formation (periosteal neostosis) in renal osteodystrophy. Relation to osteosclerosis, osteitis fibrosa, and osteoid excess. Radiology 110 (1974) 513–522

Mertz, D. P.: Gicht. Grundlagen, Klinik und Therapie, 3. Aufl. Thieme, Stuttgart 1978

Middlemiss, J. H., A. B. Raper: Skeletal changes in the haemoglobinopathies. J. Bone Jt Surg. 48 B (1966) 693–702

Milikow, E., T. Asch: Hemiangiomatosis, localized growth disturbance, and intravascular coagulation disorder presenting with an unusual arthritis resembling hemophilia. Radiology 97 (1970) 387–388

Miller, W. T., R. A. Restifo: Steroid arthropathy. Radiology 86 (1966) 652–657

Mindelzun, R., M. Elkin, I. H. Scheinberg, I. Sternlieb: Skeletal changes in Wilson's disease. A radiological study. Radiology 94 (1970) 127–132

Missmahl, H. P.: Amyloidose, Klinik, Therapie, Prognose. Fortschr. Med. 85 (1967) 621–626

Moss, A. A., F. Mainzer: Osteopetrosis: An unusual case of terminal-tuft erosion. Radiology 97 (1970) 631–632

Murray, R. O.: Steriods and skeleton. Radiology 77 (1961) 729–743

Naidich, T. P., S. S. Siegelman: Paraarticular soft tissue changes in systemic diseases. Semin. Roentgenol. 8 (1973) 101–116

Neiman, H. L., B. M. Gompels, W. Martel: Pachydermoperiostosis with bone marrow failure and gross extramedullary hematopoiesis. Report of a case. Radiology 110 (1974) 553–554

Niepel, G., D. Kostka: Die Entstehung des Pseudo-Charcot-Gelenkes nach intraartikulären Instillationen von Hydrocortison bei rheumatoider Arthritis. Fortschr. Röntgenstr. 98 (1963) 505–507

Noetzli, M., H. L. Steinbach: Subperiosteal erosion of the ribs in hyperparathyroidism. Amer. J. Roentgenol. 87 (1962) 1058–1061

Norman, A., H. Robbins, J. E. Milgram: The acute neuropathic arthropathy—a rapid, severely disorganizing form of arthritis. Radiology 90 (1968) 1159–1164

Ozonoff, M. B., A. R. Clemett: Progressive osteolysis in progeria. Amer. J. Roentgenol. 100 (1967) 75–79

Pageaut, G., M. Guidet, J.-P. Carbillet, J.-P. Paquette, A. Oppermann: Anatomie pathologique de l'ochronose (Etude d'une observation et revue générale). Rev. Rhum. 38 (1971) 277–287

Partsch, H.: Hereditäre sensorische Neuropathie (Denny-Brown). (,,Familiäre Akroosterolyse"). Wien. klin. Wschr. 82 (1970) 129–136

Partsch, H.: Ulceromutilierende Neuropathien der unteren Extremitäten. Zum Krankheitsbild der ,,Acropathie ulcéromutilante". Hautarzt 22 (1971) 283–289

Pascual Gómez, E.: Evolución anatomopatológica inducida por una toracotomia exploradora en la membrana sinovial de la osteopatia hipertrofiante. Rev. esp. Reum. 5 (1978) 83–88

Pastershank, S. P., S. P. K. Tchang: Regional enteritis and hypertrophic osteoarthropathy. J. Canad. Ass. Radiol. 23 (1972) 35

Pavlov, H., A. B. Goldman, W. D. Arnold: Haemophilic arthropathy in the joints of the hands and feet. Brit. J. Radiol. 52 (1979) 173–180

Peavy, P. W., D. J. Franco: Gout: Presentation as a popliteal cyst. Radiology 111 (1974) 103–104

Perri, G.: Widening of the radial notch of the ulna: A new articular change in haemophilia. Clin. Radiol. 29 (1978) 61–62

Peyman, M. A.: Achalasia of cardia, carcinoma of oesophagus, and hypertrophic pulmonary osteoarthropathy. Brit. med. J. 1959/I, 23–25

Pogonowska, M. J., L. C. Collins, H. L. Dobson: Diabetic osteopathy. Radiology 89 (1967) 265–271

Poser, H., P. Gabriel-Jürgens: Knochen- und Gelenkveränderungen durch Druckluft bei Tauchern und Caisson-Arbeitern. Fortschr. Röntgenstr. 126 (1977) 156–160

Prager, P., R. Singer, E. Ritz, B. Krempien: Diagnostischer Stellenwert der Lamina dura dentium beim sekundären Hyperparathyreoidismus. Fortschr. Röntgenstr. 129 (1978) 237–240

Pugh, D. G.: Subperiosteal resorption of bone. A roentgenologic manifestation of primary hyperparathyroidism and renal osteodystrophy. Amer. J. Roentgenol. 66 (1951) 577–586

Rabinov, D.: Acromutilation of the fingers following severe burns. Radiology 77 (1961) 968–973

Raschke, G.: Über den Zusammenhang der Akrodermatitis chronica atrophicans Pick-Herxheimer und der Akroosteolyse. Derm. Wschr. 137 (1958) 217–221

Reichelt, A.: Röntgenologische Frühveränderungen der idiopathischen Hüftkopfnekrose. Fortschr. Röntgenstr. 108 (1968) 649–'653

Reichelt, A.: Ätiologie und Pathogenese der Hüftkopfnekrosen des Erwachsenen. Med. Klin. 70 (1975) 1535–1545

Rienhardt, K.: Pseudozystische Aufhellungen in beiden Patellae. Osteochondronekrose. Fortschr. Röntgenstr. 111 (1969) 262–269

Resnick, D.: Erosive arthritis of the hand and wrist in hyperparathyroidism. Radiology 110 (1974) 263–269

Resnick, D., G. Niwayama: Subchondral resorption of bone in renal osteodystrophy. Radiology 118 (1976) 315–321

Riskó, T., L. Kovács: Schenkelkopfnekrose nach Steroidtherapie. Z. Orthop. 99 (1965) 413–417

Ritz, E., H. M. Kuhn, B. Krempien, F. Heuck, W. Müller, W. Kerlé, C. Aschermann: Röntgenologische Zeichen gestörten Calciumstoffwechsels bei Dialysepatienten. II. Beziehungen der Röntgensymptome zu möglichen pathogenetischen Faktoren. Fortschr. Röntgenstr. 119 (1973) 194–202

Rosin, A. J.: Ectopic calcification around joints of paralysed limbs in hemiplegia, diffuse brain damage, and other neurological diseases. Ann. rheum. Dis. 34 (1975) 499–505

Rubenstein, H. M., M. H. Brooks: Aseptic necrosis of bone in myxedema. Ann. Intern. Med. 87 (1977) 580–581

Ruderman, M., D. J. McCarty jr.: Aseptic necrosis in systemic lupus erythematosus. Report of a case involving six joints. Arthr. and Rheum. 7 (1964) 709–717

Scanlon, G. T., A. R. Clemett: Thyroid acropachy. Radiology 83 (1964) 1039–1042

Schacherl, M., F. Schilling, A. Gamp: Das radiologische Bild der Gicht. Radiologe 6 (1966) 231–238

Schanche, A. F., S. M. Bierman, R. L. Sopher, B. J. O'Loughlin: Disseminated lipogranulomatosis: Early roentgenographic changes. Radiology 82 (1964) 675–678

Schaub, M. S., R. Rosen, W. Boswell, J. Gordonson: Tibiotalar slant: A new observation in sickle cell anemia. Radiology 117 (1975) 551–552

Schechter, S. L., G. G. Bole: Hypertrophic osteoarthropathy and rheumatoid arthritis. Simultaneous occurence in association with diffuse interstitial fibrosis. Arthr. and Rheum. 19 (1976) 639–643

Schellong, G., U. Göbel: Ambulante Behandlung der Hämophilie. Dtsch. Ärztebl. 74 (1977) 743–748

Schilling, F.: Klinik und Therapie der Gicht und deren Abgrenzung von der Pseudogicht. In: Fettsucht—Gicht. Sechste Bad Mergentheimer Stoffwechseltagung, hrsg. von W. Boecker. Thieme, Stuttgart 1971 (S. 139–160)

Schlumpf, U., N. Gerber, H. Bünzli, U. Elsässer, A. Pestalozzi, A. Böni: Arthritiden bei Thalassaemia minor. Schweiz. med. Wschr. 107 (1977) 1156–1162

Schneider, R., A. B. Goldman, W. H. O. Bohne: Neuropathic injuries to the lower extremities in children. Radiology 129 (1978) 713–718

Schuckmann, W.: Die aseptische Osteonekrose im Bereich des Tuber ossis ischii. Beitr. Orthop. Traum. 20 (1973) 113–118

Schüler, K.-H., W. Laschner: Zur Differentialdiagnose osteolytischer Prozesse. Arch. orthop. Unfall-Chir. 65 (1969) 146 bis 167

Schumacher jr., H. R.: Hemochromatosis and arthritis. Arthr. and Rheum. 7 (1964) 41–50

Schumacher, H. R., R. Andrews, G. McLaughlin: Arthropathy in sickle-cell disease. Ann. intern. Med. 78 (1973) 203–211

Schumacher, H. R., B. B. Dorwart, J. Bond, A. Alavi, W. Miller: Chronic synovitis with early cartilage destruction in sickle cell disease. Ann. rheum. Dis. 36 (1977) 413–419

Schwarz, E., A. Fish: Reticulohistiocytoma: A rare dermatologic disease with Roentgen manifestations. Amer. J. Roentgenol. 83 (1960) 692–697

Schwille, P. O., H. Bünte, P. Hermanek, M. Nüvemann: Normound hypocalcämischer primärer Hyperparathyreoidismus (Pseudohypohyperparathyreoidismus). Chirurg 43 (1972) 518–521

Scott, R. B., S. McD. Elmore, N. C. Brackett jr., W. O. Harris jr., W. J. S. Still: Neuropathic joint disease (Charcot joints) in Waldenström's macroglobulinemia with amyloidosis. Amer. J. Med. 54 (1973) 549–558

Seewald, K.: Bericht über einen Fall der Dissektion des oberen Patellapoles im Verlauf einer Arthritis urica. Wien. klin. Wschr. 83 (1971) 548–549

Sella, E. J., A. H. Goodman: Arthropathy secondary to transfusion hemochromatosis. J. Bone Jt Surg. 55 A (1973) 1077–1081

Sellers, A., A. C. Winfield, S. G. Massry: Resorption of condyloid process of mandible. Arch. intern. Med. 131 (1973) 727–728

Sengupta, S., K. Prathap: Radiation necrosis of the humerus. A report of three cases. Acta radiol. Ther. Phys. Biol. 12 (1973) 313–320

Sennara, H., F. Gorry: Orthopedic aspects of sickle cell anemia and hemoglobinopathies. Clin. Orthop. 130 (1978) 154–157

Sharon, P., N. Kaplinsky, S. Leiba, O. Frankl: Aseptic necrosis of head of femur: Presenting manifestation in Cushing's disease. J. Rheumatol. 4 (1977) 73–75

Shawarby, K., M. S. Ibrahim: Pachydermoperiostosis. A review of literature and report on four cases. Brit. med. J. 1962/I, 763–766

Sherman, M.: Pathogenesis of disintegration of the hip in sickle cell anemia. Sth. med. J. (Bgham, Ala.) 52 (1959) 632–637

Singleton, E. B., Ching Tseng Teng: Pseudohypoparathyroidism with bone changes simulating hyperparathyroidism. Radiology 78 (1962) 388–393

Sommer, F., K. Reinhardt: Das Osteolysesyndrom. Arch. orthop. Unfall-Chir. 51 (1959) 69–107

Spelsberg, F., M. A. Dambacher, P. C. Scriba: Klassifikation, Diagnostik und Behandlung des primären Hyperparathyreoidismus im Umbruch. Chirurg 46 (1975) 215–221

Stecken, A.: Akroosteolysis bei einem Geiger. Fortschr. Röntgenstr. 80 (1954) 405–407

Stein, G., S. Jühe, C.-E. Lange, G. Veltman: Bandförmige Osteolysen in den Endphalangen des Handskeletts. Fortschr. Röntgenstr. 118 (1973) 60–63

Steinbach, H. L., G. S. Gordon, E. Eisenberg, J. T. Crane, S. Silverman, L. Goldman: Primary hyperparathyreoidism: A correlation of roentgen, clinical, and pathologic features. Amer. J. Roentgenol. 86 (1961) 329–343

Storey, G. O.: Bone necrosis in joint disease. Proc. roy. Soc. Med. 61 (1968) 961–969

Strauss, J., J. L. Magnet, M. Guidet, R. Paul: Les nécroses osseuses au cours des ostéomalacies. Rev. Rhum. 46 (1979) 101–109

Stuber, J. L., E. Palacios: Vertebral scalloping in acromegaly. Amer. J. Roentgenol. 112 (1971) 397–400

Sundaram, M., P. F. Joyce, J. B. Shields, M. A. Riaz, S. Sagar: Terminal phalangeal tufts: Earliest site of renal osteodystrophy findings in hemodialysis patients. Amer. J. Roentgenol. 133 (1979) 25–29

Tanaka, K. R., G. O. Clifford, A. R. Axelrod: Sickle cell anemia (homozygous S) with aseptic necrosis of femoral head. Blood 11 (1956) 998–1008

Thévenard, A.: L'acropathie ulcéro-mutilante familiale. Rev. neurol. 74 (1942) 193–212

Torg, J. S., H. H. Steel: Essential osteolysis with nephropathy. A review of the literature and case report of an unusual syndrome. J. Bone Jt Surg. 50 A (1968) 1629–1638

Torg, J. S., A. M. DiGeorge, J. A. Kirkpatrick jr., M. M. Trujillo: Hereditary multicentric osteolysis with recessive transmission: A new syndrome. J. Pediat. 75 (1969) 243–252

Torres-Reyes, E., T. W. Staple: Roentgenographic appearance of thyroid acropachy. Clin. Radiol. 21 (1970) 95–100

Trapnell, D. H., D. Jackson: Bone and joints changes following burns. Clin. Radiol. 16 (1965) 180–186

Twersky, J.: Joint changes in idiopathic hemochromatosis. Amer. J. Roentgenol. 124 (1975) 139–144

Ueberschär, K. H.: Aseptische Nekrose an der Basis des Großzehenendgliedes. Fortschr. Röntgenstr. 87 (1957) 137–138

Uehlinger, E.: Hyperostosis generalisata mit Pachydermie (Idiopathische familiäre generalisierte Osteophytose Friedreich-Erb-Arnold). Virchows Arch. path. Anat. 308 (1942) 396–444

Uehlinger, E.: Aseptische Knochennekrosen (Infarkte) nach Prednisonbehandlung. Schweiz. med. Wschr. 94 (1964) 1527–1530

Uehlinger, E.: Die Amyloid-Arthropathie. Wiss. Z. Friedr.-Schiller-Univ. Jena, Math.-Naturw. R. 20 (1971) 335–342

Uehlinger, E.: Destruktive Gelenkamyloidose (Amyloidarthrose). Verh. dtsch. Ges. Rheum. 3 (1974) 233–238

Uehlinger, E.: Die pathologische Anatomie der Gicht. Therapiewoche 25 (1975) 4400–4405

Vick, H., J. Bahlmann: Störungen des Knochenstoffwechsels bei Urämie. Therapiewoche 26 (1976) 2548–2560

Vignon, E., S. Sabeh-Ayoun, L. M. Patricot, J. Favre-Gilly, M. Arlot: Les arthropathies de l'hypoconvertinémie. A propos d'une observation. Rev. Rhum. 46 (1979) 141–145

Vinson, H. A., R. Schatzki: Roentgenologic bone changes encountered in frostbite, Korea 1950–51. Radiology 63 (1954) 685–695

Voss, D., B. A. Waaler: Congenital hypoproconvertinemia. A report on 12 cases with total deficiency and 19 cases with partial deficiency. Thrombos. Diathes. haemorrh. (Stuttg.) 3 (1959) 375–385

Wagner, A., J. Schaaf: Untersuchungen über Größe und Häufigkeit der Sesambeine bei Akromegalie. Fortschr. Röntgenstr. 99 (1963) 215–219

Weinfeld, A., M. H. Stern, L. H. Marx: Amyloid lesions of bone. Amer. J. Roentgenol. 108 (1970) 799–805

Weller, M., J. Edeiken, J. Hodes: Renal osteodystrophy. Amer. J. Roentgenol. 104 (1968) 354–363

Wharton, G. W., T. H. Morgan: Ankylosis in the paralyzed patient. J. Bone Jt Surg. 52 A (1970) 105–112

von Wichert, P.: Skelettveränderungen als paraneoplastisches Syndrom bei Lungentumoren. Dtsch. med. Wschr. 92 (1967) 2396–2398

Wiedemann, H.-R.: Zur Françoisschen Krankheit. Dystrophia dermochondrocornealis familiaris. Ärztl. Wschr. 13 (1958) 905–909

Wiedemann, H.-R.: Pyknodysostose. Fortschr. Röntgenstr. 103 (1965) 590–597

Wiernick, P. H.: Amyloid joint disease. Medicine (Baltimore) 51 (1972) 465–479

Wilde, A. H., H. J. Mankin, G. P. Rodnan: Avascular necrosis of the femoral head in scleroderma. Arthr. and Rheum. 13 (1970) 445–447

Wilke, H., H. Frahm, J. Zsernaviczky, D. von Torklus: Multiple aseptische Knochennekrosen bei Hyperlipämie, Hyperurikämie und latentem Diabetes mellitus. Dtsch. med. Wschr. 99 (1974) 1530–1532

Williams, J. L., M. M. Cliff, A. Bonakdarpour: Spontaneous osteonecrosis of the knee. Radiology 107 (1973) 15–19

Wilson, R. H., W. E. McCormick, D. F. Tatum, J. L. Creech: Occupational acroosteolysis. Report of 31 cases. J. Amer. med. Ass. 201 (1967) 577–581

Winchester, P., H. Grossman, Wan Ngo Lim, B. Shannon Danes: A new acid mucopolysaccharidosis with skeletal deformities simulating rheumatoid arthritis. Amer. J. Roentgenol. 106 (1969) 121–128

Witzel, L., F. Becker, H. F. Fuchs, J. Mockwitz: Pseudotumoren der Knochen bei Hämophilie. Dtsch. med. Wschr. 98 (1973) 206–209

Wood, K., A. Omer, M. T. Shaw: Haemophilic arthropathy. A combined radiological and clinical study. Brit. J. Radiol. 42 (1969) 498–505

Enthesopathies (fibroosteosis, fibroosteitis); diseases of bursae and tendons; calcifications of soft tissues (see also under Autoimmune diseases) including chondrocalcinosis and crystalinduced synovitis; ossifications of soft tissues (see also under Neurogenic paraosteoarthropathy); carpal tunnel syndrome (unless discussed elsewhere under the headings of its causes); synovial cysts.

Adams, J. E., M. Davies: Paravertebral and peripheral ligamentous ossification: an unusual association of hypoparathyroidism. Postgrad. med. J. 53 (1977) 167–172

Alexander, C. J.: The aetiology of juvenile spondylarthritis (discitis). Clin. Radiol. 21 (1970) 178–187

Asshoff, H., P. Böhm, E. Schoen, K. Schürholz: Klinik der hereditären Chondrocalcinosis articularis. Dtsch. med. Wschr. 92 (1967) 349–357

Bahous, I., W. Müller: Die Calcinosis periarticularis generalisata. Generalisierte Hydroxylapatitkrankheit. Schweiz. med. Wschr. 109 (1979) 502–508

Baker, W. M., 1877: zit. n. M. I. V. Jayson, A. St. J. Dixon: Valvular mechanisms in juxta-articular cysts. Ann. rheum. Dis. 29 (1970) 415–420

Barabás, Cs., J. Oláh: Wirbelsäulenverkalkung bei Jugendlichen. Fortschr. Röntgenstr. 110 (1969) 831–838

Bauer, R.: Differentialdiagnose und Therapie der Periarthritis humeroscapularis. Arch. orthop. Unfall-Chir. 65 (1969) 13–30

Bensasson, M., H. Dorfmann, M. Peres-Busquier, J. Solnica, C. Mery, M.-F. Kahn, S. de Sèze: Étude radiographique de la main dans 50 cas de chondrocalcinose articulaire primitive. Comparaison avec une série de 100 temoins. Rev. Rhum. 42 (1975) 3–11

Berger, L. S., F. M. H. Ziter jr.: Calcifications within enlarged subdeltoid bursae in rheumatoid arthritis. Brit. J. Radiol. 45 (1972) 530–531

Bilezikian, J. P., T. B. Connor, R. Aptekar, J. Freijanes, G. D. Aurbach, W. N. Pachas, S. A. Wells, J. L. Decker: Pseudogout after parathyroidectomy. Lancet 1973/I, 445–446

Birkner, R., K. Consentius: Verknöcherungen in der Wand des Foramen obturatum. Fortschr. Röntgenstr. 127 (1977) 72–74

Bléry, M., B. Barré: Maladie des calcifications tendineuses multiples. J. Radiol. Électrol. 59 (1978) 271–273

Bloch, J., F. K. Fischer: Probleme der Schultersteife. Docum. rheum. 15 (J. R. Geigy, Basel) (1958)

Bopp, J.: Calcinosis interstitialis am Unterschenkel. Fortschr. Röntgenstr. 76 (1952) 542

Bouvier, M., E. Lejeune, M. Rouillat, J. Marionnet: Les formes ulcéro-mutilantes du syndrome du canal carpien. Rev. Rhum. 46 (1979) 169–176

Caffey, J., F. N. Silverman: Pediatric X-Ray Diagnosis, 5. Aufl. Year Book Medical Publ., Chicago 1967

Campbell, F., F. Feldman: Bone and soft tissue abnormalities of the upper extremity in diabetes mellitus. Amer. J. Roentgenol. 124 (1975) 7–16

Cooper, W.: Calcareous tendinitis in the metacarpophalangeal region. J. Bone Jt Surg. 24 (1942) 114–122

Coventry, M. B.: Calcification in a cervical disc with anterior protrusion and dysphagia. A case report. J. Bone Jt Surg. 52 A (1970) 1463–1466

Crasselt, C.: Arthrozelen bei rheumatischen Kniegelenkserkrankungen. Z. Orthop. 104 (1968) 570–579

Currey, H. L. F.: Pyrophosphate arthropathy and calcific periarthritis. Clin. Orthop. 71 (1970) 70–80

Dieppe, P. A., P. Crocker, E. C. Huskisson, D. A. Willoughby: Apatite deposition disease. A new arthropathy. Lancet 1976/I, 266–269

Dihlmann, W.: Calcaneopathia rheumatica (röntgenologischer Nachweis, Differentialdiagnose). Fortscher. Röntgenstr. 107 (1967) 271–276

Dihlmann, W.: Fibroostosis und Fibroostitis (Terminologie, Röntgenmorphologie, Traceruntersuchungen). Z. Orthop. 112 (1974) 1242–1248

Dinkel, L.: Ein Zeichen der langfristigen Dihydrotachysterin-(AT10-)Überdosierung. Fortschr. Röntgenstr. 107 (1967) 494–497

Dittert, R.: Ungewöhnlicher Sitz einer Peritendinitis Calcarea. Fortschr. Röntgenstr. 90 (1959) 523–524

Djian, A., R. Ellequain, N. Beaslay: Une curieuse pubite aigue première manifestation k'une chondrocalcinose diffuse. Rev. Rhum. 45 (1978) 69

Dominok, G. W.: Die industrielle Knochenfluorose und Probleme einer Fluortherapie der Osteoporose. Z. Alternsforsch. 29 (1975) 277–283

Doppman, J. L.: Baker's cyst and the normal gastrocnemio-semimembranosus bursa. Amer. J. Roentgenol. 94 (1965) 646–652

Dorwart, B. B., H. R. Schumacher: Joint effusions, chondrocalcinosis and other rheumatic manifestations in hypothyroidism. A clinicopathologic study. Amer. J. Med. 59 (1975) 780–790

Erbe, W., B. Regler: Eine Beobachtung über den zeitlichen Verlauf der Myositis ossificans progressiva. Fortschr. Röntgenstr. 119 (1973) 374–376

Eriksen, J.: A case of carpal tunnel syndrome on the basis of an abnormally long lumbrical muscle. Acta orthop. scand. 44 (1973) 275–277

Gerster, J. C., H. Hauser, G. H. Fallet: Xeroradiographic techniques applied to assessment of Achiles tendon in inflammatory diseases. Ann. rheum. Dis. 34 (1975) 479–488

Gerster, J. C., T. L. Vischer, A. Bennani, G. H. Fallet: The painful heel. Comparative study in rheumatoid arthritis, ankylosing spondylitis, Reiter's syndrome, and generalized osteoarthrosis. Ann. rheum. Dis. 36 (1977) 343–348

Gerster, J. C., C. A. Baud, R. Lagier, I. Boussina, G. H. Fallet: Tendon calcifications in chondrocalcinosis. A clinical, radiologic, histologic, cristallographic study. Arthr. and. Rheum. 20 (1977) 717–722

Glass, J. S., R. Grahame: Chondrocalcinosis after parathyroidectomy. Ann. rheum. Dis. 35 (1976) 285

Goldman, A. B.: Myositis ossificans circumscripta: A benign lesion with a malignant differential diagnosis. Amer. J. Roentgenol. 126 (1976) 32–40

Gray, R. G., M. J. Poppo, N. L. Gottlieb: Primary familial bilateral carpal tunnel syndrome. Ann. intern. Med. 91 (1979) 37–40

Greenspan, A., A. Norman, F. Kia-Ming Tchang: „Tooth" sign in patellar degenerative disease. J. Bone Jt Surg. 59 A (1977) 483–485

Guest, C. M., H. G. Jacobson: Pelvic and estrapelvic osteopathy in rheumatoid spondylitis. A clinical and roentgenographic study of ninety cases. Amer. J. Roentgenol. 65 (1951) 760–768

Heiss, W.: Werferellbogen, diagnostik 5 (1972) 452–455

Heitzeberg, H., I. Reiner-Theisen: Die Ossifikation der Korako-Klavikularbänder. Röntgen-Bl. 31 (1978) 512–515

Holden, N. T.: Deposition of calcium salts in the popliteus tendon. J. Bone Jt Surg. 37 B (1955) 446–447

Horváth, F.: Über die auf dem sternalen Drittel und kaudal befindliche „Usuration" der Klavikula. Fortschr. Röntgenstr. 116 (1972) 836–837

Hsien-Chi Fang: Periostitis of the os calcis. An osteo-periosteal manifestation of rheumatoid arthritis. Chin. med. J. 66 (1948) 57–65

Jacobelli, S., D. J. McCarty, D. C. Silcox, J. C. Mail: Calcium pyrophosphate dihydrate crystal deposition in neuropathic joints. Four cases of polyarticular involvement. Ann. intern. Med. 79 (1973) 340–347

Jansen, H. H.: Über eine besondere Verlaufsform der Psoriasis arthropathica. Verh. dtsch. Ges. Path. 47 (1963) 203–205

Jonasch, E.: Die Verknöcherung des Ligamentum popliteum obliquum. Fortschr. Röntgenstr. 99 (1963) 695–697

Jones, G. B.: Acute episodes with calcification around the hip joint. J. Bone Jt Surg. 37 (1955) 448–452

Kempmann, G.: Verkalkte Beckenvenenthrombose und Stauungssossifikation am Unterschenkel—seltene Spätfolgen der chronischvenösen Insuffizienz. Fortschr. Röntgenstr. 127 (1977) 74–76

Klages, F.: Metaplastische Knochenneubildungen im Verlaufe einer chronischen Thalliumvergiftung. Arch. klin. Chir. 201 (1941) 663–676

Klaus, E., J. Nekula: Cervicale Bandscheibenverkalkung beim Kind. Eine röntgenologische Langzeitbeobachtung. Radiologe 15 (1975) 59–61

Kohlmann, W.: Calcinosis interstitialis localisata nach Peronäuslähmung. Fortschr. Röntgenstr. 82 (1955) 419–421

Kolář, J., R. Vrabec: Der röntgenologische Nachweis von Verkalkungen und Knochenbildung in den gelenknahen Weichteilen nach Verbrennungen. Fortschr. Röntgenstr. 87 (1957) 761–765

Kolawole, T. M., S. P. Bohrer: Tumoral calcinosis with „fluid levels" in the tumoral masses. Amer. J. Roentgenol. 120 (1974) 461–465

Krasemann, P.-H.: Calcinosis interstitialis bei Gefäßverschluß. Fortschr. Röntgenstr. 103 (1965) 113–114

Kübler, E.: Neue Gesichtspunkte bei der Beurteilung der Verlaufsformen der Myositis ossificans progressiva. Fortschr. Röntgenstr. 81 (1954) 354–371

Kumar, S. P., R. A. Kemp Harper: Fluorosis in Aden. Brit. J. Radiol. 36 (1963) 497–502

La Cava, G.: Enthesitis—traumatic disease of insertions. J. Amer. med. Ass. 169 (1959) 254–255

Laczay, A., K. Scapó: Verknöcherungen im Ligamentum patellae und die Schlatter-Osgoodsche Krankheit. Fortschr. Röntgenstr. 119 (1973) 347–351

Lagier, R., H. Ott: Place de la chondrocalcinose en pathologie articulaire. Radiol. clin. (Basel) 38 (1969) 115–131

Lányi, A., B. Geryk: Verknöcherungen der Ansatzstellen einiger Sehnen und Bänder und ihr differentialdiagnostischer Wert. Radiol. diagn. (Berl.) 11 (1970) 493–499

Lanz, U., J. Wolter: Das akute Carpaltunnelsyndrom. Chirurg 46 (1975) 32–35

Lehmann, A., U. Saxer: Der Tennis- und der Werferellbogen (Epicondylitis humeri radialis und ulnaris). Ther. Umsch. 33 (1976) 398–401

Leichner-Weil, S.: Bandscheibenverkalkung beim Kinde. Fortschr. Röntgenstr. 104 (1966) 273–274

Lutwak, L.: Myositis ossificans progressiva. Mineral, metabolic and radioactive calcium studies of the effect of hormones. Amer. J. Med. 37 (1964) 269–293

McCarty jr., D. J.: Pseudogout; articular chondrocalcinosis. Calcium pyrophosphate crystal deposition disease. In: Arthritis and Allied Conditions, 8. Aufl. hrsg. von J. L. Hollander, Lea & Febiger, Philadelphia 1972

McCarty jr., D. J., R. A. Gatter: Recurrent acute inflammation associated with focal apatite crystal deposition. Arthr. and Rheum. 9 (1966) 804–819

McCarty jr., D. J., N. N. Kohn, J. S. Faires: The significance of calcium phosphate crystals in the synovial fluid of arthritic patients: the „pseudogout syndrome". I. Clinical aspects. Ann. intern. Med. 56 (1962) 711–737

McCarty jr., D. J., J. M. Hogan, R. A. Gatter, M. Grossman: Studies on pathological calcifications in human cartilage. I. Prevalence and types of crystal deposits in the menisci of two hundred fifteen cadavera. J. Bone Jt Surg. 48 A (1966) 309–325

McNulty, J. G., P. Pim: Hyperphosphatasia. Report of a case with 30 year follow-up. Amer. J. Roentgenol. 115 (1972) 614–618

Mainzer, F.: Herniation of the nucleus pulposus. A rare complication of intervertebral-disk calcification in children. Radiology 107 (1973) 167–170

Melnick, J. C., F. N. Silverman: Intervertebral disk calcification in childhood. Radiology 80 (1963) 399–408

Menkes, C.-J., F. Simon, M. Chouraki, M. Ecoffet, B. Amor, F. Delbarre: Les arthropathies destructrices de le chondrocalcinose. Rev. Rhum. 40 (1973) 115–123

Miller, C. F.: Occupational calcareous peritendinitis of the feet. A case report. Amer. J. Roentgenol. 61 (1949) 506–510

Mohr, W., W. Dihlmann, W. Wilke, J. Hersener: Kalziumpyrophosphat-Arthropathie (CPPA). Diagnose und pathogenetische Bedeutung der Kristallablagerungen. Akt. Rheumatol. 6 (1981) 37–43

Moller, P. F.: Chronic fluorine poisoning, seen from the röntgenological standpoint. Brit. J. Radiol. 12 (1939) 13–20

Newmark III, H., D. M. Forrester, J. C. Brown, A. Robinson, S. M. Olken, R. Bledsoe: Calcific tendinitis of the neck. Radiology 128 (1978) 355–358

Niepel, G. A., D. Kostka, Š. Kopecký, Š. Manca: Enthesopathy. Acta rheum. balneol. Pistiniana 1 (1966) 1–64

Otte, P.: Verkalkungs- und Entkalkungsprozesse im Schulterbereich (Anmerkung zu Reischauers neuraler Theorie). Z. Orthop. 98 (1964) 405–419

Palmer, D. G.: Synovial cysts in rheumatoid disease. Ann. intern. Med. 70 (1969) 61–68

Parkash, S., K, Kumar: Fibrodysplasia ossificans traumatica. A case report. J. Bone Jt Surg. 54 A (1972) 1306–1308

Pedersen, H. E., J. A. Key: Pathology of calcareous tendinitis and subdeltoid bursitis. Arch. Surg. 62 (1951) 50–63

Reginato, A. J., H. R. Schumacher, V. A. Martinez: ochronotic arthropathy with calcium pyrophosphate crystal deposition. A light and electron microscopic study. Arthr. and. Rheum. 16 (1973) 705–714

Reinhardt, K.: Popliteacysten und popliteogene Unterschenkelcysten (Baker-Cysten). Radiologe 12 (1972) 77–86

Reischauer, F.: Zur Pathogenese der Epicondylitiden. Langenbecks Arch. klin. Chir. 289 (Kongreßber.) (1958) 401–410

Resnick, D., G. Niwayama: Resorption of the undersurface of the distal clavicle in rheumatoid arthritis. Radiology 120 (1976) 75–77

Resnick, D., G. Niwayama, T. G. Goergen, P. D. Utsinger, R. F. Shapiro, D. H. Haselwood, K. B. Wiesner: Clinical, radiographic and pathologic abnormalities in calcium pyrophosphate dihydrate deposition disease (CPPD): Pseudogout. Radiology 122 (1977) 1–15

Rössler, A.: Zur Kenntnis der Achillodynie. Dtsch. Z. Chir. 42 (1896) 274–291

Saporta, L., M. O. Chanzy, C. Mery, P. Jasson, F. Delbarre: Apparition de calcifications cutanées chez un sujet atteint de lupus érythémateux disséminé. Rev. Rhum. 45 (1978) 53–57

Schallock, G.: Zur Pathologie des „Weichteilrheumatismus". In: Fortbildungskurse für Rheumatologie, Bd. I. Karger, Basel 1971 (S. 18–34)

Schilling, F.: Die bei chronischen rheumatischen Erkrankungen mögliche Beteiligung des Nervensystems: Polyneuropathie, periphere und medulläre Kompressionssyndrome. Therapiewoche 24 (1974) 2950–2954

Schmied, P., P. van Rossum, R. Gabay, G. Zahnd: Etude radiologique sur la frequence de l'association entre la chondrocalcinose articulaire et le diabète. Schweiz. med. Wschr. 101 (1971) 272–276

Schneider, H.: Die Abnützungserkrankungen der Sehnen und ihre Therapie. Thieme, Stuttgart 1959

Schneider, P. G.: Der Tennisellbogen. diagnostik 5 (1972) 448–451

Schumacher, H. R., A. P. Somlyo, R. L. Tse, K. Maurer: Arthritis associated with apatite crystals. Ann. intern. Med. 87 (1977) 411–416

Seyss, R.: Zu den Verkalkungen der Gelenksbänder. Fortschr. Röntgenstr. 89 (1958) 239–240

Singh, A., R. Dass, S. Singh Hayreh, S. S. Jolly: Skeletal changes in endemic fluorosis. J. Bone Jt Surg. 44 B (1962) 806–815

Smith, R.: Myositis ossificans progressiva: A review of current problems. Semin. Arthr. and. Rheum. 4 (1975) 369–380

Sobbe, A., M. Siedek, C. P. Sodomann, A. Düx: Metastatische Verkalkungen bei chronischer Hämodialyse. Fortschr. Röntgenstr. 110 (1969) 851–862

Sonnenschein, A.: Zur Verkalkung des Nucleus pulposus. Fortschr. Röntgenstr. 81 (1954) 531–534

Spiegel, P. G., M. Ginsberg, J. L. Skosey, P. Kwong: Acute carpal tunnel syndrome secondary to pseudogout. Case report. Clin. Orthop. 120 (1976) 185–187

Srping, R.: Die „chronische Leistenzerrung" beim Spitzensportler und deren Therapie. Z. Orthop. 115 (1977) 369–371

Steinbach, H. L., F. O. Kolb, J. T. Crane: Unusual roentgen manifestations of osteomalacia. Amer. J. Roentgenol. 82 (1959) 875–886

Steinfeld, J. R., K. E. Schuit, T. E. Keats: Calcification in Cooper's ligament. Amer. J. Roentgenol. 121 (1974) 107–108

Steinitz, H.: Calcinosis circumscripta („Kalkgicht") und Calcinosis universalis. Ergebn. inn. Med. Kinderheilk. 39 (1931) 216–275

Štĕpán, J., Š, Pitrová, V. Pazderka: Cystinosis with crystal-induced synovitis and arthropathy. Z. Rheumatol. 35 (1976) 347–355

Swannell, A. J., F. A. Underwood, A. St. J. Dixon: Periarticular calcific deposits mimicking acute arthritis. Ann. Rheum. Dis. 29 (1970) 380–385

Villiaumey, J., P. Galle, J. Amouroux, B. Larget-Piet, M. Rotterdam. C. Di Menza, R. Louis, M.-C. Voisin, M. Perrigot, J.-P. Bouvet, M. Boccara, P. Pointud, D. Daupleix, B. Avouac: Athropathies lytiques et chondrocalcinose articulaire. Sem. Hôp. Paris 50 (1974) 3175–3190

Virchow, H.: Ueber den Calcaneus-Sporn. Berl. klin. Wschr. 53 (1916) 995–996

Weinberger, A., J. G. Kaplan, A. R. Myers: Extensive soft tissue calcification (calcinosis universalis) in systemic lupus erythematosus. Ann. rheum. Dis. 38 (1979) 384–386

Weston, W. J.: Peroneal tendinitis calcarea. Brit. J. Radiol. 32 (1959a) 134–135

Weston, W. J.: Tendinitis calcarea on the dorsum of the foot. Brit. J. Radiol. 32 (1959b) 495

Žitňan, D., Š. Sit'aj: Chondrocalcinosis articularis. Section I. Clinical and radiological study. Ann. rheum. Dis. 22 (1963) 142–152

Space-occupying processes; tumors, tumorlike lesions (including xanthoma and pigmented villonodular synovitis), their diagnosis, radiologic differential diagnosis and their complications (see also under Pachydermoperiostosis; Paraneoplastic diseases).

Ankerhold, J., D. von Torklus, W. Jacques: Der Zeitfaktor bei der pigmentierten villonodulären Synovitis der Gelenke. Z. Orthop. 112 (1974) 384–392

Ansell, B. M.: Case report 40. (Acute lymphoblastic leukemia). Skelet. Radiol. 2 (1977) 113–115

Bedwell, G. A., A. M. Dawson: Chronic myeloid leukaemia in a child presenting as acute polyarthritis. Arch. Dis. Childh. 29 (1954) 78–79

Bjersand, A. J.: Bone changes hypercholesterolemia. Radiology 130 (1979) 101–102

Bose, K. S., B. Chowdhuri: Observations on synovial sarcoma. J. Indian med. Ass. 39 (1962) 621–627

Braun, S., A. Chevrot, B. Tomeno, F. Delbarre, G. Pallardy, J. Moutounet, R. Kulas-Durand: A propos des ostéomes ostéoides phalangiens. (13 cas personnels). Rev. Rhum. 46 (1979) 225–233

Braunstein, E., W. Martel, L. Weatherbee: Periosteal bone apposition in chondroblastoma. Skelet. Radiol. 4 (1979) 34–36

Bussière, J.-L., B. Sauvezie, R. Lopitaux, Ph. Prin, P. Valentin, S. Rampon: Ostéom ostéoide avec synovite d'allure rhumatoide. Rev. Rhum. 43 (1976) 651–653

Committee on Bone Tumours: Radiological Atlas of Bone Tumours, Bd. II. Mouton, Den Haag 1973

DeBenedetti, M. J., C. P. Schwinn: Tenosynovial chondromatosis in the hand. J. Bone Jt Surg. 61 A (1979) 898–903

Douglas, G. W., R. H. Levin, L. Sokoloff: Infectious arthritis complicating neoplastic disease. New Engl. J. Med. 270 (1964) 299–302

Ebbinghaus, K. D.: Klinik und Pathogenese der „malignen" Synovialome. Ärztl. Wschr. 8 (1953) 1071–1076

Edeiken, J., P. J. Hodes: Roentgen diagnosis of diseases of bone, 2. Aufl. Bd. II. Williams & Wilkins, Baltimore 1973

Feist, J. H., T. G. Gibbons: Osteochondromatosis of the temporomandibular joint. Radiology 74 (1960) 291–294

Flesch, R., P. Hermanek: Fasciitis nodularis (nodular Fasciitis). Fortschr. Med. 94 (1976) 627–632

Fredrickson, D. S., R. S. Lees: A system for phenotyping hyperlipoproteinemia. Circulation 31 (1965) 321–327

Fuchs, R., D. Wahl: Beitrag zur Diagnose pseudozystischer Aufhellungen der Patella. Fortschr. Röntgenstr. 115 (1971) 320–325

Glay, A.: Destructive lesions of the clavicle. J. Canad. Ass. Radiol. 12 (1961) 117–125

Goergen, T. G., D. Resnick, G. Greenway, S. L. Saltzstein: Dorsal defect of the patella (DDP): A characteristic radiographic lesion. Radiology 130 (1979) 333–336

Goldenberg, D. L., W. Kelley, R. B. Gibbons: Metastatic adenocarcinoma of synovium presenting as an acute arthritis. Arthr. and. Rheum. 18 (1975) 107–110

Goutallier, D., J. Debeyre, B. Lassale: Chondromatose synoviale d'une articulation métacarpo-phalangienne. Rev. Chir. orthop. 64 (1978) 71–74

Green, R., R. P. Whittaker: Benign chondroblastoma. Case report with pulmonary metastasis. J. Bone Jt Surg. 57 A (1975) 418–420

Groulier, P., J.-L. Goode, L. Garbe, J.-Cl. Lapousse, H. Payan, E. Hawthorn: Synovite villo-nodulaire pigmentée. A propos de 4 observations. Rev. Rhum. 40 (1973) 329–338

Hamilton, E. B. D., E. G. L. Bywaters: Joint symptoms in myelomatosis and similar conditions. Ann. rheum. Dis. 20 (1961) 353–362

Heidenblut, A.: Malignes Synoviolom. Fortschr. Röntgenstr. 93 (1960) 809–811

Horowitz, A. L., D. Resnick, R. C. Watson: The roentgen features of synovial sarcomas. Clin. Radiol. 24 (1973) 481–484

Hull, M. T., F. Gonzalez-Crussi, G. P. DeRosa, R. S. Graul: Aggressive chondroblastoma. Report of a case with multiple bone and soft tissue involvement. Clin. Orthop. 126 (1977) 261–265

Hunder, G. G., L. E. Ward, J. C. Ivins: Rheumatoid granulomatous lesion simulating malignancy in the head and neck of the femur. Mayo Clin. Proc. 40 (1965) 766–770

Hutter, R. V. P., F. W. Foote jr., K. C. Francis, N. L. Higinbotham: Parosteal fasciitis. A self-limited benign process that simulates a malignant neoplasm. Amer. J. Surg. 104 (1962) 800–807

Jaffe, H. L., L. Lichtenstein, C. J. Sutro: Pigmented villonodular synovitis, bursitis and tenosynovitis. A discussion of the synovial and bursal equivalents of the tenosynovial lesion commonly denoted as Xanthoma, Xanthogranuloma, giant cell tumor or myeloplaxoma of the tendon sheath, with some consideration of this tendon sheath lesion itself. Arch. Pathol. 31 (1941) 731–765

Jergesen, H. E., H. J. Mankin, A. L. Schiller: Diffuse pigmented villonodular synovitis of the knee mimicking primary bone neoplasm. A report of two cases. J. Bone Jt Surg. 60 A (1978) 825–829

Kattan, K. R., D. S. Babcock, B. Felson: Solitary phalangeal defect in the hand. Report of 2 rare cases. Amer. J. Roentgenol. 124 (1975) 29–31

Kavanaugh, J. H.: Multiple myeloma, amyloidarthropathy, and pathological fracture of the femur. A case report. J. Bone Jt Surg. 60 A (1978) 135–137

Keats, T. E., R. B. Harrison: The calcaneal nutrient foramen: A useful sign in the differentiation of true from simulated cysts. Skelet. Radiol. 3 (1979) 239–240

Kimmelstiel, P., I. Rapp: Cortical defect due to periosteal desmoids. Bull. Hosp. Jt. Dis. 12 (1951) 286–297

Kovac, A., Y-Z Kuo, V. Sagar: Radiographic and radioisotope evaluation of intra-osseous xanthoma. Brit. J. Radiol. 49 (1976) 281–285

Lapayowker, M. S., W. T. Miller, W. M. Levy, R. D. Harwick: Pigmented villonodular synovitis of the temporomandibular joint. Radiology 108 (1973) 313–316

Lewis, R. W.: Roentgen diagnosis of pigmented villonodular synovitis and synovial sarcoma of the knee joint. Preliminary report. Radiology 49 (1947) 26–37

Linovitz, R. J., D. Resnick, P. Keissling, J. J. Kondon, B. Sehler, R. J. Nejdl, J. H. Rowe, L. J. Deftos: Tumor-induced osteomalacia and rickets: A surgically curable syndrome. Report of two cases. J. Bone Jt Surg. 58 A (1976) 419–423

McCarthy, E. F., T. Matsuno, H. D. Dorfman: Malignant fibrous histiocytoma of bone: A study of 35 cases. Hum. Path. 10 (1979) 57–70

McLeod, R. A., J. W. Beabout: The roentgenographic features of chondroblastoma. Amer. J. Roentgenol. 118 (1973) 464–471

Marcove, R. C., R. H. Breiberger: Osteoid osteoma of the elbow—a diagnostic problem. Report of four cases. J. Bone Jt Surg. 48 A (1966) 1185–1190

Mason, M. L.: Tumors of the hand. Surg. Gynec. Obstet. 64 (1937) 129–148

Masshoff, W., U. Schultz-Ehrenburg: Studien über die Natur der Meniskusganglien. Z. Orthop. 112 (1974) 369–382

Miehlke, K., U. Brandt: Multiples Plasmozytom mit exklusiver Lokalisation im Gliedmaßenskelett. Z. Rheumatol. 38 (1979) 199–212

Miki, T., T. Yamamuro, M. Oka, H. Urushidani, M. Itokazu: Chondrosarcoma developed in the distal phalangeal bone of the third toe. A case report. Clin. Orthop. 136 (1978) 241–243

Miyamoto, Y., T. Tani, K. Hamaya: Pigmented villonodular synovitis of the temporomandibular joint. Case report. Plast. reconstr. Surg. 59 (1977) 283–286

Morczek, A.: Aus konzentrischen Schichten bestehende freie Gelenkkörper bei einer Chondromatose des Schultergelenks. Fortschr. Röntgenstr. 79 (1953) 251

Nashel, D. J., L. W. Widerlite, T. J. Pekin jr.: IgD myeloma with amyloid arthropathy. Amer. J. Med. 55 (1973) 426–430

Nelson, S. W.: Some fundamentals in the radiologic differential diagnosis of solitary bone lesions. Semin. Roentgenol. 1 (1966) 244–267

Poynton, F. J., R. Lightwood: Lymphatic leukaemia, with infiltration of periosteum simulating acute rheumatism. Lancet 1932/I, 1192–1194

Pudlowski, R. M., L. A. Gilula, M. Kyriakos: Intraarticular lipoma with osseous metaplasia: Radiographic-pathologic correlation. Amer. J. Roentgenol. 132 (1979) 471–473

Ramon, Y., I. Horowitz, M. Oberman, A. Freedman, R. Tadmor: Osteochondroma of the coronoid process of the mandible. Oral Surg. 43 (1977) 692–697

Renier, J.-C., M. Boasson, M. Pitois: Chondromatose synoviale de la hanche aspect pseudo-kystique du col fémoral. Rev. Rhum. 40 (1973) 355–357

Riddell, R. J., C. J. Louis, N. A. Bromberger: Pulmonary metastases from chondroblastoma of the tibia. Report of a case. J. Bone Jt Surg. 55 B (1973) 848–853

Rosborough, D.: Osteoid osteoma. Report of a lesion in the terminal phalanx of a finger. J. Bone Jt Surg. 48 B (1966) 485–487

Schneider, G.: Zur Chondromatose des Kiefergelenks. Dtsch. zahnärztl. Z. (Beilage Kieferchir.) 2 (1960) 1233–1241

Scott, P. M.: Bone lesions in pigmented villonodular synovitis. J. Bone Jt Surg. 50 B (1968) 306–311

Seymour, N.: Intraosseous ganglia. Report of two cases. J. Bone Jt Surg. 50 B (1968) 134–137

Sherman, M. S.: Osteoid osteoma associated with changes in adjacent joint. Report of two cases. J. Bone Jt Surg. 29 (1947) 483–490

Simon, L., J. Claustre, J.-J. Picard, M. Marty, F. Blotman: Ostéom ostéoide intra-articulaire du coude. Rhumatologie 24 (1972) 377–382

Singh, R., D. S. Grewal, A. K. Bannerjee, V. P. Bansal: Haemangiomatosis of the skeleton. Report of a case. J. Bone Jt Surg. 56 B (1974) 136–138

Snarr, J. W., M. R. Abell, W. Martel: Lymphofollicular synovitis with osteoid osteoma. Radiology 106 (1973) 557–560

Sneider, P.: Xanthoma of the calcanous. Brit. J. Radiol. 36 (1963) 222–223

Solnica, J.: Manifestations articulaires des tumeurs carcinoides du tube digestif. Rev. Rhum. 43 (1976) 591–594

Sørensen, E. W.: Hyperlipemia. A report of an unusual case complicated by bone-lesions, macrocytic anaemia and leukemoid bone marrow. Acta med. scand. 175, fasc. 2 (1964) 207–214

Spilberg, I., G. J. Meyer: The arthritis of leukemia. Arthr. and Rheum. 15 (1972) 630–635

Stern, R. E., D. W. Gauger: Pigmented villonodular tenosynovitis. A case report. J. Bone Jt Surg. 59 A (1977) 560–561

Swee, R. G., R. A. McLeod, J. W. Beabout: Osteoid osteoma. Detection, diagnosis, and localization. Radiology 130 (1979) 117–123

Talal, N., L. Sokoloff, W. F. Barth: Extrasalivary lymphoid abnormalities in Sjögren's syndrome (reticulum cell sarcoma, „pseudolymphoma", macroglobulinemia). Amer. J. Med. 43 (1967) 50–65

Thomas, L. B., C. E. Forkner jr., E. Frei III, B. E. Besse jr., J. R. Stabenau: The skeletal lesions of acute leukemia. Cancer 14 (1961) 608–621

Uehlinger, E.: Osteofibrosis deformans juvenilis (Polyostotische fibröse Dysplasie Jaffe-Lichtenstein). Virchows Arch. path. Anat. 306 (1940) 255–299

Uehlinger, E.: Diffuse pigmentierte villonoduläre Synovitis des rechten Hüftgelenks mit Skelettbeteiligung. Arch. orthop. Unfall-Chir. 89 (1977) 319–331

Velasco Dominguez, E., M. I. Pérez Alvarez, L. Pascual Barrios, P. Andujar Ortuño: Mieloma no secretante. Rev. esp. Reum. 5 (1978) 105–116

Willson, J. K. V.: The bone lesions of childhood leukemia. A survey of 140 cases. Radiology 72 (1959) 672–681

Yaghmai, I.: Intra- and extraosseous xanthomata associated with hyperlipidemia. Radiology 128 (1978) 49–54

Yoshima, S., T. Nakamura, M. Takagi, T. Imamura, K. Okano, S. Sasaki: Benign osteoblastoma as a cause of osteomalacia. A report of two cases. J. Bone Jt Surg. 59 B (1977) 279–286

Trauma (major trauma, persistent trauma, fatigue trauma, traumas of the growth period; see also under Radiologic anatomy); posttraumatic and postoperative changes (see also under Osteoarthrosis); sympathetic reflex dystrophies.

Aitken, A. P.: The end results of the fractured distal tibial epiphysis. J. Bone Jt Surg. 18 (1936) 685–691

Alnor, P.: Die posttraumatische Osteolyse des lateralen Claviculaendes. Fortschr. Röntgenstr. 75 (1951) 364–365

Arndt, J. H., A. D. Sears: Posterior dislocation of the shoulder. Amer. J. Roentgenol. 94 (1965) 639–645

Aufdermaur, M.: Pathologische Knochenstrukturen. Fortschr. Röntgenstr. 127 (1977) 322–326

Bandi, W.: Zur Pathogenese der Osteochondritis dissecans (König). Unfallheilkunde 81 (1978) 295–298

Bargon, G., H. Henkemeyer: Ergebnisse röntgenologischer und klinischer Langzeitbeobachtungen nach operativ versorgten Läsionen der tibiofibularen Syndesmose bei Luxationsfrakturen im oberen Sprunggelenk. Fortschr. Röntgenstr. 126 (1977) 542–545

Baumann, E.: Zur Behandlung der Brüche des distalen Humerusendes beim Kind. Chir. Praxis 4 (1960) 317–324

Baumann, F., H. Ilse: Ein Beitrag zur Osteochondrosis dissecans des Os naviculare manus. Therapiewoche 28 (1978) 4466–4471

Bensasson, M., L. Lanoe, R. Assan: Un cas de syndrome algodystrophique du membre supérieur survenu après vaccination antitétanique. Sem. Hôp. Paris 53 (1977) 1965–1966

Bierling, G., D. Reisch: Über das Sudeck/Syndrom nach Frakturen. Fortschr. Röntgenstr. 82 (1955) 1–14

Blumensaat, C.: Der heutige Stand der Lehre vom Sudeck-Syndrom. Hefte Unfallheilk. 51 (1956) 1–225

Böhler, J.: Röntgenologische Darstellung von Kreuzbandverletzungen. Chirurg 16 (1944) 136–138

Böhler, L.: Die Technik der Knochenbruchbehandlung, 12. u. 13. Aufl. Bd. I. Maudrich, Wien 1953

Brauer, W.: Zur posttraumatischen Ossifikation akzessorischer Ossa. Fortschr. Röntgenstr. 90 (1959) 713–716

Buchholz, H. W.: Traumatologie des Hüftgelenkes. Die mediale Schenkelhalsfraktur und ihre Behandlung. Chirurg 41 (1970) 62–67

Buchwald, W.: Posttraumatische Verkalkung des Hoffaschen Fettkörpers. Fortschr. Röntgenstr. 103 (1965) 230–231

Bugyi, B.: Atypische Veränderungen der Handgelenksknochen bei Preßluftwerkzeugearbeitern. Fortschr. Röntgenstr. 117 (1972) 346–349

Bunnell, S., J. Böhler: Die Chirurgie der Hand. 2. Teil. Maudrich, Wien 1959

Burri, C., A. Rüter: Knorpelschaden am Knie. Springer, Berlin 1976

Canigiani, G., J. Wickenhauser, W. Czech: Beitrag zur Osteochondrosis dissecans im Foramen supratrochleare. Fortschr. Röntgenstr. 117 (1972) 66–68

Cayla, J., D. Chaouat, J. Rondier, K. Guérin, J.-C. Frugier: Les algodystrophies réflexes des membres inférieurs au cours de la grossesse. Rev. Rhum. 45 (1978) 89–94

Chiroff, R. T., C. P. Cooke III: Osteochondritis dissecans: A histologic and microradiographic analysis of surgically excised lesions. J. Trauma 15 (1975) 689–696

Cisternino, S. J., L. F. Rogers, B. C. Stufflebam, G. D. Kruglik: The trough line: A radiographic sign of posterior shoulder dislocation. Amer. J. Roentgenol. 130 (1978) 951–954

Corbett, M., J. R. Colston, A. K. Tucker: Pain in the knee associated with osteoporosis of the patella. Ann. rheum. Dis. 36 (1977) 188–191

Dahm, M.: Das Röntgenbild bei Luxation des Radius im Kleinkindesalter. (Schmerzhafte Lähmung nach Chassaignac). Fortschr. Röntgenstr. 79 (1953) 224–226

Dawarpanah, P.: Subluxation des Radiusköpfchens im Kindesalter (Subluxation capituli radii). Med. Welt 24 (1973) 1408–1410

De Cuveland, E., F. Heuck: Osteochondropathie der Spina iliaca anterior inferior unter Berücksichtigung der Ossifikationsvorgänge der Apophyse des lateralen Pfannenrandes. (Gleichzeitig ein Beitrag zur Kenntnis der normalen Anatomie dieses Skelettabschnittes im Wachstumsalter). Fortschr. Röntgenstr. 75 (1951) 430–445

Dihlmann, W.: Distensionsluxation des Hüftgelenkes durch partale Lösung der proximalen Femurepiphyse. Fortschr. Röntgenstr. 116 (1972) 559–561

Dihlmann, W.: Röntgendiagnose (Frakturen, Luxationen und Erkrankungen von Sprunggelenk und Fuß). Referat, 98. Kongreß Deutsche Ges. Chirurgie, München 22.-25. 4. 1981

Dihlmann, W.: Computertomographie des Talocruralgelenkes. Chirurg 53 (1982) 123–126

Duncan, H., B. Frame, H. M. Frost, A. R. Arnstein: Migratory osteolysis of the lower extremities. Ann. intern. Med. 66 (1967) 1165–1173

Ellis, R., A. Greene: Ischial apophyseolysis. Radiology 87 (1966) 646–648

Enes-Gaiao, F.: Die distale Radiusfraktur. Therapiewoche 24 (1974) 5492–5498

Enes-Gaiao, F., W. Müller: Die Malleolarfrakturen. Therapiewoche 24 (1974) 5578–5586

Engeloch, F., H. Stirnemann: Zur Radiusfraktur loco classico. Schweiz. Rundsch. Med. 67 (1978) 1938–1944

Fischer, E.: Posttraumatische karpale Osteolysen nach isolierter Fraktur am distalen Radius. Fortschr. Röntgenstr. 112 (1970) 541–542

Fourrier, P., M. Martini: Post-traumatic avascular necrosis of the humeral head. Int. Orthop. (SICOT) 1 (1977) 187–190

Gauwerky, F.: Traumatische Deformierungen am Humeruskopf als Folge von Schulterluxationen. Fortschr. Röntgenstr. 75 (1951) 607–627

Genant, H. K., F. Kozin, C. Bekerman, D. J. McCarty, J. Sims: The reflex sympathetic dystrophy syndrome. A comprehensive analysis using fine-detail radiography, photon absorptiometry, and bone and joint scintigraphy. Radiology 117 (1975) 21–32

Godshall, R. W., C. A. Hansen: Incomplete avulsion of a portion of the iliac epiphysis: An injury of young athletes. J. Bone Jt Surg. 55 A (1973) 1301–1302

Gorman, J. B., R. Stone, T. E. Keats: Changes in the sternoclavicular joint following radical neck dissection. Amer. J. Roentgenol. 111 (1971) 584–587

Groh, H.: Meniskusverletzungen. diagnostik 5 (1972) 455–457

Guilleminet, M., J. M. Barbier: Osteochondritis dissecans of the hip. J. Bone Jt Surg. 39 B (1957) 268–277

Haage, H.: Röntgendiagnostik der Gelenkschwellung des Ellenbogens. Fortschr. Röntgenstr. 118 (1973) 45–51

Hackenbruch, W., B. Noesberger: Die Kapselbandläsion am Sprunggelenk. Ther. Umsch. 33 (1976) 433–439

Haliburton, R. A., C. R. Sullivan, P. J. Kelly, L. F. A. Peterson: The extraosseous and intra-osseous blood supply of the talus. J. Bone Jt Surg. 40 A (1958) 1115–1120

Hamsa, W. R.: Epiphyseal injuries about the hip joint. Clin. Orthop. 10 (1957) 119–124

Hasche, H. H., W. Meyer: Idiopathische Algodystrophie der Hüfte. Z. Rheumatol. 33 (1974) 206–213

Hauer, G., Ch. Feldmeier, K. Wilhelm: Ermüdungsbrüche des Schenkelhalses. Med. Klin. 72 (1977) 125–127

Haverling, M., M. Sylvén: Soft tissue abnormalities at fracture of the scaphoid. Acta radiol. Diagn. 19 (1978) 497–501

Jonasch, E.: Das Kniegelenk. Diagnose und Therapie seiner Verletzungen und Erkrankungen. De Gruyter, Berlin 1964

Jonutis, A. J.: „Fat pad sign" und Ellenbogenverletzungen. Schweiz. med. Wschr. 104 (1974) 1158–1160

Jungbluth, K. H.: Luxationen der Handwurzel. Langenbecks Arch. klin. Chir. 334 (Kongreßbericht 1973) 199–202

Kager, H.: Zur Klinik und Diagnostik des Achillessehnenrisses. Chirurg 11 (1939) 691–695

Kaiser, H.: Medikamentös ausgelöste Algodystrophien. Verh. dtsch. Ges. Rheum. 4 (1976) 358–361

Karasik, D., J. Edeiken: Case report 19. (Transient osteoporosis with unrecognized hip fractures in pregnancy). Skelet. Radiol. 1 (1977) 181–182

Kolář, J.: Schlüsselbeinosteolyse nach einer radiogen bedingten Fraktur der Klavikula. Fortschr. Röntgenstr. 94 (1961) 486–489

Kolář, J., W. Penn: Progressive posttraumatic pelvic destructions. Radiol. clin. biol. (Basel) 42 (1973) 373–384

Korkusuz, Z., E. Karaesmen, Z. Aksan: Über Teilverrenkungen im Schlüsselbein-Brustbein-Gelenk bei Gewichthebern. Arch. orthop. Unf.-Chir. 74 (1972) 224–230

Kuner, E. H., E. Kleiser, H. L. Lindemaier: Die acromio-claviculare Luxation. Akt. Traumatol. 8 (1978) 205–209

Küntscher, G.: Praxis der Marknagelung. Schattauer, Stuttgart 1962

Langloh, N. D., G. G. Hunder, B. L. Riggs, P. J. Kelly: Transient painful osteoporosis of the lower extremities. J. Bone Jt Surg. 55 A (1973) 1188–1196

Lequesne, M.: L'algo-dystrophie d'origine chimiothérapique. Pseudorhumatisme de l'isoniazide, de l'ethionamide, du phenobarbital et de l'iode radioactif. Sem. Hôp. Paris 43 (1967) 2581–2595

Lequesne, M.: Transient osteoporosis of the hip. A nontraumatic variety of Sadeck's atrophy. Ann. rheum. Dis. 27 (1968 a) 463–471

Lequesne, M.: Étiologie et pathogénie des algodystrophies. Presse méd. 76 (1968 b) 973–954

Lequesne, M., M. Kerboull, M. Bensasson, C. Perez, R. Dreiser, A. Forest: Partial transient osteoporosis. Skelet. Radiol. 2 (1977) 1–9

Mäder, G., V. Meyer: Sportverletzungen an den Fingergelenken der vier Langfinger. Ther. Umsch. 33 (1976) 407–411

Makoski, H. B., E. Löhr: Die Volkmann'sche Kontraktur der Hand. Radiologe 12 (1972) 311–313

Matzen, P. F.: Traumatische Veränderungen im Bereich des Ellenbogengelenks. In: Handbuch der Orthopädie, Bd. III, hrsg. von G. Hohmann, M. Hackenbroch, K. Lindemann. Thieme, Stuttgart 1959 (S. 378–418)

Meves, H., F. Schneider-Sickert: Gibt es eine Osteochondrosis dissecans am Kahnbein der Hand? Z. Orthop. 113 (1975) 424–426

Meyer, A.: Luxationsfrakturen des Sprunggelenks. Neuere Gesichtspunkte zu Diagnostik und Therapie. Münch. med. Wschr. 115 (1973) 296–301

Milgram J. W.: Radiological and pathological manifestations of osteochondritis dissecans of the distal femur. Radiology 126 (1978) 305–311

Miller, D. S., G. de Takats: Posttraumatic dystrophy of the extremities. Sudecks arthropathy. Surg., Gynec., Obstet. 75 (1942) 558–582

Mindell, E. R.: Aseptic necrosis following fractures and dislocations. Surg. Clin. N. Amer. 41 (1961) 1701–1720

Mordeja, J.: Posttraumatische Osteolyse am distalen Ende des Oberarmknochens. Z. Orthop. 91 (1959) 141–145

Muhr, G.: Der frische Knorpelschaden. In: Knorpelschaden am Knie, hrsg. von C. Burri, A. Rüter. Springer, Berlin 1976 (S. 59–70)

Murray, C. R.: Fractures of the ankle. Occup. Med. 3 (1947) 376–385

Norell, H.-G.: Roentgenologic visualization of the extracapsular fat. Its importance in the diagnosis of traumatic injuries to the elbow. Acta radiol. (Stockh.) 42 (1954) 205–210

Ogden, J. A.: Subluxation and dislocation of the proximal tibiofibular joint. J. Bone Jt Surg. 56 A (1974) 145–154

Pauwels, F.: Der Schenkelhalsbruch—ein mechanisches Problem. Enke, Stuttgart 1935

Pauwels, F.: Grundsätzliches über Indikation und Technik der „Umlagerung" bei Schenkelhalspseudarthrosen. Langenbecks Arch. klin. Chir. 262 (1949) 404–422

Pöschl, M.: Wachstum an abgesprengten Epiphysen und Knochenstückchen. Fortschr. Röntgenstr. 87 (1957) 756–760

Prager, W.: Diagnostische Bedeutung von Veränderungen in den volaren Weichteilen des distalen Unterarms. Radiol. diagn. (Berl.) 9 (1968) 23–30

Rahmanzadeh, R.: Traumatologie des Hüftgelenkes. Therapiewoche 24 (1974) 5516–5533

Rauber, A.: Ein wenig bekanntes Röntgensymptom bei älteren Meniskusaffektionen. Z. Unfallmed. Berufskr. 37 (1944) 168–178

Reimers, C.: Die Brüche des fußnahen Unterschenkelabschnittes. Langenbecks Arch. klin. Chir. 276 (1953) 260–277

Riess, J.: Typische Kniescheibenveränderung beim Morbus Little, zweigeteilte Kniescheibe oder Ermüdungsbruch? Fortschr. Röntgenstr. 81 (1954) 221

Rogers, L. F., S. Malave jr., H. White, M. O. Tachdjian: Plastic bowing, torus and greenstick supracondylar fractures of the humerus: Radiographic clues to obscure fractures of the elbow in children. Radiology 128 (1978) 145–150

Rohner, E.: Pagetoider Umbau des Knochens („Remaniement pagétoide post-traumatique" von Lièvre). Virchows Arch. path. Anat. 329 (1957) 628–655

Sacks, B. A., D. I. Rosenthal, F. M. Hall: Capsular visualization in lipohemarthrosis of the knee. Radiology 122 (1977) 31–32

Salter, R. B., W. R. Harris: Injuries involving the epiphyseal plate. J. Bone Jt Surg. 45 A (1963) 587–622

Schilling, J.: Reflexdystrophien und dystrophische Pseudoarthritiden der unteren Extremitäten. Z. Rheumaforsch. 32 (1973) 375–384

Schmitt, H. G.: Luxation des Radiusköpfchens. Röntgen-Bl. 20 (1967) 383–389

Schneider, R., J. J. Kaye, B. Ghelman: Adductor avulsive injuries near the symphisis pubis. Radiology 120 (1976) 567–569

Schnek, F.: Die Verletzungen der Handwurzel. Ergebn. Chir. Orthop. 23 (1930) 1–109

Schoberth, H.: Sportverletzungen an Knie und Fuß. Z. Orthop. 110 (1972) 241–248

Scholler, J.-M., U. Saxer: Sportverletzungen des Beckens und der Hüfte. Ther. Umsch. 33 (1976) 412–418

Schulze, A. J.: Zur Osteochondrosis dissecans der Hüftpfanne. Fortschr. Röntgenstr. 97 (1962) 112–114

Scotti, D. M., K. S. Vijay, F. Heimberg, A. E. O'Hara: Osgood-Schlatter's disease, an emphasis on soft tissue changes in roentgen diagnosis. Skelet. Radiol. 4 (1979) 21–25

Solovjev, M.: Ostitis condensans claviculae. Fortschr. Röntgenstr. 125 (1976) 375–376

Steinbrück, K., G. Rompe: Sportschäden und Sportverletzungen am Ellenbogen. Dtsch. Ärztebl. 74 (1977) 431–436

Steinhardt, G.: Pathologische Veränderungen der Kiefergelenke. In: Handbuch der medizinischen Radiologie, Bd. Vii/2, hrsg. von L. Diethelm, O. Olsson, F. Strnad, H. Vieten, A. Zuppinger. Springer, Berlin 1963 (S. 867–885)

Swezey, R. L.: Transient osteoporosis of the hip, foot and knee. Arthr. and Rheum. 13 (1970) 858–868

Temesvari, M., P. Temesvari, T. L. Vischer, G. H. Fallet: L'algodystrophie décalcifiante isolée de la hanche. Schweiz. med. Wschr. 106 (1976) 699–703

Tiedtke, R., R. Rahmanzadeh, W. Schneider: Funktionelle Diagnostik der frischen Außenbandrupturen am Sprunggelenk—prä- und postoperativ—nachgewiesen mit standardisierten Parametern. In: Funktionelle Diagnostik in der Orthopädie, hrsg. von E. Morscher. Enke, Stuttgart 1979 (S. 163–165)

Treugut, H., K. Schulze, G. Neff: Apophyseolysen, Abrißfrakturen und Osteochondropathie der Spina iliaca anterior inferior. Fortschr. Röntgenstr. 130 (1979) 210–213

Viernstein, K., P. M. Jantzen: Die Verletzungen im Bereich des oberen Sprunggelenkes. Z. Orthop. 88 (1957) 87–109

Volkmann, J.: Zur Kritik des Stiedaschen Schattens. Mschr. Unfallheilk. 52 (1949) 353–362 von Laer, L., A. Schneider, L. Jani, B. Herzog: Wert und Grenzen der gehaltenen Aufnahmen bei Bandläsionen des oberen Sprunggelenkes im Wachstumsalter. In: Funktionelle Diagnostik in der Orthopädie, hrsg. von E. Morscher. Enke, Stuttgart 1979 (S. 156–159)

Vyhnánek, L., P. Teisinger, V. Eckert, R. Druga: Die Weichteilveränderungen beim Trauma des Ellbogens und der peripheren Radiusepiphyse. Fortschr. Röntgenstr. 112 (1970) 505

Weber, B. G.: Zur Behandlung kindlicher Femurschaftbrüche. Arch. orthop. Unf.-Chir. 54 (1963) 713–723

Weber, B. G.: Die Verletzungen des oberen Sprunggelenkes. Huber, Bern 1966

Weber, B. G.: Knöchel, Fußwurzel und Mittelfuß. In: Chirurgie der Gegenwart. Bd. IV, 1. Teil, hrsg. von R. Zenker, F. Deucher, W. Schink. Urban & Schwarzenberg, München 1973, 1976 (S. 1–46)

Weisman, J. A., J. A. Matison: Zur Röntgendiagnostik der habituellen Luxation des Oberarmgelenks. Fortschr. Röntgenstr. 126 (1977) 29–35

Weston, W. J.: Soft tissue signs in recent sub-luxation and dislocation of the acromio-clavicular joint. Brit. J. Radiol. 45 (1972) 832–834

Willenegger, H., B. G. Weber: Malleolarfrakturen. Langenbecks Arch. klin, Chir. 313 (1965) 489–502

Wissinger, H. A., E. J. Mcclain, J. H. Boyes: Turret exostosis: Ossifying hematoma of the phalanges. J. Bone Jt Surg. 48 A (1966) 105–110

Yousefzadeh, D. K., J. H. Jackson jr.: Lipohemarthrosis of the elbow joint. Radiology 128 (1978) 643–645

Spine, including sacroiliac joints; symphysis pubis; manubriosternal synchondrosis (see also the reference relating to individual diseases, etc.).

Abel, M. S.: Sacroiliac joint changes in traumatic paraplegics. Radiology 55 (1950) 235–239

Abel, M. S.: The unstable apophyseal joint: An early sign of lumbar disc disease. Skelet. Radiol. 2 (1977) 31–37

Abel, M. S., G. R. Smith: Visualization of the posterolateral elements of the lumbar vertebrae in the anteroposterior projection. Radiology 122 (1977) 824–825

Adams, J. E., M. Davies: Paravertebral and peripheral ligamentous ossification: An unusual association of hypoparathyroidism. Postgrad. med. J. 53 (1977) 167–172

Ahlbäck, S., S. Collert, B. Sellberg: Radiologisk—klinisk—patologisk väg till diagnos vid en sällsynt ryggsjukdom. Läkartidningen 74 (1977) 1725–1726

Alexander, C. J.: Scheuermann's disease. A traumatic spondylodystrophy? Skelet. Radiol. 1 (1977) 209–221

Allen, E. H., D. Cosgrove, F. J. C. Millard: The radiological changes in infections of the spine and their diagnostic value. Clin. Radiol. 29 (1978) 31–40

Andersson, O.: Röntgenbilden vid spondylarthritis ankylopoetica. Nord. med. T. 14 (1937) 2000–2002

Arlet, J., E. Arlet-Suau, P. Sebbag, B. Mazières, R. Durroux: Ostéite pubienne a pyocyanique. Rev. Rhum. 45 (1978) 725–728

Arlet, J., M. Pujol, A. Buc, G. Géraud, M. Gayrard, S. Latorzeff: Rôle de l'hyperostose vertébrale dans les myélopathies cervicales. Rev. Rhum. 43 (1976) 167–175

Arlet, J., J. Roulleau, J. Espagno, G. Géraud, M. Gayrard, J. Guillaume, B. Mazières: Compression médullaire dorsale au cours de l'hyperostose vertébrale. Rev. Rhum. 45 (1978) 83–87

Atero Carrasco, F., M. L. Gamir Gamir, J. Beltrán Gutiérrez, P. Fernández del Vallado, J. Gijón Baños, P. Sabando Suárez, E. Garcia de la Peña: Osteitis pubiana post-prostatectomia. Rev. esp. Reum. 3 (1976) 275–280

Aufdermaur, M.: Die pathologische Anatomie der Spondylitis ankylopoetica. Docum. rheumatol. 2. Geigy, Basel 1953

Aufdermaur, M.: Die Spondylosis cervicalis. Wirbelsäule in Forschung und Praxis 17. Hippokrates, Stuttgart 1960

Aufdermaur, M.: Zur pathologischen Anatomie der Scheuermannschen Krankheit. Schweiz. med. Wschr. 95 (1965) 264–268

Aufdermaur, M.: Die Scheuermannsche Adoleszentenkyphose. Orthopäde 2 (1973) 153–161

Aufdermaur, M.: Die pathologische Anatomie der deformen Arthrose und Spondylose. Ther. Umsch. 35 (1978) 141–146

Baastrup, Ch. I.: The diagnosis and roentgen treatment of certain forms of lumbago. Acta radiol. (Stockh.) 21 (1940) 151–163

Babin, E., P. Capesius, D. Maitrot: Signes radiologiques osseux des variétés morphologiques des canaux lombaires étroits. Ann. Radiol. 20 (1977) 491–499

Baggenstoss, A. H., W. H. Bickel, L. E. Ward: Rheumatoid granulomatous nodules as destructive lesions of the vertebrae. J. Bone. Jt Surg. 34 A (1952) 601–609

Bailey, D. K.: The normal cervical spine in infants and children. Radiology 59 (1952) 712–719

Ball, J.: Enthesopathy of rheumatoid and ankylosing spondylitis. Ann. Rheum. Dis. 30 (1971) 213–223

Ball, J., J. Sharp: Rheumatoid arthritis of the cervical spine. Mod. Trends Rheumatol. 2 (1971) 117–138

Ballou, S. P., M. A. Khan, I. Kushner: Diffuse intervertebral disk calcification in primary amyloidosis. Ann. intern. Med. 85 (1976) 616–617

Bardsley, J. L., L. G. Hanelin: The unilateral hypoplastic lumbar pedicle. Radiology 101 (1971) 315–317

Barratt, J. G.: Enlargement of cervical intervertebral foramina by coiling of the vertebral artery. Aust. Radiol. 28 (1974) 171–174

Batson, O. V.: The vertebral vein system. Amer. J. Roentgenol. 78 (1957) 195–212

Beamer Y. B., J. T. Garner, C. H. Shelden: Hypertrophied ligamentum flavum. Clinical and surgical significance. Arch. Surg. 106 (1973) 289–292

Beardwell, A.: Familial ankylosing vertebral hyperostosis with tylosis. Ann. rheum. Dis. 28 (1969) 518–523

Beeler, J. W.: Further evidence on the acquired nature of spondylolysis and spondylolisthesis. Amer. J. Roentgenol. 108 (1970) 796–798

Begg, A. C.: Nuclear herniations of the intervertebral disc. Their radiological manifestations and significance. J. Bone Jt Surg. 36 B (1954) 180–193

Berk, R., T. D. Brower: Vertebral sarcoidosis. Radiology 82 (1964) 660–663

Bhate, D. V., A. J. Pizarro, A. Seitam, E. Biduman: Axial sceletal changes in paraplegics. Radiology 133 (1979) 55–58

Billenkamp, G.: Körperliche Belastung und Spondylosis deformans. Fortschr. Röntgenstr. 116 (1972) 211–216

Blackard, W. G., R. R. Robinson, J. E. White: Familial hypophosphatemia. Report of a case, with observations regarding pathogenesis. New Engl. J. Med. 266 (1962) 899–905

Blair, J. D., P. O. Wells: Bilateral undescended scapula associated with omovertebral bone. J. Bone Jt Surg. 39 A (1957) 201–206

Böhler, J.: Morphologie der Halswirbelverletzungen nach ätiologischen Gesichtspunkten. Hefte Unfallheilk. 108 (1971) 10–13

Boijsen, E.: The cervical spinal canal in intraspinal expansive processes. Acta radiol. (Stockh.) 42 (1954) 101–115

Boltze, W. H., W. Reichenbach: Verletzungen der Halswirbelsäule bei Sportunfällen. Ther. Umsch. 33 (1976) 389–397

Bonse, G.: Über Skelettbeteiligung bei der Reiterschen Krankheit. Fortschr. Röntgenstr. 85 (1956) 675–678

Bösch, J: Die unspezifische Spondylitis nach Nukleographien und Bandscheibenoperationen. Z. Orthop. 100 (1965) 191–195

Boulet, P., J. Mirouze: Les ostéoses diabétiques (osteoporose et hyperostose). Ann. Méd. 55 (1954) 674–721

Brain, R.: Some aspects of the neurology of the cervical spine. J. Fac. Radiol. 8 (1957) 74–91

Braunstein, E. M., W. Martel, E. Stilwill, D. Kay: Radiological aspects of the arthropathy of relapsing polychondritis. Clin. Radiol. 30 (1979) 441–444

Brocher, J. E. W.: Die Wirbelsäulenleiden und ihre Differentialdiagnose, 5. Aufl. Thieme, Stuttgart 1970

Brocher, J. E. W., H.-G. Willert: Differentialdiagnose der Wirbelsäulenerkrankungen, 6. Aufl. Thieme, Stuttgart 1980

Brodey, P. A., S. M. Wolff: Radiographic changes in the sacroiliac joints in familial Mediterranean fever. Radiology 114 (1975) 331–333

Brodey, P. A., S. Pripstein, G. Strange, N. D. Kohout: Vertebral sarcoidosis. A case report and review of literature. Amer. J. Roentgenol. 126 (1976) 900–902

Brown, R. C., E. T. Evans: What causes the ,,eye in the Scotty dog" in the oblique projection of the lumbar spine? Amer. J. Roentgenol. 118 (1973) 435–437

Brügger, A.: Über vertebrale, radikuläre und pseudo-radikuläre Syndrome. Zur Differentialdiagnose rheumatologischer Erkrankungen. Teil I: Vertebrale Syndrome. Acta rheum. 18. Geigy, Basel 1960

Brun, J., H. Pozetto, J.-J. Buffat, J. Soustelle, J.-L. Vauzelle, R. Patin: Sarcoidose vertébrale et sacro-iliaque avec image de pseudo-abcès pottique. Guérison par corticotherapie. Presse méd. 74 (1966) 511–516

Bücheler, E., A. Düx, H. P. Venbrocks: Die direkte vertebrale Venographie bei lumbalen Bandscheibenhernien. Fortschr. Röntgenstr. 109 (1968) 593–603

Buetti-Bäuml, D.: Funktionelle Röntgendiagnostik der Halswirbelsäule. Thieme, Stuttgart 1954

Bunim, J. J., D. V. Kimberg, L. B. Thomas, E. J. Van Scott, G. Klatskin: The syndrome of sarcoidosis, psoriasis, and gout. Combined clinical staff conference at the National Institutes of Health. Ann. intern. Med. 57 (1962) 1018–1040

Burry, H. C., J. M. Tweed, R. G. Robinson, R. Howes: Lateral subluxations of the atlanto-axial joint in rheumatoid arthritis. Ann. rheum. Dis. 37 (1978) 525–528

Busch, R.: Sternumfrakturen bei Kindern. Kinderärztl. Prax. 34 (1966) 67–70

Buse, H.: Zur Darstellung der präsakralen Wirbelgelenke und der präsakralen Interartikularportion im schrägen Strahlengang. Fortschr. Röntgenstr. 99 (1963) 211–214

Busse, O., J. Stolke, B. U. Seidel: Die postoperative Discitis intervertebralis lumbalis. Nervenarzt 47 (1976) 604–608

Bussière, J. L., J. L. Épifanie, B. Leblanc, B. Sauvezie, D. Missioux: Maladie de Whipple et spondylarthrite ankylosante. Rev. Rhum. 47 (1980) 577–578

Butler, R. W.: Spontaneous anterior fusion of vertebral bodies. J. Bone Jt Surg. 53 B (1971) 230–235

Bywaters, E. G. L.: Rheumatoid discitis in the thoracic region due to spread from costovertebral joints. Ann. rheum. Dis. 33 (1974) 408–409

Bywaters, E. G. L.: Origin of cervical disc disease in RA. Arthr. and Rheum. 21 (1978) 737–739

Bywaters, E. G. L., A. St. J. Dixon: Paravertebral ossification in psoriatic arthritis. Ann. rheum. Dis. 24 (1965) 313–331

Bywaters, E. G. L., E. B. D. Hamilton, R. Williams: The spine in idiopathic haemochromatosis. Ann. rheum. Dis. 30 (1971) 453–465

Bywaters, E. G. L., E. Olsen: A case of early ankylosing spondylitis with fatal secondary amyloidosis. Brit. med. J. 1968/II, 412–416

Cabot, A., A. Becker: The cervical spine in rheumatoid arthritis. Clin. Orthop. 131 (1978) 130–140

Calin, A.: HLA-B 27: To type or not to type? Ann. intern. Med. 92 (1980) 208–211

Calin, A., J. F. Fries: Striking prevalence of ankylosing spondylitis in „healthy" W27 positive males and females. A controlled study. New Engl. J. Med. 293 (1975) 835–839

Cameron, H. U., V. L. Fornasier: The manubriosternal joint—anatomoradiological survey. Thorax 29 (1974) 472–474

Camus, J.-P.: Spondylarthrite ankylosante et maladie péroidique. Rev. Rhum. 32 (1965) 614–616

Candardjis, G., Ph. de Bosset. Y. Saudan: L'articulation manubriosternale normale. Technique d'examen et étude des variantes. J. Radiol. Electrol. 59 (1978a) 89–92

Candardjis, G., Y. Saudan, Ph. de Bosset: Étude radiologique de l'articulation manubrio-sternale dans la pelvispondylite rhumatismale et le syndrome de Reiter. J. Radiol. Électrol. 59 (1978b) 93–97

Caroit, M., L. Darbon, J. Villiaumey: Pelvispondylite rhumatismale et maladie périodique (atteignant séparément 2 membres d'une même fratrie. Rev. Rhum. 47 (1980) 61–62

Carroll, T. B., F. H. Gruber: Seat belt fractures. A report of two cases. Radiology 91 (1968) 517–518

Catterall, R. D., V. Wright, J. B. Cook: Arthritis and genital infection in paraplegic patients. Brit. J. vener. Dis. 43 (1967) 81–85

Cauchoix, J., M. Benoist, V. Chassaing: Degenerative spondylolisthesis. Clin. orthop. 115 (1976) 122–129

Cauchoix, J., H. Bloch-Michel, M. Benoist, V. Chassaing: Spondylolisthésis dégénérativ. Manifestations cliniques et traitement à propos de 26 cas opérés. Nouv. Presse méd. 5 (1976) 561–564

Chaiton, A., A. Fam, B. Charles: Disappearing lumbar hyperostosis

in a patient with Forestier's disease: an ominous sign. Arthr. and Rheum. 22 (1979) 799–802

Chaouat, Y., J.-P. Tormen, J. Hors, J. Dausset: HLA et maladie périodique. Rev. Rhum. 44 (1977) 703–708

Chapman, M.: Case report 6. (Congenital absence of a pedicle in cervical vertebra [C-6]). Skelet. Radiol. 1 (1976) 65–66

Chaykin, L. B., B. Frame, J. W. Sigler: Spondylitis: A clue to hypoparathyroidism. Ann. intern. Med. 70 (1969) 995–1000

Chevrot, A., G. Correas, G. Pallardy: Atteinte cervicale de la polyarthrite rhumatoide. Étude de 577 dossiers. J. Radiol. Électrol. 59 (1978) 545–550

Chevrot, A., B. Pillon, M. Revel, J. Moutounet, G. Pallardy: Phénomène radiologique du „vide discal" lombaire (Vacuum-disc). J. Radiol. Électrol. 59 (1978) 267–270

Clark, W. M., J. A. Gehweiler jr., R. Laib: Twelve significant signs of cervical spine trauma. Skelet. Radiol. 3 (1979) 201–205

Cliff, J. M.: Spinal bony bridging and carditis in Reiter's disease. Ann. rheum. Dis. 30 (1971) 171–179

Cohen, M. J., J. Ezekiel, R. H. Persellin: Costovertebral and costotransverse joint involvement in rheumatoid arthritis. Ann. rheum. Dis. 37 (1978) 473–475

Cottin, S., G. Le Gall, J. M. Lanoiselee, D. Rault: Le pseudospondylodiscites de la chondrocalcinose articulaire diffuse. Nouv. Presse Méd. 9 (1980) 1827–1830

Courtois, C., G. H. Fallet, T. L. Vischer, P. Wettstein: Erosive Spondylopathie. Ann. rheum. Dis. 39 (1980) 462–468

Davies, D.: Ankylosing spondylitis and lung fibrosis. Quart. J. Med. 41 (1972) 395–417

Decking, D., W. ter Steege: Röntgenologische Parameter der Halswirbelsäule im seitlichen Strahlengang. Wirbelsäule in Forschung u. Praxis 64. Hippokrates, Stuttgart 1975

Dequeker, J., T. Decock, M. Walravens, I. van de Putte: A systematic survey of the HLA B27 prevalence in inflammatory rheumatic diseases. J. Rheumatol. 5 (1978) 452–459

De Sèze, S., R. Claisse: Hyperostose vértébrale lombaire juvenile. Rev. Rhum. 27 (1960) 219–225

Detenbeck, L. C.: Rheumatoid arthritis of the spinal column. Pathologic aspects and treatment. Orthop. Clin. N. Amer. 2 (1971) 679–686

Dharmashi, V. B., Behrooz Azar-Kia, W. A. P. Supan: Case report 76. (Primary amyloidosis with vertebral involvement [T4 and T11]). Skelet. Radiol. 3 (1978) 193–195

Dieckmann, H.: Neurologische Syndrome bei knöchernen Fehlbildungen und Fehlbildungskrankheiten der zerviko-okzipitalen Übergangsregion. In: Wirbelsäule und Nervensystem, hrsg. von E. Trostdorf, H. St. Stender. Thieme, Stuttgart 1970

Dihlmann, W.: Typische Überlastungsschäden der vorderen ileosakralen Gelenkkapsel und ihrer Bänder. (Röntgendiagnostische Studien an den Kreuzdarmbeingelenken V). Fortschr. Röntgenstr. 99 (1963) 667–681

Dihlmann, W.: Weitere Untersuchungen zur Diagnose und Differentialdiagnose der Sacroileitis circumscripta. (Röntgendiagnostische Studien an den Kreuzdarmbeingelenken IV). Deutscher Röntgenkongreß 1963, Teil A. Thieme, Stuttgart 1964 a, S. 210–214

Dihlmann, W.: Entwicklungsstörungen der Kreuzdarmbeingelenke einschließlich der sog. Osteochondritis sacri. (Röntgendiagnostische Studien an den Kreuzdarmbeingelenken VI). Fortschr. Röntgenstr. 101 (1964 b) 285–295

Dihlmann, W.: Das Röntgenbild des atypischen Morbus Bechterew. Deutscher Röntgenkongreß 1974, Teil A. Thieme, Stuttgart 1965 a, S. 271–274

Dihlmann, W.: Die Beckenstarre. Gynäk. Rdsch. 2 (1965 b) 51–62

Dihlmann, W.: Sacroiliitis circumscripta. Beitrag zur Differentialdiagnose entzündlicher Erkrankungen der Kreuzdarmbeingelenke. Z. Rheumaforsch. 24 (1965 c) 125–129

Dihlmann, W.: Die lumbosakrale Retrolisthesis und Pseudoretrolisthesis. Fortschr. Röntgenstr. 104 (1966 a) 264–265

Dihlmann, W.: Die sog. Spondylitis anterior, Discitis und Spondylodiscitis bei Morbus Bechterew - Schlüssel zum Verständnis dieser Erkrankung. Fortschr. Röntgenstr. 104 (1966 b) 699–715

Dihlmann, W.: Spondylitis ankylopoetica - die Bechterewsche Krankheit. Thieme, Stuttgart 1968 a

Dihlmann, W.: Ausgedehnte Wirbelsklerosierung bei banaler Osteochondrose oder blande, nicht eitrige, sklerosierende Spondylitis? Fortschr. Röntgenstr. 108 (1968 b) 767–770

Dihlmann, W.: Anwendung der Röntgenbildanalyse zur Erkennung der feingeweblichen Veränderungen bei der Spondylitis ankylopoetica. Verh. dtsch. Ges. Rheum. 1 (1969) 21–32

Dihlmann, W.: Zwei Aspekte der röntgenologischen Differentialdiagnose bei der Spondylarthritis ankylopoetica. Therapiewoche 20 (1970 a) 789–795

Dihlmann, W.: Röntgenologische Untersuchung der Wirbelsäule und der Kreuz-Darmbein-Gelenke. Allgemeine Röntgenphänomenologie. Ärztl. Prax. 22 (1970 b) 1243–1245

Dihlmann, W.: Gelenke—Wirbelverbindungen. Thieme, Stuttgart 1973 (S. 470)

Dihlmann, W.: Das „bunte" Sakroiliakalbild - das röntgenologische Frühkriterium der ankylosierenden Spondylitis. Fortschr. Röntgenstr. 121 (1974) 564–570

Dihlmann, W.: Röntgendiagnostische Basisinformation: Das „bunte" Sacroiliacalbild. Akt. Rheumatol. 1 (1976 a) 17–21

Dihlmann, W.: Die Hyperostosis triangularis ilii - das sakroiliakale knöcherne Streßphänomen. 1. Teil (Terminologie, Definition, Morphologie). Fortschr. Röntgenstr. 124 (1976 b) 1–6

Dihlmann, W.: Die Hyperostosis triangularis ilii - das sakroiliakale knöcherne Streßphänomen. 2. Teil (Inzidenz, Prognose, Pathogenese, Ätiologie, Tracerstudium, Differentialdiagnose). Fortschr. Röntgenstr. 124 (1976 c) 154–160

Dihlmann, W.: Röntgendiagnostische Basisinformation: Vertebralosteophyten. Akt. Rheumatol. 2 (1977) 139–142

Dihlmann, W.: Röntgendiagnostik der Iliosakralgelenke und ihrer nahen Umgebung. Thieme, Stuttfart, 1. Aufl. 1967, 2. Aufl. 1978 (Röntgendiagnostik der Sakroiliakalgelenke und ihrer nahen Umgebung).

Dihlmann, W.: Current radiodiagnostic concept of ankylosing spondylitis. Skelet. Radiol. 4 (1979) 179–188

Dihlmann, W.: Hemispherical spondylosclerosis - a polyetiologic syndrome. Skelet. Radiol. 7 (1981) 99–106

Dihlmann, W., G. Delling: Disco-vertebral destructive lesions (socalled Andersson lesions) associated with ankylosing spondylitis. Skelet. Radiol. 3 (1978) 10–16

Dihlmann, W., W. M., Dörr: Der zervikale Pseudospalt nach D. Schoen bei der Spondylois uncovertebralis. Spezielle, weniger beachtete Röntgenbefunde am Stütz-und Gleitgewebe 1. Fortschr. Röntgenstr. 113 (1970) 522–527

Dihlmann, W., U. Freund: Die Iliosakralveränderungen bei der nichtentzündlichen Wirbelsäulenversteifung (Hyperostose ankylosante vertébrale sénile, Spondylosis hyperostotica). Z. Rheumaforsch. 27 (1968) 284–291

Dihlmann, W., G. Friedmann: Die Röntgenkriterien der juvenilrheumatischen Zervikalsynostose im Erwachsenenalter. Fortschr. Röntgenstr. 126 (1977) 536–541

Dihlmann, W., H. J. Maes: Kalziphylaxie bei sogenannter Ostitis condensans ilii et sacri? Z. Rheumaforsch. 27 (1968) 274–278

Dihlmann, W., H. J. Maes: Theorie der Syndesmophyten. Z. Rheumaforsch. 29 (1970) 219–226

Dihlmann, W., G. Müller: Iliosakralveränderungen als Frühsymptom des Hyperparathyreoidismus. Beitrag zur Differentialdiagnose der Spondylitis ankylopoetica. Fortschr. Röntgenstr. 111 (1969) 558–565

Dihlmann, W., G. Müller: Pseudo-Bechterew-Befunde beim Hyperparathyreoidismus bzw. bei der renalen Osteopathie. Z. Rheumaforsch. 31 (1972) 401–408

Dihlmann, W., G. Müller: Sacroiliacalbefunde beim Hyperparathyreoidismus (Röntgenologie, Histomorphologie). Radiologe 13 (1973) 160–163

Dihlmann, W., G. Nebel: Spinale Röntgenbefunde bei der adulten chronischen Polyarthritis. Akt. Rheumatol. 5 (1980) 67–74

Dihlmann, W., B. Schuler: Die sehr umschriebene, primär ossifizierende, nicht ankylosierende Ileosakralarthritis. (Röntgendiagnostische Studien an den Kreuzdarmbeingelenken III). Fortschr. Röntgenstr. 98 (1963) 134–140

Dihlmann, W., K.-F. Gürtler, M. Heller: Sakroiliakale Computertomographie. Fortschr. Röntgenstr. 130 (1979) 659–665

Dilsen, An.: Sacro-iliitis and ankylosing spondylitis in Behçet's disease. Scand. J. Rheumatol., Suppl. 8 (1975) 20

Dirheimer, Y.: The craniovertebral region in chronic inflammatory rheumatic diseases. Springer, Berlin 1977

Dockerty, M. B., J. G. Love: Thickening and fibrosis (so-called hypertrophy) of the ligamentum flavum: A pathologic study of fifty cases. Proc. Mayo Clin. 15 (1940) 161–166

Duus, P., G. Kahlau, W. Krücke: Allgemeinpathologische Betrachtungen über die Einengung der Foramina intervertebralia. Langenbecks Arch. klin. Chir. 268 (1951) 341–362

Edgren, W., S. Vaino: Osteochondrosis juvenilis lumbalis. Acta. chir. scand., Suppl. 227 (1957) 1–48

Ehalt, W.: Angeborenes Fehlen eines oberen Schambeinastes. Röntgenpraxis 15 (1943) 230

Eichelmann, H. J.: Beitrag zur Ätio-Pathogenese der Osteitis pubis. Zbl. Chir. 101 (1976) 1184–1189

Elsberg, C. A., C. G. Dyke: The diagnosis and localization of tumors of the spinal cord by means of measurements made on the x-ray films of the vertebrae, and the correlation of clinical and x-ray findings. Bull. neurol. Inst. N. Y. 3 (1934) 359–394

Emminger, E.: Zur pathologischen Anatomie des Schleudertraumas der Halswirbelsäule. Arch. klin. Chir. 316 (1966) 445–457

Epstein, B. S., J. A. Epstein, M. D. Jones: Lumbar spinal stenosis. Radiol. Clin. N. Amer. 15 (1977) 227–239

Epstein, J. A., B. S. Epstein, A. D. Rosenthal, R. Carras, L. S. Lavine: Sciatica caused by nerve root entrapment in the lateral recess: the superior facet syndrome. J. Neurosurg. 36 (1972) 584–589

Epstein, J. A., B. S. Epstein, L. S. Lavine, R. Carras, A. D. Rosenthal, P. Sumner: Lumbar nerve root compression at the intervertebral foramina caused by arthritis of the posterior facets. J. Neurosurg. 39 (1973) 362–369

Erdheim, J.: Über Wirbelsäulenveränderungen bei Akromegalie. Virchows Arch. path. Anat. 281 (1931) 197–296

Erdmann, H.: Grundzüge einer funktionellen Wirbelsäulen-Betrachtung. 1.-3. Teil. Man. Med. 5 (1967) 1–8; 6 (1968) 1–6; 6 (1968) 79–90

Erdmann, H.: Die Begutachtung der Wirbelsäule (Einführung in das Thema). Die Wirbelsäule in Forschung und Praxis 40. Hippokrates, Stuttgart 1968 (S. 7–24)

Erdmann, H.: Schleuderverletzung der Halswirbelsäule. Erkennung und Begutachtung. Hippokrates, Stuttgart 1973

Eyler, W. R., H. P. Doub: Extraintestinal roentgen manifestations of intentinal lipodystrophy. J. Amer. med. Ass. 160 (1956) 534–536

Feldmann, J. L., C. J. Menkès, B. Weill, F. Delrieu, F. Delbarre: Les sacro-iliites infectieuses. Étude multicentrique sur 214 observations. Rev. Rhum. 48 (1981) 83–91

Fielding, J. W., P. P. Griffin: Os odontoideum: An acquired lesion. J. Bone Jt Surg. 56 A (1974) 187–190

Fielding, J. W., R. J. Hawkins: Atlanto-axial rotatory fixation. (Fixed rotatory subluxation of the atlanto-axial joint). J. Bone Jt Surg. 59 A (1977) 37–44

Finlay, J. M., R. I. Macdonald: Acromegaly. Canad. med. Ass. J. 71 (1954) 345–353

Firooznia, H., R. S. Pinto, J. P. Lin, H. H. Baruch, J. Zausner: Chordoma: Radiologic evaluation of 20 cases. Amer. J. Roentgenol. 127 (1976) 797–805

Fischer, E.: Akzessorische freie Knochenelemente in der Umgebung des Foramen occipitale magnum. Fortschr. Röntgenstr. 91 (1959) 638–642

Fischer, E., W. Stecher: Die Hyperostose der Rippenköpfchen, ein Teilbild der perivertebralen Hyperostose. Fortschr. Röntgenstr. 117 (1972) 336–342

Fitzgerald, J. A. W., P. H. Newman: Degenerative spondylolisthesis. J. Bone Jt Surg. 58 B (1976) 184–192

Fletcher, B. D., B. G. Brogdon: Seat-belt fractures of the spine and sternum. J. Amer. med. Ass. 100 (1967) 167–168

Flournoy, J. G., R. O. Cone, J. A. Saldana, M. D. Jones: Jefferson fracture: Presentation of a new diagnostic sign. Radiology 134 (1980) 88

Fohler, N., H. P. Schwerdtner: Wirbelsäule und Kunstturnen. Orthop. Prax 11 (1975) 46–49

Ford, L. T., L. A. Gilula, W. A. Murphy, M. Gado: Analysis of gas in vacuum lumbar disc. Amer. J. Roentgenol. 128 (1977) 1056–1057

Forestier, J.: The importance of sacro-iliac changes in the early diagnosis of ankylosing spondylarthritis. Marie-Strümpell-Bechterew disease. Radiology 33 (1939) 389–402

Forestier, J., R. Lagier: Ankylosing hyperostosis of the spine. Clin. Orthop. 74 (1971) 65–83

Forestier, J., P. Robert: Ostéophytes et syndesmophytes. Gaz. méd. Fr. (Suppl. Radiol.) 1934, 192–202

Forestier, J., J. Rotès-Quérol: Hyperostose ankylosante vertébrale sénile. Rev. Rhum. 17 (1950) 525–534

Forestier, J., F. Jacqueline, J. Rotes-Querol: Ankylosing Spondylitis. Clinical Considerations. Roentgenology. Pathologic Anatomy. Treatment. Thomas, Springfield, Ill. 1956

Forestier, J., R. Lagier, A. Certonciny: Le concept d'hyperostose vertébrale ankylosante. Approche anatomo-radiologique. Rev. Rhum. 36 (1969) 655–661

Fraenkel, E.: Über chronische ankylosierende Wirbelsäulen-versteifung. Fortschr. Röntgenstr. 7 (1903/04) 62–90; 11 (1907) 171–195

Francillon, M. R.: Kongenitale Analgie und Wirbelsäule. Arch. orthop. Unfall-Chir. 67 (1970) 255–263

Frank, D. F., J. E. Miller: Hypoplasia of the lumbar vertebral body simulating spondylolisthesis. Radiology 133 (1979) 59–60

Frank, P., P. J. Prager, V. Menges, H. P. Schmitt: Klinik und Röntgendiagnostik der Fehlbildungen des craniocervicalen Überganges. Radiologe 17 (1977) 296–304

Franke, J.: Ein Beitrag zur Differentialdiagnose des Morbus Strümpell-Marie-Bechterew. Arch. orthop. Unf.-Chir. 64 (1968) 135–150

Freiberger, R. H., P. D. Wilson jr., J. A. Nicholas: Acquired absence of the odontoid process. A case report. J. Bone Jt Surg. 47 A (1965) 1231–1236

Freyschmidt, J., R. Hehrmann: Primärer Hyperparathyreoidismus als Differentialdiagnose von schweren Skelettdestruktionen. Röntgen-Bl. 31 (1978) 495–502

Friedenberg, Z. B.: Osteitis pubis with involvement of the hip joint. J. Bone Jt Surg. 32 A (1950) 924–927

Frigaard, E.: Posterior atlanto-axial subluxation in rheumatoid arthritis. Scand. J. Rheumatol. 7 (1978) 65–68

Fullenlove, T. M., J. G. Wilson: Traumatic defects of the pars interarticularis of the lumbar vertebrae. Amer. J. Roentgenol. 122 (1974) 634–638

Gaizler, Gy.: Das Treppenphänomen an der Halswirbelsäule. Fortschr. Röntgenstr. 114 (1971) 317–322

Gatzweiler, W.: Die Spondylochondrose der Halswirbelsäule. (Ein statistischer Beitrag). Z. Rheumaforsch. 14 (1955) 368–371

Gay, J. R., K. H. Abbott: Common whiplash injuries of the neck. J. Amer. med. Ass. 152 (1953) 1698–1704

Gehweiler jr., J. A., W. M. Clark, R. E. Schaaf, B. Powers, M. D. Miller: Cervical spine trauma: The common combined conditions. Radiology 130 (1979) 77–86

Geiger, L. E.: Fusion of vertebrae following resection of intervertebral disc. J. Neurosurg. 18 (1961) 79–85

Gelehrter, G.: Synchondrolysis sterni superior nach geringfügigem Trauma bei einem lljährigen Knaben. Arch. orthop. Unfall-Chir. 49 (1958) 578–580

Gelman, M. I.: Cauda equina compression in acromegaly. Radiology 112 (1974) 357–360

Gerber, N., A. von Felten, A. Böni, F. Wagenhäuser: Spondylitis ankylosans (Bechterew) und Gewebsantigen HLA-B27. III. Erblichkeit der Spondylitis ankylosans (Bechterew). Z. Rheumatol. 36 (1977) 230–238

Giedion, A., A. Prader, A. Rüttimann: Der „Tarzan-Typus". Wirbelsäulenkleinwuchs, degenerative Bandscheibenveränderungen und schmales Becken. Fortschr. Röntgenstr. 94 (1961) 472–478

Gilsanz, V., J. Miranda, R. Cleveland, U. Willi: Scoliosis secondary to fractures of the transverse processes of lumbar vertebrae. Radiology 134 (1980) 627–628

Giordano, M., M. Vatti, G. La Montagna, U. Picillo, G. Valentini: La spondilopatia iperostosica dismetabolica come problema diabetologica. Atti del 6° Congr. Nazion. Soc. Ital. Diabetol. Conti Tipocolor, Firenze 1976/77. (S. 561-574)

Glimet, T., M. Sibué, A.Ryckewaert, S. de Sèze: Les condensations vertébrales étendues des discopathies dégénératives. (Étude de 25 cas). Sem. Hôp. Paris 51 (1975) 1199–1203

Glogowski, G.: Röntgenologischer Nachweis der Entstehung erscheinungsbildlich vom Morbus Bechterew nicht zu unterscheidender Krankheitsbilder durch generalisierte Osteomyelitis. Zugleich ein Beitrag zur gutachterlichen Beurteilung des Bechterew unter Berücksichtigung neuester Erkenntnisse. Z. Orthop. 91 (1959) 50–65

Glorieux, P.: La physiologie pathologique et les diverses formes de fractures de la colonne. Fortschr. Röntgenstr. 53 (1936) 422–434

Gold, R., A. L. Metzger, J. M. Mirra, H. J. Weinberger, K. Kil-

lebrew: Multicentric reticulohistiocytosis (lipoid dermatoarthritis) an erosive polyarthritis with distinctive clinical, roentgenographic and pathologic features. Amer. J. Roentgenol. 124 (1975) 610–624

Goobar, J. E., W. S. Gilmer jr., D. S. Carroll, G. M. Clark: Vertebral sarcoidosis. J. Amer. med. Ass. 178 (1961) 1162–1163

Gougeon, J., J. Moreau-Hottin, J.-C. Etienne, J. Labeaumont: Les block vértébraux acquis dus a la maladie de Scheuermann. Rev. Rhum. 38 (1971) 179–192

Greiner, L., H. W. Pia, F. Schepelmann: Spondylitis und lumbale Bandscheibenoperation. Zbl. Neurochir. 35 (1974) 179–192

Gribovsky, E.: Dysphagia in association with hyperexostoses of the cervical vertebrae. Amer. J. Gastroent. 45 (1966) 284–286

Groher, W.: Auswirkungen des Hochleistungssports auf die Lendenwirbelsäule. Spondylolyse und Spondylolisthesis als erworbener Spätzustand nach ständig einwirkendem Mikrotrauma bei Sportlern. Hofmann, Schorndorf 1975.

Gsell, O.: Chronische idiopathische Tetanie (mit Psoriasis) (hypoparathyreoider Kretinismus). Dtsch. med. Wschr. 75 (1950) 1117–1121

Güntz, E.: Abnorme Geradehaltung der Brustwirbelsäule bei Veränderungen der Zwischenwirbelscheiben. Z. orthop. Chir. 58 (1932) 66–76

Gupta, S. K., V. Mohan: The thoracic paraspinal line: Further significance. Clin Radiol. 30 (1979) 329–335

Gutmann, G.: Die Wirbelblockierung und ihr röntgenologischer Nachweis. Die Wirbelsäule in Forschg. u. Praxis 15, Hippokrates, Stuttgart 1960 (S. 83–102)

Gutmann, G.: Röntgen-Diagnostik der Occipito-cervical-Gegend unter chirotherapeutischen Gesichtspunkten. Röntgen-Bl. 22 (1969) 267–287

Gwinn, J. L., J. L. Smith: Acquired or congenital absence of the odontoid process. Amer. J. Roentgenol. 88 (1962) 424–431

Hadley, L. A.: Roentgenographic studies of the cervical spine. Amer. J. Roentgenol. 52 (1944) 173–195

Hagenlocher, H. U., K. Ciba: Radiologische Aspekte des zervikalen Chordoms. Fortschr. Röntgenstr. 125 (1976) 228–232

Hall, M., G. Selin: Spinal involvement in gout. A case report with autopsy. J. Bone Jt Surg. 42 A (1960) 341–343

Hammerbeck, W.: Synchondrose der rechten Bogenwurzel und linksseitige Spondylolysis interarticularis des 3. Lendenwirbels neben einer Spondylolisthesis des 4. Lendenwirbels. Fortschr. Röntgenstr. 64 (1941) 72–87

Hannon, R. C., C. Limas, O. S. Cigtay, H. L. Twigg: Bone and joint involvement in primary amyloidosis. J. Canad. Ass. Radiol. 26 (1975) 112–115

Harder, J.: Osteochondritis-dissecans-artige Veränderung an einem Processus uncinatus (zugleich Studie über die sog. Uncovertebralgelenke). Fortschr. Röntgenstr. 96 (1962) 423–426

Harris, J., A. R. Carter, E. N. Glick, G. O. Storey: Ankylosing hyperostosis. I. Clinical and radiological features. Ann. rheum. Dis. 33 (1974) 210–215

Harris, N., R. O. Murray: Lesions of the symphysis in athletes. Brit. med. J. 1974/IV, 211–214

Harris, R. I., J. J. Wiley: Acquired spondylolysis as a sequel to spine fusion. J. Bone Jt Surg. 45 A (1963) 1159–1170

Hart, F. D., K. D. Robinson: Ankylosing spondylitis in women. Ann. rheum. Dis. 18 (1959) 15–23

Harvie, J. N., R. S. Lester, A. H. Little: Sacroiliitis in severe psoriasis. Amer. J. Roentgenol. 127 (1976) 579–584

Harzer, K., G. Töndury: Zum Verhalten der Arteria vertebralis in der alternden Halswirbelsäule. Fortschr. Röntgenstr. 104 (1966) 687–699

Hawkins, R. J., J. W. Fielding, W. J. Thompson: Os odontoideum: Congenital or acquired. A case report. J. Bone Jt Surg. 58 A (1976) 413

Heck, C. V.: Hoarseness and painfull deglutition due to massive cervical exostoses. Surg. Gynec. Obstet. 102 (1956) 657–660

Heller, H., J. Gafni, D. Michaeli, N. Shahin, E. Sohar, G. Ehrlich, I. Karten, L. Sokoloff: The arthritis of familial Mediterranean fever (FMF). Arthr. and Rheum. 9 (1966) 1–17

Henssge, J.: Radiologische Befunde beginnender Adoleszentenkyphosen (Morbus Scheuermann). Fortschr. Röntgenstr. 108 (1968) 58–62

Herrmann, H.-D.: Das Schleudertrauma der Halswirbelsäule. Terminologie und Diagnose. Med. Welt 1970, 1797–1800

Hilton, R. C., J. Ball, R. T. Benn: Vertebral end-plate lesions (Schmorl's nodes) in the lumbar spine. Ann. rheum. Dis. 35 (1976) 127–132

Hinck, V. C., C. E. Hopkins, B. S. Savara: Sagittal diameter of the cervical spinal canal in children. Radiology 79 (1962) 97–108

Hiramatsu, Y., T. Nobechi: Calcification of the posterior longitudinal ligament of the spine among Japanese. Radiology 100 (1971) 307–312

Hohmann, D.: Die degenerativen Veränderungen der Costotransversalgelenke. Ein Beitrag zu Diagnostik, Pathogenese und Klinik der Arthrosen und Insertions-Ligamentosen der Costotransversalgelenke im Rahmen vertebragener Krankheitsbilder. Enke, Stuttgart 1968

Hohmann, D., W. Gasteiger: Zur Röntgendiagnostik der Costotransversalgelenke. Fortschr. Röntgenstr. 112 (1970) 783–789

Holits, R.: Über die Spondylolyse. Fortschr. Röntgenstr. 50 (1934) 412

Horváth, F., L. Massányi: Über diagnostische Schwierigkeiten verursachende Formveränderungen der Wirbelgelenkfortsätze. Fortschr. Röntgenstr. 97 (1962) 757–763

Houston, C. S., W. A. Zaleski: The shape of vertebral bodies and femoral necks in relation to activity. Radiology 89 (1967) 59–66

Hubbard, D. D., D. R. Gunn: Secondary carcinoma of the spine with destruction of the intervertebral disk. Clin. Orthop. 88 (1972) 86–88

Jacqueline, F.: Destructions du rachis antérieur lombo-dorsal au cours de la spondylarthrite ankylosante (classification, interprétation). Rhumatologie 17 (1965) 223–238

Jacqueline, F.: Ossifications post-opératoires (prothèse totale) des hanches de sujets atteints d'hyperostose vertébrale ankylosante. Rev. Rhum. 46 (1979) 45–52

Jaeger, W.: Über die Spondylolisthesis. Fortschr. Röntgenstr. 52 (1935) 107–114

Janker, R.: Persistierende Apophysen der Wirbelsäule. Fortschr. Röntgenstr. 44 (1931) 519–522

Jenkner, F. L., A. Dossi: Zusammenhänge und Diskrepanzen zwischen klinischer Symptomatologie und röntgenologischen Veränderungen an der Halswirbelsäule bei Zervikalsyndrom und Arm-Schulter-Syndrom. Man. Med. 15 (1977) 118–124

Jentschura, G.: Die Frühform der juvenilen Kyphose im Röntgenbild. Z. Orthop. 94 (1961) 518–540

Jimenea, C. V., B. Frame, L. B. Chaykin, J. W. Sigler: Spondylitis of hypoparathyroidism. Clin. orthop. 74 (1971) 84–89

Jirout, J.: Die Rolle der Axis bei Seitneigung der Halswirbelsäule und die „latente Skoliose". Fortschr. Röntgenstr. 109 (1968) 74–81

Johnson, T. H., N. Mital, G. P. Rodnan, R. J. Wilson: Relapsing polychondritis. Radiology 106 (1973) 313–315

Jung, A., P. Kehr, M. Hamid: Die Unkoforaminektomie bei Läsionen der Arteria vertebralis und der Zervikalnervenwurzeln. Z. Orthop. 112 (1974) 736–740

Jung, A., P. Kehr, J. M. Nuss: Das zerviko-encephale Syndrom bei Arthrosen und Traumen der Halswirbelsäule. Z. Orthop. 112 (1974) 729–736

Jung, K., E. Schumann: Korrelation zwischen Beschwerden im Sinne eines vertebragenen Syndroms und röntgendiagnostisch nachweisbaren Veränderungen der Halswirbelsäule. Wien. med. Wschr. 125 (1975) 79–82

Junghanns, H.: Spondylolisthesen ohne Spalt im Zwischengelenkstück („Pseudospondylolisthesen"). Arch. orthop. Unfall-Chir. 29 (1930) 118–127

Junghanns, H.: s. Schmorl, G

Kaganas, G.: Zur posttraumatischen aseptischen Nekrose der Bandscheibe. In: Die Wirbelsäule in Forschung und Praxis. Bd. XXVIII, hrsg. von H. Junghanns. Hippokrates, Stuttgart 1964 (S. 95–100)

Kamakura, K., S. Nanko, T. Furukawa, T. Mannen, Y. Toyokura: Cervical radiculomyelopathy due to calcified ligamenta flava. Ann. Neurol. 5 (1979) 193–195

Kamieth, H.: Beckenring und Wirbelsäule. Arch. orthop. Unfall-Chir. 50 (1958 a) 124 bis 145

Kamieth, H.: Geburtstraumen des Beckenringes vom Standpunkt der Röntgenologie. Arch. orthop. 89 (1958 b) 694–701

Kamieth, H.: Ventrales Okzipitalwirbelrudiment, verbunden mit einer Assimilation eines Ossiculum terminale mit dem vorderen Atlasbogen. Fortschr. Röntgenstr. 119 (1973) 632–633

Kamieth, H., K. Reinhardt: Der ungleiche Symphysenstand. Ein wichtiges Symptom der Beckenringlockerung. Fortschr. Röntgenstr. 83 (1955) 530–546

Karayalcin, G., J. Dorfman, F. Rosner, A. J. Aballi: Radiological changes in 127 patients with sickle cell anemia. Amer. J. med. Sci. 271 (1976) 133–144

Karten, L.: Septic arthritis complicating rheumatoid arthritis. Ann. intern. Med. 70 (1969) 1147–1158

Katzenstein, H.-J.: Ein Beitrag zur Genese des „Stachelbekkens". Röntgenpraxis 6 (1934) 742–746

Keller, R. H.: Traumatic displacement of the cartilaginous vertebral rim: A sign of intervertebral disc prolaps. Radiology 110 (1974) 21–24

Kelly III, J. J., B. B. Weisiger: The arthritis of Whipple's disease. Arthr. and Rheum. 6 (1963) 615–632

van Kerckhove, H.: Involvement of the lateral atlanto-axial joints as first and late symptom of rheumatoid arthritis. Acta rheum. scand. 16 (1970) 197–210

Kersley, G. D., D. Mandel, M. R. Jeffrey: Gout. An unusual case with softening and subluxation of the first cervical vertebra and splenomegaly. Result of ACTH administration and eventual postmortem findings. Ann. rheum. Dis. 9 (1952) 282–304

Khan, M. A., I. Kushner, A. A. Freehafer: Sacroiliac joint abnormalities in paraplegics. Ann. rheum. Dis 38 (1979) 317–319

Killebrew, K., R. H. Gold, S. D. Sholkoff: Psoriatic spondylitis. Radiology 108 (1973) 9–16

Kirschbichler, Th.: Die paarig angelegten Processus odontoidei epistrophai - Eine seltene Fehlbildung im kraniozervikalen Übergangsbereich. Fortschr. Röntgenstr. 117 (1972) 654–658

Kittleson, A. C., L. W. Lim: Measurement of scoliosis. Amer. J. Roentgenol. 108 (1970) 775–777

Klaus, E.: Ein Fall von echter Spondylolisthesis mit Spondylolyse der Halswirbelsäule. Fortschr. Röntgenstr. 110 (1969) 277–279

Kläber, V.: Sternumfraktur bei einem Zwölfjährigen. Zbl. Chir. 104 (1979) 244–245

Knetsch, A.: Beitrag zur Osteochondrose. Fortschr. Röntgenstr. 107 (1967) 811–812

Knutsson, F.: The instability associated with disk degeneration in the lumbar spine. Acta radiol. (Stockh.) 25 (1944) 593–609

Kölle, G.: Die juvenile rheumatoide Arthritis (juvenile chronische Polyarthritis) und das Still-Syndrom. Rheuma-Forum 4, Braun, Karlsruhe 1975

Kormano, M., J. Farvonen, A. Lassus: Psoriatic lesion of the sternal synchondrosis. Acta radiol. Diagn. 16 (1975) 463–468

Krämer, J.: Bandscheibenbedingte Erkrankungen. Ursachen, Diagnose, Behandlung, Vorbeugung, Begutachtung. Thieme, Stuttgart 1978

Krebs, W.: Klinik der sogenannten rheumatischen Wirbelsäulenerkrankungen. Rheumaprobleme II. Thieme, Leipzig 1931

Krüger, V., M. Schattenkirchner: Die Spondylitis ankylosans. Klinikarzt 9 (1980) 676–688

Kuhlendahl, H.: Die neurologischen Syndrome bei der Überstreckungsverletzung der Halswirbelsäule und dem sog. Schleudertrauma. Münch. med. Wschr. 106 (1964) 1025–1030

Kuhlendahl, H.: Schleudertrauma der Halswirbelsäule. Neurochirurgische Probleme. Arch. klin. Chir. 316 (1966) 470–475

Kuhlendahl, H.: Schleudertrauma und Überstreckungsverletzung. In: Wirbelsäule und Nervensystem, hrsg. von E. Trostdorf, H. Stender. Thieme, Stuttgart 1970 (S. 72–75)

Lachapèle, A.-P.: Un moyen simple pour faciliter la lecture des radiographies vertébrales obliques de la région lombo-sacrée. Bull. Mém. Soc. radiol. méd. France (1939) 175–176

Lachapèle, A. P., C. Lagarde, R. Texier, J. Duluc: De la spondylolyse (Étude radio-clinique de 93 observations personelles). J. Radiol. Électrol. 32 (1951) 453–464

Lackner, S. Schroeder: Computertomographie der Lendenwirbelsäule. Fortschr. Röntgenstr. 133 (1980) 124–131

Laczay, A.: Die degenerativen Veränderungen der Kostotransversal- und Kostovertebralgelenke. Fortschr. Röntgenstr. 119 (1973) 108–111

Lagemann, K.: Hintere Längsbandverkalkungen kombiniert mit Wirbelkörperexkavation. Fortschr. Röntgenstr. 116 (1972) 834–835

Lagier, R., W. MacGee: Erosive intervertebral osteochondrosis in association with generalized osteoarthritis and chondrocalcinosis.

Anatomico-radiological study of a case. Z. Rheumatol. 38 (1979) 405–414

Lagier, R., G. Guelpa, J.-C. Gerster: Lumbar erosive intervertebral osteochondrosis. Anatomico-radiological study of a case. Fortschr. Röntgenstr. 130 (1979) 204–209

Lame, E. L.: Vertebral osteomyelitis following operation on the urinary tract or sigmoid. The third lesion of an uncommon syndrome. Amer. J. Roentgenol. 75 (1956) 938–952

Lame, E. L, H. Ch. Chang: Pubic and ischial necrosis following cystostomy and prostatectomy (osteitis pubis). Amer. J. Roentgenol. 71 (1954) 193–212

Laur, A., C. Keller: Wirbelosteomyelitis nach Grenzstrangblokkade. Fortschr. Röntgenstr. 77 (1952) 81–89

Lawrence, J. S.: Disc degeneration. Its frequency and relationship to symptoms. Ann. rheum. Dis. 28 (1969) 121–138

Lawrence, J.: Symposion ,,Rheumatische Krankheiten als Beispiel problemoffenen Lehr- und Lernverhaltens für Ärzte und Kranke". Med. Serv. 4, Byk Gulden, Konstanz 1975 (S. 1–11)

Lawrence, J. S., J. Sharp, J. Ball, F. Bier: Rheumatoid arthritis of the lumbar spine. Ann. rheum. Dis. 23 (1964) 205–217

Leeds, N. E., H. G. Jacobson: Plain film examination of the spinal canal. Semin. Roentgenol. 7 (1972) 179–196

Léger, J.-L., R. Bouchard, R. Maltais: Étude radiologique de 305 cas de spondylolyse avec ou sans spondylolisthesis. J. Canad. Ass. Radiol. 30 (1979) 86–89

Legueu, Rochet. Les cellulites périvésicales et pelviennes après certaines cystotomies ou prostatectomies sus-pubiennes. J. Urol. 15 (1923) 1–11

Lehmann-Facius, H.: Die Keilwirbelbildung bei der kongenitalen Skoliose. Frankf. Z. Path. 31 (1925) 489–499

Lejeune, E., A. Daumont, J. P. Deplante: Association maladie périodique - spondylarthrite ankylosante. Nouv. Presse méd. 4 (1975) 2949–2950

Lenz, H., H. Rohr: Zur radikulären Genese der sogenannten Relaxatio diaphragmatis. Fortschr. Röntgenstr. 103 (1965) 540–549

Lequesne, M., P. Cassan, J. Nallet, A. Ryckewaert, S. de Sèze: Hyperostose vértebrale et diabète sucré. Rev. Rhum. 37 (1970) 281–286

Lesoine, W.: Das Stylo-Kerato-Hyoidale Syndrom. Dtsch. Ärztebl. 73 (1976) 2381–2386

Lewit, K.: Blockierung von Atlas-Axis und Atlas-Okziput in Röntgenbild und Klinik. Z. Orthop. 108 (1970) 43–50

Lewit, K., L. Krausová, D. Kneidlová: Mechanismus und Bewegungsausmaß der Seitneigung in den Kopfgelenken. Fortschr. Röntgenstr. 101 (1964) 194–201

Liberson, M., N. Mihaldzic: Sacroiliac changes and urinary tract infection with spinal cord injuries. 11. Intern. Congr. Radiol., Rom 1965, Abstracts Intern. Congr. Series No. 89, Excerpta Med. Found., Amsterdam 1965

Lindemann, K: Über eine eigenartige Form der Wirbelsynostose bei Kyphose im Wachstumsalter. Röntgenpraxis 3 (1931) 267–272

Lindgren, E.: Röntgenologie einschließlich Kontrastmethoden. In: Handbuch der Neurochirurgie, Bd. II, hrsg. von H. Olivecrona, W. Tönnis, Springer Berlin 1954

Lissner, J.: Spondylolisthese der Halswirbelsäule. Fortschr. Röntgenstr. 84 (1956) 626–628

Lodge, T.: Bone, joint and soft tissue changes following paraplegia. Acta radiol. (Stockh.) 46 (1956) 435–445

Loewenhardt, K.: Processus paracondyloideus. Fortschr. Röntgenstr. 122 (1975) 368

Logan, W. W., I. D. Stuard: Absent posterior arch of the atlas. Amer. J. Roentgenol. 118 (1973) 431–434

Lorber, A., C. M. Pearson, R. M. Rene: Osteolytic vertebral lesions as a manifestation of arthritis and related disorders. Arthr. and Rheum. 4 (1961) 514–532

Louyot, P.: Sur l'aspect radiologique de la spondylose rhizomélique. Rev. Rhum. 21 (1954) 54–57

Lowman, R. M., F. Robinson: Progressive vertebral interspace changes following lumbar disk surgery. Amer. J. Roentgenol. 97 (1966) 664–671

Luschnitz, E., J. Riedeberger, B. Bauchspiess: Das röntgenologische Bild der Osteonecrosis pubica posttraumatica. Fortschr. Röntgenstr. 107 (1967) 113—118

Luther, R., H. Legal: Spondylolyse durch Leistungssport? Orthop. Prax. 11 (1975) 50–55

McEwen, C., D. DiTata, C. Lingg, A. Porini, A. Good, T. Rankin: Ankylosing spondylitis and spondylitis accompanying ulcerative colitis, regional enteritis, psoriasis and Reiter's disease. A comparative study. Arthr. and Rheum. 14 (1971) 291–318

McGregor, M.: The significance of certain measurements of the skull in the diagnosis of basilar impression: Brit. J. Radiol. 21 (1948) 171–181

McNulty, C. R., P. Pim: Hyperphosphatasia. Report of a case with a 30 year follow-up. Amer. J. Roentgenol. 115 (1972) 614–618

Macrae, I., V. Wright: A family study of ulcerative colitis with particular reference to ankylosing spondylitis and sacroiliitis. Ann. Dis. 32 (1973) 16–20

Mäkelä, A.-L., E. Mäkinen, K. Lorenz, H. Rikalainen: Veränderungen an der Halswirbelsäule bei juveniler rheumatoider Arthritis. Fortschr. Röntgenstr. 131 (1979) 420–427

Maldague, B. J., H. Malghem: Unilateral arch hypertrophy with spinous process tilt: A sign of arch deficiency. Radiology 121 (1976) 567–574

Maldague, B. E., H. M. Noel, J. H. Malghem: The intervertebral vacuum cleft: A sign of ischemic vertebral collaps. Radiology 129 (1978) 23–29

Mandell, G. A., M. E. Kricun: Exaggerated anterior vertebral notching. Radiology 131 (1979) 367–369

Marquardt, S.: Der Umbau des Wirbelkörpers bei Skoliosen. Fortschr. Röntgenstr. 80 (1954) 607–612

Martel, W.: A radiologically distinctive cause of low back pain. Arthr. and Rheum. 20 (1977 a) 1014–1018

Martel, W.: Pathogenesis of cervical discovertebral destruction in rheumatoid arthritis. Arthr. and Rheum. 20 (1977 b) 1217–1225

Martel, W., J. W. Page: Cervical vertebral erosions and subluxations in rheumatoid arthritis and ankylosing spondylitis. Arthr. and Rheum. 3 (1960) 546–556

Martel, W., J. M. Tishler: Observations on the spine in mongoloidism. Amer. J. Roentgenol. 97 (1966) 630–638

Martel, W., R. Abell, I. F. Duff: Cervical involvement in lipoid dermato-arthritis. Radiology 77 (1961) 613–617

Martel, W., J. F. Seeger, J. D. Wicks, R. L. Washburn: Traumatic lesions of the discovertebral junction in the lumbar spine. Amer. J. Roentgenol. 127 (1976) 457–464

Mathias, K. D., H.-J. Lössl: Symmetrische Verdoppelung des Processus articularis superior des 4. LWK. Fortschr. Röntgenstr. 123 (1975) 277–279

Mehta, M. H., R. O. Murray: Scoliosis provoked by painful vertebral lesions. Skelet. Radiol. 1 (1977) 223–230

Meijers, K. A. E., G. Th. van Beusekom, W. Luyendijk, F. Duijfjes: Dislocation of the cervical spine with cord compression in rheumatoid arthritis. J. Bone Jt Surg. 56 B (1974) 668–680

Meyerding, H. W.: Spondylolisthesis. Surg. Gynec. Obstet. 54 (1932) 371–377

Minagi, H., A. T. Gronner: Calcification of the posterior longitudinal ligament: A cause of cervical myelopathy. Amer. J. Roentgenol. 105 (1969) 365–369

Mitchell, G. E., H. Lourie, A. S. Berne: The various causes of scalloped vertebrae with notes on their pathogenesis. Radiology 89 (1967) 67–74

Moll, J. M. H., I. Haslock, I. F. Macrae, V. Wright: Associations between ankylosing spondylitis, psoriatic arthritis, Reiter's disease, the intestinal arthropathies, and Behçet's syndrome. Medicine (Baltimore) 53 (1974) 343–364

Morin, M. E., E. Palacios: The aplastic hypoplastic lumbar pedicle. Amer. J. Roentgenol. 122 (1974) 639–642

Moser, C. R., W. J. Fessel: Rheumatic manifestations of hypophosphatemia. Arch. intern. Med. 134 (1974) 674–678

Mosimann, P.: Die Histologie der Spondylolyse. Arch. orthop. Unfall-Chir. 53 (1961) 264–285

Müller, W.: Spontane seitliche Wirbelkörperverschiebungen. (Das Drehgleiten von Lendenwirbeln bei Skoliosen der älteren Leute). Z. orthop. Chir. 55 (1931) 351–364

Müller, W.: Umbauzonen an den Dornfortsätzen kyphotischer Wirbelsäulen als Ursache von Schmerzzuständen. Fortschr. Röntgenstr. 48 (1933) 639–641

Nadjmi, M., U. Wagner: Kranio-zervikale Topometrie an Schädeltomogrammen. Röntgen-Bl. 26 (1973) 145–170

Nakano, K. K., W. C. Shoene, R. A. Baker, D. M. Dawson: The cervical myelopathy associated with rheumatoid arthritis: Analysis of 32 patients, with 2 postmortem cases. Ann. Neurol. 3 (1978) 144–151

Nathan, F. F., W. H. Bickel: Spontaneous axial subluxation in a child as the first sign of juvenile rheumatoid arthritis. J. Bone Jt Surg. 50 A (1968) 1675–1678

Newman, P. H.: Stenosis of the lumbar spine in spondylolisthesis. Clin. Orthop. 115 (1976) 116–121

Niedner, F.: Zur Kenntnis der normalen und pathologischen Anatomie der Wirbelkörperrandleiste. Fortschr. Röntgenstr. 46 (1932) 628–662

Olsson, T. H., G. Selvik, S. Willner: Vertebral motion in spondylolisthesis. Acta radiol. Diagn. 17 (1976) 861–868

Onji, Y., H. Akiyama, Y. Shimomura, K. Ono., S. Hukuda, S. Mizuno: Posterior paravertebral ossification causing cervical myelopathy. A report of eighteen cases. J. Bone Jt Surg. 49 A (1967) 1314–1328

Op den Orth, J. O.: Die Verkalkung bzw. Verknöcherung des Ligamentum longitudinale posterius der Halswirbelsäule. Fortschr. Röntgenstr. 122 (1975) 442–445

Ott, V. R.: Über die Spondylosis hyperostotica. Schweiz. med. Wschr. 83 (1953) 790–799

Ott, V. R., H. Schwenkenbecher, H. Iser: Die Spondylose bei Diabetes mellitus. Z. Rheumaforsch. 22 (1963) 278–290

Palacios, E., C. E. Brackett, D. J. Leary: Ossification of the posterior longitudinal ligament associated with a herniated intervertebral disk. Radiology 100 (1971) 313–314

Park, W. M., M. O'Neill, I. W. McCall: The radiology of rheumatoid involvement of the cervical spine. Skelet. Radiol. 4 (1979) 1–7

Patton, J. T.: Differential diagnosis of inflammatory spondylitis. Skelet. Radiol 1 (1976) 77–85

Patzakis, M. J., A. Knopf, M. Elfering, M. Hoffer, J. P. Harvey, jr.: Posterior dislocation of the atlas on the axis. A case report. J. Bone Jt Surg. 56 A (1974) 1260–1262

Pauwels, F.: Gesammelte Abhandlungen zur funktionellen Anatomie des Bewegungsapparates. Springer, Berlin 1965

Payne, E. E., J. D. Spillane: The cervical spine. An anatomicopathological study of 70 specimens (using a special technique) with particular reference to the problem of cervical spondylosis. Brain 80 (1957) 571–596

Peiffer, J., Ch. Wenig, E. Mäusle: Akutes Querschnittssyndrom durch Embolien von Nucleus-pulposus-Gewebe. Dtsch. med. Wschr. 101 (1976) 583–586

Peña Arrebola, A., A. Garcia López, M. de la Prada: Revisión clinica de las osteitis condensantes del iliaco. Rev. esp. Reum. 2 (1975) 22–33

Penning, L.: Functional pathology of the cervical spine. Radiographic studies of function and dysfunction in congenital disorders, cervical spondylosis and injuries. Excerpta Medica Foundation, Amsterdam 1968

Penning, L.: Normal movements of the cervical spine. Amer. J. Roentgenol. 130 (1978) 317–326

Penning, L., J. R. Blickman: Instability in lumbar spondylolisthesis: A radiologic study of several concepts. Amer. J. Roentgenol. 134 (1980) 293–301

Peter, E.: Die Insuffizienz des Achsenorgans. Z. Rheumaforsch. 29 (1970) 227–233

Peter, E.: Die Diskusdegeneration. In: Das rheumatische Gelenk. Pathologie, Diagnose, Therapie, hrsg. von W. Dihlmann, H. Mathies. Sharp & Dohme, München 1976

Peter, E., B. Schuler, W. Dihlmann: Veränderungen der Wirbeldornfortsätze bei Arthritis mutilans. Dtsch. med. Wschr. 89 (1964) 1990–1993

Pfeil, E.: Beitrag zur konservativen Behandlung der Spondylolyse und Spondylolisthesis im Kindesalter. Beitr. Orthop. Traum. 22 (1975) 238–240

Pinckney, L. E., G. Currarino, C. L. Highgenboten: Osteomyelitis of the cervical spine following dental extraction. Radiology 135 (1980) 335–337

Pohl, W.: Hyperostosis generalisata. Fortschr. Röntgenstr. 132 (1980) 734–736

Pohl, W., H. G. Kränzlein: Über blande sklerosierende Spondylitiden. Fortschr. Röntgenstr. 119 (1973) 352–357

Polgár, F.: Über interarkuelle Wirbelverkalkung. Fortschr. Röntgenstr. 40 (1929) 292–298

Porstmann, W.: Spondylitis infectiosa im Anschluß an Verletzungen des vorderen Längsbandes (Beitrag zur Spondylitis nach Paravertebralanästhesie). Fortschr. Röntgenstr. 85 (1956) 66–75

Pučar, I., M. Smokvina, T. Dürrigl: Spondylodiscitis in rheumatoid arthritis. Liječn Vjesn. 91 (1969) 183–190

Putte, R. H., H. Tesluk: Whipple's disease. Amer. J. Med. 12 (1955) 383–400

Rana, N. A., D. O. Hancock, A. R. Taylor, A. G. S. Hill: Upward translocation of the dens in rheumatoid arthritis. J. Bone Jt Surg. 55 B (1973) 471–477

Rathke, F. W.: Über Wirbelkörperaplasie. Fortschr. Röntgenstr. 127 (1977) 248–254

Rau, N.: Röntgenologische Fragestellungen am Nativbild aus der Sicht des Neurologen. Radiologe 12 (1972) 58–62

Rawat, S. S., G. K. Jain, H. K. D. Gupta: Intra-abdominal symptoms arising from spinal osteophytes. Brit. J. Surg. 62 (1975) 320–322

Reid, G. D., R. H. Hill: Atlantoaxial subluxation in juvenile ankylosing spondylitis. J. Pediat. 93 (1978) 531–532

Reimers, C.: Die Chondrosis dissecans der Knorpeldeckplatte als Ursache des Bandscheibenvorfalles. Langenbecks Arch. klin. Chir. 267 (Verh. Dtsch. Ges. Chir.) (1951) 469–472

Reinhardt, K.: Das anatomische Substrat lochförmiger Aufhellungen in den unteren Lendenwirbelkörpern und ihre klinische Bedeutung. Fortschr. Röntgenstr. 86 (1957) 222–225

Reinhold, H.: Beitrag zur Adoleszentenkyphose (Morbus Scheuermann). Radiol. austr. 15 (1966) 249–258

Reiter, R.: Zur Kenntnis der sogenannten Chondritis und Perichondritis der oberen Synchondrose des Sternums. Z. Orthop. 87 (1956) 436–446

Renier, J.-C., Ch. Bregeon, J. Boutin: Les condensations vertébrales localisées. Étude de 37 observations; réflexions pathogéniques. Rev. Rhum. 35 (1968) 521–530

Resnick, D.: Thoracolumbar spine abnormalities in rheumatoid arthritis. Ann. rheum. Dis. 37 (1978) 389–391

Resnick, D., G. Niwayama: Intervertebral disk herniations: cartilaginous (Schmorl's) nodes. Radiology 126 (1978 a) 57–65

Resnick, D., G. Niwayama: Intervertebral disc abnormalities associated with vertebral metastasis: Observations in patients with prostatic cancer. Invest. Radiol. 13 (1978 b) 182–190

Resnick, D., S. R. Shaul, J. M. Robins: Diffuse idiopathic skeletal hyperostosis (DISH): Forestier's disease with extraspinal manifestations. Radiology 115 (1975) 513–524

Ringe, J.-D., F. Kuhlencordt, J. Kühnau jr.: Mineralgehalt des Skeletts bei Langzeitdiabetikern. Dtsch. med. Wschr. 101 (1976) 280–282

Rispoli, F. P.: Schambeinsyndrom bei Fußballspielern. Z. Orthop. 99 (1965) 87–92

Ritter, G., K. Rittmeyer, H. Ch. Hopf: Konstitutionelle Enge des zervikalen Spinalkanals. Radiologische und klinische Befunde. Dtsch. med. Wschr. 100 (1975) 358–361

Rivelis, M., R. H. Freiberger: Vertebral destruction at unfused segments in late ankylosing spondylitis. Radiology 93 (1969) 251–256

Rogers, M. H., E. N. Cleaves: The adolescent sacro-iliac joint syndrome. J. Bone Jt Surg. 17 (1935) 759–768

Romanus, R.: Pelvo-spondylitis ossificans in the male (ankylosing spondylitis, Morbus Bechterew-Marie-Strümpell) and genito-urinary infection. The aetiological significance of the latter and the nature of the disease based on a study of 117 male patients. Acta med. scand., Suppl. 280, Stockholm 1953

Romanus, R., S. Ydén: Destructive and ossifying spondylitic changes in rheumatoid ankylosing spondylitis (pelvospondylitis ossificans). Acta orthop. scand. 22 (1952) 88–99

Rosenberg, F., R. Bataille, J. Sany, D. Rau, H. Serre: Lyse de l'odontoide au cours de la polyarthrite rhumatoide. Rev. Rhum. 45 (1978) 249–257

Rosenberg, N. J.: Degenerative Spondylolisthesis. Predisposing factors. J. Bone Jt Surg. 57 A (1975) 467–474

Rosin, A. J.: Ectopic calcification around joints of paralysed limbs in hemiplegia, diffuse brain damage, and other neurological diseases. Ann. rheum. Dis. 34 (1975) 499–505

Ross, E.: Die enchondrale Dysostose der Wirbelsäule. Kritisches zur Diagnose der Scheuermannschen Erkrankung. Fortschr. Röntgenstr. 98 (1963) 578–588

Rössler, A.: Zur Kenntnis der Achillodynie. Dtsch. Z. Chir. 42 (1896) 274–291

Rovira, M., O. Torrent, J. Ruscalleda: Some aspects of the spinal cord circulation in cervical myelopathy. Neuroradiology 9 (1975) 209–214

Ruffing, L.: Versteifende Wirbelsäulenveränderungen bei der Thalidomid-Embryopathie. Verh. dtsch. Ges. Rheum. 5 (1978) 427–431

Russell, M. L., D. A. Gordon, M. A. Ogryzlo, R. S. McPhedran: The cauda equina syndrome of ankylosing spondylitis. Ann. intern. Med. 78 (1973) 551–554

Rüter, A.: Pathomechanik der Wirbelsäulenverletzung und ihre Röntgendiagnostik. Hefte Unfallheilk. 110 (1972) 28–30

Sartor, K., H. Schmidt, F. Schönberg: Über einen einseitigen Verschluß der A. vertebralis bei Atlasassimilation. Fortschr. Röntgenstr. 121 (1974) 623–629

Sassard, W. R., C. F. Heinig, W. R. Pitts: Posterior atlanto-axial dislocation without fracture. Case report with successful conservative treatment. J. Bone Jt Surg. 56 A (1974) 625–628

Sauser, D. D., A. B. Goldman, J. J. Kay: Discogenic vertebral sclerosis. J. Canad. Ass. Radiol. 29 (1978) 44–50

Schabel, S. I., T. E. Moore, G. M. Rittenberg, J. H. Stanley, L. H. Javid: Vertebral vacuum phenomenon. A radiographic manifestation of metastatic malignancy. Skelet. Radiol. 4 (1979) 154–156

Schacherl, M.: Röntgendiagnostik der Halswirbelsäule bei der chronischen rheumatischen Polyarthritis. In: Klinisch-radiologisches Seminar 3, hrsg. von W. Frommhold, P. Gerhard. Thieme, Stuttgart 1974 (S. 99–112)

Schapals, G.: Röntgenologische und klinische Untersuchungen über die krankhafte Lockerung der Beckenverbindungen. Diss., Rhein.-Westf. Techn. Hochschule, Aachen 1971

Scharfetter, F., G. Müller: Über die postoperative Discitis intervertebralis lumbalis. Schweiz. Arch. Neurol. Neurochir. Psychiat. 108 (1971) 99–111

Schatzker, J., C. H. Rorabeck, J. P. Waddell: Fractures of the dens (odontoid process). An analysis of thirty-seven cases. J. Bone Jt Surg. 53 B (1971) 392–405

Scher, A. T.: Unilateral locked facet in cervical spine injuries. Amer. J. Roentgenol. 129 (1977) 45–48

Scheuermann, H.: Kyphosis dorsalis juvenilis. Z. orthop. Chir. 41 (1921) 305–317

Schiff, D. C. M., W. W. Parke: The arterial supply of the odontoid process. J. Bone Jt Surg. 55 A (1973) 1450–1456

Schilling, F.: Das klinische Bild der Spondylitis ankylopoetica. Med. Welt 19 (1968) 2334–2344

Schilling, F.: Röntgenmorphologische Befunde bei der Spondylitis ankylopoetica. Verh. dtsch. Ges. Rheum. 1 (1969) 33–46

Schilling, F.: Spondylitis Ankylopoetica. Die sogenannte Bechterewsche Krankheit und ihre Differentialdiagnose (einschließlich Spondylosis hyperostotica, Spondylitis psoriatica und chronisches Reiter-Syndrom). In: Handbuch der medizinischen Radiologie, Bd. VI/2, hrsg. von L. Diethelm, F. Heuck, O. Olsson, K. Ranniger, F. Strnad, H. Vieten, A. Zuppinger. Springer, Berlin 1974 (S. 452–689)

Schilling, F.: Die juvenile und senile Spondylitis ankylosans. Verh. dtsch. Ges. Rheum. 5 (1978) 389–395

Schilling, F., M. Schacherl: Röntgenbefunde an der Wirbelsäule bei Polyarthritis psoriatica und Reiter-Dermatose: Spondylitis psoriatica. Z. Rheumaforsch. 26 (1967) 450–459

Schilling, F., J. P. Haas, M. Schacherl: Die spontane atlanto-axiale Dislokation (Ventralluxation des Atlas) bei chronischer Polyarthritis und Spondylitis ankylopoetica. Fortschr. Röntgenstr. 99 (1963) 518–538

Schilling, F., M. Schacherl, R. Rosenberg: Die juvenile Spondylitis ankylopoetica. Dtsch. med. Wschr. 94 (1969) 473–481

Schilling, F., M. Schacherl, A. Gamp, A. Bopp: Die Beziehungen der Spondylosis hyperostotica zur Konstitution und zu Stoffwechselstörungen. Med. Klin. 60 (1965) 165–169

Schilling, F., M. Schacherl, A. Bopp, A. Gamp, J. P. Haas: Veränderungen der Halswirbelsäule (Spondylitis cervicalis) bei der chronischen rheumatischen Polyarthritis und bei der Spondylitis ankylopoetica. Radiologe 3 (1963) 483–501

Schimmel, D. H., T. H. Newton, J. Mani: Widening of the cervical intervertebral foramen. Neuroradiology 12 (1976) 3–10

Schlegel, K. F.: Zervikaler Bockwirbel bei Osteochondrose. Fortschr. Röntgenstr. 83 (1955) 373–377

Schmidt, H., E. Fischer: Die okzipitale Dysplasie. Thieme, Stuttgart 1960

Schmitt, E.: Klinik und Prognose der Scheuermann-Skoliose. Z. Orthop. 113 (1975) 573–575

Schmitt, W. G. H., H. C. Rücker: Langzeitbeobachtungen von Überlastungsschäden an der jugendlichen Meta- und Apophyse des Dornfortsatzes des 1. Brustwirbels (Schmittsche Krankheit). Fortschr. Röntgenstr. 131 (1979) 623–631

Schmorl, G.: Über Knorpelknötchen an den Wirbelbandscheiben. Fortschr. Röntgenstr. 38 (1928) 265–279

Schmorl, G.: Über Verlagerung von Bandscheibengewebe und ihre Folgen. Arch. klin. Chir. 172 (1933) 240–276

Schmorl, G., H. Junghanns: Die gesunde und die kranke Wirbelsäule in Röntgenbild und Klinik, 5. Auflage. Thieme, Stuttgart 1968

Schneider, P. G.: Das Grazilissyndrom. Die Osteonecrosis pubica posttraumatica. Z. Orthop. 98 (1964) 43–50

Schneider, R. C.: The syndrome of acute anterior spinal cord injury. J. Neurosurg. 12 (1955) 99–122

Schneider, R. C., E. A. Kahn: Chronic neurological sequelae of acute trauma to the spine and spinal cord. Part. I. The significance of the acute-flexion or „tear drop" fracture-dislocation of the cervical spine. J. Bone Jt Surg. 38 A (1956) 985–997

Schnier, B. R.: Pseudotumor of the hypopharynx and larynx due to anterior cervical osteophytes. Amer. J. Roentgenol. 115 (1972) 544–546

Schoen, D., M. Eggstein, W. Vogt: Ist die hyperostotische Spondylosis deformans eine diabetische Osteopathie? Fortschr. Röntgenstr. 110 (1969) 524–539

Schönenberg, H.: Das Syndrom der kaudalen Hypoplasie. Helv. paediat. Acta 26 (1971) 88–97

Schröder, H., K. H. Rotte, H.-J. Eichhorn: Über die Leistungsfähigkeit tomographischer Untersuchungen zum Nachweis von osteolytischen Wirbelkörpermetastasen. Fortschr. Röntgenstr. 108 (1968) 761–766

Schulitz, K.-P.: Destruktive Veränderungen an Wirbelkörpern bei der Spondylarthritis ankylopoetica. Arch. orthop. Unfall-Chir. 64 (1968) 116–134

Schulthess, W.: Beiträge zur pathologischen Anatomie der Wirbelsäule. Arch. Orthop. Unfall-Chir. 2 (1904) 1–39

Schwarz, E., A. Fish: Reticulohistiocytosis: A rare dermatologic disease with roentgen manifestations. Amer. J. Roentgenol. 83 (1960) 692–697

Schwarz, G. S.: The width of the spinal canal in the growing vertebra with special reference to the sacrum. Maximum interpediculate distances in adults and children. Amer. J. Roentgenol. 76 (1956) 476–481

Schwerdtner, H. P., H. Schoberth: Die Spondylolyse im Hochleistungssport bei Gerätturnerinnen. Z. Orthop. 111 (1973) 934–940

Scott, S. G.: Chronic infection of the sacro-iliac joints as a possible cause of spondylitis adolescens. Brit. J. Radiol. 9 (1936) 126–131

Seaman, W. B., J. Wells: Destructive lesions of the vertebral bodies in rheumatoid disease. Amer. J. Roentgenol. 86 (1961) 241–250

Seay, A. R., F. A. Ziter, J. H. Petajan: Rigid spine syndrome. A type I fiber myopathy. Arch. Neurol. 34 (1977) 119–122

Seegelken, K., H. Keller: Retroisthmische Spalte der Lendenwirbelsäule. Fortschr. Röntgenstr. 121 (1974) 659–660

Seegelken, K., G.-A. Schulte: Spaltbildungen des Wirbelbogens (Mitteilung der Beobachtung einer retrosomatischen Spalte). Fortschr. Röntgenstr. 116 (1972) 473–477

Seibert-Daiker, F. M.: Über eine halbseitige Dornfortsatzhyperplasie des 5. Halswirbels, verbunden mit einer persistierenden Apophyse des 7. Halswirbels. Fortschr. Röntgenstr. 122 (1975) 366–367

Seljeskog, E. L., S. N. Chou: Spectrum of hangman's fracture. J. Neurosurg. 45 (1976) 3–8

Sewcz, H.-G., E.-G. Preuss: Spondylitis infectiosa nach lumbalen Grenzstrangblockaden. Rad. diagn. (Berl.) 11 (1970) 23–29

Shapiro, R., H. D. Batt: Unilateral thoracic spondylosis. Amer. J. Roentgenol. 83 (1960) 660–662

Shichikawa, K., K. Matsui, K. Oze, H. Ota: Rheumatoid spondylitis. Int. Orthop. 2 (1978) 53–60

Sicard, J. A., J. Forestier 1931: zit. nach Forestier u. Mitarb. 1956

Sim, G. P. G.: Vertebral contour in spondylolisthesis. Brit. J. Radiol. 46 (1973) 250–254

Sims-Williams, H., M. I. V. Jayson, H. Baddeley: Rheumatoid involvement of the lumbar spine. Ann. rheum. Dis. 36 (1977) 524–531

Singh, A., R. Dass, S. Singh Hayreh, S. S. Jolly: Skeletal changes in endemic fluorosis. J. Bone Jt Surg. 44 B (1962) 806–815

Smith, G. R., C. H. Northrop, J. W. Loop: Jumpers' fractures: Patterns of thoracolumbar spine injuries associated with vertical plunges. A review of 38 cases. Radiology 122 (1977) 657–663

Sorin, S., A. Askari, R. W. Moskowitz: Atlantoaxial subluxation as a complication of early ankylosing spondylitis. Two case reports and a review of the literature. Arthr. and Rheum. 22 (1979) 273–276

Stahl, Ch., F. Huth: Morphologischer Nachweis synovialer Spalträume in der Unco-Vertebral-Region zervikaler Bandscheiben. Z. Orthop. 118 (1980) 721–728

Stanbury, S. W., A. J. Popert, J. Ball: Simulation of rheumatic disorders by metabolic bone diseases. Ann. rheum. Dis. 18 (1959) 63–64

Steinbach, H. L., G. S. Gordan, E. Eisenberg, J. T. Crane, S. Silverman: Primary hyperparathyreoidism: A correlation of roentgen, clinical, and pathologic features. Amer. J. Roentgenol. 86 (1961) 329–343

Stern, N., G. Schwabauer: Über den sog. Fersenschmerz. Fortschr. Röntgenstr. 44 (1931) 459–472

Stern, W. E., P. H. Crandall: Inflammatory intervertebral disc disease as a complication of the operative treatment of lumbar herniations. J. Neurosurg. 16 (1959) 261–276

Stewart jr., G. C., J. A. Gehweiler jr., R. H. Laib, S. Martinez: Horizontal fracture of the anterior arch of the atlas. Radiology 122 (1977) 349–352

Stewart, T. D.: The age incidence of neural-arch defects in Alaskan natives, considered from the standpoint of etiology. J. Bone Jt Surg. 35 A (1953) 937–950

Stuber, J. L., E. Palacios: Vertebral scalloping in acromegaly. Radiology 112 (1971) 397–400

Stump, D., A. Spock, H. Grossman: Vertebral sarcoidosis in adolescents. Radiology 121 (1976) 153–155

Sullivan, C. R., W. H. Bickell: The problem of traumatic spondylolysis. A report of three cases. Amer. J. Surg. 100 (1960) 698–708

Sundaram, M., J. T. Patton: Paravertebral ossification in psoriasis and Reiter's disease. Brit. J. Radiol. 48 (1975) 628–633

Sutherland, R. I. L., D. Matheson: Mechanism of vertebral destruction in ankylosing spondylitis. Arthr. and Rheum. 17 (1974) 502

Swischuk, L. E., C. J. Fagan, M. Sarwar: Persistence of the dens as the body of C1. A case report of a rare anomaly. Radiology 127 (1978) 330

Tchang, S. P. K.: The cervical spino-laminar line. J. Canad. Ass. Radiol. 25 (1974) 224–226

Teichert, G.: Einige Beobachtungen nicht spondylotischer Wirbelkantenveränderungen an der oberen Halwirbelsäule. Arch. orthop. Unfall-Chir. 48 (1956) 293–296

Teplick, J. G., G. L. Head, M. E. Kricun, M. E. Haskin: Ghost infantile vertebrae and hemipelves within adult skeleton from thorotrast administration in childhood. Radiology 129 (1978) 657–660

Theiss, B., A. Böni, F. Wagenhäuser, U. W. Schnyder, K. Fehr: Psoriasis-Spondylarthritis. Z. Rheumaforsch. 28 (1969) 93–117

Théron, J., J. Moret: Spinal Phlebography. Lumbar and cervical techniques. Springer, Berlin 1978

Thorel, J. B., B. Cavelier, J. C., Bonneau, J. L. Simonin, C. Ropartz, P. Deshayes: Étude d'une population porteuse de l'antigène HLA B27 comparée a celle d'une population témoin non B 27 a la recherche de la spondylarthrite ankylosante. Rev. Rhum. 45 (1978) 275–282

Tomsick, T. A., M. E. Lebowitz, C. Campbell: The congenital absence of pedicles in the thoracic spine. Report of two cases. Radiology 111 (1974) 587–589

Töndury, G.: Zur Anatomie der Halswirbelsäule. Gibt es Uncovertebralgelenke? Z. Anat. Entwickl.-Gesch. 112 (1942/43) 448–459

von Torklus, D.: Halswirbelsäulen-Syndrom. Dtsch. med. Wschr. 101 (1976) 185

von Torklus, D., W. Gehle: Die obere Halswirbelsäule. Regionale Morphologie, Pathologie und Traumatologie. Praktischer Röntgenatlas und Systematik, 2. Auflage. Thieme, Stuttgart 1975

Tredwell, S. J., J. P. O'Brien: Avascular necrosis of the proximal end of the dens. A complication of halo-pelvic distraction. J. Bone Jt Surg. 57 A (1975) 332–336

Trostler, I. S.: Slipping sacro-iliac joints. Radiology 31 (1938) 363–364

Ullrich, C. G., E. F. Binet, M. G. Sanecki, S. A. Kieffer: Quantitative assessment of the lumbar spinal canal bei computed tomography. Radiology 134 (1980) 137–143

Vahlensieck, W., G. Scheibe: Zur sogenannten „Ostitis pubis" unter Berücksichtigung klinischer und tierexperimenteller Beobachtungen. Brun's Beitr. klin. Chir. 207 (1963) 355–369

Valentin, B., W. Putschar: Dysontogenetische Blockwirbel- und Gibbusbildung. Z. Orthop. 64 (1936) 338–369

Valergakis, F. E. G.: Cervical spondylosis: Most common cause of position and vibratory sense loss. Geriatrics 31 (1976) 51–56

Verbiest, H.: A radicular syndrome from developmental narrowing of the lumbar vertebral canal. J. Bone Jt Surg. 36 B (1954) 230–237

Verhaak, R.: Congenital defect of a lumbar vertebral pedicle with dysplasia of the intervertebral joint. Radiol. clin. biol. (Basel) 43 (1974) 127–137

Verhaeghe, A., R. Lesage, B. Delcambre, B. Gosselin: Spondylodiscites chroniques au cours de la polyarthrite rhumatoide. Rev. Rhum. 36 (1969) 124–130

Vernon-Roberts, B., C. J. Pirie, V. Trenwith: Pathology of the dorsal spine in ankylosing hyperostosis. Ann. rheum. Dis. 33 (1974) 281–288

Vinstein, A. L., E. M. Cockerill: Involvement of the spine in gout. A case report. Radiology 103 (1972) 311–312

Vogelsang, H.: Discitis intervertebralis cervicalis nach Diskographie. Neurochirurgie 16 (1973) 80–83

Voss, A.-C.: Die Verknöcherung des Ligamentum flavum. Fortschr. Röntgenstr. 117 (1972) 226–227

Wackenheim, A.: Roentgen diagnosis of the craniovertebral region. Springer, Berlin 1974

Wackenheim, A., P. Capesius: Fortschritte auf dem Gebiet der Röntgendiagnostik der Halswirbelsäule. Radiologe 15 (1975) 311–316

Wald, S. L., J. E. McLennan, R. M. Carroll, H. Segal: Extradural spinal involvement by gout. J. Neurosurg. 50 (1979) 236–239

Webb, F. W. S., J. A. Hickman, D. St. J. Brew: Death from vertebral artery thrombosis in rheumatoid arthritis. Brit. med. J. 1968/II, 537–538

Weber, G.: Über lumbale Diskushernien. Z. Rheumaforsch. 9 (1950) 223–255

Weishaar, J.: Beitrag zur partiellen Blockwirbelbildung nach isolierter Bandscheibenverletzung. Fortschr. Röntgenstr. 87 (1957) 129–130

Wellauer, J.: Die Myelographie mit positiven Kontrastmitteln. Thieme, Stuttgart 1961

Wettstein, P., W. Curati: Spondylites et spondylodiscites aiguës à germes banals. Radiol. clin. biol. (Basel) 42 (1973) 353–365

Whalen, J. P., C. L. Woodruff: The cervical prevertebral fat stripe. A new aid in evaluating the cervical prevertebral soft tissue space. Amer. J. Roentgenol. 109 (1970) 445–451

Whitley, J. E., H. F. Forsyth: The classification of cervical spine injuries. Amer. J. Roentgenol. 83 (1960) 633–644

Wholey, M. H., A. J. Bruwer, H. L. Baker jr.: The lateral roentgenogram of the neck (with comments on the atlanto-odontoid-basion relationship). Radiology 71 (1958) 350–356

Wiesmayr, W.: Über die Spondylitis tuberculosa anterior. Wien. med. Wschr. 102 (1951) 468–469

Wilkinson, R. H., J. E. Hall: The sclerotic pedicle: Tumor or pseudotumor? Radiology 111 (1974) 683–688

Williams, A. J.: Rheumatoid (Marie-Strumpell) spondylitis. Technique of examination and importance of the costal joints. Calif. Med. 70 (1949) 257–261

Williams, J. I., G. A. Moller, T. L. O'Rourke: Pseudoinfections of the intervertebral disk and adjacent vertebrae? Amer. J. Roentgenol. 103 (1968) 611–615

Wilson, C. B., H. A. Norrell jr.: Congenital absence of a pedicle in the cervical spine. Amer. J. Roentgenol. 97 (1966) 639–647

Wiltse, L. L., E. H. Widell jr., D. W. Jackson: Fatigue fracture: The basic lesion in isthmic spondylolisthesis. J. Bone Jt Surg. 57 A (1975) 17–22

Wolf, B. S., M. Khilnani, L. Malis: The sagittal diameter of the bony cervical spinal canal and its significance in cervical spondylosis. J. Mt Sinai Hosp. 23 (1956) 283–292

Wooten, W. B., T. E. Summer, J. E. Crowe, A. Ayala: Case report 64 (Ewing tumor producing sclerosis of the left pedicle of the fourth thoracic vertebra). Skelet. Radiol. 3 (1978) 65–67

Wright, V.: Seronegative polyarthritis. A unified concept. Arthr. and Rheum. 21 (1978) 619–633

Wright, V.: A unifying concept for the spondyloarthropathies. Clin. Orthop. 143 (1979) 8–14

Wright, V., R. D. Catterall, J. B. Cook: Bone and joint changes in paraplegic men. Ann. rheum. Dis. 24 (1965) 419–431

Zeitler, E., H. Markuske: Röntgenologische Bewegungsanalysen der Halswirbelsäule bei gesunden Kindern und Jugendlichen. Fortschr. Röntgenstr. 96 (1962) 87–93

Zener, J. C., M. Alpert, L. M. Klainer: Vertebral sarcoidosis. Arch. intern. Med. 111 (1963) 696–702

Zimmermann, H. B., W. J. Farrel: Cervical vertebral erosion caused by vertebral artery tortuosity. Amer. J. Roentgenol. 108 (1970) 767

Zimmermann, R., N. E. Leeds: Calvarial and vertebral sarcoidosis. Case report and review of the literature. Radiology 119 (1976) 384

Zippel, H., H. Runge: Pathologische Anatomie und Pathogenese von Spondylolyse und Spondylolisthesis im Kindesalter. Z. Orthop. 114 (1976) 189–191

Zucker, G., M. J. Marder: Charcot spine due to diabetic neuropathy. Amer. J. Med. 12 (1952) 118–124

Zukschwerdt, L., E. Emminger, F. Biedermann, H. Zettel: Wirbelgelenk und Bandscheibe. Ihre Beziehung zum vertebragenen Schmerz. Zugleich eine Stellungnahme zur Chiropraktik und Begutachtung, 2. Aufl. Hippokrates, Stuttgart 1960

Zvaifler, N. J., W. Martel: Spondylitis in chronic ulcerative colitis. Arthr. and Rheum. 3 (1960) 76–87

Index